Study Guide for

Focus on Nursing Pharmacology

Wolters Kluwer | Lippincott Williams & Wilkins
Health

Philadelphia · Baltimore · New York · London
Buenos Aires · Hong Kong · Sydney · Tokyo

Vice President and Publisher: Julie Stegman
Product Managers: Michelle Clarke and Maria McAvey
Marketing Manager: Nicole Dunlap
Editorial Assistant: Dan Reilly
Design Coordinator: Joan Wendt
Illustration Coordinator: Brett MacNaughton
Production Service: SPi Global

9 8 7 6 5 4 3 2 1

Printed in the United States

978-1-4511-5166-4

Care has been taken to confirm the accuracy of the information presented and to describe generally accepted practices. However, the author, editors, and publisher are not responsible for errors or omissions or for any consequences from application of the information in this book and make no warranty, expressed or implied, with respect to the currency, completeness, or accuracy of the contents of the publication. Application of this information in a particular situation remains the professional responsibility of the practitioner; the clinical treatments described and recommended may not be considered absolute and universal recommendations.

The author, editors, and publisher have exerted every effort to ensure that drug selection and dosage set forth in this text are in accordance with the current recommendations and practice at the time of publication. However, in view of ongoing research, changes in government regulations, and the constant flow of information relating to drug therapy and drug reactions, the reader is urged to check the package insert for each drug for any change in indications and dosage and for added warnings and precautions. This is particularly important when the recommended agent is a new or infrequently employed drug.

Some drugs and medical devices presented in this publication have Food and Drug Administration (FDA) clearance for limited use in restricted research settings. It is the responsibility of the health care provider to ascertain the FDA status of each drug or device planned for use in his or her clinical practice.

LWW.com

Preface

This Study Guide was developed to accompany the Sixth Edition of *Focus on Nursing Pharmacology,* by Amy M. Karch. The Study Guide is designed to help you practice and retain the knowledge you've gained from the textbook, and it is structured to integrate that knowledge and give you a basis for applying it in your nursing practice. The following types of exercises are provided in each chapter of the Study Guide.

■ ASSESSING YOUR UNDERSTANDING

The first section of each Study Guide chapter concentrates on the basic information of the textbook chapter and helps you to remember key concepts, vocabulary, and principles.

- Fill in the Blanks

  Fill in the blank exercises test important chapter information, encouraging you to recall key points.

- Labeling

  Labeling exercises are used where you need to remember certain visual representations of the concepts presented in the textbook.

- Match the Following

  Matching questions test your knowledge of the definition of key terms.

- Sequencing

  Sequencing exercises ask you to remember particular sequences or orders, for instance testing processes and prioritizing nursing actions.

- Short Answers

  Short answer questions will cover facts, concepts, procedures, and principles of the chapter. These questions ask you to recall information as well as demonstrate your comprehension of the information.

- Crossword Puzzles

  Crossword Puzzles also cover important facts, concepts, procedures, and principles of the chapter in a diverting exercise.

■ APPLYING YOUR KNOWLEDGE

The second section of each Study Guide chapter consists of case study–based exercises that ask you to begin to apply the knowledge you've gained from the textbook chapter and reinforced in the first section of the Study Guide chapter. A case study scenario based on the chapter's content is presented, and then you are asked to answer some questions, in writing, related to the case study. The questions cover the following areas:

- Assessment
- Planning Nursing Care
- Communication
- Reflection

■ PRACTICING FOR NCLEX

The third and final section of the Study Guide chapters helps you practice NCLEX-style questions while further reinforcing the knowledge you have been gaining and testing for yourself through the textbook chapter and the first two sections of the study guide chapter. In keeping with the NCLEX, the questions presented are multiple-choice and scenario-based, asking you to reflect, consider, and apply what you know and to choose the best answer out of those offered.

■ANSWER KEYS

The answers for all of the exercises and questions in the Study Guide are provided at the back of the book, so you can assess your own learning as you complete each chapter.

We hope you will find this Study Guide to be helpful and enjoyable, and we wish you every success in your studies toward becoming a nurse.

The Publisher

Contents

PART 1

INTRODUCTION TO NURSING PHARMACOLOGY

CHAPTER **1**
Introduction to Drugs   1

CHAPTER **2**
Drugs and the Body   4

CHAPTER **3**
Toxic Effects of Drugs   7

CHAPTER **4**
The Nursing Process in Drug Therapy
and Patient Safety   10

CHAPTER **5**
Dosage Calculations   14

CHAPTER **6**
Challenges to Effective Drug Therapy   17

PART 2

CHEMOTHERAPEUTIC AGENTS

CHAPTER **7**
Introduction to Cell Physiology   21

CHAPTER **8**
Anti-Infective Agents   25

CHAPTER **9**
Antibiotics   28

CHAPTER **10**
Antiviral Agents   31

CHAPTER **11**
Antifungal Agents   35

CHAPTER **12**
Antiprotozoal Agents   39

CHAPTER **13**
Anthelmintic Agents   42

CHAPTER **14**
Antineoplastic Agents   45

PART 3

DRUGS ACTING ON THE IMMUNE SYSTEM

CHAPTER **15**
Introduction to the Immune Response
and Inflammation   49

CHAPTER **16**
Anti-Inflammatory, Antiarthritis,
and Related Agents   52

CHAPTER **17**
Immune Modulators   56

CHAPTER **18**
Vaccines and Sera   59

PART 4

DRUGS ACTING ON THE CENTRAL AND PERIPHERAL NERVOUS SYSTEMS

CHAPTER 19
Introduction to Nerves and the Nervous System   62

CHAPTER 20
Anxiolytic and Hypnotic Agents   65

CHAPTER 21
Antidepressant Agents   68

CHAPTER 22
Psychotherapeutic Agents   72

CHAPTER 23
Antiseizure Agents   76

CHAPTER 24
Antiparkinsonism Agents   79

CHAPTER 25
Muscle Relaxants   82

CHAPTER 26
Narcotics, Narcotic Antagonists and Antimigraine Agents   86

CHAPTER 27
General and Local Anesthetic Agents   90

CHAPTER 28
Neuromuscular Junction Blocking Agents   93

PART 5

DRUGS ACTING ON THE AUTONOMIC NERVOUS SYSTEM

CHAPTER 29
Introduction to the Autonomic Nervous System   96

CHAPTER 30
Adrenergic Agonists   100

CHAPTER 31
Adrenergic Blocking Antagonists   103

CHAPTER 32
Cholinergic Agonists   107

CHAPTER 33
Anticholinergic Agents   110

PART 6

DRUGS ACTING ON THE ENDOCRINE SYSTEM

CHAPTER 34
Introduction to the Endocrine System   113

CHAPTER 35
Hypothalamic and Pituitary Agents   116

CHAPTER 36
Adrenocortical Agents   119

CHAPTER 37
Thyroid and Parathyroid Agents   122

CHAPTER 38
Agents to Control Blood Glucose Levels   126

PART 7

DRUGS ACTING ON THE REPRODUCTIVE SYSTEM

CHAPTER 39
Introduction to the Reproductive System   130

CHAPTER 40
Drugs Affecting the Female Reproductive System   134

CHAPTER **41**

Drugs Affecting the Male Reproductive System   137

PART **8**

DRUGS ACTING ON THE CARDIOVASCULAR SYSTEM

CHAPTER **42**

Introduction to the Cardiovascular System   140

CHAPTER **43**

Drugs Affecting Blood Pressure   143

CHAPTER **44**

Cardiotonic Agents   147

CHAPTER **45**

Antiarrhythmic Agents   150

CHAPTER **46**

Antianginal Agents   153

CHAPTER **47**

Lipid-Lowering Agents   156

CHAPTER **48**

Drugs Affecting Blood Coagulation   159

CHAPTER **49**

Drugs Used to Treat Anemias   163

PART **9**

DRUGS ACTING ON THE RENAL SYSTEM

CHAPTER **50**

Introduction to the Renal System   166

CHAPTER **51**

Diuretic Agents   170

CHAPTER **52**

Drugs Affecting the Urinary Tract and the Bladder   173

PART **10**

DRUGS ACTING ON THE RESPIRATORY SYSTEM

CHAPTER **53**

Introduction to the Respiratory System   176

CHAPTER **54**

Drugs Acting on the Upper Respiratory Tract   179

CHAPTER **55**

Drugs Acting on the Lower Respiratory Tract   182

PART **11**

DRUGS ACTING ON THE GASTROINTESTINAL SYSTEM

CHAPTER **56**

Introduction to the Gastrointestinal System   185

CHAPTER **57**

Drugs Affecting Gastrointestinal Secretions   189

CHAPTER **58**

Drugs Affecting Gastrointestinal Motility   192

CHAPTER **59**

Antiemetic Agents   195

ANSWER KEY   198

Introduction to Drugs

LEARNING OBJECTIVES

Upon completion of this chapter, you will be able to:

1. Define the word *pharmacology*.

2. Outline the steps involved in developing and approving a new drug in the United States.

3. Describe the federal controls on drugs that have abuse potential.

4. Differentiate between generic and brand name drugs, over-the-counter drugs, and prescription drugs.

5. Explain the benefits and risks associated with the use of over-the-counter drugs.

■ ASSESSING YOUR UNDERSTANDING

MATCHING

Select the description from column 2 that best describes the term in column 1.

Column 1

____ **1.** Pharmacology

____ **2.** Brand name

____ **3.** Chemical name

____ **4.** Generic name

____ **5.** Adverse effects

Column 2

a. The original drug designation given when the drug company applies for approval

b. The study of the biologic effects of a chemical

c. Undesirable or possibly dangerous result of a drug

d. The trade name of a drug

e. The designation for a drug that reflects chemical structure

SEQUENCING

Each of the following statements reflects a step in the process of drug evaluation. Place the number of the statement in the boxes below based on the order in which they occur.

1. Healthy male volunteers are used to test the drugs.

2. The Food and Drug Administration (FDA) approves the drug.

3. Patients with the disease receive the drug.

4. The drug is tested in the laboratory using animals.

5. Prescribers administer the drug reporting any unexpected adverse effects.

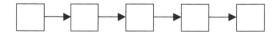

FILL IN THE BLANKS

Provide the missing term or terms in the blanks provided.

1. _____ is the branch of pharmacology that uses drugs to treat, prevent, and diagnose disease.

2. Morphine is an example of a drug derived from a _____ source.

3. Scientists produce human insulin by altering the DNA of *Escherichia coli* via a process called _____ _____.

4. During preclinical trials, a drug is considered _____ if it is found to cause adverse effects on the fetus.

5. A drug in pregnancy category _____ is considered safe for use during pregnancy because studies have shown it not to be at risk to the fetus in the first trimester or in later trimesters.

6. An _____ drug is one that has been discovered but is not considered financially viable and has not been adopted by any drug company.

■ APPLYING YOUR KNOWLEDGE

CASE STUDY

A 66-year-old man comes to the clinic for a routine visit. He has brought along a brown paper bag that contains numerous medicines. The nurse empties the bag on the table and begins to review the bottles. The patient states, "I've got so many bottles of pills here, I'm not sure what I'm supposed to take and not take." The nurse observes that several of the bottles contain the same medication.

a. How would knowledge of generic and brand names be helpful in this situation?

b. What other information would be important to obtain when taking this patient's drug history?

■ PRACTICING FOR NCLEX

Circle the letter that corresponds to the best answer for each question.

1. After administering a medication to a patient, the patient complains of an upset stomach. The nurse interprets this as a negative effect of the drug and identifies it as which of the following?
   a. Adverse effect
   b. Intended effect
   c. Teratogenic effect
   d. Therapeutic effect

2. Which of the following is a key concern related to clinical pharmacology?
   a. The biologic effect of a drug
   b. The body processes used to eliminate a drug
   c. The drug's effects on the body
   d. The proper method for administering a drug

3. Which of the following drugs may be derived from an animal source?
   a. Digitalis
   b. Opium
   c. Morphine
   d. Insulin

4. A group of students are reviewing information about the natural sources of drugs. The students demonstrate understanding of the information when they identify which of the following as a drug derived from inorganic compounds?
   a. Thyroid hormone
   b. Ferrous sulfate (iron)
   c. Codeine
   d. Castor oil

5. During a phase II study, a drug may be removed from testing for which reason?
   a. Greater than anticipated effectiveness
   b. Low risk of toxicity
   c. High benefit-to-risk ratio
   d. Unacceptable adverse effects

6. During which stage of drug development is the drug tested on laboratory animals?
   a. Preclinical trial
   b. Phase I study
   c. Phase II study
   d. Phase III study

7. While reviewing a package insert for a drug, which of the following would the nurse identify as the drug's generic name?
   a. L-thyroxine
   b. Levothyroxine sodium
   c. Levothroid
   d. Synthroid

8. Which phase of drug development is associated with continual evaluation of the drug?
   a. Phase I study
   b. Phase II study
   c. Phase III study
   d. Phase IV study

9. A nurse reviews the pregnancy risk categories for several drugs. A drug belonging to which category would the nurse identify as being safest to administer to a pregnant woman?
   a. Category X
   b. Category A
   c. Category B
   d. Category C

10. Male volunteers are usually selected for drug testing during a phase I study for which reason?
    a. Women are more unreliable in terms of adhering to the terms of the study.
    b. Men typically have a greater consistency in body build and makeup.
    c. The risk for damaging or destroying ova is too great.
    d. Men are less likely to develop toxic effects related to the drug.

11. A nurse is preparing to administer a cough syrup containing codeine to a patient. The nurse understands that this drug would be classified as which schedule of a controlled substance?
    a. C-II
    b. C-III
    c. C-IV
    d. C-V

12. Regulatory control over drug testing and evaluation by the FDA resulted from which legislation?
    a. Pure Food and Drug Act of 1906
    b. Federal Food, Drug, and Cosmetic Act of 1938
    c. Durham-Humphrey Amendment of 1951
    d. Kefauver-Harris Act of 1962

13. Which agency is responsible for the enforcement of controlled substances?
    a. FDA
    b. U.S. Department of Justice
    c. Drug Enforcement Agency
    d. Department of Health and Human Services

14. After studying the various sources of drugs, a group of students demonstrate a need for additional study when they identify which of the following as an example of a synthetic source for a drug?
    a. Plants
    b. Animals
    c. Inorganic compounds
    d. Genetic engineering

15. A nurse is administering a drug to patients who have the disease for which a drug is designed to treat. The nurse is most likely participating in which of the following?
    a. Preclinical trial
    b. Phase I study
    c. Phase II study
    d. Phase III study

Drugs and the Body

LEARNING OBJECTIVES

Upon completion of this chapter, you will be able to:

1. Describe how body cells respond to the presence of drugs that are capable of altering their function.

2. Outline the process of dynamic equilibrium that determines the actual concentration of a drug in the body.

3. Explain the meaning of half-life of a drug and calculate the half-life of given drugs.

4. List at least six factors that can influence the actual effectiveness of drugs in the body.

5. Define drug–drug, drug–alternative therapy, drug–food, and drug–laboratory test interactions.

■ ASSESSING YOUR UNDERSTANDING

SEQUENCING

The four steps of pharmacokinetics are listed below. Place the number of the step in the boxes below based on the order in which they occur.

1. Metabolism

2. Excretion

3. Absorption

4. Distribution

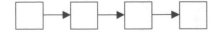

MATCHING

Select the description from column 2 that best describes the term in column 1.

Column 1

____ **1.** Critical concentration

____ **2.** Loading dose

____ **3.** First-pass effect

____ **4.** Half-life

Column 2

a. The time it takes for amount of drug in the body to decrease 50% of the peak level

b. The use of a higher dose than that which is usually used for treatment

c. The amount of drug that must be reached in tissues to cause the desired effect

d. Inactivation of an orally administered drug by liver enzymes before entering the general circulation

FILL IN THE BLANKS

Provide the missing term or terms in the blanks provided.

1. _____ refers to how a drug affects the body.

2. _____ refers to how the body acts on a drug.

3. A drug that interacts directly with receptor sites causing the same activity that natural chemicals would cause at that site is called

an _____.

4. The major process through which drugs are absorbed into the body is _____ _____.

5. Drug metabolism or _____ is the process by which drugs are changed into new, less-active chemicals.

■ APPLYING YOUR KNOWLEDGE

CASE STUDY

A 72-year-old woman comes in for a follow-up visit after being diagnosed with high blood pressure. The woman is obese and has a history of kidney disease. Her blood pressure remains elevated despite lifestyle changes. Medications to control her blood pressure are being ordered.

a. When assessing this patient, which factors possibly influencing drug effects would be most important to consider?

b. What other factors might play a role for this patient?

■ PRACTICING FOR NCLEX

Circle the letter that corresponds to the best answer for each question.

1. Which of the following would be a key element associated with pharmacodynamics?
   a. Enzyme systems
   b. Critical concentration
   c. Dynamic equilibrium
   d. Protein binding

2. When administering a drug, the nurse understands that a drug administered by which route would be absorbed most rapidly?
   a. Oral
   b. Intramuscular
   c. Intravenous
   d. Subcutaneous

3. When researching information about a drug, the nurse finds that the drug tightly binds to protein. The nurse would interpret this to mean which of the following?
   a. The drug will be released fairly quickly.
   b. The drug will have a long duration of action.
   c. The drug will be excreted quickly.
   d. The drug will lead to toxicity when given.

4. Which of the following most commonly occurs first when an oral drug is being absorbed?
   a. Liver enzymes break down the drug into metabolites.
   b. The drug is delivered to the circulatory system for transport.
   c. The drug moves from the small intestine directly into the portal venous system.
   d. A portion of the drug reaches the tissues before getting to the liver.

5. When describing biotransformation to a group of students, which of the following would the instructor include as part of phase II biotransformation?
   a. Oxidation
   b. Reduction
   c. Hydrolysis
   d. Conjugation

6. Which of the following substances would most likely inhibit the cytochrome P450 enzyme system?
   a. Nicotine
   b. Alcohol
   c. Ketoconazole
   d. Cortisone

7. Which of the following plays the largest role in drug excretion?
   a. Skin
   b. Kidneys
   c. Feces
   d. Lungs

8. A patient is receiving 250 mg of a drug that has a half-life of 8 hours. How much drug would remain after 24 hours?

   a. 125 mg

   b. 62.5 mg

   c. 31.25 mg

   d. 15.625 mg

9. A nurse administers a prescribed loading dose of digoxin based on the understanding that doing so will result in which of the following?

   a. Critical concentration being reached more quickly

   b. Enhanced absorption for effectiveness

   c. Prevention of drug breakdown by stomach acid

   d. Prolonged half-life of the administered drug

10. A nurse is preparing to administer a prescribed drug to a patient who has liver disease. The nurse expects a reduction in dosage based on the understanding that which of the following might be altered?

    a. Absorption

    b. Distribution

    c. Metabolism

    d. Excretion

11. Which mechanism is primarily responsible for drug absorption in the body?

    a. Active transport

    b. Passive diffusion

    c. Protein binding

    d. Filtration

12. When assessing a patient for possible factors that may affect the pharmacokinetics of a drug, a patient with a history of which of the following would lead the nurse to suspect that the patient may experience an alteration in the distribution of a drug?

    a. Gastrointestinal disease

    b. Liver disease

    c. Kidney disease

    d. Vascular disease

13. A nurse is reading an article that describes predictable differences in the effects of drugs in people of particular culture backgrounds due to their genetic makeup. The nurse is reading about which of the following?

    a. Pharmacogenomics

    b. Pharmacodynamics

    c. Pharmacokinetics

    d. Pharmacology

14. An instructor is describing a specific area on a cell membrane where most drugs are thought to act. The students demonstrate understanding of this information when they identify this area as which of the following?

    a. Lock

    b. Enzyme system

    c. Receptor site

    d. Agonist

15. Penicillin causes bacterial cell death without disrupting normal human cell functioning. This is an example of which of the following?

    a. Critical concentration

    b. Selective toxicity

    c. First-pass effect

    d. Enzyme induction

Toxic Effects of Drugs

Upon completion of this chapter, you will be able to:

1. Define the term *adverse drug reaction* and explain the clinical significance of this reaction.

2. List four types of allergic responses to drug therapy.

3. Discuss five common examples of drug-induced tissue damage.

4. Define the term *poison*.

5. Outline the important factors to consider when applying the nursing process to selected situations of drug poisoning.

■ ASSESSING YOUR UNDERSTANDING

MATCHING

Select the description from column 2 that best describes the term in column 1.

Column 1

_____ **1.** Anaphylactic reaction

_____ **2.** Cytotoxic reaction

_____ **3.** Serum sickness reaction

_____ **4.** Delayed allergic reaction

Column 2

a. Reaction involving antibodies that are bound to specific white blood cells

b. Reaction involving antibodies circulating in the blood and attacking antigens on cell sites, causing cell death

c. Reaction involving antibodies circulating in the blood and causing damage to tissues via deposition in blood vessels

d. Reaction involving antibody with specific sites in the body causing the release of chemicals to produce an immediate reaction

SHORT ANSWER

Supply the information requested.

1. List two reasons why adverse effects can occur.

2. Explain why it is important to always review the contraindications and cautions associated with a drug before administering it.

3. Identify the most common reason for the development of adverse effects related to drug therapy.

7

4. List the four main classifications of drug allergies.

5. Describe how superinfections occur with drug administration.

6. Define *blood dyscrasia*.

7. Name the electrolyte that when altered due to drug therapy can cause the most serious effects.

8. List four assessment findings associated with anticholinergic effects.

■ APPLYING YOUR KNOWLEDGE

CASE STUDY

The nurse is obtaining a history from a 35-year-old woman who is being scheduled for outpatient surgery. During the interview, the patient reports using an over-the-counter antihistamine for her hay fever. The nurse also asks the patient about any allergies to food or medications. The patient responds, "I'm allergic to codeine."

a. What effects might the nurse expect the patient to report with the use of antihistamines?

b. What information would the nurse need to obtain to determine if the patient has a "true allergy" to codeine?

■ PRACTICING FOR NCLEX

Circle the letter that corresponds to the best answer for each question.

1. When instructing a patient who is taking an antibiotic about the possibility of nausea and diarrhea, the nurse understands that these effects are examples of which of the following?
   a. Primary actions
   b. Secondary actions
   c. Drug allergy
   d. Hypersensitivity

2. A patient develops a cytotoxic reaction to a drug. Which of the following would the nurse expect to do?
   a. Administer prescribed epinephrine subcutaneously
   b. Encourage the use of Medic-alert identification
   c. Discontinue the drug immediately as ordered
   d. Administer antipyretics as ordered

3. When assessing a patient who has developed a serum sickness reaction, which of the following would the nurse expect to find?
   a. Hives
   b. Difficulty breathing
   c. Decreased white blood cell count
   d. Facial edema

4. A patient develops stomatitis from drug therapy. Which measure would be most appropriate for the nurse to suggest?
   a. Consumption of three large meals per day
   b. The use of an astringent mouthwash
   c. Frequent rinsing with cool liquids
   d. Brushing of teeth with a firm toothbrush

5. The nurse would assess a patient receiving which medication for possible superinfection?
   a. Antibiotics
   b. Antihistamines
   c. Antihypertensives
   d. Antineoplastics

6. Which of the following would lead the nurse to suspect that a patient has developed a blood dyscrasia related to drug therapy? Select all that apply.
   a. Thrombocytopenia
   b. Anemia
   c. Leukocytosis
   d. Dilute urine
   e. Headache
   f. Sore throat

7. The nurse is reviewing the laboratory test results of a patient receiving drug therapy. Which of the following would the nurse suspect if the results reveal an elevation in the blood urea nitrogen level and creatinine concentration?
   a. Liver injury
   b. Hypoglycemia
   c. Hyperkalemia
   d. Renal injury

8. Which of the following would the nurse include in the teaching plan for a patient who is to receive a drug that is associated with anticholinergic effects?
   a. Try to stay as warm as possible to prevent chilling.
   b. Be sure to drink plenty of fluids to prevent dehydration.
   c. Try using hard candy or lozenges to prevent dry mouth.
   d. Eat a low-fiber diet to prevent constipation.

9. Which of the following would the nurse expect to assess if a patient develops neuroleptic malignant syndrome?
   a. Mental confusion
   b. Hypothermia
   c. Hypertension
   d. Hyperactive reflexes

10. A patient exhibits muscular tremors, drooling, gait changes, and spasms. When reviewing the patient's medication history, which of the following would the nurse most likely find?
    a. Antipsychotic agent
    b. Antidiabetic agent
    c. General anesthetic
    d. Anticholinergic agent

11. An instructor is preparing a class that describes the toxic effects of drugs. Which of the following would the instructor expect to include?
    a. Many drugs are potentially harmless if used correctly.
    b. Any effect results from the alteration of several chemical factors.
    c. Most reactions occurring with present-day therapy are less severe than before.
    d. Drugs cause unexpected or unacceptable reactions despite screening and testing.

12. Which of the following is an example of a secondary action?
    a. Anticoagulant that leads to excessive and spontaneous bleeding
    b. Dizziness and weakness with a recommended dose of antihypertensive
    c. An antihistamine causes the patient to experience drowsiness
    d. Urinary retention develops in a patient with an enlarged prostate who is taking an anticholinergic

13. Which of the following would the nurse expect to assess in a patient experiencing an anaphylactic reaction? Select all that apply.
    a. Dilated pupils
    b. Feeling of panic
    c. High fever
    d. Swollen joints
    e. Difficulty breathing

14. Which of the following would the nurse expect the physician to order for a patient with a delayed allergic reaction?
    a. Epinephrine
    b. Antipyretic
    c. Anti-inflammatory
    d. Topical corticosteroid

15. A patient is receiving a drug to lower his blood glucose level. Which of the following would lead the nurse to suspect that his blood glucose level was too low?
    a. Cold, clammy skin
    b. Increased urination
    c. Fruity breath odor
    d. Increased hunger

CHAPTER 4

The Nursing Process in Drug Therapy and Patient Safety

Upon completion of this chapter, you will be able to:

1. List the responsibilities of the nurse in drug therapy.

2. Explain what is involved in each step of the nursing process as it relates to drug therapy.

3. Describe key points that must be incorporated into the assessment of a patient receiving drug therapy.

4. Describe the essential elements of a medication order.

5. Outline the important points that must be assessed and considered before administering a drug, combining knowledge about the drug with knowledge of the patient and the environment.

6. Describe the role of the nurse and the patient in preventing medication errors.

■ ASSESSING YOUR UNDERSTANDING

MATCHING

Select the description from column 2 that best describes the term in column 1.

Column 1

____ **1.** Assessment

____ **2.** Nursing diagnosis

____ **3.** Implementation

____ **4.** Evaluation

____ **5.** Nursing process

Column 2

a. Actions undertaken to meet a patient's needs

b. Information gathering

c. Determination of effectiveness

d. Problem-solving method

e. Actual or potential problem statement

SHORT ANSWER

Supply the information requested.

1. Explain what the nurse accomplishes when applying the nursing process to drug therapy.

2. List two major aspects associated with assessment.

3. Identify the seven rights to ensure safe and effective drug administration.

4. Name two areas that need to be addressed when obtaining a patient's history related to drug therapy.

5. Describe one reason why a patient may not reveal the use of over-the-counter drugs or alternative therapies during a history.

6. Explain why it is important to obtain a patient's weight before beginning drug therapy.

7. Describe the rationale for assessing physical parameters related to disease or drug effects before drug therapy begins.

8. Explain the term *placebo effect.*

LABELING

On the chart below, place the letter of the statement or phrase in the column that corresponds to the correct step of the nursing process.

Assessment	Nursing Diagnosis
Implementation	Evaluation

a. Deficient knowledge related to possible adverse effects of antihypertensive therapy

b. Diagnosed with type 2 diabetes 5 years ago

c. Administer the drug with food to minimize gastric upset

d. Takes omega-3 fish oil three times per week

e. Patient lives with husband in a two-bedroom apartment

f. Patient demonstrates independence in administering subcutaneous insulin administration

g. Obtain serum drug levels as ordered

h. Risk for injury related to drug's effect on balance and alertness

■ APPLYING YOUR KNOWLEDGE

CASE STUDY

An older adult patient is to begin drug therapy for treatment of a bacterial infection. The nurse completes an assessment and notes that the patient has a history of heart disease and diabetes. The patient, who is also somewhat underweight for his height, lives alone in a small apartment. His closest relative lives about an hour away. The patient is a native of Poland and speaks little English. He is accompanied by an older adult friend who helps explain information to him.

a. How might the patient's history of heart disease and diabetes impact his drug therapy?

b. Would the nurse expect the patient to be prescribed the typical recommended dosage? Why or why not?

c. What issues might affect the patient's ability to comply with the drug therapy regimen?

■ PRACTICING FOR NCLEX

Circle the letter that corresponds to the best answer for each question.

1. A nurse is gathering information about a patient. The nurse is participating in which step of the nursing process?
   a. Assessment
   b. Nursing diagnosis
   c. Implementation
   d. Evaluation

2. Which of the following would the nurse expect to do during implementation?
   a. Develop statements about a patient's actual problem
   b. Obtain baseline information about the patient's pattern of health care
   c. Identify the patient's social support network
   d. Provide patient teaching about a drug therapy regimen

3. A group of students are reviewing information about the nursing process and drug therapy in preparation for an examination on the material. The students demonstrate understanding of the material when they state which of the following about the nursing process?
   a. A continuous linear approach to problem solving
   b. A set of sequential steps that are dynamic in nature
   c. A method for determining a patient's priority needs
   d. A means to gather information about a patient's current status

4. During assessment, a nurse asks a patient about any chronic conditions that might have an impact on the patient's prescribed drug therapy. Which of the following, if reported by the patient, would alert the nurse to a possible problem?
   a. Two episodes of pneumonia over the last 5 years
   b. Kidney disease diagnosed 2 years ago
   c. Nearsightedness for the past 10 years
   d. Episode of gastroenteritis last month

5. Which of the following would be least important to include when teaching a patient about drug therapy?
   a. Alternative therapies to avoid
   b. Timing of administration
   c. Drug toxicity warning signs
   d. How to report a medication error

6. The nurse is reviewing several orders for medications. Which dosage would cause the nurse to be concerned?
   a. 0.5 mg
   b. 50 mg
   c. .5 mg
   d. 500 mg

7. A patient is to receive a topical drug. Which of the following would the nurse need to do?
   a. Check to see if it needs to be reconstituted
   b. Determine the possible need for skin preparation
   c. Question if the drug can be crushed
   d. Use a large amount of the drug to ensure effectiveness

8. Which of the following instructions would be most appropriate for the nurse to teach the patient to reduce the risk of medication errors in the home setting?
   a. Keep a written record of all prescription medications taken.
   b. Store the medications in the bathroom medicine cabinet.
   c. Take the medications according to what works best with the patient's schedule.
   d. Know what each drug is being used for as treatment.

9. A nurse who is caring for a patient receiving drug therapy performs the actions below. Place the actions in the proper sequence to reflect the steps of the nursing process.

    a. Teaches the patient how to minimize adverse reactions

    b. Identifies pertinent problems related to functioning

    c. Determines that the drug is therapeutically effective

    d. Questions the patient about any chronic conditions

10. After teaching the parents of a child who is receiving drug therapy, which statement indicates the need for additional teaching?

    a. "Some over-the-counter drugs contain the same ingredients, so we need to read each label closely before giving the medication."

    b. "We can use the same medications that we use for similar problems in our child, but we might need to adjust the dosage."

    c. "When measuring a liquid medication, we should use a measured device or spoon rather than a kitchen tablespoon or teaspoon."

    d. "We need to tell each health care provider about all the medications that our child is taking, even nonprescription ones."

11. Assessment of a patient receiving drug therapy reveals that the patient has been experiencing gastrointestinal upset related to the drug. The patient states, "My stomach has been so upset that all I've been able to eat is soup and dry crackers." Which nursing diagnosis would be most likely?

    a. Imbalanced nutrition: Less than body requirements

    b. Risk for imbalanced fluid volume

    c. Feeding self-care deficit

    d. Noncompliance

12. Which of the following would be least likely to occur during the assessment phase of the nursing process for drug therapy?

    a. Obtaining information about the patient's drug use

    b. Determining relevant data about financial constraints

    c. Developing outcomes for effective response to drug therapy

    d. Identifying the patient's level of understanding

13. The following are steps of the nursing process. Place the steps in the proper sequence from beginning to end.

    a. Nursing diagnosis

    b. Assessment

    c. Evaluation

    d. Implementation

14. The nurse questions a patient about the use of alternative therapies based on the understanding of which of the following?

    a. These therapies may lead to possible interactions with other drugs.

    b. The alternative therapies will need to be stopped with the newly prescribed drug.

    c. These therapies can lead to an increased risk for addiction.

    d. Alternative therapies provide information about the patient's health beliefs.

15. A nurse notes a medication error. Which action would be most appropriate?

    a. Notify the drug manufacturer.

    b. Make a report to the institution.

    c. Contact the Food and Drug Administration.

    d. Inform the Institute for Safe Medication Practices.

Dosage Calculations

Upon completion of this chapter, you will be able to:

1. Describe four measuring systems that can be used in drug therapy.

2. Convert between different measuring systems when given drug orders and available forms of the drugs.

3. Calculate the correct dose of a drug when given examples of drug orders and available forms of the drugs ordered.

4. Discuss why children require different dosages of drugs than adults.

5. Explain the calculations used to determine a safe pediatric dose of a drug.

■ ASSESSING YOUR UNDERSTANDING

FILL IN THE BLANKS

Provide the missing term or terms in the blanks provided.

1. One milliliter (mL) is equivalent to one

   _____ _____.

2. _____ rule is a method for determining the correct dose for a child based on the known adult dose.

3. One gram (g) is equivalent to _____ milligrams (mg).

4. All units in the metric system are determined as multiples of _____.

5. A _____ usually reflects the biologic activity of a drug in 1 milliliter (1 mL) of solution.

CROSSWORD

Use the clues to complete the crossword puzzle.

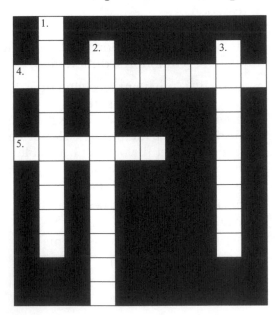

Across

4. Finding equivalent values between two systems
5. Most widely used system of measure

Down

1. Old system of measure used by pharmacists
2. Old system used when compounding medications
3. System of measure found in recipe books

■ APPLYING YOUR KNOWLEDGE

CASE STUDY

A mother brings her 3-year-old child to the clinic for evaluation of ear pain and fever. The child is diagnosed with an ear infection that is to be treated with oral antibiotics. The health care provider orders the antibiotic in suspension form. The nurse is preparing to teach the mother how to administer the antibiotic.

a. What information would be important for the nurse to obtain to ensure that the child receives the proper medication dosage?

b. What instructions would the nurse need to stress to ensure that the child receives the proper dose each time?

■ PRACTICING FOR NCLEX

Circle the letter that corresponds to the best answer for each question.

1. A group of students are reviewing the various measuring systems used for drug therapy. The students demonstrate understanding of these systems when they identify which of the following as the system used by pharmacists when they had to compound their own medications?
   a. Household system
   b. Avoirdupois system
   c. Apothecary system
   d. Metric system

2. Which of the following units of measure would a nurse expect to find when using the apothecary system?
   a. Liters
   b. Kilograms
   c. Drams
   d. Pounds

3. After teaching a group of students about measuring systems and drug calculations, the instructor determines that the teaching was successful when the students identify which system as most widely used?
   a. Metric system
   b. Apothecary system
   c. Household system
   d. Avoirdupois system

4. A nurse is using the metric system for dosage calculations. Which unit would the nurse use as the basic unit for measuring liquids?
   a. Gram
   b. Kilogram
   c. Liter
   d. Minim

5. A drug label reads "1 tablet equals 1 gr." The nurse understands that this one tablet is equivalent to how many milligrams?
   a. 30
   b. 60
   c. 240
   d. 1,000

6. A nurse needs to convert 3 fluid ounces to the metric system equivalent. The nurse performs the calculation to find which result?
   a. 90 mL
   b. 180 mL
   c. 240 mL
   d. 360 mL

7. A health care provider orders "aspirin gr x." The label on the bottle states that one tablet contains 5 grains. How many tablets would the nurse administer?
   a. 1
   b. 2
   c. 3
   d. 4

8. A physician orders 250 mg of an antibiotic suspension. The label on the suspension reads "500 mg/5 mL." How much would the nurse administer?
   a. 2.5 mL
   b. 5 mL
   c. 7.5 mL
   d. 10 mL

9. A nurse is to administer 500 mg of a drug intramuscularly. The label on the multidose vial reads 250 mg/mL. How much of the medication would the nurse prepare in the syringe?
   a. 0.5 mL
   b. 1 mL
   c. 1.5 mL
   d. 2 mL

10. The physician orders a patient to receive 1000 mL of intravenous fluid over the next 8 hours. The intravenous delivery set is a macrodrip system. The nurse would set the infusion to run at which rate?
    a. 16 gtts/min
    b. 32 gtts/min
    c. 64 gtts/min
    d. 125 gtts/min

11. A nurse needs to calculate a safe dose of medication for a child. Which of the following would be most appropriate for the nurse to use?
    a. Clark's rule
    b. Fried's rule
    c. Young's rule
    d. Body surface area

12. As part of a class exercise, an instructor asks the students to calculate a pediatric dosage using Clark's rule. Which information would be important for the students to know? Select all that apply.
    a. Weight of child in pounds
    b. Child's age in years
    c. Average adult dose
    d. Body surface area
    e. Child's height in centimeters

13. A child weighs 22 kilograms. The physician orders a drug as follows: "1.1 mg/kg by intramuscular injection." The nurse determines the proper dose as which of the following?
    a. 1.2 mg
    b. 2.4 mg
    c. 12 mg
    d. 24 mg

14. Which of the following established standards require all prescriptions to include the metric measure for quantity and strength?
    a. Food and Drug Administration
    b. U.S. Pharmacopeia Convention
    c. Drug Enforcement Agency
    d. Institute of Safe Medication Practices

15. An instructor is describing the units of measure associated with household system. Which of the following would the nurse include? Select all that apply.
    a. Teaspoon
    b. Quart
    c. Dram
    d. Ounce
    e. Cup
    f. Milliliter

CHAPTER

6

Challenges to Effective Drug Therapy

LEARNING OBJECTIVES

Upon completion of this chapter, you will be able to:

1. Discuss the impact of the media, the Internet, and direct-to-consumer advertising on drug sales and prescriptions.

2. Explain the growing use of over-the-counter drugs and the impact it has on safe medical care.

3. Discuss the lack of controls on herbal or alternative therapies and the impact this has on safe drug therapy.

4. Define the off-label use of a drug.

5. Describe measures being taken to protect the public in cases of bioterrorism.

■ ASSESSING YOUR UNDERSTANDING

MATCHING

Match the street name of the drug in column 2 with the appropriate drug in column 1.

Column 1

——— **1.** Amyl nitrate

——— **2.** Barbiturates

——— **3.** Benzodiazepines

——— **4.** Cocaine

——— **5.** MDMA

——— **6.** Heroin

——— **7.** Methamphetamine

——— **8.** Gamma-hydroxybutyrate

——— **9.** Ketamine

——— **10.** LSD

Column 2

a. Acid

b. Ecstasy

c. Blow

d. Boppers

e. Downers

f. Liquid X

g. Uncle Milty

h. Speed

i. Special K

j. Crank

SHORT ANSWER

Supply the information requested.

1. Name the one factor involved in the process for reviewing prescription drugs for possible over-the-counter (OTC) status.

2. State two reasons why patients may not mention the use of alternative therapies to health care providers.

3. Describe three areas that have impacted health care including drug therapy during the 21st century.

4. List two possible health consequences associated with the abuse of anabolic steroids.

5. Explain the term *biological weapon*.

■ APPLYING YOUR KNOWLEDGE

CASE STUDY

A patient comes to the health care clinic for a follow-up visit to evaluate his medications and control of his hypertension. During the visit he states, "My neighbor who is taking the same pills as I am for his high blood pressure has been telling me about all this information that he's gotten about his medicines on the Internet. He even said that he's found some herbs that work better than his medicines. I'm wondering if I should try these herbs too. Maybe they'll work better than what I'm using now."

a. How should the nurse respond to this patient?

b. What guidance should the nurse give to the patient about the Internet as a resource for information?

c. How should the nurse advise the patient about the use of herbs for his blood pressure?

■ PRACTICING FOR NCLEX

Circle the letter that corresponds to the best answer for each question.

1. A nurse is preparing a presentation for a local community group about various influences on drug therapy in today's health care climate. When addressing the impact of the media on drug therapy, which of the following would the nurse include?
   a. Television ads for prescription drugs is a recent development over the past 2 to 3 years.
   b. There currently are no federal guidelines as to what a company can say in an advertisement.
   c. Current medical research or reports are commonly making their way into headlines as news.
   d. Talk shows that include medical information typically present thorough and accurate information.

2. Which practice has contributed to the problem of resistant bacteria?
   a. Patients saving remaining antibiotics for the next time they feel sick
   b. The creation of matrix delivery systems for many medications
   c. The increased availability of generic-type drugs
   d. The use of drugs ordered through the Internet from foreign countries

3. A group of students ask an instructor about where to find the most updated information on biological weapons. Which of the following would the instructor recommend?
   a. Food and Drug Administration (FDA)
   b. Drug Facts and Comparisons
   c. National Center for Complementary and Alternative Medicine
   d. Centers for Disease Control

4. When describing off-label use, which of the following would the nurse need to keep in mind?
   a. Liability related to off-label use is clearly defined.
   b. Off-label drug use may lead to the discovery of a new use for the drug.
   c. Off-label drug use often involves drugs for treating heart disease.
   d. Off-label use indicates that the drug is awaiting FDA approval.

5. After reviewing the various types of street drugs frequently abused, a group of students demonstrate understanding of the information when they identify gamma-hydroxybutyrate as which class?
   a. Stimulant
   b. Hallucinogen
   c. Depressant
   d. Opioid

6. When discussing the various reasons why patients may order drugs via the Internet from other countries, which of the following would be least likely?
   a. The drugs are commonly less costly.
   b. The patient does not need to see a health care provider.
   c. The medications are delivered directly to the patient's doorstep.
   d. The drugs are the same as those the patient would get at home.

7. Which of the following would a nurse include when teaching a patient about proper drug disposal?
   a. Keep any unused or unneeded drugs in their original containers.
   b. Flush any unused medications down the toilet.
   c. Mix leftover prescription drugs with coffee grounds in a sealable bag.
   d. Crush the remaining medications in kitty litter before throwing into the trash.

8. A patient reports that he takes St. John's wort. When reviewing the patient's medication history, which of the following would be a cause of concern?
   a. Insulin
   b. Digoxin
   c. Ibuprofen
   d. Acetaminophen

9. A nurse is watching television and sees an ad for a drug. The drug's indication is mentioned in the ad. Which of the following would the nurse identify as also being required to include in the ad? Select all that apply.
   a. Adverse effects
   b. Contraindications
   c. Precautions
   d. Typical doses
   e. Route of administration

10. When describing the characteristics of the patient who comes into the health care system today, which of the following would apply?
   a. Limited exposure to other sources of health information
   b. Continued acceptance of the health care provider as omniscient
   c. Eager acceptance of the medications selected for the patient
   d. The use of a complex array of OTC and alternative therapies

11. After teaching a patient about how to evaluate an Internet site for information about health care and drug, which statement indicates that the teaching was successful?
   a. "A site is accurate if it has been updated in the last 10 years."
   b. "A commercial-type site is often the best one to use for current information."
   c. "A site that allows for feedback is more reputable than one that doesn't."
   d. "A site that gives me the information that I need is worthwhile."

12. Which of the following would be most appropriate to teach a patient about OTC drugs?

    a. They are safe when you use them as directed.

    b. There is little interaction between OTC drugs and prescription medications.

    c. Most OTC drugs have undergone stringent testing for use.

    d. OTC drugs often alert the health care provider to an underlying condition.

13. A patient arrives at the emergency department after abusing ketamine. Which of the following would the nurse expect to assess?

    a. Hallucinations

    b. Loss of sensation

    c. Memory loss

    d. Hypotension

14. A group of students are role-playing scenarios involving biological weapon exposure. Which of the following medications would the students identify as using for a patient with cutaneous anthrax?

    a. Ribavirin

    b. Ciprofloxacin

    c. Streptomycin

    d. Gentamicin

15. Which of the following drugs would be classified as a hallucinogen?

    a. Amyl nitrate

    b. Heroin

    c. Rohypnol

    d. PCP

CHAPTER 7

Introduction to Cell Physiology

LEARNING OBJECTIVES

Upon completion of this chapter, you will be able to:

1. Identify the parts of the human cell.
2. Describe the role of each organelle found within the cell cytoplasm.
3. Explain the unique properties of the cell membrane.
4. Describe three processes used by the cell to move things across the cell membrane.
5. Outline the cell cycle, including the activities going on within the cell in each phase.

MATCHING

Select the description from column 2 that best describes the term in column 1.

Column 1

____ **1.** Passive transport

____ **2.** Diffusion

____ **3.** Osmosis

____ **4.** Facilitated diffusion

____ **5.** Active transport

Column 2

a. Substance moves against a concentration gradient with the use of energy.

b. Substance moves from a region of higher concentration to a lower one via a carrier molecule.

c. Water moves from an area of low solute concentration to a higher solute concentration.

d. Substance moves across any semipermeable membrane without the use of energy.

e. Substance moves from a region of higher concentration to a lower concentration.

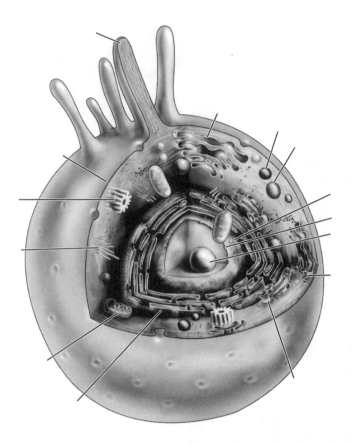

FILL IN THE BLANKS

Provide the missing term or terms in the blanks provided.

1. The _____ is the basic structural unit of the body.

2. Sequences of DNA that allow for cell division are called _____ .

3. The cell membrane is composed of _____ and _____ .

4. The cytoplasm of a cell contains many structures, called _____, which have specific functions.

5. The mitochondria produces _____ in the form of ATP for use by the cell.

6. The main goal of a cell is to maintain _____, which keeps the cytoplasm stable within the cell membrane via movement of solutes and water into and out of the cell.

7. The cell cycle consists of _____ active phases and a resting phase.

8. The _____ of a cell contains DNA and genetic material.

■ ASSESSING YOUR UNDERSTANDING

LABELING .

Use the list of terms below to label the cell.

Cell membrane
Centrioles
Cilia
Golgi apparatus
Lysosomes
Microtubules
Mitochondria
Nuclear membrane
Nuclear pore
Nucleolus
Perioxsomes
Polyribosomes
Rough endoplasmic reticulum
Smooth endoplasmic reticulum

■ APPLYING YOUR KNOWLEDGE

CASE STUDY

A group of students are working on a class assignment in which they are to present a visual demonstration of the cell cycle and events in each phase. They decide that one student will explain the cell cycle and its phases, while each of the other students will act out the events for a specific phase.

a. What events would the students need to demonstrate for each phase?

b. How might a student demonstrate the G_0 phase?

c. How might the students demonstrate the M phase?

■ PRACTICING FOR NCLEX

Circle the letter that corresponds to the best answer for each question.

1. Which of the following would be found in a cell membrane?
   a. Ribosomes
   b. Genes
   c. Cholesterol
   d. Mitochondria

2. When describing the DNA necessary for cell division, which of the following would be most accurate?
   a. It is found in long strains called *chromatin*.
   b. It is encapsulated in its own membrane.
   c. It is a series of dense fibers and proteins.
   d. It is composed of lipids and proteins.

3. The body uses which of the following to identify a cell as belonging to that individual?
   a. Receptor sites
   b. Histocompatibility antigens
   c. Channels
   d. Organelles

4. The mitochondria is responsible for which of the following functions?
   a. Protein production
   b. Cholesterol production
   c. Hormone processing
   d. Energy production

5. When preparing a class discussion about the various organelles of a cell, the instructor plans to include a description of the structure that contains digestive enzymes. Which of the following would the instructor be describing?
   a. Free ribosomes
   b. Lysosomes
   c. Golgi apparatus
   d. Endoplasmic reticulum

6. A group of students are studying for a test on cellular transport systems. The students demonstrate a need for additional study when they identify which mechanism as requiring no energy?
   a. Facilitated diffusion
   b. Osmosis
   c. Active transport
   d. Diffusion

7. A substance attaches itself to an enzyme in order to move in and out of a cell. This substance is moving via which transport mechanism?
   a. Diffusion
   b. Active transport
   c. Osmosis
   d. Facilitated diffusion

8. A solution contains the same concentration of solutes as human plasm. This solution would be classified as which of the following?
   a. Hypertonic
   b. Isotonic
   c. Hypotonic
   d. Osmotic

9. Which of the following would occur to a red blood cell if it were placed in a hypotonic solution?

   a. Burst

   b. Shrivel

   c. Shrink

   d. Remain the same

10. Which of the following statements best reflects the cell cycle?

    a. The secretion of enzymes determines the rate at which cells multiply.

    b. The reproductive rate of each cell determines the cell's life cycle.

    c. The cells found in breast tissue characteristically reproduce quickly.

    d. The life cycle of the cell involves four active phases and a resting phase.

11. Which of the following signals the end of the G_1 phase of the cell cycle?

    a. Formation of two identical daughter cells

    b. Formation of DNA

    c. Doubling of DNA

    d. Stimulation of the cell

12. Which transport mechanism is primarily used by the kidneys for drug excretion?

    a. Osmosis

    b. Facilitated diffusion

    c. Active transport

    d. Diffusion

13. A group of students are reviewing material about cell membranes in preparation for a quiz. Which statement indicates the need for additional study?

    a. The freely movable cell membrane allows the cell to repair itself.

    b. The polar regions of the cell membrane repel water.

    c. Receptor sites are located on the cell membrane.

    d. Cholesterol is found in large quantities in the cell membrane.

14. A substance being removed from a cell is being pushed through the cell membrane. What is the name of this process?

    a. Endocytosis

    b. Pinocytosis

    c. Phagocytosis

    d. Exocytosis

15. During which phase of the cell cycle is the cell at rest?

    a. G_0

    b. G_1

    c. S

    d. G_2

Anti-Infective Agents

Upon completion of this chapter, you will be able to:

1. Explain what is meant by selective toxicity and discuss its importance in anti-infective therapies.

2. Differentiate between broad-spectrum and narrow-spectrum drugs.

3. Define resistance to anti-infectives and discuss the emergence of resistant strains.

4. Explain three ways to minimize bacterial resistance.

5. Describe three common adverse reactions associated with the use of anti-infectives.

■ ASSESSING YOUR UNDERSTANDING

MATCHING

Select the drug action from column 2 that best describes the drug in column 1.

Column 1

_____ **1.** Penicillins

_____ **2.** Sulfonamides

_____ **3.** Aminoglycosides

_____ **4.** Fluoroquinolones

_____ **5.** Antifungals

Column 2

a. Interference with DNA synthesis in the cell

b. Interference with pathogen cell wall biosynthesis

c. Interference with protein synthesis

d. Prevention of invading organisms from using cellular substances

e. Alteration in the cell membrane permeability

SHORT ANSWER

Supply the information requested.

1. Identify the overall goal of anti-infective agents.

2. Explain the terms *bactericidal* and *bacteriostatic*.

3. Describe what is meant by "spectrum of activity."

4. Identify the first step in determining which anti-infective agent should be used.

5. List three ways that health care providers can help prevent the emergence of resistant strains of organisms.

■ APPLYING YOUR KNOWLEDGE

CASE STUDY

A patient comes to the clinic for a follow-up visit. On the previous visit about a week ago, the patient was prescribed penicillin to treat a staphylococcal infection of a wound on the patient's lower left leg. On this visit, the wound appears slightly smaller in size, but there is a moderate amount of purulent drainage oozing from the wound. The patient states, "It was better several days ago, about 3 days after I started taking the penicillin. Since it was better, I stopped taking the medicine."

a. What would the nurse suspect as a potential problem with the patient's wound?

b. What teaching would be most important for this patient?

■ PRACTICING FOR NCLEX

Circle the letter that corresponds to the best answer for each question.

1. A nurse is preparing a teaching plan for a patient who is receiving trimethoprim-sulfamethoxazole. Which of the following would the nurse need to keep in mind when describing how this drug works?
   a. Interfering with the pathogen cell wall
   b. Preventing the organism's cells from using substances
   c. Interfering with protein synthesis
   d. Altering the permeability of the cell membrane

2. Which of the following occurs when the normal flora is destroyed by the use of anti-infectives?
   a. Neurotoxicity
   b. Hypersensitivity
   c. Superinfection
   d. Resistance

3. A patient asks a nurse why the health care provider has prescribed two anti-infective agents. Which response by the nurse would be most appropriate?
   a. "You have a resistant strain of organism that requires the use of more than one drug."
   b. "The one drug doesn't come in a strong enough strength to clear the infection."
   c. "You need larger amounts of both drugs so you'll have fewer adverse effects."
   d. "Your infection, like many infections, is caused by more than one organism."

4. Which of the following would a nurse least expect as an adverse reaction to anti-infective agents?
   a. Kidney damage
   b. Hypersensitivity
   c. Respiratory toxicity
   d. Neurotoxicity

5. A patient is receiving an aminoglycoside antibiotic for an infection. The nurse would monitor the patient closely for which of the following?
   a. Hearing loss
   b. Lethargy
   c. Visual changes
   d. Hallucinations

6. A female patient comes to the clinic complaining of a vaginal discharge with itching. When obtaining the patient's medication history, which of the following would the nurse consider as significant?
   a. Inhaled bronchodilator for asthma
   b. Broad spectrum anti-infective for recent infection
   c. Oral contraceptive use
   d. Daily multivitamin supplement

7. A group of students are reviewing information about anti-infective agents. The students demonstrate a need for additional review when they identify which of the following as an anti-infective agent?
   a. Antibiotic
   b. Anthelmintic
   c. Antiprotozoal
   d. Anticoagulant

8. When describing an anti-infective agent with a narrow spectrum of activity, which of the following would the nurse include?

   a. The drug is effective against many different organisms.

   b. The drug is highly aggressive in killing the pathogen.

   c. The drug is selective in its action on organisms.

   d. The drug is effective in interfering with the cell's reproduction.

9. After teaching a group of students about resistance, the instructor determines that the students need additional teaching when they identify which of the following as a way that microorganisms develop resistance?

   a. Production of an enzyme that deactivates the drug

   b. Change in cellular permeability preventing drug entrance

   c. Altered binding sites that no longer accept the drug

   d. Production of a chemical to act as an agonist

10. Which of the following would contribute to drug resistance?

    a. High dosage to eradicate the organism

    b. Antibiotic prescription for viral illness

    c. Around-the-clock scheduling

    d. Prescribed duration of therapy

11. A patient is to receive penicillin. The nurse understands that this drug achieves it effect by which action?

    a. Interfering with the pathogen cell wall

    b. Not allowing the organism to use the substances it needs

    c. Disrupting the steps of protein synthesis

    d. Interfering with DNA synthesis

12. To ensure that the most appropriate drug is being used to treat a pathogen, which of the following would need to be done first?

    a. Using combination therapy

    b. Obtaining sensitivity testing

    c. Checking patient allergies

    d. Evaluating the bactericidal effects

13. A patient who is receiving anti-infective therapy is experiencing gastrointestinal toxicity. Which of the following would the nurse expect to assess?

    a. Dizziness

    b. Rash

    c. Diarrhea

    d. Vertigo

14. A patient is receiving chloroquine as part of her treatment for a rheumatic disorder. Which complaint would lead the nurse to suspect that the patient is experiencing toxicity?

    a. "I'm having trouble hearing."

    b. "My vision is getting really poor."

    c. "I feel like the room is spinning."

    d. "I get so dizzy sometimes."

15. An older adult patient is prescribed an anti-infective agent. Which of the following would the nurse need to keep in mind?

    a. Signs and symptoms of infection are the same as those for a younger patient.

    b. The patient has a lower risk for developing gastrointestinal toxicity and neurotoxicity.

    c. Liver and kidney function may be reduced, requiring cautious use.

    d. The patient will most likely want to have a rapid cure for his problem.

CHAPTER 9

Antibiotics

LEARNING OBJECTIVES

Upon completion of this chapter, you will be able to:

1. Explain how an antibiotic is selected for use in a particular clinical situation.

2. Describe therapeutic actions, indications, pharmacokinetics, contraindications, most common adverse reactions, and important drug–drug interactions associated with each of the classes of antibiotics.

3. Discuss the use of antibiotics as they are used across the lifespan.

4. Compare and contrast prototype drugs for each class of antibiotics with other drugs in that class.

5. Outline nursing considerations for patients receiving each class of antibiotic.

■ ASSESSING YOUR UNDERSTANDING

FILL IN THE BLANKS

Provide the missing term or terms in the blanks provided.

1. _____ bacteria can survive without oxygen.

2. Bacteria that are _____ - _____ are frequently associated with infections of the respiratory tract.

3. Some antibiotics are given in combination because they are _____.

4. Aminoglycosides are _____, inhibiting protein synthesis and ultimately leading to cell death.

5. The prototype cephalosporin is _____.

LABELING

Place the name of the following drugs in the appropriate box under the correct drug class.

Amikacin

Azithromycin

Erythromycin

Gemifloxacin

Gentamicin

Norfloxacin

Streptomycin

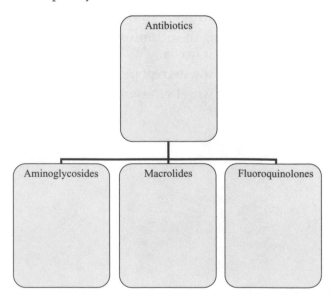

MATCHING

Match the antibiotic category with its prototype.

____ **1.** Aminoglycosides

____ **2.** Carbapenens

____ **3.** Cephalosporins

____ **4.** Fluoroquinolones

____ **5.** Macrolides

____ **6.** Penicillins

____ **7.** Sulfonamides

A. erythromycin (E-mycin)

B. ciprofloxacin (Cipro)

C. cotrimoxazole (Septra, Bactrim)

D. amoxicillin (Amoxil)

E. gentimicin (Garamycin)

F. ertapenem (Invanz)

G. cefaclor (Ceclor)

■ APPLYING YOUR KNOWLEDGE

CASE STUDY

A patient comes to the clinic complaining of urinary frequency, urgency, and pain on urination. A urine culture reveals an infection with a *Escherichia coli*. The health care provider prescribes ciprofloxacin to be taken twice daily. The patient also has a history of acid reflux for which she uses an antacid as needed.

a. Would the nurse consider this an appropriate choice for the patient's condition? Please explain.

b. When teaching the patient about this drug, how would the nurse describe the drug's action?

c. What adverse effects would the nurse need to address with this patient?

d. Would the use of antacids interfere with the prescribed drug therapy? Why or why not?

■ PRACTICING FOR NCLEX

Circle the letter that corresponds to the best answer for each question.

1. Which of the following drugs would be classified as an aminoglycoside?

   a. Levofloxacin

   b. Clarithromycin

   c. Gentamicin

   d. Cefaclor

2. A patient is receiving telithromycin. The nurse understands that this drug is structurally related to which of the following?

   a. Penicillins

   b. Macrolides

   c. Cephalosporins

   d. Lincosamides

3. A patient is prescribed streptomycin. The nurse understands that this drug can be given only by which route?

   a. Oral

   b. Intravenous

   c. Ophthalmic

   d. Intramuscular

4. A patient is to receive gentamicin for treatment of an infection. Which of the following would be most important for the nurse to assess to establish a baseline?

   a. Nutritional status

   b. Auditory function

   c. Gastrointestinal function

   d. Muscle strength

5. A group of students are reviewing information about drugs used to treat tuberculosis. The students demonstrate understanding of the material when they identify which of the following drugs as a first-line treatment option?

   a. Rifampin

   b. Kanamycin

   c. Ciprofloxacin

   d. Capreomycin

6. After teaching a group of students about carbapenems, the instructor determines the need for additional teaching when the students identify which of the following as an example?

    a. Doripenem

    b. Imipenem-cilastatin

    c. Cefuroxime

    d. Ertapenem

7. The nurse is preparing a teaching plan for a patient who is receiving cephalosporins. Which of the following would the nurse identify as the most commonly occurring adverse effects?

    a. Vomiting and diarrhea

    b. Headache and dizziness

    c. Superinfections

    d. Phlebitis

8. A patient comes to the emergency department complaining of a throbbing headache, nausea, vomiting, chest pain, dyspnea, vertigo, and blurred vision. The patient reveals that he has been taking cefaclor for an infection. Which question would the nurse ask next?

    a. "Have you had any alcohol to drink in the past 72 hours?"

    b. "Are you taking an oral anticoagulant such as warfarin?"

    c. "Did the doctor prescribe any other antibiotics with this one?"

    d. "Have you been drinking enough fluids with the medicine?"

9. A group of students are reviewing material for a test on antibiotics. They demonstrate an understanding of the material when they identify which of the following as the first antibiotic introduced for clinical use?

    a. Erythromycin

    b. Ampicillin

    c. Cephalexin

    d. Penicillin

10. After teaching a patient who is prescribed oral erythromycin, the nurse determines that the teaching was successful when the patient states which of the following?

    a. "I need to take the medicine with a meal so I don't get an upset stomach."

    b. "I should drink a full 8-oz glass of water when I take the medicine."

    c. "I might have some bloody diarrhea after using this medicine."

    d. "I only need to take one pill every day for this medicine to work."

11. A patient is receiving rifampin and isoniazid in combination for treatment of tuberculosis. Which of the following would the nurse need to monitor closely?

    a. Liver function studies

    b. Urine culture

    c. Audiometric studies

    d. Pulmonary function studies

12. Which of the following drugs would be classified as a third-generation cephalosporin?

    a. Cefazolin

    b. Cefaclor

    c. Ceftazidime

    d. Cephalexin

13. Which of the following would a nurse identify as the prototype lincosamide drug?

    a. Erythromycin

    b. Clindamycin

    c. Lincomycin

    d. Clarithromycin

14. Which of the following would be considered a penicillinase-resistant antibiotic?

    a. Amoxicillin

    b. Ticarcillin

    c. Carbenicillin

    d. Nafcillin

15. The drug's effect on which of the following best reflects the major reason for avoiding the use of tetracyclines in children under 8 years of age?

    a. Teeth

    b. Hearing

    c. Vision

    d. Kidneys

Antiviral Agents

■ASSESSING YOUR UNDERSTANDING

LABELING

Place the name of the following drugs in the appropriate box under the correct drug class.

Abacavir

Delavirdine

Indinavir

Nevirapine

Saquinavir

Zidovudine

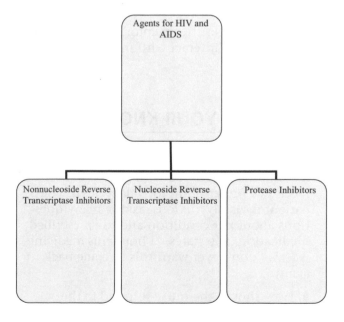

MATCHING

Select the description from column 2 that best describes the drug class in column 1.

Column 1

___ **1.** CCR5 coreceptor antagonist

___ **2.** Integrase inhibitor

___ **3.** Nucleoside reverse transcriptase inhibitor

___ **4.** Protease inhibitor

___ **5.** Nonnucleoside reverse transcriptase inhibitor

Column 2

a. Drug that directly binds to the HIV enzyme to prevent the transfer of information that would allow the virus to carry on the formation of viral DNA.

b. Drug that competes with the naturally occurring nucleosides within a human cell that the virus needs in order to develop the DNA chain.

c. Drug that interferes with the enzyme necessary for cell maturation, leaving the HIV particle immature and noninfective and unable to fuse with and inject itself into a cell.

d. Drug that interferes with the virus-specific encoded enzyme needed for viral replication, preventing the formation of the HIV-1 provirus.

e. Drug that blocks the receptor site that the HIV virus needs to interact with in order to enter the cell.

■ APPLYING YOUR KNOWLEDGE

CASE STUDY

A woman is diagnosed with genital herpes and receives a prescription for valacyclovir. The patient is visibly anxious, asking many questions about her condition and the prescribed medication. She states, "I hope this medicine works. I don't ever want this to come back again."

a. How should the nurse respond to the patient's statement?

b. What information would the nurse need to include in the teaching plan for this patient?

■ PRACTICING FOR NCLEX

Circle the letter that corresponds to the best answer for each question.

1. A patient is diagnosed with cytomegalovirus infection and is to receive foscarnet. The nurse would expect to administer this drug by which route?

   a. Oral

   b. Intramuscular

   c. Intravenous

   d. Topical

2. A patient comes to the health care facility complaining of flulike symptoms. After a thorough assessment, the patient is diagnosed with influenza and is to receive oseltamivir. The nurse understands that this drug has been prescribed because the patient been symptomatic for less than:

   a. 2 days

   b. 4 days

   c. 6 days

   d. 8 days

3. Which drug would a nurse least likely expect to be prescribed for a patient with chronic hepatitis B?

   a. Entecavir

   b. Telbivudine

   c. Adefovir

   d. Fosamprenavir

4. Which of the following was the first class of drugs developed to treat HIV infections?
   a. Protease inhibitors
   b. Nucleoside reverse transcriptase inhibitors
   c. Nonnucleoside reverse transcriptase inhibitors
   d. Fusion inhibitors

5. A nurse is explaining the rationale for the use of combination therapy in the treatment of HIV infections. Which of the following would the nurse include as the primary reason?
   a. More than one drug is needed to ensure sensitivity to the different forms of the virus.
   b. The use of multiple drugs allows attack on the virus at different points in its life cycle.
   c. One drug helps to control the virus, while the other drugs help to alleviate the adverse effects.
   d. Using several drugs at once helps to improve the patient's immune response.

6. A patient with HIV is pregnant. Which of the following agents would the nurse expect to be prescribed?
   a. Tenofovir
   b. Lamivudine
   c. Zidovudine
   d. Stavudine

7. A patient is receiving nevirapine as part of a treatment for HIV infection. The nurse would instruct the patient about which of the following adverse effects as most commonly experienced?
   a. Dry mouth and dyspepsia
   b. Light-headedness and dizziness
   c. Buffalo hump and thin extremities
   d. Paresthesias and fever

8. A patient is receiving zanamivir. When describing this drug, the nurse understands that it is absorbed through which mechanism?
   a. Gastrointestinal tract
   b. Bloodstream
   c. Respiratory tract
   d. Skin

9. Which of the following would be least likely to cause a drug interaction when rimantadine is prescribed?
   a. Atropine
   b. Acetaminophen
   c. Aspirin
   d. Ibuprofen

10. Assessment of a patient who is receiving nelfinavir reveals a severe life-threatening arrhythmia. The nurse would check the patient's history for use of which of the following?
    a. Midazolam
    b. Warfarin
    c. Clarithromycin
    d. Quinidine

11. Which of the following would a nurse identify as a CCR5 coreceptor antagonist?
    a. Enfuvirtide
    b. Maraviroc
    c. Raltegravir
    d. Didanosine

12. Which of the following would be most important to stress with a patient who is receiving adefovir for treatment of chronic hepatitis B?
    a. Possible adverse effects such as headache and dizziness
    b. Periodic follow-up renal function studies
    c. Maintenance of a continuous adequate supply of drug
    d. Measures to reduce the risk of infection transmission

13. A patient is being treated with docosanol. After teaching the patient about the drug, the nurse determines that additional instruction is needed when the patient states which of the following?
    a. "I should apply the medicine to any new open lesions that arise near the area."
    b. "I might have some burning or stinging in the area when I use the medicine."
    c. "There is little risk for absorbing the drug into my system this way."
    d. "I realize the drug won't cure me, but it should help with the discomfort."

14. A group of students are reviewing information about antiviral agents used to treat influenza and respiratory virus infections. The students demonstrate understanding of the material when they identify which drug as appropriate for treating Avian flu?

a. Amantadine

b. Oseltamivir

c. Ribavirin

d. Zanamivir

15. A patient with AIDS develops cytomegalovirus retinitis. The physician orders cidofovir. The nurse would prepare the patient for administration of the drug by which route?

a. Oral

b. Topical

c. Subcutaneous

d. Intravenous

Antifungal Agents

Upon completion of this chapter, you will be able to:

1. Describe the characteristics of a fungus and a fungal infection.

2. Discuss the therapeutic actions, indications, pharmacokinetics, contraindications, proper administration, most common adverse reactions, and important drug–drug interactions associated with systemic and topical antifungals.

3. Compare and contrast the prototype drugs for systemic and topical antifungals with the other drugs in each class.

4. Discuss the impact of using antifungals across the life span.

5. Outline the nursing considerations for patients receiving a systemic or topical antifungal.

■ ASSESSING YOUR UNDERSTANDING

CROSSWORD

Use the clues to complete the crossword puzzle.

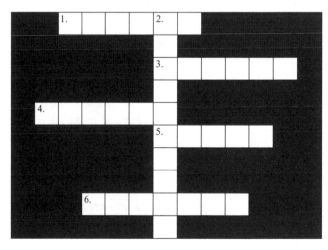

Across

1. A group of drugs used to treat fungal infections
3. An enzyme present in the fungal cell wall but not in human cells
4. A cellular organism with a hard cell wall
5. Ringworm that causes athlete's foot
6. A disease caused by a fungus

Down

2. A steroid-type protein found in fungal cell membranes

SHORT ANSWER

Supply the information requested.

1. Identify the enzyme system that is affected by ketoconazole and fluconazole.

2. Explain the reason why topical antifungals should not be used over open or draining areas.

3. Describe why the incidence of fungal infections has increased.

4. Name the three major types of local fungal infections.

5. State why a fungus is resistant to antibiotics.

6. Why should antifungal drugs be used with caution in patients with liver dysfunctions?

■ APPLYING YOUR KNOWLEDGE

CASE STUDY

During a routine physical examination of a client, the nurse notes that the skin on the patient's feet is extremely dry and cracked with areas where the skin is scaly. The area between the toes is slightly reddened, and the skin appears to be peeling. Several round 1- to 2-mm vesicles are also observed. The patient states that his feet perspire quite a bit, and they recently have become itchy. Tinea pedis is diagnosed, and topical clotrimazole as a cream is recommended.

a. How would the nurse instruct the patient to use the topical agent, and why would this be important?

b. What precautions would the nurse include about using this drug?

c. What additional instructions would be appropriate for this patient?

■ PRACTICING FOR NCLEX

Circle the letter that corresponds to the best answer for each question.

1. When describing the action of ketoconazole, which of the following would be most accurate?
   a. It inhibits the production of ergosterol.
   b. It interferes with formation of the fungal cell wall.
   c. It blocks sterol activity of the fungal cell wall.
   d. It inhibits a cytochrome P2D6 enzyme system.

2. A patient states, "My doctor said that I had mycosis, but I thought I had a fungal infection." Which response would be most appropriate?
   a. "You're both correct because mycosis means a disease is caused by a fungus."
   b. "Mycosis means that you have an underlying immune disease."
   c. "Let's talk to the doctor so that we can find out what really is going on here."
   d. "Don't worry, because mycosis is only a minor infection that is easily treatable."

3. Which of the following antifungal agents is available for systemic and topical use?
   a. Butoconazole
   b. Clotrimazole
   c. Voriconazole
   d. Ketoconazole

4. Which of the following would be most important for the nurse to monitor in a patient receiving amphotericin B?
   a. Coagulation studies
   b. Complete blood count
   c. Bowel sounds
   d. Respiratory status

5. The nurse is administering fluconazole intravenously. When would the nurse expect the drug to peak?
   a. 30 minutes
   b. 60 minutes
   c. 90 minutes
   d. 120 minutes

6. A patient is suspected of having a serious fungal infection for which systemic antifungal therapy is planned. Which of the following should be done first?
   a. Obtain a specimen for culture and sensitivity testing.
   b. Assess the patient's nutritional status.
   c. Check the results of the patient's renal function studies.
   d. Insert an intravenous access device for administration.

7. Which of the following statements best reflects topical antifungal agents?
   a. They are most effective when applied in a thick manner.
   b. They rarely cause local irritation and burning.
   c. They are too toxic to be used systemically.
   d. They are associated with many drug–drug interactions.

8. A group of students are studying for a test on antifungal agents. The students demonstrate understanding of the material when they identify which of the following as an example of an echinocandin antifungal?
   a. Terbinafine
   b. Amphotericin B
   c. Nystatin
   d. Caspofungin

9. A patient with a systemic fungal infection and a history of diabetes is to receive an antifungal agent. Based on the nurse's understanding about these agents, which agent would the nurse expect as being the least appropriate?
   a. Ketoconazole
   b. Fluconazole
   c. Itraconazole
   d. Terbinafine

10. A patient is receiving itraconazole. Which of the following drugs should be avoided? Select all that apply.
    a. Simvastatin
    b. Midazolam
    c. Warfarin
    d. Pimozide
    e. Digoxin
    f. Cyclosporine

11. A patient with migraine headaches typically uses ergot for relief. The patient now has a systemic fungal infection for which voriconazole is prescribed. Which of the following suggestions would be most appropriate for the nurse to give?
    a. "You can continue to take the ergot, but separate it from the voriconazole by at least 2 hours."
    b. "Wait until you've finished the regimen of voriconazole before using the ergot again."
    c. "Take the voriconazole with a large glass of water to promote excretion of the ergot."
    d. "The dosage of the voriconazole will need to be decreased when you take the ergot."

12. A patient is receiving flucytosine. The nurse is reviewing the patient's serum drug level. Which serum drug level would lead the nurse to suspect that the patient is developing toxicity?
    a. 22 mcg/mL
    b. 45 mcg/mL
    c. 88 mcg/mL
    d. 110 mcg/mL

13. Which of the following drugs would be contraindicated for a patient who is receiving amphotericin B?
    a. Penicillin
    b. Amantadine
    c. Gentamicin
    d. Aztreonam

14. A patient taking an oral antifungal agent reports gastrointestinal upset. Which of the following would be most appropriate to suggest?
    a. Calling the prescriber to change the drug
    b. Having the patient take the drug with food

c. Advising the patient to sit upright after taking the drug
d. Telling the patient to eat three large meals a day

15. The nurse cautions a patient taking sulconazole to limit therapy to which duration?
    a. 2 weeks
    b. 4 weeks
    c. 6 weeks
    d. 8 weeks

CHAPTER 12

Antiprotozoal Agents

LEARNING OBJECTIVES

Upon completion of this chapter, you will be able to:

1. Outline the life cycle of the protozoan that causes malaria.

2. Describe the therapeutic actions, indications, pharmacokinetics, contraindications, proper administration, most common adverse reactions, and important drug–drug interactions associated with drugs used to treat malaria.

3. Describe other common protozoal infections, including, cause and clinical presentation.

4. Compare and contrast the antimalarials with other drugs used to treat protozoal infections.

5. Outline the nursing considerations for patients receiving an antiprotozoal agent across the lifespan.

■ASSESSING YOUR UNDERSTANDING

FILL IN THE BLANKS

Provide the missing term in the blanks provided.

1. A _____ is a developing stage of a parasite.

2. *Plasmodium* is the protozoan that causes _____ in humans.

3. _____ is an infestation with a protozoan that causes vaginitis in women.

4. African sleeping sickness is called _____.

5. A _____ is a single-celled organism that passes through several stages in its life cycle.

SEQUENCING

The following are the stages in the life cycle of the plasmodium in humans. Place the number of the stage in the boxes below as they occur once a mosquito bites a human.

1. Schizont

2. Trophozoite

3. Sporozoite

4. Merozoite

5. Gametocyte

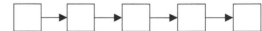

■ APPLYING YOUR KNOWLEDGE

CASE STUDY

A man comes to the urgent care center complaining of gastrointestinal distress. He states, "I've been having a fair amount of diarrhea over the past 2 days, and I have some pain in my belly." A stool specimen is obtained and sent for culture. The stool is loose, watery, and contains mucus. No blood is present. Further investigation reveals that the patient recently was camping in the mountains. Culture reports reveal giardiasis. The health care provider orders tinidazole.

a. What additional questions might the nurse ask to assist in helping the patient understand his condition? Explain why these questions would be important.

b. How would the nurse instruct the patient to take the tinidazole?

c. What specific areas need to be addressed related to this drug therapy?

■ PRACTICING FOR NCLEX

Circle the letter that corresponds to the best answer for each question.

1. Which statement best reflects the use of antimalarial agents for treatment of the protozoan?
   a. Typically, a single drug is sufficient to destroy the sporozoites in the early stages.
   b. Quinine is considered the current mainstay of treatment for malaria.
   c. Combination therapy is used to attack the parasite at various life cycle stages.
   d. The development of resistant strains of the parasite against antimalarial agents is rare.

2. When explaining the action of chloroquine to a patient, the nurse would incorporate knowledge of which of the following about the drug?
   a. Interferes with the parasites ability to reproduce
   b. Causes rupture of the cell, leading to its death
   c. Blocks the use of folic acid needed for protein synthesis
   d. Disrupts the mitochondria of the parasite

3. A patient is receiving mefloquine as part of a treatment for malaria asks the nurse about becoming pregnant. Which response by the nurse would be most appropriate?
   a. "You can plan to become pregnant once you complete the drug therapy regimen."
   b. "You need to avoid pregnancy during the therapy and for 2 months after completion."
   c. "You need to wait at least 6 months after starting the therapy before getting pregnant."
   d. "It's okay to become pregnant during therapy, but just don't plan to breast-feed."

4. A patient taking primaquine develops cinchonism. Which of the following would the nurse assess? Select all that apply.
   a. Tinnitus
   b. Vomiting
   c. Fever
   d. Dyspepsia
   e. Rash
   f. Vertigo

5. Which of the following assessments would be most important to complete for a patient who is to receive an antimalarial agent?
   a. Respiratory status
   b. Ophthalmologic evaluation
   c. Nutritional status
   d. Pupillary response

6. A patient who is receiving metronidazole therapy for trichomoniasis asks the nurse how this infection occurred. Which response by the nurse would be most appropriate?
   a. "You probably got bitten by a mosquito."
   b. "It is passed to humans by the common housefly."
   c. "The infection is spread during sexual intercourse."
   d. "You probably drank some contaminated water."

7. A patient with amebiasis is to receive metronidazole. The patient also takes warfarin for atrial fibrillation. The nurse would instruct the patient to report which of the following immediately?
   a. Abdominal cramps
   b. Ataxia
   c. Paresthesias
   d. Increased bleeding

8. A patient with *Pneumocystis carinii* pneumonia is to receive pentamidine. The nurse would expect to administer this drug most likely by which route?
   a. Oral
   b. Inhalation
   c. Transdermal
   d. Subcutaneous

9. A patient receiving which agent should be instructed to avoid alcohol consumption?
   a. Pentamidine
   b. Atovaquone
   c. Metronidazole
   d. Nitazoxanide

10. Atovaquone is indicated for use in which of the following?
    a. *Pneumocystis carinii* pneumonia
    b. Amebiasis
    c. Giardiasis
    d. Trypanosomiasis

11. Which agent would the nurse expect to administer to a patient with leishmaniasis?
    a. Metronidazole
    b. Nitazoxanide
    c. Atovaquone
    d. Pentamidine

12. A nurse is preparing a presentation for a group of individuals who are receiving prophylactic treatment for malaria in preparation for a trip to an endemic area. Which of the following would the nurse include as the underlying cause of this disorder?
    a. Bite of an infected mosquito
    b. Consumption of food from contaminated soil
    c. Consumption of unpurified spring water
    d. Bite of an infected tsetse fly

13. Which of the following would a nurse include as a major contributing factor to the development of protozoal infections?
    a. Widely scattered housing
    b. Tropical climate
    c. Adequate sanitary facilities
    d. Insect control

14. When a person is infected with malaria, the person receives which of the following?
    a. Sporozoites
    b. Schizonts
    c. Trophozoites
    d. Merozoites

15. Which agent would a nurse identify as being most schizonticidal?
    a. Chloroquine
    b. Primaquine
    c. Pyrimethamine
    d. Quinine

Anthelmintic Agents

Upon completion of this chapter, you will be able to:

1. List the common worms that cause disease in humans.

2. Describe the therapeutic actions, indications, pharmacokinetics, contraindications, most common adverse reactions, and important drug–drug interactions associated with the anthelmintics.

3. Discuss the use of anthelmintics across the lifespan.

4. Compare and contrast the prototype drug mebendazole with other anthelmintics.

5. Outline the nursing considerations, including important teaching points to stress, for patients receiving an anthelmintic.

■ ASSESSING YOUR UNDERSTANDING

SHORT ANSWER

Supply the information requested

1. List the five common types of infections by nematodes.

2. Identify the most frequent cause of helminth infection among school-age children in the United States.

3. Describe the difference between nematodes and platyhelminths.

4. Define *helminth*.

5. Name the disease that is caused by the ingestion of encysted roundworm larvae in undercooked pork.

MATCHING

Select the description of manifestations from column 2 that best reflects the infection in column 1.

Column 1

____ **1.** Pinworms

____ **2.** Whipworms

____ **3.** Threadworms

____ **4.** Hookworms

____ **5.** Cestodes

Column 2

a. Pneumonia, liver abscess

b. Weight loss, abdominal distention

c. Perianal itching, vaginal itching

d. Colic, bloody diarrhea

e. Anemia, malabsorption

■ APPLYING YOUR KNOWLEDGE

CASE STUDY

A mother brings her 7-year-old son to the office for an evaluation. The mother says that her son has been complaining of intense itching in his buttocks area over the last few days. "It's like he is scratching himself all the time." Further questioning reveals that the child attended an overnight camp about 6 weeks ago. The child is diagnosed with a pinworm infection, and drug therapy with mebendazole is prescribed. The mother says, "Oh, I'm so embarrassed. How did this happen?"

a. What factors may have contributed to the child's condition?

b. How should the nurse respond to the mother?

c. What instructions would the nurse include when teaching the mother about this drug therapy?

■ PRACTICING FOR NCLEX

Circle the letter that corresponds to the best answer for each question.

1. Which of the following would be associated with an infection caused by a flatworm?
   a. Pinworm
   b. Whipworm
   c. Ascaris
   d. Tapeworm

2. When interviewing a patient with a suspected worm infection, which of the following would lead the nurse to suspect trichinosis?
   a. Consumption of unwashed vegetables
   b. Ingestion of undercooked pork
   c. Recent insect bite
   d. Swimming in a contaminated lake

3. After reviewing class information about anthelmintic agents, a group of students demonstrate understanding of the material when they identify which drug as the prototype anthelmintic?
   a. Praziquantel
   b. Albendazole
   c. Mebendazole
   d. Pyrantel

4. Which infection would be associated with intestinal invasion by a worm?
   a. Ascaris
   b. Trichinosis
   c. Filariasis
   d. Schistosomiasis

5. A patient is prescribed pyrantel for the treatment of a roundworm infection. The nurse understands that this drug may be preferred for which reason?
   a. It is administered once a month.
   b. It completely eradicates the infection.
   c. It requires a single dose.
   d. It comes in a chewable form.

6. When describing mebendazole to a group of students, which of the following would the instructor include?

   a. Complete systemic absorption

   b. Numerous adverse effects

   c. No metabolism in the body

   d. Excretion as unchanged in urine

7. A patient is prescribed praziquantel. Which of the following would the nurse include when teaching the patient about how to take the drug?

   a. "Take the drug every morning and evening for a week."

   b. "Chew the tablet thoroughly each morning for 3 days."

   c. "Take the drug every 6 hours for three doses in 1 day."

   d. "Take the drug once in the morning."

8. Which of the following would the nurse be alert for in a patient receiving albendazole?

   a. Stevens-Johnson syndrome

   b. Bone marrow depression

   c. Diarrhea

   d. Fever

9. A patient with filariasis asks the nurse how he got the infection. The nurse would incorporate an understanding of which of the following when responding to the patient?

   a. The patient swam in a freshwater lake or pond where a snail deposited larvae.

   b. The patient consumed undercooked fish that contained the larvae of cestodes.

   c. The patient ate unwashed vegetables that were grown in contaminated soil.

   d. The patient was bitten by an insect that contained worm embryos.

10. Which drug would the nurse identify as the drug of choice for treating a threadworm infection?

    a. Pyrantel

    b. Praziquantel

    c. Albendazole

    d. Ivermectin

11. Which of the following would the nurse expect to assess in a patient with a whipworm infection?

    a. Bloody diarrhea

    b. Pneumonia

    c. Fatigue

    d. Weight loss

12. Which of the following would be most important to obtain for a patient who is suspected of having a helminthic infection?

    a. Complete blood count

    b. Urinalysis

    c. Liver function tests

    d. Stool examination

13. After teaching a local community group of students about measures to help prevent the spread of helminths, the nurse determines the need for additional teaching if the group identifies which measure?

    a. Weekly cleaning of bathroom toilets

    b. Thorough, frequent handwashing

    c. Consistent washing of fresh vegetables

    d. Using chlorine-treated water for laundry

14. Which of the following would the nurse identify as causing more damage to humans than most other helminths?

    a. Ascaris

    b. Threadworm

    c. Schistosomiasis

    d. Pinworm

15. Which of the following activities would be appropriate for a nurse to include when teaching a community group about measures to prevent trichinosis?

    a. Washing hands thoroughly after working with the soil

    b. Avoiding swimming in bodies of water that may be contaminated

    c. Ensuring that any pork products are thoroughly cooked

    d. Protecting oneself from possible insect bites

Antineoplastic Agents

Upon completion of this chapter, you will be able to:

1. Describe the nature of cancer and the changes the body undergoes when cancer occurs.

2. Describe the therapeutic actions, indications, pharmacokinetics, contraindications, most common adverse reactions, and important drug–drug interactions associated with each class of antineoplastic agents and with adjunctive therapy use with these drugs.

3. Discuss the use of antineoplastic drugs across the lifespan.

4. Compare and contrast the prototype drugs for each class of antineoplastic agents with the other drugs in that class.

5. Outline the nursing considerations and teaching needs for patients receiving each class of antineoplastic agents.

■ ASSESSING YOUR UNDERSTANDING

CROSSWORD

Use the clues to complete the crossword puzzle.

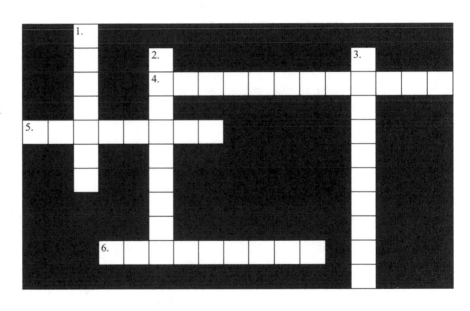

Across

4. Generation of new blood vessels
5. Hair loss
6. Loss of organization and structure

Down

1. Tumor originating in mesenchyme
2. Tumor originating in epithelial cells
3. Ability to enter circulatory or lymphatic system for travel to other areas

SHORT ANSWER

Supply the information requested.

1. Name the two major groups of cancer.

2. Explain how all cancers start.

3. List the two mechanisms by which antineoplastic drugs work.

4. Identify how or when a patient is considered to be cured of cancer.

5. Describe the reason why alkylating agents are said to be non–cell cycle specific.

6. State the phase of the cell cycle in which mitotic inhibitors act.

MATCHING

Match the antineoplastic drug category with its prototype.

____ **1.** Alkylating Agents

____ **2.** Antimetablites

____ **3.** Antineoplastic Antibiotics

____ **4.** Mitotic Inhibitors

____ **5.** Hormones and Hormone Modulators

____ **6.** Cancer Cell-Specific Agents

a. doxorubicin (Adriamycin)

b. imatinib (Gleevec)

c. chlorambucil (Leukeran)

d. tamoxifen (Soltamox)

e. vincristine (Oncovin)

f. methotrexate (Rheumatrex)

■ APPLYING YOUR KNOWLEDGE

CASE STUDY

A 75-year-old woman is diagnosed with stage IV ovarian cancer. She has undergone a total abdominal hysterectomy and is now being seen by the oncologist for follow-up chemotherapy. The oncologist plans to use cisplatin and paclitaxel. While the nurse is working with the patient to set up a schedule for the administration of the chemotherapy, the patient breaks down in tears and says, "I've heard so many horror stories about chemotherapy. I'm worried that I'll be throwing up all the time. And what am I going to do if I lose my hair?"

a. How would the nurse respond to the patient's concerns? What information should the nurse provide to the patient?

b. What issues related to scheduling would the nurse need to work out with the patient about the administration of the drugs? What suggestions would be appropriate for the nurse to make to help the patient during the visit for the chemotherapy administration?

■ PRACTICING FOR NCLEX

Circle the letter that corresponds to the best answer for each question.

1. Which drug would be classified as a mitotic inhibitor?

   a. Fluorouracil

   b. Methotrexate

   c. Chlorambucil

   d. Vincristine

2. A nurse administers ondansetron to a patient receiving chemotherapy for which reason?

   a. Reduce vomiting

   b. Prevent hypersensitivity

   c. Relieve inflammation

   d. Decrease secretions

3. A patient develops leukopenia after receiving chemotherapy. Which nursing diagnosis would be most appropriate?

   a. Disturbed body image

   b. Imbalanced nutrition

   c. Risk for infection

   d. Deficient fluid volume

4. Which agent would the nurse expect to be administered orally?

   a. Cytarabine

   b. Fluorouracil

   c. Gemcitabine

   d. Methotrexate

5. Which of the following would the nurse expect to administer to counteract the effects of methotrexate?

   a. Alprazolam

   b. Leucovorin

   c. Metoclopramide

   d. Aprepitant

6. Which of the following best reflects the action of antimetabolites?

   a. Reacts chemically with portions of RNA, DNA, or other cellular proteins

   b. Inserts itself between base pairs in the DNA chain, disrupting DNA synthesis

   c. Inhibits DNA production via replacing the natural substances needed for it

   d. Interferes with the ability of the cell to divide by blocking DNA synthesis

7. Which drug would have the least effect on healthy human cells?

   a. Etoposide

   b. Imatinib

   c. Vincristine

   d. Doxorubicin

8. A patient is receiving tamoxifen. Which adverse effect would be most specific to the action of this drug?

   a. Bone marrow suppression

   b. Gastrointestinal toxicity

   c. Hepatic dysfunction

   d. Menopausal effects

9. When planning the care for a patient receiving imatinib, the nurse would identify which nursing diagnosis as most likely?

   a. Excess fluid volume related to fluid retention

   b. Imbalanced nutrition, less than body requirements, related to severe nausea and vomiting

   c. Risk for infection related to bone marrow suppression

   d. Disturbed body image related to hair loss

10. A patient asks the nurse why the chemotherapy is often administered in cycles. Which response by the nurse would be most appropriate?

   a. "The drugs are highly toxic, so the body needs time to recover."

   b. "We want to attack the cells that might be dormant or moving into a new phase."

   c. "The cycles are the only way to guarantee a cure for the cancer."

   d. "The cycles help to prevent the drugs from destroying the healthy cells."

11. Which of the following would the nurse identify as an antineoplastic antibiotic?

   a. Mitomycin

   b. Teniposide

   c. Vinblastine

   d. Docetaxel

12. A patient is receiving bleomycin as part of his chemotherapy regimen. Which of the following would be most important for the nurse to monitor?

   a. Platelet count

   b. Electrocardiogram

   c. Chest x-ray

   d. Serum electrolytes

13. When describing the use of the various agents for combating chemotherapy-induced nausea and vomiting, the nurse understands that the majority of these agents block which of the following?

   a. Neurotransmitters

   b. Gastric acidity

   c. Gag reflex

   d. Chemoreceptor trigger zone

14. A nurse is preparing to administer imatinib to a patient. The nurse expects to administer this drug by which route?

    a. Oral

    b. Subcutaneous

    c. Intramuscular

    d. Intravenous

15. When describing the process of cancer cell growth to a patient, the nurse addresses angiogenesis. Which of the following descriptions would the nurse include?

    a. A process that involves the cells traveling to other areas of the body to develop new tumors

    b. The process of creating new blood vessels to supply oxygen and nutrients to the cells

    c. The process of growing without the usual homeostatic restrictions that regulate cells

    d. A process in which the cells lose their ability to differentiate and organize

CHAPTER 15

Introduction to the Immune Response and Inflammation

LEARNING OBJECTIVES

Upon completion of this chapter, you will be able to:

1. List four natural body defenses against infection.
2. Describe the cells associated with the body's fight against infection and their basic functions.
3. Outline the sequence of events in the inflammatory response.
4. Correlate the events in the inflammatory response with the clinical picture of inflammation.
5. Outline the sequence of events in an antibody-related immune reaction and correlate these events with the clinical presentation of such a reaction.

ASSESSING YOUR UNDERSTANDING

MATCHING

Select the description from column 2 that best describes the term in column 1.

Column 1

____ **1.** Antibody

____ **2.** Antigen

____ **3.** Calor

____ **4.** Leukocytes

____ **5.** Dolor

____ **6.** Tumor

____ **7.** Rubor

____ **8.** Pyrogen

Column 2

a. Swelling
b. Immunoglobulin
c. Heat
d. Redness
e. Foreign protein
f. Fever-causing substance
g. White blood cells
h. Pain

FILL IN THE BLANKS

Provide the missing term in the blanks provided.

1. The _____ system is activated by Hageman factor as part of the inflammatory response.

2. _____ cells are fixed basophils found in the respiratory and gastrointestinal tracts and in the skin that release chemical mediators.

3. The B-cell plasma cells produce _____ in response to a specific protein.

4. When neutrophils are drawn to an area, _____ is occurring.

5. The process of _____ involves engulfing and digesting foreign material.

■ APPLYING YOUR KNOWLEDGE

CASE STUDY

A patient comes to the clinic for evaluation. The patient is complaining of difficulty swallowing. On inspection, his throat is bright red and swollen. He has a fever and is complaining of an overall feeling of tiredness and general malaise. The patient is diagnosed with a strep throat.

a. How do the patient's signs and symptoms correlate with the events of the inflammatory response?

b. How might the immune system play a role here?

■ PRACTICING FOR NCLEX

Circle the letter that corresponds to the best answer for each question.

1. Which of the following would be considered the body's last barrier of defense?
   a. Skin
   b. Mucous membranes
   c. Gastric acid
   d. Major histocompatibility complex

2. Which of the following would be considered a lymphocyte?
   a. Neutrophils
   b. Monocytes
   c. T cells
   d. Macrophages

3. Which blood cell is responsible for phagocytosis?
   a. Neutrophils
   b. Basophils
   c. Eosinophils
   d. Macrophages

4. A group of students are reviewing class material about lymphoid tissue. The students demonstrate a need for additional teaching when they identify which of the following as lymphoid tissue?
   a. Bone marrow
   b. Thymus gland
   c. Spleen
   d. Histamine

5. Which event in the inflammatory response would the nurse correlate with the action of bradykinin?
   a. Vasoconstriction
   b. Pain
   c. Platelet aggregation
   d. Numbness

6. When describing the inflammatory response to a group of students, which of the following would the instructor include as the first event that occurs after cell injury?
   a. Activation of Hageman factor
   b. Conversion of kininogen to bradykinin
   c. Release of arachidonic acid
   d. Release of prostaglandins

7. A nurse assesses a patient and notes an area that is reddened and warm. The nurse understands that these findings are related to which of the following?
   a. Activation of nerve fibers
   b. Vasodilation
   c. Fluid leakage into tissues
   d. Release of pyrogen

8. Which cells are responsible for cell-mediated immunity?
   a. T cells
   b. B cells
   c. Neutrophils
   d. Immunoglobulins

9. Which immunoglobulin is released first when a patient encounters an antigen?
   a. Immunoglobulin M
   b. Immunoglobulin G
   c. Immunoglobulin A
   d. Immunoglobulin E

10. Which substance is responsible for stimu-lating T and B cells to initiate an immune response?
    a. Thymosin
    b. Tumor necrosis factor
    c. Interleukin-1
    d. Interferons

11. Which of the following occurs when the body produces antibodies against its own cells?
    a. Rejection
    b. Autoimmune disease
    c. Viral invasion
    d. Neoplastic growth

12. Which of the following best explains the role of mucus as a barrier for the body's defense?
    a. It promotes the removal of invaders.
    b. It sweeps away pathogens.
    c. It moves the pathogen to an area for removal.
    d. It traps the foreign material and thus inactivates it.

13. After reviewing information about the various myelocytes, the students demonstrate under-standing when they identify mast cells as which of the following?
    a. Mature leukocytes
    b. Circulating myelocytic leukocytes
    c. Fixed basophils
    d. Phagocytic neutrophils

14. Which of the following is responsible for storing a concentrated amount of white blood cells?
    a. Lymph nodes
    b. Thymus
    c. Spleen
    d. Bone marrow

15. A patient who waiting for an organ transplant asks the nurse why the donor organ must be matched. Which response by the nurse would be most appropriate?
    a. "Matching helps ensure that the proper organ is prepared."
    b. "Matching prevents you from having a reaction."
    c. "The closer the match, the less risk there is of rejection."
    d. "Matching is required by law before any transplant."

CHAPTER 16

Anti-Inflammatory, Antiarthritis, and Related Agents

Upon completion of this chapter, you will be able to:

1. Describe the sites of action of the various anti-inflammatory agents.

2. Describe the therapeutic actions, indications, pharmacokinetics, contraindications, most common adverse reactions, and important drug–drug interactions associated with each class of anti-inflammatory agents.

3. Discuss the use of anti-inflammatory drugs across the lifespan.

4. Compare and contrast the prototype drugs for each class of anti-inflammatory drugs with the other drugs in that class.

5. Outline the nursing considerations and teaching needs for patients receiving each class of anti-inflammatory agents.

■ ASSESSING YOUR UNDERSTANDING

MATCHING

Select the description from column 2 that best describes the term in column 1.

Column 1

____ **1.** Analgesic

____ **2.** Antipyretic

____ **3.** Chrysotherapy

____ **4.** Nonsteroidal anti-inflammatory drug (NSAID)

____ **5.** Anti-inflammatory agent

Column 2

a. Treatment with gold salts

b. Fever blocker

c. Pain blocker

d. Prostaglandin synthesis blocker

e. Inflammatory response blocker

SHORT ANSWER

Supply the information requested.

1. Name the prototype salicylate drug.

2. List two problems associated with the over-the-counter (OTC) use of anti-inflammatory agents.

3. Identify four signs of salicylate toxicity.

4. Describe the actions of cyclooxygenase-1 (COX-1) and cyclooxygenase-2 (COX-2).

5. Define *salicylism*.

■ APPLYING YOUR KNOWLEDGE

CASE STUDY

A 45-year-old man arrives at the clinic because he has noticed that his stools have become darker, almost black, in color and somewhat tarry. He also has noticed that his gums have started to bleed when he brushes his teeth. During the interview, the patient reveals that he takes 600 mg of ibuprofen about three times a day for a back injury that he suffered while working 2 years ago. Inspection reveals several large bruised areas—two on his left arm and one on his lower left leg. "I guess I'm a bit clumsy. I tripped and fell against my refrigerator door."

a. What other assessment information would the nurse need to gather?

b. What would the nurse need to address when teaching this patient?

■ PRACTICING FOR NCLEX

Circle the letter that corresponds to the best answer for each question.

1. Which agent would be least appropriate to administer to a patient with joint inflammation and pain?

a. Ibuprofen

b. Naproxen

c. Acetaminophen

d. Diclofenac

2. A patient is diagnosed with inflammatory bowel disease. Which agent would the nurse expect to administer?

a. Diflunisal

b. Aspirin

c. Choline magnesium trisalicylate

d. Mesalamine

3. After teaching a local community group about the use of OTC anti-inflammatory agents, the nurse determines that the group needs additional teaching when they state which of the following?

a. "These drugs are relatively safe since they don't have adverse effects."

b. "We can easily overdose on them if we don't follow the directions."

c. "Other signs and symptoms of an illness might not appear with these drugs."

d. "The drugs might interact with other drugs and cause problems."

4. A nurse suspects that a patient is experiencing salicylism. Which of the following would the nurse assess?

a. Excitement

b. Ringing in the ears

c. Tachypnea

d. Convulsions

5. Which instruction would be most important to include when teaching parents about OTC anti-inflammatory agents?
   a. "Be sure to read the label for the ingredients and dosage."
   b. "Aspirin is best for treating your child's flulike symptoms."
   c. "Make sure to give the drug on an empty stomach or before meals."
   d. "Refrain from using acetaminophen for the child's symptoms."

6. A salicylate is contraindicated in patients who have had surgery within the past week for which reason?
   a. Increased risk for allergic reaction
   b. Increased risk for toxicity
   c. Increased risk for bleeding
   d. Increased risk for fluid imbalance

7. Which of the following best describes the action of NSAIDs?
   a. Blocks prostaglandin activity
   b. Acts directly on thermoregulatory cells
   c. Inhibits phagocytosis
   d. Inhibits prostaglandin synthesis

8. A patient is to receive aurothioglucose. The nurse would administer this drug by which route?
   a. Oral
   b. Subcutaneous
   c. Intramuscular
   d. Intravenous

9. Which statement by a patient receiving gold salts indicates understanding of the drug therapy?
   a. "These drugs are used first to try to control my severe disease."
   b. "These drugs will help prevent further damage from my disease."
   c. "These drugs should help because I've had the disease for so long."
   d. "These drugs are safer than most of the other drugs for arthritis."

10. Which of the following would be appropriate to use in combination with gold salts?
    a. Penicillamine
    b. Cytotoxic agents
    c. Immunosuppressants
    d. Low-dose corticosteroids

11. After teaching a group of students about disease-modifying antirheumatic drugs, the instructor determines that the students need additional teaching when they identify which of the following as an example?
    a. Sulindac
    b. Etanercept
    c. Adalimumab
    d. Methotrexate

12. A patient is receiving anakinra as treatment for arthritis. The nurse understands that this drug acts in which manner?
    a. Interferes with free-floating tumor necrosis factor
    b. Inhibits the DHODH enzyme
    c. Blocks interleukin-1
    d. Lowers immunoglobulin M factor levels

13. A patient with severe rheumatoid arthritis of the knees has arrived at the facility for an injection of a drug into the joint. Which agent would the nurse most likely expect to be used?
    a. Auranofin
    b. Penicillamine
    c. Etanercept
    d. Sodium hyaluronate

14. A group of students are reviewing information about cyclooxygenase receptors. The students demonstrate understanding of the information when they identify which of the following as an effect of COX-2 receptors?

a. Maintenance of renal function

b. Blockage of platelet clumping

c. Provision of gastric mucosal integrity

d. Promotion of vascular hemostasis

15. A black patient is receiving a high dose of NSAID for pain relief. Which of the following would be most important for the nurse to include in the teaching plan?

a. The need to combine the drug with an OTC salicylate

b. Signs and symptoms of gastrointestinal bleeding

c. Avoidance of warm soaks for additional pain relief

d. Importance of adequate hydration

CHAPTER 17

Immune Modulators

LEARNING OBJECTIVES

Upon completion of this chapter, you will be able to:

1. Describe the sites of actions of the various immune modulators.
2. Describe the therapeutic actions, indications, pharmacokinetics, contraindications, most common adverse effects, and important drug–drug interactions associated with each class of immune stimulants and immune suppressants.
3. Discuss the use of immune modulators across the lifespan.
4. Compare and contrast the prototype drugs for each class of immune modulators with the other drugs in that class and with drugs in other classes.
5. Outline the nursing considerations and teaching needs for patients receiving each class of immune modulator.

■ ASSESSING YOUR UNDERSTANDING

LABELING

Place the name of the following drugs in the appropriate box under the correct drug class.

Adalimumab
Aldesleukin
Azathioprine
Cyclosporine
Oprelvekin
Rituximab

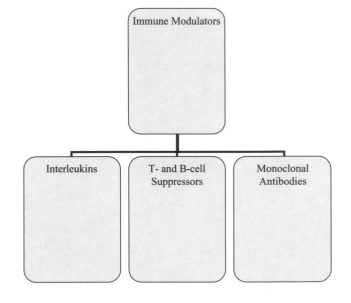

SHORT ANSWER

Supply the information requested.

1. Identify the two major classes of immune stimulants.

2. Name the interleukin receptor antagonist.

3. List the typical routes of administration for most monoclonal antibodies.

4. Describe the mechanism of action of the T- and B-cell suppressors.

5. Identify the two most serious risks associated with the use of immune suppressants.

■ APPLYING YOUR KNOWLEDGE

CASE STUDY

A patient who has been diagnosed with multiple sclerosis is experiencing an exacerbation of her symptoms. The patient reports that this has happened several times before, and the symptoms usually resolve without a problem. However, the patient has been noticing that these episodes have been occurring more often and lasting a bit longer. A decision is made to use interferon therapy. The patient asks, "What is this drug, and how will it help me?"

a. How would the nurse respond to the patient?

b. What interferons might be ordered for this patient? How are they similar, and how are they different?

c. What should the nurse include in the teaching plan about the drug therapy?

■ PRACTICING FOR NCLEX

Circle the letter that corresponds to the best answer for each question.

1. Which agent would be classified as an immune stimulant?
  a. Interferon alfa-2b
  b. Abatacept
  c. Mycophenolate
  d. Sirolimus

2. A patient is receiving oprelvekin. Which of the following would suggest that the patient is experiencing a hypersensitivity reaction?
  a. Cardiac arrhythmia
  b. Mental status change
  c. Chest tightness
  d. Fever

3. Which of the following would the nurse expect to administer orally?
  a. Alefacept
  b. Cyclosporine
  c. Glatiramer acetate
  d. Abatacept

4. A patient is experiencing flulike symptoms related to immune stimulant therapy. Which of the following instructions would be most appropriate for the patient?
  a. "Do not use acetaminophen for your fever or aches."
  b. "Keep your environment nice and warm."
  c. "You need to try and stay as busy as possible."
  d. "Drink plenty of fluids throughout the day."

5. Which monoclonal antibody is antibody specific to epidermal growth factor receptor sites?
  a. Muromonab-CD3
  b. Infliximab
  c. Cetuximab
  d. Adalimumab

6. A patient is to receive erlotinib. The nurse would expect to administer this drug by which route?
  a. Oral
  b. Subcutaneous
  c. Intramuscular
  d. Intravenous

7. Which of the following would lead the nurse to suspect that a patient receiving a monoclonal antibody is experiencing pulmonary edema?
  a. Fever
  b. Chills
  c. Myalgia
  d. Dyspnea

8. Which of the following would be most important for the nurse to do when administering gemtuzumab?
  a. Ensure that the patient's call light is readily available.
  b. Administer adequate fluids for hydration.
  c. Provide the patient with a bedside commode.
  d. Offer small frequent meals and snacks.

9. A patient is receiving mycophenolate after undergoing a liver transplant. Which of the following would be a priority nursing diagnosis?

    a. Acute pain

    b. Imbalanced nutrition

    c. Risk for infection

    d. Deficient knowledge

10. A group of students are reviewing information about immune modulators in preparation for a test. The students demonstrate understanding of the material when they identify which of the following as an immune stimulant?

    a. Monoclonal antibody

    b. Interleukin receptor antagonist

    c. T- and B-cell suppressor

    d. Interferon

11. When describing the production of interferons, the instructor discusses recombinant DNA technology. Which of the following would the instructor include as being produced this way?

    a. Interferon alfa-n3

    b. Interferon alfacon-1

    c. Interferon gamma-1b

    d. Interferon beta-1a

12. The nurse is teaching a patient receiving interferon therapy about measures to combat possible adverse effects. Which statement by the patient indicates the need for more teaching?

    a. "I need to be out in the sun so that I can get vitamin D."

    b. "I should drink plenty of liquids, including water."

    c. "I can use acetaminophen if I get a fever."

    d. "I might need some blood tests to check my blood count."

13. A patient with rheumatoid arthritis has been receiving various drug therapies for treatment but with little effect. Which of the following might the nurse expect to be used?

    a. Alefacept

    b. Azathioprine

    c. Glatiramer

    d. Abatacept

14. The nurse closely monitors a patient who is receiving anakinra and etanercept for which of the following?

    a. Anemia

    b. Severe infection

    c. Bleeding

    d. Hypersensitivity

15. After teaching a group of students about the various monoclonal antibodies, the instructor determines that the teaching was successful when the students identify muromonab-CD3 as specific to which of the following?

    a. T cells

    b. Human tumor necrosis factor

    c. Lymphocyte receptor sites

    d. Interleukin-2 receptor sites

18

Vaccines and Sera

Upon completion of this chapter, you will be able to:

1. Define the terms *active immunity* and *passive immunity*.

2. Describe the therapeutic actions, indications, pharmacokinetics, contraindications, most common adverse effects, and important drug–drug interactions associated with each vaccine, immune serum, antitoxin, and antivenin.

3. Discuss the use of vaccines and sera across the lifespan, including recommended immunization schedules.

4. Compare and contrast the prototype drugs for each class of vaccine and immune serum with others in that class.

5. Outline the nursing considerations and teaching needs for patients receiving a vaccine or immune serum.

■ ASSESSING YOUR UNDERSTANDING

FILL IN THE BLANKS

Provide the missing term or terms in the blanks provided.

1. Immune sera that contain antibodies to specific poisons produced by invaders are called _____.

2. Biologicals include _____, immune sera, and antitoxins.

3. When a host reacts to injected antibodies or foreign sera, a _____ _____ occurs.

4. _____ immunity results when preformed antibodies are injected into a host who is at high risk for exposure to a specific disease.

5. The process of artificially stimulating active immunity by exposing the body to weakened or less-toxic proteins associated with specific disease-causing organisms is called _____.

6. _____ was one of the first diseases against which children were vaccinated.

7. After an allergy shot, specific _____ antibodies appear in the serum.

8. A person who was bitten by a rattlesnake would most likely receive an _____.

SHORT ANSWER

Supply the information requested.

1. Describe the differences between active and passive immunity.

2. List two manifestations of serum sickness.

3. Describe when the vaccine against the human papilloma virus (HPV) should be given.

4. Identify the recommendations for immunizations for older adults.

5. Name the vaccine that is used throughout the world but is not routinely used in the United States.

APPLYING YOUR KNOWLEDGE

CASE STUDY

A mother brings her 14-year-old daughter to the pediatrician's office for a routine physical examination. During the visit, the mother asks the nurse practitioner about the vaccine for HPV. She states, "I've seen all those commercials on television about this vaccine, but I'm still not sure if my daughter should get it. I've heard so many stories about it. My close friend says that she doesn't want her daughter to get it because then her daughter will think that she can have sex sooner."

a. How should the nurse practitioner respond to the mother?

b. What information would be important to discuss with her?

c. If the mother decides that her daughter should be vaccinated, what would the nurse practitioner recommend?

PRACTICING FOR NCLEX

Circle the letter that corresponds to the best answer for each question.

1. When describing the use of vaccines to a local community group, which of the following would the nurse include?
   a. Vaccines are used to provide active immunity.
   b. Vaccines promote the development of antigens.
   c. Vaccines can result in signs and symptoms of the full-blown disease.
   d. Vaccines are associated with severe reactions in children.

2. A group of students are reviewing information about immunizations. The students demonstrate a need for additional study when they identify which of the following as a component of an immunization?
   a. Weakened bacterial cell membrane
   b. Viral protein coat
   c. Chemically weakened actual virus
   d. Serum with bacterial antibodies

3. A patient has been bitten by a dog, and the dog's rabies status is unknown. The nurse would expect this patient to receive which of the following?
   a. Vaccine
   b. Immune sera
   c. Antitoxin
   d. Antivenin

4. A nurse is preparing a presentation to a local community group about biological weapons. The nurse would identify which disease as lacking an available vaccine?
   a. Anthrax
   b. Plague
   c. Smallpox
   d. Botulism

5. Which of the following would the nurse identify as a vaccine that is a toxoid?
   a. Haemophilus influenza b
   b. Pneumococcal polyvalent
   c. Tetanus
   d. Hepatitis A

6. Which of the following would necessitate cautious use of a vaccine in a child? Select all that apply.
   a. Immune deficiency
   b. Allergy to a vaccine component
   c. Blood transfusion within the past 3 months
   d. History of febrile convulsions
   e. History of brain injury
   f. Acute infection

7. The nurse is teaching the parents of a child who is receiving a vaccine about possible adverse effects. Which of the following would the nurse include as necessitating an immediate call to the health care provider?
   a. Pain at the injection site
   b. Moderate fever
   c. Difficulty breathing
   d. Nodule formation at the site

8. A mother asks the nurse what she can do to help with the discomforts that her child may experience due to an immunization. Which of the following would be most appropriate?
   a. "Have him take some time to rest throughout the day."
   b. "Give him aspirin if he develops any fever."
   c. "Apply cold compresses to the injection site every 4 hours."
   d. "Encourage him to move his arm frequently during the day."

9. A patient was bitten by a poisonous snake. Which of the following would be most appropriate to administer?
   a. Antitoxin
   b. Toxoid
   c. Antivenin
   d. Immune sera

10. To prevent meningococcal infections, the nurse would administer which of the following?
    a. Vaccine
    b. Toxoid
    c. Immune globulin
    d. Antivenin

11. A nurse prepares to administer antithymocyte immune globulin. The nurse understands that this is used for which of the following?
    a. Prevent chicken pox
    b. Treat acute renal transplant rejection
    c. Provide postexposure prophylaxis for hepatitis B
    d. Prevent respiratory syncytial virus infection

12. A man who was working on his outside deck comes to the emergency department after sustaining a puncture wound of his hand from a large nail. Which of the following would the nurse expect to administer?
    a. Zoster vaccine
    b. Hepatitis A vaccine
    c. Lymphocyte immune globulin
    d. Tetanus toxoid

13. Which agent would the nurse expect to administer to a pregnant woman to prevent Rh factor sensitization?
    a. Crotalidae polyvalent immune fab
    b. Cytomegalovirus immune globulin
    c. RHO immune globulin
    d. HPV vaccine

14. The nurse is preparing to administer the rotavirus vaccine to an infant. The nurse would expect to administer this vaccine by which route?
    a. Oral
    b. Subcutaneous
    c. Intramuscular
    d. Intradermal

15. A patient who is going to college in the fall is to receive the meningococcal polysaccharide vaccine. The nurse would prepare to administer the vaccine in which site?
    a. Deep into the muscle of the lateral thigh
    b. Into the upper outer quadrant of the buttocks
    c. Directly into the dermis of the skin
    d. Into the fatty tissue of the upper arm

CHAPTER 19

Introduction to Nerves and the Nervous System

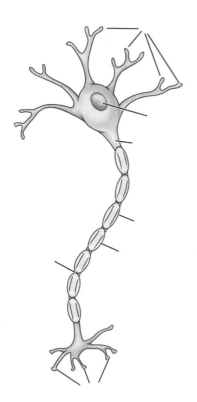

LEARNING OBJECTIVES

Upon completion of this chapter, you will be able to:

1. Label the parts of a neuron and describe the functions of each part.

2. Describe an action potential, including the roles of the various electrolytes involved in the action potential.

3. Explain what a neurotransmitter is, including its origins and functions at the synapse.

4. Describe the function of the cerebral cortex, cerebellum, hypothalamus, thalamus, midbrain, pituitary gland, medulla, spinal cord, and reticular activating system.

5. Discuss what is known about learning and the impact of emotion on the learning process.

■ ASSESSING YOUR UNDERSTANDING

LABELING

Use the list of terms below to label the neuron.

  Axon
  Dendrite
  Myelin sheath
  Neurilemma
  Nodes of Ranvier
  Nucleus
  Synaptic terminals

MATCHING

Select the description from column 2 that best describes the term in column 1.

Column 1

_____ **1.** Hindbrain

_____ **2.** Engram

_____ **3.** Dendrite

_____ **4.** Effector cell

_____ **5.** Ganglia

_____ **6.** Neuron

_____ **7.** Neurotransmitter

_____ **8.** Synapse

_____ **9.** Forebrain

_____ **10.** Axon

Column 2

a. Upper level of the brain consisting of two cerebral hemispheres

b. Short projection on a neuron that transmits information

c. Group of nerve bodies

d. Long projection from a neuron that carries information from one nerve to another

e. Most primitive area of the brain that contains the brain stem

f. Structural unit of the nervous system

g. Short-term memory made up of a reverberating electrical circuit of action potentials

h. Chemical produced by a nerve that reacts with specific receptor site

i. Muscle, gland, or another nerve stimulated by a nerve

j. Junction between a nerve and an effector

■ APPLYING YOUR KNOWLEDGE

CASE STUDY

A patient is admitted to the health care facility after experiencing a cerebrovascular accident due to a completely blocked carotid artery that has resulted in weakness of the patient's right side. His history reveals a narrowing of his carotid artery and several mini-strokes (TIAs) in which he experienced some weakness in his right arm and leg along with some numbness and tingling. These symptoms disappeared after several minutes. The patient says to the nurse, "They said I had a stroke that affected the left side of my brain, but then why is my right side so weak?"

a. How would the nurse respond to the patient?

b. What would the nurse understand about the brain's flow related to the signs and symptoms that the patient experienced with the mini-strokes?

■ PRACTICING FOR NCLEX

Circle the letter that corresponds to the best answer for each question.

1. Which of the following would be identified as the basic unit of the nervous system?

a. Synapse

b. Neurotransmitter

c. Neuron

d. Soma

2. Which of the following would a nurse identify as being responsible for carrying information from the nerve to the effector cell?

a. Dendrite

b. Axon

c. Soma

d. Ganglia

3. After teaching a group of students about the functions of the nervous system, the instructor determines that the students need additional teaching when they identify which of the following as a function?

a. Analysis of incoming stimuli

b. Control of body functions

c. Integration of responses

d. Prevention of stimulus exposure

4. Which of the following is responsible for carrying nerve impulses from the central nervous system to stimulate a muscle?

   a. Presynaptic nerve

   b. Schwann cell

   c. Efferent fibers

   d. Neurotransmitter

5. Which of the following would be most important for an action potential to occur?

   a. Sodium ions rushing into the cell

   b. Impermeability of the nerve cell membrane to potassium ions

   c. Sufficient strength of a stimulus

   d. Depolarization of the cell

6. Which of the following is considered a neurotransmitter and hormone released by the adrenal medulla?

   a. Dopamine

   b. Gamma-aminobutyric acid (GABA)

   c. Acetylcholine

   d. Epinephrine

7. A nurse is reading an article about sleep and arousal that includes a discussion of a neurotransmitter. Which neurotransmitter would most likely be discussed?

   a. GABA

   b. Serotonin

   c. Norepinephrine

   d. Dopamine

8. Which of the following best describes the blood–brain barrier?

   a. Nonfunctional boundary

   b. Defensive mechanism

   c. Blood delivery mechanism

   d. Vital function control center

9. Which of the following would a nurse identify as a component of the hindbrain?

   a. Thalamus

   b. Limbic system

   c. Brain stem

   d. Cerebrum

10. After studying for a test on the brain and spinal cord, the students demonstrate understanding when they identify the spinal cord as being made up of how many pairs of nerves?

    a. 31

    b. 24

    c. 12

    d. 8

11. When describing the function of the extrapyramidal system, which of the following would the instructor include?

    a. Regulation of motor function control

    b. Coordination of voluntary movement

    c. Processing of emotional information

    d. Coordination of position and posture

12. Stimulation of a nerve results in which of the following?

    a. Membrane potential

    b. Repolarization

    c. Depolarization

    d. Increased sodium outside the cell

13. Which of the following would be associated with the forebrain? Select all that apply.

    a. Motor neurons

    b. Cranial nerves

    c. Chemoreceptor trigger zone

    d. Speech area

    e. Spinal nerve roots

14. Which of the following would be responsible for the transmission of an electrical impulse along a nerve axon?

    a. Schwann cells

    b. Nodes of Ranvier

    c. Myelin

    d. Synapse

15. Which of the following would be found in the midbrain?

    a. Reticular activating system

    b. Respiratory control center

    c. Hypothalamus

    d. Swallowing center

Anxiolytic and Hypnotic Agents

Upon completion of this chapter, you will be able to:

1. Define the states that are affected by anxiolytic or hypnotic agents.

2. Describe the therapeutic actions, indications, pharmacokinetics, contraindications, most common adverse reactions, and important drug–drug interactions associated with each class of anxiolytic or hypnotic agent.

3. Discuss the use of anxiolytic or hypnotic agents across the lifespan.

4. Compare and contrast the prototype drugs for each class of anxiolytic or hypnotic drug with the other drugs in that class.

5. Outline the nursing considerations and teaching needs for patients receiving each class of anxiolytic or hypnotic agent.

■ ASSESSING YOUR UNDERSTANDING

FILL IN THE BLANKS

Supply the missing term in the blanks provided.

1. _____ is an unpleasant feeling of tension, fear, or nervousness in response to a real or imagined environmental stimulus.

2. Central nervous system (CNS) depression or sleep that results from extreme sedation is termed _____.

3. Sedation involves a loss of _____ and reaction to environmental stimuli.

4. Anxiety is often accompanied by signs and symptoms of the _____ stress reaction.

5. The most frequently used anxiolytic drugs are _____.

6. Hypnotics react with _____ inhibitory sites to depress the CNS.

7. A patient who consumes alcohol may experience _____ CNS depression if taken with barbiturates.

8. The drug ramelteon stimulates _____ receptors.

SHORT ANSWER

Supply the information requested.

1. Explain the reason why barbiturates are no longer considered a major drug category used to treat anxiety and promote sedation.

2. Describe the rationale for using parenteral forms of benzodiazepines only when absolutely necessary.

3. Identify the common responses that a child may exhibit after receiving an anxiolytic agent.

4. Name the site of action for drugs that are used as hypnotics.

5. Describe why blacks may require a reduced dosage of a benzodiazepine.

■ APPLYING YOUR KNOWLEDGE

CASE STUDY

A 75-year-old man is brought to the health care center by his daughter for a checkup. The daughter says that her father has been having difficulty sleeping lately. She states, "He goes to bed but then he winds up coming back downstairs and watching television. Eventually, he falls asleep a few hours later. Many times, we wake up and find him asleep on the couch." The patient says he just cannot seem to fall asleep when he goes to bed. The patient's physical examination is unremarkable, and the health care provider decides to prescribe zolpidem.

a. What additional information would be important for the nurse to obtain when assessing this patient?

b. Would the nurse expect the patient to receive the usual recommended dose for this drug? Why or why not?

c. What information would be most important for the nurse to include when teaching the patient and his daughter about this drug?

■ PRACTICING FOR NCLEX

Circle the letter that corresponds to the best answer for each question.

1. A patient is receiving ramelteon for insomnia. The nurse would instruct the patient to take the drug at which time?
   a. 2 hours before going to bed
   b. 1 hour before going to bed
   c. ½ hour before going to bed
   d. Immediately before going to bed

2. Which benzodiazepine would a nurse expect to administer as a hypnotic?
   a. Lorazepam
   b. Flurazepam
   c. Diazepam
   d. Alprazolam

3. When describing the action of benzodiazepines as anxiolytics, which of the following would the nurse need to keep in mind?
   a. Enhanced action of gamma-aminobutyric acid
   b. Effect on action potentials
   c. Depression of the cerebral cortex
   d. Depressed motor output

4. A patient received a parenteral benzodiazepine at 11 AM. The nurse would expect to allow the patient out of bed at which time?
   a. 12 PM
   b. 1 PM
   c. 2 PM
   d. 3 PM

5. Which of the following might occur if a patient inadvertently receives a benzodiazepine intra-arterially?
   a. CNS depression
   b. Blurred vision
   c. Urinary retention
   d. Arteriospasm

6. A patient is ordered to receive diazepam as part of the treatment for status epilepticus. The patient has an intravenous (IV) infusion running, which is being used to administer another drug for seizure control. The IV line is in the patient's left arm. Which action by the nurse would be most appropriate?
   a. Start another IV line in the patient's right arm.
   b. Notify the prescriber that the diazepam cannot be given.
   c. Add the diazepam to the current IV infusion.
   d. Wait until the other drug is completed to give the diazepam.

7. Which of the following would lead the nurse to suspect that a patient is experiencing withdrawal symptoms associated with benzodiazepine use?
   a. Dry mouth
   b. Nightmares
   c. Hypotension
   d. Urinary retention

8. A decrease in dosage of a prescribed benzodiazepine most likely would be necessary if a patient was also taking which of the following?
   a. Theophylline
   b. Ranitidine
   c. Oral contraceptive
   d. Alcohol

9. A patient receives a dose of diazepam at 4:00 PM. The nurse would expect to see the maximum effect of this drug at approximately which time?
   a. 4:30 PM
   b. 5:30 PM
   c. 6:30 PM
   d. 7:30 PM

10. A nurse is preparing to administer an anxiolytic to a patient. Which of the following would be most appropriate for the nurse to do before administering the drug?
    a. Raise the side rails.
    b. Institute a bowel program.
    c. Dim the lights.
    d. Have the patient void.

11. A patient has received a benzodiazepine for sedation before a diagnostic procedure. Which agent would the nurse expect the patient to receive to reverse the sedative effects?
    a. Temazepam
    b. Triazolam
    c. Flumazenil
    d. Promethazine

12. After reviewing the various drugs that are classified as barbiturates, a student demonstrates understanding when he identifies which of the following as the prototype?
    a. Amobarbital
    b. Secobarbital
    c. Pentobarbital
    d. Phenobarbital

13. A patient is receiving a barbiturate intravenously. The nurse would monitor the patient for which of the following?
    a. Hypertension
    b. Bradycardia
    c. Tachypnea
    d. Bleeding

14. A patient is prescribed an anxiolytic agent. Which of the following would be most important for the nurse to include in the teaching?
    a. "Be sure not to stop the drug abruptly."
    b. "Take the drug with meals if necessary."
    c. "Increase the amount of fiber in your diet."
    d. "Try other measures to help you relax, too."

15. Which agent has no sedative, anticonvulsant, or muscle relaxant properties but does reduce the signs and symptoms of anxiety?
    a. Diphenhydramine
    b. Zaleplon
    c. Buspirone
    d. Meprobamate

Antidepressant Agents

LEARNING OBJECTIVES

Upon completion of this chapter, you will be able to:

1. Describe the biogenic theory of depression.

2. Describe the therapeutic actions, indications, pharmacokinetics, contraindications, most common adverse reactions, and important drug–drug interactions associated with each class of antidepressant.

3. Discuss the use of antidepressants across the lifespan.

4. Compare and contrast the prototype drugs for each class of antidepressant with the other drugs in that class and with drugs in the other classes of antidepressants.

5. Outline the nursing considerations and teaching needs for patients receiving each class of antidepressant.

■ ASSESSING YOUR UNDERSTANDING

LABELING

Place the name of the following drugs in the appropriate box under the correct drug class.

Amoxapine

Citalopram

Doxepin

Fluoxetine

Nortriptyline

Phenelzine

Sertraline

Tranylcypromine

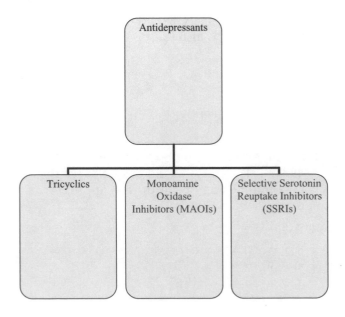

SHORT ANSWER

Supply the information requested.

1. Name the three biogenic amines implicated in depression.

2. Identify the two neurotransmitters that are affected by tricyclic antidepressants.

3. Define *affect*.

4. Describe the effect of combining foods containing tyramine with MAOIs.

5. Identify the tricyclic antidepressant that is associated with the greatest sedative and anticholinergic effects.

6. Explain why SSRIs often are a better choice for treating depression.

■ APPLYING YOUR KNOWLEDGE

CASE STUDY

A patient with a history of major depression comes to the emergency department complaining of a severe occipital headache, nausea, and vomiting. His blood pressure is extremely elevated. During the interview, the patient reports that he has taken several different drugs over the years without any real relief in his depression. He was recently started on phenelzine after having been prescribed imipramine.

a. What might the nurse suspect is happening to the patient?

b. What other assessment findings would help to confirm the suspicions?

c. Once the patient is stabilized, what information would the nurse need to include when teaching this patient about his drug therapy?

■ PRACTICING FOR NCLEX

Circle the letter that corresponds to the best answer for each question.

1. A patient is receiving an antidepressant that also aids in smoking cessation. Which drug would this most likely be?
   a. Venlafaxine
   b. Bupropion
   c. Mirtazapine
   d. Selegiline

2. A nurse is preparing a presentation about the use of antidepressants in children and adolescents. Which of the following would the nurse need to keep in mind?
   a. Studies have shown a clear link between suicide and the use of antidepressants.
   b. The majority of antidepressants approved for use in adults can be used with children.
   c. The smallest amount of drug that is feasible should be dispensed.
   d. Children typically demonstrate a predictable response to the drugs.

3. Which antidepressant would the nurse identify as being one associated with the least amount of common adverse effects?
   a. Nortriptyline
   b. Amitriptyline
   c. Clomipramine
   d. Doxepin

4. A patient is prescribed a tricyclic antidepressant. The nurse would anticipate administering this drug by which route?
   a. Oral
   b. Topical
   c. Intramuscular
   d. Intravenous

5. A group of students are reviewing information about tricyclic antidepressants and demonstrate understanding of the material when they identify which drug as also being indicated for the treatment of obsessive-compulsive disorder.
   a. Amoxapine
   b. Maprotiline
   c. Clomipramine
   d. Desipramine

6. A patient is to receive a tricyclic antidepressant. The nurse is reviewing the patient's medical record. Which of the following would alert the nurse to a possible contraindication?
   a. Glaucoma
   b. Prostatic hypertrophy
   c. Renal dysfunction
   d. Recent myocardial infarction

7. After teaching a patient who is to receive transdermal selegiline, which patient statement would indicate to the nurse that the patient has understood the instructions?
   a. "I probably won't feel drowsy, dizzy, or nauseous from this drug."
   b. "I should leave the previous patch on for an hour after applying a new one."
   c. "I can apply a new patch to my upper arm, thigh, or torso."
   d. "My skin needs to be a little damp when I apply the patch."

8. Which of the following adverse effects would the nurse instruct a patient to report to his health care provider immediately when taking trazodone?
   a. Hypertension
   b. Dizziness
   c. Sedation
   d. Painful continued erection

9. A patient is prescribed isocarboxazid. The nurse is teaching the patient about foods to avoid. Which of the following would the nurse include in the teaching? Select all that apply.
   a. Aged blue cheese
   b. Red wine
   c. Pepperoni
   d. Whole milk
   e. Fresh shellfish
   f. Sour cream

10. A patient is receiving fluoxetine. The nurse would monitor the patient for which of the following?
    a. Increased salivation
    b. Cough
    c. Improved alertness
    d. Sustained erection

11. A patient is receiving an SSRI. The nurse would inform the patient that the full benefits of the drug may not occur for which time period?
    a. 1 week
    b. 2 weeks
    c. 3 weeks
    d. 4 weeks

12. After reviewing information about the various antidepressants, a group of students demonstrate their understanding of the information when they identify which of the following as an SSRI?
    a. Doxepin
    b. Nefazodone
    c. Sertraline
    d. Bupropion

13. A patient who was previously taking paroxetine is being switched to phenelzine due to a lack of response. The nurse would expect that the phenelzine will be started at which time?

   a. Concurrently with the paroxetine as it is being tapered
   b. In 4 to 6 weeks after stopping the paroxetine
   c. Immediately upon stopping the paroxetine.
   d. Forty-eight hours after being weaned from the paroxetine

14. When teaching a patient about tricyclic antidepressants, the nurse would include which of the following? Select all that apply.

   a. Taking the drug once a day in the morning for maximum benefit
   b. Using hard candies and gums to combat dry mouth
   c. Eating a low-fiber diet
   d. Keeping the room brightly lit

15. The nurse would assess for which of the following in a patient with type 2 diabetes using an oral antidiabetic agent and receiving an MAOI?

   a. Orthostatic hypotension
   b. Diabetic ketoacidosis
   c. Hypoglycemia
   d. Renal dysfunction

CHAPTER 22

Psychotherapeutic Agents

LEARNING OBJECTIVES

Upon completion of this chapter, you will be able to:

1. Define the term psychotherapeutic agent and list conditions that the psychotherapeutic agents are used to treat.

2. Describe the therapeutic actions, indications, pharmacokinetics, contraindications, most common adverse reactions, and important drug–drug interactions associated with each class of psychotherapeutic agent.

3. Discuss the use of psychotherapeutic agents across the lifespan.

4. Compare and contrast the prototype drugs for each class of psychotherapeutic agent with other drugs in that class and with drugs in the other classes of psychotherapeutic agents.

5. Outline the nursing considerations and teaching needs for patients receiving each class of psychotherapeutic agent.

■ ASSESSING YOUR UNDERSTANDING

SHORT ANSWER

Supply the information requested.

1. Name the most common type of psychosis.

2. Describe the overall goal of psychotherapeutic agents in comparison to antidepressant agents.

3. Explain why antipsychotic agents are called *neuroleptic agents*.

4. Describe the rationale for no longer calling antipsychotic agents major tranquilizers.

5. Identify the two classifications of antipsychotic drugs.

LABELING

Place the name of each of the drugs listed below in the appropriate column of the table that identifies the neurotransmitter affected by that drug's action. Some drugs may be placed in more than one column.

Aripiprazole

Chlorpromazine

Clozapine

Lithium

Fluphenazine

Pimozide

Quetiapine

Ziprasidone

Dopamine	Serotonin	Norepinephrine

■ APPLYING YOUR KNOWLEDGE

CASE STUDY

A 32-year-old woman is brought to the emergency department by the local police after having been called to the scene by several neighbors. The neighbors reported that the patient was talking and laughing extremely loud, banging on doors, and telling everyone that she was the "queen of the world." The patient is dressed in provocative, brightly colored clothing and wearing heavy makeup.

The patient is using exaggerated gestures as she talks, quickly shifting from one topic to another. The patient, who has a history of bipolar disorder, is known to the staff in the emergency department.

a. What information would be most important for the nurse to gather in this situation, and how would the nurse go about obtaining this information?

b. What medications might the nurse expect the physician to prescribe for the patient?

c. How would the nurse approach teaching with this patient?

■ PRACTICING FOR NCLEX

Circle the letter that corresponds to the best answer for each question.

1. A patient with a history of schizophrenia has been receiving antipsychotic therapy for several years. Which of the following would indicate to the nurse that the patient is experiencing pseudoparkinsonism?
   a. Cogwheel rigidity
   b. Abnormal eye movements
   c. Neck spasms
   d. Excessive salivation

2. A nurse is reviewing a patient's serum lithium level and determines that the level is therapeutic by which result?
   a. 0.2 mEq/L
   b. 0.8 mEq/L
   c. 1.4 mEq/L
   d. 2.0 mEq/L

3. After reviewing information about antipsychotic agents, a group of students demonstrate understanding of the material when they identify which of the following as an atypical antipsychotic agent?

   a. Haloperidol

   b. Loxapine

   c. Clozapine

   d. Pimozide

4. Which of the following antipsychotics would the nurse identify as a highly potent agent?

   a. Chlorpromazine

   b. Thioridazine

   c. Prochlorperazine

   d. Fluphenazine

5. The nurse administers chlorpromazine intramuscularly to a patient. The nurse would maintain the patient in bed for at least how long after administering the drug?

   a. ½ hour

   b. 1 hour

   c. 2 hours

   d. 3 hours

6. Which of the following would be important for a nurse to include in the teaching plan for a patient taking fluphenazine?

   a. Possible development of fatal arrhythmias

   b. Urine turning pink to reddish-brown

   c. Possible severe rhinorrhea

   d. Development of diabetes mellitus

7. The nurse expects to monitor a patient's white blood count weekly when the patient is prescribed which of the following?

   a. Aripiprazole

   b. Olanzapine

   c. Clozapine

   d. Quetiapine

8. The use of which of the following would a nurse identify as placing a patient receiving lithium therapy at increased risk for toxicity?

   a. Tromethamine

   b. Thiazide diuretic

   c. Psyllium

   d. Antacids

9. A patient has a serum lithium level of 1.8 mEq/L. Which of the following would the nurse assess? Select all that apply.

   a. Electrocardiogram changes

   b. Hypotension

   c. Slurred speech

   d. Hyperreflexia

   e. Polyuria

   f. Seizures

10. A child with attention deficit hyperactivity disorder is to receive methylphenidate twice a day. The nurse would instruct the parents to administer the last dose before which time?

    a. 4 PM

    b. 5 PM

    c. 6 PM

    d. 8 PM

11. Which drug would be indicated for the treatment of narcolepsy?

    a. Atomoxetine

    b. Dexmethylphenidate

    c. Lisdexamfetamine

    d. Modafinil

12. While caring for a patient who is receiving antipsychotic therapy, the nurse observes lip smacking, a darting tongue, and slow and aimless arm movements. The nurse interprets this as which of the following?

    a. Tardive dyskinesia

    b. Akathisia

    c. Pseudoparkinsonism

    d. Dystonia

13. A nurse is assessing a patient who is receiving an antipsychotic agent for possible anticholinergic effects. Which of the following would the nurse assess?

    a. Nasal congestion

    b. Neuroleptic malignant syndrome

    c. Laryngospasm

    d. Arrhythmia

14. The parents of a child receiving a central nervous system stimulant for treatment of attention deficit disorder asks the nurse why they are stopping the drug for a time. Which statement by the nurse would be most appropriate?

a. "He probably doesn't need the medication anymore since he is getting older."

b. "We need to check and see if he still has symptoms that require drug therapy."

c. "The drug should be used for a specified period of time and then switched to another."

d. "He is prone to developing severe adverse effects if he stays on it any longer."

15. A patient is receiving haloperidol. The nurse would be most especially alert for the development of which of the following adverse effects?

a. Sedation

b. Anticholinergic

c. Extrapyramidal

d. Hypotension

16. Which of the following would a nurse identify as being used as treatment for mania as well as schizophrenia?

a. Lithium

b. Risperidone

c. Lamotrigine

d. Aripiprazole

Antiseizure Agents

Upon completion of this chapter, you will be able to:

1. Define the terms generalized seizure, tonic-clonic seizure, absence seizure, partial seizure, and status epilepticus.

2. Describe the therapeutic actions, indications, pharmacokinetics, contraindications, most common adverse reactions, and important drug–drug interactions associated with each class of antiseizure agents.

3. Discuss the use of antiepileptic drugs across the lifespan.

4. Compare and contrast the prototype drugs for each class of antiepileptic drug with the other drugs in that class and with drugs from the other classes.

5. Outline the nursing considerations and teaching needs for patients receiving each class of antiseizure agent.

■ ASSESSING YOUR UNDERSTANDING

MATCHING

Select the description from column 2 that best describes the term in column 1.

Column 1

_____ 1. Absence seizure

_____ 2. Convulsion

_____ 3. Epilepsy

_____ 4. Generalized seizure

_____ 5. Partial seizure

_____ 6. Status epilepticus

_____ 7. Tonic-clonic seizure

Column 2

a. Focal seizure

b. Syndromes characterized by seizures

c. Formerly known as grand mal seizure

d. Beginning in one area of the brain and spreading to both hemispheres

e. Rapidly recurring seizures

f. Muscular reactions to excessive electrical energy arising from nerve cells

g. Sudden temporary loss of consciousness

SHORT ANSWER

Supply the information requested.

1. Name the five types of generalized seizures.

2. Differentiate between simple and complex partial seizures.

3. List the most common adverse effect that results from the drugs used to treat generalized seizures.

4. Identify the drug class most commonly used to treat absence seizures.

5. Explain the underlying reason why phenobarbital has a slow onset and very long duration of action.

6. Identify the two ways that drugs used to control partial seizures stabilize nerve membranes.

APPLYING YOUR KNOWLEDGE

CASE STUDY

A 6-year-old child was admitted to the health care facility after experiencing a tonic-clonic seizure. His parents are at his bedside. The child was receiving phenytoin intravenously but is now being switched to oral therapy. It is expected that the child will be discharged home tomorrow. The nurse is talking with the parents about the child's drug therapy when the mother says, "It was so scary watching him like that. I just froze. What if he has another seizure, and what if it happens at school or when his friends are around?"

a. How would the nurse respond to the mother?

b. What suggestions and recommendations would be appropriate in this situation?

PRACTICING FOR NCLEX

Circle the letter that corresponds to the best answer for each question.

1. Which of the following agents would a nurse expect to administer intravenously for a partial seizure?
   a. Carbamazepine
   b. Gabapentin
   c. Levetiracetam
   d. Felbamate

2. A patient who is receiving phenytoin has a serum drug level drawn. Which result would the nurse interpret as within the therapeutic range?
   a. 4 mcg/mL
   b. 12 mcg/mL
   c. 22 mcg/mL
   d. 30 mcg/mL

3. A patient is receiving a hydantoin as treatment for tonic-clonic seizures. The nurse includes a discussion of which of the following when teaching the patient about this drug?
   a. Possible leukocytosis
   b. Physical dependence
   c. Withdrawal syndrome
   d. Gingival hyperplasia

4. When describing the action of barbiturates and barbituratelike agents in the control of seizures, which of the following would the nurse include?
   a. Promotion of impulse conduction
   b. Stimulation of the cerebral cortex
   c. Depression of motor nerve output
   d. Maintenance of cerebellar function

5. Phenobarbital is ordered for a child with status epilepticus. The nurse would anticipate administering this drug by which route?
   a. Oral
   b. Rectal
   c. Intramuscular
   d. Intravenous

6. A patient is receiving lamotrigine as treatment for partial seizures. Which assessment finding would lead the nurse to stop the drug immediately?

   a. Rash

   b. Somnolence

   c. Anorexia

   d. Confusion

7. The nurse is reviewing the medical record of a patient with partial seizures who is prescribed drug therapy. The nurse would question the order for which of the following if the nurse finds that the patient has a history of alcohol abuse?

   a. Topiramate

   b. Pregabalin

   c. Felbamate

   d. Tiagabine

8. The nurse is monitoring the serum carbamazepine level of a patient. Which result would lead the nurse to notify the prescriber that the patient most likely needs an increased dosage?

   a. 2 mcg/mL

   b. 4 mcg/mL

   c. 6 mcg/mL

   d. 8 mcg/mL

9. A patient who is receiving an antiseizure agent complains of feeling sleepy and tired and reports dizziness when standing up. Which intervention would the nurse most likely implement as the priority?

   a. Hydration therapy

   b. Safety precautions

   c. Skin-care measures

   d. Emotional support

10. A child is experiencing febrile seizures for which phenobarbital is ordered to be given intravenously. The dose is administered at 10 AM. The nurse understands that a second dose of the drug may be given at which time?

   a. 2 PM

   b. 4 PM

   c. 6 PM

   d. 10 PM

11. Which drug would the nurse expect to be ordered as the drug of choice for the treatment for myoclonic seizures?

   a. Clonazepam

   b. Diazepam

   c. Valproic acid

   d. Zonisamide

12. After teaching a class on drug classes used to treat seizures, the instructor determines that the teaching has been successful when the students identify which drug as most commonly used in the treatment of absence seizures?

   a. Mephobarbital

   b. Ethotoin

   c. Ethosuximide

   d. Primidone

13. When describing the action of zonisamide, which of the following would the nurse include?

   a. Inhibition of sodium and calcium channels

   b. Decrease in conduction through nerve pathways

   c. Depression of the cerebral cortex

   d. Depression of motor nerve output

14. A patient is to receive ethotoin. The nurse would expect to administer this drug by which route?

   a. Oral

   b. Rectal

   c. Intramuscular

   d. Intravenous

15. Which of the following would be most important to monitor in a patient receiving ethosuximide?

   a. Weight

   b. Nutritional status

   c. Electrocardiogram

   d. Complete blood count

CHAPTER 24

Antiparkinsonism Agents

LEARNING OBJECTIVES

Upon completion of this chapter, you will be able to:

1. Describe the current theory of the cause of Parkinson's disease and correlate this with the clinical presentation of the disease.

2. Describe the therapeutic actions, indications, pharmacokinetics, contraindications, most common adverse reactions, and important drug–drug interactions associated with antiparkinsonism agents.

3. Discuss the use of antiparkinsonism agents across the lifespan.

4. Compare and contrast the prototype drugs for each class of antiparkinsonism agent with the other drugs in that class and with drugs from the other classes used to treat the disease.

5. Outline the nursing considerations and teaching needs for patients receiving each class of antiparkinsonism agent.

■ ASSESSING YOUR UNDERSTANDING

FILL IN THE BLANKS

Provide the missing term or terms in the blanks provided.

1. Patients with Parkinson's disease exhibit

   _____ marked by difficulties in performing intentional movements and extreme slowness or sluggishness.

2. In Parkinson's disease, nerve cells begin to degenerate in the dopamine-rich area of the

   brain called the _____ _____.

3. Therapy for Parkinson's disease today aims at restoring the balance between the declining

   levels of _____ and the now-dominant

   _____ neurons.

4. _____ agents have been proven to

   more effective than _____ agents in the treatment of parkinsonism.

5. Patients receiving rasagiline should avoid

   _____-containing foods.

LABELING

Place the name of the following drugs listed below in the appropriate box under the correct drug class.

Amantadine   Entacapone

Benztropine   Levodopa

Trihexyphenidyl   Ropinirole

Diphenhydramine   Selegiline

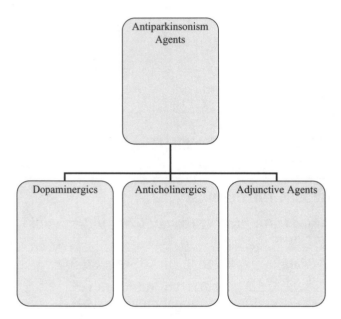

■ APPLYING YOUR KNOWLEDGE

CASE STUDY

A 65-year-old man is brought to the emergency department by his daughter, who reports that her father started complaining of a severe headache several hours ago that has not abated. He also had some nausea and vomiting and was diaphoretic. Examination reveals tachycardia and dilated pupils. The patient also reports some mild chest pain. He states, "The bright lights are really bothering me." The patient has a history of Parkinson's disease for which he takes levodopa. His daughter reports that he just started taking rasagiline about a week ago.

a. How would the nurse interpret the patient's signs and symptoms? What might be happening?

b. What additional information would the nurse need to gather from the patient and his daughter?

■ PRACTICING FOR NCLEX

Circle the letter that corresponds to the best answer for each question.

1. When describing the action of levodopa, which of the following would the nurse include?

    a. Acts like replacement therapy

    b. Increases the release of dopamine

    c. Binds directly with postsynaptic dopamine receptors

    d. Stimulates dopamine receptors

2. A patient asks the nurse why he must take his levodopa in combination with carbidopa. Which response by the nurse would be most appropriate?

    a. "The carbidopa helps the levodopa get into the brain."

    b. "The carbidopa allows a lower dose of levodopa to be used."

    c. "It boosts the action of levodopa to prevent the nerve cells from degenerating."

    d. "The carbidopa prevents too much levodopa from being excreted."

3. A patient is to receive apomorphine as treatment for Parkinson's disease. The nurse would expect to administer this drug by which route?

    a. Oral

    b. Topical

    c. Subcutaneous

    d. Intramuscular

4. When reviewing a patient's history, which of the following would the nurse identify as a contraindication to the use of levodopa?

    a. Myocardial infarction

    b. Bronchial asthma

    c. Peptic ulcer disease

    d. Suspicious skin lesions

5. Which of the following would a nurse expect to assess as a potential adverse effect of dopaminergic therapy?

   a. Sedation

   b. Muscle flaccidity

   c. Nervousness

   d. Hypertension

6. Which of the following would a nurse identify as least likely to contribute to a decrease in the effectiveness of levodopa?

   a. Pyridoxine

   b. Phenytoin

   c. Multivitamin supplement

   d. St. John's wort

7. A patient is to receive trihexyphenidyl as adjunctive treatment for Parkinson's disease. The nurse would expect to administer this drug by which route?

   a. Oral

   b. Subcutaneous

   c. Intramuscular

   d. Intravenous

8. A nurse is reviewing a patient's history for conditions that would contraindicate the use of anticholinergics for Parkinson's disease. Which of the following would cause the nurse to be concerned?

   a. Hypertension

   b. Myasthenia gravis

   c. Hepatic dysfunction

   d. Cardiac arrhythmia

9. Which of the following would lead the nurse to suspect that a patient is experiencing an adverse effect to an anticholinergic agent?

   a. Diarrhea

   b. Diaphoresis

   c. Excess salivation

   d. Agitation

10. After reviewing the drugs used to treat Parkinson's disease, the students demonstrate understanding when they identify which of the following as a dopaminergic agent?

    a. Diphenhydramine

    b. Biperiden

    c. Bromocriptine

    d. Tolcapone

11. A patient who is receiving biperiden complains of light-headedness, dizziness, and blurred vision. Which nursing diagnosis would be most appropriate?

    a. Risk for impaired thermoregulation

    b. Disturbed thought processes

    c. Deficient knowledge

    d. Risk for injury

12. When administering entacapone, the nurse understands that this drug affects which enzyme?

    a. Lactic dehydrogenase

    b. Catecholamine-O-methyl transferase

    c. Monoamine oxidase

    d. Acetylcholinesterase

13. Which action would be a priority for a patient receiving apomorphine?

    a. Giving the drug with food

    b. Monitoring cardiac status

    c. Checking for skin lesions

    d. Palpating the bladder

14. A patient is experiencing parkinsonism as a result of drug therapy with a phenothiazine. The nurse would anticipate which agent as being prescribed?

    a. Bromocriptine

    b. Pramipexole

    c. Biperiden

    d. Selegiline

15. Which of the following would be considered a peripheral anticholinergic effect of anticholinergic drug therapy?

    a. Delirium

    b. Blurred vision

    c. Agitation

    d. Memory loss

Muscle Relaxants

LEARNING OBJECTIVES

Upon completion of this chapter, you will be able to:

1. Describe a spinal reflex and discuss the pathophysiology of muscle spasm and muscle spasticity.

2. Describe the therapeutic actions, indications, pharmacokinetics, contraindications, most common adverse reactions, and important drug–drug interactions associated with the centrally acting and the direct-acting skeletal muscle relaxants.

3. Discuss the use of muscle relaxants across the lifespan.

4. Compare and contrast the prototype drugs baclofen and dantrolene with other muscle relaxants in their classes.

5. Outline the nursing considerations, including important teaching points, for patients receiving muscle relaxants as an adjunct to anesthesia.

■ ASSESSING YOUR UNDERSTANDING

CROSSWORD

Use the clues to complete the crossword puzzle.

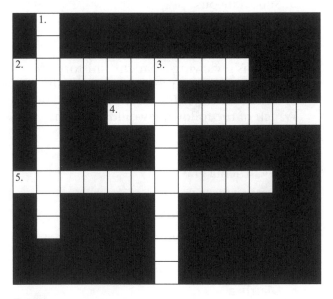

Across

2. Sustained muscle contraction
4. Tract that controls precise intentional movement
5. Structure that communicates with other neurons

Down

1. Excessive muscle response and activity
3. Lower portion of the brain that coordinates muscle movement

SHORT ANSWER

Supply the information requested.

1. Describe the type of movements associated with the pyramidal and extrapyramidal tracts.

2. Explain why muscle spasticity is a permanent condition.

3. Identify the typical cause of muscle spasm.

4. Describe the structures that regulate movement and muscle control.

5. Explain why centrally acting skeletal muscle relaxants are often referred to as spasmolytics.

6. Name the prototype centrally acting skeletal muscle relaxant.

7. Describe the action of direct-acting skeletal muscle relaxants.

8. State the drug that would be used to improve the appearance of moderate to severe glabellar lines.

■ APPLYING YOUR KNOWLEDGE

CASE STUDY

A 27-year-old man comes to the urgent care center for evaluation of his shoulder. He reports that he has been working out at the gym and may have overdone it. He is complaining of pain in the right shoulder and intense muscle spasms in the area. Diagnostic evaluation rules out any tear, dislocation, or fracture. The patient is prescribed cyclobenza-prine as a muscle relaxant.

a. What information would the nurse need to include when teaching the patient about the drug?

b. What additional information would the nurse include to help augment the effects of the prescribed drug therapy?

■ PRACTICING FOR NCLEX

Circle the letter that corresponds to the best answer for each question.

1. An older patient is to receive a centrally acting skeletal muscle relaxant. Which of the following would the nurse expect to be prescribed?
   a. Baclofen
   b. Carisoprodol
   c. Chlorzoxazone
   d. Cyclobenzaprine

2. Simple reflex arcs comprise which of the following?
   a. Pyramidal tract
   b. Extrapyramidal tract
   c. Spindle gamma loop system
   d. Basal ganglia

3. After reviewing information about skeletal muscle relaxants, a group of students demonstrate understanding of the material when they identify which drug as a direct-acting muscle relaxant?

   a. Botulinum toxin type A

   b. Diazepam

   c. Methocarbamol

   d. Orphenadrine

4. When reviewing a patient's history, which condition would the nurse identify as contraindicating the use of a centrally acting skeletal muscle relaxant?

   a. Epilepsy

   b. Cardiac disease

   c. Hepatic dysfunction

   d. Rheumatic disorder

5. A patient is receiving baclofen at 8 AM. The nurse would monitor the patient for evidence of maximum effect at which time?

   a. 9 AM

   b. 10 AM

   c. 11 AM

   d. 12 PM

6. A patient with amyotrophic lateral sclerosis is experiencing muscle spasticity. Which of the following drugs would the nurse expect the physician to order?

   a. Chlorzoxazone

   b. Metaxalone

   c. Dantrolene

   d. Methocarbamol

7. Which of the following would a nurse include when describing the action of dantrolene?

   a. Interference with calcium release from the muscles

   b. Inhibition of the release of acetycholine

   c. Interference with the reflexes causing the spasm

   d. Inhibition of presynaptic motor neurons in central nervous system

8. The nurse instructs a patient about the possibility of his urine turning orange to purple-red if the patient were receiving which of the following?

   a. Baclofen

   b. Carisoprodol

   c. Chlorzoxazone

   d. Tizanidine

9. A patient comes to the health care provider's office. The patient is to receive botulinum toxin. Which of the following, if assessed, would suggest to the nurse that the drug administration should be postponed?

   a. Recent gastrointestinal upset

   b. Infection at the intended site of administration

   c. Reports of urinary frequency

   d. Difficulty swallowing

10. Signs and symptoms of which of the following would necessitate discontinuation of dantrolene therapy?

    a. Intermittent gastrointestinal upset

    b. Visual disturbances

    c. Urinary retention

    d. Hepatic dysfunction

11. A patient with a history of malignant hyperthermia is scheduled for surgery. Which agent would the nurse most likely expect to administer?

    a. Botulinum toxin type B

    b. Dantrolene

    c. Baclofen

    d. Methocarbamol

12. Which nursing diagnosis most likely would be the priority for a patient who is receiving a centrally acting skeletal muscle relaxant as treatment for acute knee strain?

    a. Deficient knowledge

    b. Risk for injury

    c. Acute pain

    d. Disturbed thought processes

13. Which of the following would a nurse identify as increasing a patient's risk for hepatic disease with dantrolene use?

    a. Male gender

    b. Age over 35 years

    c. Respiratory disease

    d. Infection

14. A patient is receiving botulinum toxin type A as treatment for her frown lines. The nurse would instruct the patient about which of the following?

    a. Abnormal hair growth

    b. Acne

    c. Photosensitivity

    d. Drooping eyelids

15. A nurse is preparing a teaching plan for a patient who is receiving baclofen therapy. Which of the following would the nurse include as possible adverse effects? Select all that apply.

    a. Drowsiness

    b. Hypertension

    c. Urinary frequency

    d. Agitation

    e. Drooling

    f. Constipation

CHAPTER 26

Narcotics, Narcotic Antagonists and Antimigraine Agents

LEARNING OBJECTIVES

Upon completion of this chapter, you will be able to:

1. Outline the gate theory of pain and explain therapeutic ways to block pain using the gate theory.

2. Describe the therapeutic actions, indications, pharmacokinetics, contraindications, most common adverse reactions, and important drug–drug interactions associated with narcotics and antimigraine agents.

3. Discuss the use of the different classes of narcotics, narcotic antagonists, and antimigraine agents across the lifespan.

4. Compare and contrast the prototype drugs morphine, pentazocine, naloxone, ergotamine, and sumatriptan with other drugs in their respective classes.

5. Outline the nursing considerations, including important teaching points, for patients receiving a narcotic, narcotic antagonist, or antimigraine drug.

■ ASSESSING YOUR UNDERSTANDING

LABELING

Place the name of the following drugs in the appropriate box under the correct drug classification.

Butorphanol
Codeine
Fentanyl
Naloxone

Naltrexone
Pentazocine
Tapentadol

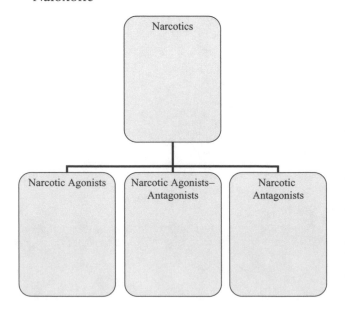

SHORT ANSWER

Supply the information requested.

1. Identify the two small-diameter sensory nerves involved in the generation of pain sensation.

2. Name the fibers that transmit sensations associated with touch and temperature.

3. Identify the type of receptors that respond to naturally occurring peptins, endorphins, and enkephalins.

4. List three factors that can play a role in pain perception.

5. Identify the functions of narcotic agonists–antagonists.

6. State the action of triptans.

7. Name the four types of opioid receptors.

■ APPLYING YOUR KNOWLEDGE

CASE STUDY

The nurse is visiting the home of a patient with cancer. The patient has been taking morphine for the relief of his pain. However, over the last 2 weeks, the patient reports that he is not experiencing the degree of relief that he had been. The patient also mentions that when he saw the physician last week, a decision was made not to pursue additional treatment.

a. What factors may be contributing to the patient's increase in pain?

b. What possible options might be appropriate for this patient?

c. What measures would the nurse suggest to enhance pain relief?

■ PRACTICING FOR NCLEX

Circle the letter that corresponds to the best answer for each question.

1. A patient is to receive a narcotic that will be applied transdermally. The nurse identifies this as which agent?
   a. Morphine
   b. Fentanyl
   c. Codeine
   d. Hydromorphone

2. A nurse is assessing a patient's pain level. Which of the following would be the most appropriate method?
   a. Ask the patient if he is experiencing any pain.
   b. Have the patient rate it on a scale of 1 to 10.
   c. Palpate the area where the patient says he has pain.
   d. Review the patient's vital signs for changes.

3. A patient is to receive a narcotic cough syrup. The nurse would expect this preparation to contain which of the following?
   a. Codeine
   b. Fentanyl
   c. Hydromorphone
   d. Meperidine

4. Which instruction would the nurse include for a patient who is prescribed extended-release oxycodone?
   a. Take the tablet as a whole tablet at one time.
   b. Cut the tablet in half, swallowing half a tablet at a time.
   c. Mix it with juice after crushing it.
   d. Chew the tablet thoroughly before swallowing it.

5. A woman who has given birth to a baby girl by cesarean delivery is experiencing abdominal pain. The patient receive a bolus dose of morphine intravenously. The nurse would recommend that the mother refrain from breast-feeding the baby for how long?
   a. 1 to 2 hours
   b. 2 to 4 hours
   c. 4 to 6 hours
   d. 6 to 8 hours

6. The nurse administers an oral dose of morphine to a patient at 3:00 PM. The nurse would expect the drug to peak at which time?
   a. 3:30 PM
   b. 4:00 PM
   c. 4:30 PM
   d. 5:00 PM

7. A patient is receiving a narcotic agonist–antagonist parenterally immediately after surgery but will be switched to the oral form when tolerating fluid and food. Which agent would most likely be preferred?
   a. Buprenorphine
   b. Butorphanol
   c. Nalbuphine
   d. Pentazocine

8. Which of the following would the nurse expect to assess in a patient receiving a narcotic for pain relief?
   a. Dilation of the pupils
   b. Diarrhea
   c. Orthostatic hypotension
   d. Tachypnea

9. A patient is experiencing significant respiratory depression and sedation related to morphine administration. The nurse would anticipate administering which of the following?
   a. Butorphanol
   b. Buprenorphine
   c. Naloxone
   d. Ergotamine

10. A patient is to receive naltrexone. The nurse would expect to administer this drug by which route?
    a. Oral
    b. Subcutaneous
    c. Intramuscular
    d. Intravenous

11. Which assessment finding would support a patient's report of migraine headaches?
    a. Severe unilateral pulsating pain
    b. Sharp steady eye pain
    c. Dull band of pain around the head
    d. Onset occurring during sleep

12. When describing the action of ergot derivatives, the nurse would incorporate understanding of which of the following?
    a. Blockage of alpha-adrenergic receptors
    b. Interference with dopamine
    c. Inhibition of opioid receptors
    d. Interference with cerebral enzyme systems

13. A patient is receiving drug therapy for prevention of an acute migraine attack. Which agent would be the most helpful?
    a. Sumatriptan
    b. Ergotamine
    c. Naloxone
    d. Eletriptan

14. A patient is prescribed dihydroergotamine. The nurse would instruct the patient to administer this drug most likely by which route?

a. Oral

b. Subcutaneous

c. Intranasal

d. Sublingual

15. A patient uses sumatriptan for treating her migraine headaches. Which statement by the patient indicates to the nurse that she understands how to take this drug?

a. "I can repeat a dose in 15 minutes for a total of four doses."

b. "I should repeat the dose in 30 minutes for a total of three doses."

c. "I can take another dose 2 hours after the first one."

d. "I can take another dose in about 4 hours, if needed."

General and Local Anesthetic Agents

LEARNING OBJECTIVES

Upon completion of this chapter, you will be able to:

1. Describe the concept of balanced anesthesia.

2. Describe the actions and uses of local anesthesia.

3. Describe the therapeutic actions, indications, pharmacokinetics, contraindications, most common adverse reactions, and important drug–drug interactions associated with general and local anesthetics.

4. Outline the preoperative and postoperative needs of a patient receiving general or local anesthesia.

5. Compare and contrast the prototype drugs thiopental, midazolam, nitrous oxide, halothane, and lidocaine with other drugs in their respective classes.

6. Outline the nursing considerations, including important teaching points, for patients receiving general and local anesthetics.

■ ASSESSING YOUR UNDERSTANDING

CROSSWORD

Use the clues to complete the crossword puzzle.

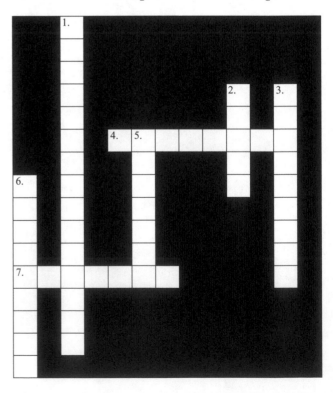

Across

4. Type of anesthesia using several different types of drugs for quick effects

7. Type of anesthesia to create analgesia, unconsciousness, and amnesia

Down

1. Loss of awareness of one's surroundings

2. Type of anesthesia via powerful nerve blockers

3. Time from beginning of anesthesia until achievement of surgical anesthesia

5. Loss of memory

6. Loss of pain sensation

SEQUENCING

Each of the following statements reflects an event in the stages of anesthesia. Place the number of the statement in the boxes below based on the order in which they occur reflecting the depth of anesthesia.

1. Combative behavior with signs of sympathetic stimulation

2. Relaxation of skeletal muscles and return of regular respirations

3. Loss of pain sensation with patient conscious

4. Deep central nervous system (CNS) depression with loss of respiratory and vasomotor center stimuli

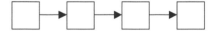

■ APPLYING YOUR KNOWLEDGE

CASE STUDY

A patient is scheduled to undergo abdominal surgery under general anesthesia and is admitted to the health care facility the night before surgery for additional diagnostic testing and preparation. In addition to laboratory tests, a chest x-ray and electrocardiogram are performed. The patient is visited by the anesthesiologist, who obtains a history and physical examination. After the anesthesiologist leaves, the patient presses her call light and wants to talk to the nurse. Upon entering the room, the patient is visibly anxious and upset and says, "Why are they checking my heart and lungs? The problem is in my belly. And who is this doctor that was just here, and why was he asking me all those questions?"

a. How would the nurse respond to the patient?

b. What information would be appropriate to provide to the patient about the events that have happened and are about to happen with surgery?

■ PRACTICING FOR NCLEX

Circle the letter that corresponds to the best answer for each question.

1. When describing the stages of anesthesia, during which stage does pupillary dilation occur?

a. Stage 1

b. Stage 2

c. Stage 3

d. Stage 4

2. The nurse is reviewing the intraoperative record of a patient who has returned from surgery. The nurse would determine that the patient will most likely need additional analgesia postoperatively due to use of which of the following?

a. Thiopental

b. Ketamine

c. Midazolam

d. Propofol

3. Which of the following would a nurse expect to assess in a patient who has had general anesthesia using methohexital?

a. Hypertension

b. Tachypnea

c. Increased gastric activity

d. Vomiting

4. A patient is receiving a narcotic after having received a barbiturate for general anesthesia. Which of the following would most likely occur?
   a. Bleeding
   b. Apnea
   c. Headache
   d. Delirium

5. After reviewing information about nonbarbiturate anesthestics, a group of students demonstrate understanding of the information when they identify which of the following as an example?
   a. Midazolam
   b. Nitrous oxide
   c. Thiopental
   d. Halothane

6. Which anesthetic is associated with a bizarre state of unconsciousness in which the patient appears to be awake and yet cannot feel pain?
   a. Propofol
   b. Droperidol
   c. Ketamine
   d. Etomidate

7. Which anesthetic would have the fastest onset of action?
   a. Droperidol
   b. Ketamine
   c. Propofol
   d. Etomidate

8. The nurse would monitor the patient for which of the following during recovery from etomidate?
   a. Chills and hypotension
   b. Respiratory depression and CNS suppression
   c. Hallucinations and cardiac arrhythmias
   d. Myoclonic movements and vomiting

9. Which agent would the nurse identify as always being given with oxygen?
   a. Thiopental
   b. Nitrous oxide
   c. Halothane
   d. Enflurane

10. After reviewing information about general anesthetics, a group of students demonstrate understanding of the information when they identify which of the following as acting like gas anesthetics?
    a. Volatile liquids
    b. Nonbarbiturate anesthetics
    c. Barbiturate anesthetics
    d. Esters

11. During recovery from general anesthesia, which of the following would be a priority?
    a. Monitoring temperature and reflexes
    b. Providing comfort measures
    c. Have emergency equipment readily available
    d. Providing pain relief as ordered

12. When a local anesthetic is administered in increasing doses, which sensation is lost first?
    a. Touch
    b. Temperature
    c. Proprioception
    d. Skeletal muscle tone

13. A patient is to have an intravenous line inserted, and the nurse prepares to apply a dermal patch to provide local anesthesia to the area. The nurse would apply the patch at which time before initiating intravenous access?
    a. 15 minutes
    b. 30 minutes
    c. 45 minutes
    d. 60 minutes

14. When preparing a patient for the application of a local anesthetic, which of the following would be most important?
    a. Inspecting the application area for intactness
    b. Checking the reflexes in that area
    c. Assessing the peripheral pulses
    d. Determining muscle tone

15. After teaching a group of students about local anesthetic agents, the instructor determines that the teaching was successful when the students identify which of the following as an example of an ester?
    a. Mepivacaine
    b. Lidocaine
    c. Benzocaine
    d. Dibucaine

Neuromuscular Junction Blocking Agents

Upon completion of this chapter, you will be able to:

1. Draw and label a neuromuscular junction.

2. Describe the therapeutic actions, indications, pharmacokinetics, contraindications, most common adverse reactions, and important drug–drug interactions associated with the depolarizing and nondepolarizing neuromuscular junction blockers.

3. Discuss the use of neuromuscular junction blockers across the lifespan.

4. Compare and contrast the prototype drugs pancuronium and succinylcholine with other neuromuscular junction blockers.

5. Outline the nursing considerations, including important teaching points, for patients receiving a neuromuscular junction blocker.

■ASSESSING YOUR UNDERSTANDING

FILL IN THE BLANKS

Provide the missing term or terms in the blanks provided.

1. Nerves communicate with muscles at a synapse

   called the _____ _____.

2. The _____, the functional unit of a muscle, is made up of light and dark filaments.

3. The striated appearance of a muscle's functional unit is due to the orderly arrangement of

   _____ and _____ molecules.

4. At the synaptic cleft, the neurotransmitter

   _____ interacts with the nicotinic cholinergic receptors to cause depolarization of the muscle membrane.

5. Drugs that act as antagonists to the neurotransmitter at the neuromuscular

   junction (NMJ) are called _____ NMJ blockers.

6. Succinylcholine is a drug classified as a

   _____ NMJ blocker.

SEQUENCING

Each of the statements below identify an event that occurs with muscle contraction based on the sliding filament theory. Place the number of the statement in the box below based on the order in which they occur.

1. Depolarization allows the release of calcium ions.

2. Acetylcholine is broken down; receptor free.

3. Nerve impulse arrives at motor nerve terminal.

4. Actin and myosin are released from binding sites.

5. Filament becomes shorter.

6. Acetylcholine interacts with nicotinic cholinergic receptors.

7. Calcium binds to troponin.

8. Muscle membrane depolarizes.

9. Actin and myosin repeatedly react with each other.

10. Acetylcholine is released into the synaptic cleft.

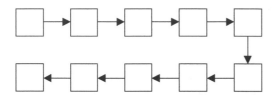

■APPLYING YOUR KNOWLEDGE

CASE STUDY

An adolescent is brought into the emergency department after being involved in a motor vehicle accident. He has sustained multiple trauma, including a fractured right femur, and is being evaluated for a possible spinal cord injury. The adolescent has a history of asthma. His respiratory status begins to deteriorate, and the decision is made to intubate him and begin mechanical ventilation. The physician administers pancuronium. His parents are at the bedside.

a. What would be the most likely rationale for using pancuronium?

b. What precautions would be necessary related to the use of this drug and the patient's history and current condition?

c. What information would be important to provide to the patient and family about this drug?

■PRACTICING FOR NCLEX

Circle the letter that corresponds to the best answer for each question.

1. After reviewing the various NMJ blockers, a group of students demonstrate understanding of the information when they identify which agent as having the longest duration?
   a. Atracurium
   b. Succinylcholine
   c. Vecuronium
   d. Cisatracurium

2. Which agent would be least appropriate to use before anesthesia induction?
   a. Atracurium
   b. Cisatracurium
   c. Pancuronium
   d. Rocuronium

3. A patient is to receive a nondepolarizing NMJ blocker. The patient also takes a calcium channel blocker. Which of the following would most likely occur?
   a. The patient would receive a cholinesterase inhibitor.
   b. The dosage of the NMJ blocker will be less.
   c. A depolarizing NMJ blocker would be used instead.
   d. The dosage of the calcium channel blocker would be increased.

4. After a patient receives succinylcholine, the nurse would assess the patient for which of the following initially?
   a. Muscle pain
   b. Hyperthermia
   c. Hypotension
   d. Respiratory depression

5. Which of the following conditions would predispose a patient to experience a prolonged action of succinylcholine?
   a. Renal failure
   b. Cirrhosis
   c. Heart disease
   d. Inflammatory bowel disease

6. After reviewing the events associated with the sliding filament theory of muscle contraction, a group students demonstrate a need for additional study when they identify which of the following?
   a. Acetylcholine interacts with muscarnic receptors.
   b. Calcium combines with tropinin.
   c. Actin and myosin, when reacting, shorten the fiber.
   d. Depolarization allows the release of calcium ions.

7. Which of the following statements best reflects the action of NMJ blockers?
   a. They cause muscle paralysis along with total central nervous system depression.
   b. They have relatively few adverse effects.
   c. Most do not affect pain perception and consciousness.
   d. They readily cross the blood–brain barrier.

8. A nurse is monitoring a patient closely for malignant hyperthermia because the patient received which NMJ blocker?
   a. Pancuronium
   b. Vecuronium
   c. Atracurium
   d. Succinylcholine

9. A patient experienced significant muscle pain after receiving an NMJ blocker for a procedure. Which of the following would be most appropriate for the nurse to administer for pain relief?
   a. Dantrolene
   b. Aspirin
   c. Morphine
   d. Naloxone

10. When a depolarizing NMJ agent is used, which of the following occurs?
    a. Prevention of depolarization
    b. Irreversible muscular contraction
    c. Enhancement of repolarization
    d. Continuous sustained muscle contraction

11. Which agent would be associated with increased intraocular pressure?
    a. Succinylcholine
    b. Vecuronium
    c. Rocuronium
    d. Pancuronium

12. A patient is receiving pancuronium. The nurse would expect to see the beginning effects of the drug in which approximate period of time?
    a. 30 to 60 seconds
    b. 1 to 2 minutes
    c. 4 to 6 minutes
    d. 8 to 10 minutes

13. A nurse understands that succinylcholine lasts for approximately how long once it is administered?
    a. 1 to 2 minutes
    b. 4 to 6 minutes
    c. 8 to 12 minutes
    d. 15 to 20 minutes

14. A nurse is reviewing a patient's history for conditions that may contraindicate the use of a nondepolarizing NMJ blocker. Which of the following would be a concern?
    a. Myasthenia gravis
    b. Cirrhosis
    c. Glaucoma
    d. Malnutrition

15. A patient who received a nondepolarizing NMJ blocker is exhibiting signs of excessive neuromuscular blockade. Which of the following would most likely be used?
    a. Peripheral nerve stimulator
    b. Direct-acting skeletal muscle relaxant
    c. Cholinesterase inhibitor
    d. Narcotic antagonist

Introduction to the Autonomic Nervous System

■ ASSESSING YOUR UNDERSTANDING

CROSSWORD

Use the clues to complete the crossword puzzle.

Across

2. Adrenergic receptor found in the heart and lungs
4. Receptor sites on effects responding to acetylcholine
6. Adrenergic receptors found in smooth muscle
8. Nervous system involved in the fight-or-flight response
9. Receptor sites on effectors responding to norepinephrine

Down

1. Enzyme important for preventing overstimulation of cholinergic receptor sites
3. Cholinergic receptors also responding to muscarine
5. A group of closely packed nerve cell bodies
7. Nervous system involved in the rest-and-digest response

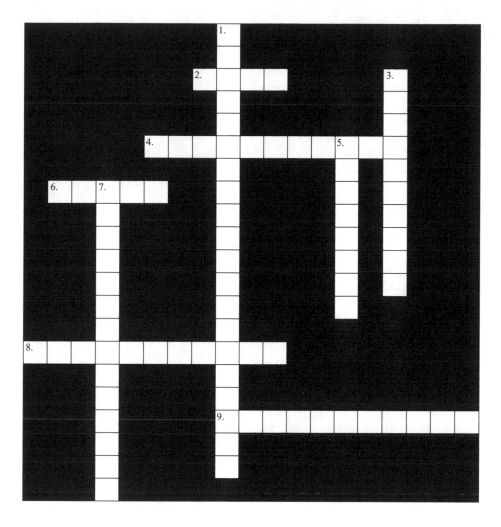

SHORT ANSWER

Supply the information requested.

1. Identify the location of the main nerve centers for the autonomic nervous system.

2. Explain how nerve impulse transmission in the autonomic nervous system is different from that of the central nervous system.

3. State the other name for the sympathetic nervous system.

4. Name the neurotransmitter released by the preganglionic nerves of the sympathetic nervous system.

5. List the four catecholamines.

6. Identify the four classifications of sympathetic nervous system adrenergic receptors.

7. Name the two classifications of parasympathetic nervous system receptors.

8. State the two enzymes involved in terminating a sympathetic nervous system response by metabolizing norepinephrine.

■ APPLYING YOUR KNOWLEDGE

CASE STUDY

A patient comes to the emergency department complaining of a very rapid heart rate and sweating. She states, "I was getting ready to do a presentation for my company, and all of a sudden I started to feel this way. I really don't like to speak in public, and I get really nervous before I do." The patient's heart rate and respiratory rate are elevated. The patient's hands are cool and clammy. Further evaluation reveals that the patient is experiencing an anxiety attack.

a. When evaluating the patient's signs and symptoms, which branch of the autonomic nervous system would the nurse suspect as predominating at this point? Correlate the patient's current manifestations with the system's action.

b. What additional signs and symptoms would the nurse most likely assess?

c. How would the nurse explain to the patient what is happening?

■ PRACTICING FOR NCLEX

Circle the letter that corresponds to the best answer for each question.

1. Which of the following would be considered functions of the autonomic nervous system? Select all that apply.
   a. Control of heart rate
   b. Maintenance of water balance
   c. Level of consciousness
   d. Sensory perception
   e. Muscle movement
   f. Regulation of respiration

2. When describing the sympathetic nervous system, the instructor would include which of the following?
   a. Cells for impulses are located primarily in the sacral area of the spinal cord.
   b. Cells typically have very long preganglionic fibers out to the synapse.
   c. The relatively long postganglionic fibers synapse with neuroeffectors.
   d. The ganglia are located close to the organ or area being affected.

3. A patient is experiencing a stress response. Which of the following would the nurse expect to assess?
   a. Bradycardia
   b. Hypotension
   c. Pupil constriction
   d. Diminished bowel sounds

4. Which of the following is secreted during the fight-or-flight response to suppress the immune and inflammatory reactions?
   a. Corticosteroid
   b. Thyroid hormone
   c. Aldosterone
   d. Glucose

5. The nurse understands that vasoconstriction that leads to a rise in blood pressure is due to stimulation of which type of receptor?
   a. Alpha-1
   b. Alpha-2
   c. Beta-1
   d. Beta-2

6. A patient is receiving a drug that helps to relax the bladder detrusor muscle. The nurse would understand that this drug is affecting which type of receptor?
   a. Alpha-1
   b. Alpha-2
   c. Beta-1
   d. Beta-2

7. Which of the following would be assessed with parasympathetic nervous system stimulation?
   a. Reduced secretions
   b. Increased gastric motility
   c. Pupillary dilation
   d. Constriction of the rectal sphincter

8. Which neurotransmitter is involved in pre- and postganglionic activity in the parasympathetic nervous system?
   a. Norepinephrine
   b. Epinephrine
   c. Acetylcholine
   d. Dopamine

9. Which of the following would be discussed when describing the parasympathetic nervous system?
   a. Vagus nerve
   b. Adrenergic receptors
   c. Norepinephrine
   d. Monoamine oxidase

10. After teaching a group of students about the differences between the sympathetic nervous system and the parasympathetic nervous system, the instructor determines that the students have understood the information when they state which of the following?
    a. Unlike the sympathetic nervous system, the parasympathetic nervous system ganglia are located in chains along the spinal cord.
    b. The sympathetic nervous system preganglionic fibers are short, while those in the parasympathetic nervous system are long.
    c. The sympathetic nervous system helps the body recuperate from the stress response of the parasympathetic nervous system.
    d. The sympathetic nervous system contains nicotinic receptors that the parasympathetic nervous system does not have.

11. Which of the following would occur if a drug stimulated beta-2 receptors?
    a. Bronchoconstriction
    b. Uterine contraction
    c. Piloerection
    d. Vasodilation

12. Which of the following receptors is found in the beta cells of the pancreas?
    a. Alpha-1
    b. Alpha-2
    c. Beta-1
    d. Beta-2

13. After reviewing the autonomic nervous system and cholinergic neurons, the students demonstrate a need for additional study when they identify which of the following as a location for cholinergic neurons?
    a. Motor nerves on skeletal muscles
    b. All preganglionic nerves
    c. Most postganglionic sympathetic nervous system nerves
    d. Postganglionic parasympathetic nervous system nerves

14. Muscarinic receptors would be found most likely at which location?
    a. Adrenal medulla
    b. Sweat glands
    c. Neuromuscular junction
    d. Central nervous system

15. Norepinephrine is made by nerve cells using which substance?
    a. Choline
    b. Tyrosine
    c. Decarboxylase
    d. Glycogen

Adrenergic Agonists

Upon completion of this chapter, you will be able to:

1. Describe two ways that sympathomimetic drugs act to produce effects at adrenergic receptors.

2. Describe the therapeutic actions, indications, pharmacokinetics, contraindications, most common adverse reactions, and important drug–drug interactions associated with adrenergic agonists.

3. Discuss the use of adrenergic agents across the lifespan.

4. Compare and contrast the prototype drugs dopamine, phenylephrine, and isoproterenol with other adrenergic agonists.

5. Outline the nursing considerations, including important teaching points, for patients receiving an adrenergic agent.

■ASSESSING YOUR UNDERSTANDING

LABELING

Place the name of the drug in the appropriate box under the correct drug class.

Albuterol   Isoproterenol

Clonidine   Phenylephrine

Dobutamine   Terbutaline

Dopamine

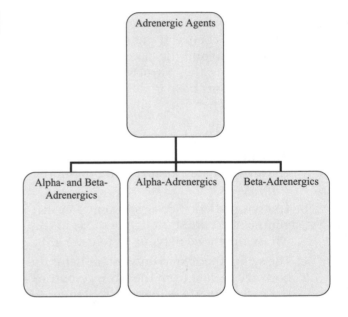

SHORT ANSWER

Supply the information requested.

1. Name the two primary actions of adrenergic agonists.

2. Explain why adrenergic agonists are also referred to as sympathomimetic agents.

3. Name the sympathomimetic drug of choice for the treatment of shock.

4. Describe the rationale for using clonidine to treat hypertension.

5. Explain the result of an interaction between a sympathomimetic agent and an adrenergic antagonist.

6. Identify the reason why adrenergic agonists should be used with caution in patients with vascular problems.

■ APPLYING YOUR KNOWLEDGE

CASE STUDY

A patient is diagnosed with hypertension, and the health care provider prescribes clonidine as a transdermal patch. The patient is concerned because the drug is in patch form instead of pill form. He states, "How will this little patch help control my blood pressure?"

a. How should the nurse respond to the patient?

b. What information would the nurse need to include when teaching the patient about this drug?

■ PRACTICING FOR NCLEX

Circle the letter that corresponds to the best answer for each question.

1. Which of the following would the nurse identify as a naturally occurring catecholamine?

a. Dobutamine

b. Dopamine

c. Ephedrine

d. Metaraminol

2. Which of the following would a nurse keep in mind about dobutamine when used to treat congestive heart failure?

a. It has slight preference for beta-1 receptor sites.

b. It causes a significant increase in the heart rate.

c. Myocardial oxygen demand is increased.

d. It rarely interacts with herbal products.

3. Which of the following would the nurse expect to assess in a patient receiving an alpha- and beta-adrenergic agonist?

a. Hypotension

b. Dyspnea

c. Diarrhea

d. Personality changes

4. A patient is experiencing shock and is extremely hypotensive. Which of the following would the nurse expect as the drug most likely to be given?

a. Ephedrine

b. Epinephrine

c. Dopamine

d. Dobutamine

5. The nurse is reviewing the medical record of a patient who is taking an alpha- and beta-adrenergic agonist. Which of the following would be of least concern to the nurse?

a. St. John's wort

b. Caffeine

c. Ma huang

d. Over-the-counter (OTC) cold preparations

6. The intravenous line of a patient receiving dobutamine infiltrates and the drug extravasates. The nurse would infiltrate the site with which of the following?

   a. Lactated Ringer's solution
   b. Hyaluronidase
   c. Sodium bicarbonate
   d. Phentolamine

7. Which of the following adverse effects might a patient receiving clonidine exhibit? Select all that apply.

   a. Photophobia
   b. Hyperglycemia
   c. Pupil constriction
   d. Personality changes
   e. Difficulty urinating

8. A patient is receiving phenylephrine via intramuscular injection. The nurse would expect the drug to begin acting in approximately which amount of time?

   a. 1 to 5 minutes
   b. 5 to 10 minutes
   c. 10 to 15 minutes
   d. 15 to 20 minutes

9. Which assessment finding would indicate to the nurse that the administered isoproterenol is effective?

   a. Decreased heart rate
   b. Bronchoconstriction
   c. Improved cardiac contractility
   d. Uterine contraction

10. Which of the following would a nurse expect to administer if a patient who is receiving isoproterenol develops a severe reaction?

    a. Beta-adrenergic blockers
    b. Sympathomimetic agents
    c. Narcotic antagonist
    d. Neuromuscular blocking agent

11. A patient is being treated for asthma. Which of the following would the nurse expect to administer?

    a. Alpha- and beta-adrenergic agonist
    b. Alpha-specific adrenergic agonist
    c. Beta-1–specific adrenergic agonist
    d. Beta-2–specific adrenergic agonist

12. The nurse is reviewing the history of a patient receiving isoproterenol. Which of the following would the nurse identify as being a contraindication?

    a. Pulmonary hypertension
    b. Glaucoma
    c. Pheochromocytoma
    d. Hypovolemia

13. Which of the following agents would the nurse expect to be used to prevent hypotension if dopamine or norepinephrine cannot be used?

    a. Dobutamine
    b. Ephedrine
    c. Norepinephrine
    d. Epinephrine

14. Which of the following would be most important for the nurse to assess in a patient receiving midodrine?

    a. Changes in respiratory rate
    b. Positional blood pressure changes
    c. Changes in urinary output
    d. Appetite changes

15. A patient is taking an OTC allergy product. The nurse would expect to find that this product most likely contains which of the following?

    a. Ephedra
    b. Phenylephrine
    c. Epinephrine
    d. Albuterol

CHAPTER 31

Adrenergic Blocking Antagonists

LEARNING OBJECTIVES

Upon completion of this chapter, you will be able to:

1. Describe the effects of adrenergic blocking agents on adrenergic receptors, correlating these effects with their clinical effects.
2. Describe the therapeutic actions, indications, pharmacokinetics, contraindications and cautions, most common adverse reactions, and important drug–drug interactions associated with adrenergic blocking agents.
3. Discuss the use of adrenergic blocking agents across the lifespan.
4. Compare and contrast the prototype drugs labetalol, phentolamine, doxazosin, propranolol, and atenolol with other adrenergic blocking agents.
5. Outline the nursing considerations, including important teaching points, for patients receiving an adrenergic blocking agent.

■ ASSESSING YOUR UNDERSTANDING

LABELING

Place the name of each drug below in the appropriate column that reflects its selectivity.

Atenolol
Carteolol
Doxazosin
Esmolol
Phentolamine
Pindolol
Propranolol
Terazosin
Timolol

Nonselective Alpha	Alpha-1 Selective	Nonselective Beta	Beta-1 Selective

FILL IN THE BLANKS

Provide the missing term in the blanks provided.

1. Adrenergic blocking agents are also called ____________ because they block the effects of the sympathetic nervous system.

2. Adrenergic blockers prevent the release of _____ from the nerve terminal or from the adrenal medulla.

3. A patient who is receiving a nonselective adrenergic blocker and an antidiabetic agent is at risk for _____.

4. Carvedilol is used to treat congestive heart failure and _____.

5. Blocking of all receptor sites within the sympathetic nervous system leads to a _____ of blood pressure.

6. Alpha-1 selective adrenergic blockers decrease blood pressure by blocking the _____ alpha-1 receptor sites.

7. Nonselective beta-adrenergic blockers are used primarily to treat _____ problems.

8. An effect associated with nonselective beta-adrenergic blockers is _____ exercise tolerance.

9. Adrenergic blocking agents should not be discontinued abruptly but rather should be gradually tapered over a period of _____ weeks.

10. The prototype beta-1 selective adrenergic blocker is _____.

■ APPLYING YOUR KNOWLEDGE

CASE STUDY

A 58-year-old patient is being seen by his cardiologist for a follow-up visit. The patient has a history of hypertension for which he is receiving carvedilol and furosemide (a diuretic). He is also receiving sotalol as treatment for atrial fibrillation. During the visit, the patient tells the physician that he has been experiencing some light-headedness. "It's mostly when I get up out of bed or when I go to stand up after I've been sitting. I have to stop and hold on for a minute or so and then it passes. I almost stopped taking the drugs because of this."

a. What might the patient be experiencing and why?

b. What information would be important to obtain to help confirm this suspicion?

c. What instructions would be important for this patient?

■ PRACTICING FOR NCLEX

Circle the letter that corresponds to the best answer for each question.

1. Which of the following would be most important to monitor in a patient receiving carvedilol?
   a. Liver function studies
   b. Renal function studies
   c. Complete blood count
   d. Coagulation studies

2. A patient is receiving sotalol. Which instruction would be most important for the nurse to provide to the patient to ensure maximum effectiveness of the drug?
   a. "Take an antacid at the same time you take the drug."
   b. "Be sure to take the drug on an empty stomach."
   c. "Eat a large meal and then take the drug."
   d. "Take the entire daily dose at one time."

3. After reviewing information about nonselective adrenergic blockers, a group of students demonstrate a need for additional teaching when they identify which of the following as an effect of these agents?
   a. Lowered blood pressure
   b. Increased pulse rate
   c. Increased renal perfusion
   d. Decreased renin levels

4. A patient with diabetes who uses insulin is also receiving labetalol. The nurse would monitor the patient closely for which of the following?
   a. Hypotension
   b. Arrhythmias
   c. Hypoglycemia
   d. Bronchospasm

5. When explaining the use of an alpha-1 selective adrenergic blocker to a patient, which of the following would the nurse need to keep in mind?
   a. Reflex tachycardia may occur.
   b. Bladder relaxation leads to improved urine flow.
   c. The overall vascular tone increases.
   d. Blood pressure decreases due to vasoconstriction.

6. After teaching a group of students about adrenergic blockers that may be used to treat benign prostatic hypertrophy, the instructor determines that the teaching has been successful when the students identify which of the following?
   a. Tamsulosin
   b. Prazosin
   c. Carteolol
   d. Amiodarone

7. A patient experiences diarrhea after receiving a nonselective adrenergic blocking agent. The nurse understands that this effect is most likely due to which of the following?
   a. Drug's effect on liver functioning
   b. Increased parasympathetic dominance
   c. Blockage of norepinephrine in the central nervous system
   d. Loss of vascular tone

8. After administering the oral form of labetalol to a patient, the nurse would monitor the patient for a peak drug effect at which time?
   a. 1 to 2 hours
   b. 2 to 3 hours
   c. 3 to 4 hours
   d. 4 to 5 hours

9. The nurse is preparing a teaching plan for a patient who is to receive a nonselective beta blocker. The nurse would make sure to address safety measures as a priority for the patient receiving which of the following?
   a. Carteolol
   b. Nadolol
   c. Sotalol
   d. Propranolol

10. Which patient statement indicates the need for additional teaching about propranolol?
    a. "I need to get up slowly after sitting or lying down."
    b. "I can stop the drug once my blood pressure is controlled."
    c. "I should space activities throughout the day."
    d. "I need to report if I have any chest pain or problems breathing."

11. A patient has a history of smoking. Which of the following agents would the nurse most likely expect to be ordered?
    a. Timolol
    b. Pindolol
    c. Nadolol
    d. Atenolol

12. Which of the following would a nurse identify as a contraindication for the use of a beta-1 selective blocker?
    a. Diabetes
    b. Thyroid disease
    c. Sinus bradycardia
    d. Chronic obstructive pulmonary disease

13. A patient is experiencing an acute myocardial infarction. The physician orders metoprolol to be given as an intravenous bolus injection. The patient responds, and the physician then orders metoprolol oral therapy. The nurse would expect to administer the first oral dose at which time after the last intravenous bolus dose?
    a. Immediately
    b. 5 minutes
    c. 10 minutes
    d. 15 minutes

14. Which agent would be the most likely drug of choice for an older adult patient with hypertension who requires an adrenergic blocker?

a. Bisoprolol

b. Betaxolol

c. Atenolol

d. Esmolol

15. A patient is receiving a beta-1 selective blocker after a myocardial infarction to prevent reinfarction. The nurse understands that the rationale for using the drug would be which of the following?

a. Improve contractility

b. Enhanced excitability

c. Decreased cardiac workload

d. Decreased blood pressure

Cholinergic Agonists

LEARNING OBJECTIVES

Upon completion of this chapter, you will be able to:

1. Describe the effects of cholinergic receptors, correlating these effects with the clinical effects of cholinergic agonists.

2. Describe the therapeutic actions, indications, pharmacokinetics, contraindications and cautions, most common adverse reactions, and important drug–drug interactions associated with the direct- and indirect-acting cholinergic agonists.

3. Discuss the use of cholinergic agonists across the lifespan.

4. Compare and contrast the prototype drugs bethanechol, donepezil, and pyridostigmine with other cholinergic agonists.

5. Outline the nursing considerations, including important teaching points, for patients receiving a cholinergic agonist.

■ASSESSING YOUR UNDERSTANDING

LABELING

Place the name of the following drugs in the appropriate box under the correct drug class.

Bethanechol
Donepezil
Edrophonium
Galantamine
Pilocarpine
Pyridostigmine

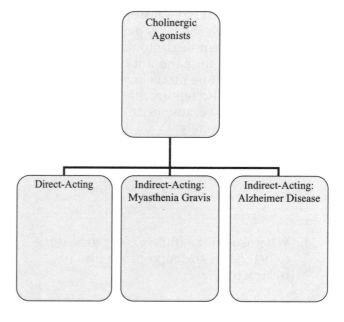

MATCHING

Select the description from column 2 that best describes the term in column 1.

Column 1

_____ 1. Acetylcholinesterase

_____ 2. Parasympathomimetic

_____ 3. Cholinergic

_____ 4. Acetylcholine

_____ 5. Nerve gas

Column 2

a. Another name for cholinergic agonists

b. Irreversible acetylcholinesterase inhibitor

c. Neurotransmitter

d. Enzyme responsible for neurotransmitter breakdown

e. Receptor sites stimulated by acetylcholine

■ APPLYING YOUR KNOWLEDGE

CASE STUDY

A 35-year-old woman is brought to the emergency department by her husband for evaluation. The patient has a history of myasthenia gravis for which she takes pyridostigmine daily. The patient began to have difficulty breathing. Her husband noticed that she was experiencing more problems swallowing and speaking. He also reports that it was difficult to see her eyes because her eyelids were drooping so severely.

a. What might be happening with this patient and why?

b. What would the nurse expect to be done to determine the appropriate plan of treatment?

c. What interventions would be instituted for this patient?

■ PRACTICING FOR NCLEX

Circle the letter that corresponds to the best answer for each question.

1. Which of the following physiologic effects would be related to the use of cholinergic agents?

   a. Pupil dilation

   b. Increased salivation

   c. Increased heart rate

   d. Decreased bladder muscle tone

2. A patient receives carbachol eye drops. Which of the following effects would the nurse expect to assess?

   a. Miosis

   b. Mydriasis

   c. Ptosis

   d. Paralysis of eye muscles

3. When assessing a patient for possible adverse effects of direct-acting cholinergic agents, which of the following might the nurse find?

   a. Tachycardia

   b. Hypertension

   c. Constipation

   d. Urinary urgency

4. A patient is experiencing urinary retention after surgery. The nurse would anticipate administering which of the following?

   a. Cevimeline

   b. Pilocarpine

   c. Bethanechol

   d. Carbachol

5. When describing the action of indirect-acting cholinergic agonists to a group of students, which of the following would the instructor include?

   a. Imitation of acetylcholine action at receptor sites

   b. Prevention of acetylcholinesterase action

   c. Reduction in the amount of acetylcholine available

   d. Occupation of acetylcholine receptor sites

6. Which of the following agents would be most appropriate to administer to a patient with Alzheimer's disease?

   a. Pyridostigmine

   b. Neostigmine

   c. Ambenonium

   d. Donepezil

7. A nurse is preparing a presentation for a local group of emergency first responders about biological and chemical weapons. The nurse is describing the effects of exposure to nerve gas. Which of the following would the nurse include?

   a. Tachycardia
   b. Pupil dilation
   c. Bronchial constriction
   d. Muscle flaccidity

8. A patient is prescribed donepezil. The nurse would expect to administer this drug at which frequency?

   a. Once a day
   b. Twice a day
   c. Three times a day
   d. Four times a day

9. The nurse would be alert for which of the following in a patient who is taking rivastigmine and ibuprofen?

   a. Fecal incontinence
   b. Abdominal cramps
   c. Gastrointestinal bleeding
   d. Diarrhea

10. Which of the following would be most important to have readily available for a patient who is receiving an indirect-acting cholinergic agonist and develops a severe reaction?

    a. Edrophonium
    b. Atropine
    c. Phentolamine
    d. Naloxone

11. A patient with myasthenia gravis is having difficulty swallowing and adhering to a routine schedule. Which agent would be the most appropriate?

    a. Ambenonium
    b. Neostigmine
    c. Pyridostigmine
    d. Rivastigmine

12. A patient is receiving galantamine as treatment for Alzheimer's disease. The nurse would instruct the patient and his family about which of the following as possible adverse effects? Select all that apply.

    a. Urinary urgency
    b. Blurred vision
    c. Constipation
    d. Hypertension
    e. Flushing

13. A patient is receiving tacrine and uses theophylline for chronic bronchospasm. Which of the following would be most important for the nurse to monitor?

    a. Respiratory status
    b. Serum theophylline levels
    c. Blood pressure
    d. Mental status

14. Which of the following would the nurse identify as a contraindication to the use of an anticholinesterase inhibitor?

    a. Asthma
    b. Peptic ulcer disease
    c. Intestinal obstruction
    d. Parkinsonism

15. When describing the action of direct-acting cholinergic agonists, which receptors would the nurse identify as being stimulated?

    a. Muscarinic
    b. Nicotinic
    c. Alpha
    d. Beta

CHAPTER 33

Anticholinergic Agents

Upon completion of the chapter, you will be able to:

1. Define anticholinergic agents.

2. Describe the therapeutic actions, indications, pharmacokinetics, contraindications and cautions, most common adverse reactions, and important drug–drug interactions of anticholinergic agents.

3. Discuss the use of anticholinergic agents across the lifespan.

4. Compare and contrast the prototype drug atropine with other anticholinergic agents.

5. Outline the nursing considerations, including important teaching points, for patients receiving anticholinergic agents.

■ ASSESSING YOUR UNDERSTANDING

FILL IN THE BLANKS

Provide the missing term in the blanks provided.

1. A plant that contains atropine as an alkaloid, _____, is used in herbal medicine today.

2. _____ agents are drugs that block the effects of acetylcholine.

3. The most widely used parasympatholytic agent is _____.

4. Relaxation of the pupil of the eye is called _____.

5. The adverse effects associated with anticholinergic agents are due to the systemic blockade of _____ receptors.

6. An antidote for atropine toxicity is _____.

7. Antihistamines _____ the adverse effects of anticholinergic agents.

8. Blockage of the parasympathetic system leads to _____ gastrointestinal (GI) activity.

MATCHING

Select the condition in column 2 that would be an indication for the drug listed in column 1.

Column 1

____ 1. Dicyclomine

____ 2. Ipratropium

____ 3. Propantheline

____ 4. Scopolamine

____ 5. Hyoscyamine

Column 2

a. Adjunct therapy for peptic ulcer disease

b. Treatment of irritable bowel

c. Maintenance treatment of bronchospasm

d. Treatment of motion sickness

e. Alleviation of GI spasms

■ APPLYING YOUR KNOWLEDGE

CASE STUDY

A 62-year-old black man comes to the clinic for an eye examination. The patient has a history of depression for which the patient takes a tricyclic antidepressant. The patient is to receive atropine eye drops in preparation for the ophthalmologic examination.

a. What issues would be important for the nurse to consider in this situation?

b. Would the nurse expect the patient to exhibit adverse effects? Why or why not?

■ PRACTICING FOR NCLEX

Circle the letter that corresponds to the best answer for each question.

1. A nurse suspects that a patient may be experiencing atropine toxicity. Which of the following would the nurse assess?
   a. Diaphoresis
   b. Excess salivation
   c. Slight cardiac slowing
   d. Cough

2. Which of the following statements best reflects the action of scopolamine?
   a. It blocks the nicotinic receptors in the parasympathetic nervous system.
   b. It exerts a major effect on the neuromuscular junction.
   c. It competes with acetylcholine at muscarinic effector sites.
   d. It acts specifically on the smooth muscles of the urinary tract.

3. Which agent would a nurse expect to administer transdermally?
   a. Atropine
   b. Scopolamine

   c. Dicyclomine
   d. Propantheline

4. A patient is prescribed propantheline. The nurse would administer this drug by which route?
   a. Oral
   b. Subcutaneous
   c. Intramuscular
   d. Intravenous

5. A patient with hypertension is to receive an anticholinergic agent. The nurse would be especially alert for which of the following?
   a. Bladder obstruction
   b. Paralytic ileus
   c. Increased intraocular pressure
   d. Increased blood pressure

6. A patient is experiencing urgency, nocturia, and frequency secondary to cystitis. Which of the following might the health care provider prescribe?
   a. Flavoxate
   b. Dicyclomine
   c. Glycopyrrolate
   d. Methscopolamine

7. An older patient is taking an anticholinergic agent. After teaching the patient about the drug, which patient statement indicates the need for additional teaching?
   a. "I should make sure that I drink plenty of fluids."
   b. "I need to exercise frequently outside in the warm weather."
   c. "I should avoid driving if I feel light-headed or dizzy."
   d. "I should eat plenty of fiber to prevent constipation."

8. A patient is diagnosed with atropine toxicity that resulted from the ingestion of herbal therapies. Which of the following would be done first?
   a. Administration of physostigmine
   b. Gastric lavage
   c. Administration of diazepam
   d. Cool sponge baths

9. Which of the following agents would be least likely to cause increased adverse effects if given with an anticholinergic agent?
   a. Antihistamines
   b. Antiparkinson agents
   c. Monoamine oxidase inhibitors
   d. Nonsteroidal anti-inflammatory drugs

10. The nurse administers atropine intramuscularly at 9:00 AM. At which time would the nurse expect the drug's peak effects to occur?
    a. 9:15 AM
    b. 9:30 AM
    c. 9:45 AM
    d. 10:00 AM

11. A patient is prescribed glycopyrrolate. The nurse understands that this drug may be administered by which route? Select all that apply.
    a. Oral
    b. Intramuscular
    c. Subcutaneous
    d. Transdermal
    e. Intravenous

12. Which of the following would the nurse expect to assess in a patient who has been given propantheline?
    a. Pupil constriction
    b. Diarrhea
    c. Bradycardia
    d. Excitement

13. A patient is using a transdermal application of scopolamine. Which of the following instructions would the nurse include when teaching the patient how to use this drug?
    a. "Shave the area where you are planning to apply the patch."
    b. "Place your fingers on the adhesive side of the patch to apply it."
    c. "Make sure the area you are using is clean, dry, and free from cuts."
    d. "Apply a new patch before you remove the old one."

14. Which agent would the nurse identify as acting specifically on the receptors in the GI tract?
    a. Ipratropium
    b. Tiotropium
    c. Trospium
    d. Hyoscyamine

15. A patient is using a scopolamine patch for treatment of motion sickness. The nurse would instruct the patient to change the patch at which frequency?
    a. Every day
    b. Every 3 days
    c. Every 5 days
    d. Every 7 days

34

Introduction to the Endocrine System

LEARNING OBJECTIVES

Upon completion of this chapter, you will be able to:

1. Label a diagram showing the glands of the traditional endocrine system and list the hormones produced by each.

2. Describe two theories of hormone action.

3. Discuss the role of the hypothalamus as the master gland of the endocrine system, including influences on the actions of the hypothalamus.

4. Outline a negative feedback system within the endocrine system and explain the ways that this system controls hormone levels in the body.

5. Describe the hypothalamic-pituitary axis and what would happen if a hormone level were altered within the hypothalamic-pituitary axis.

■ ASSESSING YOUR UNDERSTANDING

LABELING

Place the name of the hormone in the appropriate column.

Adrenocorticotropic hormone (ACTH)

Antidiuretic hormone

Follicle-stimulating hormone

Gonadotropin-releasing hormone

Growth hormone

Luteinizing hormone

Melanocyte-stimulating hormone

Oxytocin

Prolactin

Somatostatin

Thyroid-releasing hormone

Thyroid-stimulating hormone

Hypothalamus	Anterior pituitary	Posterior Pituitary

MATCHING

Select the hormone produced from column 2 that is secreted by the gland in column 1.

Column 1

____ **1.** Adrenal cortex

____ **2.** Ovaries

____ **3.** Pancreas

____ **4.** Kidney

____ **5.** Stomach

____ **6.** Testes

____ **7.** Thyroid

____ **8.** Pineal gland

Column 2

a. Erythropoietin

b. Melatonin

c. Gastrin

d. Aldosterone

e. Progesterone

f. Glucagon

g. Calcitonin

h. Testosterone

■ APPLYING YOUR KNOWLEDGE

CASE STUDY

A patient is diagnosed with a brain tumor. Diagnostic studies reveal that the tumor is located at the very back of the cerebrum (the forebrain), extending into the area between the cerebrum and the brain stem, in an area termed the *diencephalon*. The tumor is pressing on a small portion of the hypothalamus. The patient is to undergo radiation therapy to help shrink the tumor in the hopes that the tumor can then be surgically removed.

a. How might the patient's hormonal balance be affected by this condition?

b. What other effects might occur as a result of the tumor's location?

■ PRACTICING FOR NCLEX

Circle the letter that corresponds to the best answer for each question.

1. Which of the following best reflects hormones?
   a. Produced in large quantities
   b. Secreted directly into the bloodstream
   c. Require time to be broken down
   d. Travel via ducts to receptor sites

2. After reviewing the structures of the endocrine system, the students demonstrate understanding when they identify which of the following as the master gland?
   a. Thyroid
   b. Pituitary
   c. Hypothalamus
   d. Pancreas

3. A hormone that takes a while to produce an effect is most likely reacting in which manner?
   a. With a receptor on the cell membrane
   b. With a cell as it travels through the bloodstream
   c. In a specialized target area of the body
   d. Inside the cell receptor site to change messenger RNA

4. Which of the following would the nurse identify as being secreted by the hypothalamus?
   a. Somatostatin
   b. ACTH
   c. Luteinizing hormone
   d. Prolactin

5. Which of the following would be delivered by the neurologic network from the hypothalamus to the pituitary?
   a. Growth hormone-releasing hormone
   b. Gonadotropin-releasing hormone
   c. Corticotropin-releasing hormone
   d. Oxytocin

6. After teaching a group of students about the factors that affect the release of hormones from the anterior pituitary gland, the instructor determines that the students need additional teaching when they identify which of the following as a factor?

   a. Central nervous system activity

   b. Hypothalamic hormones

   c. Drugs

   d. Plasma osmolality

7. Which of the following would a nurse identify as being released from the intermediate lobe of the pituitary gland?

   a. Oxytocin

   b. Endorphins

   c. Antidiuretic hormone

   d. Melanocyte-stimulating hormone

8. Which hormone would a nurse identify as being involved in diurnal rhythm?

   a. Corticotropin-releasing factor

   b. Thyroid-stimulating hormone

   c. Growth hormone release-inhibiting factor

   d. Luteinizing hormone

9. Which hormone would be responsible for the letdown reflex in lactating women?

   a. Prolactin

   b. Follicle-stimulating hormone

   c. Oxytocin

   d. Luteinizing hormone

10. After teaching a group of students about the negative feedback system, the instructor determines that the students have understood the information when they identify which hormone as not being regulated by this mechanism?

    a. Prolactin

    b. Thyroid hormone

    c. Follicle-stimulating hormone

    d. ACTH

11. Which of the following regulates the release of parathormone?

    a. Acid in the gastrointestinal tract

    b. Calcium levels

    c. Blood pressure

    d. Blood glucose levels

12. Which hormone is released by activation of the sympathetic nervous system?

    a. Aldosterone

    b. Prostaglandin

    c. ACTH

    d. Calcitonin

13. When describing the hypothalamic-pituitary axis, which event would occur first?

    a. Anterior pituitary release of stimulating hormones

    b. Hypothalamus secretion of releasing factor

    c. Hormone secretion by the endocrine gland

    d. Rising levels of secreted hormone

14. Which of the following is a primary effect of aldosterone secretion?

    a. Increased glucose levels

    b. Increased red blood cell production

    c. Increased sodium levels

    d. Increased potassium levels

15. Stimulation of which of the following would result from thyroid hormone secretion?

    a. Stomach acid production

    b. Basal metabolic rate

    c. Male secondary sex characteristics

    d. Pancreatic juice secretion

Hypothalamic and Pituitary Agents

Upon completion of this chapter, you will be able to:

1. Describe the anatomical and physiological relationship between the hypothalamus and the pituitary gland and list the hormones produced by each.

2. Describe the therapeutic actions, indications, pharmacokinetics, contraindications, most common adverse reactions, and important drug–drug interactions associated with the hypothalamic and pituitary agents.

3. Discuss the use of hypothalamic and pituitary agents across the lifespan.

4. Compare and contrast the prototype drugs leuprolide, somatropin, bromocriptine mesylate, and desmopressin with other hypothalamic and pituitary agents.

5. Outline the nursing considerations, including important teaching points, for patients receiving a hypothalamic or pituitary agent.

■ASSESSING YOUR UNDERSTANDING

CROSSWORD

Use the clues to solve the crossword puzzle.

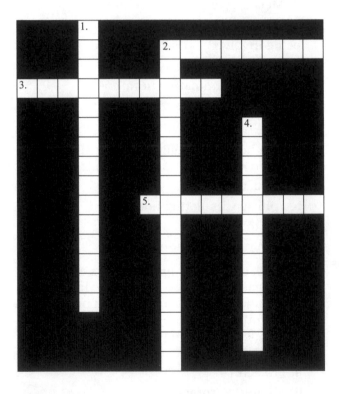

Across

2. Small stature; lack of growth hormone in children

3. Thickening of bony surfaces due to excess growth hormone after closure of the epiphyseal plates

5. Excess levels of growth hormone before closure of the epiphyseal plates

Down

1. Lack of adequate pituitary function
2. Lack of antidiuretic hormone
4. Master gland

SHORT ANSWER

Supply the information requested.

1. Describe the primary uses for hypothalamic hormones.

2. Explain the difference between gigantism and acromegaly.

3. Identify the prototype growth hormone antagonist.

4. List three signs of water intoxication that can occur with desmopressin.

5. Name two growth hormone antagonists.

■ APPLYING YOUR KNOWLEDGE

CASE STUDY

A child is to receive growth hormone therapy due to a deficiency of growth hormone. The plan is to administer somatropin, which is a synthetic human growth hormone. The child has undergone numerous screening procedures and testing. During a recent visit, he says to the nurse, "I can't wait until I start growing. I'm so tired of being the shortest one in my class."

a. How should the nurse respond to this child?

b. What psychosocial issues might arise with this therapy?

■ PRACTICING FOR NCLEX

Circle the letter that corresponds to the best answer for each question.

1. A patient is to receive nafarelin. The nurse would instruct the patient in administering this drug by which route?
   a. Oral
   b. Intranasal
   c. Intramuscular
   d. Subcutaneous

2. Which of the following would the nurse assess in a patient receiving a hypothalamic agonist?
   a. Dehydration
   b. Decreased glucose levels
   c. Impaired healing
   d. Loss of energy

3. After teaching a patient about the adverse effects of leuprolide, the nurse determines that additional teaching is needed when the patient identifies which of the following as an adverse effect?
   a. Hematuria
   b. Chills
   c. Peripheral edema
   d. Constipation

4. The nurse would know it is most important to monitor which laboratory test in a patient who is receiving lanreotide?
   a. Liver function
   b. Renal function
   c. Blood coagulation
   d. Glucose level

5. Which agent would the nurse identify as a growth hormone agonist?
   a. Bromocriptine
   b. Octreotide
   c. Somatropin
   d. Pegvisomant

6. The nurse is assessing a child who is receiving growth hormone therapy. Which of the following would the nurse identify as suggesting glucose intolerance?

a. Injection site pain

b. Fatigue

c. Thirst

d. Cold intolerance

7. The nurse is preparing to administer octreotide. The nurse expects to administer this drug by which route?

a. Oral

b. Subcutaneous

c. Intramuscular

d. Intranasal

8. A patient is receiving pegvisomant as treatment for acromegaly. Which of the following might the nurse assess as a possible adverse effect?

a. Gastrointestinal upset

b. Drowsiness

c. Postural hypotension

d. Infection

9. A patient who is receiving a growth hormone antagonist develops acute cholecystitis. Which agent would the patient most likely be receiving?

a. Bromocriptine

b. Pegvisomant

c. Somatropin

d. Octreotide

10. A patient is to undergo fertility treatment and is to receive an agent that induces ovulation because her ovaries are functioning. Which agent would this most likely be?

a. Chorionic gonadotropin

b. Corticotropin

c. Cosyntropin

d. Thyrotropin alfa

11. The nurse would administer which of the following to a patient is in labor to improve her uterine contractions?

a. Desmopressin

b. Oxytocin

c. Menotropins

d. Chorionic gonadotropin alfa

12. When describing desmopressin to a group of students, the instructor explains that it is a synthetic form of which of the following?

a. Oxytocin

b. Adrenocorticotropic hormone

c. Thyroid hormone

d. Antidiuretic hormone

13. A patient receives desmopressin intravenously at 10:00 AM. The nurse would expect the drug to begin working at which time?

a. 10:15 AM

b. 10:30 AM

c. 10:45 AM

d. 11:00 AM

14. A patient is undergoing testing for Cushing's disease and is to receive corticotropin-releasing hormone. The nurse would prepare to administer this drug as which of the following?

a. Intravenous bolus injection

b. Intramuscular injection

c. Intravenous infusion

d. Depot injection

15. After reviewing agents that act as gonadotropin-releasing hormone antagonists, the students demonstrate a need for additional study when they identify which of the following as an example?

a. Pegvisomant

b. Ganirelix

c. Goserelin

d. Degarelix

Adrenocortical Agents

Upon completion of this chapter, you will be able to:

1. Explain the control of the synthesis and secretion and the physiologic effects of the adrenocortical agents.

2. Describe the therapeutic actions, indications, pharmacokinetics, contraindications, most common adverse reactions, and important drug–drug interactions associated with the adrenocortical agents.

3. Discuss the use of adrenocortical agents across the lifespan.

4. Compare and contrast the prototype drugs prednisone and fludrocortisone with other adrenocortical agents.

5. Outline the nursing considerations, including important teaching points, for patients receiving an adrenocortical agent.

■ASSESSING YOUR UNDERSTANDING

LABELING

Place the name of the following drugs in the appropriate box under the correct drug class.

Beclomethasone   Hydrocortisone
Budesonide   Prednisone
Cortisone   Triamcinolone
Dexamethasone

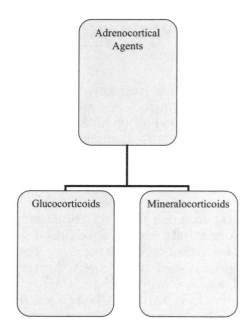

SHORT ANSWER

Supply the information requested.

1. Explain diurnal rhythm as it relates to hormonal secretion.

2. Describe the chemicals that are released by the adrenal medulla.

3. List the three types of corticosteroids produced by the adrenal cortex.

4. Explain how an adrenal crisis occurs.

5. Describe what happens with the prolonged use of corticosteroids.

6. Identify the functions of glucocorticoids in the body.

■ APPLYING YOUR KNOWLEDGE

CASE STUDY

A 9-year-old child is admitted to the facility after experiencing a severe asthmatic attack that responds to bronchodilator therapy (systemic and inhaled) and large doses of corticosteroids. The child was diagnosed with asthma at age 2¹Ú2 years and has had repeated asthmatic attacks for which he was hospitalized frequently before the age of 6 years. Since that time, the child has had two previous attacks that required hospitalization. Each time, bronchodilator and corticosteroid therapy was used as treatment. Currently, the child, who has been receiving intravenous corticosteroids, is being switched to oral therapy. The child is talking with the nurse about his condition and states, "I hate to take these steroids. My face gets all round, and I get so fat. My friends started to call me "mega Jon." Maybe I won't have to take them when I go home."

a. What effects might the child be experiencing related to his prescribed therapy?

b. How should the nurse respond to the child's statement about not taking the drugs at home?

■ PRACTICING FOR NCLEX

Circle the letter that corresponds to the best answer for each question.

1. Which of the following would a nurse identify as being secreted by the adrenal medulla?

a. Androgens
b. Neurotransmitters
c. Glucocorticoids
d. Mineralocorticoids

2. At which time would a nurse expect peak levels of adrenocorticotropic hormone to occur?

a. 10 PM to 12 AM
b. 1 AM to 3 AM
c. 6 AM to 9 AM
d. 12 PM to 3 PM

3. Which corticosteroid would a nurse identify as having the longest acting glucocorticoid effects?

a. Prednisone
b. Cortisone
c. Dexamethasone
d. Triamcinolone

4. A child is to receive a topical corticosteroid agent. Which statement by the parents indicates a need for additional teaching?

a. "We'll apply the cream in a thin layer over the area, using a small amount."
b. "We need to cover the area snugly with plastic wrap to prevent scratching."
c. "We'll keep the cream away from any open areas that might develop."
d. "We'll avoid putting the cream on any areas where the skin is abraded."

5. The nurse is preparing to administer prednisone. The nurse would expect to administer this agent by which route?

a. Oral
b. Intralesional
c. Inhalation
d. Intravenous

6. The nurse is monitoring a child who has been receiving long-term therapy with systemic corticosteroids. Which of the following would be most important for the nurse to assess?

   a. Weight changes
   b. Rectal bleeding
   c. Epistaxis
   d. Growth pattern

7. A patient receives prednisone at 7:00 AM. The nurse would expect to assess for the drug's peak effectiveness at which time after administration?

   a. 7:30 AM
   b. 8:30 AM
   c. 9:30 AM
   d. 10:30 AM

8. The nurse is teaching a patient who is receiving a glucocorticoid about the drug. Which of the following would the nurse instruct the patient to report immediately?

   a. Weight gain
   b. Abdominal distention
   c. Fever
   d. Increased appetite

9. A nurse would instruct a patient to take an oral glucocorticoid at which time?

   a. In the morning
   b. Around lunchtime
   c. Before dinner
   d. At bedtime

10. A nurse is reviewing the history of a patient who is to receive glucocorticoid therapy. Which of the following would the nurse identify as a contraindication to the drug's use?

    a. Diabetes
    b. Peptic ulcer disease
    c. Poison ivy
    d. Acute infection

11. Which glucocorticoid also exerts some mineralocorticoid effects?

    a. Triamcinolone
    b. Prednisolone
    c. Dexamethasone
    d. Betamethasone

12. After teaching a group of students about the effects of mineralocorticoids, the instructor determines that additional teaching is needed when the students identify which of the following as an effect?

    a. Increased sodium reabsorption
    b. Water retention
    c. Increased calcium retention
    d. Increased potassium excretion

13. When monitoring a patient who is receiving mineralocorticoid therapy, which assessment finding would be most important for the nurse to report?

    a. Shortness of breath
    b. Headache
    c. Weakness
    d. Slight pedal edema

14. When reviewing the serum potassium levels of a patient receiving fludrocortisone, which of the following would be a concern?

    a. 2.8 mEq/L
    b. 3.1 mEq/L
    c. 3.5 mEq/L
    d. 4.2 mEq/L

15. A group of students are reviewing material about the action of the adrenal glands and the stress response. The students demonstrate understanding of the material when they identify which of the following as a result of adrenocortical hormones?

    a. Decreased blood volume
    b. Glucose release for energy
    c. Increased protein production
    d. Stimulation of the inflammatory response

CHAPTER 37

Thyroid and Parathyroid Agents

LEARNING OBJECTIVES

Upon completion of this chapter, you will be able to:

1. Explain the control of the synthesis and secretion of thyroid hormones and parathyroid hormones, applying this to alterations in the control process (e.g., using thyroid hormones to treat obesity, Paget's disease, etc.).

2. Describe the therapeutic actions, indications, pharmacokinetics, contraindications, most common adverse reactions, and important drug–drug interactions associated with thyroid and parathyroid agents.

3. Discuss the use of thyroid and parathyroid drugs across the lifespan.

4. Compare and contrast thyroid and parathyroid prototype drugs with agents in their class.

5. Outline nursing considerations, including important teaching points, for patients receiving drugs used to affect thyroid or parathyroid function.

■ ASSESSING YOUR UNDERSTANDING

CROSSWORD

Use the clues to complete the crossword puzzle.

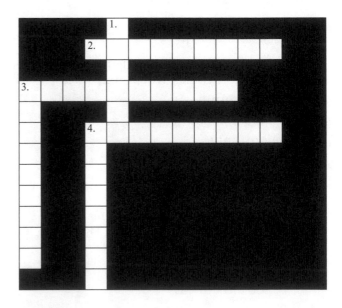

Across

2. Cells circularly arranged that form the structural unit of the thyroid gland
3. Hormone produced to counteract the effects of parathyroid hormone
4. Rate at which cells burn energy

Down

1. Dietary element used to produce thyroid hormone
3. Thyroid hormone deficiency in an infant
4. Lack of thyroid hormone in adults

LABELING

Place the following signs or symptoms in the appropriate column as indicating a deficiency or excess of thyroid hormones.

Coarse, dry skin

Tachycardia

Lethargy

Diffuse goiter

Fine, soft hair

Emotional dullness

Intolerance to heat

Weight gain

Thyroid Hormone Deficiency	Thyroid Hormone Excess

■ APPLYING YOUR KNOWLEDGE

CASE STUDY

A woman has undergone surgery to remove most of her thyroid gland as treatment for hyperthyroidism. Initially, drug therapy with methimazole was tried, but it was not effective. The patient is preparing to go home. She asks the nurse, "First I was on medicine to control my thyroid, then I had it removed. Now I have to take medicine. Now I have to take

more medicine. I thought I was done with all of this!"

a. What information would be important for the nurse to address with this patient?

b. What instructions would be important to include when teaching the patient about this drug?

■ PRACTICING FOR NCLEX

Circle the letter that corresponds to the best answer for each question.

1. Which agent would a nurse expect to administer to a patient with hypothyroidism?
   a. Levothyroxine
   b. Methimazole
   c. Propylthiouracil
   d. Calcitriol

2. Which of the following would a nurse expect to assess in a patient experiencing hyperthyroidism?
   a. Slow and deep tendon reflexes
   b. Bradycardia
   c. Flushed, warm skin
   d. Intolerance to cold

3. When describing the parafollicular cells to a group of students, which hormone would the instructor identify as being produced by these cells?
   a. Parathormone
   b. Calcitonin
   c. Levothyroxine
   d. Liothyronine

4. Which of the following would be the initial substance responsible for thyroid hormone regulation?
   a. Iodine intake
   b. Thyrotropin-releasing hormone
   c. Thyroid-stimulating hormone
   d. Levothyroxine

5. A patient is prescribed levothyroxine. The nurse understands that this drug contains which of the following?

   a. T3

   b. Iodine

   c. T4

   d. Vitamin D

6. A patient is receiving propylthiouracil. The nurse anticipates a reduction in the patient's dosage based on assessment of which of the following?

   a. Nervousness

   b. Tachycardia

   c. Weight loss

   d. Decreased appetite

7. A group of students are reviewing hypo- and hypercalcemia. The students demonstrate a need for additional review when they identify which of the following as indicating hypercalcemia?

   a. Lethargy

   b. Tetany

   c. Muscle weakness

   d. Personality changes

8. A patient is prescribed calcitriol. Which instruction would be most important for the nurse to include in the teaching plan?

   a. "Take the drug with a magnesium antacid."

   b. "Limit your intake of dairy products."

   c. "Have your calcium levels check periodically."

   d. "Take the drug with food if gastrointestinal upset occurs."

9. After teaching a group of students about bisphosphonates, the students demonstrate understanding of the information when they identify which drug as an example?

   a. Teriparatide

   b. Calcitonin-salmon

   c. Dihydrotachysterol

   d. Pamidronate

10. A patient is prescribed ibandronate. The nurse instructs the patient to take the drug at which frequency?

    a. Once a week

    b. Once every 2 weeks

    c. Once a month

    d. Once every 3 months

11. While reviewing the medication history of a patient receiving alendronate, the nurse notes that the patient also takes a multivitamin. Which instruction would be most appropriate?

    a. "Stop taking the multivitamin at once."

    b. "Take the multivitamin just before the alendronate."

    c. "Take the alendronate with an antacid before the multivitamin."

    d. "Separate taking the two drugs by about a half hour."

12. A patient is prescribed calcitonin. The nurse would teach the patient to administer the drug by which route?

    a. Oral

    b. Subcutaneous

    c. Sublingual

    d. Topical

13. Which of the following would lead a nurse to suspect that a patient receiving bisphosphonate therapy is experiencing hypercalcemia?

    a. Lethargy

    b. Paresthesias

    c. Muscle cramps

    d. Carpopedal spasms

14. A patient who is receiving a strong iodide solution, potassium iodide, develops iodism. Which of the following would the nurse expect to find?

    a. Sweet taste in the mouth
    b. Constipation
    c. Sore teeth
    d. Rash

15. A patient is to receive teriparatide. The nurse would instruct the patient in which of the following?

    a. Oral administration
    b. Subcutaneous injection
    c. Intranasal spray administration
    d. Transdermal application

Agents to Control Blood Glucose Levels

LEARNING OBJECTIVES

Upon completion of this chapter, you will be able to:

1. Describe the pathophysiology of diabetes mellitus, including alterations in metabolic pathways and changes to basement membranes.

2. Describe the therapeutic actions, indications, pharmacokinetics, contraindications, most common adverse reactions, and important drug–drug interactions associated with insulin and other antidiabetic and glucose-elevating agents.

3. Discuss the use of antidiabetic and glucose-elevating agents across the lifespan.

4. Compare and contrast the prototype drugs insulin, chlorpropamide, glyburide, and metformin with other antidiabetic agents in their class.

5. Outline the nursing considerations, including important teaching points, for patients receiving an antidiabetic or glucose-elevating agent.

■ ASSESSING YOUR UNDERSTANDING

MATCHING

Select the description from column 2 that best describes the term in column 1.

Column 1

____ 1. Glycosuria

____ 2. Insulin

____ 3. Ketosis

____ 4. Polyphagia

____ 5. Polydipsia

____ 6. Adiponectin

____ 7. Glycogen

____ 8. Incretins

Column 2

a. Increased thirst

b. Breakdown of fats for energy

c. Glucose in the urine

d. Hormone that increases insulin sensitivity

e. Peptides produced in the gastrointestinal (GI) tract

f. Hormone of the pancreatic beta cells

g. Increased hunger

h. Storage form of glucose

SHORT ANSWER

Supply the information requested.

1. Explain the role of the pancreas as an endocrine and exocrine gland.

2. Describe the action of glucagonlike polypeptide-1.

3. List four disorders that may occur as a result of diabetes.

4. Identify the test that is used to evaluate overall blood glucose level control.

5. Name the condition in which the pancreatic beta cells are no longer functioning.

6. List three manifestations of hyperglycemia.

■ APPLYING YOUR KNOWLEDGE

CASE STUDY

A 12-year-old boy is newly diagnosed with diabetes. The child is to receive insulin twice a day via subcutaneous injection. The patient also is actively involved in soccer and swimming, competing competitively and practicing four to five times a week. The parents and child are concerned about how the diabetes will affect his ability to participate in these activities.

a. How might the nurse address the child and parents' concerns related to sports?

b. What other issues might occur based on the child's developmental stage?

■ PRACTICING FOR NCLEX

Circle the letter that corresponds to the best answer for each question.

1. Which of the following would a nurse identify as an example of a sulfonylurea?
   a. Glyburide
   b. Metformin
   c. Acarbose
   d. Miglitol

2. Which agent would a nurse expect to administer as a single oral dose in the morning?
   a. Repaglinide
   b. Rosiglitazone
   c. Exenatide
   d. Miglitol

3. Which of the following would alert the nurse to suspect that a patient is developing ketoacidosis?
   a. Fluid retention
   b. Blurred vision
   c. Hunger
   d. Fruity breath odor

4. After teaching a group of students about the various insulin preparations, the instructor determines that the teaching was successful when the students identify that which type of insulin cannot be mixed with other types?
   a. Regular
   b. Lente
   c. Detemir
   d. Lispro

5. A patient receives regular insulin at 8:00 AM. The nurse would be alert for signs and symptoms of hypoglycemia at which time?

   a. Between 10:00 AM and 12:00 PM

   b. Between 8:30 AM and 9:30 AM

   c. Between 2:00 PM and 4:00 PM

   d. Between 12:00 PM and 8:00 PM

6. Which of the following would be least appropriate when administering insulin by subcutaneous injection?

   a. Using a 25 gauge ^{1}Ú$_2$ -inch needle

   b. Inserting the needle at a 45-degree angle

   c. Injecting the insulin slowly

   d. Massaging the site after removing the needle

7. A nurse is preparing a syringe that contains regular and NPH insulin. To ensure effectiveness, the nurse would administer the insulins within which time frame?

   a. 10 minutes

   b. 15 minutes

   c. 30 minutes

   d. 60 minutes

8. A patient is receiving glipizide as treatment for his type 2 diabetes. The nurse understands that this drug acts by which of the following?

   a. Binding to potassium channels on pancreatic beta cells

   b. Inhibiting alpha-glucosidase to delay glucose absorption

   c. Increasing the uptake of glucose

   d. Decreasing insulin resistance

9. A patient is taking metformin as part of his treatment for diabetes. The nurse would warn the patient that he may experience signs and symptoms of hypoglycemia within approximately which time frame?

   a. 1 hour

   b. 2 hours

   c. 3 hours

   d. 4 hours

10. A patient newly diagnosed with type 1 diabetes asks the nurse why he cannot just take a pill. The nurse would incorporate knowledge of which of the following when responding to this patient?

    a. Insulin is needed because the beta cells of the pancreas are no longer functioning.

    b. The insulin is more effective in establishing control of blood glucose levels initially.

    c. More insulin is needed than that which the patient can produce naturally.

    d. The patient most likely does not exercise enough to control his glucose levels.

11. When describing the effects of incretins on blood glucose control to a group of students, which of the following would an instructor include?

    a. Increases glucagon release

    b. Increases GI emptying

    c. Increases insulin release

    d. Increases protein building

12. A nurse is preparing an in-service presentation for a group of staff members on diabetes. Which of the following would the nurse include as the primary delivery system for insulin?

    a. Jet injector

    b. Insulin pen

    c. External pump

    d. Subcutaneous injection

13. A man is brought to the emergency department. He is nonresponsive, and his blood glucose level is 32 mg/dL. Which of the following would the nurse expect to be ordered?

    a. Insulin lispro

    b. Glucagon

    c. Diazoxide

    d. Regular insulin

14. When reviewing sites for insulin administration with a patient, which site, if stated by the patient as an appropriate site, indicates the need for additional teaching?

   a. Upper arm

   b. Abdomen

   c. Buttocks

   d. Upper thigh

15. The nurse is instructing a patient how to take his prescribed pramlintide. Which of the following would be most appropriate?

   a. "Give it by subcutaneous injection immediately before your major meals."

   b. "Take the drug orally once a day, preferably in the morning."

   c. "Give yourself an injection 1 hour before you eat breakfast and dinner."

   d. "Take the drug orally with the first bite of each meal."

CHAPTER 39

Introduction to the Reproductive System

LEARNING OBJECTIVES

Upon completion of this chapter, you will be able to:

1. Label a diagram depicting the structures of the female ovaries and male testes as part of the reproductive systems and explain the function of each structure.

2. Outline the control mechanisms involved with the male and female reproductive systems, using this outline to explain the negative feedback systems involved with each system.

3. List five effects for each of these sex hormones: Estrogen, progesterone, and testosterone.

4. Describe the changes that occur to the female body during pregnancy.

5. Describe the phases of the human sexual response and briefly describe the clinical presentation of each stage.

■ ASSESSING YOUR UNDERSTANDING

LABELING

Place the name of the structure at the appropriate location on the illustration below.

Bladder
Fallopian tube
Labia
Ovary
Uterus
Vagina
Rectum

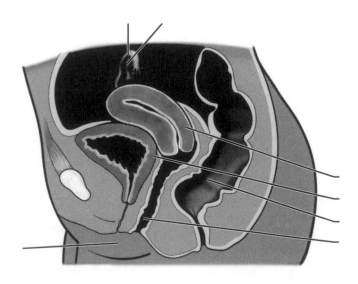

LABELING

Place the name of the structure at the appropriate location on the illustration below.

Corpus cavernosum

Corpus spongiosum

Epididymis

Glans penis

Prostate

Pubic symphysis

Rectum

Scrotum

Seminal vesicle

Testis

Ureter

Urethra

Urinary bladder

Vas deferens

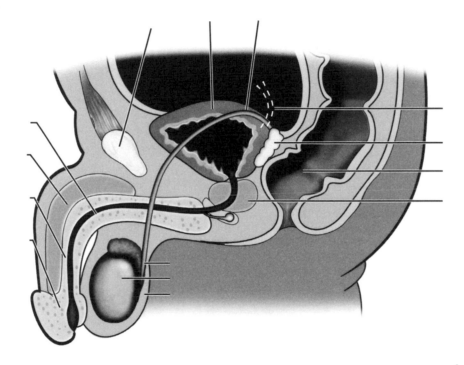

■ APPLYING YOUR KNOWLEDGE

CASE STUDY

A nurse has been invited to teach a health class to a group of freshmen girls at a local high school on the topic of female reproduction. The girls are between the ages of 13 and 14 years.

a. What topics would be most important for the nurse to address?

b. How might the age of the girls in the class influence the nurse's methods for teaching?

■ PRACTICING FOR NCLEX

Circle the letter that corresponds to the best answer for each question.

1. Which hormone would be initially responsible for hormone secretion from the ovaries and testes?
   a. Follicle-stimulating hormone
   b. Luteinizing hormone
   c. Gonadotropin-releasing hormone
   d. Interstitial cell-stimulating hormone

2. Which of the following statements about the female reproductive system structures is most accurate?
   a. A female produces ova continuously, starting from the time of birth.
   b. An ovum contains one-half of the genetic material to produce a whole cell.
   c. The fallopian tube is a muscular tube connected directly to the ovary.
   d. The uterus is responsible for producing estrogen and progesterone.

3. Which hormone is involved if a couple engages in the rhythm method of birth control?
   a. Estradiol
   b. Estrone
   c. Estriol
   d. Progesterone

4. Which of the following would a nurse attribute to estrogen?
   a. Breast growth
   b. Thickened cervical mucus
   c. Increased body temperature
   d. Increased appetite

5. After teaching a group of students about female reproductive hormones, the instructor determines that the teaching was successful when the students identify which hormone as being primarily responsible for maintaining pregnancy?
   a. Estrogen
   b. Progesterone
   c. Follicle-stimulating hormone
   d. Luteinizing hormone

6. Which hormone is responsible for ovulation?
   a. Estrogen
   b. Progesterone
   c. Follicle-stimulating hormone
   d. Luteinizing hormone

7. If an ovum is fertilized and implants into the uterine wall, which of the following would occur next?
   a. Development of the placenta
   b. Increasing production of estrogen
   c. Production of human chorionic gonadotropin
   d. Formation of corpus albicans

8. Which of the following is associated with an increase in gonadotropin-releasing hormone secretion?
   a. Stress
   b. Starvation
   c. Extreme exercise
   d. Increased light exposure

9. A group of students are reviewing information about the menstrual cycle. The students demonstrate understanding when they identify which of the following as the onset of the menstrual cycle?
   a. Puberty
   b. Menarche
   c. Andropause
   d. Menopause

10. A patient complains of menstrual cramps. The nurse understands that this is due to which of the following?
    a. High levels of plasminogen
    b. Lowered estrogen levels
    c. Prostaglandins
    d. Follicle-stimulating hormone

11. During pregnancy, which of the following becomes a massive endocrine gland?
    a. Umbilical cord
    b. Placenta
    c. Embryo
    d. Uterus

12. Which structure is responsible for producing sperm?
    a. Seminiferous tubules
    b. Leydig cells
    c. Vas deferens
    d. Prostate gland

13. Which of the following would a nurse attribute to the effect of testosterone? Select all that apply.
    a. Increased high-density lipoprotein levels
    b. Vocal cord thickening
    c. Increased hematocrit
    d. Facial hair growth
    e. Increased skin elasticity

14. When describing the human sexual response cycle, which of the following would a nurse include as occurring first?
    a. Recovery
    b. Climax
    c. Stimulation
    d. Plateau

15. Which of the following occurs during andropause?
    a. Atrophy of the seminiferous tubules
    b. Development of the interstitial cells
    c. Decreased release of follicle-stimulating hormone
    d. Increased inhibin levels

CHAPTER 40

Drugs Affecting the Female Reproductive System

LEARNING OBJECTIVES

Upon completion of this chapter, you will be able to:

1. Integrate knowledge of the effects of sex hormones on the female body to explain the therapeutic and adverse effects of these agents when used clinically.

2. Describe the therapeutic actions, indications, pharmacokinetics, contraindications, most common adverse reactions, and important drug–drug interactions associated with drugs that affect the female reproductive system.

3. Discuss the use of drugs that affect the female reproductive system across the lifespan.

4. Compare and contrast the prototype drugs estradiol, raloxifene, norethindrone, clomiphene, oxytocin, and dinoprostone with other agents in their class.

5. Outline the nursing considerations, including important teaching points to stress, for patients receiving drugs that affect the female reproductive system.

■ ASSESSING YOUR UNDERSTANDING

FILL IN THE BLANKS

Provide the missing term in the blanks provided.

1. Female sex hormones include estrogens and

   _____.

2. Drugs such as norethindrone acetate transform the proliferative endometrium

   into a _____ endometrium.

3. The combination of estrogens with

   _____ increases the risk for development of thrombi and emboli.

4. Two estrogen receptor modulators are

   _____ and toremifene.

5. The prototype fertility agent is _____.

6. _____ are a group of drugs that stimulate uterine contraction.

SHORT ANSWER

Supply the information requested.

1. Explain the two major indications for using female sex hormones.

2. Describe the characteristics of a woman who may be a candidate for the use of fertility drugs.

3. Name the drug that may be used to stimulate spermatogenesis in a male.

4. Describe the effect that may occur if a woman with ovarian cysts uses fertility drugs.

5. Identify the uterine motility agent that can be used intranasally to stimulate the letdown reflex in a lactating woman.

■ APPLYING YOUR KNOWLEDGE

CASE STUDY

A 45-year-old woman comes to the clinic for an evaluation. The woman is experiencing menopausal symptoms, complaining of extreme moodiness and hot flashes, especially during the nighttime hours and sleep. She is visibly upset about these changes. "Sometimes my hot flashes are so bad that I find myself having to change my pajamas because they get so wet. And sometimes I just feel like I want to burst into tears for no reason. I just don't know what to do. My friend said to try hormone therapy, but I'm afraid. I've heard so many stories about the side effects."

a. How should the nurse respond to this patient?

b. What information would the nurse and patient need to discuss related to the patient's current complaints and concerns?

■ PRACTICING FOR NCLEX

Circle the letter that corresponds to the best answer for each question.

1. A patient is prescribed estradiol in a vaginal ring form. The nurse would instruct the patient to insert a new vaginal ring at which frequency?
   a. Daily
   b. Weekly
   c. Monthly
   d. Every 3 months

2. When reviewing the history of a patient, which of the following would the nurse identify as a contraindication for the use of progestins?
   a. Migraine headaches
   b. Asthma
   c. Pelvic inflammatory disease
   d. Epilepsy

3. A patient is using an oral contraceptive combination that include drospirenone. The nurse would assess the patient for which of the following?
   a. Irritation
   b. Headache
   c. Abdominal pain
   d. Hyperkalemia

4. After teaching a woman who is receiving estrogen hormonal therapy about substances to avoid, the nurse determines that additional teaching is needed when the patient cites which of the following?
   a. St. John's wort
   b. Orange juice
   c. Smoking
   d. Grapefruit juice

5. A postmenopausal woman is receiving raloxifene as part of a treatment plan for osteoporosis. The nurse would instruct the patient that this drug is administered by which route?

   a. Oral
   b. Transdermal
   c. Intravaginal
   d. Intramuscular

6. A group of students are reviewing the various fertility drugs that are available. The students demonstrate understanding when they identify which drug as being administered orally?

   a. Cetrorelix
   b. Follitropin alfa
   c. Clomiphene
   d. Ganirelix

7. Which agent would a nurse expect to be ordered for a patient who experiences preterm labor?

   a. Ergonovine
   b. Oxytocin
   c. Dinoprostone
   d. Terbutaline

8. The nurse monitors a patient receiving oxytocin for water intoxication based on the understanding that this condition is the result of which of the following?

   a. Stimulation of the neuroreceptor sites
   b. Release of antidiuretic hormone
   c. Effects secondary to ergotism
   d. Blockage of estrogen receptor sites

9. A patient is beginning therapy with a combined oral contraceptive. The nurse would instruct the patient to take the first pill on which of the following?

   a. First day of menstrual bleeding
   b. Fifth day of the cycle
   c. Fourteenth day of the usual cycle
   d. First day of the next month

10. A patient who is taking oral contraceptives develops an upper respiratory infection for which a tetracycline is ordered. Which instruction would be most important for the nurse to include?

   a. Taking the tetracycline 2 hours after taking the oral contraceptive

   b. Using an alternative means of contraception while taking the tetracycline
   c. Reducing the oral contraceptive to every other day
   d. Monitoring for increased adverse effects of the oral contraceptive

11. A patient is receiving estrogen therapy. Which of the following would the nurse instruct the patient to report immediately?

   a. Abdominal bloating
   b. Weight gain
   c. Dizziness
   d. Shortness of breath

12. Which of the following would a nurse identify as a gonadotropin-releasing hormone antagonist?

   a. Cetrorelix
   b. Chorionic gonadotropin
   c. Follitropin alfa
   d. Menotropins

13. A patient is to receive lutropin alfa. The nurse would expect to administer this agent by which route?

   a. Oral
   b. Subcutaneous
   c. Intramuscular
   d. Intravaginal

14. A patient is to receive dinoprostone at 4:00 PM. The nurse would expect the patient to begin to experience uterine contractions at which time?

   a. 4:10 PM
   b. 4:15 PM
   c. 6:00 PM
   d. 7:00 PM

15. A patient who has come to the emergency department after being raped is given a dose of emergency contraception at 12 AM. The nurse would instruct the patient to take another dose of the drug at which time?

   a. 4 AM
   b. 6 AM
   c. 10 AM
   d. 12 PM

CHAPTER 41

Drugs Affecting the Male Reproductive System

LEARNING OBJECTIVES

Upon completion of this chapter, you will be able to:

1. Discuss the effects of testosterone and androgens on the male body and use this information to explain the therapeutic and adverse effects of these agents when used clinically.

2. Describe the therapeutic actions, indications, pharmacokinetics, contraindications, most common adverse reactions, and important drug–drug interactions associated with drugs affecting the male reproductive system.

3. Discuss the use of drugs that affect the male reproductive system across the lifespan.

4. Compare and contrast the prototype drugs testosterone, oxandrolone, and sildenafil with other agents in their class.

5. Outline the nursing considerations, including important teaching points, for patients receiving drugs used to affect the male reproductive system.

■ ASSESSING YOUR UNDERSTANDING

FILL IN THE BLANKS

Provide the missing term in the blanks provided.

1. Male sex hormones, or _____, are produced in the testes and adrenal glands.

2. Underdevelopment of the testes in males is called _____.

3. Testosterone is considered class _____ controlled substances.

4. Patients taking testosterone can experience _____ or increased hair distribution.

5. Anabolic steroids are known to be used illegally for the enhancement of _____ performance.

SHORT ANSWER

Supply the information requested.

1. Explain how anabolic steroids work.

2. Identify the hormones that are considered androgens.

3. List three androgenic effects associated with testosterone administration.

4. Describe the action of alprostadil.

5. Name two dietary factors that could affect the action of PDE5 inhibitors.

■ APPLYING YOUR KNOWLEDGE

CASE STUDY

A 55-year-old man comes to the clinic for a routine physical examination. During the examination, the patient mentions that he has noticed a change in his sexual activity ability. He mentions that it has been taking longer to achieve an erection and that the erection does not last as long. He also mentions that he has had several episodes where an erection did not occur. He states, "It's really embarrassing. I guess this is what it means to get old. Maybe I should try that "viva Viagra" stuff like I've seen on TV."

a. How would the nurse respond to the patient?

b. What information would be important for the nurse to gather about the patient's current condition to determine if the medication would be appropriate for this patient?

■ PRACTICING FOR NCLEX

Circle the letter that corresponds to the best answer for each question.

1. A patient is receiving a medication that has androgenic effects. Which of the following would the nurse expect to assess?
   a. Flushing
   b. Sweating
   c. Oily skin
   d. Nervousness

2. After reviewing the various methods for administering testosterone to patient, the nurse indicates a need for additional review when the nurse identifies which route as appropriate?
   a. Depot injection
   b. Transdermal patch
   c. Intramuscular injection
   d. Oral

3. The nurse is reviewing the history of a patient who is to receive testosterone. Which of the following would alert the nurse to the need for close monitoring of the patient?
   a. Prostate cancer
   b. Breast cancer
   c. Cardiovascular disease
   d. Penile implant

4. A patient has been receiving long-term testosterone therapy. The nurse would expect to monitor which of the following?
   a. Renal function studies
   b. Liver function studies
   c. Complete blood count
   d. Coagulation studies

5. A patient is using a transdermal system for androgen administration. Which drug would the patient most likely be using?
   a. Fluoxymesterone
   b. Danazol
   c. Testosterone
   d. Methyltestosterone

6. Which of the following would a nurse expect to occur with the administration of anabolic steroids?
   a. Increased catabolism
   b. Decreased hemoglobin
   c. Reduced tissue building
   d. Increased red blood cell mass

7. A 30-year-old debilitated patient is receiving anabolic steroids. Which of the following might the patient experience?
   a. Breast size reduction
   b. Priapism
   c. Testicular enlargement
   d. Excessive hair growth

8. A patient is receiving androgen therapy. Which of the following would cause the nurse the greatest concern?
   a. Decreased thyroid function
   b. Elevated liver enzyme levels
   c. Increased creatinine level
   d. Increased creatinine clearance

9. When teaching a group of high school students about using anabolic steroids, the nurse would include information that these drugs are classified as which class of controlled substances?
   a. I
   b. II
   c. III
   d. IV

10. A group of students are reviewing the drugs available for treating penile erectile dysfunction. The students demonstrate understanding when they identify which drug as a PDE5 inhibitor?
    a. Alprostadil
    b. Sildenafil
    c. Oxandrolone
    d. Danazol

11. Which agent would a patient most likely be prescribed for penile erectile dysfunction if the patient is very sexually active and the timing of sexual stimulation is not known?
    a. Sildenafil
    b. Tadalafil
    c. Vardenafil
    d. Alprostadil

12. Sildenafil may be used in women to treat which of the following?
    a. Pulmonary hypertension
    b. Sexual dysfunction
    c. Coronary artery disease
    d. Peptic ulcer disease

13. A nurse is reviewing the medication history of a patient. The nurse understands that a PDE5 inhibitor would be inappropriate for a patient taking which of the following?
    a. Ketoconazole
    b. Indinavir
    c. Nitroglycerin
    d. Erythromycin

14. A nurse is instructing a patient about vardenafil. The nurse would instruct the patient to take the drug how many minutes before sexual stimulation?
    a. 15 minutes
    b. 30 minutes
    c. 45 minutes
    d. 60 minutes

15. The nurse would instruct a patient who is using a transdermal system for testosterone administration to apply a new patch at which frequency?
    a. Every 12 hours
    b. Every day
    c. Every 3 days
    d. Every 7 days

CHAPTER 42

Introduction to the Cardiovascular System

LEARNING OBJECTIVES

Upon completion of this chapter, you will be able to:

1. Label a diagram of the heart, including all chambers, valves, great vessels, coronary vessels, and the conduction system.

2. Describe the flow of blood during the cardiac cycle, including flow to the cardiac muscle.

3. Outline the conduction system of the heart, correlating the normal electrocardiogram pattern with the underlying electrical activity in the heart.

4. Discuss four normal controls of blood pressure.

5. Describe the capillary fluid shift, including factors that influence the movement of fluid in clinical situations.

■ ASSESSING YOUR UNDERSTANDING

LABELING

Place the name of the structures listed below in the appropriate location on the illustration.

Aorta
Inferior vena cava
Left atrium
Left ventricle
Mitral valve
Pulmonary arteries
Pulmonary veins
Pulmonic valve
Right atrium
Right ventricle
Superior vena cava
Triscupid valve

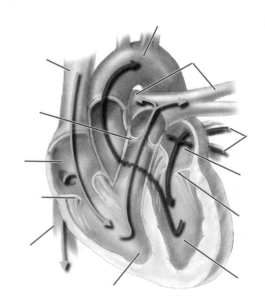

SEQUENCING

Place the number of the statement in the box based on the correct sequence of events for conduction through the heart.

1. Impulse travels via the bundle branches

2. Atrial bundles carry impulses

3. Ventricular cells are stimulated

4. Impulse reaches the atrioventricular (AV) node

5. Purkinje fibers carry the impulse

6. Sinoatrial (SA) node fires

7. Impulse travels via the bundle of His

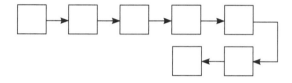

■ APPLYING YOUR KNOWLEDGE

CASE STUDY

It has been several days since a patient with a history of hypertension was admitted to the health care facility with an acute myocardial infarction. The patient has responded well to treatment and will be discharged the next day. The nurse is talking with the patient about his condition, the medications that are being prescribed, and instructions for activity and exercise. "I was taking my blood pressure medicine pretty regularly, but then I forgot to get them refilled. And when I remembered to call, I didn't pick them up right away."

a. How might the patient's history of hypertension have played a role in his myocardial infarction?

b. What would the nurse teach the patient about activity and oxygen consumption?

■ PRACTICING FOR NCLEX

Circle the letter that corresponds to the best answer for each question.

1. When describing Starling's law of the heart, the instructor compares this to which of the following?

   a. Moving up and down on a staircase
   b. Stretching of a rubber band
   c. Pushing and pulling of a rope
   d. Flowing of water through a pipe

2. Which of the following would the nurse explain as the pacemaker of the heart?

   a. SA node
   b. AV node
   c. Bundle of His
   d. Purkinje fibers

3. An instructor is describing the unique characteristic of cells of the conducting system, explaining that these cells can generate action potentials without outside stimulation. The instructor is describing which of the following?

   a. Conductivity
   b. Contractility
   c. Automaticity
   d. Capacitancy

4. Sodium ion concentrations are equal inside and outside the cell during which phase of the action potential of the cardiac muscle?

   a. Phase 0
   b. Phase 1
   c. Phase 2
   d. Phase 3

5. When explaining the contraction of the heart muscle, the instructor describes the basic unit as which of the following?

   a. Actin
   b. Myosin
   c. Troponin
   d. Sarcomere

6. After explaining an electrocardiogram to a patient, which statement indicates that the patient understands this test?

   a. "It will show the chambers of my heart in different views."

   b. "It will measure the amount of blood being pumped."

   c. "It will show how impulses are moving through my heart."

   d. "It will help to identify how my heart is working mechanically."

7. A nurse is reviewing a patient's electrocardiogram. Which of the following would the nurse identify as indicating depolarization of the bundle of His and ventricles?

   a. P wave

   b. QRS complex

   c. T wave

   d. PR interval

8. The nurse is reviewing a patient's electrocardiogram and notes that the P waves are sawtoothed in shape and there are three P waves for every QRS complex. The nurse would interpret this as suggesting which of the following?

   a. Sinus bradycardia

   b. Paroxysmal atrial tachycardia

   c. Atrial fibrillation

   d. Atrial flutter

9. When describing circulation, which of the following would a nurse include?

   a. Low to high pressure system

   b. One course of blood flow

   c. A closed system

   d. Primarily a resistance system

10. Fluid moves into the arterial end of a capillary due to which of the following?

    a. Hydrostatic pressure

    b. Fluid needs of the cells

    c. Oncotic pressure

    d. Loose endothelial cells

11. Which area of the heart is supplied by the right coronary artery?

    a. Left ventricle

    b. Right side of the heart

    c. Cardiac septum

    d. Conduction system

12. Which of the following is released initially when blood flow to the kidneys is decreased?

    a. Renin

    b. Angiotensin I

    c. Angiotensin II

    d. Aldosterone

13. Blood returning to the heart arrives at the right ventricle by way of which of the following?

    a. Aorta

    b. Pulmonary vein

    c. Vena cava

    d. Triscupid valve

14. Which of the following is responsible for transmitting the nerve impulse to the ventricular cells?

    a. AV node

    b. Bundle of His

    c. Bundle branches

    d. Purkinje fibers

15. At which area is the conduction velocity the slowest?

    a. Bundle of His

    b. AV node

    c. Purkinje fibers

    d. Bundle branches

Drugs Affecting Blood Pressure

LEARNING OBJECTIVES

Upon completion of this chapter, you will be able to:

1. Outline the normal controls of blood pressure and explain how the various drugs used to treat hypertension or hypotension affect these controls.

2. Describe the therapeutic actions, indications, pharmacokinetics, contraindications, most common adverse reactions, and important drug–drug interactions associated with drugs affecting blood pressure.

3. Discuss the use of drugs that affect blood pressure across the lifespan.

4. Compare and contrast the prototype drugs captopril, losartan, diltiazem, nitroprusside, and midodrine with other agents in their class and with other agents used to affect blood pressure.

5. Outline the nursing considerations, including important teaching points, for patients receiving drugs used to affect blood pressure.

■ ASSESSING YOUR UNDERSTANDING

LABELING

Place the name of the following drugs in the correct box for the drug class.

Captopril   Losartan

Diltiazem   Quinapril

Enalaprilat   Valsartan

Felodipine   Verapamil

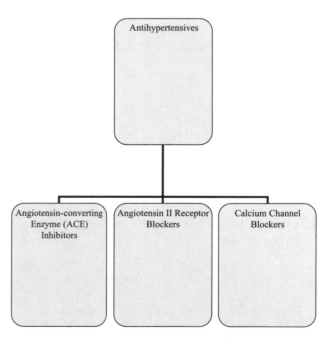

MATCHING

Match the blood pressure drug category with its prototype.

____ **1.** Angiotensin-Converting-Enzyme (ACE) Inhibitor

____ **2.** Angiotensin II-Receptor Blocker

____ **3.** Calcium Channel Blocker

____ **4.** Vasodilator

____ **5.** Alpha-Specific Adrenergic Agent

a. losartan (Cozaar)

b. nitroprusside (Nitropress)

c. midodrine (ProAmatine)

d. captopril (Capoten)

e. diltiazem (Cardizem)

SHORT ANSWER

Supply the information requested.

1. Identify the three elements that determine pressure in the cardiovascular system.

2. Name the two areas where baroreceptors are located.

3. Describe two dangers associated with hypertension.

4. List four factors that are known to increase blood pressure.

5. Explain the focus of treatment for hypertension.

6. Identify the drugs of choice for treating stage 1 hypertension in a patient who does not have any complicating conditions.

7. Describe the lifestyle modifications that are indicated as part of step 1 treatment for hypertension.

■ APPLYING YOUR KNOWLEDGE

CASE STUDY

A 58-year-old man has been diagnosed with hypertension and has been receiving carvedilol. The patient also has a history of left ventricular hypertrophy. The patient's blood pressure on the last few visits has remained somewhat elevated. The physician has decided to add quinapril to the patient's regimen. The nurse is talking with the patient about his drug therapy when the patient states, "It always seems that my pressure is much higher when I come here. I started checking my blood pressure at the local drug store, and it is usually lower than the readings here."

a. How might the nurse interpret the patient's statement? What would the nurse need to consider when responding to the patient?

b. What would the nurse need to address when teaching the patient about the new drug?

■ PRACTICING FOR NCLEX

Circle the letter that corresponds to the best answer for each question.

1. When describing the pressures in the cardiovascular system, the nurse would identify which of the following as the area of highest pressure?

a. Right atrium

b. Right ventricle

c. Left atrium

d. Left ventricle

2. Which of the following would be considered the most important factor in determining peripheral resistance?
   a. Arterioles
   b. Capillaries
   c. Arteries
   d. Veins

3. Which of the following functions continually maintain blood pressure within a predetermined range of normal?
   a. Cardiovascular center
   b. Medulla
   c. Baroreceptors
   d. Carotid arteries

4. A patient develops a severe elevation in blood pressure. The physician orders an ACE inhibitor to be given intravenously. Which agent would be most likely?
   a. Captopril
   b. Enalapril
   c. Lisinopril
   d. Enalaprilat

5. A patient receiving an ACE inhibitor reports a problem with coughing. The nurse would ask the patient if he is receiving which of the following?
   a. Ramipril
   b. Benazepril
   c. Lisinopril
   d. Quinapril

6. A patient is receiving captopril. Which of the following would be most important for the nurse to monitor?
   a. Electrocardiogram
   b. Nutritional status
   c. Complete blood count
   d. Liver function studies

7. A group of students are reviewing the various antihypertensive agents. The students demonstrate understanding of the information when they identify which of the following as an example of an angiotensin II receptor blocker?
   a. Moexipril
   b. Losartan
   c. Minoxidil
   d. Amlodipine

8. When describing the action of calcium channel blockers, which of the following would be an expected effect?
   a. Increased contractility
   b. Arterial contraction
   c. Increased venous return
   d. Slowed impulse formation

9. The nurse is teaching a patient how to take his diltiazem. Which instruction would be most appropriate?
   a. "Cut the tablet in half to make it easier to swallow."
   b. "Mix the crushed tablet with applesauce to improve the taste."
   c. "Swallow the drug whole with a large glass of water."
   d. "Chew the tablet thoroughly before swallowing."

10. A patient who has been receiving verapamil for several months comes to the clinic reporting significant dizziness, lightheadedness, and fatigue. He also reports frequent episodes of nausea and swelling of his ankles. Drug toxicity is suspected. Which question would be critical to ask the patient?
    a. "Are you taking any over-the-counter pain relievers like ibuprofen?"
    b. "Have you been drinking any grapefruit juice lately?"
    c. "Are your splitting or crushing your pills?"
    d. "When did you take the last dose of the drug?"

11. A patient is receiving nitroprusside. The nurse suspects that the patient is experiencing cyanide toxicity based on assessment of which of the following?

    a. Increased hair growth

    b. Absent reflexes

    c. Pupil constriction

    d. Chest pain

12. Which of the following agents would be used to treat hypertension by blocking the post-synaptic alpha-1 receptor sites?

    a. Prazosin

    b. Labetalol

    c. Guanabenz

    d. Nadolol

13. A patient is experiencing orthostatic hypotension that is affecting his ability to function. Which of the following medications would be most appropriate?

    a. Dopamine

    b. Methyldopa

    c. Midodrine

    d. Clonidine

14. A patient is receiving a diuretic as the first-line treatment of mild hypertension. The nurse monitors the patient for signs and symptoms of hypokalemia with which agent?

    a. Amiloride

    b. Spironolactone

    c. Triamterene

    d. Hydrochlorothiazide

15. A group of students are reviewing the various antihypertensive agents available. The students demonstrate understanding of the information when they identify which agent as an example of a renin inhibitor?

    a. Mecamylamine

    b. Aliskiren

    c. Candesartan

    d. Captopril

CHAPTER 44

Cardiotonic Agents

LEARNING OBJECTIVES

Upon completion of this chapter, you will be able to:

1. Describe the pathophysiologic process of heart failure and the resultant clinical signs.

2. Explain the body's compensatory mechanisms that occur in response to heart failure.

3. Describe the therapeutic actions, indications, pharmacokinetics, contraindications and cautions, most common adverse reactions, and important drug–drug interactions associated with the cardiotonic agents.

4. Discuss the use of cardiotonic agents across the lifespan.

5. Compare and contrast the prototype drugs digoxin and inamrinone and digoxin immune Fab.

6. Outline the nursing considerations, including important teaching points, for patients receiving cardiotonic agents.

■ ASSESSING YOUR UNDERSTANDING

MATCHING

Select the description from column 2 that best describes the term in column 1.

Column 1

____ 1. Cardiomegaly

____ 2. Heart failure

____ 3. Dyspnea

____ 4. Cardiomyopathy

____ 5. Hemoptysis

____ 6. Nocturia

____ 7. Orthopnea

____ 8. Positive inotropic

Column 2

a. Getting up to void at night

b. Effect resulting in an increased contraction force

c. Enlargement of the heart

d. Discomfort with respirations

e. Disease of the heart muscle

f. Inability of the heart to pump adequately

g. Blood-tinged sputum

h. Difficulty breathing when lying down

FILL IN THE BLANKS

Provide the missing term or terms in the blanks provided.

1. _____ drugs are used to increase the contractility of the heart muscle in patients experiencing heart failure.

2. Severe heart failure causing the left ventricle to pump inefficiently can lead to

   _____ _____ manifested by rales and wheezes.

3. In heart failure, the heart rate

   will be _____ secondary to sympathetic stimulation.

4. In left-sided heart failure, rales indicate the presence of _____ in the lung tissue.

5. In right-sided heart failure, venous return to the heart is _____ because the pressure on the right side of the heart is increased.

6. Increased _____ venous pressure is manifested by distended neck veins.

7. With right-sided heart failure, increased blood flow to the kidneys can lead to increased urination and _____.

8. Cardiotonic drugs are also called

   _____ drugs.

■ APPLYING YOUR KNOWLEDGE

CASE STUDY

A patient has a history of atrial fibrillation for which he takes amiodarone and hypertension for which he takes a thiazide diuretic. The patient comes to the office for a checkup. During the visit, the nurse notes that the patient has slight pitting edema of both lower extremities and jugular vein distention. The patient is tachypneic. Auscultation reveals rales and a third heart sound. The patient states, "Over the last week, I've noticed that I've had to sleep with two pillows instead of one. And I've been getting up at night to urinate." The physician decides to order digoxin 0.125 mg daily for the patient.

a. Based on the patient's assessment findings, what type of heart failure would this patient be experiencing?

b. What information would be crucial for the nurse to cover when teaching the patient about the newly prescribed drug?

■ PRACTICING FOR NCLEX

Circle the letter that corresponds to the best answer for each question.

1. A nurse suspects that a patient is experiencing left-sided heart failure. Which of the following would the nurse assess? Select all that apply.
   a. Tachypnea
   b. Hemoptysis
   c. Peripheral edema
   d. Hepatomegaly
   e. Orthopnea
   f. Polyuria

2. When describing how vasodilators help alleviate heart failure, which of the following would the nurse include?
   a. Increase cardiac workload
   b. Decrease afterload
   c. Increase preload
   d. Decrease blood volume

3. Which of the following would be considered a therapeutic effect of digoxin?
   a. Decreased cardiac output
   b. Increased heart rate
   c. Increased force of contraction
   d. Decreased renal perfusion

4. Which serum digoxin level would the nurse interpret as indicating digoxin toxicity?
   a. 0.6 ng/mL
   b. 1.4 ng/mL
   c. 1.8 ng/mL
   d. 2.3 ng/mL

5. A nurse is administering digoxin intravenously as ordered. The nurse would administer the drug over which time frame?
   a. 2 minutes
   b. 3 minutes
   c. 4 minutes
   d. 5 minutes

6. A patient who is prescribed digoxin asks the nurse how he should take the drug. Which instruction would be most appropriate?

   a. "Take the medicine with an antacid at any time of the day."

   b. "Take the drug after eating your breakfast."

   c. "Eat a small snack just before taking the drug."

   d. "Take the drug on an empty stomach at the same time each day."

7. A patient takes his pulse rate before taking his regular daily dose of digoxin and finds his pulse to be 52 beats/min. Which of the following would the patient do next?

   a. Take the drug as ordered and note the pulse rate in a log

   b. Hold the dose and retake the pulse in 1 hour

   c. Withhold the drug and call the doctor immediately

   d. Go the nearest emergency care facility for evaluation

8. A nurse is preparing to administer inamrinone. The nurse would administer this drug most likely by which route?

   a. Oral

   b. Subcutaneous

   c. Intramuscular

   d. Intravenous

9. A patient is receiving inamrinone. Which of the following would be most important for the nurse to monitor?

   a. Pulmonary function studies

   b. Platelet count

   c. White blood cell count

   d. Renal function studies

10. A patient received an intravenous bolus of inamrinone. The nurse would anticipate repeating the dose at which time if needed?

    a. 10 minutes

    b. 20 minutes

    c. 30 minutes

    d. 40 minutes

11. After teaching a class of students about heart failure and drug therapy, the instructor determines that the teaching has been successful when the students identify which drug as most often used as treatment?

    a. Digoxin

    b. Human B-type natriuretic peptide

    c. Nitrate

    d. Furosemide

12. Which of the following conditions would least likely contribute to the development of heart failure?

    a. Coronary artery disease

    b. Renal failure

    c. Valvular disease

    d. Hypertension

13. A patient who is taking digoxin would withhold the drug if his pulse rate were which of the following?

    a. 78 beats/minute

    b. 70 beats/minute

    c. 64 beats/minute

    d. 56 beats/minute

14. Which of the following would the nurse identify as a cardiac glycoside?

    a. Inamrinone

    b. Milrinone

    c. Digoxin

    d. Captopril

15. Which of the following would a nurse expect to assess if a patient is experiencing right-sided heart failure?

    a. Wheezing

    b. Peripheral edema

    c. Hemoptysis

    d. Dyspnea

CHAPTER 45

Antiarrhythmic Agents

LEARNING OBJECTIVES

Upon completion of this chapter, you will be able to:

1. Describe the cardiac action potential and its phases to explain the changes made by each class of antiarrhythmic agent.
2. Describe the therapeutic actions, indications, pharmacokinetics, contraindications and cautions, most common adverse reactions, and important drug–drug interactions associated with antiarrhythmic agents.
3. Discuss the use of antiarrhythmic agents across the lifespan.
4. Compare and contrast the prototype antiarrhythmic drugs lidocaine, propranolol, sotalol, and diltiazem with other agents in their class and with other classes of antiarrhythmics.
5. Outline the nursing considerations, including important teaching points, for patients receiving antiarrhythmic agents.

■ ASSESSING YOUR UNDERSTANDING

LABELING

Place the name of the drugs listed below in the proper column identifying the antiarrhythmic class.

Acebutolol
Amiodarone
Diltiazem
Disopyramide
Flecainide
Lidocaine
Mexiletine
Propafenone
Propranolol
Quinidine
Sotalol
Verapamil

Class I	Class II	Class III	Class IV

SEQUENCING

Each of the following statements describes an event in the phases of the action potential of the cardiac muscle cell. Place the number of the statement in the box based on the order in which the events occur.

1. Cell comes to rest; restoration of the resting membrane potential

2. Cells becomes stimulated and sodium gates open, allowing sodium to rush into the cell

3. Rapid repolarization occurs with sodium gates closing and potassium flowing out of the cell

4. Sodium ion concentration equalizes inside and outside the cell

5. Plateau stage with the cell membrane becoming less permeable to sodium and calcium slowly entering and potassium beginning to leave the cell

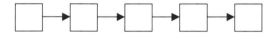

■ APPLYING YOUR KNOWLEDGE

CASE STUDY

A patient goes to see his primary care provider because he has been "feeling strange" lately. He is complaining of fatigue and lack of energy for about the past 2 weeks. "It seems like all I do is sleep. At first, I thought I had the flu or had just overdone things. But I should be rested with all the sleep I've had." Examination reveals an irregular pulse. An electrocardiogram reveals atrial fibrillation. The patient is sent to the emergency department of the local hospital for admission. Intravenous heparin is started, and sotalol is ordered. After 3 days, the sotalol is discontinued due to lack of effectiveness, and the patient is started on amiodarone. Warfarin therapy and heparin are discontinued once the patient has achieved the desired level of anticoagulation. The patient remains in atrial fibrillation and is discharged home on amiodarone and warfarin.

a. What would be the most likely reason for the use of warfarin and heparin for this patient?

b. What monitoring would be essential for this patient?

■ PRACTICING FOR NCLEX

Circle the letter that corresponds to the best answer for each question.

1. When describing the action of antiarrhythmics, which effect would most likely be included?

   a. Reduction of peripheral resistance

   b. Enhancement of automaticity

   c. Alteration in conductivity

   d. Reduction in cardiac output

2. Which arrhythmia would the nurse identify as being related to an alteration in conduction through the heart muscle?

   a. Premature atrial contraction

   b. Atrial flutter

   c. Ventricular fibrillation

   d. Heart block

3. Which of the following agents would be classified as a class Ia antiarrhythmic?

   a. Lidocaine

   b. Procainamide

   c. Mexiletine

   d. Flecainide

4. Which phase of the cardiac muscle action potential is affected by class I antiarrhythmics?

   a. Phase 0

   b. Phase 1

   c. Phase 2

   d. Phase 3

5. A patient is prescribed disopyramide. The nurse would expect to administer this drug by which route?

   a. Oral

   b. Intramuscular

   c. Subcutaneous

   d. Intravenous

6. The health care provider orders quinidine for a patient who is receiving digoxin. The nurse would monitor this patient for which of the following?

   a. Increased quinidine effect

   b. Digoxin toxicity

   c. Bleeding

   d. Renal dysfunction

7. The nurse is teaching a patient who is receiving quinidine about foods to avoid. The patient demonstrates the need for additional teaching when he identifies the need to avoid which of the following?

   a. Citrus juices

   b. Antacids

   c. Milk

   d. Apple juice

8. A patient receives lidocaine by intramuscular injection. The nurse would expect the drug to begin to exert its therapeutic effects within which time frame?

   a. 5 to 10 minutes

   b. 10 to 20 minutes

   c. 20 to 30 minutes

   d. 30 to 40 minutes

9. When describing the action of class II antiarrhythmics, which of the following would the nurse include?

   a. Membrane stabilization with depression of phase 0 action potential

   b. Blockage of beta receptors in the heart and kidneys

   c. Blockage of potassium channels during phase 3 action potential

   d. Interference with calcium ion movement across the membrane

10. A patient is to receive esmolol. The nurse would expect to administer this agent by which route?

    a. Oral

    b. Intramuscular

    c. Intravenous

    d. Subcutaneous

11. Which of the following would be a contraindication for the use of a class II antiarrhythmic?

    a. Sinus bradycardia

    b. Diabetes

    c. Thyroid dysfunction

    d. Hepatic dysfunction

12. The nurse would instruct a patient receiving acebutolol about which of the following adverse effects?

    a. Hypertension

    b. Increased libido

    c. Improved exercise tolerance

    d. Bronchospasm

13. When describing the action of dofetilide, the nurse understands that the drug affects which phase of the action potential?

    a. Phase 0

    b. Phase 1

    c. Phase 2

    d. Phase 3

14. A patient is prescribed sotalol. Which instruction would be most important?

    a. "Sit up for at least 30 minutes after taking the drug."

    b. "Be sure to take the drug on an empty stomach."

    c. "Try using an antacid along with this drug."

    d. "Hold the drug if your pulse rate is less than 60 beats per minute."

15. A patient is receiving adenosine for treatment of supraventricular tachycardia. The nurse understands that this drug results in which of the following?

    a. Increased conduction through the atrioventricular node

    b. Prolonged refractory period

    c. Increased automaticity in the atrioventricular node

    d. Slowed release of calcium leaving the cell

Antianginal Agents

■ASSESSING YOUR UNDERSTANDING

MATCHING

Select the description from column 2 that best describes the term in column 1.

Column 1

___ **1.** Atheroma

___ **2.** Atherosclerosis

___ **3.** Angina pectoris

___ **4.** Prinzmetal's angina

___ **5.** Myocardial infarction

___ **6.** Stable angina

___ **7.** Coronary artery disease

___ **8.** Unstable angina

Column 2

a. Episode of myocardial ischemia with pain due to an imbalance of myocardial oxygen supply and demand when a person is at rest

b. Drop in blood flow through coronary arteries due to vasospasm

c. Disorder involving progressive narrowing of arteries supplying the myocardium

d. Suffocation of the chest

e. Narrowing of the arteries resulting in a loss of elasticity

f. Pain due to imbalance of myocardial oxygen supply and demand that is relieved by rest

g. Plaque in the endothelial lining of the arteries

h. End result of vessel blockage leading to ischemia and then necrosis

SHORT ANSWER

Supply the information requested.

1. Identify the leading cause of death in the Western world.

2. Explain the difference in how the heart muscle receives its blood supply when compared with other tissues.

3. Describe what happens when a person with atherosclerosis experiences an increased demand on the heart.

4. List two ways that antianginal agents work to improve blood delivery to the heart.

5. Describe the action of nitrates.

■ APPLYING YOUR KNOWLEDGE

CASE STUDY

A patient comes to the clinic for an evaluation. The patient has a history of stable angina for which he has used nitroglycerin sublingually. The patient tells the nurse that he has not had any complaints of chest pain for the past 6 months or so. As the nurse is reviewing the patient's medications, the patient removes a small plastic bag from his back pants pocket that contains his nitroglycerin. He says, "See, I still have all the pills. I haven't used any for quite a while."

a. What problem would the nurse need to address with the patient?

b. What actions by the nurse would be appropriate?

■ PRACTICING FOR NCLEX

Circle the letter that corresponds to the best answer for each question.

1. When describing angina to a group of patients, which of the following would be most accurate?
   a. Pain due to lack of oxygen in the heart muscle
   b. Chest pain that occurs with exercise
   c. Damage to the heart muscle
   d. Spasm of the blood vessels

2. A patient experiences pain in the chest that radiates to the jaw, occurring when the patient is at rest. The nurse would interpret this as which of the following?
   a. Stable angina
   b. Unstable angina
   c. Prinzmetal's angina
   d. Myocardial infarction

3. When describing the effects of a myocardial infarction, the nurse understands that the majority of deaths related to this condition result from which of the following?
   a. Shock
   b. Arrhythmias
   c. Heart failure
   d. Stroke

4. Which of the following would a nurse identify as a nitrate?
   a. Metoprolol
   b. Amlodipine
   c. Nicardipine
   d. Isosorbide

5. A group of students are reviewing information about isosorbide dinitrate. The students demonstrate the need for additional study when they identify that this drug is available in which form?
   a. Oral
   b. Sublingual
   c. Intravenous
   d. Chewable tablet

6. Which of the following would contraindicate the use of nitrates?
   a. Cardiac tamponade
   b. Hypotension
   c. Cerebral hemorrhage
   d. Hepatic disease

7. A patient is using nitroglycerin in sublingual spray form. The nurse would inform the patient that the drug would begin working within which time frame?
   a. 1 minute
   b. 2 minutes
   c. 3 minutes
   d. 4 minutes

8. Which of the following indicates that a patient understands how to use sublingual nitroglycerin?
   a. "I should feel a fizzing or burning sensation."
   b. "I should put the pill between my tongue and cheek."
   c. "I need to avoid taking any sips of water before using the drug."
   d. "I can chew the tablet once it starts dissolving."

9. The nurse instructs the patient that he can repeat the dose of nitroglycerin every 5 minutes up to a maximum total of how many doses?
   a. Two
   b. Three
   c. Four
   d. Five

10. Which of the following drugs should be avoided by a patient taking nitrates?
    a. Phosphodiesterase 5 inhibitors
    b. Beta-blockers
    c. Nonsteroidal anti-inflammatory drugs
    d. Cardiac glycosides

11. After teaching a group of students about drugs used as antianginal agents, the instructor determines that the teaching was successful when the students identify which of the following as a beta-blocker antianginal agent?
    a. Amlodipine
    b. Nadolol
    c. Verapamil
    d. Ranolazine

12. A patient has had a myocardial infarction and is to receive propranolol. The nurse understands that this drug is being used to achieve which of the following?
    a. Reduce the risk for recurrent anginal attacks
    b. Control the risk for vasospasm
    c. Prevent reinfarction
    d. Prevent the development of hypertension

13. Which of the following agents would be most appropriate for a patient with Prinzmetal's angina?
    a. Nitroglycerin
    b. Metoprolol
    c. Nadolol
    d. Amlodipine

14. When describing the action of ranolazine, which of the following would be most appropriate?
    a. Shortens the QT interval
    b. Decreases myocardial workload
    c. Decreases heart rate
    d. Decreases blood pressure

15. A patient is using transdermal nitroglycerin. The nurse would instruct the patient to apply a new patch at which frequency?
    a. Each time he has chest pain
    b. Before activities that may cause chest pain
    c. Every day
    d. Every week

47

Lipid-Lowering Agents

LEARNING OBJECTIVES

Upon completion of this chapter, you will be able to:

1. Outline the mechanisms of fat metabolism in the body and discuss the role of hyperlipidemia as a risk factor for coronary artery disease.

2. Describe the therapeutic actions, indications, pharmacokinetics, contraindications and cautions, most common adverse reactions, and important drug–drug interactions associated with the bile acid sequestrants, HMG-CoA inhibitors, cholesterol absorption inhibitors, and other agents used to lower lipid levels.

3. Discuss the use of drugs that lower lipid levels across the lifespan.

4. Compare and contrast the various drugs used to lower lipid levels.

5. Outline the nursing considerations, including important teaching points, for patients receiving drugs used to lower lipid levels.

■ ASSESSING YOUR UNDERSTANDING

LABELING

Place the name of the following drugs in the appropriate box under the correct drug class.

Cholestyramine   Simvastatin

Colestipol   Ezetimibe

Fluvastatin

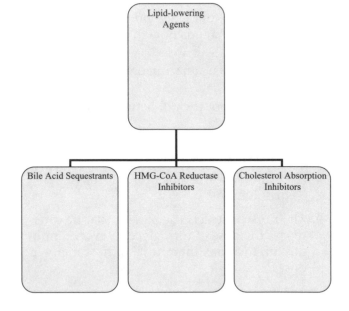

SHORT ANSWER

Supply the information requested.

1. List the six characteristics associated with metabolic syndrome.

2. Name the three nonmodifiable risk factors for coronary artery disease.

3. Explain how gout is a risk factor for coronary artery disease.

4. Describe the variations in lipoprotein levels of black Americans as compared with white Americans.

5. Identify three ways to modify risk factors for coronary artery disease.

6. Name the substance that carries micelles for absorption.

■ APPLYING YOUR KNOWLEDGE

CASE STUDY

A 55-year-old woman with a history of hyperlipidemia comes to her primary care provider's office for a checkup. The woman had been taking simvastatin for several years but was switched to atorvastatin because the simvastatin was no longer being covered by her health insurance. During the interview, the patient reports that she has been feeling tired lately, "almost like I have the flu," and is complaining of generalized muscle aches and pains. "I've been watching my diet and drinking lost of juices. I've been exercising, too, but it just seems like my muscles are getting smaller."

a. What information would be important for the nurse to obtain about the patient's diet?

b. What might the patient be experiencing, and what testing would be indicated for the patient based on her complaints?

■ PRACTICING FOR NCLEX

Circle the letter that corresponds to the best answer for each question.

1. An instructor is describing the characteristics associated with metabolic syndrome. Which of the following would the instructor include in the description? Select all that apply.
   a. Fasting blood glucose less than 110 mg/dL
   b. Waist measurement over 40 inches in men
   c. Triglyceride levels greater than 150 mg/dL
   d. Blood pressure less than 130/85 mm Hg
   e. Decreased levels of plasminogen activator

2. The nurse is reviewing the results of a patient's lipid profile. Which of the following would the nurse identify as borderline high?
   a. Total cholesterol 160 mg/dL
   b. Low-density lipoprotein (LDL) cholesterol 110 mg/dL
   c. High-density lipoprotein (HDL) cholesterol 45 mg/dL
   d. Triglycerides 180 mg/dL

3. Which substance would a group of students identify as being responsible for breaking up dietary fats into smaller units?
   a. Bile acids
   b. Cholesterol
   c. Chylomicrons
   d. Micelles

4. After reviewing information about lipoproteins, a group of students demonstrate understanding of the information when they identify which of the following as being loosely packed?
   a. LDLs
   b. HDLs
   c. Triglycerides
   d. Lipids

5. Which of the following would be classified as a bile acid sequestrant?
   a. Lovastatin
   b. Ezetimibe
   c. Cholestyramine
   d. Gemfibrozil

6. A patient who is receiving colestipol is also taking a thiazide diuretic. Which instruction would be most appropriate for the nurse to give?

   a. "Take the colestipol at the same time as the thiazide diuretic."

   b. "Take the thiazide diuretic about 4 hours before the colestipol."

   c. "Take the colestipol first and then take the diuretic a half hour later."

   d. "Take the thiazide diuretic about 1 hour before the colestipol."

7. A nurse would caution a patient receiving cholestyramine to avoid mixing the drug with which of the following?

   a. Soups

   b. Carbonated beverages

   c. Fruit juices

   d. Cereals

8. The nurse instructs a patient to take the prescribed pravastatin at bedtime based on the understanding about which of the following?

   a. Adverse effects are less likely during the night.

   b. Compliance is enhanced with nighttime administration.

   c. Greater drug effectiveness is achieved at this time.

   d. Lack of dietary intake during sleep increases absorption.

9. Which of the following best reflects the action of ezetimibe?

   a. Blocks the enzyme involved in cholesterol synthesis

   b. Binds with bile acids to form an insoluble complex for excretion

   c. Stimulates the breakdown of lipoproteins from tissues

   d. Decreases the absorption of dietary cholesterol from the small intestine

10. A patient with atrial fibrillation who is receiving oral anticoagulant therapy is receiving atorvastatin. The nurse would monitor this patient for which of the following?

    a. Abdominal pain

    b. Cataract development

    c. Liver failure

    d. Bleeding

11. A patient is being prescribed fluvastatin. The nurse reviews the patient's medical record to ensure that the patient has attempted lifestyle changes for at least a minimum of which amount of time?

    a. 2 weeks

    b. 4 weeks

    c. 8 weeks

    d. 12 weeks

12. A patient is receiving niacin as part of therapy for hyperlipoproteinemia. The nurse would explain that the lipid levels will usually begin to drop in approximately which amount of time?

    a. 3 to 5 days

    b. 5 to 7 days

    c. 7 to 10 days

    d. 10 to 14 days

13. Which agent would the nurse identify as inhibiting the release of free fatty acids from adipose tissue?

    a. Niacin

    b. Fenofibrate

    c. Gemfibrozil

    d. Fenofibric acid

14. A patient who is receiving a bile acid sequestrant is being prescribed an additional agent to lower lipid levels. Which agent would the nurse most likely expect the provider to order?

    a. Statin

    b. Fibrate

    c. Niacin

    d. Cholesterol absorption inhibitor

15. After teaching a group of students about fats and biotransformation, the instructor determines that the teaching was successful when the students identify which of the following as the storage location of bile acids?

    a. Liver

    b. Gallbladder

    c. Small intestine

    d. Stomach

Drugs Affecting Blood Coagulation

Upon completion of this chapter, you will be able to:

1. Outline the mechanisms by which blood clots dissolve in the body, correlating this information with the actions of drugs used to affect blood clotting.

2. Describe the therapeutic actions, indications, pharmacokinetics, contraindications, most common adverse reactions, and important drug–drug interactions associated with drugs affecting blood coagulation.

3. Discuss the use of drugs that affect blood coagulation across the lifespan.

4. Compare and contrast the prototype drugs aspirin, heparin, urokinase, antihemophilic factor, and aminocaproic acid with other agents used to affect blood coagulation.

5. Outline the nursing considerations, including important teaching points, for patients receiving drugs used to affect blood coagulation.

■ ASSESSING YOUR UNDERSTANDING

MATCHING

Select the description in column 2 that best describes the term in column 1.

Column 1

_____ **1.** Plasminogen

_____ **2.** Clotting factors

_____ **3.** Hageman factor

_____ **4.** Platelet aggregation

_____ **5.** Thrombolytic agents

_____ **6.** Anticoagulants

_____ **7.** Hemostatic agents

_____ **8.** Extrinsic pathway

_____ **9.** Intrinsic pathway

_____ **10.** Coagulation

Column 2

a. Drugs that stop blood loss

b. Clumping together to plug an injury to the vascular system

c. Clotting factors leading to clot formation within an injured vessel

d. Drugs that prevent or slow clot formation

e. Natural clot-dissolving substance

f. First substance activated with blood vessel or cell injury

g. Clotting factors forming a clot on the outside of the injured vessel

h. Substances formed in the liver, many of which require vitamin K

i. Drugs that lyse a formed clot

j. Blood changing from a fluid state to a solid state to plug vascular system injuries

LABELING

Place the name of the following drugs in the appropriate box under the correct drug class.

Abciximab   Heparin

Alteplase   Reteplase

Clopidogrel   Ticlopidine

Desirudin   Warfarin

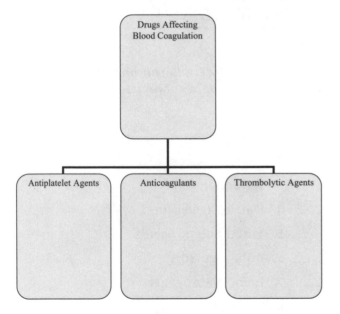

■ APPLYING YOUR KNOWLEDGE

CASE STUDY

A patient is brought to the emergency department with complaints of severe, sharp chest pain that is accompanied by diaphoresis, hemoptysis, and tachycardia. The patient has a history of deep vein thrombosis. Further assessment reveals a pulmonary embolism. The patient receives alteplase, which is followed by anticoagulant therapy with a heparin infusion. The patient improves and is started on warfarin while continuing to

receive the heparin infusion. The heparin infusion is discontinued, and the patient is being discharged on warfarin therapy.

a. What was the rationale for using alteplase?

b. Why was the patient receiving heparin and warfarin at the same time?

c. What instructions are important to include in the discharge teaching plan for this patient?

■ PRACTICING FOR NCLEX

Circle the letter that corresponds to the best answer for each question.

1. Which of the following would be considered a topical hemostatic agent?

   a. Thrombin

   b. Protamine sulfate

   c. Pentoxifylline

   d. Urokinase

2. When describing the clotting process, which step would the nurse identify as the first reaction to occur with injury to a blood vessel?

   a. Platelet aggregation

   b. Vasoconstriction

   c. Release of factor XI

   d. Thrombin formation

3. A patient is to receive clopidogrel. The nurse would expect to administer this agent by which route?

   a. Oral

   b. Intravenous

   c. Intramuscular

   d. Subcutaneous

4. The nurse would monitor the platelet levels closely for a patient receiving which of the following?
   a. Aspirin
   b. Abciximab
   c. Anagrelide
   d. Dipyridamole

5. A patient is receiving warfarin. The nurse would expect to administer this drug by which route?
   a. Oral
   b. Subcutaneous
   c. Intravenous
   d. Intramuscular

6. A patient is receiving heparin. Which of the following would the nurse use to monitor the effects of the drug?
   a. Partial thromboplastin time
   b. International normalized ratio
   c. Prothrombin time
   d. Vitamin K level

7. Which of the following would a nurse identify as inhibiting factor Xa?
   a. Heparin
   b. Warfarin
   c. Argatroban
   d. Fondaparinux

8. A patient exhibits signs and symptoms of heparin overdose. The nurse would anticipate administering which of the following?
   a. Vitamin K
   b. Protamine sulfate
   c. Urokinase
   d. Drotrecogin alfa

9. After reviewing the drugs that may interfere with warfarin, the students indicate that they need additional study when they identify which of the following as requiring a dosage increase in the warfarin?
   a. Clofibrate
   b. Quinidine
   c. Phenytoin
   d. Cefoxitin

10. A patient who is experiencing the signs and symptoms of an acute myocardial infarction says that his symptoms started at 10:00 AM this morning. It is now 11:15 AM. The nurse understands that the latest time that the patient could receive a thrombolytic agent would be which of the following?
    a. 1:00 PM
    b. 2:00 PM
    c. 3:00 PM
    d. 4:00 PM

11. A patient is started on enoxaparin immediately after hip surgery. The nurse would explain to the patient that this drug will be continued for how long?
    a. 1 to 3 days
    b. 3 to 7 days
    c. 7 to 10 days
    d. 10 to 14 days

12. The nurse is reviewing the coagulation studies of a patient who is receiving a heparin infusion. The patient's baseline partial thromboplastin time is 32 seconds. Which result would indicate therapeutic effectiveness?
    a. 32 seconds
    b. 40 seconds
    c. 64 seconds
    d. 96 seconds

13. An instructor is describing the drug drotrecogin alfa to a group of students. The instructor determines that the students need additional teaching when they state which of the following?
    a. The drug is used primarily for adults with severe sepsis.
    b. The drug is administered by intravenous infusion for a total of 4 days.
    c. The drug is fairly expensive, possibly limiting its used.
    d. The drug is associated with a high risk for embolism.

14. A patient is receiving antihemophilic factor. The nurse understands that this drug is which factor?

a. VIII

b. VIIa

c. IX

d. X

15. Which of the following would a nurse identify as a systemic hemostatic agent?

a. Absorbable gelatin

b. Aminocaproic acid

c. Human fibrin sealant

d. Thrombin

CHAPTER 49

Drugs Used to Treat Anemias

LEARNING OBJECTIVES

Upon completion of this chapter, you will be able to:

1. Explain the process of erythropoiesis and its correlation to the development of three types of anemias.

2. Describe the therapeutic actions, indications, pharmacokinetics, contraindications and cautions, most common adverse reactions, and important drug–drug interactions associated with drugs used to treat anemias.

3. Discuss the use of drugs used to treat anemias across the lifespan.

4. Compare and contrast the prototype drugs epoetin alfa, ferrous sulfate, folic acid, and hydroxocobalamin with other agents in their class.

5. Outline the nursing considerations, including important teaching points, for patients receiving drugs used to treat anemias.

■ ASSESSING YOUR UNDERSTANDING

MATCHING

Select the description in column 2 that best describes the term in column 1.

Column 1

____ **1.** Anemia

____ **2.** Plasma

____ **3.** Erythrocytes

____ **4.** Erythropoiesis

____ **5.** Erythropoietin

____ **6.** Reticulocyte

Column 2

a. Liquid portion of the blood

b. Stimulates red blood cell production in the bone marrow

c. Immature nonnucleated red blood cell

d. Cell responsible for carrying oxygen to the tissues

e. Disorder of too few or ineffective red blood cells

f. Production and life cycle of red blood cells

SHORT ANSWER

Supply the information requested.

1. Describe how erythropoietin produces a red blood cell.

2. Identify the average life span of a red blood cell.

3. List three important elements in the bone marrow needed to produce healthy red blood cells.

4. Describe the three major types of anemia.

5. Name the type of anemia that occurs when the gastric mucosa cannot produce intrinsic factor.

■APPLYING YOUR KNOWLEDGE

CASE STUDY

A patient has been undergoing cancer chemotherapy and has developed anemia. The patient has been prescribed ferrous sulfate 100 mg three times a day. He has been taking the medication for approximately 4 months, but he continues to exhibit signs and symptoms of anemia. Blood tests confirm this. The health care provider orders epoetin alfa.

a. What would be the rationale for using epoetin alfa?

b. What areas would require close monitoring of the patient receiving this drug?

■PRACTICING FOR NCLEX

Circle the letter that corresponds to the best answer for each question.

1. Which of the following would a nurse identify as the primary issue associated with anemias?
   a. Defective white blood cells
   b. Increased plasma proteins
   c. Ineffective red blood cells
   d. Lack of vitamin B_{12}

2. After reviewing the major types of anemia, students demonstrate understanding of the information when they identify which of the following as an example of a hemolytic anemia?
   a. Iron deficiency anemia
   b. Pernicious anemia
   c. Folic acid deficiency anemia
   d. Sickle cell anemia

3. Which of the following would the nurse encourage a patient to consume to prevent folic acid anemia? Select all that apply.
   a. Fruits
   b. Fish
   c. Broccoli
   d. Milk
   e. Liver

4. A patient is receiving hydroxocobalamin for treatment of pernicious anemia. The nurse would administer this agent by which route?
   a. Oral
   b. Subcutaneous
   c. Intramuscular
   d. Intravenous

5. A patient is diagnosed with sickle cell anemia. Which agent would the nurse expect to be ordered?
   a. Hydroxyurea
   b. Epoetin alfa
   c. Ferrous sulfate
   d. Iron dextran

6. A patient is receiving darbepoetin alfa. The nurse would inform the patient that he will be receiving this drug at which frequency?

   a. Once a week

   b. Two to three times/week

   c. Every other week

   d. Monthly

7. A patient is prescribed iron therapy using iron dextran. The nurse would administer this drug by which route?

   a. Oral

   b. Subcutaneous

   c. Intramuscular

   d. Intravenous

8. A patient is receiving ferrous sulfate as treatment for iron deficiency anemia. After teaching the patient, which statement indicates the need for additional teaching?

   a. "I need to take an antacid with the pill to prevent an upset stomach."

   b. "I need to make sure that I eat enough foods containing iron."

   c. "It might take several months before my iron levels get back to normal."

   d. "I need to avoid taking the drug with coffee or tea."

9. Which of the following would be appropriate for a patient who is receiving iron therapy?

   a. Ensuring that the patient consumes three large meals per day

   b. Cautioning the patient that stool may be dark or green

   c. Encouraging the patient to take the drug on an empty stomach

   d. Advising the patient to limit the amount of fiber in his diet

10. When describing the function of vitamin B_{12}, which of the following would be appropriate to include?

    a. Maintenance of myelin sheath

    b. Prevention of neural tube defects

    c. Important role in cell division

    d. Oxygen transport to the tissues

11. Which of the following would be least important in producing healthy, efficient red blood cells? Select all that apply.

    a. Iron

    b. Carbohydrates

    c. White blood cells

    d. Amino acids

    e. Plasma

12. A patient is receiving epoetin alfa. The nurse understands that this drug's duration of effect would be which amount of time?

    a. 12 hours

    b. 24 hours

    c. 36 hours

    d. 48 hours

13. A patient is experiencing iron toxicity. Which agent would the nurse expect to be given?

    a. Dimercaprol

    b. Succimer

    c. Deferoxamine

    d. Edetate calcium disodium

14. Which of the following would the nurse expect the health care provider to prescribe for a patient receiving methotrexate?

    a. Cyanocobalamin

    b. Leucovorin

    c. Hydroxyurea

    d. Iron sucrose

15. A patient is prescribed oral ferrous sulfate solution. Which statement by the patient indicates that he understands how to take the drug?

    a. "I'll mix the dose with orange juice to make it easier to swallow."

    b. "I should drink a big glass of water after swallowing the solution."

    c. "I can mix the dose with a small amount of yogurt to make it taste better."

    d. "I should drink the solution through a straw so my teeth don't get stained."

CHAPTER 50

Introduction to the Renal System

LEARNING OBJECTIVES

Upon completion of this chapter, you will be able to:

1. Review the anatomy of the kidney, including the structure of the nephron.

2. Explain the basic processes of the kidney and where these processes occur.

3. Explain the control of calcium, sodium, potassium, and chloride in the nephron.

4. Discuss the countercurrent mechanism and the control of urine concentration and dilution, applying these effects to various clinical scenarios.

5. Describe the renin-angiotensin-aldosterone system, including controls and clinical situations where this system is active.

6. Discuss the roles of the kidney with acid-base balance, calcium regulation, and red blood cell production, integrating this information to explain the clinical manifestations of renal failure.

■ ASSESSING YOUR UNDERSTANDING

MATCHING

Select the description from column 2 that best describes the term in column 1.

Column 1

___ 1. Aldosterone

___ 2. Antidiuretic hormone

___ 3. Carbonic anhydrase

___ 4. Filtration

___ 5. Reabsorption

___ 6. Secretion

___ 7. Countercurrent mechanism

___ 8. Nephron

Column 2

a. Movement of substances from the renal tubule back into vascular system

b. Catalyst that speeds up the reaction combining water and carbon dioxide

c. Hormone produced by the adrenal gland

d. Functional unit of the kidney

e. Active movement of substances from the blood into the renal tubule

f. Hormone produced by the hypothalamus

g. Passage of fluid and small components through the glomerulus into the tubule

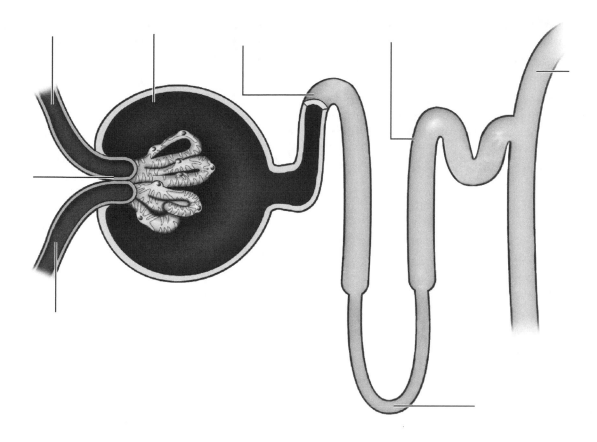

h. Process used by medullary nephrons to concentrate or dilute urine

LABELING

Place the name of the structure in the appropriate location on the illustration above.

Afferent arteriole

Bowman's capsule

Collecting duct

Distal convoluted tubule

Efferent arteriole

Glomerulus

Loop of Henle

Proximal convoluted tubule

■ APPLYING YOUR KNOWLEDGE

CASE STUDY

As part of a class assignment, a group of students are to role-play the processes that occur in the nephron. In addition, the students are to depict how the nephron

maintains the volume and composition of body fluids.

a. What processes would the student need to demonstrate, and how might they accomplish this task?

b. What key electrolytes would the students act out?

■ PRACTICING FOR NCLEX

Circle the letter that corresponds to the best answer for each question.

1. Which of the following statements best reflects information about the renal system?

a. The kidneys consist of two protective layers.

b. The system includes the kidneys and urinary tract.

c. The system is primarily involved with regulating blood pressure.

d. Most of the fluid filtered by the kidneys is excreted.

2. After reviewing the structure of the kidneys, the students demonstrate understanding of the information when they identify which of the following?

a. The renal medulla drains the urine into the ureters.

b. The renal arteries come directly off the iliac artery.

c. The medullary nephrons are able to concentrate or dilute urine.

d. Erythropoietin is produced in the glomerulus.

3. The kidneys receive approximately what percentage of the cardiac output?

a. 5%

b. 15%

c. 25%

d. 40%

4. When describing the signs and symptoms associated with renal failure, which of the following would be most important for a nurse to keep in mind?

a. A small number of nephrons usually are affected when manifestations develop.

b. Most signs and symptoms are unrelated to nephron damage.

c. Renal failure reflects injury to the protective layers of the kidneys.

d. Renal failure suggests that extensive kidney damage has already occurred.

5. An instructor is reviewing the process of tubular secretion. Which of the following would the nurse include?

a. Movement of fluid and small components through the glomerulus into the tubule

b. Active movement of substances from the blood into the renal tubule

c. Movement of substances from the tubule back into the vascular system

d. Activity to create a more concentrated or diluted urine

6. The amount of fluid excreted as urine each day averages approximately less than how many liters?

a. 1 L

b. 2 L

c. 3 L

d. 4 L

7. Which of the following substances are moved from the glomerulus into the tubule due to hydrostatic pressure?

a. Lipids

b. Proteins

c. Blood cells

d. Water

8. Sodium ions are actively reabsorbed in which location?

a. Proximal convoluted tubule

b. Loop of Henle

c. Ascending loop of Henle

d. Distal convoluted tubule

9. Which of the following would lead to a release of aldosterone?

a. Low potassium levels

b. Parasympathetic stimulation

c. Angiotensin III

d. Natriuretic hormone

10. When describing the fluid in the ascending loop of Henle, which of the following would be most accurate?

a. Highly concentrated

b. Hypotonic

c. Hypertonic

d. Osmotically balanced

11. Where is the majority of potassium that is filtered at the glomerulus reabsorbed?

a. Bowman's capsule

b. Descending loop of Henle

c. Ascending loop of Henle

d. Distal convoluted tubule

12. Which substance stimulates the reabsorption of calcium in the distal convoluted tubule?

a. Aldosterone

b. Antidiuretic hormone

c. Vitamin D

d. Parathyroid hormone

13. Which of the following is released in response to a decrease in blood flow to the nephron?
    a. Calcium
    b. Renin
    c. Angiotensinogen
    d. Aldosterone

14. The nurse is describing the need to maintain the acidity of urine based on the understanding that this is necessary for which of the following?
    a. Maintain fluid balance
    b. Destroy any bacteria that may enter
    c. Prevent loss of sphincter control
    d. Maintain peristaltic movement

15. A nurse is describing the reasons why more women than men are affected by cystitis. Which of the following would the nurse identify as a major reason?
    a. "A woman's urine has a tendency to be more alkaline."
    b. "The urethra doesn't have the protection of the prostate gland."
    c. "The urethra exits into an area rich in gram-negative bacteria."
    d. "A woman's bladder stretches to accommodate more urine."

Diuretic Agents

Upon completion of this chapter, you will be able to:

1. Define the term diuretic and list four types of diuretic drugs.

2. Describe the therapeutic actions, indications, pharmacokinetics, contraindications and cautions, most common adverse reactions, and important drug–drug interactions associated with the various classes of diuretic drugs.

3. Discuss the use of diuretic agents across the life span.

4. Compare and contrast the prototype drugs of each class of diuretic drugs with other agents in their class.

5. Outline the nursing considerations, including important teaching points, for patients receiving diuretic agents.

■ ASSESSING YOUR UNDERSTANDING

LABELING

Place the name of the following drugs in the appropriate box under the correct drug class.

Amiloride	Mannitol
Bumetanide	Spironolactone
Ethacrynic acid	Triamterene
Furosemide	

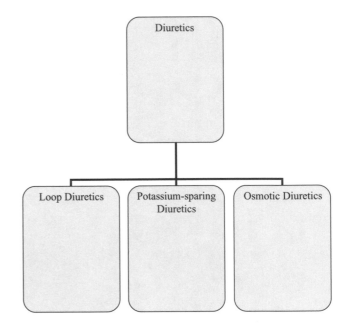

SHORT ANSWER

Supply the information requested.

1. Explain the clinical significance of the action of diuretics.

2. Describe what is meant by fluid rebound.

3. Explain how heart failure can cause edema.

4. Identify how thiazide and thiazidelike diuretics act.

5. Name the prototype loop diuretic.

6. Identify the most common use for carbonic anhydrase inhibitors.

■ APPLYING YOUR KNOWLEDGE

CASE STUDY

An older adult woman has a history of cardiovascular disease including hypertension and heart failure. The patient had been receiving furosemide. The patient developed mild hypokalemia for which a potassium supplement was prescribed. She also was instructed in measures to increase her dietary potassium intake. The hypokalemia continued, and the patient was switched to spironolactone. She arrives at the health care provider's office. During the assessment, the patient reveals that she has been experiencing nausea, abdominal cramping, and diarrhea along with some muscle cramps and weakness. Hyperkalemia is suspected.

a. What information would be most important for the nurse to obtain?

b. What should the nurse emphasize in the teaching plan for this patient?

■ PRACTICING FOR NCLEX

Circle the letter that corresponds to the best answer for each question.

1. A patient is receiving a diuretic and tells the nurse that he has decreased his fluid intake so that he does not have to make so many trips to the bathroom. The nurse interprets this information, realizing that this patient is at risk for which of the following?
   a. Hypokalemia
   b. Fluid rebound
   c. Weight loss
   d. Dehydration

2. After reviewing the different classes of diuretics available, a student demonstrates understanding when he identifies which of the following as an example of a thiazidelike diuretic?
   a. Metolazone
   b. Chlorothiazide
   c. Furosemide
   d. Triamterene

3. A patient is receiving hydrocholorothiazide. The nurse would expect to administer this drug by which route?
   a. Oral
   b. Subcutaneous
   c. Intramuscular
   d. Intravenous

4. Which of the following would contraindicate the use of indapamide?
   a. Diabetes
   b. Systemic lupus erythematosus
   c. Hypokalemia
   d. Gout

5. The nurse is monitoring the results of laboratory testing for a patient receiving chlorthalidone. Which of the following would be a cause for concern?
   a. Decreased uric acid levels
   b. Hypercalcemia
   c. Hyperkalemia
   d. Anemia

6. A patient is receiving hydrochlorothiazide. The nurse would expect this drug to begin acting within which time frame?

   a. 1 hour

   b. 2 hours

   c. 3 hours

   d. 4 hours

7. When describing where bumetanide acts, which of the following would the nurse include?

   a. Proximal convoluted tubule

   b. Loop of Henle

   c. Collecting tubule

   d. Glomerulus

8. The nurse assesses a patient receiving furosemide for which of the following?

   a. Acidosis

   b. Hypercalcemia

   c. Hypotension

   d. Hypoglycemia

9. A patient receives a dose of furosemide intravenously at 8:00 AM. The nurse would expect this drug to exert is peak effects at which time?

   a. 8:15 AM

   b. 8:30 AM

   c. 8:45 AM

   d. 9:00 AM

10. After teaching a group of students about loop diuretics, the instructor determines that the teaching has been successful when the students identify which agent as the safest for use in the home?

    a. Furosemide

    b. Ethacrynic acid

    c. Bumetanide

    d. Torsemide

11. Which of the following would the nurse expect to find in a patient receiving acetazolamide?

    a. Metabolic alkalosis

    b. Metabolic acidosis

    c. Respiratory acidosis

    d. Respiratory alkalosis

12. When describing the action of spironolactone, the nurse would explain that this drug acts by which of the following?

    a. Blocking potassium secretion through the tubule

    b. Slowing the movement of hydrogen ions

    c. Blocking the chloride pump

    d. Blocking aldosterone in the distal tubule

13. A patient is receiving triamterene. The nurse instructs the patient to avoid which of the following? Select all that apply.

    a. Bananas

    b. Prunes

    c. Lettuce

    d. Broccoli

    e. Apples

14. Which of the following instructions would be most appropriate for a patient who is taking a diuretic?

    a. "Take the daily dose around dinnertime."

    b. "It's okay to take it with food."

    c. "Lie down after taking the drug."

    d. "Limit the amount of fluids you drink."

15. A patient is diagnosed with increased intracranial pressure. Which of the following would the nurse expect to be ordered?

    a. Mannitol

    b. Furosemide

    c. Amiloride

    d. Bumetanide

Drugs Affecting the Urinary Tract and the Bladder

LEARNING OBJECTIVES

Upon completion of this chapter, you will be able to:

1. Describe four common problems associated with the urinary tract, including the clinical manifestations of these problems.

2. Describe the therapeutic actions, indications, pharmacokinetics, contraindications and cautions, most common adverse reactions, and important drug–drug interactions associated with urinary tract anti-infectives, antispasmodics, and analgesics, bladder protectants, and drugs used to treat benign prostatic hyperplasia.

3. Discuss the use of drugs affecting the urinary tract and bladder across the lifespan.

4. Compare and contrast the prototype drugs norfloxacin, oxybutynin, and doxazosin with other agents in their class.

5. Outline the nursing considerations, including important teaching points, for patients receiving drugs affecting the urinary tract and bladder.

■ ASSESSING YOUR UNDERSTANDING

MATCHING

Select the description from column 2 that best describes the term in column 1.

Column 1

___ **1.** Cystitis

___ **2.** Dysuria

___ **3.** Nocturia

___ **4.** Urgency

___ **5.** Frequency

Column 2

a. Feeling of the need to void often

b. Inflammation of the bladder

c. Getting up to void at night

d. Painful urination

e. Feeling of needing to void immediately

SHORT ANSWER

Supply the information requested.

1. Describe the difference between cystitis and pyelonephritis.

2. List the two types of urinary tract anti-infectives.

3. Explain how urinary tract antispasmodics act.

4. Identify the indication for use of pentosan polysulfate sodium.

5. Describe the two types of drugs used to treat benign prostatic hyperplasia (BPH).

6. Name the herbal therapy that may be used to relieve the symptoms of BPH.

■ APPLYING YOUR KNOWLEDGE

CASE STUDY

A 42-year-old woman comes to the clinic for an evaluation. The woman reports urgency and frequency and some stress incontinence but denies any pain or burning on urination. She states, "There are times when I literally have to run to the bathroom because I have to go so badly. It's really embarrassing. It doesn't matter how much I've had to drink. In fact, whenever I go anywhere, I find where the restrooms are first, just in case. There have been several times when I almost didn't make it to the bathroom." Further assessment and a urine culture rule out a urinary tract infection. The health care provider prescribes trospium.

a. When explaining the action of this drug, what information would the nurse need to address?

b. What information would the nurse need to include when teaching the patient about using this drug?

■ PRACTICING FOR NCLEX

Circle the letter that corresponds to the best answer for each question.

1. A group of students are reviewing the agents used as urinary tract anti-infectives. The students demonstrate understanding of the material when they cite which of the following as an example?

   a. Flavoxate

   b. Phenazopyridine

   c. Doxazosin

   d. Nitrofurantoin

2. When describing a urinary tract anti-infective, which of the following would a nurse identify as one that acidifies the urine?

   a. Cinoxacin

   b. Fosfomycin

   c. Methenamine

   d. Co-trimoxazole

3. A patient has a history of renal dysfunction. Which agent would the nurse expect to administer as the usual dosage?

   a. Cinoxacin

   b. Nitrofurantoin

   c. Norfloxacin

   d. Co-trimoxazole

4. A patient with cystitis is receiving fosfomycin. Which statement indicates that the patient has understood the instructions?

   a. "I need to drink lots of citrus juices."

   b. "I mix one packet in water to take the drug."

    c. "I can drink milk with the drug if my stomach is upset."

    d. "I have to take the drug for no less than 7 days."

5. A physician prescribes a urinary antispasmodic as a transdermal patch. The nurse identifies this as drug as which of the following?

    a. Oxybutynin

    b. Flavoxate

    c. Tolterodine

    d. Darifenacin

6. A patient who takes digoxin for heart failure is also prescribed trospium. The nurse would monitor the patient closely for which of the following?

    a. Increased central nervous system effects

    b. Signs of digoxin toxicity

    c. Excess anticholinergic effects

    d. Changes in urine color

7. A patient is receiving phenazopyridine. The nurse would inform the patient that this drug may cause the urine to become which color?

    a. Brown

    b. Dark yellow

    c. Blue-green

    d. Reddish-orange

8. A patient is prescribed oxybutynin as a transdermal patch. The nurse would instruct the patient to change the patch at which frequency?

    a. Every day

    b. Every other day

    c. Every 4 days

    d. Every 7 days

9. The nurse is reviewing the medical record of a patient who is to receive pentosan. Which of the following would alert the nurse to the need for close monitoring?

    a. Splenic dysfunction

    b. Use of anticoagulants

    c. Thrombocytopenia

    d. Recent surgery

10. When explaining the action of dutasteride as treatment for BPH, the nurse would explain that the drug acts to achieve which of the following?

    a. Blockage of alpha-1 adrenergic receptors

    b. Inhibition of testosterone conversion

    c. Buffering to control cell wall permeability

    d. Interference with DNA replication

11. A patient is prescribed tamsulosin. The nurse would instruct the patient to take the drug in which manner?

    a. At night before going to bed

    b. An hour before the same meal each day

    c. One-half hour before the same meals daily

    d. At a consistent time each day

12. The nurse would inform the patient about which of the following when dutasteride is prescribed?

    a. Hypertension

    b. Bradycardia

    c. Increased libido

    d. Impotence

13. Which of the following would be most important to monitor in a patient receiving an agent for BPH?

    a. Complete blood count

    b. Serum electrolyte levels

    c. Renal function studies

    d. Prostate-specific antigen level

14. Which of the following would lead a nurse to suspect that a patient most likely has pyelonephritis?

    a. Urinary frequency

    b. Flank pain

    c. Dysuria

    d. Urgency

15. A patient is experiencing signs and symptoms of an overactive bladder. Which agent would the nurse expect the health care provider to prescribe?

    a. Norfloxacin

    b. Methylene blue

    c. Tolterodine

    d. Terazosin

CHAPTER 53

Introduction to the Respiratory System

LEARNING OBJECTIVES

Upon completion of this chapter, you will be able to:

1. Describe the major structures of the respiratory system, including the role of each in respiration.
2. Describe the process of respiration, with clinical examples of problems that can arise with alterations in the respiratory membrane.
3. Differentiate between the common conditions that affect the upper respiratory system.
4. Identify three conditions involving the lower respiratory tract, including the clinical presentations of these conditions.
5. Discuss the process involved in obstructive respiratory diseases, correlating this to the signs and symptoms of these diseases.

ASSESSING YOUR UNDERSTANDING

LABELING

Place the name of the structure in the proper location of the respiratory tract.

Alveoli
Bronchiole
Bronchus
Larynx
Lung
Mouth
Nose
Pharynx
Sinuses
Trachea

Upper Respiratory Tract	Lower Respiratory Tract

MATCHING

Select the description from column 2 that best describes the term in column 1.

Column 1

____ **1.** Asthma

____ **2.** Chronic obstructive pulmonary disease (COPD)

_____ **3.** Atelectasis

_____ **4.** Common cold

_____ **5.** Cystic fibrosis

_____ **6.** Pneumonia

_____ **7.** Pneumothorax

_____ **8.** Respiratory distress syndrome

_____ **9.** Seasonal rhinitis

_____ **10.** Sinusitis

Column 2

a. Hay fever

b. Bacterial or viral inflammation of the lungs

c. Hereditary disease involving copious thick secretions in the lungs

d. Viral upper respiratory tract infection

e. Disorder involving recurrent episodes of bronchospasm

f. Collapse of once-expanded alveoli

g. Condition involving the destruction of respiratory defense mechanisms

h. Disorder of premature neonates related to surfactant deficiency

i. Inflammation of the epithelial lining of the air-filled passages of the skull

j. Air in the pleural space exerting high pressure against the air sacs

■ APPLYING YOUR KNOWLEDGE

CASE STUDY

The nurse is assessing a patient who had abdominal surgery 36 hours ago. Assessment reveals crackles on auscultation and diminished breath sounds at the bases. His respirations are also somewhat shallow. Oxygen saturation levels via pulse oximetry are slightly decreased. The patient is complaining of abdominal pain. The patient states that he is trying not to cough or move because it hurts too much. The patient is receiving morphine for pain.

a. What might the patient be experiencing based on his status and assessment findings and why?

b. What measures might be helpful to promote the patient's respiratory function?

■ PRACTICING FOR NCLEX

Circle the letter that corresponds to the best answer for each question.

1. Which of the following would the nurse identify as being involved with asthma?

a. Acute infection

b. Hyperactive airways

c. Alveolar collapse

d. Progressive loss of lung compliance

2. Which term would be used to describe the movement of air in and out of the body?

a. Perfusion

b. Respiration

c. Ventilation

d. Gas exchange

3. An instructor is describing the respiratory membrane at the alveolar level. Which of the following would the instructor include as a component?

a. Cilia

b. Goblet cells

c. Mast cells

d. Capillary endothelium

4. Sympathetic nervous system stimulation of the respiratory tract would result in which of the following?

a. Diaphragmatic contraction

b. Bronchoconstriction

c. Increased respiratory rate

d. Inspiratory movement

5. A nurse is describing the events associated with a common cold to a local community group. Which of the following would the nurse include?

a. Release of epinephrine

b. Shrinkage of the mucous membranes

c. Increased activity of the goblet cells

d. Invasion by a bacterium

6. A group of students are reviewing the common conditions associated with the upper respiratory tract. The students demonstrate understanding of the material when they identify which of the following as a response to a specific antigen?

   a. Asthma

   b. Seasonal rhinitis

   c. Sinusitis

   d. Pharyngitis

7. When describing the structure of the lungs, the nurse would identify the left lung as consisting of how many lobes?

   a. Two

   b. Three

   c. Four

   d. Five

8. Which mechanism is involved in the movement of oxygen and carbon dioxide at the alveolar level?

   a. Active transport

   b. Diffusion

   c. Facilitated diffusion

   d. Osmosis

9. Which of the following disorders would alter the ability to move gases in and out of the lungs? Select all that apply.

   a. Atelectasis

   b. Common cold

   c. Bronchitis

   d. Respiratory distress syndrome

   e. Sinusitis

   f. Cystic fibrosis

10. With bronchitis, proteins leak into the area due to which of the following?

    a. Swelling

    b. Increased blood flow

    c. Changes in capillary permeability

    d. Inflammatory reaction

11. With which condition are the bronchial epithelial cells replaced by a fibrous scar tissue?

    a. Asthma

    b. Bronchiectasis

    c. Bronchitis

    d. Pneumonia

12. A neonate develops respiratory distress syndrome. Which of the following would be used?

    a. Anti-infective agents

    b. Bronchodilators

    c. Surfactant replacements

    d. Antihistamines

13. After reviewing information about respiratory tract disorders, a group of students demonstrate understanding of the material when they identify which of the following as the most common cause of COPD?

    a. Infection

    b. Allergen exposure

    c. Genetic inheritance

    d. Cigarette smoking

14. A patient experiences bronchospasm with asthma. The nurse understands that this is due to which of the following?

    a. Cytokines

    b. Histamine

    c. Norepinephrine

    d. Serotonin

15. When describing the mast cells to a group of students, an instructor would include which of the following as being released by these cells? Select all that apply.

    a. Histamine

    b. Serotonin

    c. Adenosine triphosphate

    d. Epinephrine

    e. Dopamine

CHAPTER 54

Drugs Acting on the Upper Respiratory Tract

LEARNING OBJECTIVES

Upon completion of this chapter, you will be able to:

1. Outline the underlying physiologic events that occur with upper respiratory disorders.

2. Describe the therapeutic actions, indications, pharmacokinetics, contraindications, most common adverse reactions, and important drug–drug interactions associated with drugs acting on the upper respiratory tract.

3. Discuss the use of drugs that act on the upper respiratory tract across the lifespan.

4. Compare and contrast the prototype drugs with other agents in their class and with other classes of drugs that act on the upper respiratory tract.

5. Outline the nursing considerations, including important teaching points, for patients receiving drugs acting on the upper respiratory tract.

■ASSESSING YOUR UNDERSTANDING

LABELING

Place the name of the following drugs in the appropriate box under the correct classification.

Azelastine

Benzonatate

Meclizine

Chlorpheniramine

Dextromethorphan

Diphenhydramine

Fexofenadine

Hydrocodone

Hydroxyzine

Loratadine

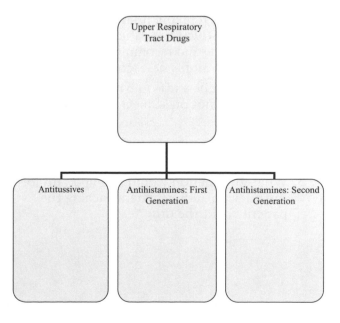

MATCHING

Select the description from column 2 that best describes the term in column 1.

Column 1

____ **1.** Antihistamine

____ **2.** Antitussive

____ **3.** Expectorant

____ **4.** Mucolytic

Column 2

a. Drug that blocks the cough reflex

b. Drug that increases a productive cough

c. Drug that blocks the action of a chemical released during inflammation

d. Drug that liquefies secretions

■ APPLYING YOUR KNOWLEDGE

CASE STUDY

A 20-year-old student comes to the campus health center. Over the past several days, he has developed nasal congestion, sneezing, and itchy and watery eyes. He had been participating in a service project in which they were cleaning up abandoned homes. The student says, "I often get this way when I'm exposed to dust. I wore a mask, but there really was a huge amount of dust flying around." The patient has a prescription for fexofenadine, which has been effective but has not been taking it lately. The nurse practitioner instructs the patient to start taking his fexofenadine and recommends the use of oxymetazoline for his nasal congestion.

a. What might be a reason why the nurse practitioner did not prescribe a nasal steroid?

b. What information would be important for the nurse to address when teaching the patient about the drug?

■ PRACTICING FOR NCLEX

Circle the letter that corresponds to the best answer for each question.

1. Which agent acts directly on the medullary cough center?

   a. Benzonatate

   b. Codeine

   c. Ephedrine

   d. Tetrahydrozoline

2. A nurse administers an antitussive agent cautiously to a patient with asthma for which reason?

   a. The airway needs to be maintained.

   b. The drug can lead to addiction.

   c. A loss of respiratory reserve can occur.

   d. The patient may experience increased sedation.

3. After teaching a patient who is receiving an antitussive about the drug, which statement indicates the need for additional teaching?

   a. "I'll get a humidifier for my bedroom."

   b. "I'll keep the room warm and toasty."

   c. "I can use some lozenges for comfort."

   d. "I need to increase the amount of fluids I drink."

4. Which agent would the nurse instruct a patient to use orally?

   a. Pseudoephedrine

   b. Phenylephrine

   c. Tetrahydrozoline

   d. Xylometazoline

5. An instructor is describing topical decongestants as belonging to which class?

   a. Adrenergic antagonists

   b. Anticholinergics

   c. Antihistamines

   d. Sympathomimetics

6. After teaching a group of parents about the use of over-the-counter cough and cold products with their children, which statement indicates the need for additional teaching?

   a. "We can use over-the-counter products for our 5-year-old but not for our 18-month-old."

   b. "We need to read the label carefully to see how often and how much to give."

   c. "We can use the adult brand, but we just have to decrease the amount."

   d. "We should use the cup that comes with the drug to measure it out."

7. A patient is taking pseudoephedrine. The nurse would assess the patient for which of the following adverse effects?

   a. Anxiety

   b. Lethargy

   c. Hypotension

   d. Dry skin

8. The nurse instructs a patient who is prescribed a nasal steroid that it may take up to how long before effects may be noted?

   a. 2 days

   b. 4 days

   c. 7 days

   d. 21 days

9. A group of students are reviewing information about antihistamines. The students demonstrate understanding of the information when they identify which agent as a second-generation antihistamine?

   a. Brompheniramine

   b. Promethazine

   c. Meclizine

   d. Loratadine

10. When describing the effects of second-generation antihistamines, which of the following would the nurse address as being decreased?

    a. Hypersensitivity

    b. Dry mouth

    c. Gastrointestinal upset

    d. Sedation

11. A patient receives diphenhydramine orally. The nurse would expect this drug to begin acting within which time frame?

    a. 15 to 30 minutes

    b. 30 to 45 minutes

    c. 45 to 60 minutes

    d. 60 to 75 minutes

12. The health care provider suggests that a patient use guaifenesin to help his cough. The nurse instructs the patient to call the health care provider if he continues to have a productive cough after which amount of time?

    a. 5 days

    b. 1 week

    c. 2 weeks

    d. 3 weeks

13. Which agent would a nurse expect the health care provider to prescribe for a patient experiencing motion sickness?

    a. Clemastine

    b. Meclizine

    c. Cyproheptadine

    d. Hydroxyzine

14. When describing the action of acetylcysteine in treating cystic fibrosis, which of the following would the nurse need to keep in mind about the drug?

    a. It binds with a heptatoxic metabolite.

    b. It separates extracellular DNA from protein in the mucus.

    c. It splits the disulfide bonds that hold mucus together.

    d. It liquefies secretions to decrease viscosity.

15. A patient is receiving dornase alfa at home. Which of the following would the nurse instruct the patient to do?

    a. "Store the drug at room temperature."

    b. "Mix the drug with tap water."

    c. "Protect the drug from light."

    d. "Take the drug orally with meals."

Drugs Acting on the Lower Respiratory Tract

Upon completion of this chapter, you will be able to:

1. Describe the underlying pathophysiology involved in obstructive pulmonary disease and correlate this information with the presenting signs and symptoms.

2. Describe the therapeutic actions, indications, pharmacokinetics, contraindications, most common adverse reactions, and important drug–drug interactions associated with drugs used to treat lower respiratory tract disorders.

3. Discuss the use of drugs used to treat obstructive pulmonary disorders across the lifespan.

4. Compare and contrast the prototype drugs used to treat obstructive pulmonary disorders with other agents in their class and with other classes of drugs used to treat obstructive pulmonary disorders.

5. Outline the nursing considerations, including important teaching points, for patients receiving drugs used to treat obstructive pulmonary disorders.

■ ASSESSING YOUR UNDERSTANDING

LABELING

Place the name of the following drugs in the appropriate box under the correct drug class.

Albuterol   Salmeterol

Aminophylline   Terbutaline

Epinephrine   Theophylline

Ipratropium   Tiotropium

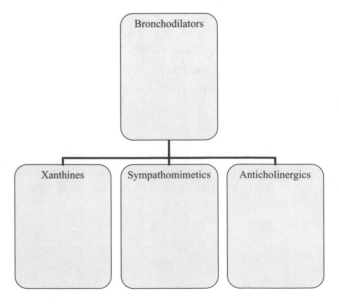

SHORT ANSWER

Supply the information requested.

1. Describe the first step in treatment for pulmonary obstructive diseases.

2. Explain the role of surfactant in the treatment of respiratory distress syndrome in a neonate.

3. Describe why xanthines are no longer considered first-line agents for asthma and bronchospasm.

4. Identify the receptor affected by sympathomimetic agents used as bronchodilators.

5. Explain the action of anticholinergics used as bronchodilators.

6. Define what is meant by the term *mast cell stabilizer*.

7. List three interventions necessary for administration of lung surfactants for an infant.

■ APPLYING YOUR KNOWLEDGE

CASE STUDY

A patient has a history of moderate persistent asthma for which he takes a combination inhaler of budesonide and formoterol. He also takes montelukast daily. His asthma has been fairly well controlled with these medications. The patient calls the health care provider's

office to report that he is experiencing some difficulty breathing and feels congested in his chest. He also reports that he is wheezing. He asks if he should use his rescue inhaler of albuterol.

a. How would the albuterol help in this situation?

b. What information would be important to include when talking with the patient?

■ PRACTICING FOR NCLEX

Circle the letter that corresponds to the best answer for each question.

1. When describing the action of mast cell stabilizers, which of the following would the nurse include as being inhibited?
   a. Epinephrine
   b. Intracellular calcium
   c. Prostaglandins
   d. Slow-reacting substance of anaphylaxis

2. After teaching a group of students about drugs as bronchodilators, the instructor determines that the teaching has been successful when the students identify which group of drugs as once being first-line agents?
   a. Mast cell stabilizers
   b. Leukotriene receptor antagonists
   c. Xanthines
   d. Sympathomimetics

3. A patient is receiving theophylline intravenously. The nurse reviews the results of his serum drug levels and notifies the physician for which result?
   a. 10 mcg/mL
   b. 15 mcg/mL
   c. 20 mcg/mL
   d. 25 mcg/mL

4. A nurse would expect to increase the dosage of theophylline if the patient has a current history of which of the following?

   a. Hyperthyroidism

   b. Cigarette smoking

   c. Gastrointestinal upset

   d. Alcohol intake

5. A nurse is administering levalbuterol to a patient. The nurse would administer this drug by which route?

   a. Oral

   b. Intravenous

   c. Inhalation

   d. Intramuscular

6. A patient is using an inhaled bronchodilator as treatment for exercise-induced asthma. The nurse would instruct the patient to use the inhaler at which time?

   a. Immediately after beginning to exercise

   b. 15 minutes before engaging in exercise

   c. Right before and after exercising

   d. Midway during the exercise routine

7. A patient who is experiencing anaphylaxis with severe wheezing receives a dose of epinephrine intravenously. The nurse would expect the drug to exert it full effects within which time frame?

   a. 5 minutes

   b. 10 minutes

   c. 15 minutes

   d. 20 minutes

8. An 8-year-old child with an acute asthmatic attack is receiving metaproterenol via nebulizer. Which of the following would be most appropriate?

   a. Have the child lie flat.

   b. Mix the drug with saline.

   c. Encourage rapid shallow breaths.

   d. Turn the device off when the mist slows.

9. While reviewing a patient's history, an allergy to which of the following would alert the nurse to a possible problem with the use of ipratropium?

   a. Eggs

   b. Dairy

   c. Peanuts

   d. Shellfish

10. Which statement by a patient who is prescribed triamcinolone indicates the need for additional teaching?

    a. "I should see some results in about 3 to 4 days."

    b. "I can't use this drug if I have an acute attack."

    c. "I might notice some hoarseness with the drug."

    d. "I should rinse my mouth after using the drug."

11. A patient is receiving ipratropium as maintenance therapy for chronic obstructive pulmonary disease. The nurse would caution the patient that up to how many inhalations may be used in 24 hours if needed?

    a. 4

    b. 8

    c. 12

    d. 16

12. Which of the following effects would result from the action of montelukast?

    a. Increased neutrophil aggregation

    b. Decreased eosinophil migration

    c. Decreased capillary permeability

    d. Increased smooth muscle contraction

13. A patient is experiencing an acute asthmatic attack. Which agent would be most effective?

    a. Inhaled steroid

    b. Leukotriene receptor antagonist

    c. Mast cell stabilizer

    d. Beta-2 selective adrenergic agonist

14. Which of the following would a nurse identify as a surfactant?

    a. Cromolyn

    b. Beractant

    c. Zileuton

    d. Theophylline

15. Which of the following would be most important to assess before administering calfactant? Select all that apply.

    a. Endotracheal tube placement

    b. Bowel sounds

    c. Lung sounds

    d. Abdominal girth

    e. Oxygen saturation levels

CHAPTER 56

Introduction to the Gastrointestinal System

LEARNING OBJECTIVES

Upon completion of this chapter, you will be able to:

1. Label the parts of the gastrointestinal (GI) tract on a diagram, describing the secretions, absorption, digestion, and type of motility that occurs in each part.
2. Discuss the nervous system control of the GI tract, including influences of the autonomic nervous system on gastrointestinal activity.
3. List three of the local GI reflexes and describe the clinical application of each.
4. Describe the steps involved in swallowing, including two factors that can influence this reflex.
5. Discuss the vomiting reflex, addressing three factors that can stimulate the reflex.

■ ASSESSING YOUR UNDERSTANDING

LABELING

Place the name of the structure in its correct location on the diagram.

Duodenum
Epiglottis
Esophagus
Gallbladder
Large intestine
Liver
Pancreas
Parotid gland
Pharynx
Rectum
Salivary glands
Small intestine
Stomach
Tongue

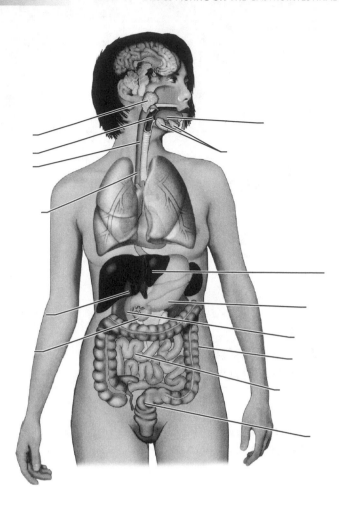

MATCHING

Select the description from column 2 that best describes the term in column 1.

Column 1

____ **1.** Chyme

____ **2.** Bile

____ **3.** Gastrin

____ **4.** Hydrochloric acid

____ **5.** Peristalsis

____ **6.** Saliva

____ **7.** Segmentation

____ **8.** Swallowing

Column 2

a. Action that moves a food bolus forward via progressive waves of muscular contraction

b. Substance released by parietal cells of the stomach

c. Fluid stored in the gallbladder

d. Fluid produced in the mouth in response to tactile stimuli and cerebral stimulation

e. Stomach contents containing ingested food and secreted enzymes, water, and mucus

f. Movement with contraction of one portion of small intestine while the next portion is relaxed

g. Substance secreted by the stomach in response to many stimuli

h. Complex reflex response to a bolus of food in the back of the throat

■ APPLYING YOUR KNOWLEDGE

CASE STUDY

A 45-year-old woman comes to the clinic complaining of right upper quadrant pain that sometimes radiates to the shoulder. She states that it seems to increase after she has eaten a heavy meal. The woman reports that her mother and sister have had gallstones, and she asks if this is what is happening.

a. Based on the nurse's understanding of the gallbladder, what information would be important to assess with this patient?

b. What might be happening that would lead to the patient's complaint of pain?

■ PRACTICING FOR NCLEX

Circle the letter that corresponds to the best answer for each question.

1. Which of the following would the nurse identify as being secreted by the exocrine pancreas?

   a. Insulin

   b. Pancreatin

   c. Gastrin

   d. Hydrochloric acid

2. Which substance is responsible for making the food bolus slippery?
   a. Saliva
   b. Bile
   c. Chyme
   d. Pancrelipase

3. Which structure would a nurse identify as being responsible for the mechanical breakdown of food?
   a. Mouth
   b. Stomach
   c. Small intestine
   d. Pancreas

4. Which layer of the gastrointestinal tract is innermost?
   a. Mucosal layer
   b. Muscularis layer
   c. Nerve plexus layer
   d. Adventitia

5. Which substance is secreted by the chief cells of the stomach?
   a. Gastrin
   b. Hydrochloric acid
   c. Pepsin
   d. Bile

6. After reviewing the process of secretion, a group of students demonstrate understanding when they identify which pancreatic enzyme as being secreted to break down sugars?
   a. Chymotrypsin
   b. Trypsin
   c. Sodium bicarbonate
   d. Amylase

7. Which process is used by the small intestine for motility?
   a. Peristalsis
   b. Churning
   c. Segmentation
   d. Mass movement

8. After teaching a group of students about the reflexes involved in the gastrointestinal tract, the instructor determines that the teaching

has been successful when the students identify which of the following as a central reflex?
   a. Gastroenteric
   b. Somatointestinal
   c. Vomiting
   d. Ileogastric

9. When auscultating bowel sounds on a patient who has had abdominal surgery, the nurse finds that they are absent. The nurse interprets this as indicating a disruption in which of the following?
   a. Ileogastric reflex
   b. Intestinointestinal reflex
   c. Gastroenteric reflex
   d. Gastrocolic reflex

10. Which of the following occurs first when pressure receptors in the back of the throat and pharynx send impulses to the medulla to stimulate nerves?
    a. Soft palate elevates
    b. Larynx rises
    c. Glottis closes
    d. Pharyngeal constrictor muscles contract

11. Which of the following would facilitate the swallowing reflex?
    a. Applying heat to the tongue
    b. Turning the head to one side
    c. Using different textured foods
    d. Providing foods of similar temperature

12. Upon stimulation of the chemotrigger receptor zone, which of the following occurs next?
    a. Increased production of mucus
    b. Increased salivation
    c. Decreased acid production
    d. Increased sweating

13. Which of the following best reflects the gastrointestinal system?
    a. It is one of only a few body systems open to the external environment.
    b. It plays a major role in waste excretion.
    c. It is comprised of one continuous, long tube.
    d. It is subject to high levels of friction with movement.

14. Which of the following would be least likely to increase gastrin secretion?

a. Alcohol

b. Caffeine

c. Proteins

d. High acid levels

15. Which substances are primarily absorbed by the large intestine? Select all that apply.

a. Alcohol

b. Drugs

c. Water

d. Sodium

e. Vitamins

CHAPTER 57

Drugs Affecting Gastrointestinal Secretions

Upon completion of this chapter, you will be able to:

1. Describe the current theories on the pathophysiologic process responsible for the signs and symptoms of peptic ulcer disease.

2. Describe the therapeutic actions, indications, pharmacokinetics, contraindications and cautions, most common adverse reactions, and important drug–drug interactions associated with drugs used to affect gastrointestinal (GI) secretions.

3. Discuss the drugs used to affect GI secretions across the life span.

4. Compare and contrast the prototype drugs used to affect GI secretions with other agents in their class and with other classes of drugs used to affect GI secretions.

5. Outline the nursing considerations, including important teaching points, for patients receiving drugs used to affect GI secretions.

■ ASSESSING YOUR UNDERSTANDING

LABELING

Place the name of the following drugs in the box corresponding to the correct drug class.

Cimetidine   Omeprazole

Esomeprazole   Ranitidine

Nizatidine   Sucralfate

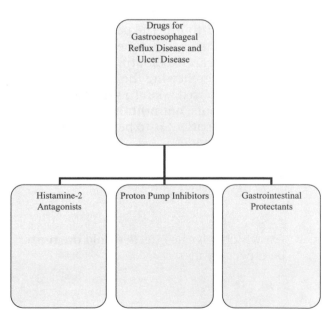

FILL IN THE BLANKS

Provide the missing term or terms in the blanks provided.

1. Histamine-2 receptor antagonists block the release of _____ _____ in response to gastrin.

2. _____ ulcers are often seen in situations such as trauma, burns, or prolonged illness.

3. The only histamine-2 receptor antagonist approved for use in children is _____.

4. The reflex response of the stomach to lower more than normal acid levels is called acid _____ .

5. Antacids _____ stomach acid.

6. An antacid of calcium carbonate often causes _____ and acid rebound; magnesium salt antacids often cause _____.

7. Proton pump inhibitors are typically administered _____ meals.

8. The only gastrointestinal protectant currently available is _____.

■ APPLYING YOUR KNOWLEDGE

CASE STUDY

A 62-year-old man comes to the clinic complaining of heartburn. The patient tells the nurse that he has acid, frequently experiencing a sour taste in his mouth. He states, "I was using Tums and chewing them almost all the time. Then I started taking a liquid antacid like every 2 hours, but nothing seems to be helping." The patient is to be evaluated by the health care provider.

a. What might be happening with this patient and why?

b. For which adverse effects would the nurse be especially alert?

c. What teaching would be important for this patient?

■ PRACTICING FOR NCLEX

Circle the letter that corresponds to the best answer for each question.

1. Which agent would a nurse identify as inhibiting the secretion of gastrin?
   a. Histamine-2 receptor antagonist
   b. Proton pump inhibitor
   c. Antacid
   d. Prostaglandin

2. Which agent would a nurse identify as the prototype histamine-2 receptor antagonist?
   a. Cimetidine
   b. Ranitidine
   c. Famotidine
   d. Nizatidine

3. A nurse is reviewing information about proton pump inhibitors. The nurse recognizes that which of the following is available as an over-the-counter agent?
   a. Lansoprazole
   b. Omeprazole
   c. Rabeprazole
   d. Esomeprazole

4. Which of the following would a nurse expect as most likely to be used in combination with antibiotics for treatment of *Helicobacter pylori* infection?
   a. Famotidine
   b. Calcium carbonate
   c. Omeprazole
   d. Sucralfate

5. A patient is taking an antacid that contains aluminum salts. The nurse would monitor the patient for which of the following?
   a. Diarrhea
   b. Hypercalcemia
   c. Acid rebound
   e. Hypophosphatemia

6. Which of the following would a nurse expect to administer intravenously?

   a. Esomeprazole

   b. Omeprazole

   c. Rabeprazole

   d. Dexlansoprazole

7. Which instruction would be most important to give to a patient who is receiving omeprazole?

   a. "Chew the tablet thoroughly before swallowing."

   b. "Open the capsule and sprinkle it on applesauce."

   c. "Swallow the tablet whole with a large glass of water."

   d. "Take an antacid immediately before taking the drug."

8. After teaching a patient who is receiving sucralfate about the drug, which statement indicates that the teaching has been successful?

   a. "I need to limit my fluid intake."

   b. "I should eat a high-fiber diet."

   c. "I may need something to control diarrhea."

   d. "I need to avoid sugarless lozenges."

9. A patient is receiving pancrelipase. The nurse would expect to administer this drug at which time?

   a. 1 hour before meals

   b. With meals and snacks

   c. At bedtime

   d. First thing on arising

10. Which of the following best reflects the rationale for using histamine-2 receptor antagonists for stress ulcer prophylaxis?

    a. Reduces the overall acid level, promoting healing and comfort

    b. Blocks the overproduction of hydrochloric acid

    c. Decreases the acid being regurgitated into the esophagus

    d. Protects the stomach lining via acid blockage

11. Which agent is associated with antiandrogenic effects?

    a. Ranitidine

    b. Famotidine

    c. Cimetidine

    d. Nizatidine

12. A patient has a history of liver dysfunction. Which histamine-2 receptor antagonist would the nurse expect to be prescribed?

    a. Cimetidine

    b. Famotidine

    c. Ranitidine

    d. Nizatidine

13. A patient is receiving sodium bicarbonate orally. Which of the following would lead the nurse to suspect that the patient is developing systemic alkalosis? Select all that apply.

    a. Headache

    b. Constipation

    c. Confusion

    d. Irritability

    e. Tetany

14. When describing the possible adverse effects associated with omeprazole therapy, which of the following would the nurse identify as least common?

    a. Dizziness

    b. Headache

    c. Alopecia

    d. Cough

15. A patient is receiving sucralfate. The nurse understands that this drug would begin to act within which time frame?

    a. 15 minutes

    b. 30 minutes

    c. 45 minutes

    d. 60 minutes

CHAPTER 58

Drugs Affecting Gastrointestinal Motility

LEARNING OBJECTIVES

Upon completion of this chapter, you will be able to:

1. Describe the underlying processes in diarrhea and constipation and correlate this with the types of drugs used to treat these conditions.

2. Describe the therapeutic actions, indications, pharmacokinetics, contraindications and cautions, most common adverse reactions, and important drug–drug interactions associated with laxatives and antidiarrheal drugs.

3. Discuss the use of laxatives and antidiarrheal agents across the lifespan.

4. Compare and contrast the prototype laxatives and antidiarrheals with other agents in their class and with other classes of laxatives and antidiarrheals.

5. Outline the nursing considerations, including important teaching points, for patients receiving laxatives and antidiarrheal agents.

■ ASSESSING YOUR UNDERSTANDING

LABELING

Place the name of the following drugs in the appropriate box under the correct drug class.

Bisacodyl   Glycerin

Cascara   Lactulose

Castor oil   Magnesium citrate

Docusate   Psyllium

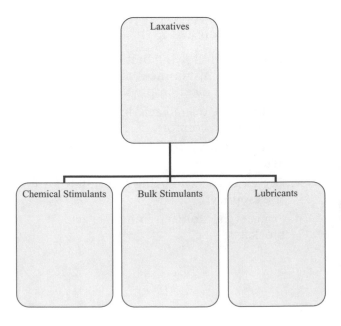

SHORT ANSWER

Supply the information requested.

1. Describe how gastrointestinal (GI) stimulants work.

2. Explain the three methods of action of antidiarrheal agents.

3. Define the term *lubricant* as it refers to GI motility.

4. Compare the action of chemical stimulant laxatives with bulk laxatives.

5. Explain what is meant by cathartic dependence.

6. Describe the action of docusate.

■ APPLYING YOUR KNOWLEDGE

CASE STUDY

A 78-year-old woman comes to the health care agency for a routine checkup. She lives alone in a small two-bedroom senior apartment. During the visit, the patient states that she is "constipated." Further inquiry reveals that she has not had a bowel movement for 2 days. The health care provider recommends psyllium.

a. What factors may be contributing to the patient's constipation?

b. What information would be important to stress with this patient about psyllium?

■ PRACTICING FOR NCLEX

Circle the letter that corresponds to the best answer for each question.

1. A patient is receiving metoclopramide intravenously prior to cancer chemotherapy. The nurse would expect this drug to begin acting within which time frame?
   a. 1 to 5 minutes
   b. 5 to 15 minutes
   c. 15 to 30 minutes
   d. 30 to 45 minutes

2. A group of students are reviewing information about the indications for laxatives. The students demonstrate understanding of the information when they identify which of the following as an indication?
   a. Adjunct to peptic ulcer therapy to eradicate *Helicobacter pylori*
   b. Enhance straining efforts after surgery
   c. Remove ingested poisons from the lower GI tract
   d. Increase secretions and overall activity of the GI tract

3. After teaching a group of students about laxatives, the instructor determines that the teaching has been successful when the students identify which agent as an example of a bulk laxative?
   a. Bisacodyl
   b. Senna
   c. Docusate
   d. Polycarbophil

4. A patient is taking bisacodyl to treat constipation. The nurse suggests that the patient take the drug at which time?
   a. In the morning before breakfast
   b. After eating lunch
   c. At any time during the day
   d. Before going to bed

5. The nurse is preparing to administer cascara to a patient. The nurse anticipates administering this drug by which route?
   a. Oral
   b. Rectal, via enema
   c. Rectal, via suppository
   d. Intramuscular

6. When reviewing the medical record of a patient who is to receive a chemical stimulant laxative, the nurse would monitor the patient closely if he had which condition?
   a. Appendicitis
   b. Diverticulitis
   c. Coronary artery disease
   d. Ulcerative colitis

7. A patient is prescribed polyethylene glycol–electrolyte solution in preparation for a colonoscopy. The nurse would instruct the patient to do which of the following?
   a. "Take one glassful of the liquid."
   b. "Mix a packet in a glass of cold water."
   c. "Take one to eight spoonfuls in a day."
   d. "Drink 8 ounces every 10 minutes."

8. A patient who is taking magnesium citrate experiences sweating, palpitations, and flushing. The nurse understands that this is most likely related to which of the following?
   a. Direct stimulation of the nerve plexus in the abdominal wall
   b. Sympathetic stress reaction due to intense GI tract neurostimulation
   c. Detergent action on the surface of the intestinal bolus
   d. Formation of a slippery coat on the contents of the intestinal tract

9. The nurse is teaching the patient about possible adverse effects associated with mineral oil. Which of the following would be most important for the nurse to include?
   a. Leakage
   b. Abdominal cramping
   c. Diarrhea
   d. Sweating

10. The nurse is preparing to administer dexpanthenol to a patient based on the understanding that this drug acts in which manner?
    a. Blocking dopamine receptors
    b. Increasing acetylcholine levels
    c. Exerting an osmotic pull on fluids
    d. Acting directly on the muscles of the GI tract

11. Which of the following would the nurse expect to administer to a patient with traveler's diarrhea?
    a. Metoclopramide
    b. Loperamide
    c. Bismuth subsalicylate
    d. Opium derivative

12. After describing the drugs used to treat irritable bowel syndrome, the students demonstrate understanding of the information when they identify alosetron as which of the following?
    a. Anticholinergic
    b. Serotonin antagonist
    c. Chloride channel activator
    d. Selective opioid antagonist

13. A patient is diagnosed with traveler's diarrhea, and the health care provider prescribes rifaximin. The nurse describes this drug as which of the following?
    a. Antidiarrheal
    b. GI stimulant
    c. Antibiotic
    d. Opium derivative

14. A patient who is diagnosed with terminal cancer has been using opioids for pain relief and experiencing constipation despite numerous drug therapies and interventions for relief. The nurse anticipates the use of which agent for this patient?
    a. Lubiprostone
    b. Psyllium
    c. Mineral oil
    d. Methylnaltrexone

15. After teaching a class about irritable bowel syndrome, which statement indicates that the teaching has been successful?
    a. The disorder is relatively rare.
    b. It occurs more often in women than in men.
    c. Diarrhea is the predominant complaint.
    d. The cause is primarily stress related.

Antiemetic Agents

Upon completion of this chapter, you will be able to:

1. Outline the vomiting reflex, including factors that stimulate it and mechanisms for measures used to block it.

2. Describe the therapeutic actions, indications, pharmacokinetics, contraindications and cautions, most common adverse reactions, and important drug–drug interactions associated with each of the classes of antiemetic agents.

3. Discuss the use of antiemetics across the lifespan.

4. Compare and contrast the prototype antiemetics with other agents in their class and with other classes of antiemetics.

5. Outline the nursing considerations, including important teaching points, for patients receiving antiemetics.

■ ASSESSING YOUR UNDERSTANDING

LABELING

Place the name of the following drugs in the appropriate box under the correct drug class.

Buclizine	Ondansetron
Dolasetron	Perphenazine
Meclizine	Prochlorperazine

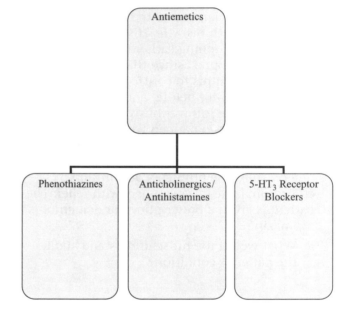

SHORT ANSWER

Supply the information requested.

1. Name the two most common phenothiazines used as antiemetics.

2. Describe the two ways that antiemetics achieve their action.

3. Explain the action of cyclizine.

4. Identify the drug that is used in combination with aprepitant.

5. Name the two drugs that contain the active ingredient of cannabis.

■ APPLYING YOUR KNOWLEDGE

CASE STUDY

A 54-year-old man comes to the emergency department with his wife. His wife states that he started hiccupping earlier that afternoon and has not stopped since that time despite numerous attempts to control the hiccups. "He had this twice before, and they gave him something intravenously and it worked. It always seems to happen when he gets stressed." The patient also has a history of gastroesophageal reflux for which he takes omeprazole. The physician administers chlorpromazine intravenously with relief. The patient is given a prescription for oral chlorpromazine.

a. What would the nurse understand about the patient's condition?

b. What information would be important for the nurse to include when teaching the patient and his wife about chlorpromazine?

■ PRACTICING FOR NCLEX

Circle the letter that corresponds to the best answer for each question.

1. After reviewing the various agents used as antiemetics, a group of students demonstrate understanding of the information when they identify which agent as a 5-HT$_3$ receptor blocker?
   a. Chlorpromazine
   b. Cyclizine
   c. Granisetron
   d. Aprepitant

2. When describing the action of prochlorperazine, which of the following would the nurse include as being affected?
   a. Local response to stimuli
   b. Chemoreceptor trigger zone
   c. Cerebrum
   d. Medulla

3. When reviewing the medical record of a patient who is to receive promethazine, which of the following would indicate to the nurse that the patient needs to be monitored closely?
   a. Active peptic ulcer disease
   b. Severe hypotension
   c. Brain injury
   d. Coma

4. A patient is receiving a phenothiazine antiemetic. The nurse instructs the patient to use the call light if he needs to get out of bed to go to the bathroom based on the understanding that this group of drugs is associated with which of the following?
   a. Gastrointestinal overstimulation
   b. Central nervous system effects
   c. Urinary abnormalities
   d. Endocrine effects

5. A patient is receiving an antiemetic. Which of the following would be most appropriate to facilitate the patient's comfort?
   a. Offering carbonated drinks
   b. Encouraging rapid, shallow breaths
   c. Distracting the patient with activities
   d. Offering mouth care every 4 to 6 hours

6. A patient receives prochlorperazine rectally at 6:00 PM. The nurse would expect the drug to begin acting at approximately which time?
   a. 6:15 PM
   b. 6:45 PM
   c. 7:15 PM
   d. 8:00 PM

7. A patient is to start receiving chemotherapy at 10:00 AM. The patient has an order for intravenous metoclopramide. The nurse would expect to give the drug at which time?

   a. 9:00 AM

   b. 9:30 AM

   c. 10:15 AM

   d. 11:00 AM

8. The nurse would expect a patient with motion sickness to receive which of the following?

   a. Promethazine

   b. Dolasetron

   c. Perphenazine

   d. Cyclizine

9. A patient is receiving meclizine. The nurse would caution the patient to avoid which of the following?

   a. Caffeine

   b. Chocolate

   c. Alcohol

   d. Aged cheese

10. A patient who received palonosetron prior to a chemotherapy session asks the nurse if she can have a prescription for this drug in case she has nausea and vomiting over the next several days. Which of the following would the nurse need to keep in mind when responding to the patient?

    a. Seven days must pass before a repeat dose can be given.

    b. The drug is a controlled substance.

    c. The drug is limited to the days that chemotherapy is given.

    d. The drug can be given for two or three more doses.

11. The nurse is assessing a patient who is receiving aprepitant for adverse effects. Which of the following would the nurse expect to find? Select all that apply.

    a. Dizziness

    b. Dry mouth

    c. Constipation

    d. Anorexia

    e. Headache

    f. Irritability

12. Which agent would the nurse identify as acting directly in the central nervous system to block receptors associated with nausea and vomiting with little to no effect on serotonin, dopamine, or corticosteroid receptors?

    a. Metoclopramide

    b. Aprepitant

    c. Meclizine

    d. Granisetron

13. A patient is receiving palonosetron. The nurse would expect to administer this drug by which route?

    a. Oral

    b. Intramuscular

    c. Subcutaneous

    d. Intravenous

14. After reviewing information about various antiemetic agents, a group of students demonstrate understanding of the information when they identify which drug as similar to antihistamines but not as sedating?

    a. Hydroxyzine

    b. Nabilone

    c. Trimethobenzamide

    d. Dronabinol

15. When describing dronabinol to a group of students, the instructor emphasizes that this antiemetic is classified as which class of controlled substance?

    a. C-I

    b. C-II

    c. C-III

    d. C-IV

Answers

CHAPTER 1

■ ASSESSING YOUR UNDERSTANDING

MATCHING

1. b   **2.** d   **3.** e   **4.** a   **5.** c

SEQUENCING

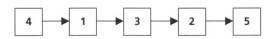

FILL IN THE BLANKS

1. Pharmacotherapeutics
2. Plant
3. Genetic engineering
4. Teratogenic
5. A
6. Orphan

■ APPLYING YOUR KNOWLEDGE

CASE STUDY

a. Knowledge of generic and brand names would help the nurse identify if any of the medications were duplicates of the same drug. Some prescribers specify that a drug prescription be "dispensed as written" such that the brand-name product be used. If the patient was taking medications that were the same but one was a generic form while another was the brand-name form, then he would be at high risk for overdose or toxicity.

b. It would be important to obtain a thorough drug history for this patient. Of special emphasis would be his use of any over-the-counter (OTC) medications. Often patients do not consider OTC drugs to be medications. However, OTC drugs can mask signs and symptoms of underlying disease. They also can cause drug interactions and interfere with drug therapy when taken with prescription drugs. Moreover, not taking these drugs as indicated could result in serious overdoses.

■ PRACTICING FOR NCLEX

1. **Answer: a**
   RATIONALE: An adverse effect is considered a negative effect of a drug, one that is undersirable or potentially dangerous. The intended or therapeutic effect is the response that occurs when the drug is given—that is, the helpful effect. A teratogenic effect is a negative effect on a fetus that occurs when a drug is given.

2. **Answer: c**
   RATIONALE: Clinical pharmacology or pharmacokinetics addresses two key concerns: The drug's effects on the body and the body's response to the drug. The biologic effect of chemicals or drugs relates to pharmacology, which also involves the administration of drugs and the processes used by the body to handle the drugs, such as elimination.

3. **Answer: d**
   RATIONALE: Insulin for treating diabetes was obtained exclusively from the pancreas of cows and pigs, but now genetic engineering has allowed scientists to produce human insulin by altering *Escherichia coli* bacteria. Digitalis, opium, and morphine are derived from plant sources.

4. **Answer: b**
   RATIONALE: Ferrous sulfate, or iron, is a drug derived from the iron salt, an inorganic compound. Thyroid hormone, although created synthetically, may be obtained from animal thyroid tissue. Codeine is obtained from the poppy plant; castor oil is derived from *Ricinus communis*, also a plant.

5. **Answer: d**
   RATIONALE: A drug may be removed from further testing during a phase II study if it produces unacceptable adverse effects, is less effective than anticipated, is too toxic when used with patients, and has a low benefit-to-risk ratio.

6. **Answer: a**
   RATIONALE: During preclinical trials, drugs are tested on laboratory animals. A phase I study uses human volunteers for testing. A phase II study allows investigators to try out the drug in patients who have the disease that the drug is designed to treat. A phase III study involves the use of the drug in a vast clinical market.

7. **Answer: b**
   RATIONALE: Levothyroxine sodium is the generic name. L-thyroxine would be the chemical name; Levothroid or Synthroid would be the brand names.

8. **Answer: d**
   RATIONALE: Phase IV study is a phase of continual evaluation in which prescribers are obligated to report to the Food and Drug Administration (FDA) any untoward or unexpected adverse effects associated with the drugs being used. A phase I study uses human volunteers for testing. A phase II study allows investigators to try out the drug in patients who have the disease that the drug is designed to treat. A phase III study involves the use of the drug in a vast clinical market.

9. **Answer: b**
   RATIONALE: A drug identified as category A would be safest because studies of such a drug have not demonstrated a risk to the fetus in the first trimester of pregnancy and no evidence of risk in later trimesters. A category X drug is one in which studies have demonstrated fetal abnormalities or adverse reactions with reported evidence of fetal

risks. A category B drug is one in which animal studies have not demonstrated a risk to the fetus but there are no adequate studies in pregnant women, or animal studies have shown an adverse effect but adequate studies in pregnant women have not demonstrated a risk to the fetus during the first trimester of pregnancy and there is no evidence of risk in later trimesters. A category C drug is one in which animal studies have shown an adverse effect on the fetus, but there are no adequate studies in humans.

10. **Answer: c**
    RATIONALE: Women are not good candidates for phase I studies because the chemicals may exert unknown and harmful effects on a woman's ova, and too much risk is involved in taking a drug that might destroy or alter the ova. Women do not make new ova after birth. Men produce sperm daily, so there is less potential for complete destruction or alteration of the sperm. Women are not more unreliable, and men are not more consistent in body build or less likely to develop toxic effects.

11. **Answer: d**
    RATIONALE: Small amounts of narcotics such as codeine used as antitussives (cough suppressants) or antidiarrheal agents are classified as schedule V (C-V) controlled substances, which indicates that there is little abuse potential. Schedule II (C-II) drugs, such as narcotics, amphetamines, and barbiturates, have a high abuse potential. Schedule III (C-III) drugs, such as nonbarbiturate sedatives or nonamphetamine stimulants, have less abuse potential than C-II. Schedule IV (C-IV) drugs, such as some sedatives, antianxiety agents, and nonnarcotic analgesics, have less abuse potential than C-III drugs.

12. **Answer: d**
    RATIONALE: The Kefauver–Harris Act of 1962 gave the FDA regulatory control over the testing and evaluating of drugs and set standards for efficacy and safety. The Pure Food and Drug Act of 1906 prevented the marketing of adulterated drugs and required labeling to eliminate false or misleading claims. The Federal Food, Drug, and Cosmetic Act of 1938 mandated tests for drug toxicity and provided means for recall of drugs and gave the FDA the power of enforcement. The Durham–Humphrey Amendment of 1951 tightened control over certain drugs and required specification of drugs to be labeled "may not be distributed without a prescription."

13. **Answer: c**
    RATIONALE: The Drug Enforcement Agency, a part of the U.S. Department of Justice, is the agency responsible for enforcing the control of substances with abuse potential. The FDA, an agency in the U.S. Department of Health and Human Services, is responsible for studying drugs and determining their abuse potential.

14. **Answer: d**
    RATIONALE: Genetic engineering is a technologically advanced technique that allows drugs to be created. Plants, animals, and inorganic compounds are examples of natural sources for drugs.

15. **Answer: c**
    RATIONALE: In a phase II study, clinical investigators try out the drug in patients who have the disease that the drug is designed to treat. Preclinical trials involve the use of animal testing of a drug. A phase I study involves the use of human volunteers, usually healthy young men, to test a drug. A phase III study involves the use of the drug in a vast clinical market.

CHAPTER 2

■ ASSESSING YOUR UNDERSTANDING
SEQUENCING

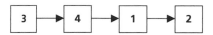

MATCHING
1. c   2. d   3. b   4. a

FILL IN THE BLANKS
1. Pharmacodynamics
2. Pharmacokinetics
3. Agonist
4. Passive diffusion
5. Biotransformation

■ APPLYING YOUR KNOWLEDGE
CASE STUDY

a. Several factors would be most important for the nurse to consider. First, the patient's age may affect all aspects of pharmacokinetics due to the myriad physical changes that occur as part of the aging process. Second, the patient's weight may be a factor necessitating a larger dose to obtain a therapeutic effect. Third, the patient's history of kidney disease may be a factor necessitating a lower dose due to possible interference with the drug's excretion.

b. Other factors that might play a role include the patient's gender (women have more fat cells than men do; thus, drugs depositing in fat may be slowly released and cause prolonged effects); physiologic factors such as hydration status, which could affect the way a drug works on the body; and environmental factors, which could exacerbate or decrease the effectiveness of the drug, in particular antihypertensive agents. In addition, the genetic, immunologic, and psychological factors may play a role in altering the effectiveness of the prescribed therapy.

■ PRACTICING FOR NCLEX

1. **Answer: a**
   RATIONALE: Pharmacodynamics, or how drugs affect the body, involves the action of enzyme systems and receptor sites. Critical concentration, dynamic equilibrium, and protein binding are associated with pharmacokinetics.

2. **Answer: c**
   RATIONALE: Generally, drugs given by the oral route are absorbed more slowly than those given parenterally. Of the parenteral routes, intravenously administered drugs are absorbed the fastest.

3. **Answer: b**
   RATIONALE: Drugs that are tightly bound to protein are released very slowly and have a very long duration of action because they are not free to be broken down or excreted. Drugs that are loosely bound tend to act quickly and to be excreted quickly. Drugs that compete with each other for protein binding sites alter the effectiveness or cause toxicity when the two drugs are given together.

4. **Answer: c**
   RATIONALE: Drugs that are taken orally are usually absorbed from the small intestine directly into the portal venous system (the blood vessels that flow through the liver on their way back to the heart). The portal veins deliver these absorbed molecules into the liver, which immediately transforms most of the chemicals delivered to it by a series of liver enzymes that break the drug into

metabolites, some of which are active and cause effects in the body and some of which are deactivated and can be readily excreted from the body. As a result, a large percentage of the oral dose is destroyed at this point and never reaches the tissues. This phenomenon is known as the first-pass effect. The portion of the drug that gets through the first-pass effect is delivered to the circulatory system for transport throughout the body. Injected drugs and drugs absorbed from sites other than the gastrointestinal tract undergo a similar biotransformation when they pass through the liver. However, some of the active drug already has had a chance to reach the reactive tissues before reaching the liver.

5. **Answer: d**
RATIONALE: Phase II biotransformation usually involves a conjugation reaction that makes the drug less polar and more readily excreted by the kidneys. Phase I biotransformation involves oxidation, reduction, or hydrolysis of the drug via the cytochrome P450 system of enzymes.

6. **Answer: c**
RATIONALE: Ketoconazole is an example of a drug that inhibits the activity of the cytochrome P450 enzyme system. Nicotine, alcohol, and glucocorticoids, such as cortisone, increase the activity of this enzyme system.

7. **Answer: b**
RATIONALE: Although the skin, saliva, lungs, bile, and feces are some of the routes used to excrete drugs, the kidneys play the most important role in drug excretion.

8. **Answer: c**
RATIONALE: For each 8 hours, the drug would be reduced by one-half. Thus, after 8 hours, there would be 125 mg remaining; after the next 8 hours (16 hours later), there would be 62.5 mg (125/2) remaining; and after the next 8 hours (or 24 hours later), there would be 31.25 mg (62.5/2) remaining.

9. **Answer: a**
RATIONALE: A loading dose, which is used to obtain needed effects quickly, uses a higher dose than usual to reach critical concentration. A loading dose does not enhance absorption, prevent drug breakdown by stomach acid, or prolong the half-life.

10. **Answer: c**
RATIONALE: The liver is the single most important site of drug metabolism. If it is not functioning properly, the drug may not be metabolized correctly and may reach toxic levels in the body. Liver disease does not affect absorption or distribution. Kidney disease would affect drug excretion.

11. **Answer: b**
RATIONALE: Passive diffusion is the major process through which drugs are absorbed into the body. Active transport, although not very important in the absorption of most drugs, is very important in drug excretion. Filtration also is an important process used in drug excretion, not absorption. Protein binding is an important mechanism involved in distribution of a drug.

12. **Answer: d**
RATIONALE: A patient with a history of vascular disease or low blood pressure may experience an alteration in the distribution of a drug, preventing it from being delivered to the reactive tissue. A history of gastrointestinal disorders can affect the absorption of many drugs; liver disease may affect the way a drug is biotransformed; and kidney disease may affect the way a drug is excreted.

13. **Answer: a**
RATIONALE: Pharmacogenomics is a new area of study that explores unique differences in response to drugs that an individual possesses based on genetic makeup. Pharmacodynamics refers to how the drug affects the body; pharmacokinetics refers to how the body acts on drugs. Pharmacology refers to the study of the biologic effects of chemicals.

14. **Answer: c**
RATIONALE: The receptor site is the area on a cell membrane where many drugs are thought to act. The process is similar to how a key works in a lock, where the chemical (the key) approaches a cell membrane and finds a perfect fit (the lock) at a receptor site. The enzyme system acts as a catalyst for various chemical reactions. An agonist is a drug that interacts directly with receptors sites to cause the same activity that natural chemicals would cause at this site.

15. **Answer: b**
RATIONALE: Penicillin affecting only bacterial cells is an example of selective toxicity, the property of a drug that affects only systems found in foreign cells without affecting healthy human cells. Critical concentration is the concentration a drug must reach in the tissues that respond to the particular drug to cause the desired effect. First-pass effect is a phenomenon in which drugs given orally are carried directly to the liver after absorption, where they may be largely inactivated by liver enzymes before they can enter the general circulation. Enzyme induction is the process by which the presence of a chemical that is biotransformed by a particular enzyme system in the liver causes increased activity of that enzyme system.

CHAPTER 3

■ ASSESSING YOUR UNDERSTANDING

MATCHING

1. d   2. b   3. c   4. a

SHORT ANSWER

1. Reasons that adverse effects may occur include the following: The drug may have other effects on the body besides the therapeutic effect; the patient is sensitive to the drug being given; the drug's action on the body causes other responses that are undesirable or unpleasant; or the patient is taking too much or too little of the drug, leading to adverse effects.

2. Before administering any drug to a patient, it is important to review the contraindications and cautions associated with that drug as well as the anticipated adverse effects of the drug. This information will direct your assessment of the patient, helping you to focus on particular signs and symptoms that would alert you to contraindications or to proceed cautiously and to establish a baseline for that patient so that you will be able to identify adverse effects that occur.

3. One of the most common occurrences in drug therapy is the development of adverse effects from simple overdosage. In such cases, the patient suffers from effects that are merely an extension of the desired effect.

4. Drug allergies fall into four main classifications: anaphylactic reactions, cytotoxic reactions, serum sickness, and delayed reactions.

5. One of the body's protective mechanisms is the wide variety of bacteria that live within or on the surface of the body. This bacterial growth is called *normal flora*. The normal flora protect the body from invasion by other bacteria, viruses, fungi, and so on. Several kinds of drugs (especially antibiotics) destroy the normal flora, leading to

the development of superinfections or infections caused by the usually controlled organisms.

6. Blood dyscrasia refers to bone marrow depression caused by drug effects on the rapidly multiplying cells of the bone marrow.

7. The electrolyte that can cause the most serious effects when it is altered, even a little, is potassium.

8. Anticholinergic effects may include dry mouth, altered taste perception, dysphagia, heartburn, constipation, bloating, paralytic ileus, urinary hesitancy and retention, impotence, blurred vision, cycloplegia, photophobia, headache, mental confusion, nasal congestion, palpitations, decreased sweating, and dry skin.

■ APPLYING YOUR KNOWLEDGE

CASE STUDY

a. The use of antihistamines is associated with the development of anticholinergic effects. These may include dry mouth, altered taste perception, dysphagia, heartburn, constipation, bloating, paralytic ileus, urinary hesitancy and retention, impotence, blurred vision, cycloplegia, photophobia, headache, mental confusion, nasal congestion, palpitations, decreased sweating, and dry skin. The nurse should focus the assessment on these effects.

b. The nurse would need to question the patient further about what signs and symptoms she experienced specifically related to the use of codeine. For example, the nurse could ask, "What exactly happens when you take codeine?" Many people state that they have a drug allergy because of the effects of the drug. For example, a rash may suggest an allergy, but sleepiness or sedation may reflect the therapeutic effect or, if excessive, a hypersensitivity to the drug's effect. Additional questions may include asking the patient how often she has taken the codeine and whether this (these) reaction(s) occurred only once or with subsequent use. For a true allergy, the patient develops antibodies to a particular drug.

■ PRACTICING FOR NCLEX

1. **Answer: b**
   RATIONALE: Secondary actions are effects that are inevitable and undesired but not related to the desired pharmacologic effects. Nausea and diarrhea are examples of secondary actions due to an antibiotic's effect on the gastrointestinal tract. Primary actions are those associated with the therapeutic effect. Drug allergy involves the formation of antibodies to a particular drug. Hypersensitivity refers to an excessive response to either primary or secondary effects of a drug.

2. **Answer: c**
   RATIONALE: For a patient experiencing a cytotoxic reaction, the prescriber is notified and the drug is discontinued. Subcutaneous epinephrine is used to treat an anaphylactic reaction. The patient is also encouraged to wear some type of Medic-alert identification denoting the allergy. Antipyretics would be used to treat serum sickness reaction.

3. **Answer: d**
   RATIONALE: Serum sickness reaction is manifested by an itchy rash, high fever, swollen lymph nodes, swollen and painful joints, and edema of the face and limbs. Hives and difficulty breathing would be associated with an anaphylactic reaction. Decreased white blood cell count would be associated with a cytotoxic reaction.

4. **Answer: c**
   RATIONALE: For stomatitis, the nurse should recommend frequent mouth care with a nonirritating solution. This may include frequent rinsing with cool liquids. The patient should consume frequent small meals rather than three large meals. An astringent mouthwash or a firm toothbrush would be too irritating.

5. **Answer: a**
   RATIONALE: Superinfection is caused by several kinds of drugs, especially antibiotics (which destroy the normal flora). Antihistamines, antihypertensives, and antineoplastics are not typically associated with superinfection.

6. **Answer: a, b, f**
   RATIONALE: Manifestations of blood dyscrasia include anemia, thrombocytopenia, sore throat, fever, chills, back pain, dark urine, leukopenia, and a reduction of all cellular elements of the complete blood count.

7. **Answer: d**
   RATIONALE: Renal injury is reflected by elevated blood urea nitrogen and creatinine concentration. Liver injury would be reflected by elevated liver enzymes such as aspartate aminotransferase (AST) and alanine aminotransferase (ALT). Hypoglycemia would be indicated by decreased blood glucose levels. Hyperkalemia would be reflected by elevated potassium levels (greater than 5.0 mEq/L).

8. **Answer: b**
   RATIONALE: Drugs with anticholinergic effects often cause dry mouth, constipation, dehydration, and decreased sweating. The patient should be instructed to drink fluids to prevent dehydration and to avoid overly warm or hot environments. In addition, the patient should use sugarless lozenges and perform frequent mouth care to combat dry mouth. A high-fiber diet would be indicated to prevent constipation. Diarrhea is an anticholinergic effect.

9. **Answer: c**
   RATIONALE: Neuroleptic malignant syndrome is manifested by extrapyramidal symptoms, including slowed reflexes, rigidity, and involuntary movements; hyperthermia; and autonomic disturbances, such as hypertension, fast heart rate, and fever.

10. **Answer: a**
    RATIONALE: The manifestations exhibited reflect Parkinson-like syndrome commonly associated with many of the antipsychotic and neuroleptic drugs. These symptoms are not associated with antidiabetic agents, general anesthetics, or anticholinergic agents.

11. **Answer: d**
    RATIONALE: All drugs are potentially dangerous. Even though chemicals are carefully screened and tested in animals and in people before they are released as drugs, drug products often cause unexpected or unacceptable reactions when they are administered. Drugs are chemicals, and the human body operates by a vast series of chemical reactions. Consequently, many effects can be seen when just one chemical factor is altered. Today's potent and amazing drugs can cause a great variety of reactions, many of which are more severe than ever seen before.

12. **Answer: c**
    RATIONALE: A patient taking an antihistamine who experiences drowsiness is an example of a secondary action. The antihistamine is very effective in drying up secretions and helping breathing—the therapeutic effect. Bleeding associated with anticoagulant therapy or a patient taking a recommended dose of antihypertensive who becomes dizzy or weak is an example of a primary action. Urinary

retention in a patient with an enlarged prostate taking an anticholinergic agent is an example of hypersensitivity.

13. Answer: a, b, e

RATIONALE: Anaphylactic reaction would be manifested by hives, rash, difficulty breathing, increased blood pressure, dilated pupils, diaphoresis, panic feeling, increased heart rate, and respiratory arrest. High fever and swollen joints would be associated with serum sickness reaction.

14. Answer: d

RATIONALE: A delayed allergic reaction is manifested by rash, hives, and swollen joints, similar to the reaction to poison ivy. Skin care, comfort measures, antihistamines, or topical steroids may be used. Epinephrine would be used to treat an anaphylactic reaction. Antipyretics and anti-inflammatory agents may be used to treat serum sickness reaction.

15. Answer: a

RATIONALE: Signs of hypoglycemia, or low blood glucose level, include fatigue; drowsiness; hunger; anxiety; headache; cold, clammy skin; shaking and lack of coordination (tremulousness); increased heart rate; increased blood pressure; numbness and tingling of the mouth, tongue, and/or lips; confusion; and rapid and shallow respirations. In severe cases, seizures and/or coma may occur. Increased urination, fruity breath odor, and increased hunger are signs of hyperglycemia.

CHAPTER 4

■ ASSESSING YOUR UNDERSTANDING

MATCHING

1. b   **2.** e   **3.** a   **4.** c   **5.** d

SHORT ANSWER

1. Application of the nursing process with drug therapy ensures that the patient receives the best, safest, most efficient, scientifically based, holistic care.

2. Two major aspects associated with assessment are the patient's history (past illnesses and the current problem) and examination of his or her physical status.

3. The seven rights are as follows: right drug, right storage, right route, right dosage, right preparation, right time, and right recording.

4. Areas to address when obtaining a patient's history include chronic conditions, drug use, allergies, level of education and understanding, social supports, financial supports, and pattern of health care.

5. Patients often neglect to mention over-the-counter drugs or alternative therapies because they do not consider them to be actual drugs or they may be unwilling to admit their use to the health care provider.

6. A patient's weight helps determine whether the recommended drug dosage is appropriate. Because the recommended dosage typically is based on a 150-pound adult male, patients who are much lighter or much heavier often need a dosage adjustment.

7. The specific parameters that need to be assessed depend on the disease process being treated as well as the expected therapeutic and adverse effects of the drug therapy. Assessing these factors before drug therapy begins provides a baseline level to which future assessments can be compared to determine the effects of drug therapy.

8. The placebo effect refers to the anticipation that a drug will be helpful.

LABELING

Assessment	Nursing Diagnosis
b, d, e	a, h
Implementation	**Evaluation**
c, g	f

■ APPLYING YOUR KNOWLEDGE

CASE STUDY

a. The patient's history of heart disease and diabetes are possible factors that could affect the pharmacokinetics and pharmacodynamics of a drug. The nurse would need to research the specific drug to determine if these conditions would be contraindications to use or require cautious use.

b. The patient is somewhat underweight for his height. Thus, the typical recommended dose may be too great for this patient. The nurse would need to obtain the patient's weight and compare it with the standard weight (150 pounds) used for drug therapy. If the patient's weight is much lighter, a dosage reduction might be necessary.

c. Several issues may affect the patient's compliance. The patient's ability to understand explanations and teaching may be hampered by his limited ability to speak English. The nurse would need to include the patient's friend in any teaching and explanation to ensure that the patient understands the information. The patient also has limited social supports, such that he lives alone and the nearest relative is about an hour away. Financial supports also may be limited.

■ PRACTICING FOR NCLEX

1. Answer: a

RATIONALE: Gathering information is the first step—assessment—of the nursing process. Nursing diagnosis is a statement about the patient's status from a nursing perspective. Implementation involves planning patient care and intervening. Evaluation determines the effectiveness of the care and therapy.

2. Answer: d

RATIONALE: Implementation involves planning patient care and intervention. Providing patient teaching would be a part of implementation. Developing a problem statement is done during the nursing diagnosis step. Obtaining baseline information about the patient's health patterns and identifying the patient's social support system would be completed during assessment.

3. Answer: b

RATIONALE: The nursing process is a continual dynamic cyclical process of problem solving that occurs as series of steps to ensure that a patient receives the best, safest, most efficient, scientifically based, holistic care. It is not static or linear. Assessment, one step of the nursing process, allows information to be obtained to determine the patient's current status, priority needs, and problems.

4. Answer: b

RATIONALE: Chronic conditions, such as renal disease, heart disease, diabetes, or chronic lung disease, can affect the pharmacokinetics and pharmacodynamics of a drug and may be contraindications to the use of a drug. Or, these conditions may require cautious use or dosage adjustment when administering a certain drug. Pneumonia, near sightedness, or an episode of gastroenteritis would not be as significant as a history of kidney disease.

5. Answer: d
RATIONALE: Patients typically are not involved with reporting medication errors. Reporting is the responsibility of national- and institutional-level agencies; thus, this information would not be included in patient teaching about drug therapy. Alternative therapies to avoid, timing of administration, and drug toxicity warning signs would be important points to cover in a patient teaching program.

6. Answer: c
RATIONALE: A drug order should never be written as .5 mg because it could be interpreted as 5 mg, which would be 10 times the ordered dose. The proper dosage would be 0.5 mg. An order for 5.0 mg also requires caution because it could be interpreted as 50 mg.

7. Answer: b
RATIONALE: When administering a topical drug, the nurse needs to determine if the skin needs to be prepared in a specific way because topical agents may require specific handling. Reconstitution would apply to parenteral drugs. Crushing refers to oral drugs. The nurse should always apply the ordered dose or amount.

8. Answer: d
RATIONALE: The patient should know what each of the drugs is being used to treat to ensure a better understanding of what to report, what to watch for, and when to report to the health care provider if the drug is not working. The patient should keep a list of all drugs taken, including prescription, over-the-counter, and herbal medications. Medications should be stored in a dry place, away from children or pets. Storage in the bathroom, which may be hot and humid, may cause drugs to break down faster. The patient should read the labels and follow the directions so that if there are specific times to take the drug, they are followed.

9. Answer: d, b, a, c
RATIONALE: Applying the nursing process steps, the nurse would first question the patient about any chronic conditions, then identify problems related to functioning, then teach the patient about ways to minimize adverse effects, and finally determine that the drug is being effective.

10. Answer: b
RATIONALE: Adult medications should never be used to treat a child. The body organs and systems of children are very different from those of an adult. Parents should read all labels before giving a child a drug, especially over-the-counter products because many of these may contain the same ingredients, thereby accidently overdosing the child. Liquid medications should be measured with appropriate measuring devices such as a measured dosing device or spoon from a measuring set. The parents should never use a flatware teaspoon or tablespoon to measure a child's drugs. Health care providers do not always know what a child is taking, so parents need to keep a list of all medications given to a child, including prescription, over-the-counter, and herbal medicines.

11. Answer: a
RATIONALE: The patient is reporting a problem with ingesting adequate food and nutrients. Therefore, imbalanced nutrition: Less than body requirements would be most appropriate. Risk for imbalanced fluid volume may be a problem if the patient were experiencing vomiting or diarrhea that could lead to excess fluid loss. The patient is not verbalizing a problem with feeding himself. Rather, he is reporting difficulty in eating or consuming adequate food. The patient is taking the medication, so he is not noncompliant.

12. Answer: c
RATIONALE: Developing outcomes is a component of the implementation phase of the nursing process. Obtaining information about the patient's drug use, data about financial constraints, and information about the patient's level of understanding are important aspects of the assessment phase.

13. Answer: b, a, d, c
RATIONALE: The nursing process consists of four major steps in this order: assessment, nursing diagnosis, implementation, and evaluation. The steps overlap and are continuous and dynamic.

14. Answer: a
RATIONALE: The nurse questions the patient about the use of alternative therapies because they can interact with prescribed drugs, causing unwanted or even dangerous drug–drug interactions. Depending on the prescribed drug, the alternative therapy may or may not need to be stopped. There is no evidence to support that alternative therapies increase the risk for addiction. Although the patient's use of alternative therapies may provide some clues as to the patient's health beliefs, this is not the reason for questioning the patient about them as they relate to drug therapy.

15. Answer: b
RATIONALE: If a nurse sees or participates in a medication error, the nurse needs to report it to the institution and then report it to the national reporting program. This report would then be shared with the appropriate agencies, such as the Food and Drug Administration, the drug manufacturer, and the Institute for Safe Medication Practices.

CHAPTER 5

■ ASSESSING YOUR UNDERSTANDING
FILL IN THE BLANKS
1. Cubic centimeter
2. Clark's
3. 1,000
4. Ten
5. Unit

CROSSWORD

■ APPLYING YOUR KNOWLEDGE

CASE STUDY

a. The nurse needs to determine if the mother understands the need for accurate dosage and the prescribed dosage amount to be given to minimize the risk to the child. In addition, the nurse needs to determine if the mother has an appropriate measuring device (a standardized measuring device) in the home for accurate dosage. The nurse should question the mother about what she uses to give liquid medications to her child.

b. The nurse would need to emphasize the need for using a standardized measuring device for the dosage. The nurse should explain that the typical flatware teaspoon or tablespoon or drinking cup varies tremendously in the volume contained. The nurse needs to urge the mother not to use these devices for measuring. Instead, the nurse should instruct the mother to use a standardized measuring device. If the mother does not have one, then the nurse could suggest to the mother where to obtain one or, if appropriate, supply the mother with one. The nurse could also contact the pharmacy where the prescription will be filled to ask if one could be provided with the prescription or assist the mother in finding one. Usually, most pharmacies have these relatively inexpensive devices readily available.

■ PRACTICING FOR NCLEX

1. **Answer: b**
   RATIONALE: The avoirdupois system is an older system that was very popular when pharmacists routinely had to compound medications on their own. The household system of measurement is the system that is commonly found in recipe books. The apothecary system is a very old system of measurement specifically developed for use by apothecaries or pharmacists. The metric system is the most widely used system of measure.

2. **Answer: c**
   RATIONALE: The apothecary system includes units such as grain, dram, ounce, minim, fluidram, and fluid ounce. Liters and kilograms are units in the metric system. Pound is a unit in the household system.

3. **Answer: a**
   RATIONALE: The metric system is the most widely used system of measure. The apothecary system and avoirdupois system are rarely used in the clinical setting. The household system is the measuring system found in most recipe books used at home.

4. **Answer: c**
   RATIONALE: In the metric system, the basic unit of liquid measure is the liter; the basic unit of solid measure is the gram. The kilogram is another unit used for solid measure in the metric system. The minim is the basic unit of liquid measure in the apothecary system.

5. **Answer: b**
   RATIONALE: One grain in the apothecary system of measure is equivalent to 60 mg. Fifteen grains would be equivalent to 1 g or 1,000 mg. One-half grain would be equivalent to 30 mg. Eight fluid ounces would be equivalent to 240 mL in the metric system.

6. **Answer: a**
   RATIONALE: To convert 3 fluid ounces to the metric system, the nurse would set up the following ratio and proportion using the equivalent of 1 fluid ounce = 30 mL:

   $$1/30 = 3/X$$

   Cross multiplying: $1X = 90$; $X = 90$

7. **Answer: b**
   RATIONALE: To determine the amount to give, the nurse would set up the following ratio and proportion using Amount of drug available/One tablet or capsule = Amount of drug prescribed/Number of tablets/Capsules to give:

   $$5 \text{ gr}/1 \text{ tablet} = 10 \text{ gr}/X$$

   Cross multiplying: $5X = 10$; solving for X: $X = 2$

8. **Answer: a**
   RATIONALE: To determine the amount to give, the nurse would set up the following ratio and proportion using Amount of drug available/Volume available = Amount of drug prescribed/Volume to administer:

   $$500 \text{ mg}/5 \text{ mL} = 250 \text{ mL}/X$$

   Cross multiplying: $500X = 1,250$; solving for X: $X = 2.5 \text{ mL}$

9. **Answer: d**
   RATIONALE: To determine the amount to give, the nurse would set up the following ratio and proportion using Amount of drug available/Volume available = Amount of drug prescribed/Volume to administer:

   $$500 \text{ mL}/1 \text{ mL} = 250 \text{ mL}/X$$

   Cross multiplying: $250X = 500$; solving for X: $X = 2$

10. **Answer: b**
    RATIONALE: To determine the flow rate (gtts/minute), the nurse would set up the following ratio using mL of solution prescribed per hour × Drops delivered per mL/60 minutes/1 hour:

    $$X = \frac{1,000 \text{ mL}/8 \text{ hours} \times 15 \text{ gtts/minute}}{60 \text{ minutes}/1 \text{ hour}}$$

    $$X = \frac{125 \text{ mL/hour} \times 15 \text{ gtts/minute}}{60 \text{ minutes/hour}}$$

    $$X = \frac{1,875 \text{ drops/hour}}{60 \text{ minutes/hour}}$$

    $X = 31.25$ gtts/minute or 32 gtts/minute

11. **Answer: d**
    RATIONALE: Today, the body surface area (nomogram) is considered the most accurate way for determining dosages. The Clark, Fried, and Young rules are rarely used today.

12. **Answer: a, c**
    RATIONALE: To use Clark's rule (Weight of child in pounds/150 pounds X Average adult dose), the nurse needs to know the child's weight in pounds and average adult dose. The child's age in years would be important for using Young's rule. The child's height in centimeters is needed to determine body surface area. Body surface area is not used with the Fried, Clark or Young rules. It is a separate method for calculating pediatric dosages.

13. **Answer: d**
    RATIONALE: Using the mg/kg method, the nurse would set up the problem as follows:

    $$1.1 \text{ mg}/1 \text{ kg} = X \text{ mg}/22 \text{ kg}$$

    Cross multiplying: $1X = 24.2$; solving for X: $X = 24.2$, which would be rounded down to 24 mg.

14. **Answer: b**
    RATIONALE: In 1995, the U.S. Pharmacopeia Convention established standards requiring that all prescriptions, regardless of the system used in drug dosage, include the metric measure for quantity and strength. The Food and Drug Administration and the Institute for Safe Medication Practices are involved with medication errors. The Drug Enforcement Agency enforces control over drugs with abuse potential.

15. Answer: a, b, d, e
   RATIONALE: Units in the household system of measurement include pint, quart, gallon, ounces, cups, tablespoons, teaspoons, drops, and pounds. Dram is a unit of measure in the apothecary system. Milliliter is a unit of measure in the metric system.

CHAPTER 6

■ ASSESSING YOUR UNDERSTANDING

MATCHING

1. d	**2.** e	**3.** g	**4.** c	**5.** b
6. j	**7.** h	**8.** f	**9.** i	**10.** a

SHORT ANSWER

1. One factor involved in the review process is the ability of the patient for self-care, which is the act of self-diagnosing and determining one's own treatment needs.

2. Patients often do not mention the use of alternative therapies to the health care provider. Some patients believe that the health care provider will disapprove of the use of these products and do not want to discuss it; others believe that these are just natural products and do not need to be mentioned.

3. Areas impacting health care including drug therapy in the 21st century include consumers having access to medical and pharmacologic information from many sources and taking steps to demand specific treatments and considerations; offering and advertising of alternative therapies at a record pace, causing people to rethink their approach to medical care and the medical system; financial pressures leading to early discharge of patients from health care facilities and to provision of outpatient care for patients who, in the past, would have been hospitalized and monitored closely; health care providers being pushed to make decisions about patient care and prescriptions based on finances in addition to medical judgment; events of 9/11 and the increased threat of terrorism leading to serious concerns about dealing with exposure to biological or chemical weapons; increasing illicit drug use (at an all-time high), bringing increased health risks and safety concerns; and increasing concerns about the environment and the need to protect it from contamination.

4. Possible health consequences of anabolic steroid abuse include hypertension, hyperlipidemia, acne, cancer, and cardiomyopathy.

5. A biological weapon, or germ warfare, uses bacteria, viruses, and parasites on a large scale to incapacitate or destroy a population.

■ APPLYING YOUR KNOWLEDGE

CASE STUDY

a. The nurse needs to caution the patient about the information he received from his neighbor. Each person responds to medications differently, so what might seem to work for one patient might not work for another. In addition, the nurse needs to talk with the patient about the Internet as a source for information, informing the patient that not all information presented is accurate or reputable.

b. The nurse should help the patient sift through the information to determine if it is appropriate or relevant to this patient. The nurse also could provide the patient with a list of reputable Internet resources that the patient can use to search for information. In addition, the nurse should provide the patient with tips for evaluating Web sites—for example, the way to identify appropriate sources through their Web address, recent updates of information, information that is supported by other sites, and credentials of the author or contributor.

c. The nurse must inform the patient that herbal remedies are not controlled or tested by the Food and Drug Administration (FDA) and as such are considered dietary supplements. Other concerns that need to be addressed include lack of testing of the active ingredients in these products and that if test results are available, they typically were for only a very small number of people with no reproducible results; lack of information about the incidental ingredients in many of these products (some may come directly from plants or from a natural state, the fertilizer used for the plant, the time of the year when the plant was harvested, and the other ingredients that are compounded with the product), which have a direct effect on efficacy; and the increased risk for possible interactions or serious complications when used with prescription medications.

   If the patient wishes to use an alternative therapy with the medication regimen prescribed, then the patient and nurse need to talk with the health care prescriber because drug dosages or timing of the various drugs may need to be changed.

■ PRACTICING FOR NCLEX

1. Answer: c
   RATIONALE: It is not unusual for the media to make current medical research or reports into news. Advertisements of prescription drugs directly to the public became legal in the 1990s. Federal guidelines are present to determine what can be said in an advertisement, but in some cases this further confuses the issue for many consumers. Many standard talk shows include a medical segment that presents just a tiny bit of information frequently out of context—for example, the "disease of the week," which opens a whole new area of interest for the viewer.

2. Answer: a
   RATIONALE: Due to cost, patients may be tempted to stop taking an antibiotic in order to save the remaining pills for the next time they feel sick and to save the costs of another health care visit and a new prescription. This practice has contributed to the problem of resistant bacteria, which is becoming more dangerous all the time. The creation of a matrix delivery system for many medications can lead to toxicity or ineffectiveness if the patient attempts to split the drug. Generic drug availability in many cases reduces the cost of a drug but is unrelated to the development of resistant bacteria. Drugs obtained via the Internet may be cheaper, but the FDA has found many discrepancies between what was ordered and what is in the product.

3. Answer: d
   RATIONALE: The Centers for Disease Control and Prevention (CDC) posts regularly updated information on signs and symptoms of infection by various biological agents, guidelines for management, and ongoing research. The FDA Web site would be helpful for information about

drugs, including those obtained via the Internet and off-label use of drugs. Drug Facts and Comparisons provides a cost comparison of drugs in each class. The National Center for Complementary and Alternative Medicine is a reputable source for information on alternative therapies.

4. **Answer: b**
RATIONALE: Using a drug for off-label use involves using the drug for a situation not on the approved list for which it may be effective. Such use may eventually lead to a new approval of the drug for the new indication. Liability surrounding off-label use is unclear. Drugs often used for off-label indications include the drugs used to treat various psychiatric problems. Off-label use occurs after the drug has received FDA approval for the specific therapeutic indications and then is used for situations that are not part of those stated for approval.

5. **Answer: c**
RATIONALE: Gamma-hydroxybutyrate, or GHB, is a depressant. Cocaine or methamphetamine is considered a stimulant. LSD or MDMA is considered a hallucinogen. Fentanyl, morphine, or OxyContin is an opioid.

6. **Answer: d**
RATIONALE: Although ordering drugs on the Internet (often from other countries) may be cheaper, do not require the patient to see a health care provider (many of these sites simply have customers fill out a questionnaire that is reviewed by a doctor), and are delivered right to the patient's door, there are many discrepancies in these drugs when compared with those obtained through usual methods, such as a pharmacy.

7. **Answer: c**
RATIONALE: The patient should take any unused, unneeded, or expired prescription drugs out of their original containers, mix them with an undesirable substance (such as coffee grounds or kitty litter), and put them in an impermeable, nondescript container such as an empty can or sealable bag and then throw the closed container in the trash. Prescription drugs should be flushed only if the patient information specifically instructs that this is safe to do.

8. **Answer: b**
RATIONALE: St. John's wort, a highly advertised and popular alternative therapy, has been found to interact with oral contraceptives, digoxin (a heart medication), the selective serotonin reuptake inhibitors (used for depression), theophylline (a drug used to treat lung disease), various antineoplastic drugs used to treat cancer, and the antivirals used to treat AIDS. It has not been shown to interact with acetaminophen or ibuprofen. Insulin or other antidiabetic agents interact with juniper berries, ginseng, garlic, fenugreek, coriander, dandelion root, and celery to cause hypoglycemia.

9. **Answer: a, b, c**
RATIONALE: If a drug advertisement states what the drug is used for, it must also state adverse effects, contraindications, and precautions. Doses and route of administration are not required to be included.

10. **Answer: d**
RATIONALE: Gone is the era when the health care provider was seen as omniscient and always right. The patient now comes into the health care system burdened with the influence of advertising, the Internet, and a growing alternative therapy industry. Many patients no longer calmly accept whatever medication is selected for them. They often come with requests and demands, and they partake of a complex array of over-the-counter (OTC) and alternative medicines that further complicate the safety and efficacy of standard drug therapy.

11. **Answer: c**
RATIONALE: When using the Internet, sites that are reputable or accurate are ones in which there is a mechanism for feedback or interaction, the preparer is listed with his or her qualifications, the site has been reviewed and recently updated (more than in the last 10 years), and the information is supported by other sites and is in agreement with other sources reviewed.

12. **Answer: a**
RATIONALE: OTC drugs are safe when used as directed, but many times the directions are not followed or even read. However, they can mask the signs and symptoms of an underlying problem, making it difficult to arrive at an accurate diagnosis if the condition persists. OTC drugs do interact with prescription drugs. Many OTC drugs were "grandfathered in" as drugs when stringent testing and evaluating systems became law and have not been tested or evaluated to the extent that new drugs are tested or evaluated today.

13. **Answer: b**
RATIONALE: A patient who abuses ketamine experiences paralysis, loss of sensation, disorientation, and psychic changes. Hallucinations, memory loss, and hypotension would be assessed in a patient abusing MDA (Ecstasy).

14. **Answer: b**
RATIONALE: For cutaneous anthrax, ciprofloxacin or doxycycline would be used. Ribavirin would be used for hemorrhagic fever; streptomycin or gentamicin would be used for tularemia.

15. **Answer: d**
RATIONALE: PCP is a hallucinogen. Amyl nitrate is a stimulant; heroin is an opioid; and rohypnol is an amnesiac.

CHAPTER 7

■ ASSESSING YOUR UNDERSTANDING
LABELING

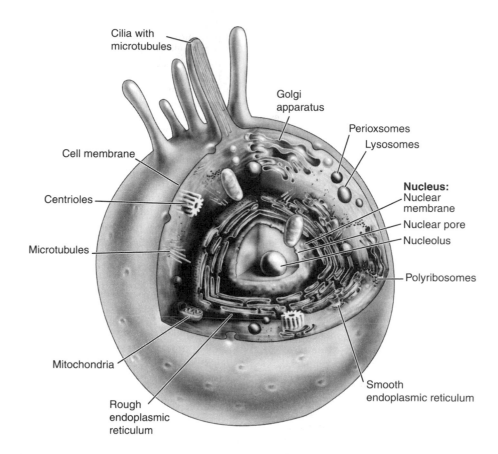

Cilia with microtubules

Golgi apparatus

Perioxsomes

Lysosomes

Cell membrane

Centrioles

Microtubules

Nucleus:
Nuclear membrane

Nuclear pore

Nucleolus

Polyribosomes

Mitochondria

Rough endoplasmic reticulum

Smooth endoplasmic reticulum

FILL IN THE BLANKS
1. Cell
2. Genes
3. Lipids, proteins
4. Organelles
5. Energy
6. Homeostasis
7. Four
8. Nucleus

MATCHING
1. d   2. e   3. c   4. b   5. a

■ APPLYING YOUR KNOWLEDGE
CASE STUDY

a. The students would need to demonstrate the four active phases and the resting phase. For the resting phase, the students would demonstrate typical functioning of the cell or the cell going about its usual actions; for the G_1 phase, the students would show synthesis of substances for DNA formation, collecting materials to make these substances; for the S phase, the students would show DNA synthesis, including doubling of DNA; for the G_2 phase, the students would show production of substances needed for making the mitotic spindles; and for the M phase, the students would show cell division.

b. The students could demonstrate the G_0 phase by walking around and performing usual activities, such as moving

substances, getting nutrition and oxygen, repairing things, and so forth.

c. The students could demonstrate the M phase by having two students side by side and then separating to show the creation of two identical daughter cells or by having a student hold two identical items attached and then splitting the items into two identical ones.

■ PRACTICING FOR NCLEX

1. **Answer: c**
   RATIONALE: The cell membrane contains cholesterol, along with phospholipids and glycolipids as well as proteins. Ribosomes are membranous structures involved in protein production within a cell; free ribosomes are found floating free in the cytoplasm, while others are attached to the surface of the endoplasmic reticulum. Genes are located in the nucleus. The mitochondria are found within the cytoplasm and produce energy as adenosine triphosphate (ATP).

2. **Answer: a**
   RATIONALE: DNA necessary for cell division is found on long strains called *chromatin*. The nucleus is encapsulated in its own membrane. A series of dense fibers and proteins are found within the nucleolus and eventually will become ribosomes. The cell membrane is composed of lipids and proteins.

3. **Answer: b**
   RATIONALE: Histocompatibility antigens or human leukocyte antigens (HLAs) are proteins that the body uses to

identify a cell as a self-cell or one belonging to that individual. Receptor sites react with a specific chemical outside the cell to stimulate a reaction. Channels allow for the passage of small substances in and out of the cell. Organelles, located in the cytoplasm, are structures with specific functions.

4. **Answer: d**
   RATIONALE: The mitochondria is responsible for energy production to allow the cell to function. Proteins are produced by the endoplasmic reticulum and free ribosomes. Cholesterol is produced by the endoplasmic reticulum. Hormone processing occurs in the Golgi apparatus.

5. **Answer: b**
   RATIONALE: Lysosomes contain specific digestive enzymes that can break down proteins, nucleic acids, carbohydrates, and lipids and are responsible for digesting worn or damaged sections of a cell when the membrane ruptures and the cell dies. Free ribosomes produce proteins that are important to the cell's structure. The Golgi apparatus prepares hormones or other substances for secretion by processing them and packaging them in vesicles to be moved to the cell membrane for excretion. The endoplasmic reticulum (ER) functions to produce proteins, phospholipids, and cholesterol (rough ER) and to produce lipid and cholesterol and cell products (smooth ER).

6. **Answer: c**
   RATIONALE: Active transport requires the expenditure of energy to transport substances. Facilitated diffusion, osmosis, and diffusion are passive transport mechanisms that require no energy for transport.

7. **Answer: d**
   RATIONALE: Facilitated diffusion involves the use of a carrier molecule such as an enzyme to move in and out of a cell. Diffusion is the movement of a substance from an area of higher concentration to a lower one due to the concentration gradient. No carrier molecule is needed. Active transport requires the use of energy to move a substance against a concentration gradient. Osmosis is the movement of water from an area of low solute concentration to a higher solute concentration.

8. **Answer: b**
   RATIONALE: An isotonic solution has the same solute concentration as human plasma. A hypertonic solution is one that contains a higher concentration of solutes than human plasma. A hypotonic solution contains a lower concentration of solutes than human plasma. Osmotic is not a classification for solutions or fluids.

9. **Answer: a**
   RATIONALE: If a red blood cell were placed in a hypotonic solution, the cell would swell and burst because water moves from the solution into the cell. If the cell were placed in a hypertonic solution, the cell would shrink and shrivel because the water inside the cell diffuses out of the cell into the solution. A red blood cell placed in an isotonic solution would remain the same.

10. **Answer: d**
    RATIONALE: The life cycle of a cell consists of four active phases and a resting phase. The genetic makeup of a cell determines the rate at which the cells can multiply. Regardless of the rate of reproduction, each cell has approximately the same life cycle. The cells found in breast milk reproduce very slowly, usually over a few months.

11. **Answer: b**
    RATIONALE: The G_1 phase starts with stimulation of the cell and ends with the formation of DNA. The formation of two identical daughter cells after cell division occurs in the M phase. Doubling of DNA marks the end of the S phase.

12. **Answer: c**
    RATIONALE: Cells in the kidneys use active transport to excrete drugs from the body. Osmosis, facilitated diffusion, and diffusion are not used.

13. **Answer: b**
    RATIONALE: Polar regions of the cell membrane (of the phospholipid layer) mix well with water, while the nonpolar regions lying within the cell repel water. The freely moving nature of the cell membrane allows it to adjust to the changing shape of the cell for areas of the membrane to move together to repair itself. Receptor sites are located on the cell membrane, and cholesterol is found in large quantities in the cell membrane, working to keep the phospholipids in place and the cell membrane stable.

14. **Answer: d**
    RATIONALE: Exocytosis involves the removal of substances from a cell by pushing them through the cell membrane. Endocytosis involves the incorporation of material into the cell by extending the cell membrane around the substance. Pinocytosis refers to the engulfing of specific substances that have reacted with a receptor site on the cell membrane. Phagocytosis allows the cell to engulf bacterium or a foreign protein and destroy it within the cell by secreting digestive enzymes into the area.

15. **Answer: a**
    RATIONALE: The G_0 phase is the resting phase when the cell is stable. The G_1 phase lasts from the time of stimulation from the resting phase until the formation of DNA. The S phase involves the actual synthesis of DNA. In the G_2 phase, the cell produces all substances needed for manufacture of the mitotic spindles.

CHAPTER 8

■ ASSESSING YOUR UNDERSTANDING

MATCHING

1. b	2. d	3. c	4. a	5. e

SHORT ANSWER

1. The overall goal of anti-infective agents is to interfere with the normal function of the invading organism to prevent it from reproducing and to cause cell death without affecting the host cell.
2. Bactericidal refers to agents that actually cause the death of the cells that they affect. Bacteriostatic refers to agents that interfere with the ability of the cells to reproduce or divide.
3. Spectrum of activity refers to the effectiveness against invading organisms. Some agents, those with a narrow spectrum of activity, are highly selective in their action, making them effective against only a few microorganisms with a very specific metabolic pathway or enzyme. Other agents, those with a broad spectrum of activity, interfere with the biochemical reactions in many different kinds of microorganisms, making them useful in the treatment of a wide variety of infections.
4. The correct identification of the organism causing an infection is an important first step in determining which anti-infective agent should be used.
5. Health care providers can help prevent the emergence of resistant strains by not using antibiotics inappropriately; assuring that the anti-infective is taken at a high enough dose for a long enough period of time; and avoiding the use of newer, powerful anti-infectives if other drugs would be just as effective.

■ APPLYING YOUR KNOWLEDGE

CASE STUDY

a. The patient's wound, which according to the patient was healing, now does not appear to be healing. There is purulent drainage coming from the wound, suggesting that an infection is still present. The wound should probably be recultured to determine if the infection is the same as on the previous visit or if the patient has developed another infection or possibly an infection involving a resistant organism. If a new or resistant infection has developed, then the anti-infective agent may need to be changed.

b. The patient needs to understand the prescribed medication therapy regimen, especially the need to take the medication exactly as prescribed for the time period prescribed to ensure complete eradication of the infection. In addition, the nurse needs to stress to the patient that he is to continue the medication even if he is feeling better or the wound looks better.

■ PRACTICING FOR NCLEX

1. **Answer: b**
   RATIONALE: Trimethoprim-sulfamethoxazole prevents the cells of the invading organism from using substances essential to their growth and development, leading to an inability to divide and eventually to cell death. Penicillins interfere with the bacterial cell wall. Aminoglycosides, macrolides, and chloramphenicol interfere with protein synthesis. Some antibiotics, antifungals, and antiprotozoal drugs alter the permeability of the cell membrane.

2. **Answer: c**
   RATIONALE: Destruction of the normal flora by anti-infectives commonly leads to superinfection, an infection that occurs when opportunistic pathogens that were kept in check by the normal bacteria have the opportunity to invade the tissues. Neurotoxicity involves damage or interference with the function of nerve tissue, usually in areas where drugs tend to accumulate in high concentrations. Hypersensitivity or allergic reactions result from antibody formation. Resistance refers to the ability over time to adapt to an antibiotic and produce cells that are no longer affected by a particular drug.

3. **Answer: d**
   RATIONALE: Combination therapy may be used when an infection is caused by more than one organism and each pathogen may react to a different anti-infective agent. Combined effects of different drugs sometimes delay the emergence of resistant strains. Typically, combination therapy involves the use of a smaller dosage of each drug, leading to fewer adverse effects while still having a therapeutic impact on the pathogen. Some drugs are synergistic, meaning that they are more powerful when given in combination.

4. **Answer: c**
   RATIONALE: The least commonly encountered adverse effect associated with the use of anti-infective agents is respiratory toxicity. The most commonly encountered adverse effects are direct toxic effects on the kidney, gastrointestinal tract, and nervous system along with hypersensitivity and superinfections.

5. **Answer: a**
   RATIONALE: Aminoglycosides collect in the eighth cranial nerve and can cause hearing loss, dizziness, and vertigo. Lethargy and hallucinations may be associated with other anti-infective agents. Visual changes such as blindness are associated with chloroquine use.

6. **Answer: b**
   RATIONALE: The use of broad-spectrum anti-infectives may result in superinfections—infections occurring when opportunistic pathogens kept in check by normal flora invade the tissues. The patient's complaint of vaginal discharge with itching suggests a superinfection. Bronchodilator therapy, oral contraceptives, and multivitamins would be unrelated to the patient's current complaint.

7. **Answer: d**
   RATIONALE: An anticoagulant interferes with blood clotting and is not an anti-infective agent. Antibiotics, anthelmintics, antiprotozoals, antivirals, and antifungals are all anti-infective agents.

8. **Answer: c**
   RATIONALE: An anti-infective with a narrow spectrum of activity is selective in its action; thus, it is effective against only a few microorganisms with a very specific metabolic pathway or enzyme. Broad-spectrum activity refers to effectiveness against a wide variety of pathogens. Bactericidal refers to a highly aggressive drug that causes cell death. Bacteriostatic refers to a drug's effectiveness in interfering with a cell's ability to reproduce or divide.

9. **Answer: d**
   RATIONALE: Microorganisms develop resistance by producing a chemical that acts as an antagonist to the drug. In addition, the microorganism can produce an enzyme that deactivates the drug, change cellular permeability so that the drug cannot enter the cell, and alter binding sites to no longer accept the drug.

10. **Answer: b**
    RATIONALE: The use of antibiotic prescription for viral illnesses or infections is a contributing factor to the development of resistance. A high enough drug dosage and long enough duration of therapy helps to ensure complete eradication of even slightly resistant organisms. Around-the-clock dosage scheduling eliminates peaks and valleys in drug concentration and helps to maintain a constant therapeutic level to prevent the emergence of resistant microbes.

11. **Answer: a**
    RATIONALE: Penicillins interfere with the biosynthesis of the pathogen cell wall. Sulfonamides, antimycobacterial drugs, and trimethoprim-sulfamethoxazole prevent the cells of the invading organism from using substances essential to their growth and development, leading to cell death. Aminoglycosides and macrolides interfere with the steps involved in protein synthesis. Fluoroquinolones interfere with DNA synthesis in the cell.

12. **Answer: b**
    RATIONALE: Performing sensitivity testing on cultured microbes is important to evaluate the bacteria and determine which drugs are capable of controlling the particular organism. Once the sensitivity testing is completed, then the decision for the drug can be made. Combination therapy is used when appropriate after culture and when sensitivity testing has been completed. Checking patient allergies also would be done after sensitivity testing but before administering the drug. The bactericidal effects of a drug may or may not play a role in the selection of the drug.

13. **Answer: c**
    RATIONALE: Gastrointestinal toxicity would be manifested by diarrhea, nausea, vomiting, or stomach upset. Dizziness and vertigo would reflect neurotoxicity. Rash may suggest a hypersensitivity or allergic reaction.

14. Answer: b
RATIONALE: Chloroquine can accumulate in the retina and optic nerve and cause blindness. Therefore, a patient complaining of changes in vision would be a cause for concern. Trouble hearing, feeling like the room is spinning, and dizziness are associated with problems involving the eighth cranial nerve.

15. Answer: c
RATIONALE: Anti-infectives that adversely affect the liver and kidneys must be used with caution in older patients, who may have decreased organ function. Older patients often do not present with the same signs and symptoms of infection that are seen in younger people. The older patient is susceptible to severe adverse gastrointestinal, renal, and neurologic effects and must be monitored for nutritional status and hydration during drug therapy. Adults, not older adults, often demand anti-infectives for a "quick cure" of various signs and symptoms.

CHAPTER 9

■ ASSESSING YOUR UNDERSTANDING

FILL IN THE BLANKS

1. Anaerobic
2. Gram-positive
3. Synergistic
4. Bactericidal
5. Cefaclor

LABELING

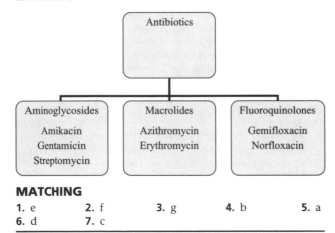

MATCHING

1. e	**2.** f	**3.** g	**4.** b	**5.** a
6. d	**7.** c			

■ APPLYING YOUR KNOWLEDGE

CASE STUDY

a. Ciprofloxacin, a fluoroquinolone, is indicated for treatment of infections caused by susceptible strains of gram-negative bacteria, such as *Escherichia coli*. These infections commonly include the urinary tract, respiratory tract, and skin infections.

b. Ciprofloxacin belongs to the group of antibiotics known as fluoroquinolones. This group acts by entering the bacterial cell by passive diffusion through channels in the cell membrane. Once inside, the drug interferes with the action of DNA enzymes that are necessary for the bacteria's growth and reproduction. This leads to cell death because the bacterial DNA is damaged and the cell cannot be maintained.

c. Although the adverse effects associated with ciprofloxacin are relatively mild, the nurse would still need to address the most common ones, such as headache, dizziness, insomnia, nausea, vomiting, and dry mouth. The nurse would also need to caution the patient about possible

bone marrow suppression and photosensitivity, urging the patient to report any signs and symptoms of an infection, to avoid sun and ultraviolet light exposure, and to wear protective clothing and use sunscreens.

d. Antacids can interfere with the therapeutic effect of the drug, making it less effective. Therefore, the nurse should instruct the patient to make sure that at least 4 hours have passed between the time she takes the ciprofloxacin and the antacid.

■ PRACTICING FOR NCLEX

1. Answer: c
RATIONALE: Gentamicin is classified as an aminoglycoside. Levofloxacin is a fluoroquinolone; clarithromycin is a macrolide; and cefaclor is a cephalosporin.

2. Answer: b
RATIONALE: Telithromycin is a ketolide, which is structurally similar to macrolides. It is not structurally related to penicillins, cephalosporins, or lincosamides.

3. Answer: d
RATIONALE: Streptomycin is an aminoglycoside that is available only for intramuscular use.

4. Answer: b
RATIONALE: Gentamicin, like other aminoglycosides, can cause ototoxicity leading to irreversible hearing loss. Therefore, it would be most important to determine the patient's auditory function to establish a baseline for comparison. Gentamicin can affect the gastrointestinal (GI) tract, leading to nausea, vomiting, diarrhea, and weight loss, which in turn can affect nutrition. However, the patient's GI function and nutritional status would be less of a priority to assess. Gentamicin may cause numbness, tingling, and weakness. However, assessing the patient's muscle strength would be a lower priority.

5. Answer: a
RATIONALE: Rifampin, along with isoniazid, pyrazinamide, ethambutol, streptomycin, and rifapentine, are considered first-line agents for treating tuberculosis. Kanamycin, ciprofloxacin, and capreomycin are second-line agents.

6. Answer: c
RATIONALE: Cefuroxime is a cephalosporin. Doripenem, imipenem-cilastatin, and ertapenem are carbapenems.

7. Answer: a
RATIONALE: Although headache and dizziness, superinfections, and phlebitis (with intravenous administration) can occur, the most common adverse effects of cephalosporins involve the GI tract and include vomiting, diarrhea, nausea, anorexia, abdominal pain, and flatulence.

8. Answer: a
RATIONALE: The patient is exhibiting signs and symptoms of a disulfiramlike reaction that occurs when a cephalosporin such as cefaclor interacts with alcohol. Concurrent use of cefaclor with an oral anticoagulant may increase the patient's risk for bleeding. Concurrent use of cefaclor with another antibiotic such as an aminoglycoside can increase the patient's risk for nephrotoxicity. Adequate fluid intake, although important in maintaining hydration and nutrition, is unrelated to what the patient is experiencing.

9. Answer: d
RATIONALE: Penicillin was the first antibiotic introduced for clinical use. Sir Alexander Fleming produced the original penicillin in the 1920s.

10. Answer: b
RATIONALE: Food in the stomach decreases the absorption of oral macrolides such as erythromycin. Therefore, the drug should be taken on an empty stomach with a full,

8-oz glass of water, 1 hour before or at least 2 to 3 hours after meals. The patient may experience diarrhea with this drug, but it should not be bloody. Bloody diarrhea is associated with pseudomembranous colitis, which needs to be reported to the health care provider immediately. Due to its long half-life, azithromycin is usually ordered as a once-daily dose.

11. **Answer: a**
RATIONALE: When rifampin and isoniazid are used in combination, the possibility of toxic liver reactions increases, requiring close monitoring. Urine culture would not need to be monitored. Audiometric studies would be monitored for patients receiving ototoxic drugs such as aminoglycosides. Although pulmonary function studies may
be indicated to evaluate the patient's respiratory function, these would not be as important as monitoring liver function studies.

12. **Answer: c**
RATIONALE: Ceftazidime is considered a third-generation cephalosporin. Cefazolin and cephalexin are considered first-generation cephalosporins. Cefaclor is a second-generation cephalosporin.

13. **Answer: b**
RATIONALE: Clindamycin is considered the prototype lincosamide. Erythromycin and clarithromycin are macrolide antibiotics. Lincomycin is also a lincosamide but not the prototype.

14. **Answer: d**
RATIONALE: Nafcillin and oxacillin are penicillinase-resistant antibiotics. Amoxicillin, ticarcillin, and carbenicillin are penicillins.

15. **Answer: a**
RATIONALE: Tetracyclines should be used with caution in children younger than age 8 years because the drugs can potentially damage developing teeth and bones. They do not affect hearing or vision. They are excreted in the urine, so caution is necessary if the patient has underlying renal dysfunction; however, this is not the main reason for avoiding use in children.

CHAPTER 10

■ ASSESSING YOUR UNDERSTANDING

LABELING

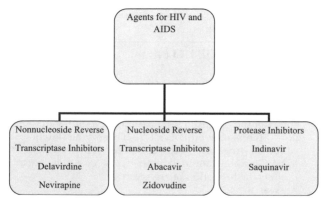

MATCHING
1. e **2.** d **3.** b **4.** c **5.** a

■ APPLYING YOUR KNOWLEDGE

CASE STUDY

a. The nurse needs to explain to the patient about her condition in a calm, nonjudgmental, supportive manner. The nurse must emphasize that although the medication can help alleviate the current infection, it does not cure the condition.

b. The nurse needs to instruct the patient that she should take the medication exactly as prescribed for the exact duration of therapy, usually 5 days. In addition, the nurse needs to teach the patient about her infection, including the fact that the drug is not curative. The nurse also should instruct the patient about possible adverse effects, most commonly, nausea, vomiting, headache, depression, paresthesias, neuropathy, rash, and hair loss. Offering suggestions as to how to cope with these effects, such as maintaining adequate food and fluid intake, would be important. The nurse needs to emphasize avoiding sexual activity during a current outbreak and to use safe sex practices to prevent disease transmission.

■ PRACTICING FOR NCLEX

1. **Answer: c**
RATIONALE: Foscarnet is available only for intravenous use.

2. **Answer: a**
RATIONALE: Oseltamivir is used as treatment for influenza if the patient has been symptomatic for fewer than 2 days.

3. **Answer: d**
RATIONALE: Fosamprenavir is a protease inhibitor that may be indicated as part of combination therapy for symptomatic HIV infection. Entecavir, telbivudine, and adefovir are indicated for the treatment of chronic hepatitis B.

4. **Answer: b**
RATIONALE: Nucleoside reverse transcriptase inhibitors, such as didanosine and zidovudine, were the first class of drugs developed to treat HIV infection. Of the classes listed, fusion inhibitors would be the newest class of drugs developed for HIV infection.

5. **Answer: b**
RATIONALE: HIV mutates over time, presenting a slightly different configuration with each new generation. Thus, multiple drugs are used to attack the virus at various points in the life cycle to achieve the maximum effectiveness with the least amount of toxicity. Sensitivity is not an issue. The virus needs to enter the cell to cause infection. Adverse effects are numerous with anti-HIV drugs and the use of combination therapy can increase the patient's risk for these adverse effects, including further depression of the immune response.

6. **Answer: c**
RATIONALE: Of the drugs listed, only zidovudine has been proven safe for use during pregnancy.

7. **Answer: a**
RATIONALE: Nevirapine is associated with gastrointestinal-related effects, most commonly, dry mouth, dyspepsia, constipation or diarrhea, nausea, and abdominal pain. Rimantadine is more commonly associated with light-headedness and dizziness. Tenofovir and fosamprenavir are associated with changes in body fat distribution, leading to buffalo hump and thin arms and legs. Maraviroc is associated with paresthesias and fever.

8. **Answer: c**
RATIONALE: Zanamivir is delivered by a Diskhaler device and is absorbed through the respiratory tract.

9. Answer: d

RATIONALE: Ibuprofen has not been found to interact with rimantadine. However, anticholinergics such as atropine and drugs such as acetaminophen and aspirin have been associated with an increase in anticholinergic effects and decreased effectiveness, respectively.

10. Answer: a

RATIONALE: Nelfinavir, if used with midazolam, pimozide, rifampin, or triazolam, can lead to severe toxic effects and life-threatening arrhythmias. Delavirdine, if used with warfarin, clarithromycin, or quinidine, can lead to life-threatening effects.

11. Answer: b

RATIONALE: Maraviroc is classified as a CCR5 co-receptor antagonist. Enfuvirtide is categorized as a fusion inhibitor; raltegravir is categorized as an integrase inhibitor; and didanosine is categorized as a nucleoside reverse transcriptase inhibitor.

12. Answer: c

RATIONALE: Although patient teaching about adverse effects, follow-up laboratory testing, and measures to reduce infection transmission are important, it is essential that the patient ensure that he or she has a continuously available and adequate supply of the drug because there is a risk for an acute exacerbation of hepatitis B when the drug is stopped.

13. Answer: a

RATIONALE: If the patient develops a severe local reaction or if open lesions occur near the site of administration, then the drug needs to be stopped to prevent systemic absorption and adverse effects. Localized burning, stinging, and discomfort are associated with the use of docosanol. Since the drug is applied locally, it is not absorbed systemically. The drug does not cure the disease but should help alleviate discomfort.

14. Answer: b

RATIONALE: Oseltamivir is the only antiviral agent found to be effective in the treatment of Avian flu.

15. Answer: d

RATIONALE: Cidofovir is given by intravenous infusion over 1 hour. It is not given orally, topically, or subcutaneously.

CHAPTER 11

■ ASSESSING YOUR UNDERSTANDING

CROSSWORD

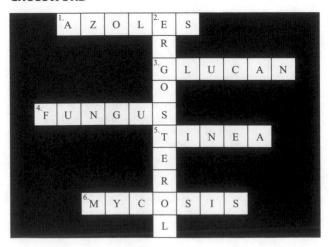

SHORT ANSWER

1. Ketoconazole and fluconazole strongly inhibit the cytochrome P450 (CYP450) enzyme system in the liver.
2. Topical antifungal agents should not be used over open or draining areas, because doing so increases the risk for systemic absorption.
3. The incidence of fungal infections has increased due to the rising number of immunocompromised individuals, such as those with AIDS and AIDS-related complex, those taking immunosuppressant drugs, those who have undergone transplant surgery or cancer treatment, and those with advancing age (the growing number of older adults) who are no longer able to protect themselves from the many fungi found throughout the environment.
4. Three major types of local fungal infections include vaginal infections, oral yeast infections, and a variety of tinea infections.
5. The composition of the protective layer of the fungal cell (the rigid cell wall of chitin and polysaccharides and cell membrane containing ergosterol) makes the organism resistant to antibiotics.
6. The antifungals are metabolized extensively in the liver and have been associated with liver toxicity; therefore, these drugs should be used with caution in patients with liver dysfunction.

■ APPLYING YOUR KNOWLEDGE

CASE STUDY

a. The nurse should instruct the patient to apply the cream to the affected area in a thin layer twice a day for approximately 2 to 4 weeks. The cream is available over the counter, so it would be essential to ensure that the patient understands how to use the medication properly to avoid possible systemic absorption.

b. The nurse should reinforce the need for the patient to use the cream exactly as recommended and to follow the manufacturer's instructions about use. In addition, the nurse should tell the patient not to apply an occlusive dressing over the area, because this would increase the risk for systemic absorption. The nurse should also tell the patient not to apply the cream to any open or weeping areas and to stop using the drug if he develops blisters or a rash that is severe.

c. Additional instructions would include proper foot-care measures, including cleaning the feet with soap and water and patting them dry before applying the cream; wearing clean, dry cotton socks and keeping the feet dry; avoiding scratching of the area; and using cool compresses to help decrease the itching.

■ PRACTICING FOR NCLEX

1. **Answer: c**

RATIONALE: Ketoconazole blocks the activity of a sterol in the fungal wall. Posaconazole and voriconazole inhibit the synthesis of ergosterol, which in turn leads to an inability of the fungus to form a cell wall, resulting in cell death. Terbinafine inhibits a CYP2D6 enzyme system, which may make it a better choice for patients who need to take drugs metabolized by the CYP450 system; it also inhibits the formation of ergosterol.

2. **Answer: a**

RATIONALE: *Mycosis* is a term used to describe a disease that is caused by a fungus. So both parties are correct, and the nurse's response appropriately addresses the patient's concerns. Mycosis may be related to immunosuppression, but it refers to the disease caused by a fungus.

Suggesting that the nurse and patient talk to the doctor indicates that there is some discrepancy between what the doctor said and what the patient thought, which is not the case. Although the infection may be minor and treatable, telling the client not to worry does not address his concerns.

3. **Answer: d**
RATIONALE: Ketoconazole can be used systemically and topically to treat fungal infections. Butoconazole and clotrimazole are for topical use only. Voriconazole is for systemic use only.

4. **Answer: b**
RATIONALE: Amphotericin B is associated with bone marrow suppression, so it would be especially important for the nurse to monitor the patient's complete blood count for changes. The drug does not affect coagulation. Although the drug can cause gastrointestinal (GI) irritation with nausea, vomiting, and potentially severe diarrhea, monitoring bowel sounds would not be as important as monitoring the blood count. Amphotericin B does not affect respiratory function.

5. **Answer: b**
RATIONALE: Fluconazole, when given intravenously, peaks in 1 hour (60 minutes) and has a duration of action of 2 to 4 hours.

6. **Answer: a**
RATIONALE: The nurse should arrange for an appropriate culture and sensitivity test before beginning the therapy to ensure that the appropriate drug is being used. This should be done first. Once the specimen has been obtained, the nurse would evaluate renal and hepatic function test to determine baseline function and to determine the risk for possible toxicity during therapy. Not all systemic antifungals are administered intravenously, so inserting an intravenous access device may or may not be necessary.

7. **Answer: c**
RATIONALE: Topical antifungal agents are agents that are too toxic to be used systemically but are effective in the treatment of local infections. Typically, topical agents should be applied as a thin film. These agents can cause serious local irritation, burning, and pain. Systemic, not topical, antifungal agents are associated with many drug–drug interactions.

8. **Answer: d**
RATIONALE: Caspofungin is an example of an echinocandin antifungal. Terbinafine is an example of an azole antifungal agent. Nystatin and amphotericin B are examples other antifungals.

9. **Answer: a**
RATIONALE: Ketoconazole is not the drug of choice for patients with endocrine problems such as diabetes or those with fertility problems. Fluconazole is not associated with the endocrine problems seen with ketoconazole. Itraconazole and terbinafine are associated with liver failure and toxicity.

10. **Answer: a, b, d**
RATIONALE: Itraconazole has a black box warning regarding the potential for serious cardiovascular effects if it is given with simvastatin, midazolam, pimozide, lovastatin, triazolam, or dofetilide. Increased serum level of warfarin, digoxin, and cyclosporine occur when they are administered with ketoconazole due to the drug's strong inhibition of the cytochrome P450 enzyme system.

11. **Answer: b**
RATIONALE: Voriconazole should not be used with ergots alkaloids because ergotism can occur. In this situation, the nurse should recommend that the patient not use the ergot until the antifungal therapy is finished.

12. **Answer: d**
RATIONALE: Serum flucytosine levels greater than 100 mcg/mL are associated with toxicity.

13. **Answer: c**
RATIONALE: Patients receiving amphotericin B should not take other nephrotoxic drugs such as gentamicin unless absolutely necessary because of the increased risk of severe renal toxicity. Penicillin, amantadine, and aztreonam are not associated with an increased risk for renal dysfunction if given with amphotericin B.

14. **Answer: b**
RATIONALE: If the patient experiences GI upset, the nurse should suggest that the patient take the drug with food or meals and to try eating small frequent meals instead of three large meals. There is no need to call the prescriber to change the drug unless the patient experiences severe nausea and vomiting, which could interfere with his nutritional status. Advising the patient to sit upright may or may not be helpful.

15. **Answer: c**
RATIONALE: Sulconazole should not be used longer than 6 weeks due to the risk of adverse effects and possible emergency of resistant strains of fungi. Naftifine, oxiconazole, sertaconazole nitrate, and terbinafine should not be used longer than 4 weeks.

CHAPTER 12

■ ASSESSING YOUR UNDERSTANDING

FILL IN THE BLANKS

1. Trophozoite
2. Malaria
3. Trichomoniasis
4. Trypanosomiasis
5. Protozoan

SEQUENCING

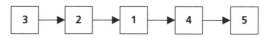

■ APPLYING YOUR KNOWLEDGE

CASE STUDY

a. The nurse needs to ask the patient about what he had to drink and eat during his camping trip. Giardiasis is transmitted through contaminated water or food. It would be important to find out if the patient had consumed unpurified water or contaminated food, such as fish from a contaminated stream or river or if he used the local water for cooking. The nurse also needs to inquire about hygiene facilities when camping because personal hygiene measures are essential to prevent the transmission of disease.

b. Tinidazole typically is ordered as a one-time single dose of 2 g. The nurse would need to instruct the patient to take this medication as a single dose with food.

c. The nurse should warn the patient not to consume alcohol with this drug to prevent severe adverse effects (disulfiram reaction). The nurse should advise the patient to avoid alcohol for at least 3 days after taking the single dose. Other areas to address include measures to ensure adequate fluid and nutritional intake, such as clear fluids initially and then gradually advancing diet as tolerated, with an emphasis on increased fluid intake and small frequent meals; possible adverse effects such as central nervous system effects; and warning signs that need to be reported, such as an increase in his gastrointestinal (GI) symptoms or development of signs and symptoms of another infection, like fever and chills.

■ PRACTICING FOR NCLEX

1. Answer: c
RATIONALE: Antimalarial drugs are usually given in combination form to attack the parasite at various stages of its life cycle, thereby preventing the acute malarial reaction in individuals who have been infected with the parasite. Currently, chloroquine is the mainstay of antimalarial treatment. Quinine was the first drug found to be effective against malaria, but it is no longer available. Combination therapy is recommended because many strains of the parasite are developing resistance to chloroquine.

2. Answer: a
RATIONALE: Chloroquine enters the human red blood cells and changes the metabolic pathways necessary for reproduction. It is also directly toxic to the parasites that absorb it and, due to its acidity, decreases the ability of the parasite to create DNA. Mefloquine increases the acidity of the plasmodial food vacuoles, causing cell rupture and death. Pyrimethamine blocks the use of folic acid in protein synthesis. Primaquine disrupts the mitochondria.

3. Answer: b
RATIONALE: Pregnancy should be avoided during treatment with any of the antimalarial agents. For mefloquine, the patient should avoid pregnancy during therapy and for 2 months after the completion of therapy. Antimalarial agents are contraindicated for use with lactating women, so another method of feeding should be chosen if treatment is absolutely necessary.

4. Answer: a, b, f
RATIONALE: Cinchonism may occur with high levels of primaquine and is manifested by tinnitus, vomiting, vertigo, and nausea. Fever, dyspepsia, and rash are adverse effects associated with antimalarial agents not suggestive of cinchonism.

5. Answer: b
RATIONALE: Ophthalmologic evaluation would be most important, because these drugs are associated with visual changes including possible blindness due to retinal damage from the drug. Assessment of the patient's respiratory status and pupillary response would not be crucial. Assessing the patient's nutritional status would be helpful to establish a baseline if the patient experiences adverse GI effects. However, this assessment would be a lower priority than an ophthalmologic evaluation.

6. Answer: c
RATIONALE: Trichomoniasis is usually spread during sexual intercourse by men who have no signs and symptoms of the infection. A mosquito bite can transmit malaria. The common housefly is responsible for transmitting Chagas' disease. Drinking contaminated water is associated with giardiasis.

7. Answer: d
RATIONALE: Metronidazole combined with oral anticoagulants can lead to increased bleeding, necessitating dosage adjustments with the anticoagulant. Abdominal cramps, ataxia, and peripheral neuropathy (as manifested by paresthesias) are adverse effects that are associated with antiprotozoal agents and are unrelated to the use of the warfarin.

8. Answer: b
RATIONALE: Pentamidine is given as an inhalation or intramuscular or intravenous injection. It is not given orally, transdermally, or subcutaneously.

9. Answer: c
RATIONALE: A patient should not consume alcohol if he or she is taking metronidazole or tinidazole. Interaction with alcohol is not associated with pentamidine, atovaquone, or nitazoxanide use.

10. Answer: a
RATIONALE: Atovaquone is indicated for the prevention and treatment of *Pneumocystis carinii* pneumonia (PCP). Metronidazole or tinidazole is used to treat giardiasis, amebiasis, and trichomoniasis. Pentamidine can be used to treat trypanosomiasis.

11. Answer: d
RATIONALE: Leishmaniasis is treated with systemic pentamidine. Amebiasis is treated with metronidazole or tinidazole. Giardiasis may be treated with nitazoxanide. PCP is treated with oral atovaquone.

12. Answer: a
RATIONALE: Malaria results from the bite of an infected mosquito, most specifically the *Anopheles* mosquito. Consuming food grown in contaminated soil can lead to amebiasis. Consumption of unpurified spring water is associated with giardiasis. The bite of an infected tsetse fly leads to trypanosomiasis (African sleeping sickness).

13. Answer: b
RATIONALE: Protozoal infections are most common in tropical areas, where many people experience multiple infestations at the same time. Protozoa also survive and reproduce in any area where people live in very crowded and unsanitary conditions. Insect control has helped to control the various insects associated with these infections; however, the rise of insecticide-resistant insects such as mosquitoes has allowed the infections to continue to flourish.

14. Answer: a
RATIONALE: The person who is bitten by an infected mosquito is injected with thousands of sporozoites that then undergo asexual cell division and reproduction. Trophozoites form, which lead to the formation of schizonts and then merozoites, which enter the circulation and invade red blood cells.

15. Answer: a
RATIONALE: Chloroquine is considered a potent schizonticidal agent. Primaquine is considered a portent gametocytocidal agent. Primaquine and pyrimethamine are considered important prophylactic agents. Quinine is rarely used today to treat malaria.

CHAPTER 13

■ ASSESSING YOUR UNDERSTANDING

SHORT ANSWER

1. Infections by nematodes include pinworms, whipworms, threadworms, Ascaris, and hookworms.
2. Pinworms are the most common helminthic infection in school-age children in the United States.
3. Nematodes are roundworms; platyhelminths are flatworms. Both cause intestine-invading worm infections.
4. A helminth is a worm that can cause disease by invading the body.
5. Trichinosis is the disease that is caused by the ingestion of the encysted larvae of the roundworm in undercooked pork.

MATCHING

1. c 2. d 3. a 4. e 5. b

■ APPLYING YOUR KNOWLEDGE

CASE STUDY

a. Pinworms spread rapidly among children in schools, summer camps, and other institutions. Inadequate hygiene measures at the summer camp and the close proximity of children in the camp, possibly sharing clothing or other items, may have contributed to the transmission of the infection. The worm eggs are ingested either from transfer by touching the eggs when they are shed to clothing, toys, or bedding or by inhaling the eggs that become airborne and then are swallowed.

b. The nurse needs to respond to the mother in a supportive and nonjudgmental manner, emphasizing that the infection is not a reflection of hygiene measures or lifestyle. The nurse needs to clarify any misconceptions that the mother may have, reminding the mother that pinworms is the most common helminthic infection among school-age children.

c. The child is to receive mebendazole (available in chewable form), which is given orally in the morning and evening for three consecutive days. If necessary, the nurse should assist the mother in making up a schedule to ensure compliance with the therapy, informing the mother that the regimen may need to be repeated in 3 weeks if the infection does not clear. In addition, the nurse should review the common adverse effects of the drug, such as abdominal discomfort, diarrhea, or pain and suggest to the mother to give the drug with meals or food to minimize any gastrointestinal upset that may occur. Other instructions should address hygiene measures such as frequent hand washing, especially after using the toilet; keeping the child's nails short; showering in the morning to remove any eggs deposited in the anal area; changing and washing undergarments, bed linens, and other clothing every day; and disinfecting the toilet facilities.

■ PRACTICING FOR NCLEX

1. **Answer: d**
   RATIONALE: Tapeworms are cestodes—segmented flatworms that cause infection. Pinworms, whipworms, and Ascaris are roundworm infections.

2. **Answer: b**
   RATIONALE: Trichinosis is caused by the ingestion of encrusted larvae of the roundworm in undercooked pork. Consumption of unwashed vegetables would lead to Ascaris. A recent insect bite would be associated with causing filariasis. Swimming in a contaminated lake could lead to schistosomiasis.

3. **Answer: c**
   RATIONALE: Mebendazole is considered the prototype anthelmintic agent.

4. **Answer: a**
   RATIONALE: Ascaris is an intestinal-invading worm infection. Trichinosis, filariasis, and schistosomiasis are examples of tissue-invading worm infections.

5. **Answer: c**
   RATIONALE: Pyrantel may be preferred especially for patients who have trouble remembering to take medications or following drug regimens because it is administered as a single one-time dose. It is not administered monthly. All anthelmintic agents are effective in eradicating the infection. Mebendazole is available in chewable form.

6. **Answer: c**
   RATIONALE: Mebendazole is not metabolized in the body. Very little of the drug is absorbed systemically, so adverse effects are few. Most of the drug is excreted unchanged in the feces.

7. **Answer: c**
   RATIONALE: Praziquantel is administered orally in three doses every 4 to 6 hours over a period of 1 day. Mebendazole, a chewable tablet, is administered every morning and evening for a period of 3 days. Ivermectin and pyrantel are administered as a single one-time dose.

8. **Answer: b**
   RATIONALE: Albendazole is associated with bone marrow depression and renal failure. Stevens–Johnson syndrome is associated with thiabendazole use. Diarrhea and fever are adverse effects associated with mebendazole and pyrantel.

9. **Answer: d**
   RATIONALE: Filariasis occurs when worm embryos enter the body via insect bites. Swimming in contaminated water with snail-deposited larvae causes schistosomiasis. Consuming undercooked fish containing the larvae of cestodes leads to a tapeworm infection. Eating unwashed vegetables grown in contaminated soil can cause Ascaris.

10. **Answer: d**
    RATIONALE: The drug of choice for treating a threadworm infection is ivermectin. Albendazole is used to treat pork tapeworms. Pyrantel is used to treat pinworms and roundworms. Praziquantel is used to treat a wide number of schistosomes or flukes.

11. **Answer: a**
    RATIONALE: With a whipworm infection, bloody diarrhea and colic may be noted. Pneumonia is associated with a threadworm infection. Fatigue suggests a hookworm infection. Weight loss is associated with a tapeworm infection.

12. **Answer: d**
    RATIONALE: For proper diagnosis of a helminthic infection, a stool examination for ova and parasites is essential. A complete blood count may help to identify anemia associated with a hookworm infection. A urinalysis may be done to establish a baseline but would provide no information about the infection. Liver function tests would be appropriate before administering therapy to ensure adequate liver function and evaluate for possible toxicity related to drug therapy but would not provide information about the helminthic infection.

13. **Answer: a**
    RATIONALE: Toilets should be cleaned daily. Other measures including thorough and frequent hand washing, especially after using the bathroom; consistently washing any fresh fruits and vegetables, and using hot, chlorine-treated water for laundering clothes and bed linens.

14. **Answer: b**
    RATIONALE: Threadworm infections can cause more damage to the human than most other helminths, possibly leading to death from pneumonia or from lung or liver abscesses that result from larval invasion. Ascaris is the most prevalent helminthic infection worldwide. Schistosomiasis is a common problem in parts of Africa, Asia, and certain South American and Caribbean countries. Pinworm infection is the most common helminthic infection among school-age children.

15. **Answer: c**
    RATIONALE: Trichinosis is caused by the ingestion of undercooked pork, so the nurse should emphasize the need to thoroughly cook any pork products. Washing hands after working with soil would help to minimize the risk for threadworm or whipworm infections. Avoiding swimming in waters that may be contaminated would be helpful in preventing schistosomiasis. Protection from insect bites would be helpful in preventing filariasis.

CHAPTER 14

■ ASSESSING YOUR UNDERSTANDING

CROSSWORD

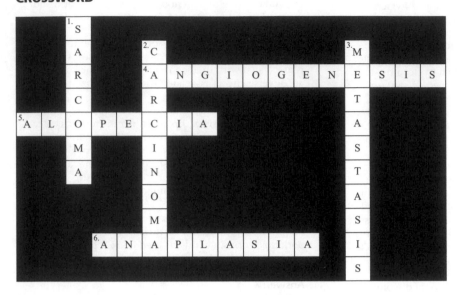

SHORT ANSWER

1. The two major groups of cancer are solid tumors and hematologic malignancies.
2. All cancers start with a single cell that is genetically different from other cells in the surrounding tissue. The cell divides, passing it abnormalities to daughter cells and eventually producing a tumor or neoplasm that has characteristics quite different from the original tissue.
3. Antineoplastic drugs work by affecting cell survival or by boosting the immune system in its efforts to combat abnormal cells.
4. Most cancer patients are not considered cured until they have been cancer free for a period of 5 years due to the possibility that cancer cells will emerge from dormancy to cause new tumors or problems. No cells yet have been identified that can remain dormant for longer than 5 years, so the chances of the emergence of one after that time are very slim.
5. Alkylating agents can affect cells even in the resting phase of the cell cycle, thus they are said to be non–cell cycle specific.
6. Mitotic inhibitors kill cells as the process of mitosis begins in the M phase of the cell cycle.

MATCHING

1. c   2. f   3. a   4. e   5. d
6. b

■ APPLYING YOUR KNOWLEDGE

CASE STUDY

a. The nurse needs to respond to the patient's concerns honestly and with empathy. The nurse should acknowledge the patient's concern and then provide the patient with information about the possible adverse effects of the two drugs. Cisplatin is an alkylating agent; paclitaxel is a mitotic inhibitor. Both are associated with neurologic adverse effects and hypersensitivity reactions. Alopecia and bone marrow suppression may occur with both drugs. In addition, cisplatin can be nephrotoxic, and paclitaxel can be cardiotoxic.

The patient is visibly anxious, so it would be appropriate to provide the patient with written handouts and pamphlets about her therapy so that the patient can review them and then ask questions on the next visit. The patient also needs information about the usual protocol, including how the drugs will be given and any special devices, such as a central venous access device (port) that may need to be inserted for administration. The nurse also needs to provide the patient with information about measures to address the typical adverse effects such as frequent rest periods, small frequent meals, increased fluid intake, and scarves/wigs for hair loss. In addition, the nurse should explain any medications that may be ordered to manage the adverse effects, such as using antiemetics before chemotherapy sessions to reduce the risk of nausea and vomiting and the use of amifostine to protect the healthy cells from the toxic effects of cisplatin. Some protocols also include the use of intravenous fluids to ensure adequate hydration and antihistamines to reduce the risk of hypersensitivity reactions. The nurse should review the protocols with the patient.

b. Cisplatin is given intravenously every 3 weeks; paclitaxel is administered intravenously over 3 hours every 3 weeks. Therefore, the nurse needs to explain the schedule to the patient and assist her in estimating the amount of time that will be required for the chemotherapy sessions, possibly suggesting some activity such as reading or listening to music to help pass the time. Since the patient may experience some fatigue related to the therapy, it might be helpful for the nurse to suggest that someone be available to transport the patient to and from the facility where the therapy will be administered.

■ PRACTICING FOR NCLEX

1. **Answer: d**
   RATIONALE: Vincristine is classified as a mitotic inhibitor. Fluorouracil and methotrexate are classified as antimetabolites. Chlorambucil is classified as an alkylating agent.

2. Answer: a
RATIONALE: Odansetron blocks serotonin receptors in the chemoreceptor trigger zone (CTZ) and is one of the most effective antiemetics. Antihistamines help to reduce the risk of hypersensitivity reactions and decrease secretions; corticosteroids help to relieve inflammation and may aid in reducing possible hypersensitivity.

3. Answer: c
RATIONALE: Leukopenia indicates that the number of white blood cells is low. Subsequently, the patient is at risk for infection because adequate white blood cells are not present to mount a response. Disturbed body image might result from alopecia or significant weight loss. Imbalanced nutrition may be appropriate for the patient who is unable to consume adequate calories or nutrients secondary to nausea and vomiting. Deficient fluid volume would be appropriate for a patient who is experiencing an increase in fluid loss through vomiting or diarrhea or who is unable to consume adequate amounts of fluid by mouth due to nausea or vomiting.

4. Answer: d
RATIONALE: Methotrexate is absorbed well from the gastrointestinal (GI) tract and can be administered orally. Cytarabine, fluorouracil, and gemcitabine must be administered parenterally because they are not absorbed well from the GI tract.

5. Answer: b
RATIONALE: Leucovorin is administered to counteract the effects of treatment with methotrexate. Alprazolam, metoclopramide, and aprepitant are used to help alleviate the nausea and vomiting associated with chemotherapy.

6. Answer: c
RATIONALE: Antimetabolites inhibit DNA production in cells that depend on certain natural metabolites to produce DNA, replacing the needed metabolites, which prevents normal cellular function. Alkylating agents react chemically with portions of the RNA, DNA, or other cellular proteins. Antineoplastic antibiotics interfere with cellular DNA synthesis by inserting themselves between base pairs in the DNA chain. Mitotic inhibitors interfere with the ability of a cell to divide, blocking or altering DNA synthesis.

7. Answer: b
RATIONALE: Imatinib belongs to the group of drugs called *protein tyrosine kinase inhibitors*, which do not affect healthy human cells. Etoposide and vincristine, both mitotic inhibitors, and doxorubicin, an antineoplastic antibiotic, damage both healthy and cancer cells.

8. Answer: d
RATIONALE: Tamoxifen belongs to the group of drugs that are hormones or hormone modulators. These agents are hormone specific. This drug competes with estrogen at the receptor sites, ultimately blocking estrogen. The adverse effects specific to this action would involve menopause-associated effects. Bone marrow suppression, GI toxicity, and hepatic dysfunction occur with this drug, but these are not specific to the drug's action.

9. Answer: a
RATIONALE: The adverse effects associated with imatinib include GI upset, muscle cramps, heart failure, fluid retention, and skin rash. Thus a nursing diagnosis of excess fluid volume would be most likely. The severe bone marrow suppression, alopecia, and severe GI effects associated with the more traditional antineoplastic therapy do not occur.

10. Answer: b
RATIONALE: Cancer cells tend to move through the cell cycle at about the same rate as their cells of origin. Malignant cells that remain in a dormant phase for long periods are difficult to destroy. These cells can emerge long after cancer treatment has finished—after weeks, months, or years—to begin their division and growth cycle all over again. Therefore, antineoplastic agents are often given in sequence over periods of time, in the hope that the drugs will affect the cancer cells as they emerge from dormancy or move into a new phase of the cell cycle. The use of cycles is unrelated to allowing the body to recover. A person is said to be cured of cancer only after a 5-year period of being cancer free. Most antineoplastic agents destroy healthy and cancer cells.

11. Answer: a
RATIONALE: Mitomycin is an example of an antineoplastic antibiotic. Teniposide, vinblastine, and docetaxel are examples of mitotic inhibitors.

12. Answer: c
RATIONALE: Bleomycin is associated with pulmonary fibrosis. Therefore, the nurse would need to monitor the patient's chest x-ray periodically. Although bone marrow suppression can occur, monitoring the patient's platelet count would be less of a concern when compared to the risks associated with pulmonary fibrosis. The drug is not associated with cardiac toxicity, so monitoring the patient's electrocardiogram would not be warranted. Monitoring serum electrolyte levels may be indicated if the patient is experience severe GI effects, but this would not take priority over the chest x-rays.

13. Answer: d
RATIONALE: The majority of agents used to control nausea and vomiting secondary to chemotherapy directly block the CTZ. They do not affect neurotransmitters, gastric acidity, or the gag reflex.

14. Answer: a
RATIONALE: Imatinib is administered orally.

15. Answer: b
RATIONALE: Angiogenesis refers to the process in which abnormal cells release enzymes that generate blood vessels in the area to supply both oxygen and nutrients to the cells. Metastasis refers to process of traveling from the place of origin to develop new tumors in other areas of the body. Autonomy refers to the process of growing without the usual homeostatic restrictions that regulate cell growth and control. Anaplasia refers to the process in which the cells lose their ability to differentiate and organize, which leads to a loss in their ability to function normally.

CHAPTER 15

■ ASSESSING YOUR UNDERSTANDING

MATCHING

1. b	**2.** e	**3.** c	**4.** g	**5.** h
6. a	**7.** d	**8.** f		

FILL IN THE BLANKS
1. Kinin
2. Mast
3. Antibodies or immunoglobulins
4. Chemotaxis
5. Phagocytosis

■ APPLYING YOUR KNOWLEDGE

CASE STUDY

a. The patient is exhibiting three of the four cardinal signs of an inflammatory reaction. The patient's throat is red (rubor), swollen (tumor), and he has pain (dolor). The throat is not touched to determine if it is warm (calor). In addition, the patient also has a fever, which is most likely due to the release of a natural pyrogen by the neutrophils engulfing and digesting the invader. In addition, leukotrienes are being released to induce slow-wave sleep as an energy conservation measure, which is reflected by the patient's malaise and complaints of feeling tired.

b. Pathogens introduced in the body via the respiratory tract will meet up with B cells in the tonsils and begin an immune response. Other mediators also may be involved. For example, interleukins, which stimulate the T and B cells, also cause fever and slow-wave sleep induction.

■ PRACTICING FOR NCLEX

1. Answer: d
RATIONALE: The major histocompatibility complex is the body's last barrier of defense, which involves the ability to distinguish between self-cells and foreign cells. The skin is considered the body's first line of defense. The mucous membranes and gastric acid are also two other body defenses.

2. Answer: c
RATIONALE: Lymphocytes include T cells, B cells, and natural killer cells. Neutrophils and monocytes or macrophages are types of myelocytes.

3. Answer: a
RATIONALE: Neutrophils are capable of engulfing and digesting foreign material, or phagocytosis. Basophils contain chemical mediators important for initiating and maintaining an immune or inflammatory response. The exact function of eosinophils is unknown. Macrophages release chemicals necessary to elicit a strong inflammatory reaction.

4. Answer: d
RATIONALE: Histamine is a substance released when a cell membrane is injured and is not considered lymphoid tissue. Bone marrow, the thymus gland, and the spleen are lymphoid tissues.

5. Answer: b
RATIONALE: Bradykinin causes local vasodilation and also stimulates nerve endings to cause pain, not numbness. Vasoconstriction and platelet aggregation result from the action of thromboxanes.

6. Answer: a
RATIONALE: Cell injury causes activation of the Hageman factor, which in turn activates kallikrein, leading to the conversion of kininogen to bradykinin. Bradykinin causes the release of arachidonic acid, which also causes the release of autocoids, such as prostaglandins, leukotrienes, and thromboxanes.

7. Answer: b
RATIONALE: Warmth or heat and redness are due to vasodilation. Activation of the nerve fibers would be noted as pain. Fluid leakage into tissues would be assessed as swelling. Pyrogen release would result in a fever.

8. Answer: a
RATIONALE: T cells provide cell-mediated immunity. B cells provide humoral immunity, which involves antibody or immunoglobulin production. Neutrophils are not associated with either cell-mediated or humoral immunity.

9. Answer: a
RATIONALE: Immunoglobulin M is the first immunoglobulin released and contains antibodies produced at the first exposure to the antigen. Immunoglobulin G contains antibodies made by the memory cells. Immunoglobulin

A is secreted by plasma cells in the gastrointestinal and respiratory tracts and in epithelial cells. Immunoglobulin E appears to be involved with allergic responses and activation of mast cells.

10. Answer: c
RATIONALE: Interleukin-1 stimulates T and B cells to initiate an immune response. Thymosin is a thymus hormone that is important in the maturation of T cells and cell-mediated immunity. Tumor necrosis factor is a chemical released by macrophages that inhibits tumor growth. Interferons are chemicals secreted by cells that have been invaded by viruses to prevent viral replication and also suppress malignant cell replication and tumor growth.

11. Answer: b
RATIONALE: Autoimmune disease occurs when the body responds to specific self-antigens to produce antibodies or cell-mediated immune responses against its own cells. Rejection occurs in response to foreign cells introduced into the body. Viral invasion results in an alteration of the cell membrane and antigenic presentation of the cell. Neoplastic growth occurs when mutant cells escape the normal surveillance of the immune system and begin to grow and multiply.

12. Answer: d
RATIONALE: Mucus is sticky and traps invaders and inactivates them for later destruction and removal by the body. It does not promote their removal. Cilia sweep away captured pathogens and also move them to an area, causing irritation and leading to removal by coughing or sneezing.

13. Answer: c
RATIONALE: Mast cells are basophils that are fixed and do not circulate. Mature leukocytes are monocytes or macrophages. Eosinophils are circulating myelocytic leukocytes. Neutrophils are phagocytes.

14. Answer: a
RATIONALE: The lymph nodes store concentrated populations of neutrophils, basophils, eosinophils, and lymphocytes in areas of the body that facilitate their surveillance for and destruction of foreign proteins. The thymus gland is responsible for the final differentiation of T cells and for regulating the actions of the immune system. The bone marrow plays a role in differentiating the cellular components.

15. Answer: c
RATIONALE: All transplants, except autotransplantation, produce an immune response. Therefore, matching a donor's HLA markers as closely as possible to those of the recipient for histocompatibility is essential. The more closely the foreign cells can be matched, the less aggressive the immune reaction will be to the donated tissue.

CHAPTER 16

■ ASSESSING YOUR UNDERSTANDING

MATCHING

1. c   **2.** b   **3.** a   **4.** d   **5.** e

SHORT ANSWER

1. The prototype salicylate drug is aspirin.
2. Because many anti-inflammatory drugs are available over the counter (OTC), there is a potential for abuse and overdosing. They also block the signs and symptoms of

a present illness, thus potentially causing the misdiagnosis of a problem. Patients also may combine these drugs and unknowingly induce toxicity.

3. Signs of salicylate toxicity include hyperpnea; tachypnea; hemorrhage; excitement; confusion; pulmonary edema; convulsions; tetany; metabolic acidosis; fever; coma; and cardiovascular, renal, and respiratory collapse.

4. Cyclooxygenase-1 (COX-1) is present in all tissues and seems to be involved in many body functions, including blood clotting, protecting the stomach lining, and maintaining sodium and water balance in the kidneys. COX-1 turns arachidonic acid into prostaglandins as needed in a variety of tissues. Cyclooxygenase-2 (COX-2) is active at sites of trauma or injury when more prostaglandins are needed, but it does not seem to be involved in the other tissue functions.

5. Salicylism is a syndrome that is associated with high levels of salicylates.

■ APPLYING YOUR KNOWLEDGE

CASE STUDY

a. The nurse needs to find out if the patient is experiencing any other signs and symptoms of bleeding, including any prolonged bleeding from cuts, nosebleeds, or upper gastrointestinal (GI) bleeding. The nurse should also test the patient's stool for blood to determine if there is blood in the stool. Changes in stool color may be related to other factors such as food. Additionally, the nurse should inquire about the duration of use for the ibuprofen and the actual frequency as well as how the patient takes the drug. For example, does the patient routinely take the drug every day, three times a day? How long has he been taking it? Does the patient take the drug on an empty stomach, or does he take it with food? The nurse also needs to inquire about any other drugs that the patient may be using that could interact with the ibuprofen. Moreover, the nurse would need to assess the patient's vital signs for changes and monitor laboratory test results, such as complete blood count, and coagulation studies to determine if the patient is experiencing blood loss leading to anemia or to evaluate his clotting abilities.

b. Teaching should address administration measures such as taking the drug with food or meals to prevent gastric irritation, safety measures to prevent injury and bruising, oral care measures such as using a soft toothbrush and gentle brushing, and danger signs and symptoms such as increased bleeding as well as any follow-up laboratory testing that may be necessary. Depending on the evaluation, the ibuprofen may need to be stopped, and another analgesic may need to be prescribed. If this is the case, then patient teaching would focus on the new drug and the reasons for stopping the ibuprofen.

■ PRACTICING FOR NCLEX

1. **Answer: c**
   RATIONALE: Acetaminophen has analgesic and antipyretic properties but does not exert an anti-inflammatory effect. Therefore, it would not be indicated for joint inflammation. Ibuprofen, naproxen, and diclofenac have anti-inflammatory properties and would be appropriate for use.

2. **Answer: d**
   RATIONALE: Mesalamine or olsalazine would be appropriate for a patient with inflammatory bowel disease. Diflunisal is indicated for the treatment of moderate pain and arthritis in adults; aspirin is used for the treatment of fever, pain, and inflammatory conditions. Choline

magnesium trisalicylate is indicated for the relief of mild pain, fever, and arthritis.

3. **Answer: a**
   RATIONALE: All anti-inflammatory drugs available OTC have adverse effects that can be dangerous if toxic levels of the drug circulate in the body. Since these drugs are available OTC, there is a potential for abuse and overdosing. In addition, these drugs block the signs and symptoms of a present illness. OTC agents, if combined with other drugs, can induce toxicity.

4. **Answer: b**
   RATIONALE: Salicylism can occur with high levels of aspirin and be manifested by ringing in the ears, dizziness, difficulty hearing, nausea, vomiting, diarrhea, mental confusion, and lassitude. Excitement, tachypnea, and convulsions suggest acute salicylate toxicity.

5. **Answer: a**
   RATIONALE: Care must be taken to make sure that the child receives the correct dose of any anti-inflammatory agent. This can be a problem because many of these drugs are available in OTC pain, cold, flu, and combination products. Parents need to be taught to read the label to find out the ingredients and the dosage they are giving the child. Aspirin for flulike symptoms in children is to be avoided due to the increased risk for Reye's syndrome. Children are more susceptible to the GI and central nervous system effects of these drugs, so the drugs should be given with food or meals. Acetaminophen is the most used anti-inflammatory drug for children. However, parents need to be cautioned to avoid overdosage, which can lead to severe hepatotoxicity.

6. **Answer: c**
   RATIONALE: Salicylates are contraindicated for patients who have had surgery within the past week because of the increased risk for bleeding. Their use in patients with an allergy to salicylates or tartrazine would increase the risk for an allergic reaction. Their use in patients with impaired renal function may increase the risk for toxicity because the drug is excreted in the urine. There is no associated risk for fluid imbalance and salicylate therapy.

7. **Answer: d**
   RATIONALE: Nonsteroidal anti-inflammatory drugs (NSAIDs) inhibit prostaglandin synthesis. Salicylates block prostaglandin activity. Acetaminophen acts directly on thermoregulatory cells in the hypothalamus. Gold salts inhibit phagocytosis.

8. **Answer: c**
   RATIONALE: Aurothioglucose is administered by intramuscular injection. Auranofin is given orally. Anakinra and etanercept are administered subcutaneously. None of the antiarthritic drugs are given intravenously.

9. **Answer: b**
   RATIONALE: Gold salts do not repair damage but rather help to prevent further damage. They are indicated for patients whose disease has been unresponsive to standard therapy. They are most effective if used early in the disease. Gold salts are highly toxic.

10. **Answer: d**
    RATIONALE: Gold salts should not be combined with penicillamine, cytotoxic drugs, immunosuppressive agents, or antimalarials other than low-dose corticosteroids because of the potential for severe toxicity.

11. **Answer: a**
    RATIONALE: Sulindac is an NSAID. Etanercept, adalimumab, and methotrexate are classified as disease-modifying antirheumatic drugs.

12. Answer: c

RATIONALE: Anakinra blocks the increased interleukin-1 responsible for the degradation of cartilage in rheumatoid arthritis. Etanercept reacts with free-floating tumor necrosis factor released by active leukocytes in autoimmune inflammatory disease to prevent damage caused by tumor necrosis factor. Leflunomide directly inhibits an enzyme, dihydroorotate dehydrogenase (DHODH), that is active in the autoimmune process. Penicillamine lowers immunoglobulin M rheumatoid factor levels.

13. Answer: d

RATIONALE: Hyaluronidase derivatives, such as sodium hyaluronate and hylan G-F 20, have elastic and viscous properties. These drugs are injected directly into the joints of patients with severe rheumatoid arthritis of the knee. Auranofin is administered orally. Penicillamine is administered orally, and etanercept is administered subcutaneously.

14. Answer: b

RATIONALE: COX-2 receptors block platelet clumping. COX-1 receptors maintain renal function, provide for gastric mucosal integrity, and promote vascular hemostasis.

15. Answer: b

RATIONALE: Although adequate hydration is important to promote renal function and drug excretion, it would be more important to instruct the patient in the signs and symptoms of GI bleeding. Blacks have a documented decreased sensitivity to the pain-relieving effects of many anti-inflammatory agents and have an increased risk of developing GI adverse effects to these drugs. Increased dosages may be needed to achieve pain relief, but the increased dosage increases the patient's risk for developing adverse GI effects. The drug should not be combined with an OTC salicylate, as this would further increase the patient's risk for adverse GI effects. The patient should be instructed to use nonpharmacologic measures to relieve pain, such as warm soaks and positioning.

CHAPTER 17

■ ASSESSING YOUR UNDERSTANDING

LABELING

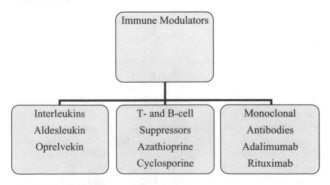

SHORT ANSWER

1. Immune stimulants include the interferons and interleukins.
2. The interleukin receptor antagonist is anakinra.
3. With the exception of erlotinib, which is given orally, all of the monoclonal antibodies are injected either intramuscularly, intravenously, or subcutaneously.
4. The exact mechanism of action of the T- and B-cell suppressors is not clearly understood. It has been shown that

they do block antibody production by B cells, inhibit suppressor and helper T cells, and modify the release of interleukins and T-cell growth factor.

5. Patients receiving immune suppressants have an increased susceptibility to infection and an increased risk of neoplasm.

■ APPLYING YOUR KNOWLEDGE

CASE STUDY

a. The nurse would need to explain to the patient that interferons are considered immune stimulants, and they act like the substances naturally produced and released by the cells in response to a virus or other stimuli. The nurse needs to correlate the drug's action with the underlying pathophysiologic events associated with multiple sclerosis as an autoimmune disorder. In addition, the nurse would explain that these drugs may help to reduce the frequency and duration of the episodes.

b. One of two interferons may be prescribed: interferon beta-1a or interferon beta-1b. Interferon beta-1a is administered intramuscularly once a week; interferon beta-1b is administered subcutaneously every other day.

c. Patient teaching should include information about the drug, its actions, and the method for administration. The patient may need to learn how to self-administer the injection, if indicated. In addition, the nurse needs to teach the patient about possible adverse effects, such as flulike symptoms (due to stimulation of the immune and inflammatory response), and other effects, such as headache, dizziness, bone marrow depression, depression, suicidal ideation, photosensitivity, and liver impairment. If the patient is of childbearing age, the nurse needs to recommend the use of barrier contraception to avoid pregnancy.

■ PRACTICING FOR NCLEX

1. Answer: a

RATIONALE: Interferon alfa-2b would be classified as an immune stimulant. Abatacept, mycophenolate, and sirolimus are T- and B-cell suppressors that are immune suppressants.

2. Answer: c

RATIONALE: Oprelvekin has been associated with severe hypersensitivity reactions, as manifested by chest tightness, difficulty breathing or swallowing, or swelling. Cardiac arrhythmias and mental status changes are adverse effects associated with interleukin therapy and do not suggest hypersensitivity. Fever is associated with the flulike adverse effects of interleukin therapy, not hypersensitivity.

3. Answer: b

RATIONALE: Cyclosporine is administered orally. Alefacept is administered as an intravenous bolus or intramuscularly; glatiramer acetate is administered subcutaneously; and abatacept is given intravenously.

4. Answer: d

RATIONALE: Supportive care and comfort measures are appropriate, including drinking plenty of fluids, using acetaminophen for fever or aches and pains, maintaining a comfortable environment such as one that is neither too warm nor too cool, and getting plenty of rest.

5. Answer: c

RATIONALE: Cetuximab is antibody specific to epidermal growth factor receptor sites. Muromonab-CD3 is a T-cell–specific antibody. Infliximab and adalimumab are antibodies specific for human tumor necrosis factors.

6. Answer: a
RATIONALE: Erlotinib, a monoclonal antibody, is administered orally. All other monoclonal antibodies are administered parenterally.

7. Answer: d
RATIONALE: Pulmonary edema would be manifested by dyspnea, chest pain, and wheezing. Fever, chills, and myalgia suggest the development of a flulike adverse effect.

8. Answer: b
RATIONALE: Although safety measures and nutrition are important, it is essential to ensure that the patient is well hydrated because gemtuzumab is associated with fever after the infusion of the drug. A bedside commode would be appropriate if the patient experienced diarrhea and had difficulty getting to the bathroom.

9. Answer: c
RATIONALE: Mycophenolate is a T- and B-cell suppressor that is used in patients having transplants to reduce the risk of rejection. Subsequently, the patient is at high risk for infection. Acute pain, imbalanced nutrition, and deficient knowledge may be appropriate, but the risk for infection would be the priority.

10. Answer: d
RATIONALE: Interferons and interleukins are immune stimulants; monoclonal antibodies, interleukin receptor antagonists, and T- and B-cell suppressors are immune suppressants.

11. Answer: b
RATIONALE: A number of interferons are produced by recombinant DNA technology, including interferon alfacon-1 (Infergen), interferon alfa-2b (Intron A), peginterferon alfa-2a (Pegasys), peginterferon alfa-2b (PEG-INTRON), and interferon beta-1b (Betaseron). Interferon alfa-n3 (Alferon N) is produced by harvesting human leukocytes. Interferon gamma-1b (Actimmune) is produced by *Escherichia coli* bacteria. Interferon beta-1a (Avonex) is produced from Chinese hamster ovary cells.

12. Answer: a
RATIONALE: Photosensitivity is a possible adverse effect, so the patient should avoid exposure to the sun and ultraviolet light, if possible, and wear protective clothing when outside. Fluid intake, use of acetaminophen, and follow-up laboratory testing are appropriate for a patient receiving interferons.

13. Answer: d
RATIONALE: Abatacept is indicated for a reduction in the signs and symptoms and the slowing of structural damage in adults with rheumatoid arthritis who have had inadequate response to other drugs. Alefacept is appropriate for patients with moderate to severe chronic plaque psoriasis who are candidates for systemic therapy. Azathioprine is indicated for the prevention of transplant rejection. Glatiramer is used to reduce the number of relapses in multiple sclerosis patients.

14. Answer: b
RATIONALE: Patients receiving anakinra and etanercept must be monitored closely for severe and even life-threatening infections. The combination is not associated with anemia, bleeding, or hypersensitivity.

15. Answer: a
RATIONALE: Muromonab-CD3 is a T-cell–specific antibody. Adalimumab, certolizumab, and infliximab are antibodies specific for human tumor necrosis factor. Alemtuzumab is an antibody specific for lymphocyte receptor sites. Basiliximab and daclizumab are specific to interleukin-2 receptor sites on activated T cells.

CHAPTER 18

■ ASSESSING YOUR UNDERSTANDING

FILL IN THE BLANKS
1. Antitoxins
2. Vaccines
3. Serum sickness
4. Passive
5. Immunization
6. Smallpox
7. Immunoglobulin G
8. Antivenin

SHORT ANSWER
1. Active immunity occurs when the body recognizes a foreign protein and begins producing antibodies to react with that specific protein or antigen. After plasma cells are formed to produce antibodies, specific memory cells that produce the same antibodies are created. If the specific foreign protein is introduced into the body again, these memory cells react immediately to release antibodies. This type of immunity is thought to be lifelong. Passive immunity occurs when preformed antibodies are injected into the system and react with a specific antigen. These antibodies come from animals that have been infected with the disease or from humans who have had the disease and have developed antibodies. The circulating antibodies act in the same manner as those produced from plasma cells, recognizing the foreign protein and attaching to it, rendering it harmless. Unlike active immunity, passive immunity is limited. It lasts only as long as the circulating antibodies last because the body does not produce its own antibodies.
2. Serum sickness is manifested by fever, arthritis, flank pain, myalgia, and arthralgia.
3. The human papilloma virus (HPV) vaccine, Gardasil, is recommended for girls ages 9 to 26 years, being most effective when given before HPV infection occurs. It is best given before a girl becomes sexually active.
4. Older adults should receive yearly flu and pneumococcal vaccines as well as a tetanus booster every 10 years.
5. The bacillus Calmette-Guérin (BCG) vaccine for tuberculosis is widely used throughout the world, in countries with a high incidence of tuberculosis to limit the spread of the disease. However, the vaccine is not routinely used in the United States because the incidence of tuberculosis is relatively low, and it can induce false-positive tuberculin skin test results.

■ APPLYING YOUR KNOWLEDGE

CASE STUDY
a. There is some controversy surrounding the HPV vaccine. The nurse needs to listen to the mother's concerns and address each of them, specifically providing the mother with accurate information about the vaccine.
b. The nurse should inform the mother that the vaccine is effective against certain but not all types of HPV (types 16 and 18, which account for 70% of cervical cancers, and types 6 and 11, which are responsible for 90% of genital warts). In addition, it is only effective if it is given before HPV infection occurs. The nurse would need to stress that HPV infection is highly prevalent and does not always cause symptoms. Other information that the nurse needs to address is that the vaccine, which requires a series of

three injections, can be expensive. Additionally, the nurse needs to address the questions posed by others such as the long-term effects and effectiveness of the vaccine, the belief that the vaccine will cause women to stop getting annual pelvic exams and Pap smears, and the misconception that the vaccine will lead to earlier or more frequent sexual activity among women who have had the vaccination.

c. The girl is within the recommended age for the vaccine. The vaccine is administered in a series of three injections. The nurse practitioner could administer the first dose with this visit, then administer the second dose in approximately 2 months, followed by the third dose in about 6 months.

■ PRACTICING FOR NCLEX

1. **Answer: a**
   RATIONALE: Vaccines provide active immunity. They promote the formation of antibodies against a specific disease. The person experiences an immune response without having to suffer the full course of the disease. Severe reactions are rare.

2. **Answer: d**
   RATIONALE: The protein of an immunization could be an actual weakened bacterial cell membrane, the protein coat of a virus, or an actual virus (protein coat with the genetic fragment that makes up a virus) that has been chemically weakened and thus cannot cause disease. Immune sera refers to sera that contains antibodies to specific bacteria or viruses.

3. **Answer: b**
   RATIONALE: The patient would receive an immune sera, most specifically rabies immune globulin. A vaccine would be used to stimulate active immunity due to exposure to a specific disease. An antitoxin would be used to protect the person from toxins released by invading pathogens. Antivenin is used to protect against spider or snake bites.

4. **Answer: b**
   RATIONALE: There is no vaccine available for plague. There is a vaccine for anthrax, but it is available only for military use. There is a vaccine for smallpox and a botulinum toxoid for botulism.

5. **Answer: c**
   RATIONALE: The vaccine for tetanus is a toxoid. The vaccines for haemophilus influenza B and pneumococcal polyvalent are bacterial vaccines. Hepatitis A is a viral vaccine.

6. **Answer: d, e, f**
   RATIONALE: Caution should be used any time a vaccine is given to a child with a history of febrile convulsions or brain injury or in any condition in which a potential fever would be dangerous. Caution also should be used in the presence of any acute infection. An immune deficiency, allergy to a vaccine component, and a blood transfusion within the past 3 months are contraindications to the use of vaccines.

7. **Answer: c**
   RATIONALE: Difficulty breathing may be a sign of a hypersensitivity reaction and should be reported immediately.

Pain or nodule formation at the injection site and moderate fever are common and expected adverse effects that do not require notification of the health care provider.

8. **Answer: a**
   RATIONALE: The nurse should instruct the mother to ensure that the child has ample rest time during the day. Acetaminophen, not aspirin, should be used for fever. Aspirin masks the signs of Reye's syndrome. Warm compresses, not cold, would be better for any pain at the injection site. The child should also rest his arm and avoid overuse.

9. **Answer: c**
   RATIONALE: Antivenin is used to treat snake bites. An antitoxin would be used to treat poisonous substances released by invading pathogens. Toxoids are vaccines. Immune sera typically refers to sera that contain antibodies to specific bacteria or viruses.

10. **Answer: a**
    RATIONALE: Meningococcal infections would be prevented by a vaccine. A toxoid is a type of vaccine made from the toxins produced by the organism. Immune globulins and antivenin are examples of immune sera.

11. **Answer: b**
    RATIONALE: Antithymocyte immune globulin is used to treat acute renal transplant rejection. The varicella virus vaccine would be used to prevent varicella (chicken pox). Hepatitis B immune globulin would be used for postexposure prophylaxis for hepatitis B. Respiratory syncytial virus (RSV) immune globulin would be used to prevent RSV in children younger than 2 years of age with bronchopulmonary dysplasia or premature birth.

12. **Answer: d**
    RATIONALE: Tetanus toxoid is used to provide passive immunization against tetanus as the result of an injury that could potentially precipitate a tetanus infection, such as a puncture wound by a nail. Zoster vaccine would be indicated to prevent herpes zoster (shingles) in a person over age 60 years. Hepatitis A vaccine is indicated for prevention of hepatitis A infection. Lymphocyte immune globulin is indicated for the management of allograft rejection in a patient with renal transplantation.

13. **Answer: c**
    RATIONALE: To prevent Rh factor sensitization, the woman would receive RHO immune globulin (RhoGAM). Crotalidae polyvalent immune fab would be used to treat rattlesnake bites. Cytomegalovirus immune globulin would be used to lessen primary cytomegalovirus disease after renal transplantation. The HPV vaccine would be used to prevent human papilloma virus infection.

14. **Answer: a**
    RATIONALE: The rotavirus vaccine is only administered orally.

15. **Answer: d**
    RATIONALE: The meningococcal polysaccharide vaccine is administered subcutaneously, often into the fatty (adipose) tissue layer of the upper arm. Deep into the muscle of the lateral thigh or upper outer quadrant of the buttocks reflects intramuscular administration. Directly into the dermis layer of the skin reflects intradermal administration.

CHAPTER 19

■ ASSESSING YOUR UNDERSTANDING

LABELING

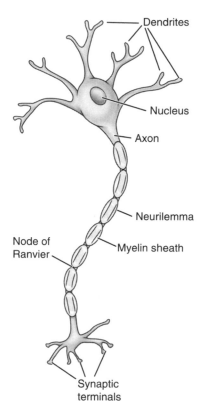

Dendrites

Nucleus

Axon

Neurilemma

Node of
Ranvier

Myelin sheath

Synaptic
terminals

MATCHING

1. e	**2.** g	**3.** b	**4.** i	**5.** c
6. f	**7.** h	**8.** j	**9.** a	**10.** d

■ APPLYING YOUR KNOWLEDGE

CASE STUDY

a. The nurse would need to explain to the patient that motor fibers from the brain cross to the other side of the spinal cord before emerging to interact with effector cells in the periphery such as the muscles. As a result, injury to the left side of the brain would lead to motor problems on the opposite side. Thus, the patient's right side is affected.

b. Blood flow to the brain is supplied by the carotid and vertebral arteries, which deliver blood to a common vessel at the bottom of the brain (the circle of Willis). This vessel then distributes blood to the brain as needed. With the mini-strokes, one of the carotid arteries was narrowed, thus supplying less blood to the circle of Willis. Although the blood flow was decreased, the areas of the brain on that side still have an adequate blood supply because the circle of Willis is able to provide blood to the area. The signs and symptoms most likely reflect a slight reduction in blood flow initially, but their quick resolution suggests that the circle of Willis was able to compensate and re-establish adequate blood flow.

■ PRACTICING FOR NCLEX

1. Answer: c
   RATIONALE: The neuron is the basic structural unit of the nervous system. The synapse refers to the junction between a nerve and an effector, such as a gland, muscle, or another nerve. Neurotransmitter is a chemical produced by a nerve and released when the nerve is stimulated. Soma refers to the cell body of a neuron.

2. Answer: b
   RATIONALE: The axon carries information from a nerve to be transmitted to effector cells. The dendrite brings information into the neuron from other neurons. The soma is the cell body of the neuron. Ganglia are groups of nerve bodies located in specific areas.

3. Answer: d
   RATIONALE: The nervous system does not prevent stimulus exposure. Rather, the nervous system is responsible for analyzing incoming stimuli, controlling the functions of the human body, and integrating internal and external responses.

4. Answer: c
   RATIONALE: Efferent fibers are nerve axons that carry nerve impulses from the central nervous system to the peripheral to stimulate muscles or glands. The presynaptic nerve is the nerve that releases a chemical, a neurotransmitter, into the synaptic cleft. Schwann cells are cells located at specific intervals along nerve axons to allow nerve conduction.

5. Answer: c
   RATIONALE: For an action potential to occur, a stimulus of sufficient strength must be present and the nerve membrane must be able to respond—that is, when it has repolarized. Sodium ions rush into the cell when the neuron is stimulated, termed *depolarization*. The nerve cell membrane is permeable to potassium ions when the cell is at rest.

6. Answer: d
   RATIONALE: Epinephrine and norepinephrine are catecholamines released by nerves in the sympathetic branch of the autonomic nervous system and are classified as hormones when released by the adrenal medulla. Dopamine is a neurotransmitter involved with the coordination of motor and intellectual impulses and responses. Gamma-aminobutyric acid (GABA) inhibits nerve activity. Acetylcholine aids in communication between nerves and muscles.

7. Answer: b
   RATIONALE: Serotonin is an important neurotransmitter involved in arousal and sleep. GABA is important in preventing overexcitability or stimulation of nerve activity. Norepinephrine is a catecholamine involved in the fight-or-flight response. Dopamine is involved in the coordination of impulses and responses, both motor and intellectual.

8. Answer: b
   RATIONALE: The blood–brain barrier is a functioning boundary that keeps toxins, proteins, and other large structures out of the brain and prevents their contact with the sensitive and fragile neurons. It is not the mechanism for blood delivery to the brain or the center responsible for controlling vital functions.

9. Answer: c
   RATIONALE: The hindbrain contains the brain stem, where the pons and medulla oblongata are located. The thalamus and limbic system are part of the midbrain. The cerebrum is part of the forebrain.

10. **Answer: a**
    RATIONALE: The spinal cord is made up of 31 pairs of spinal nerves.

11. **Answer: d**
    RATIONALE: The extrapyramidal system coordinates unconscious motor activity that regulates control of posture and position. Motor function control is regulated by sensory nerves and motor nerves along with the pyramidal system, which coordinates voluntary movement, and the extrapyramidal system. The cerebral cortex is involved in processing intellectual and emotional information, but the exact mechanism is not known.

12. **Answer: c**
    RATIONALE: Stimulation of a neuron causes depolarization, which allows sodium to rush into the cell, changing the resting membrane potential (cell is relatively negative [containing more potassium ions] compared to the outside of the cell [containing more sodium ions]). This sudden reversal creates an action potential, leading to repolarization, which returns the cell to its resting membrane potential.

13. **Answer: a, d**
    RATIONALE: The cerebrum contains motor and sensory neurons and the speech/communication areas. Cranial nerves and the chemoreceptor trigger zone are part of the hindbrain. Spinal nerve roots are found in the spinal cord.

14. **Answer: b**
    RATIONALE: The nodes of Ranvier are areas of uncovered nerve membrane that allow electrical impulses to "leap" or be conducted along the fiber. Schwann cells are myelinated areas along nerve axons that are resistant to electrical stimulation. Myelin is a substance that speeds electrical conduction and protects the nerves from fatigue due to frequent formation of action potentials. Synapse is the area where nerves communicate with each other.

15. **Answer: c**
    RATIONALE: The midbrain contains the hypothalamus, thalamus, and midbrain. The hindbrain contains the reticular activating system, respiratory control center, and swallowing center.

CHAPTER 20

■ ASSESSING YOUR UNDERSTANDING

FILL IN THE BLANKS

1. Anxiety
2. Hyponosis
3. Awareness
4. Sympathetic
5. Benzodiazepines
6. Gamma-aminobutyric acid (GABA)
7. Increased
8. Melatonin

SHORT ANSWER

1. Barbiturates, once the mainstay for the treatment of anxiety as well as for sedation and sleep induction, are not used frequently today because they are associated with potentially severe adverse effects and many drug–drug interactions. In addition, the risk for addiction and dependence is high.

2. Parenteral forms of benzodiazepines place the patient at increased risk for adverse effects, especially central nervous system (CNS) depression. The patient should be switched to oral forms as soon as possible.

3. The response of a child to anxiolytic may be unpredictable. Commonly, inappropriate aggressiveness, crying, irritability, and tearfulness can occur.

4. Drugs used as hypnotics act on the reticular activating system and block the brain's response to incoming stimuli.

5. Some blacks are genetically predisposed to delayed metabolism of benzodiazepines, leading to increased serum drug levels and increased sedation and incidence of adverse effect.

■ APPLYING YOUR KNOWLEDGE

CASE STUDY

a. The nurse would need to gather information related to the patient's usual routine and sleep hygiene activities. For example, the nurse should question the patient about naps during the day, level of activity and exercise, use of stimulants such as caffeine (including when and how much), and usual routine before going to bed.

b. The patient is an older adult who will probably need a dosage reduction for several reasons. He may have age-related changes in liver and/or renal function that may increase his risk for toxicity related to the drug. Older adult patients also have been found to be especially sensitive to this drug, thus necessitating a lower dosage.

c. Education should include the following: information about the drug, such as the drug name, dosage, and time for administration (taking the drug before bed); need to ensure at least 4 to 8 hours for sleep; signs and symptoms of adverse drug effects; safety measures to reduce the risk for injury; need for daily exercise and avoidance of daytime naps; and sleep hygiene measures such as a consistent routine, use of warm milk before bed, avoidance of caffeine-containing products after dinner, and avoidance of stimulating activities.

■ PRACTICING FOR NCLEX

1. **Answer: c**
   RATIONALE: Ramelteon should be taken $^1Ú_2$ hour before going to bed.

2. **Answer: b**
   RATIONALE: Flurazepam would be used as a hypnotic. Lorazepam, diazepam, and alprazolam would be use as anxiolytics.

3. **Answer: a**
   RATIONALE: Benzodiazepines make GABA more effective, which leads to the anxiolytic effect. The drug does not affect action potentials. Depression of the cerebral cortex and motor output are associated with the use of barbiturates.

4. **Answer: c**
   RATIONALE: Patients who receive parenteral benzodiazepines should be monitored in bed for a period of at least 3 hours. Thus, the patient would be allowed out of bed at approximately 2 PM.

5. **Answer: d**
   RATIONALE: Intra-arterial administration of benzodiazepines would result in arteriospasm and gangrene. CNS depression, blurred vision, and urinary retention are adverse effects associated with benzodiazepines in general.

6. **Answer: a**
   RATIONALE: When giving diazepam intravenously, it should not be mixed in solution with any other drugs. Therefore, it would be best to start an intravenous line in another

area, such as the opposite arm, so that the patient can receive the full benefits of both drugs. Notifying the prescriber that the diazepam cannot be given or waiting until the other drug is completed before giving the diazepam is inappropriate. Adding it to the current infusion is inappropriate because potentially serious drug–drug interactions can occur.

7. **Answer: b**
   RATIONALE: Signs and symptoms of benzodiazepine withdrawal include nightmares, nausea, headache, and malaise. Dry mouth, hypotension, and urinary retention are adverse effects associated with benzodiazepine use.

8. **Answer: c**
   RATIONALE: The effects of benzodiazepines are increased when taken with oral contraceptives, necessitating a change in dosage of the benzodiazepine. The effects of benzodiazepines are decreased when taken with theophylline and ranitidine, which might result in the need for an increased dosage of the benzodiazepine. Alcohol should not be used with benzodiazepines because the combination increases the risk of CNS depression.

9. **Answer: b**
   RATIONALE: Diazepam peaks in approximately 1 to 2 hours, so the maximum effect of the drug would be seen between 5 and 6 PM.

10. **Answer: d**
    RATIONALE: It would be appropriate to have the patient void before administering the medication to reduce the patient's risk for injury if the patient attempts to get out of bed after the drug is given. Raising the side rails, instituting a bowel program, and dimming the lights would be appropriate after giving the drug.

11. **Answer: c**
    RATIONALE: Flumazenil is the antidote for benzodiazepines and is used to reverse the sedation of benzodiazepines used for diagnostic procedures. Temazepam and triazolam are benzodiazepines used as hypnotics. Promethazine is an antihistamine with sedative effects.

12. **Answer: d**
    RATIONALE: Phenobarbital is considered the prototype barbiturate.

13. **Answer: b**
    RATIONALE: When given intravenously, barbiturates can result in bradycardia, hypotension, hypoventilation, respiratory depression, and laryngospasm. Bleeding is not associated with barbiturate therapy.

14. **Answer: a**
    RATIONALE: Although taking the drug with meals, increasing fiber intake (to prevent constipation), and using additional measures to promote relaxation would be helpful instructions, it would be most important for the nurse to warn the patient not to stop the drug abruptly. There is a risk for withdrawal if anxiolytics, both benzodiazepines and barbiturates, are stopped abruptly.

15. **Answer: c**
    RATIONALE: Buspirone has no sedative, anticonvulsant, or muscle relaxant properties, but it does reduce the signs and symptoms of anxiety. Diphenhydramine is an antihistamine that can be sedating. Zaleplon causes sedation and is used for short-term treatment of insomnia. Meprobamate has some anticonvulsant properties and CNS-relaxing effects.

CHAPTER 21

■ ASSESSING YOUR UNDERSTANDING
LABELING

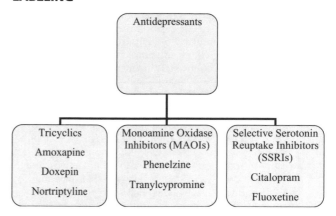

SHORT ANSWER

1. The three biogenic amines are norepinephrine, dopamine, and serotonin.
2. Tricyclic antidepressants all reduce the uptake of serotonin and norepinephrine.
3. Affect refers to the feelings that people experience when they respond emotionally.
4. When ingested while taking MAOIs, tyramine may be absorbed in high concentrations, resulting in increased blood pressure. In addition, tyramine causes the release of stored norepinephrine from nerve terminals, which contributes to high blood pressure and hypertensive crisis.
5. Amitriptyline is associated with a marked sedative and anticholinergic effect.
6. SSRIs do not have the many adverse effects associated with tricyclic antidepressants and MAOIs.

■ APPLYING YOUR KNOWLEDGE
CASE STUDY

a. The nurse would most likely suspect that the patient is experiencing a hypertensive crisis due to ingestion of foods containing tyramine while receiving MAOIs or a possible drug–drug interaction with the patient's current MAOI and a tricyclic antidepressant (imipramine).

b. The nurse would need to assess for additional manifestations of hypertensive crisis, including palpitations, neck stiffness, sweating, dilated pupils, photophobia, tachycardia, and chest pain. In addition, the nurse needs to gather information about the patient's recent food intake to determine if the patient ingested foods containing tyramine, which can precipitate a hypertensive crisis with MAOIs. Another area that the nurse needs to investigate is if the patient is still taking the imipramine, a tricyclic antidepressant with phenelzine. These drugs can interact, leading to hypertensive crisis. In addition, the nurse should obtain information about any other medications that the patient may be taking—for example, sympathomimetics, which could lead to an increase in sympathomimetic effects such as vasoconstriction, pupillary dilation, and increased heart rate as well as increased blood pressure.

c. The nurse would need to teach the patient to check with his health care provider before taking any other over-the-counter drugs or prescription medications because MAOIs interact with many of them. If the patient was still taking the imipramine, then the nurse would need to tell the patient to stop the drug to prevent further interaction. In addition, the nurse needs to teach the patient about foods that contain tyramine and the importance of avoiding them. The nurse could give the patient a written list of the foods so that he can refer to it in the future.

■ PRACTICING FOR NCLEX

1. **Answer: b**
RATIONALE: Bupropion is an antidepressant that is also used for smoking cessation in lower dosages. Venlafaxine is used to treat and prevent depression in generalized anxiety disorder, as treatment for social anxiety disorder, and to help decrease addictive behaviors. Mirtazapine and selegiline are used to treat depression.

2. **Answer: c**
RATIONALE: Although studies have been done, the Food and Drug Administration has concluded that there is not enough evidence to link suicidal ideation to antidepressant use. However, all of the drugs should be used with caution, and prescriptions should be written in the smallest quantity feasible. Only a few tricyclic antidepressants have established pediatric dosages for children over age 6 years; the use of MAOIs should be avoided; and SSRIs are associated with serious adverse effects in children. Antidepressant use with children is challenging because the child's response is unpredictable.

3. **Answer: a**
RATIONALE: The adverse effects of nortriptyline, such as sedation, anticholinergic effects, hypotension, and cardiovascular effects, are negligible. Amitriptyline exhibits marked sedation, anticholinergic effects, and hypotension. Clomipramine is associated with moderate sedation, anticholinergic effects, hypotension, and cardiovascular effects. Doxepin is associated with moderate sedative and anticholinergic effects as well as mild hypotension and cardiovascular effects.

4. **Answer: a**
RATIONALE: Tricyclic antidepressants are administered in oral form.

5. **Answer: c**
RATIONALE: Only clomipramine is indicated for the treatment of obsessive-compulsive disorder.

6. **Answer: d**
RATIONALE: A recent myocardial infarction would be a contraindication for use because of the potential occurrence of reinfarction or extension of the infarction due to the drug's cardiac effects. Cautious use and close monitoring would be appropriate for the patient with glaucoma and prostatic hypertrophy due to the anticholinergic effects. Cautious use in renal dysfunction also is warranted because the drugs are excreted in the urine.

7. **Answer: c**
RATIONALE: Transdermal selegiline should be applied to dry intact skin on the upper arm, upper thigh, or upper torso. The patient should always remove the old patch before applying a new one to prevent inadvertent overdose. Transdermal selegiline is associated with central nervous system (CNS) and gastrointestinal (GI) effects.

8. **Answer: d**
RATIONALE: Trazodone is associated with a risk for low blood pressure and priapism (a sustained, painful erection). CNS effects, such as dizziness and sedation, occur with this drug but are not a cause for notifying the health care provider.

9. **Answer: a, b, c, f**
RATIONALE: Isocarboxazid is an MAOI, which necessitates avoiding foods containing tyramine such as aged cheeses, red wines, smoked meats (i.e., pepperoni), and sour cream.

10. **Answer: b**
RATIONALE: Fluoxetine is associated with respiratory changes such as cough, GI effects such as dry mouth, CNS effects such as drowsiness, and genitourinary effects such as impotence.

11. **Answer: d**
RATIONALE: It may take up to 4 weeks before the full effect of an SSRI is noted.

12. **Answer: c**
RATIONALE: Sertraline is an SSRI. Doxepin is a tricyclic antidepressant. Nefazodone and bupropion are other antidepressants that are not classified as tricyclic antidepressants, SSRIs, or MAOIs.

13. **Answer: b**
RATIONALE: Paroxetine, a SSRI, and phenelzine, an MAOI, should not be given together because of the risk for serotonin syndrome. At least 4 to 6 weeks should be allowed between the use of the two drugs when switching from one to the other.

14. **Answer: a, b**
RATIONALE: The nurse should inform the patient to take the tricyclic antidepressant once daily in the morning as prescribed to ensure the maximum benefit. The dosage could be divided if the patient experiences severe GI effects. Sugar-free hard candies and gums would help to alleviate the dry mouth that may occur. A high-fiber diet would be appropriate if the patient develops constipation. The nurse should instruct the patient to control the lighting, temperature, and stimuli of the environment to address possible CNS effects.

15. **Answer: c**
RATIONALE: MAOIs interact with oral antidiabetic agents, increasing the patient's risk for hypoglycemia. Diabetic ketoacidosis would be associated with hyperglycemia. Orthostatic hypotension, urinary retention, dysuria, and incontinence may occur with MAOI therapy, but these are not associated with the interaction of an oral antidiabetic agent and an MAOI.

CHAPTER 22

■ ASSESSING YOUR UNDERSTANDING

SHORT ANSWER

1. The most common type of psychosis is schizophrenia.
2. Psychotherapeutic agents are used to treat perceptual and behavioral disorders, targeting action at thought processes rather than affective states. They do not cure the disorder but help patients function in a more acceptable manner and carry out activities of daily living.
3. Antipsychotic agents are called neuroleptic agents because of the associated neurologic adverse effects.
4. Antipsychotic agents are no longer called major tranquilizers because the primary action of these drugs is not sedation but a change in neuron stimulation and response.
5. Antipsychotic drugs are classified as typical or atypical antipsychotics.

LABELING

Dopamine	Serotonin	Norepinephrine
Aripiprazole	Aripiprazole	Lithium
Chlorpromazine	Clozapine	
Clozapine	Quetiapine	
Lithium	Ziprasidone	
Fluphenazine		
Pimozide		
Quetiapine		
Ziprasidone		

■ APPLYING YOUR KNOWLEDGE

CASE STUDY

a. Since the patient is experiencing mania, obtaining the information from the patient at this time would probably be quite difficult. The nurse could question the patient but would need to keep in mind that the patient may not be a reliable source of information. Since the patient is known to the staff, the nurse could review the patient's medical record to gather information about the patient's medications (including herbal therapies such as psyllium, which could interact with lithium and lead to nontherapeutic drug levels) and previous episodes. In addition, the medical record could provide the nurse with the name of a family member or contact person who could help provide information. If the nurse determines that the patient has been taking lithium in the past, the nurse could obtain a serum drug level to determine if the drug level was therapeutic. If the level was not therapeutic, then the nurse might conclude that the patient had stopped taking the medication.

b. In most cases, the drug of choice would be lithium. However, other agents can be used for acute manic episodes such as olanzapine or ziprasidone.

c. The nurse would need to provide clear, simple explanations to the patient at the present time, emphasizing what is being done and why. Any other teaching would need to be postponed until the patient's mania is controlled. Once this occurs, the nurse would need to implement a teaching plan that addresses the medication prescribed, including the importance of compliance and follow-up to monitor drug levels. The nurse may need to involve a family member or support person in this teaching to ensure that the patient understands the information. It may be necessary to initiate a social service referral to assist the patient in complying with the therapy.

■ PRACTICING FOR NCLEX

1. **Answer: a**
   RATIONALE: Pseudoparkinsonism is manifested by cogwheel rigidity, muscle tremors, drooling, a shuffling gait, and slow movements. Abnormal eye movements, neck spasms, and excessive salivation would suggest dystonia.

2. **Answer: b**
   RATIONALE: Therapeutic serum lithium levels range from 0.6 mEq/L to 1.2 mEq/L, so a level of 0.8 mEq/L would be considered therapeutic. A level of 0.2 mEq/L would be nontherapeutic. Levels above 1.2 mEq/L would be considered toxic.

3. **Answer: c**
   RATIONALE: Clozapine is classified as an atypical antipsychotic. Haloperidol, loxapine, and pimozide are considered typical antipsychotics.

4. **Answer: d**
   RATIONALE: Fluphenazine is considered a highly potent antipsychotic. Chlorpromazine, thioridazine, and prochlorperazine are considered low-potent antipsychotics.

5. **Answer: a**
   RATIONALE: After administering parenteral forms of antipsychotic agents, the nurse should keep the patient recumbent for approximately $\frac{1}{2}$ hour to reduce the risk of orthostatic hypotension.

6. **Answer: b**
   RATIONALE: Phenothiazines such as fluphenazine often turn the urine pink to reddish-brown as a result of excretion. Fatal arrhythmias are associated with thioridazine, mesoridazine, and ziprasidone. Nasal congestion, not rhinorrhea, is a possible adverse effect. The risk for developing diabetes is associated with atypical antipsychotics. Fluphenazine is a typical antipsychotic.

7. **Answer: c**
   RATIONALE: Clozapine is associated with significant leukopenia. Subsequently, is it available only through the Clozaril Patient Management System, which involves monitoring white blood cell count and compliance issues with only a 1-week supply being given at a time. Aripiprazole, olanzapine, and quetiapine are not associated with leukopenia.

8. **Answer: b**
   RATIONALE: A thiazide diuretic–lithium combination increases the risk of lithium toxicity because sodium is lost and lithium is retained. Lithium effectiveness is decreased with tromethamine and antacids. Psyllium interferes with the absorption of lithium, leading to nontherapeutic levels.

9. **Answer: a, c, e**
   RATIONALE: A patient with a serum lithium level between 1.5 to 2.0 mEq/L would exhibit central nervous system (CNS) problems such as slurred speech. The patient may also exhibit electrocardiogram changes and polyuria. Hypotension, hyperreflexia, and seizures would be assessed with levels between 2.0 to 2.5 mEq/L.

10. **Answer: c**
    RATIONALE: The last dose of methylphenidate should be administered before 6 PM to reduce the incidence of insomnia.

11. **Answer: d**
    RATIONALE: Modafinil would be indicated for the treatment of narcolepsy. Atomoxetine, dexmethylphenidate, and lisdexamfetamine are indicated for the treatment of attention deficit disorders.

12. **Answer: a**
    RATIONALE: Tardive dyskinesia involves abnormal muscle movements such as lip smacking, tongue darting, slow and aimless arm and leg movements, and chewing movements. Akathisia is manifested by continued restlessness and an inability to sit still. Pseudoparkinsonism is manifested by muscle tremors, cogwheel rigidity, drooling, shuffling gait, and slow movements. Dystonia is manifested by spasms of the tongues, neck, back, and legs.

13. **Answer: a**
    RATIONALE: Nasal congestion is a manifestation of anticholinergic effects. Neuroleptic malignant syndrome reflects the drug's effect on the CNS. Laryngospasm is a respiratory effect; arrhythmia is a cardiovascular effect.

14. **Answer: b**
    RATIONALE: Periodically, the drug therapy needs to be interrupted to determine if the child experiences a recurrence of symptoms, which would indicate the need for continued treatment.

15. Answer: c
RATIONALE: Haloperidol is associated with the greatest increased risk of extrapyramidal adverse effects. Sedation, anticholinergic effects, and hypotension can occur, but the risk for these is much less when compared with the risk for extrapyramidal effects.

16. Answer: d
RATIONALE: Aripiprazole is indicated for the treatment of mania and schizophrenia. Lithium and lamotrigine are indicated only for the treatment of mania. Risperidone is indicated only for the treatment of schizophrenia.

CHAPTER 23

■ ASSESSING YOUR UNDERSTANDING

MATCHING

1. g   **2.** f   **3.** b   **4.** d   **5.** a
6. e   **7.** c

SHORT ANSWER

1. The five types of generalized seizures are tonic-clonic, absence, myoclonic, febrile, jacksonian, and psychomotor.

2. Simple partial seizures occur in a single area of the brain and may involve a single muscle movement or sensory alteration. Complex partial seizures involve a series of reactions or emotional changes, complex sensory changes such as hallucinations, mental distortion, changes in personality, loss of consciousness, and loss of social inhibitions. Motor changes may include involuntary urination, chewing motions, diarrhea, and so on. The onset of complex partial seizures usually occurs by the late teens.

3. Drugs used to treat generalized seizures most often lead to sedation and other central nervous system (CNS) effects.

4. The succinimides and drugs that modulate gamma-aminobutyric acid (GABA) are most frequently used to treat absence seizures.

5. Phenobarbital has very low lipid solubility, giving it a slow onset and very long duration of action.

6. The drugs used to control partial seizures stabilize nerve membranes in two ways—either directly, by altering sodium and calcium channels, or indirectly, by increasing the activity of GABA, an inhibitory neurotransmitter, and thereby decreasing excessive activity.

■ APPLYING YOUR KNOWLEDGE

CASE STUDY

a. The nurse needs to allow the mother and father to verbalize their concerns and fears and then correct any misconceptions that they may have about their son's condition. The nurse also would then begin to teach the parents about the disorder and his treatment, including the drug therapy regimen, emphasizing that consistency and compliance with the therapy is essential in controlling the disorder. In addition, the nurse would begin teaching the parents how to manage a seizure if it does occur to avoid injury to the child while at the same time remaining calm. Written instructions in this case would probably be very helpful so that the parents can review the information and then ask questions that they may have. Information about the drug's adverse effects and the need for follow-up testing of serum drug levels would be important. Knowing that the child's drug level is therapeutic is helpful in alleviating some of the anxiety related to the child having another seizure.

b. The nurse would recommend that the child wear Medic-alert identification that lists his condition and the therapy he is taking. Additional recommendations and suggestions may include having the parents talk with parents of other children with seizures as well as having the parents join a support group. In addition, the nurse would encourage the parents to talk with child's teacher and school nurse about dealing with the seizures as well as talk with the child's classmates and friends about his condition and what to do if a seizure occurs. Talking with the school nurse would be very important because the child may need to take medication while at school.

■ PRACTICING FOR NCLEX

1. Answer: c
RATIONALE: Levetiracetam is available for oral or intravenous use. Carbamazepine, gabapentin, and felbamate are administered orally.

2. Answer: b
RATIONALE: The therapeutic serum phenytoin levels range from 10 to 20 mcg/mL. Thus, a level of 12 mcg/mL would fall within this range.

3. Answer: d
RATIONALE: Hydantoins may cause gingival hyperplasia, severe liver toxicity, and bone marrow suppression. Physical dependence and withdrawal syndrome are associated with benzodiazepines.

4. Answer: c
RATIONALE: The barbiturates and barbituratelike drugs depress motor nerve output, inhibit impulse conduction in the ascending reticular activating system (RAS), depress the cerebral cortex, and alter cerebellar function. They stabilize nerve membranes throughout the CNS directly by influencing ionic channels in the cell membrane, thereby decreasing excitability and hyperexcitability to stimulation.

5. Answer: d
RATIONALE: Although phenobarbital is available in oral and parenteral forms, status epilepticus is an emergency situation that requires the drug to be given intravenously to achieve a rapid onset of action.

6. Answer: a
RATIONALE: Lamotrigine has been associated with very serious to life-threatening rashes, and the drug should be discontinued at the first sign of any rash. Somnolence and confusion are typical CNS effects; anorexia is a common gastrointestinal effect.

7. Answer: b
RATIONALE: Pregabalin has a controlled substance rating of category V because it causes feelings of well-being and euphoria. Subsequently, its use should be limited in patients who have a history of abuse of medications and alcohol. Increased CNS depression would occur if the patient ingested alcohol with either topiramate, felbamate, or tiagabine.

8. Answer: a
RATIONALE: Therapeutic serum carbamazepine levels range from 4 to 12 mcg/mL. Therefore, a level under 4 mcg/mL would suggest that the drug has not reached therapeutic levels, so the dosage may need to be increased.

9. Answer: b
RATIONALE: The patient is experiencing CNS effects that could lead to injury. Therefore, the nurse would need to implement safety precautions as the priority. Hydration may be needed if the patient were experiencing vomiting

or diarrhea. Skin-care measures would be appropriate for the development of a rash. Emotional support would be appropriate if the patient had verbalized difficulty coping with the condition or drug therapy.

10. Answer: b
RATIONALE: When phenobarbital is given to a child intravenously for treatment of a febrile seizure, a second dose may be repeated in 6 hours, which in this situation would be 4 PM.

11. Answer: c
RATIONALE: Valproic acid is considered the drug of choice for myoclonic seizures and a second choice drug for absence seizures. Clonazepam may be used for myoclonic seizures, but it is not considered the drug of choice. Diazepam and zonisamide are not used for treating myoclonic seizures.

12. Answer: c
RATIONALE: Ethosuximide is most frequently used to treat absence seizures. Mephobarbital, ethotoin, and primidone are typically used for tonic-clonic seizures.

13. Answer: a
RATIONALE: Zonisamide inhibits voltage-sensitive sodium and calcium channels, thus stabilizing the nerve cell membranes and modulating calcium-dependent presynaptic release of excitatory neurotransmitters. Hydantoins decrease the conduction through nerve pathways. Barbiturates and barbituratelike agents depress the cerebral cortex and motor nerve output.

14. Answer: a
RATIONALE: Ethotoin is administered orally.

15. Answer: d
RATIONALE: Although weight loss and anorexia may occur, ethosuximide is associated with bone marrow suppression, including potentially fatal pancytopenia, so it would be most important for the nurse to monitor the patient's complete blood count. The drug is not associated with any cardiovascular effects that would necessitate an electrocardiogram.

CHAPTER 24

■ ASSESSING YOUR UNDERSTANDING

FILL IN THE BLANKS

1. Bradykinesia
2. Substantia nigra
3. Dopamine, cholinergic
4. Dopaminergic, anticholinergic
5. Tyramine

LABELING

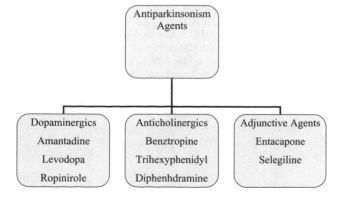

■ APPLYING YOUR KNOWLEDGE

CASE STUDY

a. The nurse might interpret these signs and symptoms as being related to a possible hypertensive crisis that can occur with rasagiline and the ingestion of foods containing tyramine, some drugs, and some herbal preparations.

b. The nurse would need to investigate if the patient has taken any herbal preparations such as St. John's wort or medications such as meperidine or other analgesics. In addition, the nurse would need to ask the patient and his daughter about ingestion of tyramine foods such as aged cheeses; red wine; smoked or pickled meats or fish; certain dairy products, such as sour cream or yogurt; chocolate; or certain fruits, such as figs, raisins, grapes, pineapples, or oranges.

■ PRACTICING FOR NCLEX

1. Answer: a
RATIONALE: Levodopa is a precursor of dopamine that crosses the blood–brain barrier, where it is converted to dopamine, acting like a replacement therapy. Amantadine increases the release of dopamine. Apomorphine directly binds with postsynaptic dopamine receptors. Ropinirole directly stimulates dopamine receptors.

2. Answer: b
RATIONALE: When levodopa is used in combination with carbodopa, the enzyme dopa is inhibited in the periphery, diminishing the metabolism of levodopa in the gastrointestinal tract and in peripheral tissues, thereby leading to higher levels crossing the blood–brain barrier. Because the carbidopa decreases the amount of levodopa needed to reach a therapeutic level in the brain, the dosage of levodopa can be decreased, which reduces the incidence of adverse side effects.

3. Answer: c
RATIONALE: Apomorphine is administered subcutaneously. The other dopaminergic agents are administered orally.

4. Answer: d
RATIONALE: Levodopa is contraindicated in patients with suspicious skin lesions because the drug is associated with the development of melanoma. Cautious use is recommended for patients with myocardial infarction, bronchial asthma, and peptic ulcer disease, as these conditions could be exacerbated by dopamine receptor stimulation.

5. Answer: c
RATIONALE: Adverse effects associated with dopaminergics usually result from stimulation of dopamine receptors and may include nervousness, anxiety, confusion, mental changes, muscle twitching, ataxia, and hypotension.

6. Answer: d
RATIONALE: St. John's wort can lead to hypertensive crisis if taken with rasagiline, not levodopa. Decreased effectiveness of levodopa is seen with the use of pyridoxine (vitamin B₆), phenytoin, and multivitamin supplements.

7. Answer: a
RATIONALE: Trihexyphenidyl is available only in an oral form.

8. Answer: b
RATIONALE: Anticholinergics are contraindicated for patients with myasthenia gravis, which could be exacerbated by the blocking of acetylcholine receptor sites at the neuromuscular synapses. Hypertension, hepatic dysfunction, and cardiac arrhythmia would require cautious use.

9. Answer: d
RATIONALE: Agitation would be noted due to the blocking of central acetylcholine receptors. Constipation, reduced sweating, and dry mouth may be noted as well.

10. Answer: c
RATIONALE: Bromocriptine is classified as a dopaminergic agent. Diphenhydramine and biperiden are classified as anticholinergics. Tolcapone is considered an adjunctive agent.

11. Answer: d
RATIONALE: The patient is experiencing central nervous system (CNS) effects related to drug therapy, which could predispose the patient to falls. Thus, a risk for injury would be appropriate. Risk for impaired thermoregulation would be related to blockage of reflex sweating mechanism. Disturbed thought processes would be reflected by disorientation, confusion, and memory loss. Deficient knowledge would be appropriate if the patient were asking questions about the drug therapy.

12. Answer: b
RATIONALE: Entacapone inhibits catecholamine-O-methyl transferase, which eliminates catecholamines including dopamine. Lactic dehydrogenase is a liver enzyme. Rasagiline inhibits monoamine oxidase type B. Acetylcholinesterase breaks down acetylcholine.

13. Answer: b
RATIONALE: Apomorphine is associated with a risk for hypotension and a prolonged QT interval. Therefore, the priority would be to monitor the patient's cardiac status closely. The drug is given by subcutaneous injection, not oral administration. Checking for skin lesions would be appropriate for a patient receiving levodopa due to its association with melanoma. Palpating the bladder would be appropriate for any dopaminergic agent because of the risk for urinary retention. However, this would not be the priority.

14. Answer: c
RATIONALE: Biperiden is indicated for the treatment of drug-induced parkinsonism resulting from the drug effects of phenothiazines. Bromocriptine and pramipexole are indicated for the treatment of idiopathic Parkinson's disease. Selegiline is indicated for the treatment of idiopathic Parkinson's disease with levodopa-carbidopa in patients whose response to therapy has decreased.

15. Answer: b
RATIONALE: Blurred vision is considered a peripheral anticholinergic effect. Delirium, agitation, and memory loss are considered central effects affecting the CNS.

CHAPTER 25

■ ASSESSING YOUR UNDERSTANDING
CROSSWORD

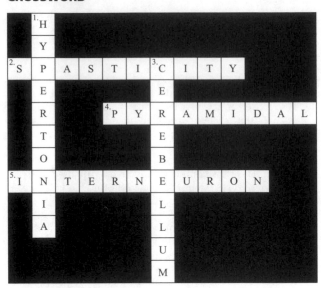

SHORT ANSWER

1. The pyramidal tract controls precise intentional movement; the extrapyramidal tract coordinates unconsciously controlled muscle activity and allows the body to make automatic adjustments in posture or position and balance.
2. Muscle spasticity is caused by nerve damage in the central nervous system (CNS).
3. Muscle spasm often results from injury to the musculoskeletal system.
4. Movement and muscle control are regulated by spinal reflexes and the upper CNS, including the basal ganglia, cerebellum, and cerebral cortex.
5. Centrally acting skeletal muscle relaxants are often referred to as spasmolytics because they lyse or destroy spasm by interfering with the reflexes that are causing the spasm.
6. Baclofen is the prototype centrally acting skeletal muscle relaxant.
7. Direct-acting skeletal muscle relaxants enter the muscle to prevent muscle contraction directly.
8. Botulinum toxin type A is used to improve the appearance of moderate to severe glabellar lines.

■ APPLYING YOUR KNOWLEDGE
CASE STUDY

a. Cyclobenzaprine is a centrally acting skeletal muscle relaxant that is used to relieve the discomfort of acute musculoskeletal conditions. The nurse would need to determine if the patient is to receive the regular or the controlled-release form so that the appropriate schedule can be determined. Typically, the controlled-release form is taken at the same time each day to ensure consistent drug levels. In addition, the nurse would need to teach the patient about the commonly occurring adverse effects such as CNS depression; gastrointestinal (GI) upset, including dry mouth, nausea, and constipation; and urinary frequency and urgency. The nurse would also need to instruct the patient to avoid alcohol and other CNS depressants.

b. The nurse would also need to include instructions for care of the injured area such as rest, support for the injured area, heat application, and the use of anti-inflammatory agents. As the area heals, physical therapy may be indicated to help the muscle return to its normal tone. In addition, the nurse should teach the patient about ways to minimize injury in the future, including adequate warm-ups and not overdoing it.

■ PRACTICING FOR NCLEX

1. Answer: b
RATIONALE: Carisoprodol is the centrally acting skeletal muscle relaxant of choice for older patients because it is considered safer than the other agents.

2. Answer: c
RATIONALE: Simple reflex arcs involve sensory receptors in the periphery and spinal motor nerves. Such reflex arcs make up what is known as the spindle gamma loop system. The pyramidal tract is part of the CNS that controls precise intentional movement. The extrapyramidal tract, also a part of the CNS, controls unconscious muscle activity. The basal ganglia is the portion of the brain that is associated with unconscious muscle movements.

3. Answer: a
RATIONALE: Botulinum toxin type A is classified as a direct-acting skeletal muscle relaxant. Diazepam, methocarbamol, and orphenadrine are centrally acting skeletal muscle relaxants.

4. Answer: d
RATIONALE: Centrally acting skeletal muscle relaxants would be contraindicated for treatment of muscle spasms related to a rheumatic disorder. Epilepsy, cardiac disease, or hepatic function would necessitate cautious use.

5. Answer: b
RATIONALE: Baclofen peaks in 2 hours after administration, so maximum effectiveness would be noted at this time, which in this case would be 10 AM.

6. Answer: c
RATIONALE: Dantrolene is indicated for the control of spasticity resulting from upper motor neuron disorders such as amyotrophic lateral sclerosis. Chlorzoxazone, metaxalone, and methocarbamol are used to treat acute musculoskeletal conditions.

7. Answer: a
RATIONALE: Dantrolene interferes with the release of calcium from the muscle tubules, preventing the fibers from contracting. Botulinum toxins A and B bind directly to the receptor sites of motor nerve terminals and inhibit the release of acetylcholine. Centrally acting skeletal muscle relaxants interfere with the reflexes that are causing the muscle spasm. Tizanidine is thought to increase inhibition of presynaptic motor neurons in the CNS.

8. Answer: c
RATIONALE: Chlorzoxazone may discolor the urine, becoming orange to purple-red in color. Baclofen, carisoprodol, and tizanidine do not discolor urine.

9. Answer: b
RATIONALE: Botulinum toxin is administered as an injection and should not be given if there is active infection at the site of the intended injection.

10. Answer: d
RATIONALE: Dantrolene therapy must be discontinued at any sign of liver dysfunction. Intermittent GI upset,

visual disturbances, and urinary retention are associated adverse effects of the drug and, although problematic, do not necessitate discontinuing the drug.

11. Answer: b
RATIONALE: Dantrolene is the drug that would be used as prevention and treatment of malignant hyperthermia.

12. Answer: c
RATIONALE: Although deficient knowledge, risk for injury, and disturbed thought processes may apply, the patient with an acute knee strain most likely would be experiencing pain as well as muscle spasms further contributing to the pain, subsequently leading to the use of a centrally acting skeletal muscle relaxant. Thus, a nursing diagnosis of acute pain would be the priority.

13. Answer: b
RATIONALE: The risk for hepatocellular disease is increased in women and all patients over the age of 35 years. Respiratory disease could be exacerbated with the use of dantrolene. Acute infection would be a contraindication to the use of botulinum toxins.

14. Answer: d
RATIONALE: The use of botulinum toxin type A is associated with droopy eyelids (in severe cases), headache, respiratory infections, flulike syndrome, pain, redness, and muscle weakness, which are usually temporary. Abnormal hair growth, acne, and photosensitivity may be associated with dantrolene.

15. Answer: a, c, f
RATIONALE: Adverse effects associated with baclofen therapy include drowsiness, urinary frequency, constipation, hypotension, fatigue, weakness, and dry mouth.

CHAPTER 26

■ ASSESSING YOUR UNDERSTANDING

LABELING

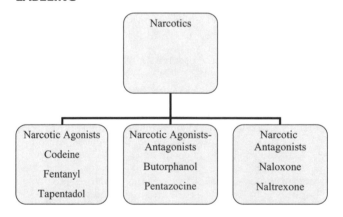

SHORT ANSWER

1. Two small-diameter sensory nerves, called the A-delta and C fibers, respond to stimulation by generating nerve impulses that produce pain sensations.
2. A fibers transmit sensations associated with touch and temperature.
3. Opioid receptors respond to naturally occurring peptins, endorphins, and enkephalins.
4. The three factors may include past experience with pain, learned response, and environmental setting.
5. The three functions of narcotic agonists-antagonists include relief of moderate to severe pain, adjunct to general anesthesia, and pain relief during labor and delivery.

6. Triptans cause cranial vascular constriction and relief of migraine headaches.
7. The four types of opioid receptors are mu, kappa, beta, and sigma.

■ APPLYING YOUR KNOWLEDGE

CASE STUDY

a. The patient's increase in pain may be due to several factors. The patient's cancer may be progressing, which most likely would increase the amount of pain that he is experiencing. The patient also may be developing a tolerance for the medication, necessitating a larger dose or a more frequent dosing schedule. Additionally, psychological factors may be involved since the patient will not be receiving any further treatment, thus dispelling any hopes for a remission or cure.

b. Possible options include increasing the dosage of the morphine or administering it by another route that may be more effective. Another drug such as fentanyl may be added to the regimen to address the breakthrough pain that the patient is experiencing.

c. The nurse would suggest comfort measures to promote the effectiveness of the medication. For example, the nurse might suggest back rubs or massages, heat or cold therapy, relaxation techniques, and complementary therapies such as music therapy or aromatherapy to aid in relaxation. In addition, it would be important for the nurse to encourage the patient to verbalize his feelings and concerns related to his prognosis so that the patient's pain is not exacerbated by anxiety, fear, or depression. Support groups and hospice care may be appropriate suggestions.

■ PRACTICING FOR NCLEX

1. **Answer: b**
   RATIONALE: Fentanyl is available as a transdermal patch.
2. **Answer: b**
   RATIONALE: The most appropriate method for assessing pain is to have the patient rate his pain by using some type of scale. This provides objective evidence of the severity of the pain and provides a basis for comparison later on.
3. **Answer: a**
   RATIONALE: Typically, codeine or hydrocodone are used to relieve coughing.
4. **Answer: a**
   RATIONALE: Extended-release preparations should be taken as a whole tablet—not cut, crushed, or chewed. Doing so with oxycodone would allow release of the entire drug dose at one time instead of the gradual release over time, as would be appropriate with an extended-release form.
5. **Answer: c**
   RATIONALE: Many sources recommend waiting 4 to 6 hours to breast-feed a baby after receiving a narcotic.
6. **Answer: b**
   RATIONALE: Oral morphine peaks in approximately 1 hour; in this situation, it would be 4:00 PM.
7. **Answer: d**
   RATIONALE: Pentazocine is available in parenteral and oral forms, making it the preferred choice for patients who will be switched from parenteral to oral forms after surgery.
8. **Answer: c**
   RATIONALE: Narcotics are associated with orthostatic hypotension, pupil constriction, constipation, and respiratory depression with apnea.
9. **Answer: c**
   RATIONALE: Naloxone is a narcotic antagonist that is used to reverse the effects of narcotics such as morphine.

Butorphanol and buprenorphine are narcotic agonists-antagonists that are used for moderate to severe pain relief. Ergotamine would be used to prevent and treat migraine attacks.

10. **Answer: a**
    RATIONALE: Naltrexone is administered orally.
11. **Answer: a**
    RATIONALE: Migraine headaches are associated with severe unilateral pulsating pain on one side of the head. Sharp steady eye pain with an onset usually during sleep is associated with cluster headaches. A dull band of pain around the head suggests a tension headache.
12. **Answer: a**
    RATIONALE: Ergot derivatives block alpha-adrenergic and serotonin receptor sites in the brain to cause constriction of cranial vessels, a decrease in cranial artery pulsation, and a decrease in the hyperperfusion of the basilar artery bed.
13. **Answer: b**
    RATIONALE: Ergotamine, an ergot derivative, would be most appropriate for the prevention and treatment of an acute migraine attack. Triptans such as sumatriptan and eletriptan are used for treatment of an acute migraine but not prevention. Naloxone is used to reverse the effects of opioids.
14. **Answer: c**
    RATIONALE: Dihydroergotamine is administered intranasally or intramuscularly at the first sign of a headache. Ergotamine could be administered sublingually or via inhalation. All triptans are administered orally except for sumatriptan, which could be administered orally, subcutaneously, or by nasal spray.
15. **Answer: c**
    RATIONALE: With sumatriptan, the patient should take the first dose at the first sign of a headache and then repeat the dose, if needed, in approximately 2 hours.

CHAPTER 27

■ ASSESSING YOUR UNDERSTANDING

CROSSWORD

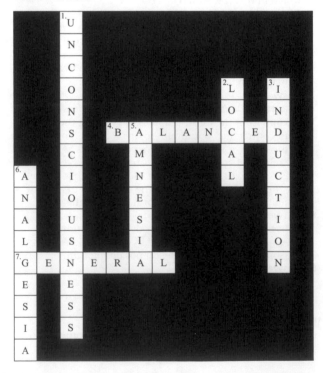

SEQUENCING

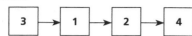

■ APPLYING YOUR KNOWLEDGE

CASE STUDY

a. The nurse needs to approach the patient in a supportive, nonjudgmental manner and slowly explain the events of the day. The nurse needs to determine what the patient knows about the surgical experience and then reinforce this information, correcting any misconceptions or misinformation that she may have. If necessary, the nurse may need to go step-by-step as to what to expect so that the patient does not experience any additional upset or stress. In addition, the patient is visibly anxious, so the nurse need to provide the patient with support to help alleviate her anxiety. Explanations geared to the patient's level of understanding would be the most effective.

b. The nurse needs to underscore the importance of the history and physical examination as well as the tests being done to ensure that the most appropriate choices for anesthesia are used—that is, ones that would be the most effective without causing her undue harm. Information about underlying medical conditions and the use of other drugs is important to prevent additional adverse effects and drug–drug interactions. The anesthesiologist or certified nurse anesthetist is the individual who will decide which anesthetics the patient will receive. It might be helpful to have the anesthesiologist return to talk with the patient about what to expect. This may have already been done, but it does not seem that the patient has understood or heard what was told to her. The nurse would also explain the use of any preoperative sedation that may be given and how that might make her feel as well as what will happen when she is transported to the surgical suite.

■ PRACTICING FOR NCLEX

1. **Answer: c**
   RATIONALE: Pupillary dilation occurs during stage 3 of surgical anesthesia.
2. **Answer: a**
   RATIONALE: Although ketamine, midazolam, and propofol exert only mild analgesic effects, thiopental has no analgesic properties, indicating that the patient may need additional analgesics after surgery.
3. **Answer: d**
   RATIONALE: Methohexital is associated with nausea and vomiting during the recovery period. Adverse effects include hypotension, suppressed respirations, and decreased gastrointestinal activity.
4. **Answer: b**
   RATIONALE: Combinations of barbiturate anesthestics and narcotics may produce apnea more commonly than with other analgesics.
5. **Answer: a**
   RATIONALE: Midazolam is an example of a nonbarbiturate anesthetic. Nitrous oxide is an anesthetic gas. Thiopental is a barbiturate anesthetic. Halothane is a volatile liquid anesthetic.
6. **Answer: c**
   RATIONALE: Ketamine is associated with a bizarre state of unconsciousness in which the patient appears to be awake but is unconscious and cannot feel pain. Propofol produces much less of a hangover effect. Droperidol

produces a state of mental detachment. Etomidate is sometimes used to sedate patients receiving mechanical ventilation.
7. **Answer: b**
   RATIONALE: Ketamine has an onset of action within 30 seconds; droperidol's onset is within 3 minutes; etomidate's onset occurs within 1 minute; and propofol's onset occurs within 30 to 60 seconds.
8. **Answer: d**
   RATIONALE: During recovery from etomidate, myoclonic and tonic movements, nausea, and vomiting may occur. Chills, hypertension, hallucinations, and cardiac arrhythmias can occur during recovery from droperidol. Respiratory depression and central nervous system suppression may occur during recovery from midazolam.
9. **Answer: b**
   RATIONALE: Nitrous oxide can block the reuptake of oxygen after surgery and cause hypoxia. Subsequently, it is always given in combination with oxygen.
10. **Answer: a**
    RATIONALE: Volatile liquids are liquids that are unstable at room temperature and release gases that are inhaled by the patient, as are gas anesthetics.
11. **Answer: c**
    RATIONALE: Although monitoring temperature and reflexes, providing comfort measures, and providing pain relief are important, the priority is to ensure that emergency equipment is readily available to allow for prompt intervention should problems arise.
12. **Answer: b**
    RATIONALE: In increasing concentrations, local anesthetics also cause the loss of the following sensations in this order: temperature, touch, proprioception, and skeletal muscle tone.
13. **Answer: b**
    RATIONALE: The dermal patch is applied 20 to 30 minutes before the procedure.
14. **Answer: a**
    RATIONALE: When a local anesthetic is to be applied, it is important to ensure that the area is intact and free of breakdown to prevent inadvertent systemic absorption of the drug.
15. **Answer: c**
    RATIONALE: Benzocaine is an example of an ester. Mepivacaine, lidocaine, and dibucaine are examples of amide local anesthetic agents.

CHAPTER 28

■ ASSESSING YOUR UNDERSTANDING

FILL IN THE BLANKS

1. Neuromuscular junction (NMJ)
2. Sarcomere
3. Actin, myosin
4. Acetylcholine
5. Nondepolarizing
6. Depolarizing

SEQUENCING

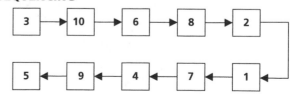

■ APPLYING YOUR KNOWLEDGE

CASE STUDY

a. The patient is to be intubated; the pancuronium would be used to facilitate passage of the endotracheal tube during the intubation procedure and to minimize the patient's attempt to fight or resist mechanical ventilation.

b. The patient has a history of asthma, which could be exacerbated by the use of pancuronium due to the paralysis of the respiratory muscles altering perfusion and respiratory function. In addition, the drug can cause respiratory obstruction with wheezing and bronchospasm. Therefore, his respiratory status and oxygenation would need to be monitored very closely as he is mechanically ventilated. Also, measures to prevent aspiration would be important to prevent drug-related gastrointestinal effects from further compromising the patient's respiratory status. As a victim of multiple trauma, it is likely that his fluid and electrolyte balanced would be altered. This could affect membrane stability and subsequent muscular function. In addition, hyperkalemia can occur due to changes in the muscle membrane. Close monitoring of fluid and electrolyte status would be essential. Monitoring for hypotension and cardiac arrhythmias would be necessary to determine the patient's ability to adapt to the drugs. Moreover, the drug does not alter the pain perception, so the nurse would need to assess the patient's level of pain frequently.

c. The drug does not allow muscle contraction, so the nurse needs to inform the patient and family that the patient's muscles will be paralyzed. However, the patient may still feel pain and be conscious because the drug does not affect pain perception or consciousness. The nurse needs to work with the patient and family in setting up a means to communicate his needs or changes in his condition because the patient is unable to speak since he is intubated and receiving mechanical ventilation. Additionally, the nurse would inform the patient and family about the need for frequent turning and repositioning to prevent skin breakdown and the use of periodically evaluating muscle response and recovery, including the use of a peripheral nerve stimulator to assess the degree of neuromuscular blockade.

■ PRACTICING FOR NCLEX

1. **Answer: d**
   RATIONALE: Of the NMJ blockers, cisatracurium has the longest duration of action.

2. **Answer: a**
   RATIONALE: Atracurium should not be used before induction of anesthesia.

3. **Answer: b**
   RATIONALE: Calcium channel blockers may greatly increase the paralysis caused by nondepolarizing NMJ blockers. If used together, the dose of the nondepolarizing NMJ agent would be decreased. Cholinesterase inhibitors would decrease the effectiveness of the nondepolarizing NMJ agent. Depolarizing NMJ blockers also interact with calcium channel blockers.

4. **Answer: a**
   RATIONALE: The body's initial reaction to succinylcholine is muscle pain that occurs with the initial muscle contraction reaction. Hyperthemia would suggest malignant hyperthermia but does not occur as a first response. Hypotension and respiratory depression also occur, but these would not be an initial assessment finding.

5. **Answer: b**
   RATIONALE: Conditions associated with a decreased production of cholinesterase, the enzyme necessary to break down succinylcholine, include cirrhosis, metabolic disorders, cancer, burns, dehydration, malnutrition, hyperpyrexia, thyrotoxicosis, collagen diseases, and exposure to neurotoxic insecticides.

6. **Answer: a**
   RATIONALE: According to the sliding filament theory, acetylcholine interacts with nicotinic receptors, not muscarinic receptors. Acetylcholine is broken down by acetylcholinesterase, freeing the receptor for further stimulation which when stimulated causes depolarization that leads to the release of calcium. Calcium combines with troponin, which then causes the release of actin and myosin binding sites, allowing them to react together. This repeated reaction leads to fiber shortening and muscle contraction.

7. **Answer: c**
   RATIONALE: NMJ blockers, in most cases, do not affect pain perception and consciousness. They cause muscle paralysis without total central nervous system depression and are associated with serious adverse effects. They do not readily cross the blood–brain barrier.

8. **Answer: d**
   RATIONALE: Succinylcholine is associated with the development of malignant hyperthermia in susceptible patients. Pancuronium, vecuronium, and atracurium are not associated with the development of this condition.

9. **Answer: b**
   RATIONALE: Aspirin is useful in relieving the muscle pain that occurs with administration of a NMJ blocker, specifically succinylcholine. Dantrolene would be used to treat malignant hyperthermia that may occur with succinylcholine. Morphine would not be used to alleviate this muscle pain. Naloxone is used to reverse the depression associated with narcotic overdoses.

10. **Answer: d**
    RATIONALE: Depolarizing NMJ blockers cause stimulation of the muscle cell, stay on the receptor site, and prevent repolarization, resulting in muscle paralysis with a muscle that is in a constant contracted state. Nondepolarizing NMJ blockers prevent depolarization of the muscle cells.

11. **Answer: a**
    RATIONALE: Succinylcholine is the only NMJ blocker that may cause increased intraocular pressure.

12. **Answer: c**
    RATIONALE: Pancuronium has an onset of action of approximately 4 to 6 minutes.

13. **Answer: b**
    RATIONALE: Succinylcholine has a short duration of action, lasting approximately 4 to 6 minutes after administration.

14. **Answer: a**
    RATIONALE: Myasthenia gravis would be a contraindication for the use of a nondepolarizing NMJ blocker because blockage of the acetylcholine cholinergic receptors would aggravate the neuromuscular disease. Cirrhosis and malnutrition would require extremely cautious use of succinylcholine, which is a depolarizing NMJ blocker. Glaucoma would be a contraindication to the use of succinylcholine due to the increased intraocular pressure that occurs.

15. **Answer: c**
    RATIONALE: A cholinesterase inhibitor is used to overcome the excessive neuromuscular blockade of a nondepolarizing NMJ blocker. A direct-acting skeletal muscle relaxant, such as dantrolene, would be used to treat malignant hyperthermia associated with a depolarizing NMJ blocker. A peripheral nerve stimulator is used to assess the degree of neuromuscular blockade. A narcotic antagonist would be used to reverse a narcotic's effect.

CHAPTER 29

■ ASSESSING YOUR UNDERSTANDING

CROSSWORD

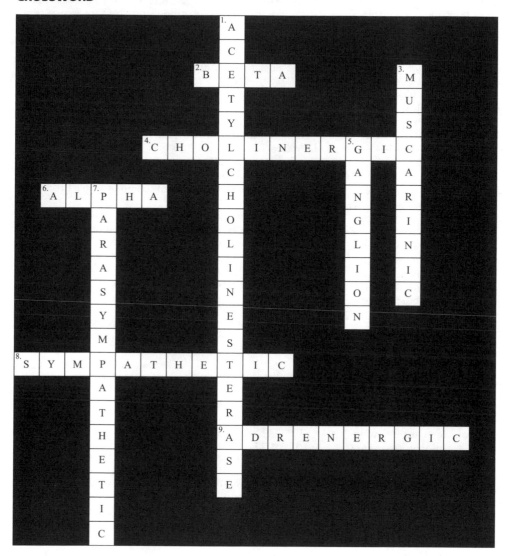

SHORT ANSWER

1. The main nerve centers are located in the hypothalamus, medulla, and spinal cord.
2. Throughout the autonomic nervous system (ANS), nerve impulses are carried from the central nervous system (CNS) to the outlying organs by way of a two-neuron system. In most peripheral nervous system activities, the CNS nerve body sends an impulse directly to an effector organ or muscle. The ANS does not send impulses directly to the periphery. Instead, axons from CNS neurons end in ganglia, or groups of nerve bodies that are packed together, located outside the CNS. These ganglia receive information from the preganglionic neuron that started in the CNS and relay that information along postganglionic neurons. The postganglionic neurons transmit impulses to the neuroeffector cells—muscles, glands, and organs.
3. The sympathetic nervous system (SNS) is also called the thoracolumbar system.
4. Acetylcholine is the neurotransmitter released by the preganglionic nerves of the SNS.
5. The catecholamines include norepinephrine, dopamine, serotonin, and epinephrine.
6. Sympathetic adrenergic receptors are classified as alpha-1, alpha-2, beta-1, and beta-2.
7. Parasympathetic nervous system (PNS) receptors are classified as muscarinic or nicotinic.
8. The two enzymes involved are monoamine oxidase (MAO), and catechol-O-methyl transferase.

■ APPLYING YOUR KNOWLEDGE

CASE STUDY

a. The patient is experiencing an anxiety attack, which in most instances would be similar to a fight-or-flight response. Thus, the patient's SNS is predominating at this point. The patient's heart rate and respiratory rate are increased, and she is experiencing sweating due to the increase in metabolic activity that is occurring. The patient's cool and clammy hands are most likely related to the vasoconstriction and diversion of blood away from the area to more vital centers.

b. Additional signs and symptoms would include increased blood pressure, increased depth of respirations, bronchial dilation, pupillary dilation, piloerection, decreased bowel sounds, and decreased urination.

c. The nurse would explain the fight-or-flight response as the basis for what she is experiencing, correlating her anxiety level as a stimulus for the response. The nurse could liken the response to an accelerator that speeds things up for action. The nurse needs to emphasize that this response is a normal body response but that if the body becomes over-stimulated, it can lead to system overload and disorders.

■ PRACTICING FOR NCLEX

1. **Answer: a, b, f**
   RATIONALE: The ANS functions to control heart rate, water balance, and respiration. Level of consciousness, sensory perception, and muscle movement are functions of the CNS.

2. **Answer: c**
   RATIONALE: The SNS has short preganglionic nerve fibers and long postganglionic nerve fibers that synapse with neuroeffectors. The cells are located primarily in the thoracic and lumbar sections of the spinal cord. The ganglia are located in chains running alongside the spinal cord.

3. **Answer: d**
   RATIONALE: In the stress or fight-or-flight response, the nurse would assess diminished bowel sounds, tachycardia, hypertension, and pupil dilation.

4. **Answer: a**
   RATIONALE: The release of adrenal hormones, including cortisol, suppress the immune and inflammatory reactions to preserve energy during the fight-or-flight response. Thyroid hormone increases metabolism and efficient use of energy. Aldosterone causes sodium and water retention and potassium excretion. Glucose is formed by glycogenolysis to increase the blood glucose level and provide energy.

5. **Answer: a**
   RATIONALE: Alpha-1 stimulation leads to vasoconstriction and increased peripheral vascular resistance resulting in a rise in blood pressure. Alpha-2 stimulation prevents overstimulation of effector sites and moderate insulin release by the beta cells of the pancreas. Beta-1 stimulation increases myocardial activity. Beta-2 stimulation causes vasodilation and bronchodilation.

6. **Answer: d**
   RATIONALE: Relaxation of the urinary detrusor muscle occurs with stimulation of beta-2 receptors. Alpha-1 receptor stimulation would promote closure of the urinary sphincter. Alpha-2 stimulation prevents overstimulation of effector sites and moderate insulin release by the beta cells of the pancreas. Beta-1 stimulation increases myocardial activity.

7. **Answer: b**
   RATIONALE: With parasympathetic nervous stimulation, gastric motility increases, secretions increase, pupils constrict, and the rectal and urinary sphincters relax to allow elimination.

8. **Answer: c**
   RATIONALE: In the PNS, the neurotransmitter involved in pre- and postganglion activity is acetylcholine. Norepinephrine is involved in postganglionic activity of the SNS. Epinephrine is involved in the adrenergic response, being secreted directly into the bloodstream by the adrenal medulla. Dopamine is converted to norepinephrine in the adrenergic cells.

9. **Answer: a**
   RATIONALE: The vagus nerve, originating in the cranium, is one of the most important parts of the PNS. Adrenergic receptors, norepinephrine, and MAO are aspects that would be included in the discussion of the SNS.

10. **Answer: b**
    RATIONALE: The SNS preganglionic fibers are short; the PNS preganglionic fibers are long. The SNS ganglia are located in chains along the spinal cord; those of the PNS are located close to or within the effector tissue. The SNS is the system involved in the stress response, while the PNS is the rest and digest system. The PNS contains nicotinic and muscarinic receptors.

11. **Answer: d**
    RATIONALE: Vasodilation, as well as bronchodilation and uterine relaxation, occur as a result of beta-2 stimulation. Piloerection results from stimulation of alpha-1 receptors.

12. **Answer: b**
    RATIONALE: Alpha-2 receptors are found in the beta cells of the pancreas. Alpha-1 receptors are found in blood vessels, the iris, and urinary bladder. Beta-1 receptors are found in cardiac tissue. Beta-2 receptors are found in the smooth muscle of the blood vessels, bronchi, periphery, and uterine muscle.

13. **Answer: c**
    RATIONALE: Cholinergic nerves are located on all preganglionic nerves in the ANS, postganglionic nerves of the PNS and a few SNS nerves, motor nerves on skeletal muscles, and cholinergic nerves within the CNS.

14. **Answer: b**
    RATIONALE: Muscarinic receptors are located in visceral effector organs such as the gastrointestinal tract, bladder, and heart; in sweat glands; and in some vascular smooth muscle. Nicotinic receptors would be found in the adrenal medulla, neuromuscular junction, and CNS.

15. **Answer: b**
    RATIONALE: Norepinephrine is made by the nerve cells using tyrosine, which is obtained in the diet. Dihydroxyphenylalanine (dopa) is produced by a nerve, using tyrosine from the diet and other chemicals. With the help of the enzyme dopa decarboxylase, the dopa is converted to dopamine, which in turn is converted to norepinephrine in adrenergic cells.

CHAPTER 30

■ ASSESSING YOUR UNDERSTANDING
LABELING

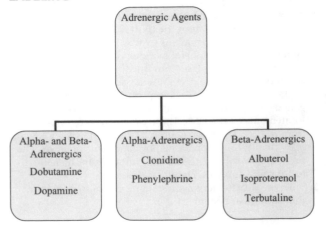

SHORT ANSWER

1. Adrenergic agonists stimulate the adrenergic receptors of the sympathetic nervous system directly by reacting with receptor sites or indirectly by increasing norepinephrine levels.
2. Adrenergic agonists are also referred to as sympathomimetic agents because they mimic or produce the same effects of the sympathetic nervous system.
3. Dopamine is the sympathomimetic drug of choice for treating shock.
4. Clonidine specifically stimulates alpha-2 receptors and is used to treat hypertension because its action blocks release of norepinephrine from nerve axons.
5. A sympathomimetic agent (adrenergic agonist) will lose effectiveness if it is combined with any adrenergic antagonist.
6. Adrenergic agonists cause vasoconstriction. In patients with vascular problems, their use could exacerbate the underlying vascular problem due to the systemic vasoconstriction that occurs.

■ APPLYING YOUR KNOWLEDGE

CASE STUDY

a. The nurse should respond to the patient in a nonjudgmental and supportive manner. The nurse should investigate further about the underlying reasons for the patient's statements. For example, is the patient concerned that there is not a sufficient dosage contained in the patch? Or is the patient more comfortable with taking pills? Possibly, the patient may be anxious about how to apply the patch or apply the patch correctly. He might believe that it is easier to just take a pill.

b. The nurse needs to instruct the patient how the patch works, providing a gradual release of the drug that lasts 7 days, and about how to apply the patch, once every 7 days to a hairless area of the body, such as the upper arm or chest. The nurse also needs to reinforce the need to apply the patch to intact, clean, dry skin and to remove the patch before applying a new one. Additional instructions also should address not stopping the patch abruptly because of possible rebound hypertension. The nurse also needs to warn the patient about possible adverse effects, including central nervous system effects such as bad dreams, sedation, drowsiness, fatigue, and headache. Safety measures including changing positions slowly, lifestyle modifications to control blood pressure, the importance of avoiding over-the-counter (OCT) cold preparations, and compliance with regular follow-ups to evaluate blood pressure would be essential.

■ PRACTICING FOR NCLEX

1. **Answer: b**
   RATIONALE: Dopamine is a naturally occurring catecholamine. Dobutamine, ephedrine, and metaraminol are synthetic catecholamines.
2. **Answer: a**
   RATIONALE: Dobutamine, although it acts at both receptor sites, has a slight preference for beta-1 receptor sites. It is used in the treatment of congestive heart failure because it can increase myocardial contractility without much change in rate and does not increase the oxygen demand of the cardiac muscle. There is an increased risk for hypertension if any alpha- and beta-adrenergic agonist is used with herbal therapies and OTC preparations.

3. **Answer: b**
   RATIONALE: Adverse effects of alpha- and beta-adrenergic agonists include dyspnea, hypertension, and constipation. Personality changes are associated with alpha-specific adrenergic agonists.
4. **Answer: c**
   RATIONALE: The drug of choice for treating shock is dopamine because it stimulates the heart and blood pressure and also causes a renal and splanchnic arteriole dilation that increases blood flow to the kidney, preventing diminished renal blood supply and possible renal shutdown that can occur with epinephrine or norepinephrine. Ephedrine is used to treat hypotensive episodes, but its use is declining because of the availability of less-toxic drugs with more predictable onset and action. Dobutamine is used to treat congestive heart failure.
5. **Answer: a**
   RATIONALE: Alpha- and beta-adrenergic agonists interact with caffeine, ma huang, and OTC cold preparations, increasing the risk for hypertension. St. John's wort has not been shown to interact with these agents.
6. **Answer: d**
   RATIONALE: If extravasation occurs, the nurse should infiltrate the site with 10 mL of saline containing 5 to 10 mg of phentolamine. Hyaluronidase and sodium bicarbonate may be used for extravasation of certain antineoplastic agents. Lactated Ringer's solution would be inappropriate.
7. **Answer: a, d, e**
   RATIONALE: Clonidine is an alpha-specific adrenergic agonist that may cause sensitivity to light (photophobia), personality changes, difficulty urinating, and pupil dilation. Hyperglycemia may occur if the patient has diabetes and takes clonidine.
8. **Answer: c**
   RATIONALE: Intramuscular phenylephrine has an onset of action within 10 to 15 minutes.
9. **Answer: c**
   RATIONALE: The desired effects of isoproterenol include improved contractility and conductivity, increased heart rate, bronchodilation, relaxation of the uterus, and increased blood flow to skeletal muscles and splanchnic beds.
10. **Answer: a**
    RATIONALE: To counteract the effects of isoproterenol, a beta-specific adrenergic agonist, the nurse would administer a beta-adrenergic blocker.
11. **Answer: d**
    RATIONALE: Most of the beta-specific adrenergic agonists are beta-2–specific adrenergic agonists, which are used to treat and manage bronchial spasm, asthma, and other obstructive pulmonary conditions.
12. **Answer: a**
    RATIONALE: Pulmonary hypertension would be a contraindication for isoproterenol because the drug could exacerbate the condition. Glaucoma would be a contraindication for the use of an alpha-specific adrenergic agonist. Pheochromocytoma and hypovolemia would be contraindications for the use of alpha- and beta-adrenergic agonists.
13. **Answer: c**
    RATIONALE: If dopamine could not be used to prevent hypotension, then norepinephrine would be the drug of choice. It increases myocardial contractility and causes peripheral vasoconstriction.

14. Answer: b

RATIONALE: Midodrine is associated with a serious supine hypertension. Therefore, monitoring blood pressure changes in different positions (standing, sitting, and supine) would be most important. The drug is not associated with respiratory adverse effects. Decreased urinary output and anorexia may occur, but these would not be as important as monitoring the changes in the patient's blood pressure.

15. Answer: b

RATIONALE: Phenylephrine is a common agent found in many OTC cold and allergy products. Ephedra has been banned by the Food and Drug Administration as a drug. Neither epinephrine nor albuterol are found in OTC products.

CHAPTER 31

■ ASSESSING YOUR UNDERSTANDING

LABELING

Nonselective Alpha	Alpha-1 Selective	Nonselective Beta	Beta-1 Selective
Phentolamine	Doxazosin Terazosin	Carteolol Pindolol Propranolol	Atenolol Esmolol

FILL IN THE BLANKS

1. Sympatholytics
2. Norepinephrine
3. Hypoglycemia
4. Hypertension
5. Lowering
6. Postsynaptic
7. Cardiovascular
8. Decreased
9. Two
10. Atenolol

■ APPLYING YOUR KNOWLEDGE

CASE STUDY

a. The patient is receiving carvedilol, a nonselective adrenergic blocker, as well as sotalol, a nonselective beta blocker. Both agents lower blood pressure. The diuretic promotes fluid loss, which also aids in lowering blood pressure. The fluid loss associated with diuretic therapy also may be contributed to possible dehydration, which could lower the blood pressure further. The patient may be experiencing orthostatic hypotension, which is a drop in blood pressure that occurs with position changes.

b. It would be important to obtain additional information by obtaining the following: vital signs; blood pressure evaluation in the lying, sitting, and standing positions (to evaluate any changes in readings with position changes); electrocardiogram (to rule out any underlying cardiac changes that might be contributing to the patient's complaints); evaluation of hydration status (skin turgor, review of fluid intake, and electrolyte levels). In addition, it would be important to ask the patient about any alcohol ingestion, which can contribute to hypotension.

c. The patient needs instructions related to safety measures, such as rising slowly from a sitting position or sitting at the edge of the bed for a few minutes before arising. In addition, the patient needs to ensure that he is taking in adequate amounts of fluid to prevent any dehydration that would further compound the hypotension. Additionally, the patient should be instructed not to stop taking the drugs abruptly because of the possible serious adverse effects that might occur. Additionally, emphasis on compliance with the therapy and follow-up is essential to ensure that the patient's needs and concerns are addressed and to ensure maximum drug therapy effectiveness with the least amount of adverse effects.

■ PRACTICING FOR NCLEX

1. Answer: a

RATIONALE: Monitoring liver function studies would be most important because carvedilol has been associated with hepatic failure. Renal function studies may be appropriate to evaluate for possible renal dysfunction that might necessitate a change in drug dosage, but this would not be the priority. Monitoring complete blood count and coagulation studies would not be necessary.

2. Answer: b

RATIONALE: Sotalol absorption is decreased by the presence of food; to ensure maximum effectiveness of the drug, the patient should take it on an empty stomach, not with an antacid or after a large meal. The dose is typically divided during the day and should not be taken all at once.

3. Answer: b

RATIONALE: Nonselective adrenergic blockers block the effects of norepinephrine at the alpha and beta receptors in the sympathetic nervous system, leading to a slower pulse rate, lowering of blood pressure, increased renal perfusion, and decreased renin levels.

4. Answer: c

RATIONALE: Labetalol, a nonselective adrenergic blocker, increases the effectiveness of antidiabetic agents leading to an increased risk for hypoglycemia. Hypotension would occur if the drug were combined with other drugs that are known to lower blood pressure. Arrhythmias and bronchspasm are adverse effects of nonselective adrenergic blockers and are unrelated to the combination of labetalol and insulin.

5. Answer: b

RATIONALE: Alpha-1 selective adrenergic blockers cause a decrease in vascular tone and vasodilation, which leads to a fall in blood pressure. Because these drugs do not block the presynaptic alpha-2 receptor sites, the reflex tachycardia that accompanies a fall in blood pressure does not occur. They also block smooth muscle receptors in the prostate, prostatic capsule, prostatic urethra, and urinary bladder neck, which lead to a relaxation of the bladder and prostate and improved flow of urine in males.

6. Answer: a

RATIONALE: Tamsulosin, an alpha-1 selective adrenergic blocker, is used for the treatment of benign prostatic hypertrophy. Prazosin, also an alpha-1 selective blocker, is used to treat hypertension. Carteolol, a nonselective beta blocker, is used for the treatment of hypertension. Amiodarone, a nonselective adrenergic blocker, is reserved for use in treating arrhythmias.

7. Answer: b

RATIONALE: Adverse gastrointestinal (GI) effects are associated with the loss of the balancing sympathetic effect on the GI tract and the increased parasympathetic dominance. The drug's effect on liver function would be associated with the development of liver dysfunction and failure. Blockage of norepinephrine in the central nervous system (CNS) would lead to adverse effects such as dizziness, paresthesias, insomnia, fatigue, and vertigo. Loss of vascular tone would be associated with hypotension, heart failure, pulmonary edema, and cerebrovascular accident.

8. Answer: a

RATIONALE: Oral labetalol peaks in 1 to 2 hours.

9. Answer: d

RATIONALE: Although safety measures are important part of the teaching plan for any nonselective beta blocker, they would be a priority for a patient receiving propranolol. The drug crosses the blood–brain barrier, leading to the development of CNS effects. Carteolol, nadolol, and sotalol do not cross the blood–brain barrier; thus, the risk for CNS effects would be less.

10. Answer: b

RATIONALE: A patient receiving propranolol should understand that the drug should not be stopped abruptly but rather should be tapered over a period of 2 weeks. Getting up slowly, spacing activities, and reporting any chest pain or difficulty breathing demonstrate an understanding of the possible adverse effects of the drug and measures to address them.

11. Answer: d

RATIONALE: Atenolol is a beta-1 selective adrenergic blocker. This agent would be preferred for the patient who smokes because the drug does not usually block beta-1 receptor sites. Subsequently, it does not block the sympathetic bronchodilation that would be important for this patient. Timolol, pindolol, and nadolol are nonselective beta-adrenergic blockers that would block this sympathetic bronchodilation.

12. Answer: c

RATIONALE: Beta-1 selective blockers are contraindicated in patients with sinus bradycardia. Diabetes, thyroid disease, and chronic obstructive pulmonary disease are conditions that require cautious use of beta-1 selective blockers.

13. Answer: d

RATIONALE: For acute myocardial infarction, metoprolol is given via intravenous bolus. Three doses, each given at 2-minute intervals, are used and then the patient is started on oral therapy, which is started 15 minutes after the last intravenous dose.

14. Answer: a

RATIONALE: Bisoprolol is often the drug of choice for older patients who require an adrenergic blocker for hypertension because it is not associated with as many problems in this age group and regular dosing profiles may be used.

15. Answer: c

RATIONALE: A beta-1 selective blocker is helpful after a myocardial infarction because it decreases the cardiac workload and myocardial oxygen demand. The drug decreases contractility, excitability, and the heart rate. Although it also decreases blood pressure, it is not this effect that makes it a useful in preventing reinfarction.

CHAPTER 32

■ ASSESSING YOUR UNDERSTANDING
LABELING

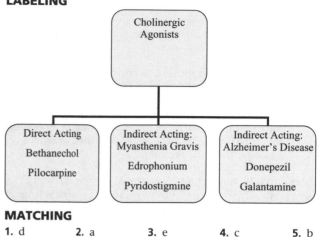

MATCHING

1. d	2. a	3. e	4. c	5. b

■ APPLYING YOUR KNOWLEDGE
CASE STUDY

a. The patient is most likely experiencing either a myasthenic crisis in which she needs additional medication or a cholinergic crisis or cholinergic overdose, necessitating withdrawal of the medication. Myasthenia gravis is a condition that is characterized by periods of exacerbations and remissions that are highly unpredictable. Too much pyridostigmine can lead to a cholinergic crisis, whereas as not enough pyridostigmine can lead to a myasthenic crisis. Both conditions are manifested by increasing muscle weakness.

b. To determine whether the patient is experiencing a myasthenic or cholinergic crisis, an edrophonium challenge test would be used. *If* the patient improves after injection of the edrophonium, then she most likely is experiencing a myasthenic crisis. In this case, additional cholinergic medication would be given. If the patient's signs and symptoms do not improve or actually become worse with edrophonium, then the patient most likely is experiencing a cholinergic crisis. In this situation, the pyridostigmine would be stopped.

c. If the patient is experiencing a myasthenic crisis, additional pyridostigmine may be ordered or possibly another indirect-acting cholinergic agonist might be used. The patient would require close monitoring to evaluate for resolution of the signs and symptoms, such as improved swallowing, speech, and breathing. For example, if an increased dosage of pyridostigmine were ordered, improved signs and symptoms would be seen within 5 minutes of intravenous administration and within 35 to 45 minutes of oral administration.

If the patient were experiencing a cholinergic crisis, then the pyridostigmine would be stopped immediately and supportive intensive care, including possible intubation and mechanical ventilation, is necessary to ensure adequate respiratory function.

■ PRACTICING FOR NCLEX

1. Answer: b

RATIONALE: Cholinergic agents cause increased salivation, pupil constriction, decreased heart rate, and increased bladder muscle tone.

2. Answer: a
RATIONALE: When administered ophthalmically, carbachol results in miosis. It does not cause ptosis (drooping) or paralysis of the eye muscles.

3. Answer: d
RATIONALE: Adverse effects associated with direct-acting cholinergic agents include urinary urgency, bradycardia, hypotension, and diarrhea.

4. Answer: c
RATIONALE: For nonobstructive postoperative urinary retention, bethanechol may be ordered. Cevimeline is used to treat dry mouth associated with Sjorgren's syndrome. Pilocarpine is used to relieve intraocular pressure of glaucoma (ophthalmic form) or to treat dry mouth associated with Sjorgren's syndrome. Carbachol is used to relieve increased intraocular pressure.

5. Answer: b
RATIONALE: Indirect-acting cholinergic agonists react chemically with acetylcholinesterase to prevent it from breaking down acetylcholine. This leads to an accumulation of acetylcholine. Direct-acting cholinergic agonists occupy receptor sites for acetylcholine on the membranes of the effectors cells. Cholinergic agonists in general act at the same site as the neurotransmitter acetylcholine and are often called *parasympathomimetic* because their action mimics that of the parasympathetic nervous system.

6. Answer: d
RATIONALE: Donepezil is an indirect-acting cholinergic agent used to treat Alzheimer's disease. Pyridostigmine, neostigmine, and ambenonium would be used to treat myasthenia gravis.

7. Answer: c
RATIONALE: Exposure to nerve gas would be manifested by the following: bronchial and pupil constriction, slow heart rate, muscle contraction, and increased gastrointestinal (GI) activity and secretions.

8. Answer: a
RATIONALE: Donepezil has a 70-hour half-life and is usually given in a once-a-day dosing. Galantamine and rivastigmine are usually taken twice a day. Tacrine must be taken four times a day.

9. Answer: c
RATIONALE: There is an increased risk of GI bleeding if indirect-acting cholinergic agonists such as rivastigmine are used with nonsteroidal anti-inflammatory drugs (NSAIDs) such as ibuprofen because of the combination of increased GI secretions and GI mucosal erosion associated with the use of NSAIDs. Fecal incontinence, abdominal cramps, and diarrhea are adverse effects associated with indirect-acting cholinergic agonists.

10. Answer: b
RATIONALE: Atropine should be readily available to counteract the severe effects of an indirect-acting cholinergic agonist. Edrophonium is used as the antidote for nondepolarizing neuromuscular junction (NMJ) blockers. Phentolamine is used to as treatment for extravasation of intravenous norepinephrine or dopamine. Naloxone is used to treat narcotic overdose.

11. Answer: c
RATIONALE: Pyridostigmine is available in oral and parenteral forms; the parenteral form can be used if the patient is having trouble swallowing. In addition, the drug has a longer half-life than neostigmine and thus can be given less frequently. Ambenonium is available only in oral form and would be inappropriate for a patient who is having difficulty swallowing. Rivastigmine is used to treat Alzheimer's disease, not myasthenia gravis.

12. Answer: a, b, e
RATIONALE: Possible adverse effects related to anticholinesterase agents include urinary urgency, blurred vision, flushing, diarrhea, and hypotension.

13. Answer: b
RATIONALE: Although respiratory status and mental status would be important areas to monitor, it would be most important to evaluate serum theophylline levels because these levels can be increased up to twofold when combined with tacrine, placing the patient at high risk for theophylline toxicity.

14. Answer: c
RATIONALE: Intestinal obstruction would be a contraindication to the use of anticholinesterase inhibitors. Asthma, peptic ulcer disease, and parkinsonism would require cautious use and close monitoring.

15. Answer: a
RATIONALE: Direct-acting cholinergic agonists usually stimulate muscarinic receptors within the parasympathetic nervous system. Alpha and beta receptors are found in the sympathetic nervous system and are affected by adrenergic agents.

CHAPTER 33

■ ASSESSING YOUR UNDERSTANDING

FILL IN THE BLANKS

1. Belladonna
2. Anticholinergic
3. Atropine
4. Mydriasis
5. Cholinergic
6. Physostigmine
7. Increase
8. Decreased

MATCHING

1. b   **2.** c   **3.** e   **4.** d   **5.** a

■ APPLYING YOUR KNOWLEDGE

CASE STUDY

a. The patient is black, so he may require an additional length of time for the mydriatic effect of atropine to occur. Or, the patient may require a larger dose to achieve mydriasis. The patient also is taking a tricyclic antidepressant, which may interact with atropine and increase possible anticholinergic effects. However, systemic absorption of the atropine is less likely when given ophthalmically.

b. Instillation of the eye drops would lead to localized adverse effects such as blurred vision, pupil dilation, and subsequent photophobia. However, the nurse would need to be alert for systemic adverse effects as well. Inadvertent systemic absorption may occur with the instillation of eye drops. Thus, the nurse would need to assess the patient for systemic adverse effects, such as weakness, dizziness, mental confusion, dry mouth, constipation, tachycardia, urinary retention, and decreased sweating. These effects may be exacerbated by the interaction of the atropine (absorbed systemically) with the tricyclic antidepressant.

■ PRACTICING FOR NCLEX

1. Answer: c
RATIONALE: Atropine toxicity is dose related. Typically, slight cardiac slowing, inhibition of sweating, and dry mouth are seen with 0.5 mg of atropine. Cough would not be associated with atropine toxicity.

2. Answer: c
RATIONALE: Scopolamine blocks only the muscarinic effectors in the parasympathetic nervous system and those few cholinergic receptors in the sympathetic nervous system. It does not block the nicotinic receptors and has little or no effect at the neuromuscular junction.

3. Answer: b
RATIONALE: Only scopolamine is available as a transdermal system.

4. Answer: a
RATIONALE: Propantheline is available only in oral form.

5. Answer: d
RATIONALE: A patient with hypertension who receives an anticholinergic is at risk for additive hypertensive effects due to the dominance of the sympathetic system with parasympathetic blockage. Bladder obstruction, paralytic ileus, and increased intraocular pressure are contraindications for the use of an anticholinergic agent.

6. Answer: a
RATIONALE: Flavoxate may be ordered to provide symptomatic relief of dysuria, urgency, nocturia, suprapubic pain, frequency, and incontinence associated with cystitis. Dicyclomine is used to treat irritable or hyperactive bowel. Glycopyrrolate is used to decrease secretions before surgery or intubation and as an adjunct for treatment of ulcers. Methscopolamine is used as an adjunct treatment for peptic ulcers.

7. Answer: b
RATIONALE: The patient should avoid temperature extremes and exertion in warm temperatures because of possible heat intolerance, which could be more severe in older patients. Drinking fluids is important to maintain hydration and prevent heat intolerance. Avoiding driving is an appropriate safety measure. Constipation may occur with an anticholinergic; therefore, increased fiber intake would be appropriate.

8. Answer: b
RATIONALE: If atropine toxicity is due to ingestion, immediate gastric lavage is performed to limit absorption of the drug. Physostigmine would then be given as an antidote. Diazepam may be used if the patient experiences seizures. Cool sponge baths would be used as additional support measure to relieve fever and hot skin.

9. Answer: d
RATIONALE: When used with anticholinergic agents, increased anticholinergic effects can occur with antihistamines, antiparkinson agents, and monoamine oxidase inhibitors. Nonsteroidal anti-inflammatory drugs are not known to interact with anticholinergic agents.

10. Answer: b
RATIONALE: When given intramuscularly, atropine peaks in approximately 30 minutes; for this situation, the peak effects would be noted at approximately 9:30 AM.

11. Answer: a, b, c, e
RATIONALE: Glycopyrrolate can be given orally, intramuscularly, subcutaneously, and intravenously.

12. Answer: d
RATIONALE: Excitement is a possible adverse central nervous system effect associated with anticholinergic agents. Pupil dilation, constipation, and tachycardia are other adverse effects.

13. Answer: c
RATIONALE: The patch should be applied to a clean, dry, intact, and hairless area of the body. The area should not be shaved, as this could abrade the skin and lead to increased absorption. Hair may be clipped if necessary. The backing is peeled off without touching the adhesive side of the patch, and the patch is placed at a new site each time to avoid skin irritation or degradation. The old patch is removed and the area is cleaned before a new patch is applied.

14. Answer: d
RATIONALE: Hyoscyamine acts more specifically on the receptors of the gastrointestinal tract. Ipratropium and tiotriopium act more specifically to decreased respiratory secretions and cause bronchodilation. Trospium acts more specifically on the smooth muscle of the urinary tract.

15. Answer: b
RATIONALE: A scopolamine patch is changed every 3 days.

CHAPTER 34

■ ASSESSING YOUR UNDERSTANDING

LABELING

Hypothalamus	Anterior Pituitary	Posterior Pituitary
Gonadotropin-releasing hormone Somatostatin Thyroid-releasing hormone	Adrenocorticotropic hormone (ACTH) Follicle-stimulating hormone Growth hormone Luteinizing hormone Melanocyte-stimulating hormone Prolactin Thyroid-stimulating hormone	Antidiuretic hormone Oxytocin

MATCHING

1. d **2.** e **3.** f **4.** a **5.** c
6. h **7.** g **8.** b

■ APPLYING YOUR KNOWLEDGE

CASE STUDY

a. The tumor pressing on a small portion of the patient's hypothalamus can result in numerous hormonal problems because the hypothalamus is considered the master gland. It acts as the coordinating center. Hormonally, the secretion of the various releasing hormones may be affected, thereby disrupting the function of the pituitary gland and eventually the target organ function. In addition, this disruption would also interfere with the functioning of the hypothalamic-pituitary axis and the negative feedback system that maintains homeostasis. Depending on the areas of the hypothalamus that are involved, the patient may experience too much secretion of certain releasing hormones and not enough of others. In turn, the secretion of hormones by the pituitary also would be altered.

b. The hypothalamus also plays a role in neurologic function and is the site of various neurocenters. Depending on the neurocenters that may be affected by the tumor, the patient may experience problems with the regulation of various body functions such as body temperature, thirst, hunger, water balance, blood pressure, respirations, reproduction, and emotional reactions. It also receives input from virtually all other areas of the brain, including the limbic system and cerebral cortex. Alterations in limbic system function can affect the neurotransmitters of epinephrine, norepinephrine, and serotonin, which in turn could affect the patient's expression of emotion. Additionally, the hypothalamus plays a role in the autonomic nervous system, which could lead to alterations in the sympathetic and parasympathetic nervous system control of body functions. The tumor's extension toward the cerebrum could impact the patient's sensory capabilities and motor function along with speech and communication.

■ PRACTICING FOR NCLEX

1. **Answer: b**
   RATIONALE: Hormones are chemical substances that are produced in small quantities, are secreted directly into the bloodstream, travel through the blood to specific receptor sites, and are immediately broken down.

2. **Answer: c**
   RATIONALE: Although traditionally the pituitary gland was considered the master gland, current thought is that the hypothalamus is the master gland because it is responsible for coordinating the nervous and endocrine responses to internal and external stimuli.

3. **Answer: d**
   RATIONALE: A hormone that takes a while to produce its effect is most likely entering the cell and reacting with a receptor site inside the cell to change messenger RNA, ultimately affecting cellular DNA and the cell's function. Reaction with a receptor on the cell membrane usually results in an immediate hormonal effect. Hormones do not react with a cell as it travels through the bloodstream or in a specialized target area of the body.

4. **Answer: a**
   RATIONALE: The hypothalamus secretes the releasing and inhibiting hormones such as somatostatin, or growth hormone inhibiting factor. ACTH, luteinizing hormone, and prolactin are secreted by the anterior pituitary gland.

5. **Answer: d**
   RATIONALE: Oxytocin and antidiuretic hormone are delivered by the neurologic network that connects the hypothalamus to the pituitary gland. The releasing hormones are delivered by the vascular network.

6. **Answer: d**
   RATIONALE: Plasma osmolality affects the release of antidiuretic hormone from the posterior pituitary gland. Central nervous system activity, hypothalamic hormones, and drugs can affect the release of hormones from the anterior pituitary gland.

7. **Answer: b**
   RATIONALE: Endorphins and enkephalins are released by the intermediate lobe of the pituitary gland. Oxytocin and antidiuretic hormone are released by the posterior pituitary gland. Melanocyte-stimulating hormone is released from the anterior pituitary gland.

8. **Answer: a**
   RATIONALE: Diurnal rhythm occurs when the hypothalamus begins secretion of corticotropin-releasing factor in the evening.

9. **Answer: c**
   RATIONALE: Oxytocin stimulates uterine smooth muscle contraction in late pregnancy and also causes the milk release or letdown reflex in lactating women. Prolactin is the hormone responsible for milk production. Follicle-stimulating hormone and luteinizing hormone are responsible for the initial events of the menstrual cycle.

10. **Answer: a**
    RATIONALE: Prolactin and growth hormone are two anterior pituitary hormones that do not have a target organ to produce hormones for regulation by a negative feedback mechanism. Thyroid hormone, follicle-stimulating hormone, and ACTH are regulated by a negative feedback mechanism.

11. **Answer: b**
    RATIONALE: Parathormone release is regulated by calcium levels. Acid in the gastrointestinal (GI) tract helps regulate GI hormones. Blood pressure aids in the regulation of erythropoietin release by the juxtaglomerular cells of the kidneys. Blood glucose levels regulate the release of insulin, glucagon, and somatostatin from the pancreas.

12. **Answer: c**
    RATIONALE: Activation of the sympathetic nervous system directly causes the release of ACTH. Aldosterone is released in response to ACTH and also is released directly in response to high potassium levels. Prostaglandins are released in response to local stimuli in the tissues that produce them. Calcitonin is released in response to serum calcium levels.

13. **Answer: b**
    RATIONALE: The initiating event in the hypothalamic-pituitary axis is the hypothalamic secretion of releasing factors, which leads to the anterior pituitary secreting the stimulating hormone, which in turn leads to the secretion of the hormone by the gland. Rising levels of the hormone cause the hypothalamus to cease secretion of the releasing hormone.

14. **Answer: c**
    RATIONALE: Aldosterone leads to sodium retention and thus increasing serum sodium levels and increased potassium excretion. Increased glucose levels result from cortisol secretion; increased red blood cell production results from secretion of erythropoietin.

15. **Answer: b**
    RATIONALE: Thyroid hormone secretion stimulates the basal metabolic rate. Gastrin stimulates stomach acid production; testosterone stimulates male secondary sex characteristics. Secretin and cholecystokinin stimulate pancreatic juice and bile secretion.

CHAPTER 35

■ ASSESSING YOUR UNDERSTANDING

CROSSWORD

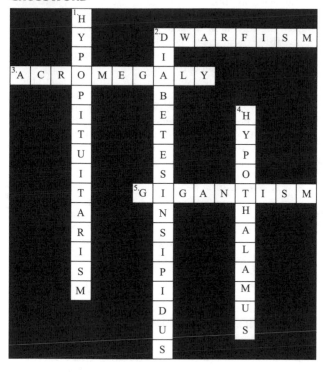

SHORT ANSWER

1. Hypothalamic hormones are not all available for pharmacologic use. Ones that are available are used mostly for diagnostic testing, for treating some forms of cancer, or as adjuncts in fertility programs.
2. Gigantism is due to hypersecretion of growth hormone that occurs before the epiphyseal plates of the long bones fuse, causing an acceleration in linear skeletal growth; acromegaly is used to describe the onset of excessive growth hormone secretion that occurs after puberty and epiphyseal plate closure.
3. The prototype growth hormone antagonist is bromocriptine mesylate.
4. Signs of water intoxication include drowsiness, light-headedness, headache, coma, and convulsions related to the shift to water retention and resulting electrolyte imbalance; and tremor, sweating, vertigo, and headache related to water retention.
5. Growth hormone antagonists include octreotide and bromocriptine.

■ APPLYING YOUR KNOWLEDGE

CASE STUDY

a. The nurse needs to use a nonjudgmental and empathetic approach with the child, encouraging the child to verbalize his feelings about being the "shortest one" in the class. This information might help to provide clues from which the nurse could plan specific measures to assist the child in coping with the upcoming changes. The nurse also can gain insight into coping mechanisms that the child has used in the past, encouraging the child to use the ones that were effective in dealing with this situation.

b. Growth hormone does promote growth, and this is a benefit that the child is expecting. However, the child will also need to learn how to cope with the changes that will be occurring in his body because the changes can happen suddenly. In addition, there are times when growth may not occur, which could cause significant upset for the child who is expecting growth. Somatropin is associated with thyroid dysfunction manifested by thinning hair and puffy skin. The nurse needs to address these possibilities with the child so that he is aware that they may occur and is prepared if they do happen.

■ PRACTICING FOR NCLEX

1. **Answer: b**
   RATIONALE: Nafarelin is given in nasal form.
2. **Answer: c**
   RATIONALE: Hypothalamic agonists are associated with impaired healing, fluid retention, elevated glucose levels, and electrolyte imbalance. Hypothalamic antagonists can lead to a decrease in testosterone levels leading to a loss of energy.
3. **Answer: b**
   RATIONALE: Leuprolide causes hot flashes, not chills. Other adverse effects include hematuria, peripheral edema, and constipation.
4. **Answer: d**
   RATIONALE: Patients who are receiving lanreotide must have careful monitoring of glucose levels. Liver function, renal function, and blood coagulation do not need close monitoring when taking this medication.
5. **Answer: c**
   RATIONALE: Somatropin is considered a growth hormone agonist. Bromocriptine, octreotide, and pegvisomant are growth hormone antagonists.
6. **Answer: c**
   RATIONALE: Signs of glucose intolerance include thirst, hunger, and voiding pattern changes. Injection site pain is an adverse effect of the therapy. Fatigue and cold intolerance suggest thyroid dysfunction.
7. **Answer: b**
   RATIONALE: Octreotide must be administered subcutaneously.
8. **Answer: d**
   RATIONALE: Pegvisomant may lead to increased incidence of infection, nausea, diarrhea, and changes in liver function. Gastrointestinal upset, drowsiness, and postural hypotension are associated with bromocriptine.
9. **Answer: d**
   RATIONALE: Octreotide is associated with the development of acute cholecystitis; bromocriptine and pegvisomant are not. Somatropin is a growth hormone agonist.

10. **Answer: a**
   RATIONALE: Chorionic gonadotropin would be used to induce ovulation in females with functioning ovaries. Corticotropin and cosyntropin are used to diagnose adrenal function. Thyrotropin alfa is used as adjunctive treatment for radioiodine ablation of thyroid tissue for thyroid cancer.

11. **Answer: b**
   RATIONALE: Oxytocin is a posterior pituitary hormone that is used to promote uterine contractions. Desmopressin is used to treat diabetes insipidus. Menotropins and chorionic gonadotropin alfa are fertility agents.

12. **Answer: d**
   RATIONALE: Desmopressin is a synthetic antidiuretic hormone.

13. **Answer: b**
   RATIONALE: Intravenous desmopressin has an onset of action of 30 minutes, or in this case, the drug would begin to work at approximately 10:30 AM.

14. **Answer: c**
   RATIONALE: Corticotropin-releasing hormone is administered as an intravenous infusion of the drug diluted in 500 mL of 5% dextrose in water (D5W) over 8 hours.

15. **Answer: c**
   RATIONALE: Goserelin is a gonadotropin-releasing hormone agonist, actually an analog of gonadotropin-releasing hormone. Ganirelix and degarelix are gonadotropin-releasing hormone antagonists. Pegvisomant is a growth hormone agonist.

CHAPTER 36

■ ASSESSING YOUR UNDERSTANDING

LABELING

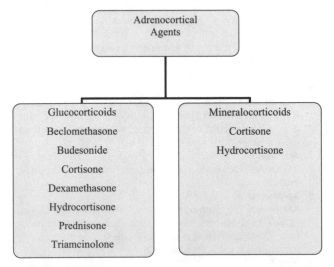

SHORT ANSWER

1. Diurnal rhythm is the response of the hypothalamus and then the pituitary and adrenal glands to wakefulness and sleeping. Normally, the hypothalamus begins secretion of corticotropin-releasing factor (CRF) in the evening, peaking at about midnight; adrenocortical peak response is between 6 and 9 AM; and levels fall during the day until evening, when the low level is picked up by the hypothalamus and CRF secretion begins again.

2. The adrenal medulla is actually part of the sympathetic nervous system (SNS). It is a ganglion of neurons that releases the neurotransmitters norepinephrine and epinephrine into circulation when the SNS is stimulated. The secretion of these neurotransmitters directly into the bloodstream allows them to act as hormones, traveling from the adrenal medulla to react with specific receptor sites throughout the body.

3. The three types of corticosteroids are androgens, glucocorticoids, and mineralocorticoids.

4. People with adrenal insufficiency are exposed to extreme stress such as a motor vehicle accident, a surgical procedure, or a massive infection. Because they are not able to supplement the energy-consuming effects of the sympathetic reaction, they enter an adrenal crisis, which can include physiologic exhaustion, hypotension, fluid shift, shock, and even death.

5. Prolonged use of corticosteroids suppresses the normal hypothalamic–pituitary axis and leads to adrenal atrophy from lack of stimulation.

6. Glucocorticoids stimulate an increase in glucose levels for energy. They also increase the rate of protein breakdown and decrease the rate of protein formation from amino acids, which is another way of preserving energy. Glucocorticoids also cause lipogenesis, or the formation and storage of fat in the body. This stored fat will then be available to be broken down for energy when needed.

■ APPLYING YOUR KNOWLEDGE

CASE STUDY

a. Systemically administered corticosteroids are associated with weight gain, increased appetite, and sodium and fluid retention. They cause lipogenis (formation and storage of fat in the body), which might be seen as an increase in size, primarily in the abdominal area. The round face is most likely due to changes in fluid balance. His friends' comment about "mega Jon" most likely reflects the fluid retention and weight gain associated with corticosteroid use.

b. The child has taken corticosteroids before, so he probably has experienced various adverse effects, especially with his previous history of hospitalizations for exacerbations. The nurse also should remember that the child is a preadolescent, and body image and peers are extremely important to him. The nurse should encourage the child to talk about how he feels and what he has used in the past to cope with his disorder and the effects of drug therapy. The nurse also needs to teach the child about how the corticosteroid acts so that he can have a better understanding for why he needs the medication. The nurse can help the child develop effective strategies for dealing with the therapy and for dealing with his friends' statements. The nurse also needs to reinforce with the child that he needs to take the medication exactly as prescribed and not to stop the drug abruptly to prevent adrenal insufficiency. Rather, the dose needs to be tapered over a period of time.

■ PRACTICING FOR NCLEX

1. **Answer: b**
   RATIONALE: The adrenal medulla secretes the neurotransmitters epinephrine and norepinephrine. Androgens, glucocorticoids, and mineralocorticoids are secreted by the adrenal cortex.

2. **Answer: c**
   RATIONALE: A peak response of increased adrenocortico-tropic hormone and adrenocortical hormones occurs sometime early in the morning, about 6 AM to 9 AM. The corticosteroid levels fall to low levels by evening. Then, the hypothalamus and pituitary sense low levels of the hormones and begin the production and release of corticotropin-releasing hormone usually during sleep, around midnight.

3. **Answer: c**
   RATIONALE: Dexamethasone exerts the longest-acting glucocorticoid effects followed by triamcinolone, prednisone, and then cortisone.

4. **Answer: b**
   RATIONALE: Covering the area with a dressing or diaper would increase the risk for systemic absorption of the drug and should be avoided. Topical corticosteroids should be used sparingly and should not be applied to any open lesions or excoriated areas to reduce the risk for systemic absorption.

5. **Answer: a**
   RATIONALE: Prednisone is available for oral use only.

6. **Answer: d**
   RATIONALE: Long-term systemic corticosteroid therapy in children can increase the child's risk for growth retardation; therefore, this would be most important to assess. Weight gain is associated with corticosteroid use but would not be as critical to monitor as the child's growth pattern. Rectal bleeding can occur with corticosteroids administered via a retention enema. Epistaxis can occur with the use of intranasal corticosteroids.

7. **Answer: b**
   RATIONALE: Prednisone peaks in 1 to 2 hours after administration. In this situation, peak effects would occur between 8 and 9 AM.

8. **Answer: c**
   RATIONALE: Glucocorticoids interfere with the immune and inflammatory reactions of the body, increasing a patient's risk for infection. Thus, fever would need to be reported immediately. Weight gain, abdominal distention, and increased appetite are adverse effects that can occur and do not need to be reported immediately.

9. **Answer: a**
   RATIONALE: Typically, a glucocorticoid is taken in the morning around 8 or 9 AM to mimic the normal peak diurnal concentration levels and thereby minimize suppression of the hypothalamic-pituitary axis.

10. **Answer: d**
    RATIONALE: Glucocorticoids are contraindicated in patients with acute infection because the infection could become serious or even fatal if the immune and inflammatory responses are blocked. Cautious use is necessary in patients with diabetes because glucose control can be upset or peptic ulcer disease because steroid use is associated with the development of peptic ulcers. It is the recommended treatment for an inflammatory disorder such as poison ivy or an allergic reaction to a medication.

11. **Answer: b**
    RATIONALE: Prednisolone exerts some mineralocorticoid effects. Triamcinolone, dexamethasone, and betamethasone exert no mineralocorticoid effects.

12. **Answer: c**
    RATIONALE: Mineralocorticoids increase sodium reabsorption in the renal tubules, leading to sodium and water retention and increased potassium excretion. Calcium is not affected by mineralocorticoids.

13. **Answer: a**
    RATIONALE: Shortness of breath may be a sign of heart failure and needs to be reported immediately. Headache and weakness are general signs and common adverse effects. The nurse would report these if the patient complained that they were getting worse or interfering with the patient's activities of daily living. Slight pedal edema may or may not be significant.

14. **Answer: a**
    RATIONALE: Fludrocortisone can lead to hypokalemia. A serum potassium level less than 3.0 mEq/L (normal K+ level is 3.5-5.0 mEq/L) would suggest hypokalemia.

15. **Answer: b**
    RATIONALE: Adrenocortical hormones cause the release of glucose for energy, increase the blood volume (aldosterone effect), slow the rate of protein production, and block the activities of the inflammatory and immune systems.

CHAPTER 37

■ ASSESSING YOUR UNDERSTANDING

CROSSWORD

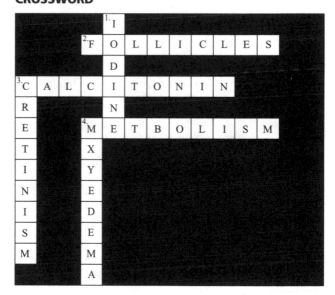

LABELING

Thyroid Hormone Deficiency	Thyroid Hormone Excess
Coarse, dry skin	Tachycardia
Lethargy	Diffuse goiter
Emotional dullness	Fine, soft hair
Weight gain	Intolerance to heat

■ APPLYING YOUR KNOWLEDGE

CASE STUDY

a. The nurse needs to explain to the patient that with the removal of part or all of the thyroid gland, hormone production will be deficient. This is unlike what she experienced before when her thyroid gland was producing too much hormone. In addition, the nurse needs to emphasize that adequate levels of the hormone are necessary to maintain normal body function and metabolism.

b. The patient needs information about how to take the drug, as a single dose before breakfast each day. Doing so will help to maintain consistent therapeutic levels. The nurse should also encourage the patient to take the dose with a full glass of water to prevent any difficulty in swallowing the drug. Additionally, the nurse should teach the patient about the delicate balance between deficient and excess amounts of the hormone and the possibility that symptoms of hyperthyroidism (similar to what she experienced when she was first diagnosed) may occur until the patient's dose is regulated. The nurse also needs to provide information about periodic follow-up testing of thyroid function and hormone levels to evaluate the patient's condition and effectiveness of therapy.

■ PRACTICING FOR NCLEX

1. **Answer: a**
   RATIONALE: Levothyroxine would be used to treat a deficiency of thyroid hormone or hypothyroidism. Methimazole and propylthiouracil are antithyroid agents used to treat hyperthyroidism. Calcitriol is an anithypocalcemic agent used to treat hypoparathyroidism.

2. **Answer: c**
   RATIONALE: Patients with hyperthyroidism typically exhibit flushed, warm skin; hyperactive deep tendon reflexes; tachycardia; and intolerance to heat.

3. **Answer: b**
   RATIONALE: The parafollicular cells of the thyroid produce calcitonin. Parathormone is produced by the parathyroid glands. Levothyroxine and liothyronine are produced by the thyroid gland and stored in the follicular cells.

4. **Answer: b**
   RATIONALE: The initial substance responsible for thyroid hormone release is thyrotropin-releasing hormone from the hypothalamus. This hormone then stimulates the anterior pituitary to release thyroid-stimulating hormone, which in turn causes the release of thyroid hormones. Levothyroxine is one of the thyroid hormones. Iodine is needed to produce the thyroid hormones.

5. **Answer: c**
   RATIONALE: Levothyroxine is a synthetic salt of T4; desiccated thyroid contains both T3 and T4. Liothyronine contains T3. Iodine is an antithyroid agent. Calcitriol is a form of vitamin D.

6. **Answer: d**
   RATIONALE: Propylthiouracil can cause thyroid suppression leading to signs and symptoms of hypothyroidism such as decreased appetite. Nervousness, tachycardia, and weight loss would suggest hyperthyroidism.

7. **Answer: b**
   RATIONALE: Tetany is an indication of hypocalcemia. Lethargy, muscle weakness, and personality changes occur with hypercalcemia.

8. **Answer: c**
   RATIONALE: Calcitriol increases serum calcium levels; therefore, periodic monitoring is important to ensure effectiveness of therapy without causing hypercalcemia. Antacids containing magnesium should be avoided due to the increased risk for hypermagnesemia. Calcitriol is often combined with dietary supplementation of calcium. Dairy products are a good source of calcium and should not be limited. The drug can cause nausea, vomiting, and dry mouth. Taking the drug with food may help alleviate these effects.

9. **Answer: d**
   RATIONALE: Pamidronate is an example of a bisphosphonate. Teriparatide and dihydrotachysterol are antihypocalcemic agents. Calcitonin-salmon is a calcitonin used to treat hypercalcemia.

10. **Answer: c**
    RATIONALE: Ibandronate is taken once a month on the same day each month.

11. **Answer: d**
    RATIONALE: Alendronate can interact with a multivitamin, decreasing the absorption of the bisphosphonate. Therefore, the drugs should be separated by at least a half hour. The multivitamin does not need to be stopped. The alendronate should be taken on arising in the morning before anything else. Antacids also can decrease the absorption of alendronate, and these should also be separated by at least a half hour.

12. **Answer: b**
    RATIONALE: Calcitonin is administered subcutaneously, intramuscularly, or intranasally.

13. **Answer: a**
    RATIONALE: Lethargy would suggest hypercalcemia. Paresthesias, muscle cramps, and carpopedal spasms suggest hypocalcemia.

14. **Answer: c**
    RATIONALE: Signs and symptoms of iodism include sore teeth and gums, metallic taste and burning in the mouth, diarrhea, cold symptoms, and stomach upset. Rash is an adverse effect that is not indicative of iodism.

15. **Answer: b**
    RATIONALE: Teriparatide is administered subcutaneously.

CHAPTER 38

■ ASSESSING YOUR UNDERSTANDING

MATCHING

1. c   2. f   3. b   4. g   5. a
6. d   7. h   8. e

SHORT ANSWER

1. The pancreas is both an endocrine gland, producing hormones, and an exocrine gland, releasing sodium bicarbonate and pancreatic enzymes directly into the common bile duct to be released into the small intestine, where

they neutralize the acid chyme from the stomach and aid digestion. The endocrine part of the pancreas produces hormones in collections of tissue called the islets of Lang-erhans. These islets contain endocrine cells that produce specific hormones. The alpha cells release glucagon in direct response to low blood glucose levels. The beta cells release insulin in direct response to high blood glucose levels. Delta cells produce somatostatin in response to very low blood glucose levels. Somatostatin blocks the secretion of both insulin and glucagon.

2. Glucagonlike polypeptide-1 (GLP-1) increases insulin release and decreases glucagon release (in preparation for the nutrients that will soon be absorbed). GLP-1 also slows gastrointestinal (GI) emptying to allow more absorp-tion of nutrients and stimulates the satiety center in the brain to decrease the desire to eat since food is already in the GI tract.

3. Disorders that may result from diabetes include athero-sclerosis, retinopathy, neuropathies, and nephropathy.

4. The glycosylated hemoglobin level (HbA1c) test provides a 3-month average of glucose levels.

5. Type 1 diabetes (insulin-dependent diabetes) involves pancreatic beta cells that are no longer functioning.

6. Clinical signs and symptoms include fatigue, lethargy, irritation, glycosuria, polyphagia, polydipsia, and itchy skin (from accumulation of wastes that the liver cannot clear).

■ APPLYING YOUR KNOWLEDGE

CASE STUDY

a. The nurse would need to reinforce the benefits of activity and exercise in maintaining health. However, the nurse would need to emphasize consistency in administering the insulin and ensuring adequate nutrition as well as being alert to the signs and symptoms of hypoglycemia and knowing how to prevent and/or properly intervene if they occur. The nurse would work with the patient and family to develop an appropriate schedule to reduce the child's risks. A referral to a dietician or nutritionist would be help-ful in devising an appropriate plan for nutritional intake, especially at times when the child will be participating in the sports activity. The nurse would encourage the child and parents to talk with child's coaches to ensure that they too are knowledgeable of the child's condition, signs and symptoms that require intervention, and appropriate emergency treatment measures.

b. The child is an adolescent and as such can pose a chal-lenge to managing diabetes. The desire to be "normal" often leads to a resistance to dietary restrictions and insu-lin injections. The child may feel a need to exert indepen-dence. The metabolism of the teenager is also in flux, lead-ing to complications in regulating insulin dosage. A team approach, including the child, family members, teachers, coaches, and even friends, may be the best way to help the child deal with the disease and the required therapy. New delivery methods for insulin may help this age group cope with the drug therapy in the future.

■ PRACTICING FOR NCLEX

1. **Answer: a**
   RATIONALE: Glyburide is an example of a sulfonylurea. Metformin is classified as a biguanide. Acarbose and miglitol are alpha-glucosidase inhibitors.

2. **Answer: b**
   RATIONALE: Rosiglitazone would be administered as a single oral dose. Repaglinide is used orally before meals. Exenatide is administered by subcutaneous injection within 60 minutes before morning and evening meals. Miglitol is given with the first bite of each meal.

3. **Answer: d**
   RATIONALE: Fruity breath odor would be noted as ketones build up in the system and are excreted through the lungs. Dehydration would be noted as fluid and electro-lytes are lost through the kidneys. Blurred vision and hunger would be associated with hypoglycemia.

4. **Answer: c**
   RATIONALE: Insulin detemir cannot be mixed in solution with any other drug, including other insulins. Regular, lente, and lispro can be mixed.

5. **Answer: a**
   RATIONALE: Regular insulin peaks in 2 to 4 hours, so the nurse would be alert for signs and symptoms of hypo-glycemia at this time, which would be between 10:00 AM and 12:00 PM. If insulin lispro were administered, peak effects would occur in 30 to 90 minutes or between 8:30 AM and 9:30 AM. If insulin detemir were given, peak effects would occur in 6 to 8 hours, or between 2:00 PM and 4:00 PM. If NPH insulin were given, peak effects would occur in 4 to 12 hours, or between 12:00 PM and 8:00 PM.

6. **Answer: d**
   RATIONALE: Gentle pressure should be applied to the injection after the needle is withdrawn. Massaging could contribute to erratic or unpredictable absorption.

7. **Answer: b**
   RATIONALE: To ensure therapeutic effectiveness and appro-priate suspension of the mixed insulin, the nurse would need to administer the injection within 15 minutes of mixing the insulins in the syringe.

8. **Answer: a**
   RATIONALE: Glipizide is a second-generation sulfonylurea that binds to potassium channels on the pancreatic beta cells to improve insulin binding to insulin receptors and increase the number of insulin receptors. Acarbose and miglitol inhibit alpha-glucosidase, thereby delaying the absorption of glucose. Metformin increases the uptake of glucose. Thiazolidinediones such as rosiglitazone decrease insulin resistance.

9. **Answer: b**
   RATIONALE: Metformin peaks in approximately 2 to $2\frac{1}{2}$ hours; thus, the patient should be alert for possible signs and symptoms of hypoglycemia.

10. **Answer: a**
    RATIONALE: Insulin is needed in type 1 diabetes because the beta cells of the pancreas are no longer functioning. With type 2 diabetes, insulin is produced, but perhaps not enough to maintain glucose control or the insulin receptors are not sensitive enough to insulin.

11. **Answer: c**
    RATIONALE: Incretins increase insulin release, decrease glu-cagon release, slow GI emptying, and stimulate the satiety center. Growth hormone increases protein building.

12. **Answer: d**
    RATIONALE: Although other delivery systems are available for insulin administration such as the jet injector, insulin pen, and external pump, subcutaneous injection remains the primary delivery system.

13. Answer: b
RATIONALE: The patient is significantly hypoglycemic and needs emergency treatment. Glucagon would be the agent of choice to raise the patient's glucose level because it can be given intravenously and has an onset of approximately 1 minute. Diazoxide can be used to elevate blood glucose levels, but it must be given orally. Lispro and regular insulin would be used to treat hyperglycemia.

14. Answer: c
RATIONALE: The buttocks would be an inappropriate site for administering insulin subcutaneously. The best sites include the upper arm, abdomen, and upper thigh.

15. Answer: a
RATIONALE: Pramlintide is administered subcutaneously immediately before major meals. Numerous antidiabetic drugs are taken orally, often once a day in the morning. Exenatide is given subcutaneously within 1 hour before the morning and evening meals. Miglitol should be taken orally with the first bite of each meal.

CHAPTER 39

■ ASSESSING YOUR UNDERSTANDING

LABELING

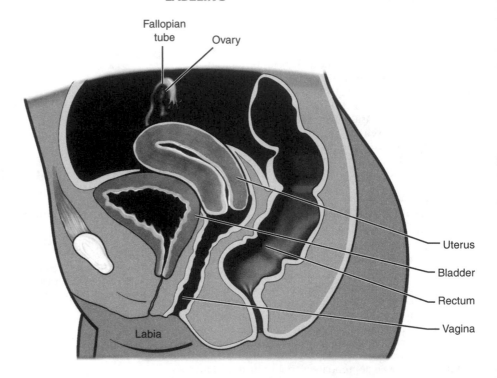

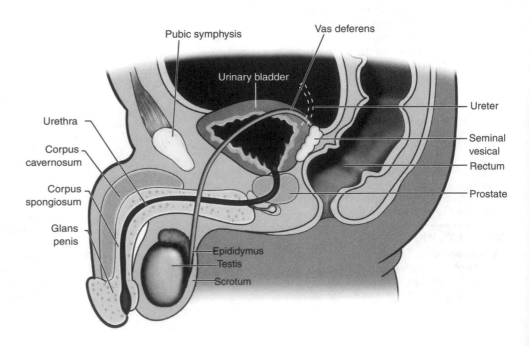

■ APPLYING YOUR KNOWLEDGE

CASE STUDY

a. The nurse would need to provide a review of the various structures involved in reproduction, including the ovaries, fallopian tubes, and uterus, and the hormones involved in the everyday function of the female reproductive system. The nurse also would need to explain the menstrual cycle, correlating the hormones involved with the events that occur, such as ovulation and menstruation. In addition, the nurse would need to review what happens with the system during pregnancy, beginning with fertilization and ending with the birth of the fetus.

b. The girls are adolescents, many of whom have already experienced menarche. So, rather than providing a straight lecture-type presentation on the menstrual cycle, it might be helpful for the nurse to engage the students in a discussion of the topic, either as a class or in small groups, or role-play different scenarios. The nurse could also incorporate visual methods, such as slide shows, videos, posters, or handouts to describe the structures of the system and the events of pregnancy. Independence is a key issue for adolescents. Therefore, the nurse should use methods that foster this independence while at the same time provide the girls with important information so that they are well informed.

■ PRACTICING FOR NCLEX

1. **Answer: c**
   RATIONALE: The gonadotropin-releasing hormone (GnRH) is the hormone responsible for the sequence of events that eventually lead to hormonal secretion from the ovaries and testes. GnRH released from the hypothalamus stimulates the release of follicle-stimulating hormone (FSH) and luteinizing hormone (LH; sometimes referred to as the interstitial cell-stimulating hormone in males) from the anterior pituitary gland. These in turn stimulate the male and female glands to secrete their hormones.

2. **Answer: b**
   RATIONALE: An ovum contains one-half of the genetic material to produce a whole cell. At birth, a female's ovaries contain all of the ova that a woman will have. The fallopian tube is a muscular tube that lies very near to each ovary but is not connected directly to it. The ovaries are responsible for producing estrogen and progesterone.

3. **Answer: d**
   RATIONALE: Progesterone's effects on body temperature are monitored in the rhythm method of birth control to indicate that ovulation has occurred. Estradiol, estrone, and estriol are estrogens produced by the ovaries.

4. **Answer: a**
   RATIONALE: Although progesterone plays a role in breast growth to prepare for lactation, estrogen plays a major role in breast growth overall. Progesterone is responsible for thickened cervical mucus, increased body temperature, and increased appetite.

5. **Answer: b**
   RATIONALE: Progesterone is the hormone responsible for maintaining pregnancy.

6. **Answer: d**
   RATIONALE: A massive release of luteinizing hormone or its surge causes one of the developing follicles to burst and release the ovum. This is called ovulation.

7. **Answer: c**
   RATIONALE: Fertilization of the ovum and implantation in the uterine wall results in the production of human chorionic gonadotropin, which stimulates the corpus luteum to continue to produce estrogen and progesterone until the placenta develops and becomes functional, producing these hormones at a level high enough to sustain the pregnancy. If pregnancy does not occur, the corpus luteum involutes and becomes a white scar on the ovary, called the *corpus albicans*.

8. **Answer: d**
   RATIONALE: Increased light exposure has been found to boost the release of FSH and LH through earlier GnRH release by the hypothalamus. Stress, starvation, and extreme exercise are associated with a decrease in reproductivity related to the controls of the hypothalamus.

9. **Answer: b**
   RATIONALE: The onset of the menstrual cycle at puberty is called *menarche*. Puberty refers to the point at which the hypothalamus starts releasing gonadotropin-releasing hormone to stimulate the release of FSH and LH and begins sexual development. Andropause refers to a decrease in gonadal function in males. Menopause refers to the cessation of menstruation in a female when female ova are depleted.

10. **Answer: c**
    RATIONALE: Prostaglandins in the uterus stimulate uterine contraction to clamp off vessels as the lining sheds away during menstruation. This causes menstrual cramps. High levels of plasminogen in the uterus prevent clotting of the lining as the vessels shear off. Lowered estrogen and progesterone levels trigger the release of FSH and LH and cause the inner lining of the uterus to slough off because it is no longer stimulated by the hormones.

11. **Answer: b**
    RATIONALE: The placenta serves as a massive endocrine gland during pregnancy, maintaining high levels of estrogen and progesterone to support the uterus and developing fetus. The umbilical cord is important for nutrient and oxygen exchange between the fetus and the mother. The embryo implants in the wall of the uterus and becomes the developing fetus. The uterus provides the area for implantation of the embryo and growth of the fetus.

12. **Answer: a**
    RATIONALE: The seminiferous tubules produce sperm. The Leydig cells produce testosterone. The vas deferens stores the produced sperm and carries it from the testes for ejaculation. The prostate gland produces enzymes to stimulate sperm maturation and lubricating fluid.

13. **Answer: b, c, d**
    RATIONALE: Testosterone leads to the following: thickening of the vocal cords, increased hematocrit, and facial hair growth. Increased high-density lipoprotein levels and skin elasticity are associated effects of estrogen.

14. **Answer: c**
    RATIONALE: The human sexual response cycle begins with stimulation, which is followed by a plateau stage, climax, and then recovery or resolution.

15. **Answer: a**
    RATIONALE: During andropause, the seminiferous tubules and interstitial cells atrophy. The hypothalamus and anterior pituitary gland put out larger amounts of GnRH, FSH, and LH in an attempt to stimulate the gland. If no increase in testosterone or inhibin occurs, levels of GnRH, FSH, and LH return to normal.

CHAPTER 40

■ ASSESSING YOUR UNDERSTANDING

FILL IN THE BLANKS

1. Progestins
2. Secretory
3. Nicotine
4. Raloxifene
5. Clomiphene
6. Oxytoxics

SHORT ANSWER

1. Female sex hormones are used to replace hormones that are missing or to act on the control mechanisms of the endocrine system to decrease the release of endogenous hormones.
2. Women without primary ovarian failure who cannot get pregnant after 1 year of trying may be candidates for the use of fertility drugs.
3. Menotropins also stimulate spermatogenesis in men with low sperm counts and otherwise normally functioning testes.
4. A woman with ovarian cysts who uses a fertility drug may experience an increase in the size of the cysts due to stimulation from the drugs.
5. Oxytocin is available in a nasal form to stimulate the letdown reflex in a lactating woman.

■ APPLYING YOUR KNOWLEDGE

CASE STUDY

a. The nurse needs to listen to the patient's complaints and provide nonjudgmental acceptance and support. While talking with the patient, the nurse may note areas in which clarification or correction is needed because of myths and misconceptions that the patient may relate. These areas provide opportunities for teaching to help the patient better understand what is happening in her body. The nurse also needs to emphasize that they will work together to find a suitable solution. Doing so helps to alleviate any feelings that the patient may have about being alone in dealing with these changes.

b. First, the nurse needs to assess the patient's concerns about hormone replacement therapy. Then, the nurse would address these concerns and provide the patient with information about hormone replacement therapy, including the risks and benefits. The nurse also would need to obtain a complete family and personal history of cancer and coronary artery disease risk factors as well as the use of any other medications or herbal therapies to provide additional information for the patient to weigh the pros and cons about therapy. Once the information has been obtained and the patient understands it, then the patient can make an informed decision about the therapy with the support and guidance from the nurse.

■ PRACTICING FOR NCLEX

1. **Answer: d**
   RATIONALE: The vaginal ring formulation of estradiol is applied once every 3 months.
2. **Answer: c**
   RATIONALE: Progestins are contraindicated in patients with pelvic inflammatory disease because progestins affect the vasculature of the uterus. Cautious use is necessary for women with migraine headaches, asthma, and epilepsy due to possible exacerbation of these conditions with the use of progestins.
3. **Answer: d**
   RATIONALE: Drospirenone used in combination contraceptives has antimineralocorticoid activity and can block aldosterone, leading to increased potassium levels. Irritation is associated with transdermal or vaginal use. Headache is associated with vaginal gel use. Abdominal pain may be due to intrauterine system administration.
4. **Answer: b**
   RATIONALE: Orange juice does not need to be avoided with estrogen hormonal therapy. However, St. John's wort, smoking, and grapefruit juice should be avoided.
5. **Answer: a**
   RATIONALE: Raloxifene is administered only by the oral route.
6. **Answer: c**
   RATIONALE: Clomiphene is administered orally. Cetrorelix, follitropin alfa, and ganirelix are administered parenterally.
7. **Answer: d**
   RATIONALE: Terbutaline, a beta-2 selective adrenergic agonist, is used as a uterine motility agent to relax the gravid uterus to prolong pregnancy and prevent premature labor and delivery. Ergonovine and oxytocin would be used to stimulate uterine contractions. Dinoprostone would be used to terminate a pregnancy of 12 to 20 weeks.
8. **Answer: b**
   RATIONALE: Oxytocin can cause severe water intoxication, which is thought to occur because of related effects of antidiuretic hormone, which may be released in response to oxytocin activity. Oxytocin does stimulate neuroreceptor sites but this is not the reason for the development of water intoxication. Ergonovine and methylergonovine can produce ergotism. Blockage of estrogen receptor sites occurs with estrogen receptor modulators.
9. **Answer: b**
   RATIONALE: Oral contraceptives are started on the fifth day of the cycle for 21 days; the inert tablets, or no tablets, are taken for the next 7 days. Then, a new course of 21 days is started.
10. **Answer: b**
    RATIONALE: Certain drugs such as tetracyclines and penicillins can reduce the effectiveness of progestins. Therefore, the patient needs to use an alternative means of contraception while taking the tetracycline. There is no need to separate administration times of the drug. Reducing the oral contraceptive to every other day further reduces the drug's effectiveness. An increase in adverse effects is not associated with the use of tetracyclines and oral contraceptives.
11. **Answer: d**
    RATIONALE: Estrogens are associated with the development of thrombi and emboli. Complaints of shortness of breath may indicate a possible pulmonary embolism necessitating emergency treatment. Abdominal bloating, weight gain, and dizziness are common adverse effects of estrogen therapy that should be reported, but it is not necessary to report them immediately.
12. **Answer: a**
    RATIONALE: Cetrorelix inhibits premature luteinizing hormone (LH) surges in women undergoing controlled ovarian stimulation by acting as a gonadotropin-releasing hormone (GnRH) antagonist. Chorionic gonadotropin acts like GnRH. Follitropin alfa is a follicle-stimulating molecule. Menotropins are a purified gonadotropin similar to follicle-stimulating hormone and LH.

13. **Answer: b**
RATIONALE: Lutropin alfa is a fertility drug that is administered subcutaneously with follitropin alfa.

14. **Answer: b**
RATIONALE: Dinoprostone begins to act in 10 minutes, reaching a peak action in 15 minutes with a duration of action of 2 to 3 hours.

15. **Answer: d**
RATIONALE: With emergency contraception, the first dose is started within 72 hours after unprotected intercourse; then, a follow-up dose of the same dosage must be taken 12 hours after the first dose.

CHAPTER 41

■ ASSESSING YOUR UNDERSTANDING

FILL IN THE BLANKS

1. Androgens
2. Hypogonadism
3. III
4. Hirsutism
5. Athletic

SHORT ANSWER

1. Anabolic steroids promote body tissue–building processes, reverse catabolic or tissue-destroying processes, and increase hemoglobin and red blood cell mass.
2. Androgens are male sex hormones and include testosterone produced in the testes and the androgens produced in the adrenal glands.
3. Androgenic effects include acne, edema, hirsutism (increased hair distribution), deepening of the voice, oily skin and hair, weight gain, decrease in breast size, and testicular atrophy.
4. When injected directly into the cavernosum, alprostadil acts locally to relax the vascular smooth muscle and allows filling of the corpus cavernosum, causing penile erection.
5. Patients using PDE5 inhibitors should avoid drinking grapefruit juice when taking the drug as well as avoid taking the drug with or just after a high-fat meal.

■ APPLYING YOUR KNOWLEDGE

CASE STUDY

a. The nurse needs to maintain a nonjudgmental approach with the patient and allow him to verbalize his feelings and concerns, especially in relation to his complaints, his feelings about himself, his sexual ability, and aging (self-esteem, body image, maleness). When responding to the patient, the nurse should be honest with the patient and inform him that the medication may or may not be appropriate for him, depending on a variety of factors. The nurse also needs to review the normal physiologic changes that occur with aging while at the same time reinforce that help is available.

b. The nurse needs to obtain a complete history and physical examination of the patient. It would be essential to find out if there are any underlying medical conditions that may be affecting the patient's status. Information about the use of any medications or herbal therapies also would be important because numerous agents have adverse effects on sexual functioning. In addition, the nurse needs to inquire about other areas, such as stresses that could affect neuroendocrine function and disrupt the hypothalamic-pituitary axis.

■ PRACTICING FOR NCLEX

1. **Answer: c**
RATIONALE: Androgenic effects include oily skin and hair. Flushing, sweating, and nervousness are antiestrogenic effects.

2. **Answer: d**
RATIONALE: Testosterone can be administered as a depot injection, transdermal patch, or intramuscular injection. It is not administered orally.

3. **Answer: c**
RATIONALE: Patients with a history of cardiovascular disease need to be monitored closely when receiving testosterone because the disorder could be exacerbated by the hormone's effect. Prostate or breast cancer would be contraindications to the use of testosterone. Penile implant would be a contraindication for the use of drugs for treating penile erectile dysfunction.

4. **Answer: b**
RATIONALE: A potentially life-threatening effect associated with long-term testosterone use is hepatocellular cancer. Patients should have liver function studies monitored regularly, before beginning therapy and every 6 months during therapy.

5. **Answer: c**
RATIONALE: Testosterone is available in a transdermal form. Fluoxymesterone, danazol, and methyltestosterone are administered orally.

6. **Answer: d**
RATIONALE: Anabolic steroids increase red blood cell mass and hemoglobin, reverse catabolic or tissue-destroying processes, and promote body tissue–building processes.

7. **Answer: b**
RATIONALE: Postpubertal males may experience priapism, gynecomastia, testicular atrophy, balding, inhibition of testicular function, and change in libido with anabolic steroids.

8. **Answer: b**
RATIONALE: Elevated liver enzyme levels indicated impaired hepatic function that could be related to the development of hepatocellular cancer—a potential and life-threatening effect associated with androgen therapy. Decreased thyroid function and increased creatinine and creatinine clearance levels are not associated with disease states and can last for up to 2 weeks after discontinuing therapy.

9. **Answer: c**
RATIONALE: Anabolic steroids are classified as a class III controlled substance.

10. **Answer: b**
RATIONALE: Sildenafil is a PDE5 inhibitor used to treat penile erectile dysfunction. Alprostadil is a prostaglandin. Oxandrolone is an anabolic steroid. Danazol is an androgen.

11. **Answer: b**
RATIONALE: Tadalafil is approved for daily use in men who are very sexually active. This drug may be selected if the timing of sexual stimulation is not known and may be several hours away. Sidenafil and vardenafil must be taken approximately 1 hour before sexual stimulation. Alprostadil is injected directly into the cavernosum.

12. **Answer: a**
RATIONALE: Sildenafil is used in women for the treatment of pulmonary arterial hypertension. It is not used for sexual dysfunction in women. Coronary artery disease and peptic ulcer disease are conditions that require cautious use of the drug in men.

13. Answer: c

RATIONALE: The PDE5 inhibitors cannot be taken in combination with any organic nitrates or alpha-adrenergic blockers because serious cardiovascular effects may occur, including death. Increased PDE5 inhibitor levels and effects may be seen with ketoconazole, indinavir, and erythromycin; the dosage of the inhibitor would need to be reduced.

14. Answer: d

RATIONALE: Vardenafil should be taken 60 minutes before sexual stimulation.

15. Answer: b

RATIONALE: Transdermal testosterone patches are replaced daily.

CHAPTER 42

■ ASSESSING YOUR UNDERSTANDING

LABELING

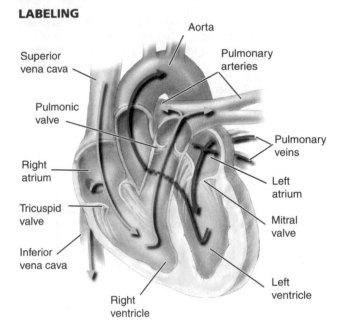

Aorta
Superior vena cava
Pulmonary arteries
Pulmonic valve
Pulmonary veins
Right atrium
Left atrium
Tricuspid valve
Mitral valve
Inferior vena cava
Left ventricle
Right ventricle

SEQUENCING

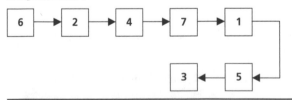

■ APPLYING YOUR KNOWLEDGE

CASE STUDY

a. If constant and excessive, hypertension can damage the inner fragile lining of the blood vessels and disrupt the flow of blood to the tissues. These vessels can include the coronary vessels. Hypertension also puts a tremendous strain on the heart muscle, increasing myocardial oxygen consumption and putting the heart itself at risk. The patient acknowledges some noncompliance with his antihypertensive medications that could have allowed his blood pressure to rise, causing excess demand on the heart. Blood pressure is a measure of afterload, and the higher the resistance in the system, the harder the heart will have

to contract to pump blood. Chronic hypertension also can overstretch the heart muscle, interfering with the heart's ability to pump effectively. Ultimately, the coronary arteries can be affected.

b. The patient needs to learn to balance activity and rest periods so that he does not overtax the heart. In addition, energy conservation measures would be helpful to minimize the amount of oxygen needed and used to perform certain activities. In addition, measures to control his blood pressure can help to minimize the oxygen demand as well as reduce the workload of the heart.

■ PRACTICING FOR NCLEX

1. Answer: b

RATIONALE: Starling's law of the heart is often compared with the stretching of a rubber band, such that the heart returns to its normal size after it is stretched—the further it is stretched, the stronger is the spring back to normal.

2. Answer: a

RATIONALE: The sinoatrial (SA) node acts as the pacemaker of the heart. The atrioventricular (AV) node, bundle of His, and Purkinje fibers are part of the conduction system.

3. Answer: c

RATIONALE: Automaticity is the cells' ability to generate action potentials or electrical impulses without being excited to do so by external stimuli. Conductivity refers to the ability of the cells to conduct this action potential. Contractility refers to the unified contraction of the atria and ventricles to move blood through the vascular system. Capacitancy refers to the venous system, which is distensible and flexible and able to hold large amounts of blood.

4. Answer: b

RATIONALE: During phase 1, sodium ion concentrations are equal inside and outside the cell. During phase 0, the cell reaches a point of stimulation with sodium rushing into the cell (depolarization). During phase 2, the cell membrane becomes less permeable to sodium, and calcium slowly enters the cell and potassium begins to leave (repolarization). During phase 3, rapid repolarization occurs, as the gates close and potassium rapidly moves out of the cell.

5. Answer: d

RATIONALE: The basic structural unit of cardiac muscle is the sarcomere, which contains the proteins actin and myosin. These proteins are kept apart by the protein troponin.

6. Answer: c

RATIONALE: An electrocardiogram is a recording of the patterns of electrical impulses as they move through the heart. It is a measure of electrical activity and provides no information about the mechanical function of the heart.

7. Answer: b

RATIONALE: The QRS complex represents depolarization of the bundle of His (Q) and the ventricles (RS). The P wave indicates impulses originating in the SA node as they pass through atrial tissue. The T wave represents repolarization of the ventricles. The PR interval reflects the normal delay of conduction at the AV node.

8. Answer: d

RATIONALE: Atrial flutter is characterized by sawtooth-shaped P waves, often with two or three P waves occurring for every QRS complex. Sinus bradycardia would be characterized by a normal-appearing electrocardiogram but with a rate usually less than 60 beats/minute. Paroxysmal atrial tachycardia would be characterized by sporadically occurring runs of rapid heart rate. Atrial fibrillation would be characterized by many irregular

P waves, depicting bombardment of the AV node in an unpredictable number causing the ventricles to beat in a fast, irregular, and often inefficient heart manner.

9. **Answer: c**
RATIONALE: Circulation is a closed, high- to low-pressure system that can follow two courses (systemic and pulmonary) and involves a resistance system (arterial) and a capacitance (venous) system.

10. **Answer: a**
RATIONALE: Hydrostatic pressure regulates the movement of fluids at the arterial end of the capillary; entotic pressure regulates this movement at the venous end of the capillary. It is the pressure that directs flow through the loosely connected endothelial cells of the capillary.

11. **Answer: b**
RATIONALE: The right coronary artery supplies most of the right side of the heart, including the SA node. The left circumflex artery supplies most of the left ventricle. The left anterior descending artery feeds the septum and anterior areas, including much of the conduction system.

12. **Answer: a**
RATIONALE: When blood flow to the kidneys is reduced, the cells in the kidney release renin, which then converts angiotensinogen to angiotensin I. This is converted by angiotensin-converting enzyme to angiotensin II, which reacts with specific receptor sites on blood vessels to cause vasoconstriction. Angiotensin II also causes the release of aldosterone.

13. **Answer: c**
RATIONALE: The superior vena cava brings blood from the head and arms to the right ventricle and the inferior vena cava brings blood from the lower body back to the heart. The aorta delivers blood to the systemic circulation. The pulmonary vein returns blood from the lungs to the left atrium. The triscupid valve separates the right atrium from the right ventricle.

14. **Answer: d**
RATIONALE: The Purkinje fibers deliver the impulse to the ventricular cells. The AV node receives the impulse from the atrial bundles and moves it to the bundle of His and then into the bundle branches.

15. **Answer: b**
RATIONALE: The conduction velocity is the slowest in the AV node and the fastest in the Purkinje fibers.

CHAPTER 43

■ ASSESSING YOUR UNDERSTANDING

LABELING

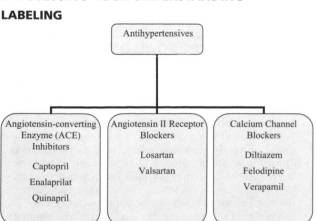

MATCHING
1. d   **2.** a   **3.** e   **4.** b   **5.** c

SHORT ANSWER

1. The pressure in the cardiovascular system is determined by heart rate, stroke volume, and total peripheral resistance.
2. Baroreceptors are located in the aortic arch and carotid arteries.
3. The underlying danger of hypertension of any type is the prolonged force on the vessels of the vascular system. The muscles in the arterial system eventually thicken, leading to a loss of responsiveness in the system. The left ventricle thickens because the muscle must constantly work hard to expel blood at a greater force. The thickening of the heart muscle and the increased pressure that the muscle has to generate every time it contracts increase the workload of the heart and the risk of coronary artery disease (CAD) as well. The force of the blood being propelled against them damages the inner linings of the arteries, making these vessels susceptible to atherosclerosis and to narrowing of the lumen of the vessels (see Chapter 46). Tiny vessels can be damaged and destroyed, leading to losses of vision (if the vessels are in the retina), kidney function (if the vessels include the glomeruli in the nephrons), or cerebral function (if the vessels are small and fragile vessels in the brain).
4. Factors that are known to increase blood pressure in some people include high levels of psychological stress, exposure to high-frequency noise, a high-salt diet, lack of rest, and genetic predisposition.
5. Because an underlying cause of hypertension is usually unknown, altering the body's regulatory mechanisms is the best treatment currently available. Drugs used to treat hypertension work to alter the normal reflexes that control blood pressure.
6. A patient with stage 1 hypertension without complicating conditions may receive thiazide diuretics most often. ACE inhibitors, angiotensin receptor blockers, beta blockers, or calcium channel blockers may be used alone or in combination.
7. Lifestyle modifications include weight reduction, smoking cessation, moderation of alcohol intake, reduction of salt in the diet, and increase in physical activity.

■ APPLYING YOUR KNOWLEDGE

CASE STUDY

a. The patient may be describing what is known as "white coat syndrome"—a condition in which the patient is hypertensive only when in the doctor's office having the blood pressure measured. This has been correlated to a sympathetic stress reaction and a tendency to tighten the muscles while waiting to be seen and during the blood pressure measurement. Although this may be occurring to some degree with the patient, his blood pressure has been elevated for a sustained period, which has led to his diagnosis of hypertension. In addition, the patient also has a history of left ventricular hypertrophy, which has caused the heart muscle to be stretched, ultimately causing the heart to work harder to contract. Also, blood pressure machines in grocery stores and pharmacies are not always accurate and can mislead patients. Thus, the nurse would need to address these issues when responding to the patient.

b. The nurse would need to explain that the quinapril is an ACE inhibitor that is relatively well tolerated and not associated with as many adverse effects as other drugs in this class. However, the nurse still needs to review possible adverse effects such as reflex tachycardia, gastrointestinal irritation, constipation, renal problems, and photosensitivity. In addition, the nurse needs to address possible effects related to the combination of carvedilol, an alpha- and beta blocker. These might include orthostatic hypotension, dizziness, or the development of possible arrhythmias. Instructions on safety measures and danger signs and symptoms to report would be important.

■ PRACTICING FOR NCLEX

1. Answer: d
RATIONALE: The area of highest pressure in the system is always the left ventricle during systole. This pressure propels the blood out of the aorta and into the system.

2. Answer: a
RATIONALE: The small arterioles are thought to be the most important factor in determining peripheral resistance. Because they have the smallest diameter, they are able to almost stop blood flow into the capillary beds when they constrict, building up tremendous pressure in the arteries behind them as they prevent the blood from flowing through.

3. Answer: c
RATIONALE: The baroreceptor reflex functions continually to maintain blood pressure within a predetermined range of normal. Input from the baroreceptors is received by the medulla in the cardiovascular center. Baroreceptors are located in the carotid arteries.

4. Answer: d
RATIONALE: Enalaprilat is an ACE inhibitor that is administered intravenously. Captopril, enalapril, and lisinopril are administered orally.

5. Answer: b
RATIONALE: Benazepril is associated with an unrelenting cough. Ramipril, lisinopril, and quinapril are not associated with this adverse effect.

6. Answer: c
RATIONALE: Captopril is associated with a sometimes fatal pancytopenia, so it would be most important for the nurse to monitor the patient's complete blood count for changes. Monitoring the electrocardiogram would be important to detect arrhythmias but not as important as monitoring for bone marrow suppression. Nutritional status and liver function studies would be lower priorities for monitoring.

7. Answer: b
RATIONALE: Losartan is an example of an angiotensin II receptor blocker. Moexipril is an ACE inhibitor. Minoxidil is a vasodilator. Amlodipine is a calcium channel blocker.

8. Answer: d
RATIONALE: Calcium channel blockers slow cardiac impulse formation in the conductive tissues, depress myocardial contractility, and relax and dilate arteries, leading to a fall in blood pressure and a decrease in venous return.

9. Answer: c
RATIONALE: Diltiazem, like other calcium channel blockers, should be swallowed whole with a large glass of water. The tablet should not be split in half, crushed, or chewed.

10. Answer: b
RATIONALE: Verapamil, like other calcium channel blockers, interacts with grapefruit juice, increasing the concentration of calcium channel blockers and leading to toxicity. Calcium channel blockers do not interact with ibuprofen. Splitting or crushing the pills could lead to a release of the drug all at once, but this is more common when the drug is first taken. Asking about the time the patient last took the drug might be important, but

it would not address the problem associated with the significant adverse effects.

11. Answer: b
RATIONALE: Manifestations of cyanide toxicity include absent reflexes, dilated pupils, dyspnea, headache, vomiting, dizziness, ataxia, loss of consciousness, imperceptible pulse, pink color, distant heart sounds, and shallow breathing. Hair growth is an adverse effect of minoxidil. Chest pain is an adverse effect associated with vasodilator therapy related to changes in blood pressure.

12. Answer: a
RATIONALE: Prazosin is an alpha-1 blocker that is used to treat hypertension. Labetolol and guanabenz are alpha- and beta blockers used to treat hypertension. Nadolol is a beta blocker used to treat hypertension.

13. Answer: c
RATIONALE: Midodrine is an alpha-specific adrenergic agent that is used to treat orthostatic hypotension. Dopamine is a sympathomimetic agent that is used to treat shock. Methyldopa and clonidine are alpha-2 blockers used to treat hypertension.

14. Answer: d
RATIONALE: Hydrochlorothiazide is a thiazide diuretic that promotes the loss of sodium as well as potassium from the body. Subsequently, the patient is at risk for hypokalemia. Amiloride, spironolactone, and triamterene are potassium-sparing diuretics. The patient using these diuretics would need to be monitored for hyperkalemia because potassium is not lost along with sodium.

15. Answer: b
RATIONALE: Aliskiren is a renin inhibitor. Mecamylamine is a ganglionic blocker. Candesartan is an angiotensin II receptor blocker; captopril is an ACE inhibitor.

CHAPTER 44

■ ASSESSING YOUR UNDERSTANDING

MATCHING

1. c	**2.** f	**3.** d	**4.** e	**5.** g
6. a	**7.** h	**8.** b		

FILL IN THE BLANKS

1. Cardiotonic
2. Pulmonary edema
3. Rapid
4. Fluid
5. Decreased
6. Jugular
7. Nocturia
8. Inotropic

■ APPLYING YOUR KNOWLEDGE

CASE STUDY

a. The patient is experiencing signs and symptoms of both right-sided heart failure and left-sided heart failure. Right-sided heart failure is evidenced by the pitting edema, jugular vein distention, and nocturia. Left-sided heart failure is evidenced by the patient's tachypnea, rales, third heart sound, and orthopnea (the need to sleep on two pillows).

b. The nurse would need to instruct the patient to take the digoxin at the same time each day on an empty stomach to ensure adequate absorption of the drug. In addition, the nurse needs to teach the patient about signs and symptoms of digoxin toxicity especially because digoxin interacts with amiodarone, which could lead to an increase in digoxin levels. The combination of digoxin and the thiazide diuretic increases the risk for arrhythmias, so the nurse needs to teach the patient to report if he notices any changes in his heart rhythm, such as palpitations. The patient also needs to have his serum potassium levels checked periodically because the thiazide diuretic can lead to excess potassium loss (hypokalemia) further contributing to the risk for arrhythmias and digoxin toxicity. The patient also needs instruction in how to monitor his apical pulse rate and to hold the drug if the pulse rate is less than 60 beats/minute and notify the prescriber.

■ PRACTICING FOR NCLEX

1. **Answer: a, b, e, f**
   RATIONALE: Left-sided heart failure would be indicated by tachypnea, hemoptysis, orthopnea, increased urine output (polyuria), nocturia, dyspnea, and cough. Peripheral edema and hepatomegaly suggest right-sided heart failure.

2. **Answer: b**
   RATIONALE: Vasodilators decrease cardiac workload, relax vascular smooth muscle to decrease afterload, and allow pooling in the veins thereby decreasing preload. Decreased blood volume results from the use of diuretics.

3. **Answer: c**
   RATIONALE: Digoxin increases the force of myocardial contraction, increases cardiac output and renal perfusion, and slows the heart rate.

4. **Answer: d**
   RATIONALE: Therapeutic digoxin levels range from 0.5 ng/mL to 2.0 ng/mL. A level above 2.0 ng/mL would indicate toxicity.

5. **Answer: d**
   RATIONALE: Intravenous digoxin must be administered slowly over at least 5 minutes to prevent cardiac arrhythmias and adverse effects.

6. **Answer: d**
   RATIONALE: Food and antacids interfere with the absorption of the drug. Digoxin should be taken on an empty stomach at approximately the same time each day. *If* the patient takes an antacid, the patient should separate the dose of antacid and digoxin by 2 to 4 hours.

7. **Answer: b**
   RATIONALE: If the pulse rate is below 60 beats/minute, the patient should hold the dose and recheck his pulse in 1 hour. Then, if the pulse is still low, he make a note of it, withhold the drug, and notify the prescriber. The prescriber can then determine the next action.

8. **Answer: d**
   RATIONALE: Inamrinone is administered only by the intravenous route.

9. **Answer: b**
   RATIONALE: Although renal function studies may be appropriate to monitor and evaluate the need for possible dosage changes, inamrinone is associated with thrombocytopenia. Therefore, it would be most important for the nurse to monitor the patient's platelet count. Inamrinone is not associated with changes in pulmonary function or white blood cell counts.

10. **Answer: c**
    RATIONALE: After the initial bolus dose of inamrinone, the dose may be repeated in 30 minutes as needed.

11. **Answer: a**
    RATIONALE: Digoxin is the drug most often used to treat heart failure. Human B-type natriuretic peptide, nitrate, or furosemide also may be used, but these drugs are not the ones most commonly used.

12. **Answer: b**
    RATIONALE: Renal failure would be least likely to contribute to the development of heart failure. Coronary artery disease, valvular disease, hypertension, and cardiomyopathy are commonly associated with heart failure.

13. **Answer: d**
    RATIONALE: If a patient's pulse rate is less than 60 beats/minute, the drug should be withheld and the pulse retaken in 1 hour. If the pulse is still below 60 beats/minute, the dose is held and the prescriber should be notified.

14. **Answer: c**
    RATIONALE: Digoxin is a cardiac glycoside. Inamrinone and milrinone are phosphodiesterase inhibitors. Captopril is an angiotensin-converting enzyme inhibitor.

15. **Answer: b**
    RATIONALE: Peripheral edema would be noted in patients with right-sided heart failure. Wheezing, hemoptysis, and dyspnea would suggest left-sided heart failure.

CHAPTER 45

■ ASSESSING YOUR UNDERSTANDING

LABELING

Class I	Class II	Class III	Class IV
Disopyramide Flecainide Lidocaine Mexiletine Propafenone Quinidine	Acebutolol Propranolol	Amiodarone Sotalol	Diltiazem Verapamil

SEQUENCING

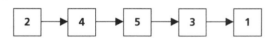

■ APPLYING YOUR KNOWLEDGE

CASE STUDY

a. Atrial fibrillation is associated with the development of blood clots due to the uncoordinated pumping, which leads to blood stagnating in the auricles. If the atria would contract properly, these clots would then travel to the lungs, brain, or periphery. Initially, heparin is used to initiate coagulation because warfarin is an oral agent that takes several days to reach therapeutic level.

b. The patient most definitely needs electrocardiogram monitoring to evaluate the current rhythm status and to determine if the amiodarone is effective in converting the arrhythmia. In addition, this monitoring is important to evaluate for the development of other arrhythmias (proarrhythmic effect) that may pose danger to the patient. Amiodarone also interacts with oral anticoagulants, so the nurse needs to assess the patient for signs and symptoms of bleeding once warfarin therapy is initiated. The nurse would need to inspect the patient for bruising and petechiae, check invasive device insertion sites for oozing, and urge the patient to report any frank or occult blood in his urine or stool. The nurse would also need to institute bleeding precautions to reduce the patient's risk for bleeding.

■ PRACTICING FOR NCLEX

1. Answer: c
RATIONALE: Antiarrhythmic agents alter the conductivity or suppress automaticity of the heart.

2. Answer: d
RATIONALE: Heart block is an arrhythmia related to an alteration in conduction through the muscle. Premature atrial contraction, atrial flutter, and ventricular fibrillation are arrhythmias due to stimulation from an ectopic focus.

3. Answer: b
RATIONALE: Procainamide is a class Ia antiarrhythmic agent. Lidocaine and mexiletine are classified as class Ib antiarrhythmics. Flecainide is a class 1c antiarrhythmic.

4. Answer: a
RATIONALE: Class I antiarrhythmics stabilize the cell membrane by binding to sodium channels, depressing phase 0 of the action potential.

5. Answer: a
RATIONALE: Disopyramide is administered orally.

6. Answer: b
RATIONALE: Quinidine interacts with digoxin, possibly leading to increased digoxin levels and digoxin toxicity. The effects of digoxin, not quinidine, are increased. Bleeding may occur if class I antiarrhythmics are given with oral anticoagulants such as warfarin. Renal dysfunction is unrelated to the use of both drugs.

7. Answer: d
RATIONALE: Quinidine requires a slightly acidic urine for excretion. Patients receiving quinidine should avoid foods that alkalinize the urine, such as citrus juices, antacids, milk products, and vegetables.

8. Answer: a
RATIONALE: Lidocaine, when given by intramuscular injection, has an onset of action between 5 to 10 minutes and peaks in 5 to 15 minutes.

9. Answer: b
RATIONALE: Class II antiarrhythmics are beta-adrenergic blockers that block the beta receptor sites in the heart and kidneys. Membrane stabilization and phase 0 depression occurs with class I antiarrhythmics. Blockage of potassium channels during phase 3 of the action potential occurs with class III antiarrhythmics. Blockage of calcium ion movement occurs with class IV antiarrhythmics.

10. Answer: c
RATIONALE: Esmolol, a class II agent, is administered intravenously.

11. Answer: a
RATIONALE: Class II antiarrhythmics are contraindicated in sinus bradycardia but should be used cautiously in patients with diabetes, thyroid dysfunction, and hepatic dysfunction.

12. Answer: d
RATIONALE: Bronchospasm is a possible adverse effect of acebutolol, a class II antiarrhythmic. Other effects include hypotension, decreased libido, and decreased exercise tolerance.

13. Answer: d
RATIONALE: Dofetilide is a class III antiarrhythmic that blocks potassium channels and slows the outward movement of potassium during phase 3 of the action potential.

14. Answer: b
RATIONALE: Sotalol absorption is decreased by the presence of food, so it should be taken on an empty stomach to maximize absorption. There is no need to sit up after taking the drug. Antacids would interfere with the absorption. Holding the drug if the pulse rate is less than 60 beats/minute applies to digoxin.

15. Answer: b
RATIONALE: Adenosine slows conduction through the atrioventricular node, prolongs the refractory period, and decreases automaticity through the atrioventricular node. Digoxin used as an antiarrhythmic slows calcium from leaving the cell, prolonging the action potential and slowing conduction and heart rate.

CHAPTER 46

■ ASSESSING YOUR UNDERSTANDING

MATCHING

1. g	**2.** d	**3.** e	**4.** b	**5.** h
6. f	**7.** c	**8.** a		

SHORT ANSWER

1. Coronary artery disease is the leading cause of death in the Western world.

2. Unlike other tissues in the body, the heart muscle receives its blood supply during diastole while it is at rest. This is important because when the heart muscle contracts, it becomes tight and clamps the blood vessels closed, rendering them unable to receive blood during systole, which is when all other tissues receive fresh blood.

3. The person with atherosclerosis has a classic supply-and-demand problem. The heart may function without problem until increases in activity or other stresses place a demand on it to beat faster or harder. Normally, the heart would stimulate the vessels to deliver more blood when this occurs, but the narrowed vessels are not able to respond and cannot supply the blood needed by the working heart. The heart muscle then becomes hypoxic.

4. Antianginal drugs can work to improve blood delivery to the heart muscle in one of two ways: by dilating blood vessels (i.e., increasing the supply of oxygen) or by decreasing the work of the heart (i.e., decreasing the demand for oxygen).

5. Nitrates act directly on smooth muscle to cause relaxation and to depress muscle tone. Because the action is direct, these drugs do not influence any nerve or other activity, and the response is usually quite fast.

■ APPLYING YOUR KNOWLEDGE

CASE STUDY

a. Nitroglycerin sublingual tablets should be kept in the original dark container in which they were dispensed because the drugs need to be protected from light. Otherwise, they will lose their potency. In addition, keeping the tablets in the original container allows the nurse and the patient to check the expiration date to ensure that the tablets are still usable. The tablets also need to be stored in a cool, dry place. The patient's back pants pocket is not such a place.

b. The nurse needs to teach the patient about proper storage of the drug, including the need to keep the drug in its dark container to protect it from light and to store the drug in a cool, dry place. The nurse also needs to emphasize that the patient check the expiration date so that the patient has access to medication that is still potent. Since there is no way to tell if the tablets have expired and since they have not been protected from light and heat, it would be appropriate for the nurse to obtain a new prescription for the patient so that he can have a fresh supply should he need them. The nurse could also instruct the patient to note if the tablet fizzles or burns when he uses them, as this would indicate potency.

■ PRACTICING FOR NCLEX

1. **Answer: a**
   RATIONALE: Angina is most accurately described as the body's response to a lack of oxygen in the heart muscle. It commonly is manifested as chest pain, but it can occur at rest or with activity. Angina does not necessarily indicate damage to the heart muscle. Ischemia leads to damage. Prinzmetal's angina is a type of angina that is due to vessel spasm.

2. **Answer: b**
   RATIONALE: Unstable angina is chest pain that occurs when the patient is at rest. Stable angina is chest pain that occurs with activity and is relieved by rest. Prinzmetal's angina is chest pain due to vessel spasm. Myocardial infarction indicates ischemia and subsequent necrosis of the heart muscle.

3. **Answer: b**
   RATIONALE: Most of the deaths caused by myocardial infarction occur as a result of fatal arrhythmias.

4. **Answer: d**
   RATIONALE: Isosorbide is classified as a nitrate. Metoprolol is a beta-blocker. Amlodipine and nicardipine are calcium channel blockers.

5. **Answer: c**
   RATIONALE: Isosorbide dinitrate is available as an oral agent, sublingual tablet, and chewable tablet. It cannot be given intravenously.

6. **Answer: c**
   RATIONALE: Nitrates would be contraindicated in patients with cerebral hemorrhage because the relaxation of the cerebral vessels could cause intracranial bleeding. Cardiac tamponade, hypotension, and hepatic disease require cautious use of nitrates.

7. **Answer: b**
   RATIONALE: Nitroglycerin sublingual spray begins to act in approximately 2 minutes.

8. **Answer: a**
   RATIONALE: A fizzing or burning sensation indicates that the tablet is potent. The patient should place the tablet under his tongue and away from any lesions or abrasions. If needed, the patient can take a sip of water to moisten the mucous membranes so that the tablet will dissolve quickly. After placing the tablet under the tongue, the patient should close his mouth and wait until the table has dissolved.

9. **Answer: b**
   RATIONALE: Nitroglycerin can be repeated every 5 minutes if relief is not felt for a total of three doses.

10. **Answer: a**
    RATIONALE: Phosphodiesterase 5 inhibitors, such as sildenafil, tadalafil, or vardenafil used to treat erectile dysfunction, should be avoided if the patient is taking nitrates due to the risk of severe hypotension and cardiovascular events. Beta-blockers in combination with nitrates may cause hypotension and should be used cautiously together. Nitrates do not interact with nonsteroidal anti-inflammatory drugs or cardiac glycosides.

11. **Answer: b**
    RATIONALE: Nadolol is a beta-blocker used as an antianginal agent. Amlodipine and verapamil are calcium channel blocker antianginal agents. Ranolazine is classified as a piperazine acetamide.

12. **Answer: c**
    RATIONALE: Propranolol is used after a myocardial infarction to prevent reinfarction. The drug could cause vasospasm and as such would not be indicated for the treatment of Prinzmetal's angina.

13. **Answer: d**
    RATIONALE: Calcium channel blockers such as amlodipine are indicated as treatment for Prinzmetal's angina because they relieve coronary artery vasospasm. Nitroglycerin is indicated for acute angina attacks. Metoprolol and nadolol would be contraindicated for patients with Prinzmetal's angina.

14. **Answer: b**
    RATIONALE: Although the exact mechanism of action of the drug is not understood, it does prolong the QT interval. It does not decrease heart rate or blood pressure but does decrease myocardial workload, bringing the supply and demand for oxygen back into balance.

15. **Answer: c**
    RATIONALE: Transdermal nitroglycerin is applied once daily. The patch has a duration of 24 hours. Isosorbide dinitrate can be used before an activity that may cause chest pain. Sublingual, translingual spray, or buccal nitroglycerin is used with episodes of acute angina.

CHAPTER 47

■ ASSESSING YOUR UNDERSTANDING

LABELING

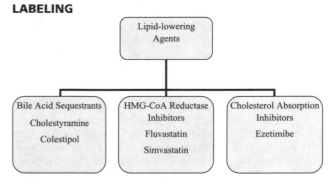

SHORT ANSWER

1. Metabolic syndrome is characterized by increased insulin resistance, high blood pressure, altered lipid levels, abdominal obesity, proinflammatory state, and prothrombotic state.
2. Nonmodifiable risk factors for coronary artery disease include family history, age, and gender.
3. Gout increases uric acid levels, which seem to injure vessel walls.
4. Black Americans have lower serum cholesterol levels, higher high-density lipoprotein (HDL) levels, and lower low-density lipoprotein (LDL) levels, and their HDL to cholesterol level is less when compared with white Americans.
5. Ways to modify risk factors include decreasing dietary fats, losing weight, eliminating smoking, increasing exercise levels, and decreasing stress as well as treating hypertension, gout, and diabetes.
6. Chylomicrons are a package of fats and proteins on which micelles are carried to allow absorption.

■ APPLYING YOUR KNOWLEDGE

CASE STUDY

a. First, the nurse would need to investigate exactly what types of fruit juices the patient is drinking. Grapefruit juice should be avoided in patients who are taking HMG-CoA inhibitors because it alters the metabolism of the drug, leading to an increased serum drug level and increased risk for adverse effects, including rhabdomyolysis.

b. The patient may be experiencing early signs of rhabdomyolysis, especially if the patient has been drinking grapefruit juice while taking the drug. She needs to have some laboratory testing done to determine if she is experiencing problems with any liver or renal dysfunction and to evaluate for possible rhabdomyolysis. It would be important to obtain specimens to evaluate muscle and liver enzyme levels for increases that may suggest rhabdomyolysis. Muscle and liver enzymes such as creatine kinase, lactic dehydrogenase, aspartate aminotransferase, and alanine aminotransferase levels may be elevated to three times the normal level with rhabdomyolysis. In addition, renal function studies would be important because the breakdown of muscle results in the waste products injuring the glomerulus leads to renal failure.

■ PRACTICING FOR NCLEX

1. **Answer: b, c**
   RATIONALE: Characteristics of metabolic syndrome include waist measurement over 40 inches in men; triglyceride levels greater than 150 mg/dL or HDL levels less than 40 mg/dL in men or less than 50 mg/dL in women; fasting blood glucose levels greater than 110 mg/dL; blood pressure greater than 130/85 mm Hg; increased plasminogen activator levels; and increased macrophages, levels of interleukin-6, and tumor necrosis factor.

2. **Answer: d**
   RATIONALE: A triglyceride level of 180 mg/dL is considered borderline high (normal or desirable would be less than 150 mg/dL). A total cholesterol of 160 mg/dL and an LDL cholesterol of 110 mg/dL would be considered normal or desirable. An HDL level of 45 mg/dL would be considered normal; levels above 60 mg/dL would be considered high.

3. **Answer: a**
   RATIONALE: Bile acids act like a detergent in the small intestine and break up fats into small units. These small units are called *micelles*. High levels of cholesterol are part of bile acids. Chylomicrons are carriers for micelles.

4. **Answer: b**
   RATIONALE: HDLs are loosely packed lipids that are used for energy and to pick up remnants of fats and cholesterol left in the periphery by the breakdown of LDLs. LDLs are tightly packed cholesterol, triglycerides, and lipids that are carried by proteins that enter the circulation to be broken down for energy or stored for future use as energy.

5. **Answer: c**
   RATIONALE: Cholestyramine is classified as a bile acid sequestrant. Lovastatin is a HMG-CoA reductase inhibitor. Ezetimibe is a cholesterol absorption inhibitor. Gemfibrozil is classified as a fibrate.

6. **Answer: d**
   RATIONALE: The absorption of thiazide diuretic can be decreased or delayed with colestipol, a bile acid sequestrant.

Therefore, the diuretic should be taken 1 hour before or 4 to 6 hours after the colestipol.

7. **Answer: b**
   RATIONALE: Cholestyramine should not be mixed with carbonated beverages. Soups, fruit juices, cereals, liquids, or pulpy fruit are acceptable alternatives.

8. **Answer: c**
   RATIONALE: The drug is administered at bedtime because the highest rates of cholesterol synthesis occur between 12 and 5 AM, and the drug should be taken when it will be most effective.

9. **Answer: d**
   RATIONALE: Ezetimibe is a cholesterol absorption inhibitor that works in the brush border of the small intestine to decrease absorption of dietary cholesterol from the small intestine. HMG-CoA reductase inhibitors block the enzyme involved in cholesterol synthesis. Bile acid sequestrants block bile acids to form insoluble complexes for excretion in the feces. Fibrates stimulate the breakdown of lipoproteins from the tissues and their removal from the plasma.

10. **Answer: d**
    RATIONALE: Increased serum levels and resultant toxicity can occur if a statin is combined with warfarin, an oral anticoagulant. This would increase the patient's risk for bleeding. Abdominal pain and cataract development are related to the use of atorvastatin alone. Liver failure also is associated with atorvastatin use alone.

11. **Answer: d**
    RATIONALE: To ensure the need for the drug therapy, the patient needs to have attempted lifestyle modifications including a cholesterol-lowering diet and exercise program for at least 3 to 6 months.

12. **Answer: b**
    RATIONALE: The initial effect on lipid levels is usually seen within 5 to 7 days of starting niacin therapy.

13. **Answer: c**
    RATIONALE: Niacin acts to inhibit the release of free fatty acids from adipose tissue, increases the rate of triglyceride removal from the plasma, and generally reduces LDL and triglyceride levels and increases HDL levels. Fenofibrate inhibits triglyceride synthesis in the liver, resulting in a reduction of LDL levels. Gemfibrozil inhibits the peripheral breakdown of lipids, reduces the production of triglycerides and LDLs, and increases HDL concentrations. Fenofibric acid activates a specific hepatic receptor that results in increased breakdown of lipids, elimination of triglyceride-rich particles from the plasma, and reduction in the production to an enzyme that naturally inhibits lipid breakdown.

14. **Answer: c**
    RATIONALE: Although any combinations may be used, niacin is often combined with bile acid sequestrants for increased effects.

15. **Answer: b**
    RATIONALE: The presence of fatty acids, lipids, and cholesterol in the duodenum stimulates contraction of the gallbladder and the release of bile, which contains bile acids. Once their action is completed, they are reabsorbed and recycled to the gallbladder, where they remain until the gallbladder is stimulated again.

CHAPTER 48

■ ASSESSING YOUR UNDERSTANDING

MATCHING
1. e   **2.** h   **3.** f   **4.** b   **5.** i
6. d   **7.** a   **8.** g   **9.** c   **10.** j

LABELING

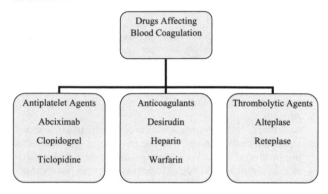

■ APPLYING YOUR KNOWLEDGE

CASE STUDY

a. The patient had an acute embolism or blood clot that had traveled to the lungs. The alteplase was used to dissolve the clot and restore blood flow.

b. Heparin was used to prevent the formation of any new clots. Warfarin also was used to prevent blood clots. The patient was receiving both drugs because warfarin's onset of action typically takes approximately 3 days. Once therapeutic levels of warfarin are achieved (prothrombin time [PT] 1.5 to 2.5 times the control or international normalized ratio [INR] of 2 to 3), then the heparin is stopped.

c. The patient needs instructions about the following: appropriate administration, including the need to use the same formulation of the drug and possible dosage adjustments; follow-up laboratory testing of coagulation status; bleeding precautions; safety measures, including ways to avoid injury that could lead to bruising; measures to stop bleeding, such as ice and direct pressure; importance of reporting any blood in urine or stool; the use of a Medic-alert bracelet; foods containing vitamin K such as green leafy vegetables and the importance of maintaining consistent use of these foods to prevent decreasing the effectiveness of warfarin; and measures to prevent recurrent deep vein thrombosis and pulmonary embolism.

■ PRACTICING FOR NCLEX

1. Answer: a
RATIONALE: Thrombin is a topical hemostatic agent. Protamine sulfate is the antidote for heparin. Pentoxifylline is a hemorheologic agent (one that can induce hemorrhage). Urokinase is a thrombolytic agent.

2. Answer: b
RATIONALE: The first reaction to a blood vessel injury is local vasoconstriction. In addition, injury then exposes blood to the collagen and other substances under the endothelial lining of the vessel, causing platelet aggregation. Release of factor XI occurs in response to activation of the Hageman factor. Thrombin formation occurs at the end of the intrinsic pathway.

3. Answer: a
RATIONALE: Clopidogrel is administered orally.

4. Answer: c
RATIONALE: Anagrelide decreases the production of platelets in the bone marrow, necessitating close monitoring of platelet levels for thrombocytopenia.

5. Answer: a
RATIONALE: Warfarin is administered orally.

6. Answer: a
RATIONALE: Heparin's effectiveness is monitored by the results of the partial thromboplastin time. The INR and PT are used to monitor warfarin. Vitamin K is the antidote for warfarin, and levels are not monitored to evaluate the effects of any anticoagulant.

7. Answer: d
RATIONALE: Fondaparinux inhibits factor Xa and blocks the clotting cascade to prevent clot formation. Heparin and argatroban block the formation of thrombin from prothrombin. Warfarin decreases the production of vitamin K–depending clotting factors in the liver.

8. Answer: b
RATIONALE: Protamine sulfate is the antidote for heparin overdose. Vitamin K is the antidote for warfarin overdose. Urokinase is a thrombolytic. Drotrecogin alfa is a C reactive protein that has anticoagulant effects.

9. Answer: c
RATIONALE: When combined with phenytoin, warfarin leads to a decrease in anticoagulant effect, which would necessitate an increase in the dosage of the warfarin. Clofibrate, quinidine, and cefoxitin increase the risk of bleeding with warfarin; thus, a decreased dose of warfarin would be indicated.

10. Answer: d
RATIONALE: Treatment with a thrombolytic must be instituted within 6 hours of the onset of symptoms of an acute myocardial infarction to achieve maximum therapeutic effectiveness. In this case, 4 PM would be the latest.

11. Answer: c
RATIONALE: When used for hip surgery, enoxaparin typically is administered for 7 to 10 days to prevent deep vein thrombosis that may lead to pulmonary embolism after hip replacement.

12. Answer: c
RATIONALE: Therapeutic range for heparin would be 1.5 to 2.5 times the patient's baseline. For a baseline value of 32 seconds, this would range from 48 to 80 seconds. A value of 64 seconds would be considered therapeutic.

13. Answer: d
RATIONALE: Drotrecogin alfa is approved for use in adults with severe sepsis who are at high risk for death. The usual dose is given by intravenous infusion for a total of 96 hours. It is associated with a high risk for bleeding, which requires extremely close patient monitoring. It is a very expensive drug, which may be a factor in limiting its use.

14. Answer: a
RATIONALE: Antihemophilic factor is factor VIII, which is the factor missing in classic hemophilia. Coagulation factors VIIa and IX are separate clotting factors. Factor IX complex contains plasma fractions of many of the clotting factors and increases blood levels of factors II, VII, IX, and X.

15. Answer: b
RATIONALE: Aminocaproic acid is the only systemic hemostatic agent available. Absorbable gelatin, human fibrin sealant, and thrombin are topical hemostatic agents.

CHAPTER 49

■ ASSESSING YOUR UNDERSTANDING

MATCHING

1. e   2. a   3. d   4. f   5. b
6. c

SHORT ANSWER

1. Erythropoietin is released from the kidneys in response to decreased blood flow or decreased oxygen tension in the kidneys. Under the influence of erythropoietin, an undifferentiated cell in the bone marrow becomes a hemocytoblast. This cell uses certain amino acids, lipids, carbohydrates, vitamin B_{12}, folic acid, and iron to turn into an immature red blood cell (RBC). In the last phase of RBC production, the cell loses its nucleus and enters the circulation. This cell, called a *reticulocyte*, finishes its maturing process in the circulation.
2. The average life span of an RBC is 120 days.
3. The bone marrow must have adequate amounts of iron, which is used in forming hemoglobin rings to carry the oxygen; minute amounts of vitamin B_{12} and folic acid to form a strong supporting structure that can survive being battered through blood vessels for 90–120 days; and essential amino acids and carbohydrates to complete the hemoglobin rings, cell membrane, and basic structure.
4. A deficiency anemia occurs when the diet cannot supply enough of a nutrient or enough of the nutrient cannot be absorbed; fewer RBCs are produced, and the ones that are produced are immature and inefficient iron carriers. Megaloblastic anemia involves decreased production of RBCs and ineffectiveness of those RBCs that are produced (they do not usually survive for the 120 days that is normal for the life of an RBC). Hemolytic anemia involves a lysing of RBCs because of genetic factors or from exposure to toxins.
5. Pernicious anemia occurs when the gastric mucosa cannot produce intrinsic factor and vitamin B_{12} cannot be absorbed.

■ APPLYING YOUR KNOWLEDGE

CASE STUDY

a. Epoetin alfa is indicated for the treatment of anemia associated with cancer chemotherapy when the bone marrow is suppressed. It acts like the natural glycoprotein erythropoietin to stimulate production of the RBCs in the bone marrow.
b. Epoetin alfa is associated with a possible decrease in the normal levels of erythropoietin. Administration to a patient with normal renal function can actually cause a more severe anemia if endogenous levels fall and no longer stimulate RBC production. The patient's blood count needs to be monitored closely because of the risk for developing pure red cell aplasia secondary to erythropoietin; neutralizing antibodies can occur. In addition, the drug should not be used if the patient's hemoglobin is above 12 g/dL because of the risk of cardiovascular events and increased rates of tumor progression death in cancer patients. Other areas that need close monitoring include the patient's cardiovascular and central nervous system status for possible adverse effects.

■ PRACTICING FOR NCLEX

1. **Answer: c**
   RATIONALE: Anemias are disorders that involve too few or ineffective RBCs that alter the ability of the blood to carry oxygen. White blood cells are associated with the immune response. Plasma proteins are important in the immune response and blood clotting. Lack of vitamin B_{12} is associated with a specific type of anemia.
2. **Answer: d**
   RATIONALE: Sickle cell anemia is an example of a hemolytic anemia that involves lysing of RBCs because of genetic factors or from exposure to toxins. Iron deficiency anemia is a deficiency anemia. Pernicious anemia and folic acid deficiency anemia are examples of megaloblastic anemia.
3. **Answer: c, d, e**
   RATIONALE: Folic acid is found in green leafy vegetables such as broccoli, milk, liver, and eggs. Fruits and fish are not good sources of folic acid.
4. **Answer: c**
   RATIONALE: Hydroxocobalamin is administered intramuscularly for 5 to 10 days and then monthly.
5. **Answer: a**
   RATIONALE: Hydroxyurea is indicated for the treatment of sickle cell anemia to increase the amount of fetal hemoglobin produced in the bone marrow and to dilute the formation of abnormal hemoglobin S in adults who have sickle cell anemia. Epoetin alfa is indicated for treatment of anemia associated with renal failure and those on dialysis and for patients with anemia associated with AIDS therapy and cancer chemotherapy. Ferrous sulfate and iron dextran are indicated for the treatment of iron deficiency anemia.
6. **Answer: a**
   RATIONALE: Darbepoetin alfa is administered once a week. Epoetin alfa is administered three times/week. Methoxy polyethylene glycol–epoetin alfa is administered once every 2 weeks or once a month.
7. **Answer: c**
   RATIONALE: Iron dextran is administered by intramuscular injection using the Z-track technique. Ferrous gluconate, fumarate, and sulfate are administered orally. Iron sucrose and sodium ferric gluconate complex are given intravenously.
8. **Answer: a**
   RATIONALE: Iron is not absorbed if taken with antacids, so the patient should avoid this combination. Adequate iron intake is necessary to assist in regaining a positive iron balance. It can take 2 to 3 weeks to see an improvement and up to 6 to 10 months to return to a stable iron level once a deficiency exists. Iron absorption also is altered if it is taken with milk, eggs, coffee, or tea. These substances should be avoided.
9. **Answer: b**
   RATIONALE: The patient needs to be informed that his stools may become dark or green. Small frequent meals with snacks can help minimize nausea. The patient may take the drug with meals as long as those meals do not include eggs, milk, coffee, or tea. Constipation is possible, so the patient needs to increase the fiber in his diet.
10. **Answer: a**
    RATIONALE: Vitamin B_{12} is important for maintaining the myelin sheath. Folic acid is important in preventing neural tube defects and is essential for cell division in all types of tissues. RBCs are important for transporting oxygen to the tissues.
11. **Answer: a, b, d**
    RATIONALE: The bone marrow uses iron, carbohydrates, amino acids, folic acid, and vitamin B_{12} to produce healthy, efficient RBCs.
12. **Answer: b**
    RATIONALE: Epoetin alfa has a duration of effect of usually 24 hours.

13. Answer: c

RATIONALE: Deferoxamine is the antidote for iron toxicity. Dimercaprol is used for arsenic, gold, or mercury poisoning. Succimer and edetate calcium disodium can be used to treat lead poisoning.

14. Answer: b

RATIONALE: Leucovorin is used as a rescue following methotrexate therapy. Cyancobalamin is used to treat megaloblastic anemia. Hydroxyurea is used to treat sickle cell anemia. Iron sucrose is indicated for treatment of iron deficiency anemia.

15. Answer: d

RATIONALE: Oral liquid iron solution can stain the teeth; therefore, it should be taken through a straw to prevent this from occurring. Orange juice is acidic, and although it may enhance the absorption of the medication, it should not be used concurrently. The risk of staining would still be present. Drinking a big glass of water after swallowing the solution would not reduce the risk of staining the teeth. The dose should not be mixed with other foods, especially dairy products such as yogurt, which can interfere with absorption.

CHAPTER 50

■ ASSESSING YOUR UNDERSTANDING
LABELING

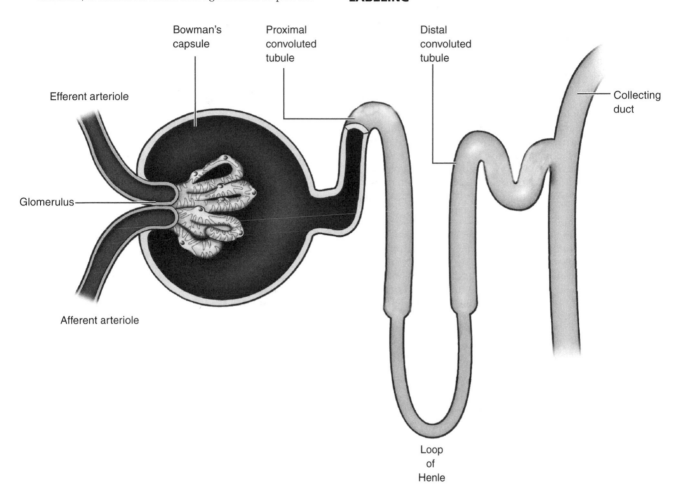

MATCHING

1. c **2.** f **3.** b **4.** g **5.** a
6. e **7.** h **8.** d

■ APPLYING YOUR KNOWLEDGE
CASE STUDY

a. The students would need to demonstrate glomerular filtration, tubular secretion, and tubular reabsorption. The students could arrange themselves as the glomerulus, Bowman's capsule, proximal convoluted tubule, descending loop of Henle, loop of Henle, ascending loop of Henle, distal convoluted tubule, and collecting duct. The students could be connected by rope, tubing, or other item to illustrate the "tubule," such as a noodle commonly found in swimming pools. Other props could be used to represent sodium, water, calcium, potassium, chloride, aldosterone, and antidiuretic hormone. These props could then be moved back and forth along the "tubule" to illustrate secretion and reabsorption.

b. The students would need to address water, sodium, chloride, potassium, and calcium. When demonstrating the movement of sodium, chloride would need to go hand in hand with the sodium. The students could use the props identified above to act out the movement of the various electrolytes along the tubule and the countercurrent mechanism.

■ PRACTICING FOR NCLEX

1. Answer: b
RATIONALE: The renal system consists of the kidneys and structures of the urinary tract: ureters, bladder, and urethra. The kidneys have three protective layers. The system has four major functions: maintaining the volume and composition of body fluids, regulating vitamin D activation, regulating blood pressure, and regulating red blood cell production. Most of the fluid that is filtered by the kidneys is returned to the body.

2. Answer: c
RATIONALE: All nephrons filter and make urine, but only the medullary nephrons can concentrate or dilute urine. The renal pelvises drain the urine into the ureters. The renal arteries come directly off the aorta. Erythropoietin is produced by a small group of cells called the *juxtaglomerular apparatus.*

3. Answer: c
RATIONALE: The kidneys receive approximately 25% of the cardiac output.

4. Answer: d
RATIONALE: It is estimated that only about 25% of the total number of nephrons are necessary to maintain healthy renal function. This means that the renal system is well protected from failure with a large backup system. However, it also means that by the time a patient manifests signs and symptoms suggesting failure of the kidneys, extensive kidney damage has already occurred.

5. Answer: b
RATIONALE: Tubular secretion involves the active movement of substances from the blood into the renal tubule. Movement of fluid and other elements through the glomerulus into the tubule describes glomerular filtration. The movement of substances from the tubule back into the vascular system describes tubular reabsorption. The process of concentrating or diluting urine refers to the countercurrent mechanism.

6. Answer: b
RATIONALE: Approximately 1% of the filtrate or less than 2 L of fluid is excreted each day in the form of urine.

7. Answer: d
RATIONALE: The glomerulus acts as an ultrafine filter for all of the blood that flows into it. The semipermeable membrane keeps lipids, proteins, and blood cells inside the vessel, whereas the hydrostatic pressure from the blood pushes water and smaller components of the plasma into the tubule.

8. Answer: a
RATIONALE: Sodium is filtered through the glomerulus and enters the renal tubule, where it is actively reabsorbed in the proximal convoluted tubule to the peritubular capillaries.

9. Answer: c
RATIONALE: Aldosterone is released into the circulation in response to angiotensin III, high potassium levels, or sympathetic stimulation. Aldosterone stimulates a sodium–potassium exchange pump in the cells of the distal tubule, causing reabsorption of sodium in exchange for potassium. As a result of aldosterone stimulation, sodium is reabsorbed into the system and potassium is lost in the filtrate. Natriuretic hormone causes a decrease in sodium reabsorption from the distal tubules with a resultant dilute urine or increased volume. Natriuretic hormone is released in response to fluid overload or hemodilution.

10. Answer: b
RATIONALE: The fluid in the ascending loop of Henle is hypotonic in comparison to the hypertonic situation in the peritubular tissues. The filtrate in the descending loop is highly concentrated in comparison to the rest of the filtrate.

11. Answer: a
RATIONALE: About 65% of the potassium that is filtered at the glomerulus is reabsorbed at Bowman's capsule and the proximal convoluted tubule. Another 25% to 30% is reabsorbed in the ascending loop of Henle.

12. Answer: d
RATIONALE: Parathyroid hormone stimulates the reabsorption of calcium in the distal convoluted tubule to increase serum calcium levels when they are low. Aldosterone is important in adjusting sodium levels. Antidiuretic hormone is important in maintaining fluid balance and is released in response to falling blood volume, sympathetic stimulation, or rising sodium levels. Vitamin D regulates the absorption of calcium from the gastrointestinal tract.

13. Answer: b
RATIONALE: Whenever blood flow or oxygenation to the nephron is decreased (due to hemorrhage, shock, congestive heart failure, or hypotension), renin is released from the juxtaglomerular cells. Calcium is not involved. Renin activates angiotensinogen. After subsequent conversions, angiotensin III ultimately stimulates the release of aldosterone from the adrenal gland.

14. Answer: b
RATIONALE: Urine is usually a slightly acidic fluid; this acidity helps to maintain the normal transport systems and to destroy bacteria that may enter the bladder. The acidity does not play a role in maintaining fluid balance or affect sphincter control. Peristaltic movement is necessary to push urine down from the ureters into the bladder.

15. Answer: c
RATIONALE: In the female, the urethra is a very short tube that leads from the bladder to an area populated by normal flora, including *Escherichia coli*, which can cause frequent bladder infections or cystitis. In the male, the urethra is much longer and passes through the prostate gland, a small gland that produces an alkaline fluid that is important in maintaining the sperm and lubricating the tract. Neither the prostate nor the fluid has any effect on the development of cystitis. The urinary bladder does stretch, but the amount of stretch is highly variable.

CHAPTER 51

■ ASSESSING YOUR UNDERSTANDING

LABELING

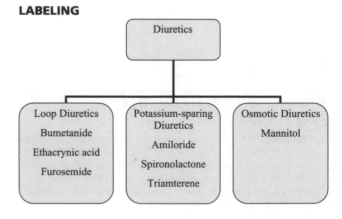

SHORT ANSWER

1. Diuretic agents are commonly thought of simply as drugs that increase the amount of urine produced by the kidneys. Most diuretics do increase the volume of urine produced to some extent, but the greater clinical significance of diuretics is their ability to increase sodium excretion. Most diuretics prevent the cells lining the renal tubules from reabsorbing an excessive proportion of the sodium ions in the glomerular filtrate. As a result, sodium and other ions (and the water in which they are dissolved) are lost in the urine instead of being returned to the blood, where they would cause increased intravascular volume and therefore increased hydrostatic pressure, which could result in leaking of fluids at the capillary level.

2. Fluid rebound is a reflex reaction of the body to the loss of fluid or sodium; the hypothalamus causes the release of antidiuretic hormone, which retains water, and stress related to fluid loss combines with decreased blood flow to the kidneys to activate the renin-angiotensin-aldosterone system, leading to further water and sodium retention.

3. Heart failure can cause edema as a result of several factors. The failing heart muscle does not pump sufficient blood to the kidneys, causing activation of the renin-angiotensin system and resulting in increases in blood volume and sodium retention. Because the failing heart muscle cannot respond to the usual reflex stimulation, the increased volume is slowly pushed out into the capillary level as venous pressure increases because the blood is not being pumped effectively.

4. Thiazide and thiazidelike diuretics act to block the chloride pump. Chloride is actively pumped out of the tubule by cells lining the ascending limb of the loop of Henle and the distal tubule. Sodium passively moves with the chloride to maintain an electrical neutrality. (Chloride is a negative ion, and sodium is a positive ion.) Blocking of the chloride pump keeps the chloride and the sodium in the tubule to be excreted in the urine, thus preventing the reabsorption of both chloride and sodium in the vascular system. Because these segments of the tubule are impermeable to water, there is little increase in the volume of urine produced, but it will be sodium rich, which is a saluretic effect.

5. The prototype loop diuretic is furosemide.

6. Most often, carbonic anhydrase inhibitors are used to treat glaucoma because the inhibition of carbonic anhydrase results in decreased secretion of aqueous humor of the eye.

■ APPLYING YOUR KNOWLEDGE

CASE STUDY

a. It would be important to investigate if the patient is continuing to take her potassium supplement even though the furosemide has been stopped. It would also be important to ask the patient about the foods that she is eating. For example, she may still be eating foods that are high in potassium, inadvertently thinking that she still needs to do so. The nurse also needs to determine the patient's understanding of her current drug therapy. It is possible that the patient understands that she is still taking a "diuretic" but does not understand that spironolactone is different from furosemide.

b. The nurse should relate to the patient that the spironolactone is a potassium-sparing diuretic, emphasizing that she is not losing potassium like she had been with the furosemide. In addition, the nurse needs to instruct the patient to watch her intake of high-potassium foods to avoid raising her potassium level too high. Moreover, the nurse should make sure that the patient is no longer using the potassium supplement. Other teaching should address the signs and symptoms of hypo- and hyperkalemia so that the patient can contact the health care provider should any occur. Hyperkalemia can cause lethargy, confusion, ataxia, muscle cramps, and cardiac arrhythmias, the latter being especially problematic for the patient with a history of hypertension and heart failure.

■ PRACTICING FOR NCLEX

1. **Answer: b**
   RATIONALE: If a patient decreases his fluid intake to decrease the number of trips to the bathroom, the patient is at risk for fluid rebound, which leads to water retention. Fluid retention, leading to weight gain, would occur. Hypokalemia and dehydration would not be associated effects.

2. **Answer: a**
   RATIONALE: Metolazone is an example of a thiazidelike diuretic. Chlorothiazide is a thiazide diuretic; furosemide is a loop diuretic; and triamterene is a potassium-sparing diuretic.

3. **Answer: a**
   RATIONALE: Hydrochlorothiazide is only available as an oral preparation. Only chlorothiazide can be given by intravenous infusion.

4. **Answer: c**
   RATIONALE: Indapamide would be contraindicated in a patient with hypokalemia because any fluid and electrolyte imbalance could be potentiated by the changes caused by the diuretic. Indapamide would be used cautiously in patients with diabetes, systemic lupus erythematosus, or gout.

5. **Answer: b**
   RATIONALE: Chlorthalidone is a thiazidelike diuretic that may lead to hypercalcemia (due to decreased calcium excretion), hyperuricemia (increased levels of uric acid due to decreased uric acid secretion), and hypokalemia. Anemia is not associated with this drug.

6. **Answer: b**
   RATIONALE: Hydrochlorothiazide has an onset of action of 2 hours, peaking in 4 to 6 hours, and lasting approximately 6 to 12 hours.

7. **Answer: b**
   RATIONALE: Bumetanide is a loop diuretic that blocks the chloride pump in the ascending loop of Henle. It also has a similar effect in the descending loop and in the distal convoluted tubule.

8. **Answer: c**
   RATIONALE: Use of furosemide can lead to hypotension due to fluid loss, alkalosis due to loss of bicarbonate, hypocalcemia due to loss of calcium, and hyperglycemia (with long-term use) due to diuretic effect on glucose levels.

9. **Answer: b**
   RATIONALE: Furosemide, when given intravenously, begins to act in 5 minutes, reaching peak effects in 30 minutes. In this case, this would be 8:30 AM.

10. **Answer: a**
    RATIONALE: Furosemide is less powerful than bumetanide and torsemide and therefore has a larger margin of safety for home use (see the Critical Thinking Scenario in this chapter for additional information about using furosemide in heart failure). Ethacrynic acid is used less frequently in the clinical setting because of the improved potency and reliability of the newer drugs.

11. Answer: b
RATIONALE: Metabolic acidosis is a relatively common and potentially dangerous effect that occurs when bicarbonate is lost due to the action of carbonic anhydrase inhibitors. Metabolic alkalosis would occur if bicarbonate were retained. No respiratory acid-base imbalances are associated with this drug.

12. Answer: d
RATIONALE: Spironolactone acts as an aldosterone antagonist blocking the actions of aldosterone in the distal tubule. Amiloride and triamterene block potassium secretion through the tubule. Carbonic anhydrase inhibitors slow the movement of hydrogen ions. Loop diuretics block the chloride pump.

13. Answer: a, b, d
RATIONALE: Foods high in potassium should be avoided. These would include bananas, prunes, and broccoli.

14. Answer: b
RATIONALE: Instructions for a patient taking a diuretic include taking the drug with food or meals if gastrointestinal upset occurs, taking the dose early in the morning to prevent interfering with sleep, implementing safety precautions if dizziness or weakness is a problem, and ensuring adequate fluid intake to prevent fluid rebound. It is not necessary to lie down after taking the drug.

15. Answer: a
RATIONALE: Mannitol is a powerful osmotic diuretic that is used to treat increased intracranial pressure. It is given intravenously and begins to work in 30 to 60 minutes. Furosemide, amiloride, and bumetanide are not indicated for the treatment of increased intracranial pressure.

CHAPTER 52

■ ASSESSING YOUR UNDERSTANDING

MATCHING

1. b   **2.** d   **3.** c   **4.** e   **5.** a

SHORT ANSWER

1. Cystitis is an infection of the bladder. Blockage anywhere in the urinary tract can lead to backflow problems and the spread of bladder infections into the kidneys resulting in pyelonephritis.

2. The two types of urinary anti-infectives include antibiotics that are particularly effective against the gram-negative bacteria that cause most urinary tract infections (UTIs) and drugs that work to acidify the urine.

3. The urinary tract antispasmodics relieve these spasms by blocking parasympathetic activity, thus suppressing overactivity, which leads to relaxation of the detrusor and other urinary tract muscles.

4. Pentosan polysulfate sodium is used specifically to decrease the pain and discomfort associated with interstitial cystitis.

5. Two types of drugs are currently used to relieve the symptoms of benign prostatic hyperplasia (BPH). These drugs include the alpha-adrenergic blockers and drugs that block testosterone production.

6. Saw palmetto is an herbal therapy that has been used very successfully for the relief of symptoms associated with BPH.

■ APPLYING YOUR KNOWLEDGE

CASE STUDY

a. Trospium is an anticholinergic that relieves the overactive bladder by blocking parasympathetic activity, thereby suppressing overactivity. As a result, the detrusor and other urinary tract muscles relax. The drug specifically blocks muscarinic receptors and reduces bladder muscle tone.

b. Patient teaching should include how to take the drug (at least 1 hour before meals, usually twice a day); possible adverse effects including anticholinergic effects such as dry mouth, dizziness, photophobia (due to pupil dilation), nausea, constipation, decreased sweating, and tachycardia and palpitations as well as measures to address these, such as using sugarless hard candy and frequent sips of water (for dry mouth), safety measures (for dizziness and photophobia), increased fiber intake (for constipation), avoidance of overactivity or heat extremes (for decreased sweating); importance of adequate fluid intake to prevent urinary stasis and possible UTIs; and the need to check with her health care provider before using any over-the-counter cold remedies or antihistamines, as these could increase the risk of anticholinergic effects.

■ PRACTICING FOR NCLEX

1. Answer: d
RATIONALE: Nitrofurantoin is considered a urinary tract anti-infective. Flavoxate is an antispasmodic; phenazopyridine is a urinary tract analgesic; and doxazosin is an alpha-adrenergic blocker used for treating BPH.

2. Answer: c
RATIONALE: Methenamine works to acidify the urine. Cinoxacin, fosfomycin, and co-trimoxazole act against the gram-negative bacteria that cause most UTIs.

3. Answer: b
RATIONALE: Nitrofurantoin does not need a dosage adjustment when used for patients with renal dysfunction. Dosage adjustments would be necessary for cinoxacin, norfloxacin, and co-trimoxazole.

4. Answer: b
RATIONALE: Fosfomycin is administered as one packet dissolved in water. It is used as a one-time dose, so it does not need to be continued for 7 to 14 days like most anti-infectives. Citrus juices and milk should be avoided because these cause the urine to be alkaline and promote bacterial growth. Rather, the patient should drink fluids that make the urine more acidic.

5. Answer: a
RATIONALE: Oxybutynin is available as a transdermal patch as well as in an oral form. Flavoxate, tolterodine, and darifenacin are available only in oral form.

6. Answer: b
RATIONALE: Trospium interacts with digoxin, leading to increased serum levels of digoxin. Therefore, the nurse would need to monitor the patient for signs and symptoms of digoxin toxicity. Levels of trospium would not increase, so increased central nervous system effects or excess anticholinergic effects would most likely not occur. The combination of tropsium and digoxin does not change the color of urine.

7. Answer: d
RATIONALE: Phenazopyridine can cause the urine to turn a reddish-orange. Nitrofurantoin can cause the urine to change to brown or dark yellow. Methylene blue can cause the urine to become blue-green.

8. Answer: c
RATIONALE: When given by the transdermal patch, oxybutynin has a duration of 96 hours; thus, the patch should be replaced every 4 days.

9. **Answer: a**
   RATIONALE: Pentosan should be used cautiously in patients with splenic dysfunction because of the drug's heparinlike actions. The drug is contraindicated in patients with conditions involving an increased risk for bleeding, such as use of anticoagulants, thrombocytopenia, and recent surgery.

10. **Answer: b**
    RATIONALE: Dutasteride blocks testosterone production by inhibiting the intracellular enzyme that converts testosterone to a potent androgen, DHT, on which the prostate gland depends for its development and maintenance. Doxazosin, tamsulosin, alfuzosin, and terazosin are alpha-adrenergic blockers used to treat BPH. Pentosan, a urinary bladder protectant acts as a buffer to control cell permeability. Urinary anti-infectives such as norfloxacin interfere with DNA replication in susceptible gram-negative bacteria leading to cell death.

11. **Answer: c**
    RATIONALE: Tamsulosin should be taken one-half hour after the same meal each day.

12. **Answer: d**
    RATIONALE: Dutasteride is associated with impotence, decreased libido, and sexual dysfunction, all of which are related to decreased levels of DHT. Hypotension and tachycardia are associated with the use of alpha-adrenergic blockers such as alfuzosin, doxazosin, or terazosin.

13. **Answer: d**
    RATIONALE: Periodically, a patient receiving an agent for BPH should have his prostate-specific antigen level evaluated to reconfirm that the enlargement is not due to cancer. Other testing such as a complete blood count, serum electrolyte levels, and renal functions studies would not be as important.

14. **Answer: b**
    RATIONALE: Flank pain, chills, fever, and tenderness are indicative of pyelonephritis. Urinary frequency, dysuria, and urgency are associated with cystitis.

15. **Answer: c**
    RATIONALE: Tolterodine is a urinary antispasmodic used to treat overactive bladder. Norfloxacin and methylene blue are urinary anti-infectives used to treat UTIs. Terazosin is an alpha-adrenergic blocker used to treat BPH.

CHAPTER 53

■ ASSESSING YOUR UNDERSTANDING

LABELING

Upper Respiratory Tract	Lower Respiratory Tract
Larynx	Alveoli
Mouth	Bronchiole
Nose	Bronchus
Pharynx	Lung
Sinuses	
Trachea	

MATCHING

1. e	**2.** g	**3.** f	**4.** d	**5.** c
6. b	**7.** j	**8.** h	**9.** a	**10.** i

■ APPLYING YOUR KNOWLEDGE

CASE STUDY

a. The patient is most likely experiencing atelectasis based on the decreased aeration of the lungs at the bases, crackles, decreased oxygen saturation levels, and lack of coughing. In addition, the patient has had anesthesia for surgery and is receiving morphine for pain, which can also depress respiratory function. The lack of coughing also is impairing the patient's ability to move secretions, which are preventing air from entering the alveoli.

b. Since pain is interfering with his ability to cough and move, administering the morphine would be appropriate so that the patient can accomplish these actions with minimal discomfort. Although morphine can lead to respiratory depression, its use here would facilitate measures to help move secretions and thus be beneficial to the patient. In addition, the nurse can have the patient splint his incision to assist in coughing. Frequent turning, deep breathing, and the use of incentive spirometry to maximize lung expansion would be helpful. Elevating the head of the bed also would allow for increased chest expansion with each breath. Depending on his oxygen saturation levels, oxygen administration may be needed to ensure adequate tissue oxygenation.

■ PRACTICING FOR NCLEX

1. **Answer: b**
   RATIONALE: Asthma is characterized by reversible bronchospasm, inflammation, and hyperactive airways. Sometimes an infection may be a trigger, but it is not always associated with asthma. Alveolar collapse refers to atelectasis, which might occur with asthma if the airways become blocked with secretions. Progressive loss of lung compliance is associated with acute respiratory distress syndrome.

2. **Answer: c**
   RATIONALE: Ventilation refers to the movement of air in and out of the body. Perfusion refers to the delivery of oxygen via the blood to tissues and cells. Respiration refers to the act of breathing to allow gas exchange and to the exchange of gases at the alveolar level.

3. **Answer: d**
   RATIONALE: The respiratory membrane is made up of the capillary endothelium, capillary basement membrane, interstitial space, alveolar basement membrane, alveolar epithelium, and surfactant layer. Cilia, goblet cells, and mast cells are found along the upper respiratory tract.

4. **Answer: c**
   RATIONALE: Sympathetic stimulation leads to an increased rate and depth of respiration and bronchodilation. Parasympathetic stimulation including the vagus nerve would lead to stimulation of diaphragmatic contraction, bronchoconstriction, and inspiratory movement.

5. **Answer: c**
   RATIONALE: With the common cold, numerous viruses can invade the tissue, initiating the release of histamine and prostaglandins causing an inflammatory response. The mucous membranes become engorged with blood, the tissues swell, and goblet cells increase the production of mucus.

6. Answer: b
RATIONALE: Seasonal rhinitis, or hay fever, is a condition of the upper respiratory tract that involves a response to an antigen such as pollen or dust. Asthma affects the lower respiratory tract and can be associated with a response to an antigen. Sinusitis results from inflammation of the sinus cavities due to irritation or infection. Pharyngitis involves a bacterial or viral infection.

7. Answer: a
RATIONALE: The left lung consists of two lobes, and the right lung consists of three lobes.

8. Answer: b
RATIONALE: At the alveolar level, oxygen and carbon dioxide move via diffusion. Active transport involves the use of energy to move substances. Facilitated diffusion requires the use of a carrier molecule. Osmosis refers to the movement of water.

9. Answer: a, c, d, f
RATIONALE: Disorders affecting the lower respiratory tract such as atelectasis, bronchitis, respiratory distress syndrome, and cystic fibrosis all involve, to some degree, an alteration in the ability to move gases in and out of the lungs. The common cold and sinusitis are upper respiratory tract disorders that typically are not associated with altered gas exchange.

10. Answer: c
RATIONALE: Although an inflammatory reaction occurs leading to swelling and increased blood flow with bronchitis, it is the change in the capillary permeability that allows proteins to leak into the area.

11. Answer: b
RATIONALE: Bronchiectasis is a chronic disease characterized by dilation of the bronchial tree and chronic inflammation of the bronchial passages. The chronic inflammation leads to replacement of the bronchial epithelial cells by fibrous scar tissue. Asthma is an obstructive disorder characterized by reversible bronchospasm, inflammation, and hyperactive airways.
Bronchitis is an acute inflammation of the bronchi. Pneumonia is an inflammation of the lungs.

12. Answer: c
RATIONALE: With respiratory distress syndrome, there is a surfactant deficiency necessitating the use of surfactant replacement. Anti-infectives would be used to treat infections; bronchodilators would be used to relieve bronchospasm; and antihistamines may be used to address allergic reactions.

13. Answer: d
RATIONALE: Cigarette smoking is most commonly associated with chronic obstructive pulmonary disease. The patient may be at greater risk for infection, but infection is not an underlying factor contributing to the disorder. Allergen exposure is more commonly related to seasonal rhinitis or asthma. Genetic inheritance is associated with cystic fibrosis.

14. Answer: b
RATIONALE: The bronchospasm associated with asthma is due to the immediate release of histamine.

15. Answer: a, b, c
RATIONALE: Mast cells release histamine, serotonin, adenosine triphosphate, and other chemicals to ensure a rapid and intense inflammatory reaction to any cell injury. Release of epinephrine and dopamine are not associated with mast cells.

CHAPTER 54

■ ASSESSING YOUR UNDERSTANDING
LABELING

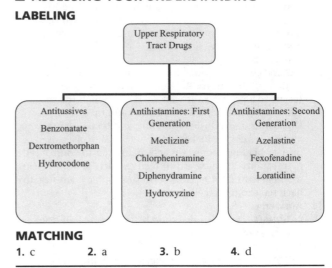

MATCHING
1. c   **2.** a   **3.** b   **4.** d

■ APPLYING YOUR KNOWLEDGE
CASE STUDY

a. Nasal steroids typically are ordered for patients with allergic rhinitis who are no longer getting a response with other decongestants. The patient stopped taking his fexofenadine, which he admits to being effective. So it would be appropriate to restart the fexofenadine rather than add another drug to the regimen. Also, this type of agent does not work immediately; it may take up to 1 week before effects are seen. The patient needs fairly prompt relief.

b. The patient needs instructions in how to use the nasal spray properly (sitting upright with a finger over one of the nares, holding the bottle upright and placing the tip about $\frac{1}{2}$ inch into the open nares, and firmly squeezing the bottle to deliver the drug but not too forcefully), to use the spray exactly as recommended, not to use the spray for longer than recommended to prevent rebound congestion, general respiratory hygiene measures, and measures to reduce the risk of exposure to allergens.

■ PRACTICING FOR NCLEX

1. Answer: b
RATIONALE: Codeine, a centrally acting antitussive, works directly on the medullary cough center. Benzonatate provides local anesthetic action on the respiratory passages, lungs, and pleurae. Ephedrine and tetrahydrozoline are topical nasal decongestants.

2. Answer: c
RATIONALE: Antitussives are used cautiously in patients with asthma because cough suppression can lead to accumulation of secretion and a loss of respiratory reserve. Airway maintenance is important for patients who have had surgery and need a cough to maintain the airway. Antitussives such as codeine and hydrocodone must be used cautiously in patients with a history of addiction. Increased sedation can be problematic for patients who need to drive or be alert.

3. Answer: b
RATIONALE: Measures to assist with cough control when using antitussives include cool temperatures, humidification, lozenges, and increased fluids.

4. Answer: a
RATIONALE: Pseudoephedrine is the only oral decongestant. Phenylephrine, tetrahydrozoline, and xylometazoline are topical decongestants.

5. Answer: d
RATIONALE: Topical decongestants are sympathomimetic, imitating the effects of the sympathetic nervous system to cause vasoconstriction. Pseudoephedrine has adrenergic properties. Topical decongestants are not anticholinergics or antihistamines or adrenergic antagonists.

6. Answer: c
RATIONALE: Parents should use the children's, pediatric, or infant formulations of the drug. Over-the-counter cough and cold preparations should not be used in children under the age of 2 years. The parents need to read the label carefully to determine the dosage and frequency, and they need to use the device that comes with the drug to ensure a proper dosage.

7. Answer: a
RATIONALE: Adverse effects related to the sympathomimetic effects of pseudoephedrine are more likely to occur, including feelings of anxiety, restlessness, hypertension, sweating, tenseness, tremors, arrhythmias, and pallor.

8. Answer: c
RATIONALE: The onset of nasal steroids is not immediate, and it may take up to 7 days before any changes occur. If no effect occurs within 21 days, the drug should be discontinued.

9. Answer: d
RATIONALE: Loratadine is a second-generation antihistamine. Brompheniramine, promethazine, and meclizine are considered first-generation antihistamines.

10. Answer: d
RATIONALE: The adverse effects most often seen with antihistamine use are drowsiness and sedation. However, second-generation antihistamines are less sedating in many people. The anticholinergic effects associated with both generations include drying of the respiratory and gastrointestinal mucous membranes, gastrointestinal upset and nausea, arrhythmias, dysuria, urinary hesitancy, and skin eruption and itching associated with dryness.

11. Answer: a
RATIONALE: The onset of oral diphenhydramine is 15 to 30 minutes.

12. Answer: b
RATIONALE: Guaifenesin should not be used for more than 1 week; if the cough persists, encourage the patient to seek health care.

13. Answer: b
RATIONALE: Meclizine is used to relieve the nausea and vomiting associated with motion sickness. Clemastine, cyproheptadine, and hydroxyzine are used to provide relief of seasonal and perennial allergic rhinitis.

14. Answer: c
RATIONALE: In treating cystic fibrosis, acetylcysteine splits apart the disulfide bonds that are responsible for holding the mucus material together. When used to treat acetaminophen toxicity, the drug protects liver cells from damage because it normalizes hepatic glutathione levels and binds with a reactive hepatotoxic metabolite

of acetaminophen. Dornase alfa selectively breaks down respiratory tract mucus by separating extracellular DNA from proteins. Expectorants liquefy secretions.

15. Answer: c
RATIONALE: Patients receiving dornase alfa should be cautioned to store the drug in the refrigerator, protected from light. The nurse also needs to review how to administer the drug using a nebulizer.

CHAPTER 55

■ ASSESSING YOUR UNDERSTANDING

LABELING

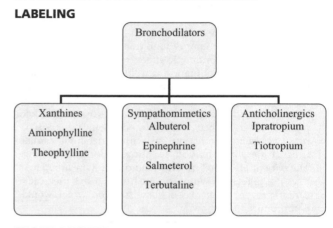

SHORT ANSWER

1. The first step for treatment of pulmonary obstructive diseases includes reducing environmental exposure to irritants such as stopping smoking, filtering allergens from the air, and avoiding exposure to known irritants and allergens.

2. The obstruction of respiratory distress syndrome in the neonate is related to a lack of the lipoprotein surfactant, which leads to an inability to maintain an open alveolus. Surfactant is essential in decreasing the surface tension in the tiny alveolus, allowing it to expand and remain open. If surfactant is lacking, the alveoli collapse and gas exchange cannot occur. Pharmacologic therapy for respiratory distress syndrome involves instilling surfactant into the alveoli.

3. Xanthines have a relatively narrow margin of safety, and they interact with many other drugs. Therefore, they are no longer considered the first-choice bronchodilators.

4. Most of the sympathomimetics used as bronchodilators are beta-2 selective adrenergic agonists. That means that at therapeutic levels, their actions are specific to the beta-2 receptors found in the bronchi. This specificity is lost at higher levels.

5. Anticholinergics are used as bronchodilators because of their effect on the vagus nerve, which is to block or antagonize the action of the neurotransmitter acetylcholine at vagal-mediated receptor sites. Normally, vagal stimulation results in a stimulating effect on smooth muscle, causing contraction. By blocking the vagal effect, relaxation of smooth muscle in the bronchi occurs, leading to bronchodilation.

6. A mast cell stabilizer prevents the release of inflammatory and bronchoconstricting substances when the mast cells are stimulated to release these substances because of irritation or the presence of an antigen.

7. Administration of lung surfactants requires proper placement of an endotracheal tube, suctioning the infant before administration (but not for 2 hours after administration unless necessary), and careful monitoring and support of the infant to ensure lung expansion and proper oxygenation.

■ APPLYING YOUR KNOWLEDGE

CASE STUDY

a. Albuterol is a sympathomimetic agent that is used to provide relief for acute bronchospasm. It is a beta-2 selective adrenergic agent that will dilate the bronchi and increase the rate and depth of respiration. The drug is absorbed rapidly into the lungs, so it would be helpful in a relatively short period of time.

b. The patient needs to understand that he may experience increased sympathomimetic effects related to the use of the albuterol in combination with his usual maintenance inhaler, which includes formoterol—also a sympathomimetic agent. Although little of the drug is absorbed, the patient is receiving two drugs of the same class, increasing his risk for possible adverse effects. These effects may include central nervous system stimulation, gastrointestinal upset, cardiac irregularities, hypertension, sweating, pallor, and flushing. The patient also needs to understand that if the albuterol does not relieve his symptoms, he needs to seek medical care to prevent further bronchoconstriction, which would compromise his airflow.

■ PRACTICING FOR NCLEX

1. **Answer: d**
   RATIONALE: Mast cell stabilizers work at the cellular level to inhibit the release of histamine and the release of slow-reacting substance of anaphylaxis. Epinephrine is not affected by mast cell stabilizers. Xanthines are thought to work by directly affecting the mobilization of calcium within the cell by stimulating two prostaglandins.

2. **Answer: c**
   RATIONALE: Xanthines were once the main treatment choices for asthma and bronchospasm; however, due to their narrow range of safety and interaction with many other drugs, they are no longer considered first-line bronchodilators.

3. **Answer: d**
   RATIONALE: A serum theophylline level greater than 20 mcg/mL is considered toxic.

4. **Answer: b**
   RATIONALE: Nicotine increases the metabolism of xanthines; therefore, an increased dosage would be necessary. Hyperthyroidism, gastrointestinal, upset or alcohol intake requires cautious use of the drug because these conditions may be exacerbated by the systemic effects of the drug. The drug dosage may need to be decreased in these situations.

5. **Answer: c**
   RATIONALE: Levalbuterol is administered only as an inhalant by nebulizer.

6. **Answer: b**
   RATIONALE: The patient should use the inhaler approximately 15 minutes before exercising to achieve the maximum therapeutic effects.

7. **Answer: d**
   RATIONALE: When given intravenously, epinephrine peaks in approximately 20 minutes. It would be at this time that the drug is most effective.

8. **Answer: b**
   RATIONALE: Metaproterenol is mixed with saline in the nebulizer chamber for administration. The child should sit upright or be in a semi-Fowler's position. He should breathe slowly and deeply during the treatment. The treatment is completed when all of the solution (liquid) is gone from the chamber.

9. **Answer: c**
   RATIONALE: The use of ipratropium is contraindicated in the presence of known allergy to the drug or to peanuts or soy products because the vehicle used to make ipratropium, an aerosol, contains a protein associated with peanut allergies.

10. **Answer: a**
    RATIONALE: Inhaled steroids, such as triamcinolone, can take from 2 to 3 weeks to reach effective levels, so the patient should be encouraged to take them to reach and then maintain the effective levels. The drug is not effective for acute attacks. It can cause hoarseness and sore throat. The patient should rinse his mouth after using the inhaler to decrease the risk of systemic absorption and decrease gastrointestinal upset and nausea.

11. **Answer: c**
    RATIONALE: With ipratropium, the usual dosage is 2 inhalations four times/day for a total of 8 inhalations. However, the patient can use up to 12 inhalations if needed in 1 day.

12. **Answer: b**
    RATIONALE: Montelukast selectively and competitively blocks receptors for the production of leukotrienes D4 and E4, which are components of slow-reacting substance of anaphylaxis. As a result, the drug blocks many of the signs and symptoms of asthma, such as neutrophil and eosinophil migration, neutrophil and monocyte aggregation, leukocyte adhesion, increased capillary permeability, and smooth muscle contraction.

13. **Answer: d**
    RATIONALE: A beta-2 selective adrenergic agonist or sympathomimetic would be most appropriate because these agents are rapidly distributed after injection and rapidly absorbed after inhalation. An inhaled steroid would require 2 to 3 weeks to reach effective levels. Leukotriene receptor antagonists and mast cell stabilizers do not have immediate effects.

14. **Answer: b**
    RATIONALE: Beractant is a lung surfactant. Cromolyn is a mast cell stabilizer. Zileuton is a leukotriene receptor antagonist. Theophylline is a xanthine.

15. **Answer: a, c, e**
    RATIONALE: Before administering calfactant, it would be important to ensure proper endotracheal tube placement because the drug is instilled directly into the trachea. In addition, lung sounds and oxygen saturation levels would be important as a baseline to evaluate effectiveness of the drug.

CHAPTER 56

■ ASSESSING YOUR UNDERSTANDING
LABELING

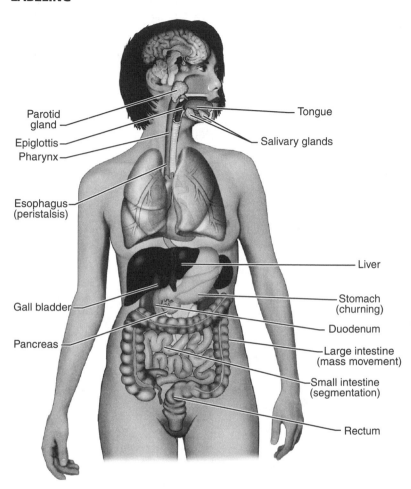

Parotid gland

Epiglottis

Pharynx

Esophagus (peristalsis)

Gall bladder

Pancreas

Tongue

Salivary glands

Liver

Stomach (churning)

Duodenum

Large intestine (mass movement)

Small intestine (segmentation)

Rectum

MATCHING

1. e	**2.** c	**3.** g	**4.** b	**5.** a
6. d	**7.** f	**8.** h		

■ APPLYING YOUR KNOWLEDGE
CASE STUDY

a. The gallbladder stores bile that is produced in the liver. Bile is very important in the digestion of fats and is deposited into the small intestine when the gallbladder is stimulated to contract by the presence of fats. Once bile is delivered to the gallbladder for storage, it is concentrated; water is removed by the walls of the gallbladder. It would be important for the nurse to obtain more information about the types of food eaten during a meal in which the woman then develops pain afterward. In addition, it would be important for the nurse to investigate the patient's history a bit further to gather data about the signs and symptoms that her mother and sister experienced when they had their gallstones.

b. The patient's pain might be related to the contraction of the gallbladder in response to fatty foods that the patient may have ingested. If the patient has gallstones, then the concentrated bile has crystallized. The stones can move down the duct, causing severe pain. If large enough, the stones can block the duct, preventing bile from reaching its intended target.

■ PRACTICING FOR NCLEX

1. Answer: b
   RATIONALE: The exocrine pancreas secretes pancreatin and pancrelipase. Insulin is secreted by the beta cells of the endocrine pancreas. Gastrin and hydrochloric acid are secreted by the stomach.

2. Answer: a
   RATIONALE: Saliva is the fluid produced by the salivary glands in the mouth that makes the food bolus slippery and easier to swallow. Bile is stored in the gallbladder and released to break down fats. Chyme refers to the contents of the stomach containing ingested food and secreted enzymes, water, and mucus. Pancrelipase is a pancreatic enzyme.

3. Answer: b
   RATIONALE: The stomach is responsible for the mechanical and chemical breakdown of foods into useable nutrients. The mouth initiates secretion of saliva that contains water and digestive enzymes to begin the digestive process. The small intestine is responsible for absorption of nutrients.

The pancreas secretes enzymes and sodium bicarbonate into the beginning of the small intestine to neutralize acid from the stomach and further facilitate digestion.

4. Answer: a
RATIONALE: The mucosal layer is the innermost layer of the gastrointestinal (GI) tract, followed by the circular muscularis layer, the nerve plexus, the longitudinal muscularis, and finally the adventitia.

5. Answer: c
RATIONALE: Pepsin is secreted by the chief cells of the stomach in response to gastrin, which is secreted when the food arrives at the stomach. Gastrin also stimulates the parietal cells of the stomach to secrete hydrochloric acid. Bile is secreted by the gallbladder in response to fats in the bolus.

6. Answer: d
RATIONALE: Amylase is secreted by the pancreas to break down sugars. Chymotrypsin and trypsin break down proteins into amino acids; sodium bicarbonate is secreted to neutralize the acid bolus.

7. Answer: c
RATIONALE: The small intestine uses a process of segmentation with an occasional peristaltic wave to clear the segment. Peristalsis is seen in the esophagus. Churning occurs in the stomach. Mass movement with an occasional peristaltic wave occurs in the large intestine.

8. Answer: c
RATIONALE: Vomiting is a central reflex. Gastroenteric, somatointestinal, and ileogastric are local reflexes.

9. Answer: b
RATIONALE: Absence of bowel sounds or intestinal activity secondary to abdominal surgery indicates a disruption of the intestinointestinal reflex, which occurs due to intense irritation from handling of the intestines. The continued stretch of the ileum with constipation is associated with the ileogastric reflex. The gastroenteric reflex occurs with stimulation of the stomach by stretching, the presence of food, or cephalic stimulation. The gastrocolic reflex involves stimulation of the stomach that also causes increased activity in the colon.

10. Answer: a
RATIONALE: The swallowing reflex is stimulated whenever a food bolus stimulates pressure receptors in the back of the throat and pharynx. These receptors send impulses to the medulla, which stimulates a series of nerves that cause the following actions: The soft palate elevates and seals off the nasal cavity; respirations cease in order to protect the lungs; the larynx rises and the glottis closes to seal off the airway; and the pharyngeal constrictor muscles contract and force the food bolus into the top of the esophagus, where pairs of muscles contract in turn to move the bolus down the esophagus and into the stomach.

11. Answer: c
RATIONALE: The swallowing reflex can be facilitated in a number of ways if swallowing (food or medication) is a problem. Icing the tongue by sucking on an ice pop or an ice cube blocks external nerve impulses and allows this more basic reflex to respond. Icing the sternal notch or the back of the neck, although not as appealing, has also proved effective in stimulating the swallowing reflex. In addition, keeping the head straight (not turned to one side) allows the muscle pairs to work together and helps the process. Providing stimulation of the receptors in the mouth through temperature variations and textured foods helps initiate the reflex.

12. Answer: b
RATIONALE: Once the chemotrigger receptor zone is stimulated, a series of reflexes occurs. Salivation increases, and there is a large increase in the production of mucus in the upper GI tract, which is accompanied by a decrease in gastric acid production. This action protects the lining of the GI tract from potential damage by the acidic stomach contents. The sympathetic system is stimulated, with a resultant increase in sweating, increased heart rate, deeper respirations, and nausea.

13. Answer: c
RATIONALE: The GI system is comprised of one continuous, long tube and is the only body system that is open to the external environment with an opening at the mouth and again at the anus. It is responsible for only a very small part of waste excretion; the kidneys and lungs are responsible for excreting most of the waste products of normal metabolism. It is protected from friction with movement by the peritoneum that lines the abdominal wall and viscera with a small free space between the two layers.

14. Answer: d
RATIONALE: High levels of acid decrease the secretion of gastrin. Alcohol, caffeine, proteins, and calcium increase gastrin secretion.

15. Answer: c, d
RATIONALE: The large intestine absorbs mostly water and sodium. The lower end of the stomach absorbs mostly water and alcohol. The small intestine absorbs drugs, nutrients, anything that is taken into the GI tract, and secretions.

CHAPTER 57

■ ASSESSING YOUR UNDERSTANDING
LABELING

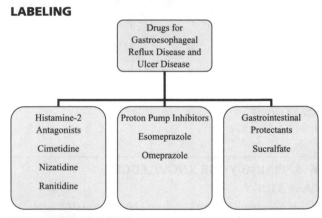

FILL IN THE BLANKS
1. Hydrochloric acid
2. Acute (or stress)
3. Famotidine
4. Rebound
5. Neutralize
6. Constipation, diarrhea
7. Before
8. Sucralfate

■ APPLYING YOUR KNOWLEDGE
CASE STUDY

a. The patient may be experiencing acid rebound because of his frequent use of antacids. The stomach produces more acid in response to the alkaline environment. Neutralizing the stomach contents to an alkaline level stimulates gastrin production to cause an increase in acid production and return the stomach to its normal acidic state. In many cases, the acid rebound causes an increase in symptoms, which results in an increased intake of the antacid. This leads to more acid production and an ongoing cycle.

b. When more and more antacid is used, the risk for systemic effects rises. Alkalosis with resultant metabolic changes (nausea, vomiting, neuromuscular changes, headache, irritability, muscle twitching, and even coma) may occur. The use of calcium salts, such as TUMS may lead to hypercalcemia and milk-alkali syndrome (seen as alkalosis, renal calcium deposits, or severe electrolyte disorders). Constipation or diarrhea may result, depending on the antacid being used. The nurse would need to determine the type of liquid antacid used because a magnesium salt antacid would lead to diarrhea, magaldrate may result in alkalosis, and an aluminum salt antacid could lead to hypophosphatemia and altered systemic calcium levels.

c. The patient needs to understand how to use over-the-counter antacids properly and that continued used can lead to a vicious cycle due to acid rebound. In addition, the patient needs to understand that systemic adverse effects are possible if antacids are overused. The nurse should also remind the patient that if his symptoms do not improve after a period of time using the antacid, he should see his health care provider.

■ PRACTICING FOR NCLEX

1. **Answer: d**
   RATIONALE: Prostaglandins inhibit the secretion of gastrin and increase the secretion of the mucous lining of the stomach, providing a buffer. Histamine-2 antagonists block the release of hydrochloric acid in response to gastrin; proton pump inhibitors suppress the secretion of hydrochloric acid into the lumen of the stomach, and antacids interact with acids at the chemical level to neutralize them.

2. **Answer: a**
   RATIONALE: Cimetidine is considered the prototype histamine-2 receptor antagonist.

3. **Answer: b**
   RATIONALE: Omeprazole is available over the counter; lansoprazole, rabeprazole, and esomeprazole are prescription medications.

4. **Answer: c**
   RATIONALE: Proton pump inhibitors such as omeprazole are used as part of combination therapy with antibiotics for treatment of *Helicobacter pylori* infection.

5. **Answer: d**
   RATIONALE: Aluminum binds dietary phosphates and causes hypophosphatemia, but they do not cause acid rebound like other antacids. Magnesium antacids cause diarrhea; calcium salts cause hypercalcemia.

6. **Answer: a**
   RATIONALE: Esomeprazole is available in intravenous preparations and delayed-release oral forms. Omeprazole, rabeprazole, and dexlansoprazole are available in delayed-release oral forms only.

7. **Answer: c**
   RATIONALE: The medication should be swallowed whole with a large glass of water. It should not be chewed, crushed, or opened. Antacids, if prescribed, should be taken 1 hour before or 2 hours after the omeprazole.

8. **Answer: b**
   RATIONALE: Constipation is the most frequently seen adverse effect; thus, the patient should increase his fiber intake to prevent constipation. Diarrhea is possible, but constipation is more likely. The patient should drink fluids and use sugarless lozenges to help with a dry mouth. Fluid intake also will help to prevent constipation.

9. **Answer: b**
   RATIONALE: Pancrelipase is given with meals and snacks so that the enzyme is available when it is needed.

10. **Answer: d**
    RATIONALE: Histamine-2 receptor antagonists are used for stress ulcer prophylaxis because the drugs block the production of acid thereby protecting the stomach lining, which is at risk because of decreased mucus production. Reducing the overall acid level is the rationale for use as short-term treatment of active duodenal ulcer. Blocking the overproduction of hydrochloric acid is the rationale for treatment of pathologic hypersecretory conditions. Decreasing the acid being regurgitated into the esophagus is the rationale for treatment of erosive gastroesophageal reflux.

11. **Answer: c**
    RATIONALE: Cimetidine was the first drug in this class to be developed and has been associated with antiandrogenic effects including gynecomastia and galactorrhea. Ranitidine, famotidine, and nizatidine are not associated with these effects.

12. **Answer: d**
    RATIONALE: Nizatidine is the drug of choice for patients with liver dysfunction because it does not undergo first-pass metabolism in the liver like the other histamine-2 receptor antagonists such as cimetidine, famotidine, or ranitidine.

13. **Answer: a, c, d, e**
    RATIONALE: Indications of systemic alkalosis include headache, confusion, irritability, tetany, nausea, and weakness.

14. **Answer: c**
    RATIONALE: Alopecia can occur with proton pump therapy, but it is not a common adverse effect. Common adverse effects include dizziness, headache, and cough.

15. **Answer: b**
    RATIONALE: Sucralfate has an onset of action of 30 minutes and a duration of 5 hours.

CHAPTER 58

■ ASSESSING YOUR UNDERSTANDING

LABELING

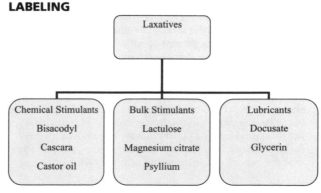

SHORT ANSWER

1. Gastrointestinal (GI) stimulants stimulate parasympathetic activity within the GI tract, resulting in increased GI secretions and motility on a general level throughout the tract. They do not have the local effects of laxatives to increase activity only in the intestines.

2. Antidiarrheal agents slow the motility of the GI tract through direct action on the lining of the GI tract to inhibit local reflexes (bismuth subsalicylate), through direct action on the muscles of the GI tract to slow activity (loperamide), or through action on central nervous system centers that cause GI spasm and slowing.

3. A lubricant is an agent that increases the viscosity of the feces, making it difficult to absorb water from the bolus and easing movement of the bolus through the intestines.

4. Chemical stimulants directly stimulate the nerve plexus in the intestinal wall, causing increased movement and the stimulation of local reflexes. Bulk stimulants (also called *mechanical stimulants*), are rapid-acting, aggressive laxatives that cause the fecal matter to increase in bulk. They increase the motility of the GI tract by increasing the fluid in the intestinal contents, which enlarges bulk, stimulates local stretch receptors, and activates local activity.

5. Cathartic dependence is a reaction that occurs when patients use laxatives over a long period and the GI tract becomes dependent on the vigorous stimulation of the laxative. Without this stimulation, the GI tract does not move for a period of time (i.e., several days), which could lead to constipation and drying of the stool and ultimately to impaction.

6. Docusate has a detergent action on the surface of the intestinal bolus, increasing the admixture of fat and water and making a softer stool.

■ APPLYING YOUR KNOWLEDGE

CASE STUDY

a. Various factors may be contributing to this older adult's constipation. These may include a lack of exercise or activity (the patient lives alone and may not be getting out often), low intake of fiber foods and adequate fluids (the patient is living alone and may not be eating nutritious meals or consuming enough food), prescribed medications being used for other underlying medical conditions, or development of new medical conditions that could be affecting the GI tract.

b. The nurse would need to instruct the patient to drink plenty of fluids with the psyllium to prevent problems that can occur if the drug starts to pull in fluid while still in the esophagus. Additionally, the nurse should recommend that the patient use the psyllium exactly as directed and to check with the health care provider before taking any other over-the-counter products. Other instructions would include teaching the patient about possible adverse effects and making sure that if she is taking any other prescribed medications that she separate their administration by at least 30 minutes to prevent interfering with the timing or absorption of these medications. The nurse would also encourage the patient to increase her fiber intake, providing her with suggestions for high-fiber foods, and to increase her fluid intake (if not contraindicated by underlying medical conditions). Additionally, the nurse would suggest ways that the patient can increase her activity level.

PRACTICING FOR NCLEX

1. **Answer: a**
   RATIONALE: When given intravenously, metoclopramide has an onset of action of 1 to 5 minutes.

2. **Answer: c**
   RATIONALE: Laxative, or cathartic, drugs are indicated to remove ingested poisons from the lower GI tract; as an adjunct in anthelmintic therapy when it is desirable to flush helminths from the GI tract; to prevent straining when it is clinically undesirable (such as after surgery, myocardial infarction, or obstetric delivery); for the short-term relief of constipation; and to evacuate the bowel for diagnostic procedures. Lubricants ease defecation without stimulating the movement of the GI tract. GI stimulants provide more generalized GI stimulation, resulting in an overall increase in GI activity and secretions.

3. **Answer: d**
   RATIONALE: Polycarbophil is an example of a bulk laxative. Bisacodyl and senna are examples of chemical stimulant laxatives. Docusate is an example of a lubricant laxative.

4. **Answer: d**
   RATIONALE: Although bisacodyl can be taken at any time, the drug has an onset of action of 6 to 8 hours, making it preferable for the drug to work overnight and seeing the effects in the morning.

5. **Answer: a**
   RATIONALE: Cascara is administered orally. Senna may be administered orally or as a rectal suppository. Bisacodyl is given orally or rectally. No laxative is given intramuscularly.

6. **Answer: c**
   RATIONALE: Chemical stimulant laxatives are used cautiously in patients with coronary artery disease and heart block because these conditions could be affected by the decrease in absorption and changes in electrolytes that can occur. Acute abdominal disorders such as appendicitis, diverticulitis, and ulcerative colitis would be contraindications to the use of chemical stimulants.

7. **Answer: d**
   RATIONALE: Polyethylene glycol–electrolyte solution is dispensed as 4 L of solution, and the patient is to take 240 mL (8 ounces) of the solution every 10 minutes until the solution is finished. Mixing a packet in a glass of cold water would be appropriate for psyllium.

8. **Answer: b**
   RATIONALE: The patient's symptoms are most likely related to a sympathetic stress reaction due to intense neurostimulation of the GI tract or to the loss of fluid and electrolyte imbalance. Direct stimulation refers to the action of chemical stimulant laxatives. Detergent action is related to the use of docusate. Formation of a slippery coat relates to the use of mineral oil.

9. **Answer: a**
   RATIONALE: Although abdominal cramping, diarrhea, and sweating may occur with lubricant laxatives such as mineral oil, it would be especially important to inform the patient about possible leakage and staining with mineral oil, which occurs because the stool cannot be retained by the external sphincter.

10. **Answer: b**
    RATIONALE: Dexpanthenol works by increasing acetylcholine levels and stimulating the parasympathetic system. Metoclopramide works by blocking dopamine receptors and making the GI cells more sensitive to

acetylcholine. Bulk laxatives exert an osmotic pull on fluids. Loperamide acts directly on the muscles of the GI tract to slow activity.

11. **Answer: c**
    RATIONALE: Bismuth subsalicylate is indicated for the treatment of traveler's diarrhea and in preventing cramping and distention associated with dietary excess and some viral infections. Loperamide is indicated for the short-term treatment of diarrhea associated with dietary problems and some viral infections. Opium derivatives are indicated for the short-term treatment of cramping and diarrhea.

12. **Answer: b**
    RATIONALE: Alosetron is classified as a serotonin 5-HT antagonist. Hyoscyamine is an anticholinergic agent that may be used to treat irritable bowel syndrome. Lubiprostone is a locally acting chloride channel activator used for treatment of chronic, idiopathic constipation and for treatment of irritable bowel syndrome with constipation in women. Methylnaltrexone is a selective antagonist to opioid binding at the mu-receptors.

13. **Answer: c**
    RATIONALE: Rifaximin is the first antibiotic approved by the Food and Drug Administration specifically for treating traveler's diarrhea, acting against noninvasive strains of *Escherichia coli*, which is the most common cause of traveler's diarrhea.

14. **Answer: d**
    RATIONALE: Patients with advanced disease who are receiving palliative care and no longer are responsive to traditional laxatives may receive methylnaltrexone for treatment of opioid-induced constipation. Lubiprostone is a locally acting chloride channel activator used for treatment of chronic, idiopathic constipation and for treatment of irritable bowel syndrome with constipation in women. Psyllium or mineral oil probably would have been tried earlier on and most likely would be ineffective because the patient's constipation is opioid induced.

15. **Answer: b**
    RATIONALE: Irritable bowel syndrome is a very common disorder, striking three times as many women as men and reportedly accounting for half of all referrals to GI specialists. The disorder is characterized by abdominal distress, bouts of diarrhea or constipation, bloating, nausea, flatulence, headache, fatigue, depression, and anxiety. No anatomical cause has been found for this disorder. Underlying causes might be stress related.

CHAPTER 59

■ ASSESSING YOUR UNDERSTANDING

LABELING

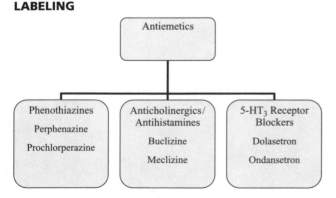

SHORT ANSWER

1. The two phenothiazines used most commonly as antiemetics are prochlorperazine and promethazine.
2. Antiemetics work by reducing the hyperactivity of the vomiting reflex in one of two ways: locally, to decrease the local response to stimuli that are being sent to the medulla to induce vomiting, or centrally, to block the chemoreceptor trigger zone (CTZ) or suppress the vomiting center directly.
3. Cyclizine is an anticholinergic/antihistamine that blocks the transmission of impulses to the CTZ.
4. Aprepitant is given orally in combination with dexamethasone.
5. Dronabinol and nabilone contain the active ingredient of cannabis (marijuana).

■ APPLYING YOUR KNOWLEDGE

CASE STUDY

a. The patient is most likely experiencing intractable hiccups, which occur when the diaphragm is repetitively stimulated, leading to persistent diaphragmatic spasm.
b. The nurse would need to instruct the patient to take the medication as prescribed and to be alert for possible adverse effects, primarily central nervous system (CNS) effects such as drowsiness, dizziness, weakness, headache, and tremor. The risk for drowsiness, dizziness, and headache may be increased because these adverse effects also occur with omeprazole. The nurse should instruct the patient in safety measures to reduce the risk of injury related to CNS effects and to avoid alcohol intake with this drug, which would potentiate the CNS effects. The nurse would also need to inform the patient about dry mouth and relief measures such as frequent sips of fluid, ice chips, and sugarless hard candies. Other adverse effects to address include nasal congestion, sweating, and possible urinary retention. Photosensitivity is possible, so the nurse should encourage the use of protective clothing and sunscreen when outside. Chlorpromazine is associated with the development of neuroleptic malignant syndrome. The nurse should review the signs and symptoms of this disorder (hyperpyrexia, muscle rigidity, altered mental status, irregular pulse or blood pressure, diaphoresis, and arrhythmias) and emphasize the need for immediate medical care.

■ PRACTICING FOR NCLEX

1. **Answer: c**
   RATIONALE: Granisetron is classified as a 5-HT₃ receptor blocker. Chlorpromazine is a phenothiazine; cyclizine is an anticholinergic/antihistamine; and aprepitant is a substance P/neurokinin-1 receptor antagonist.
2. **Answer: b**
   RATIONALE: Phenothiazines are centrally acting antiemetics that block the CTZ in the medulla. Antacids, local anesthetics, absorbents, and gastrointestinal (GI) protectants act locally.
3. **Answer: a**
   RATIONALE: Promethazine should be used cautiously in patients with active peptic ulcer disease. The drug would be contraindicated in patients with severe hypotension (possibly interfering with drug metabolism) or patients with brain injury or coma due to the risk of further CNS depression.
4. **Answer: b**
   RATIONALE: CNS effects, especially dizziness and drowsiness, are associated with phenothiazines and necessitate safety measures such as assistance with ambulation. GI

overstimulation could result in diarrhea or additional vomiting, which might require the patient to use the bathroom but not be the basis for assisting the patient. The nurse's actions are not related to urinary abnormalities or endocrine effects.

5. **Answer: a**
   RATIONALE: Offering carbonated drinks can help to promote the patient's comfort. Deep breathing, a quiet restful environment, and frequent mouth care such as every 2 hours or as needed would be appropriate.

6. **Answer: c**
   RATIONALE: When given rectally, prochlorperazine has an onset of action of 60 to 90 minutes. In this situation, the time of 7:15 PM would be most appropriate.

7. **Answer: b**
   RATIONALE: Metoclopramide is given intravenously 30 minutes before chemotherapy.

8. **Answer: d**
   RATIONALE: Cyclizine is indicated for the treatment of motion sickness. Promethazine is used to prevent and control nausea and vomiting associated with anesthesia and surgery. Dolasetron is indicated for treatment of nausea and vomiting associated with emetogenic chemotherapy and for the prevention of postoperative nausea and vomiting. Perphenazine is indicated for the treatment of severe nausea and vomiting and intractable hiccups.

9. **Answer: c**
   RATIONALE: There is an increased risk of sedation if meclizine is combined with other CNS depressants such as alcohol. The patient should be instructed to avoid this combination. Meclizine does not interact with caffeine or chocolate. Aged cheese should be avoided by patients taking monoamine oxidase inhibitors.

10. **Answer: a**
    RATIONALE: Palonosetron cannot be repeated for 7 days. The drug is not a controlled substance. Granisetron is used only on the days that chemotherapy is given. Metoclopramide typically is given as one dose 30 minutes before chemotherapy, then every 2 hours for two doses, then every 3 hours for three doses.

11. **Answer: c, d, e**
    RATIONALE: Aprepitant is associated with constipation, anorexia, headache, diarrhea, gastritis, nausea, and fatigue.

12. **Answer: b**
    RATIONALE: Aprepitant acts directly in the CNS to block receptors associated with nausea and vomiting with little to no effect on serotonin, dopamine, or corticosteroid receptors. Metoclopramide reduces the responsiveness of the nerve cells in the CTZ to circulating chemicals that induce vomiting. Meclizine blocks cholinergic receptors in the vomiting center. Granisetron blocks the 5-HT$_3$ receptors associated with nausea and vomiting in the CTZ and locally.

13. **Answer: d**
    RATIONALE: Palonosetron is available for intravenous use only.

14. **Answer: c**
    RATIONALE: Trimethobenzamide is similar to the antihistamines but is not associated with as much sedation and CNS depression, making it a drug of choice.

15. **Answer: c**
    RATIONALE: Dronabinol is classified as a category C-III controlled substance. Nabilone is a category C-II substance. Both drugs are approved for use only in managing the nausea and vomiting associated with cancer chemotherapy in cases that have not responded to other treatment.

Crossroads of Continents

CULTURES OF SIBERIA AND ALASKA

William W. Fitzhugh and Aron Crowell

Special thanks are due to the I. E. Repin Institute of Painting, Sculpture, and Art, USSR Academy of Sciences, Leningrad, and Aurora Press for photography and use of Mikhail Tikhanov illustrations.

Previous pages: ''Aleut Hunting'' (Mikhail Tikhanov, 1817, RIPSA 2126

Cover Illustration: Tasseled Shaman's Hat, Yukaghir culture, Siberia. Collected by Cottle. Accessioned by American Museum of Natural History in 1907. AMNH 70-387 (fig. 333). Ceremonial Dance Mask, Koniag Eskimo, Kodiak Island, Alaska. Collected by I. G. Voznesenskii in the 1840s. Museum of Anthropology and Ethnography, MAE 571-12 (fig. 368).
Photograph by Dane A. Penland.

© 1988 Smithsonian Institution
All rights reserved
Manufactured in the United States

Jeanne M. Sexton, editor
Alex and Caroline Castro, art direction and book design

Library of Congress Cataloging-in-Publication Data

Crossroads of continents.

''Crossroads of continents is also the title of an exhibition organized by the National Museum of Natural History and circulated by the Smithsonian Traveling Exhibition Service (SITES)''
   Bibliography: p.
   1. Ethnology—Siberia (R.S.F.S.R.)—Exhibitions.   2. Indians of North America—Alaska—Exhibitions.   3. Eskimos—Alaska—Exhibitions.   4. Siberia (R.S.F.S.R.)—Social Life and customs—Exhibitions.   5. Alaska—Social life and customs—Exhibitions.
I. Fitzhugh, William W., 1943– . II. Crowell, Aron, 1952– . III. National Museum of Natural History (U.S.)
GN635.S5C75 1988   306'.0957   88-42630
ISBN 0-87474-442-3 (alk. paper)
ISBN 0-87474-435-0 (pbk. : alk. paper)

The paper in this book meets the guidelines for permanence and durability of the Committee on Production Guidelines for Book Longevity of the Council on Library Resources.

INSTITUTIONAL ABBREVIATIONS
(Captions and Checklist)

AMHA	Anchorage Museum of History and Art (Anchorage)
AMNH	American Museum of Natural History (New York)
BCPM	British Columbia Provincial Museum (Victoria, B.C.)
CMC	Canadian Museum of Civilization (Ottawa)
FM	Field Museum of Natural History (Chicago)
GNHL	Grove National Historic Landmark (Chicago)
MAE	Museum of Anthropology and Ethnography (Leningrad)
MIHPP	Museum of History and Culture of the Peoples of Siberia and the Far East, USSR Academy of Sciences (Novosibirsk)
NMAH	National Museum of American History (Washington, D.C.)
NMNH	National Museum of Natural History (Washington, D.C.)
NPG	National Portrait Gallery (Washington, D.C.)
PMH	Peabody Museum of Archaeology and Ethnology, Harvard University (Cambridge, Massachusetts)
PMS	Peabody Museum (Salem, Massachusetts)
RIPSA	I. E. Repin Institute of Painting, Sculpture, and Architecture (Leningrad)
SA	Smithsonian Archives (Washington, D.C.)
SI-NAA	National Anthropological Archives, Smithsonian Institution (Washington, D.C.)
SKRM	Sakhalin Regional Museum (Iuzhno-Sakhalinsk, USSR)
SRM	State Russian Museum (Leningrad)
UAFM	University of Alaska Museum (Fairbanks)
UBCMA	University of British Columbia, Museum of Anthropology (Vancouver)
UMA	University Museum of Anthropology (Philadelphia)
UWL	University of Washington Libraries (Seattle)

TRANSLATOR'S NOTE

The transliteration of Russian cyrillic script is not entirely consistent. The Library of Congress transliteration, in its simplified form (without diacritics), has been used in the references, and in the text for most Russian and Soviet proper names, geographical locations on the Soviet territory, as well as for technical terms from languages of Soviet nationalities—except when commonly transliterated otherwise in English.

Set in Egyptian Light by Monotype Composition Company, Inc., Baltimore, Maryland
Printed and bound by Arcata Graphics, Kingsport, Tennessee
on 80 lb. Mountie Matte by Northwest Paper
Edited by Jeanne M. Sexton
Designed by Castro/Hollowpress

Published by the Smithsonian Institution Press
September 1988

Contents

Statement by the Secretary of the Smithsonian Institution   6
   Robert McC. Adams

**Statement by the Director of the Institute of Ethnography,
USSR Academy of Sciences**   7
   Iu. V. Bromlei

INTRODUCTION

Crossroads of Continents: Beringian Oecumene   9
   William W. Fitzhugh and Aron Crowell
Ethnic Connections Across Bering Strait   17
   I. S. Gurvich

PEOPLES OF SIBERIA AND ALASKA

Peoples of the Amur and Maritime Regions   24
   Lydia T. Black
Koryak and Itelmen: Dwellers of the Smoking Coast   31
   S. A. Arutiunov
Even: Reindeer Herders of Eastern Siberia   35
   S. A. Arutiunov
Chukchi: Warriors and Traders of Chukotka   39
   S. A. Arutiunov
Eskimos: Hunters of the Frozen Coasts   42
   William W. Fitzhugh
Aleut: Islanders of the North Pacific   52
   Lydia T. Black and R. G. Liapunova
Tlingit: People of the Wolf and Raven   58
   Frederica de Laguna
Northern Athapaskans: People of the Deer   64
   James W. VanStone

STRANGERS ARRIVE

The Story of Russian America   70
   Lydia T. Black
Treasures by the Neva: The Russian Collections   83
   G. I. Dzeniskevich and L. P. Pavlinskaia
Baird's Naturalists: Smithsonian Collectors in Alaska   89
   William W. Fitzhugh
The American Museum's Jesup North Pacific Expedition   97
   Stanley A. Freed, Ruth S. Freed, and Laila Williamson
Young Laufer on the Amur   104
   Laurel Kendall

CROSSCURRENTS OF TIME

Beringia: An Ice Age View   106
   Steven B. Young
Ancient Peoples of the North Pacific Rim   111
   Christy G. Turner II
Prehistory of Siberia and the Bering Sea   117
   S. A. Arutiunov and William W. Fitzhugh
Prehistory of Alaska's Pacific Coast   130
   Aron Crowell

THEMATIC VIEWS

Raven's Creatures   142
   Milton M. R. Freeman
Many Tongues—Ancient Tales   145
   Michael E. Krauss
Maritime Economies of the North Pacific Rim   151
   Jean-Loup Rousselot, William W. Fitzhugh, and Aron Crowell
Hunters, Herders, Trappers, and Fishermen   173
   James W. VanStone
Economic Patterns in Northeastern Siberia   183
   I. I. Krupnik
Economic Patterns in Alaska   191
   William W. Fitzhugh
Dwellings, Settlements, and Domestic Life   194
   Aron Crowell
Needles and Animals: Women's Magic   209
   Valérie Chaussonnet
War and Trade   227
   Ernest S. Burch, Jr.
Guardians and Spirit-Masters of Siberia   241
   S. Ia. Serov
Eye of the Dance: Spiritual Life of the Bering Sea Eskimo   256
   Ann Fienup-Riordan
Potlatch Ceremonialism on the Northwest Coast   271
   Frederica de Laguna
Art and Culture Change at the Tlingit-Eskimo Border   281
   Bill Holm
Comparative Art of the North Pacific Rim   294
   William W. Fitzhugh

NEW LIVES FOR ANCIENT PEOPLES

Siberian Peoples: A Soviet View   314
   V. V. Lebedev
Alaska Natives Today   319
   Rosita Worl
Alaska Native Arts in the Twentieth Century   326
   Margaret B. Blackman and Edwin S. Hall, Jr.

Appendix I   Beads and Bead Trade in the
North Pacific Region   341
   Peter Francis, Jr.

Appendix II   List of Illustrations   342

Appendix III   Exhibition Checklist   344

Notes   353

References   354

Credits   359

Acknowledgments   360

Statement by the Secretary
of the Smithsonian Institution

Robert McC. Adams

The opening of the *Crossroads* exhibition gives cause for reflection on the history of Russian/ Soviet and American research and on the prospects for future collaboration in the decades and centuries ahead. As we embark on this exploration of our common ancestry—not only of New World peoples but of the shared histories of our North Pacific Native peoples over thousands of years—certain facts are inescapable.

The Smithsonian, like the Museum of Anthropology and Ethnography in Leningrad and the American Museum of Natural History in New York, has a long history of North Pacific research. Pioneering efforts begun by the Smithsonian's Spencer F. Baird, who began probing the relationships of animals, plants, and humans between North America and Asia in the early 1850s, initiated a research tradition that contributed to the purchase of Alaska from Russia in 1867 and to the United States's first concerted national research program—the documentation of Alaska's resources and peoples, a project that served both scientific and administrative needs into the 20th century. The collections obtained and the publications issued during that period still constitute the basic reference data for much modern biological and anthropological research in this region. These resources, be they biological type specimens, extinct elephant teeth, archeological specimens, or fragments of native oral traditions, need to be protected in the same way we should protect marine mammals, native cultures, and natural environments that fall in the path of northern industrial development today. This exhibition and the synthesis it achieves would not have been possible without the concerted efforts of research institutions to collect, analyze, preserve, and disseminate knowledge about arctic regions where the national interests of the Soviet Union and the United States, to note only the major contenders, have overlapped since the early 19th century.

As the world collectively turns away from the more highly developed portions of the Earth and toward the less well developed regions—such as those of the North Pacific Rim, the Arctic, and the Antarctic—we find the world a smaller place than it used to be. The days of Iuri Lisianskii's multiyear voyage of discovery from St. Petersburg to Alaska in 1803–06 are over. Remoteness no longer is a cause for neglect of distant regions today. It is in this spirit that the United States has recently passed an Arctic Research Policy Act (*) that promotes northern research and international cooperation. Northern nations, like traditional native cultures, have worked out different solutions to problems of northern environments. History suggests that comparative studies of historical and contemporary issues would be both interesting and beneficial to mankind.

Crossroads of Continents testifies to the importance of geographically convergent themes. Many of the basic problems concerning the origins of man in the New World remain unsolved, together with the history of cultural relationships across Bering Strait over thousands of years. None of these problems can be settled without an active, collective discourse among scholars across Bering Strait. That these efforts may take time should not be of concern, given that we are only now brushing off the dust from the Jesup Expedition notes of 1897-1903.

The results of this joint research and exhibition point the way toward greater future collaboration and better understandings on the history and future economic potential of the North Pacific region, the Soviet Union, Canada, and the United States. As we enter a new age of Pacific and Arctic enterprises, and a greater awareness of native cultures and northern peoples, we look forward to closer contacts with our Soviet colleagues and to future joint research and educational programs.

Knud Rasmussen, the famous Danish arctic explorer, charted the needs of arctic research at the end of his long career in a talk to the Pacific Science Congress in 1933, calling for a multinational archeological program in Northeastern Siberia and Alaska: "I am quite aware that a task like this cannot be brought to realization in the twinkling of an eye. . . . It is, however, my firm conviction that one day there will be a great co-operative undertaking of this kind, and that this plan will be carried out at that time." Although a motion to this effect was passed by the Congress, the proposal languished, a victim of Rasmussen's death and political upheavals. The problems are as fresh now as they were 55 years ago. Today the signs are hopeful, and the need is great. Perhaps *Crossroads of Continents* and the "glasnost" era will bring Rasmussen's dream to life.

(*) *United States Arctic Research Plan.* Interagency Arctic Research Policy Committee, July 1987. (Division of Polar Programs, National Science Foundation, Washington, D.C. 20550)

Statement by the Director of the Institute of Ethnography, USSR Academy of Sciences

Iu. V. Bromlei

Scholars have not reached agreement yet about the question of when and where precisely the first human foot stepped into the New World. But practically all agree that the migration from Asia through the area covered by the exhibition *Crossroads of Continents* played an extremely important role in the peopling of America. Although we know—and must acknowledge we know—very little about these first steps on the crossroads of the two major continents, this fact alone makes it fascinating for a contemporary audience to experience visually the traditional aboriginal cultures that developed and lived in these lands on each side of the North Pacific Ocean. Comparison of these cultures, which developed in immense territories sharing comparable natural and climatic conditions on the neighboring continents of Asia and America, is also a subject of enduring interest.

It is as though history had made in the Beringian region an experiment of testing cultural variations and similarities. The contacts between the two mainlands across the Bering Strait were very intense in ancient times; later they were reduced almost exclusively to contacts between Asiatic and American Eskimo, simultaneously with the emergence of a highly developed and very specific culture of maritime Eskimo sea hunters. But even during the periods of minimal cross-continental contact, the universal historical laws favored the formation of similar economic and cultural types and comparable cultural forms on both sides of the Pacific Ocean. There were, however, differences, and these are significant as well. The most striking example was the evolution from subsistence economy in Chukotka, with its deep roots in Eurasia, into a more complex economy involving large-scale reindeer herding, whereas in Alaska and Canada nothing similar happened.

The material displayed in this exhibition demonstrates once again that the origins and the process of formation of the peoples of North America cannot be completely understood without corresponding information of the peoples and cultures of Northeastern Siberia, and vice versa. The importance given by the Soviet regime since its presence in the Soviet North to the study of the traditional cultures and the ways of life of the Small Peoples of the North; the growing interest shown in the United States and Canada in the study and support of traditional aboriginal cultures; and, now, the generally promising opportunities opening in Soviet-American scientific cooperation—all of these conditions urge us to devote our energy toward the development of further coordination of research in ethnology, anthropology, and archeology of the peoples of the northern parts of the Old and the New Worlds.

Another important circumstance of this exhibition should be noted here. Historically the peoples of Alaska and the Aleutian Islands were first studied by Russian scientists. In the 18th and early 19th centuries, they gathered unique collections of artifacts, made drawings, sketches, and paintings, and compiled written data that Canadians and Americans did not have access to. On the other hand, Northeast Siberia, particularly Chukotka, remained little studied in anthropological terms until the beginning of the 19th century. The best data on the peoples of Northeast Siberia were collected mainly in 1900–1901 by the Jesup Expedition, organized by the American Museum of Natural History in New York with the participation of the Russian Academy of Sciences in St. Petersburg, in which eminent Russian scientists, namely W. Bogoras and W. Jochelson, took part.

The present exhibition and publication, *Crossroads of Continents*, in which Soviet and North American artifacts have been combined for the first time, represent another example of the fruitful cooperation between anthropologists and museums of the two continents.

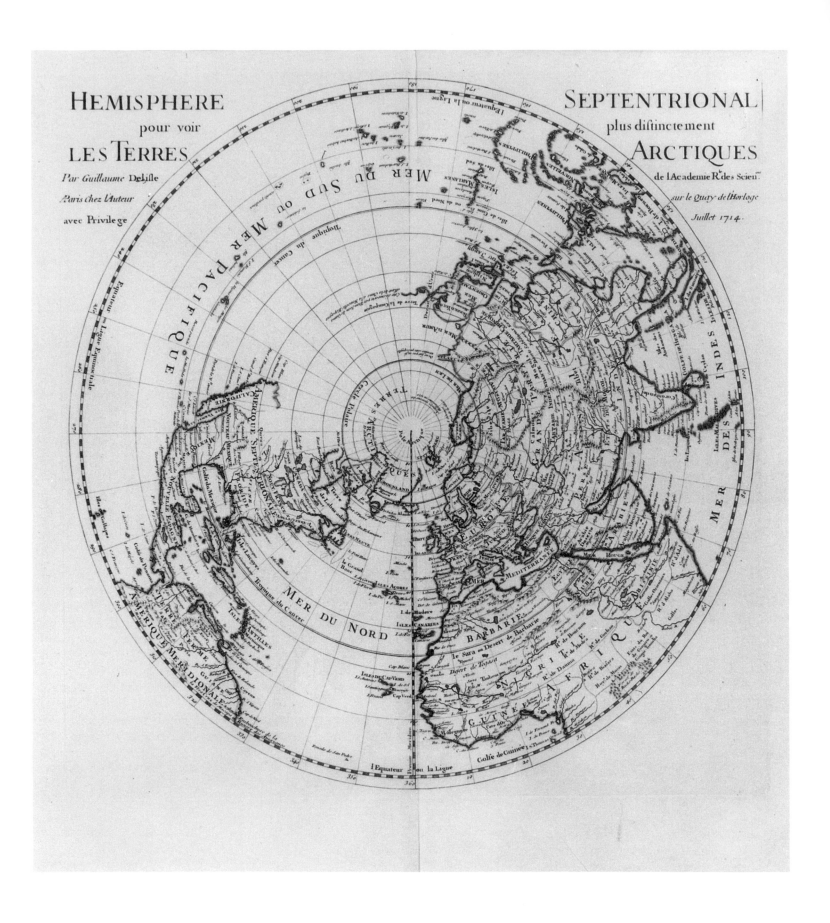

8

Crossroads of Continents: Beringian Oecumene

William W. Fitzhugh and Aron Crowell

Northeastern Siberia and Alaska—the rugged and remote lands that rim the North Pacific— were among the last regions on earth to be described by Western explorers and cartographers, or to be coveted in the courts of Europe and Russia. The North Pacific remained a great blank on world maps well into the 18th century,

then began a long and complex process of cultural change, adaptation, and diversification which generated the brilliant spectrum of hunting, fishing, and herding cultures in place at the time of first contact with explorers.

The 18th century explorations of Vitus Bering, James Cook, Joseph Billings, and other naviga-

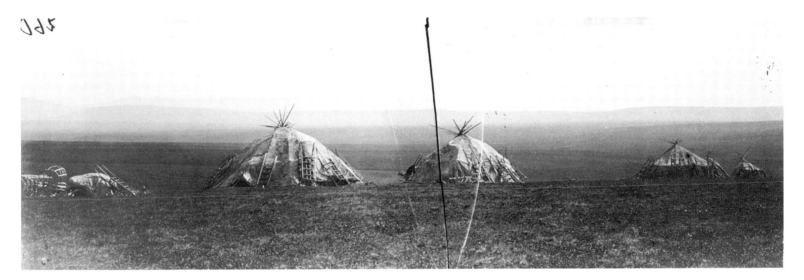

Reindeer Herders' Camp
Reindeer Chukchi: AMNH neg. 11153
During the late winter and spring some Reindeer Chukchi grazed their herds in the grassy tundra along the Kolyma River. The Kolyma District was also important because of the Aniui trade fair established here in 1788 after pacification following the Chukchi-Cossack wars (fig. 316). This photograph is a summer scene showing an abandoned camp.

Circumpolar Map
Guillaume Deslisle, 1714
AMHA B85.55
The North Pacific is a great blank, and Alaska does not exist on this early 18th-century French map. Based on the best information then available, it shows detailed geographical knowledge of the areas of North America claimed by England, France, and Spain. The Siberian coast is poorly known, and the lands of Yeso and Terre de la Campagne (Company Land) north and east of Japan are geographic phantoms.

less known to outsiders than the unexplored heart of Africa. Yet this vast northern wilderness of mountains, forests, tundra, and ice, geographically linking the continents of Eurasia and North America, was in no sense an uninviting wasteland. Sea mammals and fish abound in its cold but nutrient-rich ocean waters, and its rivers run red and silver each summer with surging millions of salmon. Caribou, moose, beaver, and dozens of other species live off the resources of the land year-round, while whales and streaming flocks of migratory birds arrive each year to reap the nightless arctic summer's burst of plant and plankton growth. This environment, harsh as it is climatically, offers a bountiful living to human beings culturally prepared to take advantage of its natural resources for food, clothing, and shelter. Human populations began moving into Northeastern Siberia over 16,000 years ago from the more temperate regions of eastern Asia, spreading north and east with the passing of the last Ice Age until they crossed into the Americas via Alaska. That great migration was only the beginning of the story, for the populations that had settled in the North Pacific region

tors, and the penetration of Siberia and then Alaska by Russian fur traders, marked the beginning of a period of intensive (and increasingly destructive) contact with North Pacific peoples that held more than a few surprises for the Europeans. From Kamchatka to the Arctic Ocean, from the Aleutian Islands to the mountainous, fjorded coasts of British Columbia, these explorers found the North Pacific Rim inhabited by peoples well and warmly dressed and housed, equipped with ingenious and effective tools and weapons, organized in large groups with wide-ranging political and economic contacts, and possessed of complex religious beliefs, striking artistic traditions, often elaborate social institutions, and a vast practical knowledge of the environment. Most Europeans in the North Pacific during the early historical period seem to have been blinded by their own cultural prejudices, unable to appreciate the wonder of what they witnessed, yet some had open eyes. Martin Sauer, a member of the Billings Expedition sent to northern Russia and America by Russia's Catherine the Second in 1785–94, wrote:

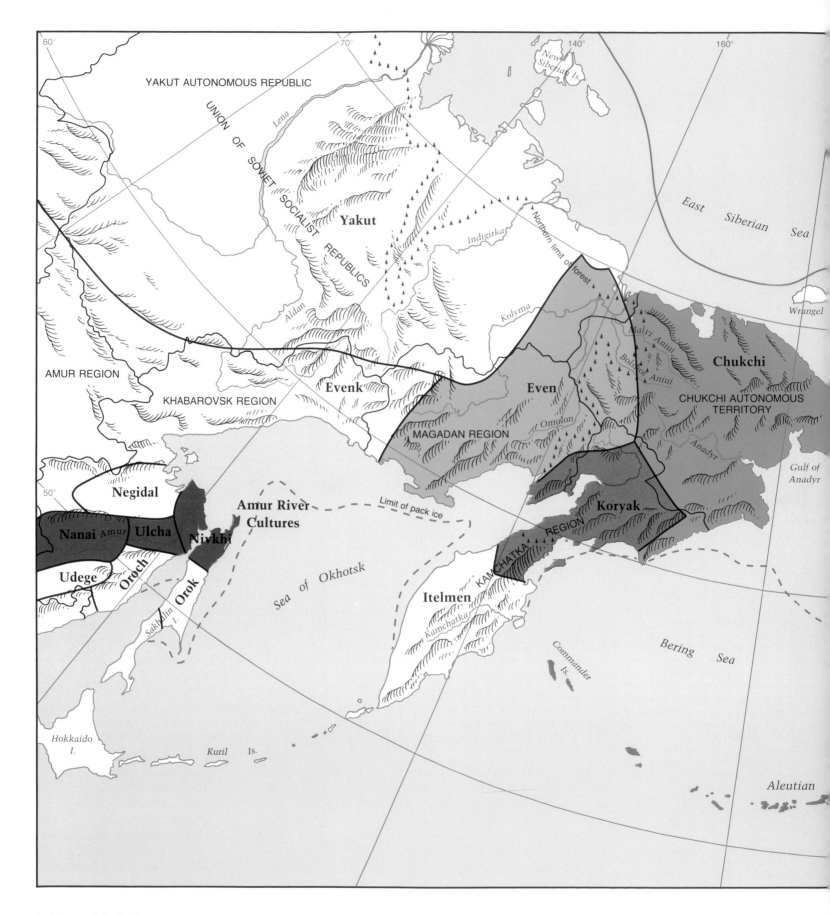

1. Cultures of the North
Pacific–Bering Sea Region ca. 1900

10

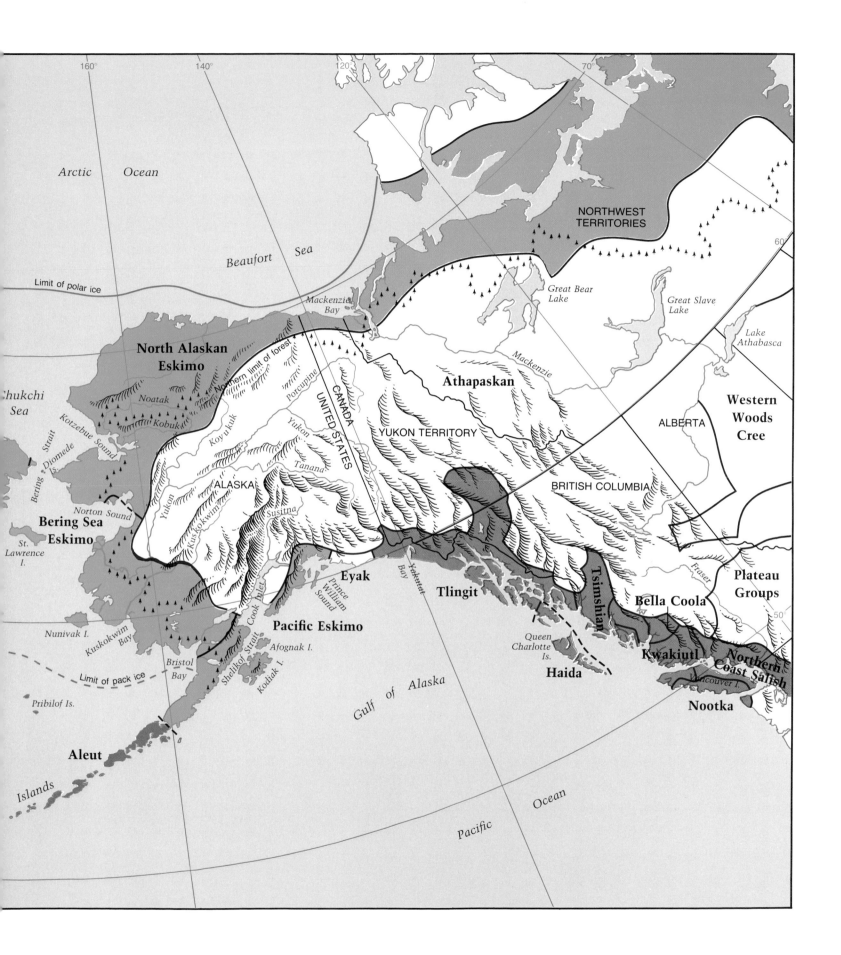

Arctic Ocean

Beaufort Sea

Limit of polar ice

NORTHWEST TERRITORIES

Mackenzie Bay

Great Bear Lake

Great Slave Lake

Lake Athabasca

North Alaskan Eskimo

Northern limit of forest

Noatak

Kobuk

Koyukuk

Porcupine

Yukon

Athapaskan

Mackenzie

CANADA

UNITED STATES

Western Woods Cree

ALBERTA

Chukchi Sea

Bering Strait

Diomede Is.

Kotzebue Sound

Norton Sound

Bering Sea Eskimo

St. Lawrence I.

ALASKA

Tanana

YUKON TERRITORY

BRITISH COLUMBIA

Susitna

Kuskokwim

Yukon

Nunivak I.

Kuskokwim Bay

Cook Inlet

Eyak

Prince William Sound

Yakutat Bay

Tlingit

Tsimshian

Bella Coola

Plateau Groups

Fraser

Pacific Eskimo

Shelikof Strait

Afognak I.

Bristol Bay

Limit of pack ice

Kodiak I.

Haida

Queen Charlotte Is.

Kwakiutl

Northern Coast Salish

Vancouver I.

Pribilof Is.

Gulf of Alaska

Nootka

Aleut

Islands

Pacific Ocean

11

The capacity of the natives of these islands [the Aleutians] infinitely surpasses every idea that I had formed of the abilities of savages . . . Their behaviour . . . is not rude or barbarous, but mild, polite, and hospitable. At the same time, the beauty, proportion, and art with which they make their boats, instruments, and apparel evince that they by no means deserve to be termed stupid; an epithet so liberally bestowed upon those whom Europeans call savages (Sauer 1802:273-74).

Sauer's sentiments reflect the beginnings of interest in the North Pacific as a unique and fascinating cultural realm, from which flowed the early collection of "curiosities"—masks, robes, weapons, and diverse other examples of native art and design—that were deposited in fledgling Russian and European museums. The Russian Academy of Science's early 19th century sponsorship of systematic, scientifically oriented collecting among the North Pacific peoples opened up a new era of museum-based anthropological research in the region. The Smithsonian Institution, the American Museum of Natural History, and other American and Canadian museums continued this tradition after Russia's sale of Alaska to the United States in 1867, culminating in the American Museum's Jesup North Pacific Expedition to Siberia and the Northwest Coast (1897–1903).

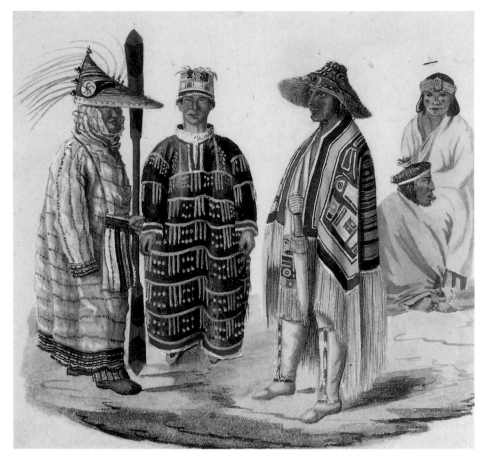

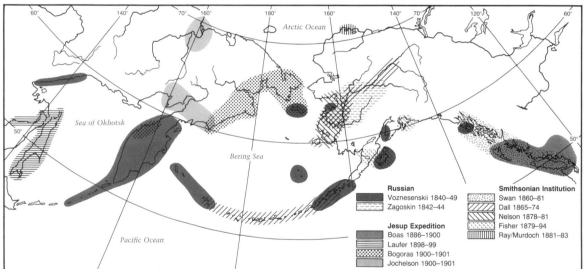

3. Anthropological Research and Collecting, 1840-1901

Finds of imported objects in archeological sites around the North Pacific Rim document prehistoric interest in "foreign" cultures. The first-known ethnographic observations by Europeans were those made by Dezhnev in 1648 and Steller in 1741 (Golder 1914; Ray 1975). The earliest extant ethnographic objects connected with known expeditions are those collected by James Cook's 1778 visit and the Billings-Sarychev Expedition of 1785-94. After 1800, recognition of the importance of documentation and preservation increased the value of ethnographic collections and set in motion the great collecting era of the 19th century. This map indicates the major collectors and study regions represented in the Crossroads exhibition.

Crossroads of Continents combines modern research in North Pacific anthropology and archeology with the presentation of many important objects from these early collections. This book and exhibition attempt to capture the wide diversity of North Pacific cultures as well as their historical development from the end of the last Ice Age to the modern day. Individual cultures are considered both in particular and as components of a pan-North Pacific "oecumene"—an ensemble of related peoples integrated by trade, migration, warfare, and the cross-fertilization of ideas, oral traditions, and art into a large cultural universe. Cross-cultural topics considered at this level include economy, technology, housing, clothing, religion, and art. Against this ancient tradition of trans-Beringian interchange, periods of political isolation, such as experienced recently, have been transient. The long historical tradition of linkages provides a compelling rationale for combining Soviet and American collections and scholarship in an exhibition and publication broad enough in scope to examine the North Pacific as a whole, with the ultimate goal of achieving new understandings both of and between peoples on both sides of Bering Strait.

North Pacific Peoples and Environments

Crossroads of Continents focuses on the arc of lands and islands that surrounds the northern reaches of the Pacific Ocean and its component and adjacent seas: the Sea of Okhotsk, the Bering Sea, and, north of Bering Strait, the Chukchi Sea (fig. 1). Located between 50 to 70 degrees North latitude, these regions experience a great variety of climatic regimes ranging from extremely cold arctic coast and inland continental climates to more moderate subarctic maritime climates that are foggy and stormy but rarely below freezing.

Archeological data presented in this catalogue demonstrate the early development of complex and diverse cultures around the North Pacific Rim as the first occupants adapted to these regional environments. The primary focus of *Crossroads*, however, is on the ethnographic peoples of the 18th–19th centuries. Unfortunately, it has not been possible to extend the full coverage given to the early ethnographic period into the 20th century, although the latter period is treated in essays dealing with Siberian and Alaskan social, political, and cultural developments.

Cultures of Northeastern Siberia are represented by four groups, the southwesternmost a composite of Chinese and Japanese influenced cultures (Gilyak, Nanai, and others) living along the lower Amur River and nearby maritime regions (fig. 1). The remaining Northeast Siberian cultures, originally designed linguistically as Paleoasiatic peoples, include the Even (formerly called Lamut), a reindeer herding culture living west of the Sea of Okhotsk; the Koryak and Itelmen (Kamchadal) of Kamchatka and adjacent maritime regions; and, farthest to the northeast, the Chukchi, who like the Koryak, were divided between reindeer breeders on the interior and maritime sea mammal hunters on the coast. These groups are to be distinguished from the central Siberian Evenk (Tungus) and Yakut, who bordered the Northeastern Siberian Paleoasiatics on the west and from whom the latter had acquired many features of their technology, clothing, art, as well as their reindeer-breeding economy.

North Amercian cultures are represented by four groups: Eskimo and Aleut, and two Indian groups, Tlingit and Athapaskan. Although Eskimo cultures extend into Canada and Greenland, only the Alaskan groups (North Alaskan, Asiatic, Bering Sea, and Pacific Eskimo) are discussed here. Also represented are the Aleut, whose occupation of the Aleutian Island chain made them the most maritime adapted of all North Pacific peoples. Of the many Northwest Coast Indian groups, we concentrate on the northernmost, the Tlingit, and refer occasionally to Haida, Tsimshian, Kwakiutl, Nootka, and Makah. The final group is made up of the many tribes of Alaskan Athapaskan Indians, forest dwellers whose life was based on hunting, trapping, and fishing.

Geographic patterning is a notable feature of the economies and culture types of these North Pacific groups. On both sides of Bering Strait, the southern limit of the greater North Pacific culture area discussed here was dominated by cultures with salmon fishing economies. To the north, the coastal economies of Siberia and Alaska were increasingly oriented toward a combination of salmon fishing and sea mammal hunting, with the hunting of the large sea mammals (whales) most characteristic of Bering Strait and North Alaskan Eskimo and Chukchi. Away from the coast, where ease of travel and similar environmental conditions over wide areas promoted cultural diffusion and convergence, economies differed dramatically. Siberian interior groups had adopted reindeer breeding as their economic mainstay, while in Alaska, Athapaskan people retained a traditional hunting and fishing economy without any domestic animals except dogs.

These patterns were strongly conditioned by ecological boundaries, especially the northern forest and shrub limit on land and the seasonally moving southern boundary of the arctic pack ice, which extends into the southern Okhotsk Sea and Bering Sea in winter and in summer withdraws to the northern Chukchi Sea. The association of animals adapted to particular ecological zones, together with the annual migration of other species across these boundaries, established the basic parameters for human life. Year-round adaptation to the most severe arctic conditions was a challenge that took Beringian peoples ten thousand years to perfect but which eventually led to human expansion into arctic regions north of Bering Strait —the last area of the world to be settled by preindustrial peoples.

Finally, a significant feature of the Beringian region is the meeting here of converging circumpolar bands of tundra and boreal ecological zones and their intersection with the biologically rich coasts of the North Pacific and Arctic Ocean. As a result of this convergence, ways of life adapted to different circumpolar and northern maritime zones converged on Bering Strait, where they mixed and were transformed (Gjessing 1944; Moberg 1960; Fitzhugh 1975).

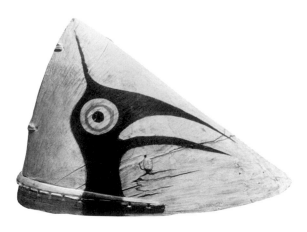

Research Themes

Interest in the culture history of Siberian and American peoples began with speculation on the origin of the American Indian even before knowledge of the Pacific Ocean and Bering Strait existed (Acosta 1598). The first records on Northeastern Siberian people date to the mid-17th century (Golder 1914). Direct observations on Siberian and American cultural relationships, however, date to the early 18th century when Stepan Krasheninnikov in 1735–41 and Georg Wilhelm Steller in 1741 noted specific similarities between these regions (Okladnikova 1987:220). Possibly these reports influenced Thomas Jefferson's (1787) ideas about the Asian origin of American Indians. Samuel Haven was the first to identify the probability of a Bering Strait entry route (Haven 1856). At this time the notion of Beringian interchange was also being pursued by American naturalists, among them the Smithsonian's Spencer F. Baird, who initiated collecting projects in northwestern North America in the 1850s. However, it was not until Franz Boas was appointed curator at the American Museum of Natural History in New York in 1896 that scientific study of cultural relationships across Bering Strait came clearly into focus.

Believing that Bering Strait must have been the source of ethnic connections between Asia and the Americas, Boas proposed studies ranging across the North Pacific in the regions closest to their point of contact. Avoiding Alaska, which had been studied by Smithsonian naturalists, Boas proposed research in the remaining gaps. Unknown Northeastern Siberia and the Northwest Coast received the greatest attention. Boas's Jesup North Pacific Expedition, named after its benefactor, American Museum President Morris K. Jesup, was an anthropological tour de force, a grandiose, brilliantly conceptualized, and masterfully orchestrated attack on one of the most important problems in American anthropology. At its heart was a close collaboration between the American Museum of Natural History and the Imperial Russian Academy of Sciences and its Museum of Anthropology and Ethnography.

The Jesup Expedition (1897–1903) produced a vast body of ethnographic, linguistic, folkloric, and physical anthropological data (Boas 1903). Based on these data, Boas and his Russian collaborators, ethnologists Waldemar Bogoras and Waldemar Jochelson, concluded that the North Pacific groups studied were of a single racial type; that they held many cultural, linguistic, and folkloristic elements in common; and that these elements indicated a common cultural base, formerly more widespread than at present, encompassing northeastern Asia, Alaska, and the Northwest Coast. Ties between Siberians and Northwest Coast groups with Alaskan Eskimos were seen as being weaker, with Aleuts intermediate between the two. Boas (1905:99) decided that "Chukchee, Koryak, Kamchadal and Yukaghir must be classed with the American race rather than with the Asiatic race."

These observations were later explained in a three-stage reconstruction of historical events, the first being the initial peopling of the New World across Bering Strait at the end of the Ice Age. The second involved a back-migration of American cultures into Northeastern Siberia (Boas 1910:534), later designated the Americanoid theory (Boas 1925, 1933; Bogoras 1902; Jochelson 1905). Boas proposed to account for the lack of evidence of close ties between the North Pacific groups and Eskimo culture as a result of the Eskimos' recent arrival in western Alaska from Canada (Boas 1905:99), a theory that later became known as the "Eskimo wedge" hypothesis (Collins 1937:4).

These conclusions were offered as preliminary findings, and because Boas never wrote the concluding volume anticipated in the Jesup Expedition series the full results of this project have never been synthesized. Despite attention to some of these questions (Boas 1925, 1933; Chowning 1962; Count 1949; Levin 1958; Hatt 1949; Jochelson 1925, 1926a; Leroi-Gourhan 1946; Michael and VanStone 1983), the study of North Pacific culture history in the 20th century has declined, victimized by the break in political relations between the Soviet Union and Western nations. Today many of the conclusions

4. Bentwood Hunting Hat
Bering Sea Eskimo: NMNH 38717
This hunting hat collected by Edward W. Nelson from Kaialigamut in the Yukon-Kuskokwim Delta depicts a bird spirit with supernaturally spiked head and red-circled eye against a white background. The spirit portrayed may be Raven, the trickster and demiurge prominent in Siberian and Alaskan mythology. Similarities in Raven mythology were cited by Boas and his Jesup Expedition collaborators as an indication of ethnic links between Siberian and North American cultures. Raven images are rare in Bering Sea Eskimo art, perhaps because of the powerful and unpredictable nature of this being.

5. Quivers and Arrows
Chukchi: AMNH 70-6980a. Athapaskan: MAE 5801-2; NMNH 43352 (arrows)
Similar types of material culture show that Bering Strait was not a physical barrier to communication between cultures of the North Pacific Rim. Objects of similar type were used in both Siberia and Alaska, and these types often exhibit clinal variation, gradual change in form and design from one region to the next.

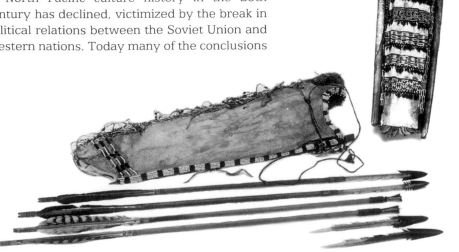

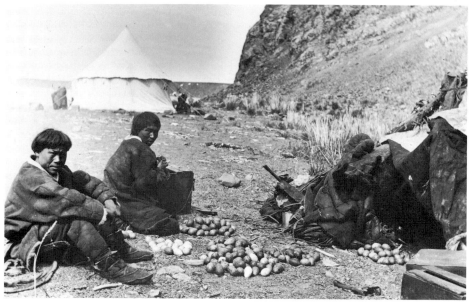

6. Koryak Egg Gatherers
AMNH neg. 22094, Jesup Exp.

Eggs are an important source of fresh food for northern peoples when the birds return to nest in early summer. Some birds, like gulls and eiders, nest in open country, and their eggs fall prey to foxes and other birds. The best egg collecting, however, is found at bird cliffs where huge numbers of birds nest in dense colonies over the water.

7. Koryak Shaman
AMNH neg. 42119, Jesup Exp.

Shamanism, the art of influencing events by the manipulation of guardian spirits, is one of the oldest and most basic forms of religious expression and was the dominant form of religious practice among North Pacific peoples. As curers, diviners, and intermediaries between people and spirits, shamans were a powerful force in society.

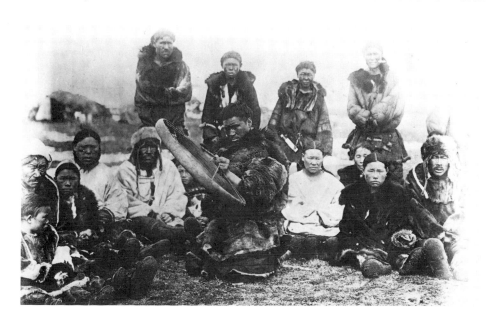

from the Jesup Expedition have been replaced by new theories in which a combination of local development and diffusion have replaced migration as the major explanation for North Pacific and Beringian culture change, while many of the ethnographic and folklore links remain unexplored and unexplained.

Crossroads of Continents: Project History

In 1977 initiatives were taken in discussions between Iu.V. Bromlei, Director of the Institute of Ethnography of the Soviet Academy of Sciences, and William W. Fitzhugh and William C. Sturtevant of the Smithsonian Institution. Although Soviet-Amercian exchange symposia on Beringian cultural interactions had been held, they did not involve collections research or exhibition work, and the results were not subject to wide public dissemination. These discussions soon led to the idea for an exhibition of North

Pacific ethnography and archeology to be assembled jointly from the earliest and most important collections of the Soviet Union and the United States. This was a project that neither country could hope to mount independently due to the scattered distribution of the necessary collections. Rather than simply exchanging objects, as is the norm for most international exhibitions, *Crossroads* would be assembled as a single, fully integrated exhibition, jointly researched and curated by American and Soviet scholars.

A unique feature of the project was the unusual history of North Pacific and Beringian ethnological studies. The earliest Alaskan ethnographic collections came from 18–19th century efforts of Russian explorers and scientists during the days when Alaska was part of the Russian colony known as Russian America (1741–1867). These collections have resided for more than a century in the Museum of Anthropology and Ethnography in Leningrad, where they have not been readily accessible to American and Canadian scholars, nor have they been available to the American public or to the native peoples whose ancestors made them. Similarly, because early Russian ethnographic collecting was conducted primarily in the territories of Russian America, Soviet institutions do not have large, early Siberian ethnological collections that can compare with those assembled in New York as a result of the Jesup Expedition. *Crossroads* created a structure for research and exhibition of these alienated and remarkable collections and provided an opportunity to view the anthropology and history of the North Pacific in the original Boasian vision of an integrated geographic and cultural realm.

In this sense, *Crossroads of Continents* as an exhibition and a publication may be viewed as a slightly delayed summary volume of Franz Boas's Jesup Expedition series. But more importantly, we see *Crossroads* as a beginning, not an end. We propose no final solutions to the problems of Siberian-American culture links; our intent has been simply to document, as fully and currently as possible, the diversity of and interrelationships between Siberian and American cultures. Final answers to the problems of the peopling of the New World and subsequent thousands of years of Siberian-American cultural interchange await future research. Study of the enthnography, folklore, and culture history of this region is in an early developmental stage; each year brings major new understandings and new problems.

In keeping with the spirit of Franz Boas and Morris K. Jesup, who in their day created a program of international research to generate

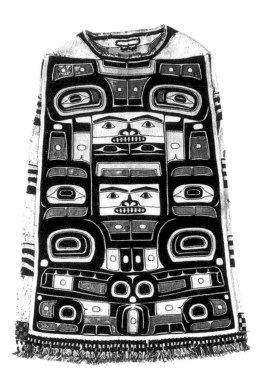

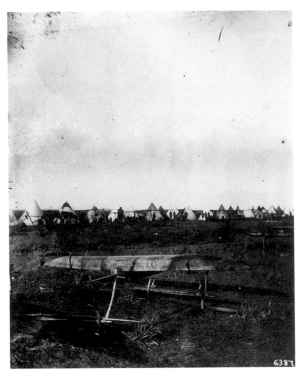

new understandings of this unique region, we dedicate this volume to hopes for future collaboration and contacts among scholars, native peoples, and the wider public interested in northern studies, and we plea for the preservation and care of ancient historical objects and information, the basic documents of the region's unwritten culture history. As we enter a new age, in which Pacific and Arctic regions are assuming great importance in the world at large and our Eurocentric and Atlantic outlook is being modified toward a dawning age of the Pacific,

we look forward to better understanding of cultural origins, more respect for cultural diversity, and more open communication, exchange, and research. Once again we hope to see these northern peoples and cultures as through the eyes of Martin Sauer. In this celebration of diversity and common ties, so evident in the pages that follow, we look forward to an era symbolized today by the historic reopening of direct contacts between the peoples of Alaska and Siberia that is taking place even as this book goes to press.

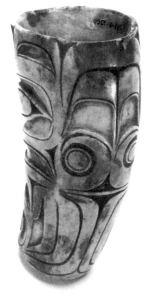

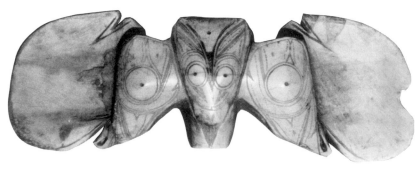

Ethnic Connections Across Bering Strait

I. S. Gurvich

12. Birdskin Parka

St. Lawrence Island Eskimo: NMNH 418612

Birdskin clothing was light, durable, waterproof, and warm. More common in Alaska than Siberia, it was most important on St. Lawrence, Nunivak, and Kodiak islands, and in the Aleutian chain, where caribou—which provided the warmest fur—were not present. This parka was made from the skins of more than 75 crested auklets, which breed in large colonies in the cliffs of St. Lawrence Island. It is trimmed with a fur ruff.

13. Ivory Bolas

Norton Sound Eskimo: NMNH 38444

One of many implement types shared by peoples of Alaska and Siberia, the bolas was used to hunt ducks and other waterfowl. Its distribution was confined largely to Eskimo areas and to coastal groups in Northeastern Siberia, where it may have been introduced by contact with Eskimo peoples. During bird hunting season, men wore the bolas wound around their heads where it could be grasped and thrown at a moment's notice. Eskimo bolas usually have four to eight weights whose lines are attached to a central knot or to a feather quill handle. Feather ornaments are common and probably had ritual function.

This bolas was collected from Inupiat Eskimos of eastern Norton Sound. Its red incised decoration includes the raven's foot motif commonly used in western Alaskan Eskimo art. The image of Raven himself, however, is almost never figured, perhaps out of respect for his powerful and unpredictable spirit.

Raven mythology is even more widely distributed among peoples of the North Pacific than the bolas and has been cited as important evidence of ethnological connections between the cultures of North America and Northeastern Siberia.

Similarities between the cultures of northern Siberia and northwestern North America have long attracted the attention of archeologists, ethnographers, and historians. These similarities provide important information on relationships and development of both ancient and historical cultures, and on the ethnic groups that inhabit this huge region. Obviously, in the Bering Sea region, not only in remote antiquity but in times relatively close to our own, trade between individual ethnolinguistic groups took place as well as shifts in population resulting from changes in economic conditions. Certainly, Bering Strait, which separates northeastern Asia from North America by a width of 56 miles, did not present a significant barrier to contacts between the populations of the adjacent regions.

Ethnographic literature frequently contains evidence on Eskimo-Koryak and Eskimo-Chukchi linguistic conformities, suggesting that these reciprocal influences date from ancient times (Bogoraz 1935:357, 1939:27, 96; Vdovin 1961:27–63). Thus, for example, not only along the seacoast of Kamchatka but in the region of the Tauisk inlet, Eskimo place-names occur (Vdovin 1973:265), even though Eskimo people do not now occupy these regions. Such place-names suggest a former Eskimo occupation of this region during the Thule or Punuk whaling period when Eskimo toggling harpoons, seal nets made from thong, skin-covered kayaks and umiaks, waterproof gutskin garments, and other items were carried from Bering Strait south into Chukotka and Kamchatka by Eskimo peoples who later became assimilated into other societies. At the same time, the northern cultures contain features characteristic of southern regions, such as braiding of grass nets, mats, and baskets and use of bird skins for clothing and boot insoles.

The peoples of Northeastern Siberia known as the Paleoasiatics (Koryak, Chukchi, Yukaghir, Itelmen, and Nivkhi) used certain hunting tools widespread among Eskimo populations in North America but little known in the rest of northern Asia. Among these are bolas with their feather handles, spear-throwers, and fishnets woven from reindeer sinew, grass, and baleen. Shared elements also include certain kinds of dugout canoes and the method of weir fishing found among the Itelmen, peoples of the Amur, and river fishermen of North America. Methods of cleaning fish and preserving meat by fermentation are also similar.

Certain types of transportation equipment are distributed across Bering Strait. Snowshoes played an important role among peoples of the North Pacific Rim (Levin and Potapov 1961:82–85) and were used by Paleoasiatic groups (including the Amur River Nivkhi), Asiatic Eskimo, and many groups in northern North America. However, snowshoes were not used in historical times by Asiatic peoples distant from coastal zones, where their place was taken by skis. On distributional evidence it has been suggested that snowshoes were brought to northeastern Asia and North America by an early wave of peoples and that skis replaced snowshoes in north-central Siberia more recently. The use of snow goggles, to protect the eyes from being burned by the bright late-winter sun reflecting on the snow, is also seen on both sides of Bering Strait. The presence of such equipment as snowshoes and snow goggles can be explained, in part, by similarities in physical conditions and by similar economic circumstances of the peoples using them; but in

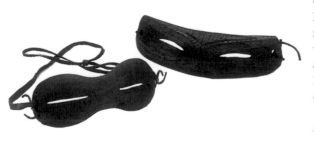

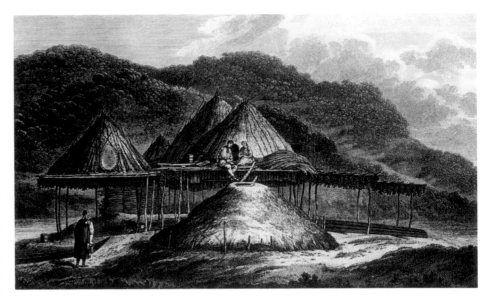

many instances reciprocal influences must also have been involved.

Archeological materials and information from explorers and ethnographers document the use of a special type of dwelling by a variety of North Pacific peoples. This type of house is semisubterranean, excavated below ground level, with walls arranged in a four-cornered plan and made of a combination of logs covered with earth or sod, which acted as insulation from the cold. Two forms of sod houses were used in the North Pacific, one by the Eskimos and another by the peoples of the Aleutian Islands and Kamchatka. Sod houses with side or underground entrances through the floor were used by Eskimo groups on both sides of Bering Strait but were abandoned in the historical period of the Asian side. The Aleut-Kamchatka–style sod house had an entrance through the center of the roof. Similarities between Asian and Alaskan Eskimo houses certainly result from historical contacts between these culturally similar neighboring regions. Similarities between the Aleut and Kamchatka houses are more difficult to explain and have been cited for many years as evidence of direct contacts between these peoples.

The North Pacific coast also saw the development of distinctive forms of clothing. Anthropologists, following the detailed analyses of Gudmund Hatt, have long noted similarities in both the general cut and detailed patterns of northern clothing and boots linking Paleoasiatics with Asiatic, Alaskan, and Greenlandic Eskimos, and with Aleut, Tlingit, and Athapaskan peoples. Details in clothing testify to the close cultural connections between peoples of this region.

Thus, for example, Koryak and Chukchi parkas are equipped with small fur bibs to protect the

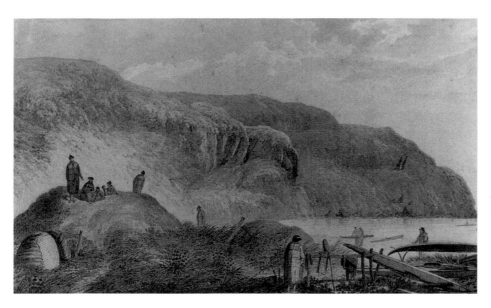

16. "Natives of Oonalaschka, and their Habitations"
John Webber. PMH 41-72-10/506

Aleut people lived nearly entirely from the resources of the sea, their islands having no land animals larger than foxes. In this regard, they were the most completely maritime of all North Pacific peoples. Early explorers were struck by their highly developed society, which included refined technology and art, complex social and ceremonial life, and elaborate systems of knowledge. The Aleut lived in large groups in permanent villages near productive fishing and sea mammal hunting locations. They were skilled boatsmen, and their kayaks won accolades from European mariners for lightness, grace, and speed.

Like Koryak dwellings, Aleut houses were semisubterranean and were entered by ladders through holes in the roof. But in other respects, scholars see few similarities between these ethnographic cultures today. Little is known of Aleut prehistory. Studies of interaction between Siberian and Alaskan peoples focus especially on the Eskimos of Bering Strait and the Aleuts, whose island habitat extends to within a few hundred miles of Kamchatka.

fur near the throat from freezing with moisture from one's breath (figs. 272, 341). Similar bibs are found in the clothing of certain groups of Eskimos, Tlingit, and Plains Indians. The sleeveless suede vest used by the Koryak in summer, a type of poncho with fringes, not sewn up under the arms, is analogous to garments used by various tribes in the Americas. And until recent times, a "tail"—an extension of the back flap—was an obligatory design feature of the Koryak funeral parka. This flap was richly ornamented with reindeer hair embroidery and, more recently, with beads. Such a tail was not found among the nearest neighbors of the Koryak but was present among the Chukchi and in circular or trapezoidal form among Asiatic Eskimos. The tail had a functional purpose in being drawn tightly between the legs and fastened in front at the belt, protecting the hunter from cold when sitting on the ice for long periods. Among the Koryak this functional aspect of design had been lost and was preserved in funeral dress. Among Canadian and Greenland Eskimos a tail flap was found only on female dress.

In Soviet literature in recent decades considerable attention has been focused on ornamentation as an important historical-ethnographic source. Study of traditional ornamental art shows it to be distinguished by significant stability, frequently dating to distant times. Long ago, Sternberg (1931) established that the strip ornamentation made from reindeer hair was present among many Asian peoples, including Chukchi, Koryak, Yukaghir, Even, Nivkhi, and American Eskimo, and also among American Athapaskans, who used porcupine quill instead of reindeer hair. Similarities in designs themselves have also been pointed out (fig. 295).

Detailed comparisons between the ornaments of the peoples of Northeast Siberia and northwest America carried out by S. V. Ivanov showed that the so-called northern Siberian straight-lined geometric ornament of strips, squares, and rectangles, known to all northeastern Paleoasiatics, Asiatic Eskimos, Aleut, and Yukaghir, was also widespread among American Eskimo. The northern Asiatic type of ornament, the composition of which includes concentric circles and semicircles, star rosettes, and ovals, was also quite characteristic of western American Eskimos and Aleuts, and in Siberia of the Even and Dolgan (Ivanov 1963:242). All of these examples testify to the presence of ancient cultural connections between the peoples of the North Pacific Rim.

Common elements are found in the traditional spiritual culture of the northeastern Paleoasiatics and their neighbors on the American shore. Seasonal animal harvest festivals of the Itelmen, Koryak, Chukchi, and Asiatic Eskimos, which are connected with the "rebirth" of game and continuance of economic success, have close counterparts among the Eskimo, Tlingit, Athapaskans, and other tribes. In both Siberia and North America, these ceremonies included dances in which people wore anthropomorphic and zoomorphic masks made of leather, wood, or bark, although masking traditions in Siberia were much less elaborate than those in northwestern North America.

Along the North Pacific Rim and adjacent areas, improvisational dances with rhythmic expressive movements of the arms and body were widely used to imitate animals. The performers imitated the behavior of seals, running deer, or peculiarities of bird habits. Dances were accompanied by drum or tambourine, frequently with vocal melodies, during festivals attended by guests from neighboring villages or from further afield. Trade and other social and economic activities took place at such times.

Mythological legends about Raven are among the strongest evidence of contacts between Itelmen, Chukchi, and Koryak on the one hand and peoples of western Alaska and the Northwest Coast on the other. Ancient Itelmen representations of Raven as a hero-creator, often transformed into its antithesis, a traitor and liar, correspond to Raven stories of the Tlingit (Meletinskii 1963) and Bering Sea Eskimo. Many other Siberian folkloristic details also correspond with North American ones. The well-known investigator W. I. Jochelson believed that mythological evidence was strong enough to support the proposition that the Koryak and Chukchi had resettled northeastern Asia from Alaska (Jochelson 1907), even though he adduced little

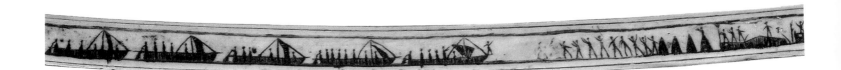

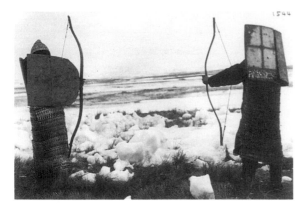

other proof of this hypothesis. Contemporary specialists do not support Jochelson's view (Levin 1958).

As is well known, customs associated with funerals and human burial are often distinguished by archaic or conservative practices. This is also an area exhibiting striking similarities between Siberian and American cultures. Both Chukchi and Eskimo had a custom of leaving their dead out on the tundra to be eaten by the foxes; a similar custom among the Itelmen is paralleled by the Athapaskan Indians. Such a list of similar practices and customs could easily be expanded. For example, peoples on both sides of Bering Strait, from the Lena River to the eastern Aleutians, had a mortuary practice of ritually dissecting the corpse and carrying out mummification on parts of the body. Such ideas must have been communicated through reciprocal influences established in antiquity between North Asia and America.

The indisputable similarity of many cultural phenomena among the peoples who have, from ancient times, inhabited the regions adjacent to the North Pacific Rim is undoubtedly the result of multiple causes. Among them should be mentioned the long period of adaptation, lasting many centuries if not millennia, during which the aboriginal population accustomed itself to the specific geographical surroundings and the climate; the similar origins of some of the ethnic groups concerned; ethnic mixing and its opposite, diversification; and, lastly, migration of peoples and their mutual influences upon each other.

According to historical evidence dating back to the 18th century, the population of the maritime settlements of Chukotka since early times had contact with the inhabitants of Alaska. Thus, Asiatic Eskimos and coastal Chukchi frequently visited settlements on the other side of the Bering Strait to trade and participate in festivals. As a consequence, they knew the Alaskan village locations and set out each spring for them by foot or dogsled (Merck 1978:54).

Sometimes, peaceful relations degenerated into predatory campaigns. "Where there is trade—there is plunder," wrote Merck, a participant in the North-Eastern Geographic Expedition of 1785–98, who noted that the Chukchi crossed over to America in their *baidaras* (umiaks) and attacked the nomadic camps of the Alaskans, killing the men and taking the women and children prisoner. One of the principal objects of these raids was the acquisition of Alaskan furs, which they then traded to the Russians (Merck 1978:121). Such warfare had a negative effect on trade across Bering Strait between Chukchi and Alaskan Eskimos. In 1891, for example, Chukchi went to the American coast and found only empty dwellings abandoned by the inhabitants because the latter feared vengeance for having slaughtered three boatloads of Chukchi who had been cast upon the American coast in a storm. At the end of the 18th century, after the Tsar's government refused to subjugate the Chukchi by force, there being few financial benefits for such a course, the relations between the Chukchi and their nearest neighbors—the Koryak and Yukaghir—began to take the form of peaceful trade. This apparently affected the contacts between the Chukchi and Asiatic Eskimos on the one hand and the population of Alaska on the other. Thus in 1789, according to the information of the Russian Lieutenant of Cossacks I. Kobelev, Chukchi in ten *baidaras*, numbering about 150 men, set out for Alaska. The goal of

17. Trade and War

Drillbow, Cape Nome Eskimo: NMNH 44399. AMNH neg. 1545, Jesup Exp.

Relations across Bering Strait probably always featured both trade and war. These activities are documented in exploration literature, in Chukchi and Eskimo oral history, and on artifacts. This drillbow engraving depicts the greeting of Siberian traders at an Alaskan Eskimo village. Annual trade fairs were the chief means of exchanging Alaskan and Siberian products.

Peaceful relations often degenerated into conflict over resources or trading rights. Evidence of warfare is known for the past 2,000 years in the North Pacific region. Its technology, including use of fortified sites, slat armor, shields, and sinew-backed bows, was introduced from Asia. Jochelson's posed photograph showing Koryak men dressed in iron plate armor, helmets, and shields illustrates typical Siberian war regalia.

18. Tobacco Pipe and Pouch

Even: AMNH 70-5623a,b

The tobacco, beads, and iron associated with this Even pipe kit were among the most important commodities traded from Siberia to Alaska. Because these products were distributed from trading centers in western Siberia, they commanded high prices in Alaska, where they were exchanged for furs, jade, and ivory (fig. 316).

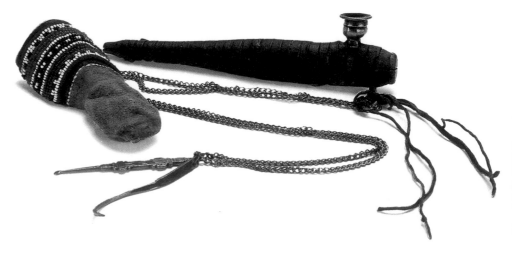

this trip was trade. Like the Chukchi, the Alaskans carried arms and wore armor. However, as Kobelev noted, both sides were armed not for battle but "as an example."

The principal items of trade included furs, Russian goods, beads, iron plates, knives, axes, harpoon heads, and copper caldrons (fig. 316). On the Asiatic coast there even was a sample price list for prisoners. Reindeer Chukchi gave 10–12 caribou cows for an American female prisoner, or two draft reindeer; children were cheaper. The Chukchi used women prisoners to

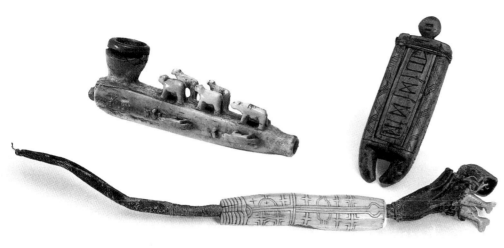

do much of the drudgery involved in camp life, sometimes beat them, dressed them in shabby clothes, and put them at the disposal of visitors. Frequently women slaves acted as translators in the barter trade.

In the first half of the 19th century a significant influence on the peaceful relations between the native populations of Chukotka and Alaska was the establishment of the Russian trade fair on the Aniui River, an eastern tributary of the Kolyma. This fair was held each winter. Fixed prices were introduced for Russian goods. Trade on credit and the petty trade of the Cossacks and industrialists were forbidden. A measure of the economic success of this fair can be seen in the value turnover during the second decade of the 19th century, which reached 200,000 rubles ($100,000). In 1837, 100 beavers, 305 marten, 30 lynx, 31 sets of marten clothes, 13 sets of desman (Eurasian muskrat) clothes, and so forth were sold here (Bogoraz 1934:81). Beaver, marten, and lynx furs came to the Chukotka fair from Alaska. In this trade, the Chukchi acted as intermediaries between Russian traders and the inhabitants of Alaska.

In his report, the companion of Capt. F. P. Wrangel, F. F. Matiushkin, provided a detailed description of this fair. "The Chukchi," he wrote, "in our time are only intermediaries in the trade

between the Russians and Americans: they put few of their own products into circulation, other than reindeer hides. . . . The path of this people into Ostrovnoe is quite remarkable: at first the Chukchi cross from the Chukchi zone to America, and having acquired furs and walrus bones there, they set out for Ostrovnoe with their wives, children, weapons, goods, reindeer and houses—a real migration of peoples on a small scale. . . . On the coast of the Chaunsk inlet they trade their tired reindeer with nomadic tribes there and continue further. . . . The Chukchi arrive in Ostrovnoe at the end of January or beginning of February. Here they stay for nine or ten days and then they turn back on the same path. Usually their caravan consists of 300 men, including 100 or 150 warriors."

After the sale of Alaska in 1867 the penetration of American whalers, traders, and spirit haulers into the Bering Sea area increased, and the turnover of the Chukotka fair began to decline and lost significance. The connections of the continental regions of Chukotka with the population of Alaska weakened from this point on.

In the 1890s American entrepreneurs brought 1,280 domestic reindeer and a number of Chukchi herders from Chukotka to Alaska with hopes of establishing a domestic reindeer economy. It happened that the plan did not work out, mostly because the Eskimos, being hunters unaccustomed to guarding and pasturing tame reindeer, did not adopt this type of life, nor did they take advantage of the methods of Chukchi herders, such as the sledge, harness, and *iaranga* (reindeer herders' tent). In addition, hostile relations existed between the local Eskimos and the immigrant Chukchi, who left Alaska and were later replaced by Saami (Lapp) herders from Scandinavia. Further difficulties were encountered because the Chukchi were reluctant to sell live reindeer, thinking this would bring them bad luck in their future relations with this animal. This experiment to introduce domestic reindeer breeding into Alaska showed that the adjustment of hunters to a new economic occupation is a complex process requiring special conditions and a long period of time.

On the whole, the traditional material culture of the peoples of the northern part of the Pacific region, as seen from the evidence provided, represents a complex phenomenon. It arose in the setting of primitive natural economies and communal relations when individual ethnic groups formed under the influence of isolation. Nevertheless, these ethnic groups interacted and influenced one another. And during a lengthy historical development in the northern part of the Pacific Ocean, a chain of interconnected traditional cultures became established.

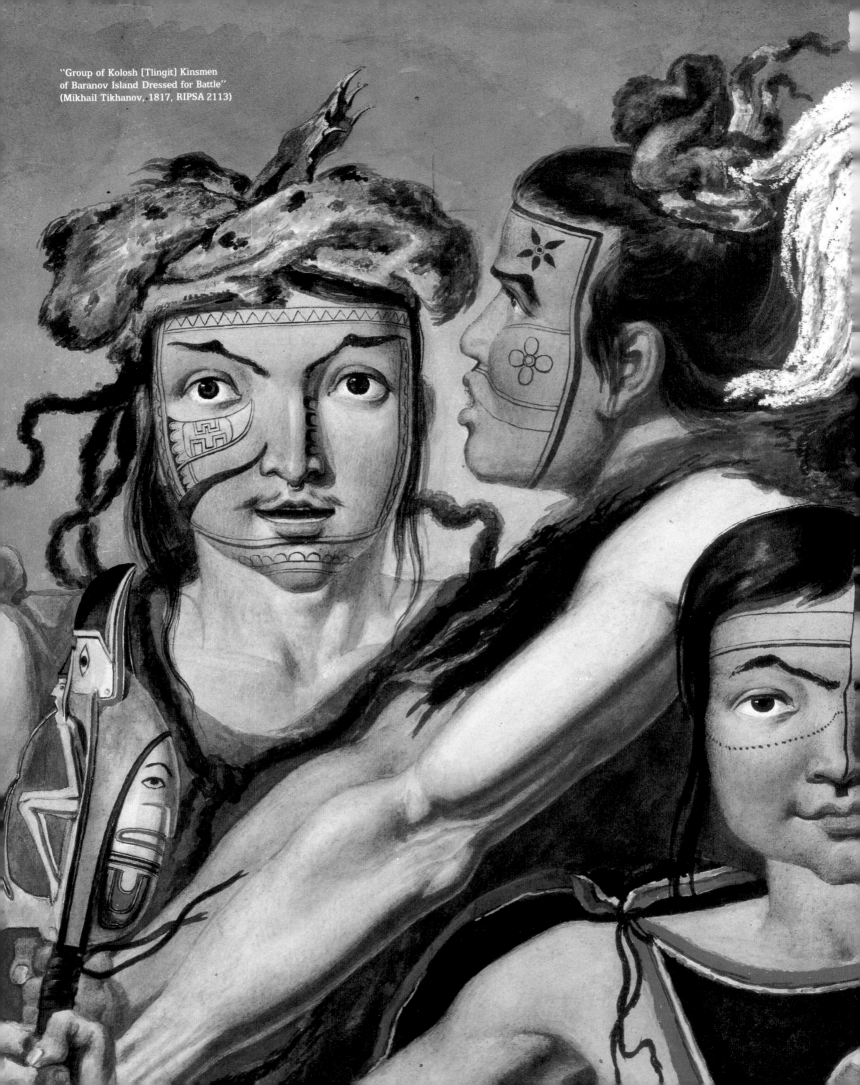

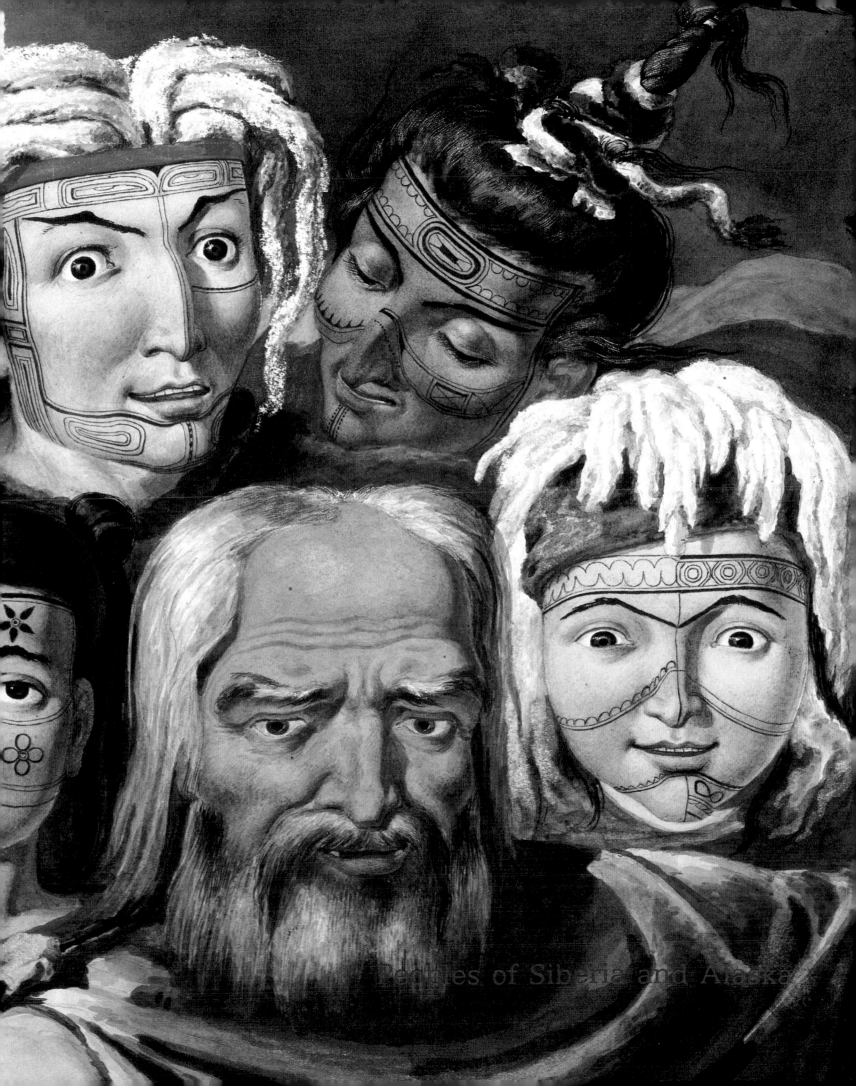

Peoples of the Amur and Maritime Regions

Lydia T. Black

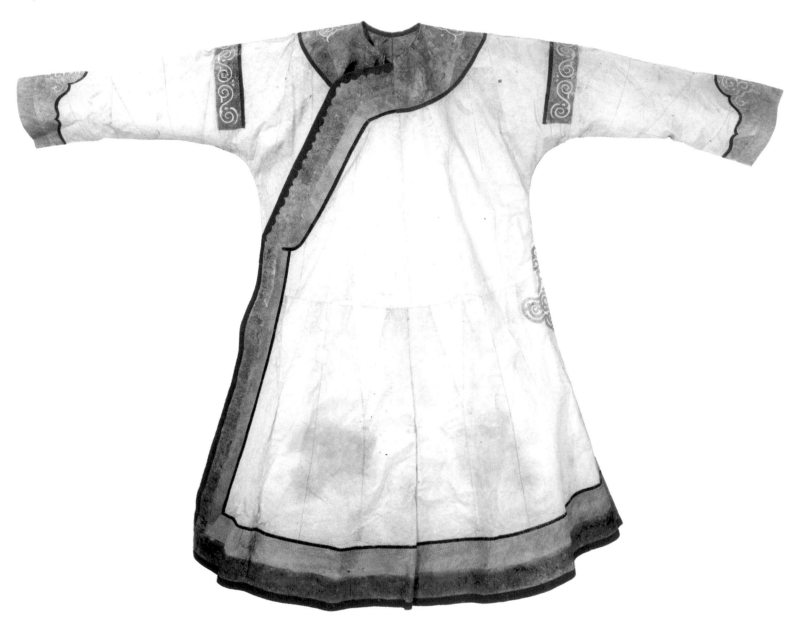

21. Nanai Woman's Coat

Decorative salmonskin coats were worn as summer garments by peoples of the Lower Amur River. Those worn by women were especially elaborate. Decoration on the fronts of these coats was limited to border designs; those on their backs were more complex, composed of symmetrical band and figure decor, often representing abstract cocks and fish (fig. 414). Designs were made with patterns and stencils (fig. 287) that were passed down from mother to daughter. The designs and wraparound cut of Lower Amur area garments reflect Chinese rather than Siberian stylistic influence. AMNH 70-628

The Lower Amur basin and the Maritime Provinces of the Soviet Far East, the Primorie, were, in all probability, one of the major staging areas from which groups of Asiatic Mongoloids spread to the American continents in remote antiquity and from which small groups continued to spread to the Asian northeast in much more recent periods. Ancient trade routes from China and Mongolia passed through this region. The Amur, "the great river," one of the largest rivers of the world, served as the highway along which the populations moved and as the major route of communication that bound together the Asiatic interior and the Polar and Pacific shores. Since time immemorial, the Amur basin was the meeting ground of peoples speaking various languages and of most diverse cultural backgrounds: peoples speaking Turkic, Mongolian, and Manchu-Tungus moved through the basin, expanding into other areas or losing ground, sometimes to fade from the pages of history forever. Since the 17th century, the Chinese and the Russian empires contested for dominion over the region. In the 19th century, Russia finally won control over the Amur, from the confluence of the Shilka with the Argun to the Pacific, and over the Ussuri River southward to the modern Bay of Peter the Great, where the ports of Vladivostok and, more recently, Nakhodka were built.

The several indigenous groups that live in the area today speak, with the exception of the Nivkhi (Gilyak) whose language has not been so far related to any language family, Manchu-

Tungus languages. The speakers of the Southern Tungusic languages, all closely related, are the Nanai (Gold), of whom a small number resides within the territory of China, while more than 10,000 live within the USSR, and the small ethnic groups of the Ulcha on the Amur, the Oroch and Udege of the Primorie, the Oroch occupying coastal areas, and the Udege inhabiting the taiga of the Ussuri River basin and the Sikhote-Alin mountain range. The Orok, a very small group resident on the island of Sakhalin, also speak a Southern Tungusic language. The Negidal, who in the 19th century migrated down the Amgun and then the Amur rivers, speak a Northern Tungusic language closely related to that of the Evenk. The Nivkhi, whose language is an isolate, occupy the mouth of the Amur and a stretch of the coastal area of the Okhotsk Sea to the north of it, and parts of Sakhalin Island. The Ainu occupied a small area on southern Sakhalin until the 1940s. The latter group, like the Nivkhi, speak a language that is an isolate. It is believed that the Ainu formerly occupied territories on the mainland that they gave up under pressure from the Manchu-Tungus speaking groups.

All these groups interacted with each other, and all were subject to the same or similar pressures from their more powerful and much more numerous neighbors and overlords: the Manchu, the Chinese, the Japanese, the Koreans,

and then, much more recently, the Russians. Through the centuries, they borrowed from each other not only items of material culture but also aspects of belief and ritual, while maintaining and, in some cases, developing (as was the case of the Ulcha) independent ethnic identities.

For all groups, their economic mainstay was fishing and hunting, both of land animals for their own use and for trade of pelts to the Chinese and the Russians, and, along the Pacific shore, of the marine mammals. Those groups that controlled good riverine fishing grounds, such as the Nanai and the Nivkhi, were sedentary, occupying permanent winter and summer villages and following a seasonal transhumance cycle. This mode of life may be traced in this area to the Neolithic. Other groups, such as the Evenk-descended Negidal, in the past had a nomadic lifestyle oriented to taiga hunting and to some degree reindeer breeding, and they adopted permanent village life (as well as the Chinese-style dwelling with interior heating system) only after they moved to the Amur and settled near and among the Nanai and Nivkhi. The Orok have remained to the present oriented toward a reindeer economy. The Nanai, on the other hand, among whom certain lineages claimed to be aboriginal and some could be traced to Ainu (probably the oldest population of the area), occupied areas along the southern Amur tributaries, especially along the Sungari. Here they

22. Nanai Family Group
AMNH neg. 41614, Jesup Exp.

Reviewing Berthold Laufer's first attempts at field photography, Franz Boas recommended he hire a professional next time. The result was a series of studio portraits, including this Nanai (Gold) group. Nanai and other ethnic groups of the Lower Amur and Sakhalin have stronger cultural relationships with eastern Asian peoples than with northeastern Siberians. Conical hats, wraparound garments, and scroll decoration are obvious markers of this affiliation.

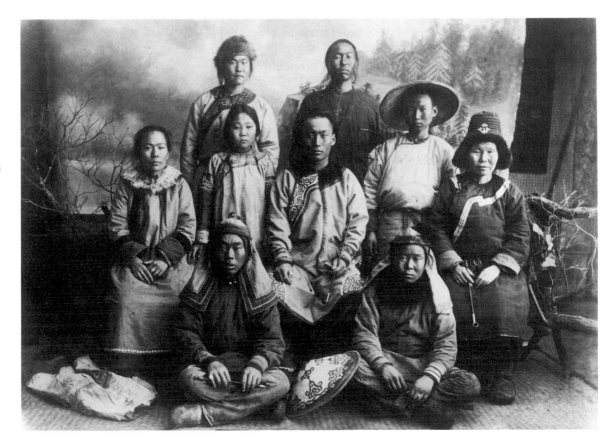

came in close contact with the Chinese and even mixed with them. Nanai (and the Nivkhi) paid tribute to the Chinese tax collectors, traded with the Chinese merchants (and to a somewhat lesser extent with the Japanese via Sakhalin), and from Chinese settlers in their territory learned agriculture and domestic animal keeping, including horse breeding. Both the Nanai and the Nivkhi were master metal workers; the craft was introduced from China by Manchu. They did not smelt ores themselves but made iron weapons, spears, knives, and daggers, as well as iron slat armor and battle helmets, to suit their taste from metal scraps obtained elsewhere. These weapons, especially spearheads, were often elaborately inlaid.

Boat building was well developed among all of the riverine and Pacific shore groups, and a variety of watercraft was used, from birchbark canoes, some of them covered and approaching the skin kayak in shape and in manner of construction, to large plank boats. The Nanai used a double-bladed paddle, much like the kayak paddle of the Aleuts, to propel their birchbark canoes.

Dog breeding was highly developed, especially among the Nivkhi, and dog transport was the preferred mode of transportation in winter (in summer, dogs were sometimes harnessed to boats and towed them upstream). Dogs were also used in hunting. In addition, men used a variety of skis, reindeer or seal skin lined. All men owned several pairs of skis, each pair designed to meet specific snow conditions.

Woodworking was a major craft in which a large tool inventory was employed, with metal tools imported from Japan, China, and later

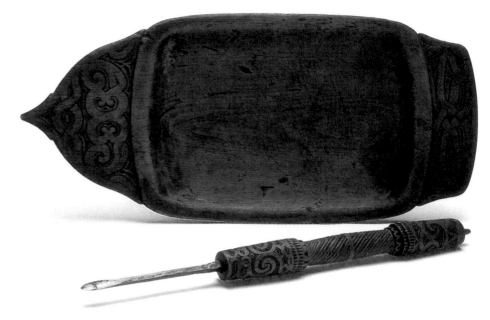

Russia. Wood was used for dwellings, sleds, boats, domestic utensils, and so on. Carved wooden dishes produced for festival use are considered today works of art. Finely carved boxes and cradles were made, though cradles of birch bark were also used. Innumerable were the wooden talismans for warding off illness or bad luck. Dwellings, especially the permanent winter dwellings, and grave houses were elaborately ornamented. Bentwood technology was also employed, especially for skis and sledge runners but also for containers.

Birch bark was an important technological material, used to cover summer dwellings, to make hunting huts and blinds, to cover boat cargo, and for summer bedding and various small items, including women's tool bags and patterns for appliqué embroidery. Women produced decorated birch-bark baskets, trays, and summer hats of exquisite beauty. Twined basketry was made of a variety of materials, predominantly grass, and mats and cordage were made of nettle and other vegetable fibers.

The fishing technology was highly developed, and several fishing methods were employed. Salmon, and in earlier times sturgeon, provided the basis of their economy, though other species, such as carp, pike, and catfish, were also taken. Fish were taken at weirs, by floating nets, seines, dip nets, and lines and hooks. Spearing of fish was also practiced. Fish, fresh, dried, smoked, salted, and soured (fermented), provided staple food. Fish skin was a basic technological material used for clothing and footwear, window and skylight coverings (instead of window glass), waterproof cargo covers on sleds and boats, and various small items, such as pouches. Fish glue

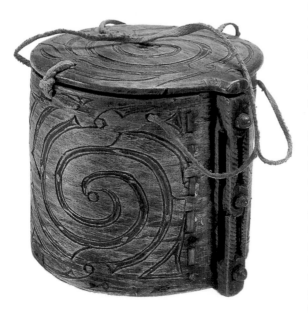

23. Wood Box
Nivkhi: AMNH 70-870a,b

Laufer was interested primarily in the art of the Amur region and published a slender volume on this subject. As he never published a full ethnographic report, little is known of the functions and details of the objects he collected. Laufer did note that most of the decorated pieces he obtained were from remote villages and had long been in use. Losing their ritual association, decorated objects were being replaced by undecorated utiliarian pieces.

This storage box illustrates the prominence of spiral motifs in Amur art. Generally absent in the Eskimo area, spirals are common in Aleut material culture (fig. 75).

24. Nivkhi Woodworking
AMNH 70-871 (tray), 70-881 (drill)

Peoples of the Amur region were masters of woodcraft art. Working with a few simple tools, they made a wide variety of wood artifacts, including boats, most of which were ornamented with interlocking scrolls and spirals cut into the surface in low relief. Drills like the one illustrated here, operated by two men with a socket and bow cords, were used for doweling wooden boats. Use of iron nails in boats was ritually prohibited. Nivkhi boats carried stylized representations of seabirds on their prows (Black 1973; Shrenk 1899:251).

was an important product, used in production of fishskin clothing and footwear and in boat building, gluing birch-bark covers, for example. The fishskin clothing, especially garments made for festive occasions, such as wedding costumes, or shaman's robes, in many colors, with complex designs that have much in common with Chinese and Manchu decorative arts, are outstanding examples of the technological sophistication and aesthetic achievement of the Amur peoples (Shrenk 1883–1903; Laufer 1902).

For the riverine populations, land mammal hunting was a subsidiary, though important, enterprise, both in terms of economics and social prestige. Others, such as the Udege, relied primarily on hunting. Animals such as elk and deer were hunted for meat. Small game and game birds were also hunted for food. Sable, marten, and raccoon were hunted for their furs, for trade. Udege also took wild boars and wolves and occasionally, in self-defense, tigers—a creature not normally hunted but often conceptualized as a manifestation of the supernatural. Bears, also associated with the supernatural, were hunted by all groups. Bear hunting was a high-prestige enterprise, accompanied by elaborate ritual, especially among the Nivkhi. Capture of live bears or bear cubs, to be reared in the settlement and later ritually killed in the course of the bear festival commemorating deceased ancestors, had an extremely great social value among the Nivkhi and the Ainu. A man could go against the bear alone or in a group.

Men hunted with bow and arrow and with a spear. Spears and the bows were often elaborately worked and decorated, conferring prestige on the owner. Some men owned powerful composite sinew-backed bows with baleen or horn and silver insets, a conspicuous status marker.

In more recent times firearms came into wide use. However, most animals were taken by traps.

Trap technology was most elaborate, ranging from deadfalls, to nets, to nooses, to forked sticks, to pit traps, and to "automats": crossbows triggered when an animal disturbed a line. Udege took deer and elk by means of fence traps supplemented with pits dug or automats placed at the openings in the fences.

Those people who occupied territories along the shores of the Pacific Ocean hunted sea mammals: bearded seal, seal, and, among the Nivkhi, white whales. Sea mammals provided an important source of food and technological materials. They were also a trade item in the intergroup barter.

Marine mammal hunting was a collective enterprise. The animals were taken on shore, on the ice, from boats, and on floating ice floes. When hunting by boat, harpoons were used. The Ulcha developed a unique weapon (described by A. V. Smoliak 1966:40–41), a kind of floating harpoon, with a wooden "rudder" attached to the harpoon head and the rudder affixed to a 100-foot-long rod, composed of six to eight long poles. This harpoon could be directed by an experienced hunter in any direction he desired. It was also used to take from shore sea mammals on floating ice. Clubbing of animals hauled out on large ice floes was also practiced. The sea mammal carcasses were divided among the hunting crew, but there were variations in the rules for the division from group to group.

The Nivkhi preferred open-sea hunting, which commenced when the rituals directed at the Master of the Waters (begun at the breaking up of winter ice) were completed and the sea was relatively free of ice. The owner of a large boat

25. Knife and Sheath
Nivkhi: MAE 36-162a,b

The Nivkhi were also known for their excellent metalwork, which they forged from iron, brass, copper, and silver stock obtained from the Japanese and Chinese. According to Shrenk, knowledge of metallurgy was hereditary and privileged. Certain towns specialized in the production of metal implements, and its producers became wealthy. This specimen is inlaid with lead, copper, and brass and carries band and fishscale pattern designs. Its sheath is made of embossed sturgeon skin.

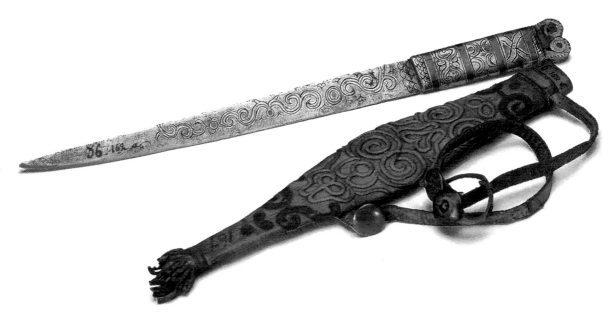

organized the crew and took care of the boat's equipment and provisioning. Affines were as a rule chosen for the crew, which had to consist of strong oarsmen, a good helmsman, and a good shot who took up his position in the bow. During the hunt, all men (and their wives at home) observed elaborate rituals and behavioral prescriptions. All animals taken were ritually treated before being dressed, such as being "fed" with special grasses brought along for that purpose.

Hunting the white whale (and rarely whales of other species) was a special enterprise among the Nivkhi. The animal, driven into shallow water, was hunted with harpoons equipped with floats, played out, then dispatched, ideally by a single thrust of a spear to the breathing hole. The carcass was then towed to the village, where it was met by drumming on a wooden board by an old woman. The boat bringing in the whale was beached bow first—the opposite of the usual practice. The head of the white whale was laid on the board that had been used for drumming the whale in. The carcass was "fed" and then divided among the entire village. The eyes were buried, together with certain ritual grasses, near shore, near the village, at a place dedicated to the Master of the Waters.

We can conclude this brief overview of the material culture and subsistence activities of the peoples of the Amur with the observation that variations in microenvironment and ideological orientation of the group resulted in significant differences in the way people made their living and in customs associated with subsistence activities.

The main organizing principle of the social structure of the peoples of the Lower Amur was the principle of agnatic kinship. An individual was born into a named exogamous patrilineal lineage or clan. Each named kin group was associated with the lineage or clan fire (which only males could handle, with the oldest male of the lineage guarding the clan fire-making apparatus used in religious ceremonies), clothing, and other symbols of clan unity. Among the Nivkhi, and apparently in the past also among the Tungusic-speaking peoples of this region, there were prescriptive rules of marriage, which specified the clans from which a young man could take a spouse. Among the Nivkhi, a clearly articulated rule prescribed marriage with mother's brother's daughter; that is, a man always took a bride from a lineage from which his father's, paternal grandfather's, and uncles' wives came. This resulted in a permanent alliance of lineages bound by the ties of affinity. Among the Tungusic-speaking peoples of this area, there were permanent alliances of clans (sometimes

called phratry, or locally, *dokha*). Marriage between clans of a *dokha* was not permitted. It is not clear if the *dokha* was analogous to the moiety organization known from the Northwest Coast of America and from South America. Among the Ulcha, the dual division by residence on the right and left riverbank developed, but it may not coincide with clan and *dokha* membership.

Marriages were polygynous, and a household consisted of an extended family; that is, of an older male, his spouses and children, his younger brothers and their spouses and children, and their sons with their spouses and children. The levirate was practiced by all groups—that is, when a man died, his lineage "brothers" took on his widows as wives and adopted the children. A form of avunculate existed: the mother's brother or, as among the Ulcha, mother's father's brother was responsible for training of the boys in all essential skills, specifically hunting and fishing skills. At the boy's wedding, this uncle presented the young man with a gift of an ornamented bow and spear and addressed the young couple with a stylized oration on their duties and proper conduct in life.

A young man's kinsmen offered bridewealth to the bride's family; the bride, in turn, brought to her new family a dowry. Only the poor men performed bride service for their bride's parents in her village. In exceptional circumstances, such a poor man could join the residential unit of his wife. Normally, the bride moved into her husband's father's house. She was subject to supervision and often control by her mother-in-law, and in the case of the junior wife, by the senior wives, unless the latter were childless or had no sons. Although the women had relative freedom, their lot was not always easy, and protest suicide by young women was not infrequent.

Among the Nivkhi, members of a lineage and, among the Tungusic-speaking peoples, members of the *dokha* or clan alliance were responsible for joining in retaliation for injury done to any of the kin-group members. Feuds persisted for several generations. However, mediation was possible and was frequently resorted to. Among some of the Tungusic-speaking groups there were formal interclan courts; among others, as among the Nivkhi, well-known mediators were called to negotiate the case, with the injured party receiving recompense for losses suffered.

The clans and lineages were associated, in ideology, with territory, and each clan or lineage had its own hunting and fishing grounds, the title validated by use. This was reflected in the clan and lineage names, which were derived from localities historically occupied by the given

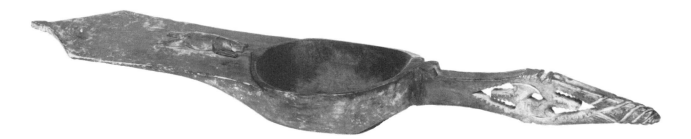

26. Bear Festival Bowl
Nivkhi: MAE 5536-165

Bear ceremonialism was an important feature in the ritual life of many Siberian peoples, and was particularly strong in the Amur region. Similar in many ways to Northwest Coast potlatches, Amur bear ceremonies were performed in honor of a deceased lineage member and took several years to prepare for. First a bear was captured and reared—using long-handled spoons—within the lineage house. After its sacrifice, the bear was eaten by the assembled guests with specially prepared utensils.

Symbolic designs on this bowl include representation of the flight of a bear spirit whose tracks and trail are shown as gouges and grooves on the left handle; notches, spirals, and cutouts decorate the other.

27. Festival Spoon and Amulet
Nivkhi: ANMH 70-891, 70-1205

Ornamented spoons made by designated specialists were used in ritual observances prior to the bear festival. These spoons were carved with representations of bears, sun, and moon, linked by spiral bands. The spoon illustrated here has two bear cubs at its end—a reference to the capture and rearing of a particular set of animals. Other spoons in the set portray other events in a bear festival. The bowl of the spoon is decorated with a sun and a swastika-like image of unknown meaning.

The small bearlike amulet represents a class of evil spirits known as *mil'k* that often appear in the guise of lizards, frogs, and toads.

group. In reality, the settlements were multi-lineage ones, and residential ties were often stressed in actual situations, such as recruitment of hunting crews for big land or marine game.

The clan structure was emphasized in religious rituals. The belief and ritual systems of all the Amur peoples were complex and, in recent historic times, syncretic. In the 19th century, most of the Amur groups were officially Orthodox Christians, but shamanism and the complex of beliefs associated with the environment—such as Master of the Mountain/Forest and Master of the Waters, belief in the material form of animals and their essence, conceptualized as anthropomorphic—persisted. Among many of the Tungusic-speaking peoples, especially the Nanai, Oroch, and Udege, the tiger was especially revered. The bear, among all the Amur peoples, like the tiger, was associated with males. The bear was subject to numerous ritual observances, but some groups, the Nanai for example, had no bear festival, so characteristic an observance among the Nivkhi and the Ainu.

Among the latter, the bear symbolized simultaneously the unity of agnates from generation to generation, the deceased ancestors who have entered, after death, the lineage of the Master of the Mountain/Forest, and the Master of the Mountain/Forest himself, who provided the abundance of land animals. As do all focal

symbols, the bear communicated many meanings, depending on the context in which the symbol was used.

The bear, seen in many aspects as human-like, was subject to ambivalent attitudes: mainly, he was seen as a stand-in for benevolent supernaturals, but sometimes also as a dangerous and at times a vindictive and harmful one. Consequently, rituals associated with the bear image could be eucharistic, as were the Nivkhi and Ainu bear festivals, or when individuals invoked the bear's aid against illness or for assistance with fishing, as among the Nanai, or apotropaic, when the aid of the shamans was needed for protection against malevolent powers loosed against an individual by the bear. A great number of amulets, therefore, represent stylized images of bears, but it is seldom possible to know if their function was eucharistic or apotropaic and which concepts associated with the bear image these figurines represented (Ivanov 1937).

The bear, like the tiger in Nanai ideology, could transform himself into a human form and enter into sexual relations with humans. Among the Nivkhi, one of a pair of twins was believed to be a bear-child. Among the Ainu of Sakhalin, the bear was considered the supernatural ancestor of certain lineages, and according to an early ethnographer of the Nanai and Oroch (Lopatin

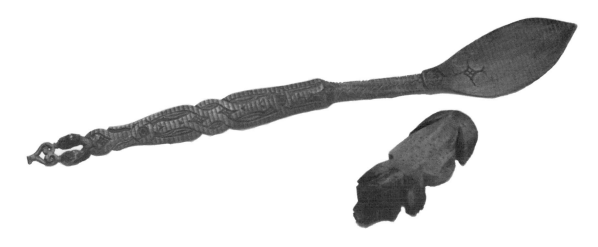

1922, 1925), similar beliefs were found among the latter groups. Arsen'ev (1926) reported analogous beliefs among the Udege. Among the Nanai, the bear was one of the most powerful, if not the most powerful, spirit-helper of the shamans. Among the Nivkhi, shamans were barred from participation in the bear festival. Nevertheless bear talismans are found among the shamans' paraphernalia, and bears are pictured on the covers of the shamans' drums; but the shaman costume, among all peoples of the Lower Amur, does not have bear pendants.

It was mentioned above that among the Nivkhi the bear could represent the Master of the Mountain/Forest who sends to the Nivkhi all the land animals they use. Among the Tungusic-speaking peoples, the Master of the Mountain/Forest sends them only bears. Clearly, the conceptualization of the bear as a supernatural varied between the Tungusic-speaking groups of the Lower Amur and among the older populations of this area, the Nivkhi and the Ainu. The bear rituals among the Tungusic-speaking peoples were hunting rituals. Among the Nivkhi and the Ainu, the bear ritual was a clan or lineage festival in which the unity of ancestors and descendants was reaffirmed and the kinship links through males stressed. The festivals were given by the agnatic lineage and attended by members of other lineages tied to the feast givers by affinity. Among the Nivkhi, it was the affinal male relatives who killed the bear by bow and arrows at the ritual killing ground. It was a festival celebrating the unity of the male kinsmen, both the agnates and the affinally linked ones. Women, among the Nivkhi, had a subordinate role in the festival; they danced a bear dance, though, and drummed the bear in, and when the bear, before being ritually slaughtered, was led through the settlement from house to house, women, like men, dressed in festive clothing, formed part of the crowd that escorted the animal. Among the Ainu, women's participation in the bear festival was somewhat greater; particularly, they lamented the coming sacrifice of the animal they had raised from a cub. They were, however, absent from the act of killing the bear.

The bear festivals of the Nivkhi and Ainu were of two kinds; scheduled ones, given in winter, when bears either reared or kept in captivity for some time were ritually killed; and occasional ones, when a bear had been killed by the hunters. The latter were much less elaborate than the regularly scheduled winter festival.

To sum up, the ritual and belief systems of the peoples of the Lower Amur combine elements of ancestor veneration and abundance rites directed to the forces of nature (defined by their complex cosmology into the forces of the above and the below, the land and the sea or water).

Among the Tungusic-speaking peoples the unity of the above and below, the heavens and waters, is symbolized by the image of the spider-woman. In these beliefs the aid of benevolent ancestors is also invoked.

The protective rituals directed against malevolent spirits (symbolized among the Nivkhi by insects) were performed by the shamans. Shamanistic rites included curing, divination, rituals averting misfortune or restoring harmony (following a disaster or unhappy experience), and many others. A shaman could also invoke the aid of malignant spirits to inflict misfortune on an enemy.

Among all groups, mortuary rituals were characterized by complexity. Death demanded special rituals and clothes. Among the Nivkhi, the manner of death determined the destination and fate of the soul in the afterworld. Therefore, funeral rites differed for those who died of old age, illness, by drowning, in war or by violence, or for those who were killed by bears, and so on.

In the course of history, Chinese and Manchu (and Korean) and eventually Orthodox Christian influences were very important, and many imported notions were incorporated by all groups into their worldview and ritual practices. The clothing of the Amur peoples' shamans closely resembled those of the Manchu shamans. Nanai celebrated the Chinese New Year, incorporated aspects of some Chinese cults, and used Chinese icons, so that some of the shaman's spirit images look conspicuously like Buddhist pictures on fabric (Levin and Potapov 1964:714). Shamanism and membership in the Orthodox Church were often perceived as compatible. It is not clear if any revitalization cults emerged in this area, but the reported appearance among the Tungusic speakers of an interclan cult focused on an interclan deity (Kheri Mapa) in the beginning of the 20th century points in that direction (Levin and Potapov 1964:714).

After the commencement of the Soviet reconstruction in 1924, the traditional life of the peoples of the Amur underwent rapid and fundamental changes. Their economy is now based on collective farm organization, from agricultural collectives among the Nanai to hunting collectives among the Nivkhi, and fishing and reindeer-breeding collectives elsewhere. A significant portion of the population has been integrated into the wage labor economy of the overarching society. There was a significant shift of the population from traditional small ethnic or clan settlements to larger cities and towns and to multiethnic settlements focused on state-supported economic enterprises. The trend is toward assimilation into the larger society, though ethnic identity is still expressed specifically through local, ethnic arts that are marketed through state-supported cooperatives, wearing of ethnic clothes on civil festival occasions, and so on. The Nivkhi won the right to conduct the winter bear festival, but under governmental pressure the timing of it is supposed to coincide with the anniversary of the Bolshevik revolution in November. The complex art of the people of the Amur is widely publicized, and so is the folklore, published in the Russian language and translated into several European languages (Nagiskin 1980).

Through education, employment, introduction of modern medical care, the Soviet local governance pattern through the village council or soviet, and through contact with the ever increasing number of permanent settlers from other areas of the USSR, the traditional life of the peoples of the Amur has undergone a dramatic change, and the direction of this change seems to lead toward eventual assimilation into the mainstream society.

Koryak and Itelmen: Dwellers of the Smoking Coast

S. A. Arutiunov

28. Imported Technology
Koryak: AMNH 70/3655a,b (upper, with sheath); 70/3441 (lower)

These knives were made by local Koryak blacksmiths who had only recently begun to practice this art. The large knife was the utilitarian side arm of the region, having been formerly used as a weapon of war. In peacetime it served as an all-purpose knife and hatchet for chopping wood and frozen meat. Its handle is of whalebone; its sealhide sheath was worn across the shoulders. The designs on the blades came from Amur River prototypes and are based on opposed cocks, a Chinese emblem passed to the Koryak through Evenk (Tungus) hands. The design of the handle on the small knife is a Yakut motif that Jochelson was told represented a stylized larch tree.

Two ethnic groups occupied the peninsula of Kamchatka. The first section of this essay concerns the Koryak, who inhabit the northern regions of Kamchatka and adjacent mainland; and the second, the Itelmen, who dwell in the southern part of the blade of the peninsula, near the Ainu.

The Koryak, the Chukchi's closest southern neighbors, did not display the latter's ethnic homogeneity. The Reindeer Koryak, closest to the Chukchi, represented almost half of the Koryak population. "Koryak" is not a native ethnonym but was created by the Russians from the root *kor*, meaning "reindeer," originally as *korak*, he "who owns reindeer." The Koryak did not have a global name for the ethnic group as a whole. Reindeer Koryak called themselves Chavchuv, in the same way that the Reindeer Chukchi called themselves Chauchu, whereas the Maritime Koryak called themselves Numulu, "the village inhabitants."

The Koryak consisted of eight territorial groups, speaking morphologically and phonetically very different dialects. Because of the mobility of the Reindeer Koryak, their dialect was the lingua franca and was chosen as the standard dialect for the modern written language.

The Chavchuv Koryak practiced reindeer herding on foot, like the Chukchi. Every year the herd moved to the rich mountain pastures for the summer. The nomadic camp was set by a river rich in fish, since fishing was an important resource, even for Reindeer Koryak.

The Aliutor Koryak, living in the Kamchatkan isthmus, combined small-scale reindeer herding with sea hunting and fishing. In the summer, during the spawning season of the salmon, the population migrated to the river mouths and left the herd to young herders.

Maritime Koryak hunted seal on the ice with dogsleds or in polynyas from kayaks and umiaks similar to those of the Eskimo, but shorter and wider. Besides kayaks and umiaks, dugout canoes (*bats*) were used on rivers, and sometimes two of them were joined as a catamaran and used boldly on the open sea. Accounts from the 18th century describe how the Koryak hunted small whales with these catamarans and umiaks in the past, chasing the whale into a large net of thong secured to the shore and then attacking it with spears and harpoons.

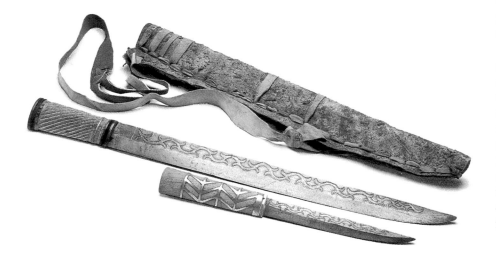

Fishing played an important role among all Koryak. Fish were caught, mainly, with fish traps in weirs, but at the beginning of the spawning run, when the weirs were not yet built, fish were harpooned with a hooked harpoon, or *marik,* known among the peoples of the Amur and the Ainu under the same name, and with hand nets. Fish was dried in large quantities for both people and dogs, and also (mainly for dogs) was fermented in pits.

The staple food for the Reindeer Koryak was boiled reindeer meat. Marrow, kidneys, and cartilage were eaten raw. As among the Chukchi, Reindeer Koryak traded with Maritime Koryak for sea mammal meat and fat and dried fish. Fish was the staple food among the Maritime Koryak, who ate it boiled in summer and dried and fermented in winter. Fish heads, brain, cartilage, and eyes were eaten raw. The favorite food was seal and beluga meat and fat.

The Koryak ate a large quantity of vegetable foods. Among the peoples of Northeast Siberia, only the Itelmen surpassed them in this respect. Roots of the wild lily, roots and sprouts of *Carex,* leaves of wild *Rumex,* young sprouts of *Epilobium,* and many others were eaten as an accompaniment to fish and meat dishes. *Empetrum nigrum* and *Vaccinium uliginosum* berries were added to reindeer and seal meat together with wild roots, as in American Indian pemmican. The *Vaccinium* berry was the basis of a slightly intoxicating beverage, but a strong intoxication, leading to the shamanistic trance, was provoked by chewing the mushroom *Amanita muscaria,* also known as fly agaric.

Reindeer were the property of the family, and so was reindeer meat. But seal meat and fat were equally distributed between all the members of the village at the return of the hunters, and only the seal skin remained the property of the hunter who struck the seal.

Working tools like canoes and traps were family property. They could be sold between families. But large fishing nets were often collective property of related families.

As in the case of the Chukchi, there were no clan divisions among the Koryak. But some customs are considered remains of this division, for example the prohibition against transferring fire to a family of another kin, certain kinds of cooperation between related families, blood revenge, and others.

There was, in Maritime Koryak settlements, as in Eskimo settlements, and partly in Maritime Chukchi settlements, a ''keeper of the place,'' *numelgenan* in Koryak or *nunalik* in Yupik Eskimo, who was also the keeper of traditions and tales. He was always a direct descendant of the

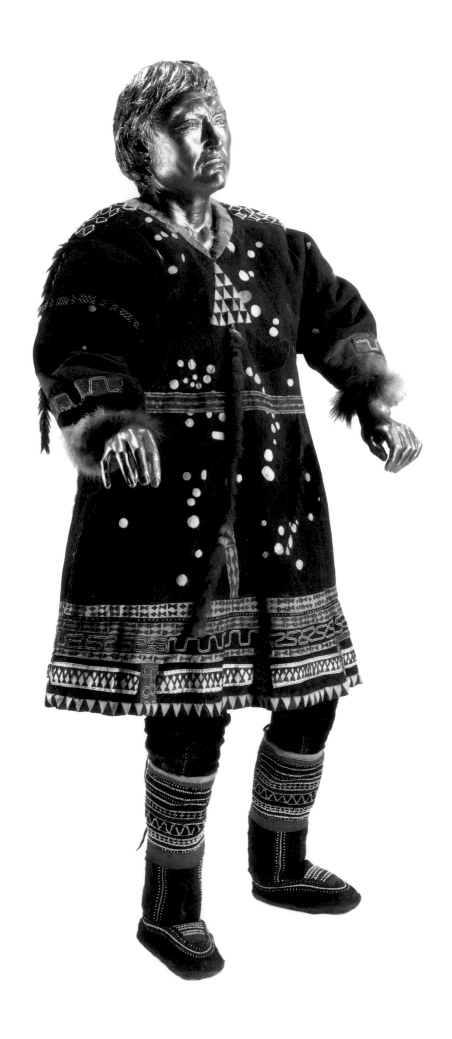

29. Koryak Dancer

Dancing was an important part of Koryak social and religious life, and special costumes were created for this purpose. This Koryak man is seen dancing in a coat of tanned reindeer skin ornamented with tassels and embroidered designs. The spots may represent stars. Tassels, celestial bodies, and information given to Jochelson suggest this garment may have belonged to an Aliutor shaman. Leggings and boots are decorated with Venetian trade beads. AMNH 70-3892 (coat),-5185a,b (pants), -5260a,b (boots)

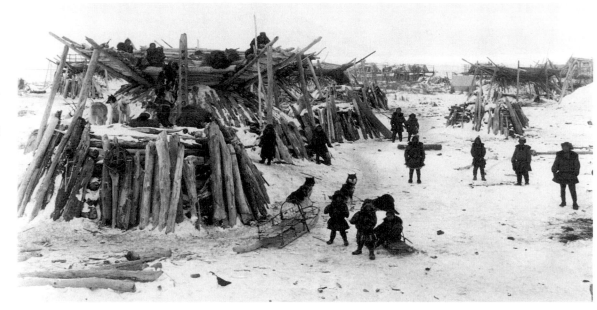

30. Koryak Winter Villages

AMNH negs. 4123 (above), 4139 (right), Jesup Exp.

These two photographs of the Maritime Koryak villages of Kuel (*above*) and Big Itkana (*right*) were taken by Jochelson in the spring of 1901. Koryak houses were octagonal in plan and were built partially underground with log crib walls. In winter, entrance was by ladder through a hole in the center of the roof. A "storm roof" in the form of an inverted cone kept snow from covering the dwelling and served as a storage area and open-air workplace in good weather. Side entrances were used in summer. Storage structures were positioned around the periphery of the dwellings. Three to five such houses constituted a typical Maritime Koryak winter village.

founder of the village. The group, led by a *numelgenan*, had a *numelgen*, a wooden representation of the totemic zoomorphic type, which was worshiped. The places where the spirits lived, such as rocks, waterfalls, remains of ancient dwellings, were cult objects as well. In addition, each family maintained a cord to which were attached seated wooden figurines representing the ancestors, each with a hole in the place of the mouth so that they could be "fed" with fat during celebrations.

The Koryak myth cycle is comparable to that of the Chukchi and Itelmen and very close to Eskimo mythology. Heroes of the myths are Raven and a series of half-human, half-beast creatures, such as bear, wolf, and fox creatures, and also people-roots, woman-grass, and others. Each Koryak group had its own cycle of heroic legends of warfare with their neighbors, although some of these were common to all Koryak.

Practically the entire Koryak population lives today in the Koryak Autonomous Territory. The same ancient tribes contributing to the origins of the Chukchi played a role in the ethnogenesis of the Koryak, but in the case of the Koryak, these were influenced by the maritime proto-Eskaleut substratum of northern Kamchatka. The spreading of the Even on the Okhotsk Sea coast reduced considerably the territory of the Mari-

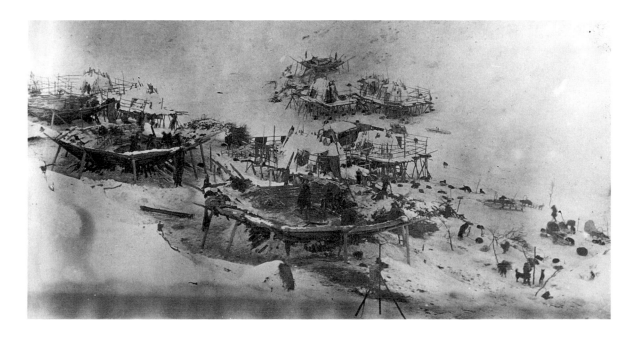

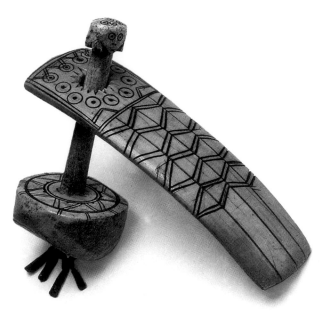

Nivkhi suggest that at least some of the ancestors of these groups were originally geographically close to one another, most probably along the Okhotsk coast, later occupied by the Koryak. Numerous examples of Koryak ornamentation, in particular on sewing reels, are reminiscent of Nivkhi and Ainu style. It is useful to recall, though, that until the 18th century the Ainu population was partly settled in southern Kamchatka as well and undoubtedly left its influence on aspects of Koryak culture.

The primary inhabitants of southern Kamchatka, however, were the Itelmen. The contemporary Itelmen retained their language and ethnic identity only in a few villages in the south of the Koryak Autonomous Territory.

The Itelmen were once a large people, which was almost completely assimilated in the 19th century by the descendants of the Russian Cossacks and peasants who had settled in Kamchatka in the 18th century. The result of this

time Koryak and forced part of them to shift to reindeer breeding. The part of the population of Koryak reindeer herders who were former maritime people immediately came in conflict with the Reindeer Chukchi, who set raids against them and stole their herds, and captured prisoners too, especially women. A reverse tendency was observed among the Chukchi, where many reindeer herders joined the maritime population after they lost their animals.

The Koryak traditional territory encompasses the land originally inhabited by proto-Eskaleut tribes, before their migration to eastern Chukotka and Alaska, and the land along the Okhotsk Sea coast bordering these ancient proto-Eskaleut tribes and a population of Nivkhi, who occupied then a much larger territory than today. It is difficult to find the direct heritage of the Eskaleut substratum in the contemporary Koryak culture, although harpoon technology, the kayak, and the sea hunting tradition in general were possibly part of it. Other remains of this ancient heritage can be found, for example, in the clothing. The ethnic Koryak clothing did not resemble that of the Eskimo, but the Koryak funeral outfit, made out of white reindeer fur with a ''tail'' in the back, was similar to that of ancient and ethnographic Eskimo clothing.

Nowadays, the Koryak culture zone lies between Eskimo and Aleut territory on the one hand and Ainu and Nivkhi territory on the other. The distance between these is so great, even on the Siberian scale, that the idea of common ethnic origins may seem odd. However, many features of mythology, belief, ritual, and social structure linking the Eskimo and Aleut to the

assimilation was an ethnographic group of Russians known as Kamchadal.

In the past, a variety of distinct Itelmen dialects existed with three main subgroups, northern, southern, and western. Only two dialects of the western group, strongly influenced by the Koryak language, survive to this day. Although Itelmen language is classified as a ''northern paleoasiatic language,'' like the Koryak and Chukchi languages, linguists believe there is no original relationship between Itelmen and Koryak or Chukchi and that the elements they hold in common are a result of mutual contact and borrowing from each other.

31. Spinner
Koryak: AMNH 70-6303
This walrus ivory object is described by Jochelson as a spinning game, but no further details are provided. Four faces decorate the spindle head; tin tinklers are attached to the base; and ratchet grooves ring the spinner hole. Edward Nelson (1899: fig. 31) described similar, but undecorated, implements from St. Lawrence Island as mechanical devices used to twist sinew thread. Perhaps Koryak women learned to enliven their laborious task with a game.

32. Koryak Jewelry
(Clockwise from upper left) MAE 442-7/7, 442-7/5; AMNH 70-3684; MAE 442-6/5
Koryak blacksmiths made ornaments from iron, brass, and copper using cold-working techniques. Unlike their neighbors to the south and west, Koryak women had not yet developed a taste for silver, and even wealthy reindeer breeders' wives still preferred baser metals and lively sounds. These Maritime Koryak bracelets have tin tinklers, whaletails, and other ornaments attached. Earrings and a crescent pendant complete the set.

The fundamental source of information on the ethnography of the Itelmen of the 18th century was written by Stepan Krasheninnikov, who participated in the Second Kamchatka Expedition under Vitus Bering between 1737 and 1742 (Krasheninnikov 1972).

As far as subsistence is concerned, the Itelmen were first of all fishermen, using hooks and nets of nettle fiber. During the spawning season they dried and fermented large amounts of fish, primarily salmon. Fermented fish heads were considered a delicacy. Land-animal and sea-mammal hunting had little significance, but seals and sea otters were occasionally caught. In southern Kamchatka a mixed Ainu-Itelmen population hunted whales with poisoned points like the Aleut. Food gathering was much more developed among the Itelmen than among any other northeastern Siberian group. Roots of wild lily and other roots, edible grass and leaves, pine nuts, and others were collected in great quantity. Dogsleds of a characteristic type were the main means of winter transportation, and dugout canoes (*bats*) and catamarans made of sets of these boats, similar to those of the Koryak, were used on rivers and on the sea.

Several Itelmen villages were organized on a clan basis and were often in conflict with one another.

The migration of the ancestors of the Itelmen from the west of Kamchatka took place during the Climatic Optimum, during the Siberian neolithic period, long before the ancestors of the Chukchi and Koryak arrived, according to N. N. Dikov, who also believes this may explain the traditional importance of vegetable-gathering in Itelmen culture.

Today, the Itelmen fish, hunt furbearers, breed milk cattle and horses, and practice garden agriculture. Economically and in their way of life, the Itelmen are no different from their neighbors, the Russian population of Kamchatka.

33. Pendants
Even: MAE 445-6/1 (left), 445-6/3
Even jewelery demonstrates more refinement than seen among the Koryak, who were at the fringe of expanding metallurgical knowledge. Brass, in particular, was more common to the west, and these Even pendants, called "throat medals" and believed to ward off colds, follow styles popular among Yakut and Tungus groups. Together with the profusion of beaded decoration on Even clothing, they indicate the social attraction of new technologies that were spreading into Northeastern Siberia.

Even: Reindeer Herders of Eastern Siberia

S. A. Arutiunov

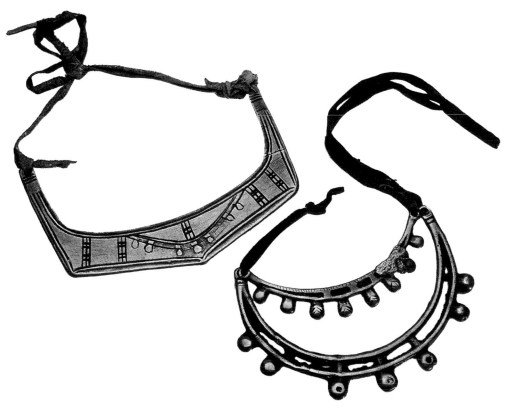

In prerevolutionary literature, and in most western literature, the Even are known as Lamut. The name "Lamut" was originally given to the Even by the Yakut people, whereas "Even" is an autonym, a name used to describe themselves. In the Tungus languages, *lamu* means "sea," in particular the Okhotsk Sea, and this is probably the root of the name "Lamut."

The Even are closely related to the Evenk group (formerly called Tungus), who are widely spread in Siberia between the Ob and Amur basin regions but separated from the Even by the Yakut ethnic mass. The Even are mainly settled on the northern coast of the Okhotsk Sea, in the middle and southern part of the Indigirka and Kolyma river basins, and in northern Kamchatka. Their neighbors are the Yakut to the west, the Yukaghir to the north, the Chukchi to the northeast, and the Koryak to the east and southeast.

In the 19th century, the Even were regarded as a local group of Evenk. Seventeenth-century sources, indeed, called the same groups indistinctly Lamut or Tungus. It is difficult to draw the boundary between Evenk and Even clan and tribal names. However, the Even language, despite dialect variations, is characterized by certain features that differentiate it from the language of the Evenk, in particular the dropping of the last vowel and consonant of the word. The formation of the Even as a separate ethnic entity probably is related to the absorption of a large number of early Yukaghir, Koryak, and possibly some local peoples by a group of northeastern Evenk. The contemporary prominent specialist on the Evenk, V. A. Tugolukov, believes that the Even first originated around the confluence of the Lena and Aldan rivers when an ancient local Uralic population even older than the Yukaghir shifted to a Tungus language. Pushed by the arrival of the Yakut in the 13th century, the eastern Even migrated to the north and lost their ethnic identity by merging with local groups to constitute the Nganasan and Dolgan peoples.

The present ethnic boundaries of the Even territory are fairly recent. The northern coast of the Okhotsk Sea was still occupied by the Koryak in the 18th century, and the Even settled in Kamchatka only 150 years ago. The Even as an ethnic entity were finally established during the 15th through 17th centuries in the basins of the Indigirka and Kolyma rivers as a result of the merging of the immigrant eastern Tungus element with the local Yukaghir substratum. Thus, although the Even per se are a fairly recent ethnic group, their cultural heritage encompasses features of ancient Siberian groups.

Even culture and economy are based on reindeer herding and hunting. The Even raised a much smaller number of reindeer than the Chukchi and Koryak and valued them most of all as means of transportation. Milking of reindeer was known only to southwestern Even, who lived in close contact with the Yakut. Lamut reindeer were larger and much stronger than Chukchi and Koryak reindeer. The Chukchi and Koryak were eager to exchange two of their reindeer for one Lamut reindeer. The sledge was relatively rare among the Even in the past, since it had been borrowed quite recently either from the Yakut or from the Koryak and Chukchi, and existed only among Even having close contacts with these groups. This type of reindeer breeding (i.e., initially exclusively for transportation, for hunting expeditions, and also frequently as

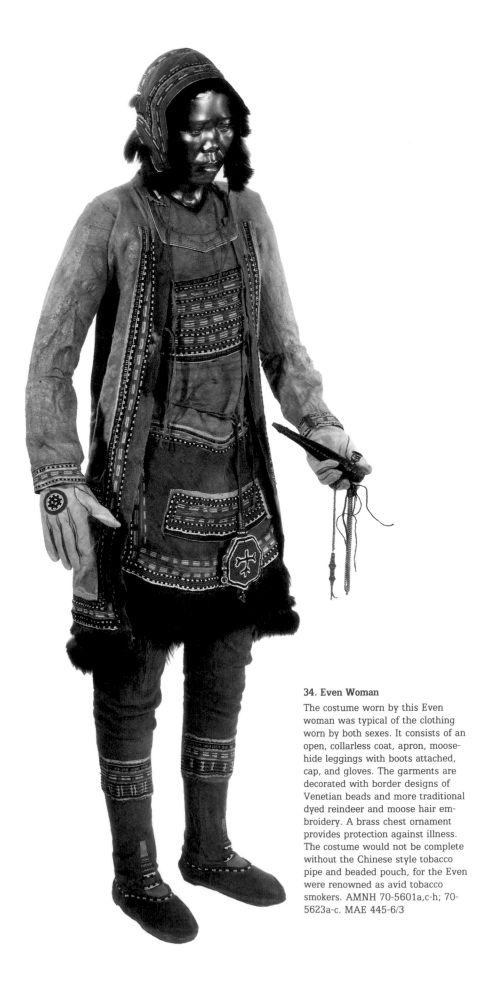

34. Even Woman

The costume worn by this Even woman was typical of the clothing worn by both sexes. It consists of an open, collarless coat, apron, moose-hide leggings with boots attached, cap, and gloves. The garments are decorated with border designs of Venetian beads and more traditional dyed reindeer and moose hair embroidery. A brass chest ornament provides protection against illness. The costume would not be complete without the Chinese style tobacco pipe and beaded pouch, for the Even were renowned as avid tobacco smokers. AMNH 70-5601a,c-h; 70-5623a-c. MAE 445-6/3

a lure for wild reindeer hunting) represents an archaic stage of reindeer breeding, perhaps close to the form of this complex when it originated. Soviet scholars believe that reindeer breeding originated around A.D. 0 among the Tungus-speaking ancestors of the modern Even and possibly also simultaneously among the Southern Samoyed, their close neighbors, in the Sayan Highlands region in the south and west of Lake Baikal. Here the complex emerged as a result of contact with the horse-breeding cultures of the ancient Turks and Mongols of Central Asia or, possibly, also with the last remains of Indo-European cattle breeders and horse breeders of Central Asia, the eastern Scythian or Massaget of the Altai.

Having borrowed the horse from the latter groups but experiencing difficulties with horses in the tundra, the ancient Tungus tried to use horse saddles on the domestic reindeer, which they already had at the time but used only as lures in hunting. The experience proved successful, and the saddle reindeer was born.

Milking of reindeer was practiced only by reindeer breeders who lived in close contact with peoples who were engaged in milk cattle breeding, such as the Yakut. As far as large-scale reindeer breeding is concerned (i.e., when reindeer were raised mainly for meat and hides), this was possible only in the large pastures of the tundra and mixed-forest tundra and, in general, did not begin in Northeastern Siberia before the 17th and 18th centuries. Among the Even, it was fully developed only at the end of the 19th century and in the 20th century.

In the 19th century, even, the Even did not slaughter their reindeer for meat under normal conditions, since their herds were quite small and represented too valuable an economic asset. The basic source of subsistence was hunting game: wild reindeer, fox, and mountain sheep. Wild reindeer were taken by individual hunters on skis with a dog or more often mounted on a saddle reindeer. After contact with Russians, the main source of cash income became the fur trade, especially squirrel pelts. Hunting dogs of the Even were highly valued in Kamchatka and Chukotka, but they were not used in herding. As among the Chukchi, dogs were tied up when near the reindeer herd, since they would otherwise scare the herd or attack the animals. The only case of dogs being used in herding was when the herd entered an area where mushrooms abounded. Such areas are common in tundra and forest tundra, and the herders particularly dislike them. Reindeer are so fond of mushrooms that in searching for them, the animals would spread out in every direction, becoming completely dispersed. When this occurred, the herder tied the dog to a long leash and made it bark, which scared the reindeer and made them quickly gather together again. The Even also fished in rivers and lakes, but not significantly. Until the development of collective cooperatives, fishing interfered with herding activity. Fishing requires a long stay in an appropriate spot, whereas herding is a nomadic activity with constant moving. Therefore fishing remained secondary for most of the Even and became important only among the Even of the Okhotsk Sea coast, who fished with nets made of nettle fibers, fish spears, and hooks for dog salmon when they ascended the adjacent rivers to spawn.

Today, large-scale herding is still the main activity of the Even, and fishing the main activity of the Okhotsk Sea Even. These two enterprises are financially very rewarding. However, many families also rely on fur trade to provide cash income.

The traditional dwellings, clothing, and utensils of the Even differ significantly from those of

35. Apron
Even: MAE 454-3

In cut and function, Even aprons closely resemble European aprons. Set within dyed reindeer skin borders, a delicate geometric design has been created in this garment by weaving strips of dark skin through slits in undyed skin, and by lines of dyed reindeer hair embroidery bounded by a blue and white beaded border. Siberian reindeer hair embroidery produced similar visual effects to that seen in moosehair and porcupine quill embroidery in New World clothing decoration (fig. 298).

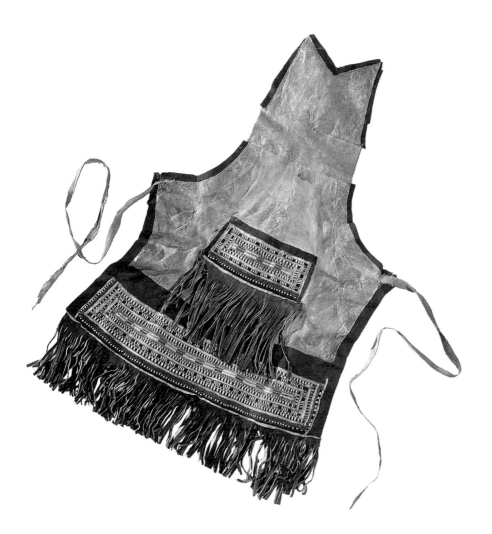

the Chukchi and Koryak. At the same time, the Even preserved archaic features characteristic of the pedestrian (as opposed to reindeer-riding) hunters of the taiga, which disappeared among the Koryak and Chukchi who used the reindeer sled as their predominant means of transportation. Examples of these archaic features are the opened coat with the breast piece and apron, richly ornamented with beads, and the conical dwelling known as the *chum*, similar in form to the American tepee.

The Lamut had several types of dwellings. The most ancient and simple one, the *chum*, or *diu* in Even, similar to the Evenk *chum*, had a conical structure covered with hides or birch bark. The *chorama-diu* was more complicated (fig. 257). The structure of the *chorama-diu* was erected in a circle with an even number (8, 10, 12, or 14) of bipods, each of which consisted of a pair of 1-meter-long poles. Horizontal beams were placed on the tops of the bipods, forming a circle on which the poles for the conical roof were tied. The *chorama-diu* is a transitional form between the *chum* and the *iaranga*, the typical dwelling of the Koryak and Chukchi. The structure was covered with processed reindeer hides. The Okhotsk Sea Even also used fish skin. In the 18th century the semisedentary Maritime Even lived in semisubterranean houses with an entrance on the side or through the roof and, in the summer, in dwellings made of larch bark. The latter were of the same construction as the *chorama-diu*, but since bark is not flexible, they were octagonal rather than round. These dwellings had two entrances, one facing the east, one facing the west. Wooden planks were used to make a floor from one entrance to the other, delimiting the central hearth from the lateral sleeping areas, which were covered with skins.

Even households, utilizing common nomadic pastures, hunting, and fishing grounds, were united in a nomadic group. Each family looked after the common herd in turn. In the summer, some families traveled with the animals, while the other part of the group caught fish and made dried fish reserves, which were later distributed to all members of the nomadic group. The Even practiced ancient customs in distributing game, more particularly a custom common to every Tungus group, called *nimat*. The principle of *nimat* is that neither the hunter who caught a land animal nor his family could keep the game for themselves. The hunter had to present the game to another family of the camp, who distributed the meat between the families, giving to the hunter's family their own share. *Nimat* was partly extended to sea game, birds, and, to a certain extent, fur animals, despite the fact that pelts were a trade item and played a role as a standard of exchange. When two hunters hunted together, the hunter killing the fur animal had to give it to his partner, no matter how valuable the pelt was. The obligation, of course, was reciprocal. This custom was strictly observed in bear hunting. The man receiving the bear as a *nimat* present organized a general feast in which the bear was eaten. The meat of the head and the front part of the body of the bear was boiled and consumed exclusively by men. The bones were disposed in anatomical order on a platform, and the skull was tied to the top of a tree.

Even folklore included genres such as tales, realistic stories, songs, and riddles. The heroes of the songs were animals and birds and stereotyped human characters, such as an old couple quarreling, for example. Part of these tales belongs to the Tungus oral traditions, and the other part is closer to Chukchi and Koryak tales. The Even liked to dance circle dances at festivals. The only musical instrument used was the Jew's harp.

Until the 20th century, the Even were divided in exogamic patrilineal clans, some of obvious Yukaghir origin, others of Koryak origin. The members of one clan might be scattered over a huge territory in various nomadic groups composed of members of several clans.

In conclusion, the Even are a relatively recent ethnic formation who became distinct from the Tungus only a few centuries ago. Local Even groups experienced intensive ethnocultural contacts with Yakut, Yukaghir, Chukchi, and Koryak, from whom they borrowed numerous cultural features without losing their ethnic identity and distinguishing characteristics. At the same time, there is no doubt that very ancient pre-Yukaghir elements from the Uralic linguistic branch, the descendants of the neolithic inhabitants of northeast Asia, played as important a role in the ethnic formation of the Even as they did in the Tungus branch. This ancient heritage can still be observed in the Even way of life nowadays.

36. Chukchi Woman and Child

This Chukchi woman wears the V-necked, hoodless reindeer fur "combination suit", or *khonba*, that was her principal garment, winter and summer. Her tattoos protect her against harmful spirits and sterility, and her bracelet and beads reflect contacts with Russian traders and American whaling ships. The child's combination suit is fitted with a moss or hair diaper. AMNH: 70-7267a,b (earrings). MAE: 256-17 (boots), 395-11 (child's suit), 395-8b (woman's suit).

Chukchi: Warriors and Traders of Chukotka

S. A. Arutiunov

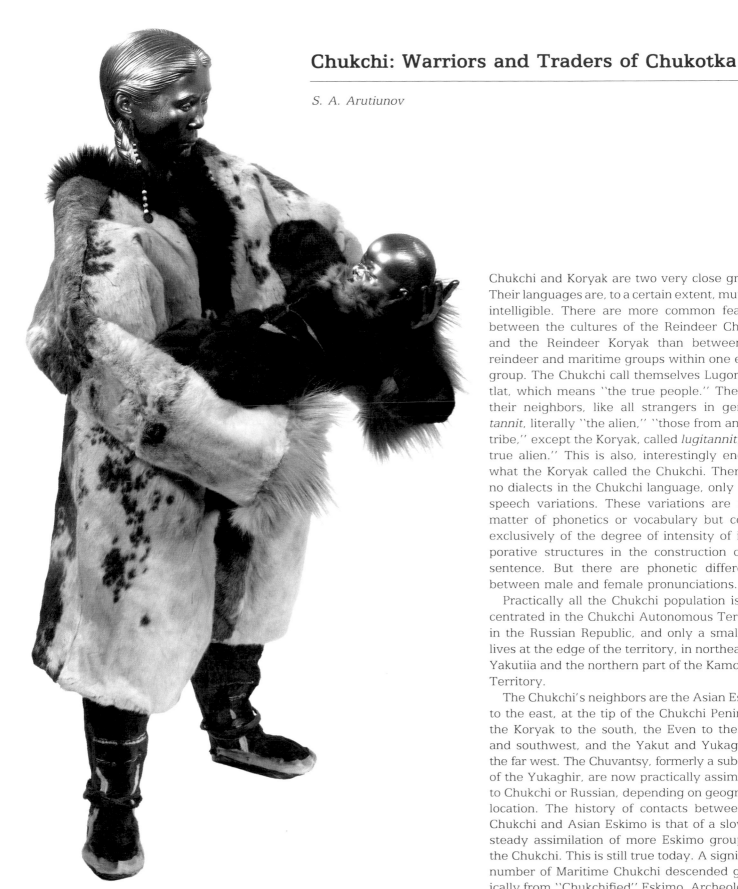

Chukchi and Koryak are two very close groups. Their languages are, to a certain extent, mutually intelligible. There are more common features between the cultures of the Reindeer Chukchi and the Reindeer Koryak than between the reindeer and maritime groups within one ethnic group. The Chukchi call themselves Lugora Vetlat, which means "the true people." They call their neighbors, like all strangers in general, *tannit*, literally "the alien," "those from another tribe," except the Koryak, called *lugitannit*, "the true alien." This is also, interestingly enough, what the Koryak called the Chukchi. There are no dialects in the Chukchi language, only slight speech variations. These variations are not a matter of phonetics or vocabulary but consist exclusively of the degree of intensity of incorporative structures in the construction of the sentence. But there are phonetic differences between male and female pronunciations.

Practically all the Chukchi population is concentrated in the Chukchi Autonomous Territory in the Russian Republic, and only a small part lives at the edge of the territory, in northeastern Yakutiia and the northern part of the Kamchatka Territory.

The Chukchi's neighbors are the Asian Eskimo to the east, at the tip of the Chukchi Peninsula, the Koryak to the south, the Even to the west and southwest, and the Yakut and Yukaghir to the far west. The Chuvantsy, formerly a subgroup of the Yukaghir, are now practically assimilated to Chukchi or Russian, depending on geographic location. The history of contacts between the Chukchi and Asian Eskimo is that of a slow but steady assimilation of more Eskimo groups by the Chukchi. This is still true today. A significant number of Maritime Chukchi descended genetically from "Chukchified" Eskimo. Archeological evidence suggests that around A.D. 0 the entire coast of Chukotka, at least east of 170 degrees longitude, was occupied by the Eskimo. But as far as can be seen, the Chukotkan Eskimo, unlike American Eskimo, never existed as an interior caribou-hunting people. The interior regions of Chukotka were probably occupied by hunters of wild reindeer, the ancestors of the Chukchi and Koryak, by at least 3,000 years ago.

Waldemar Jochelson developed a theory, based on the study of numerous mythological themes (more particularly the Raven cycle among the North American Indians and the Koryak, Chukchi, and Itelmen), according to which there was initially a continuous link between American Indians, on one side, and the Chukchi, Koryak, and Itelmen on the other. In this theory, which was part of Boas's "Eskimo wedge" hypothesis, the Eskimo settled in their present habitat later, disturbing the former continuity of Asian-American coastal peoples. It is, as a matter of fact, reasonable to consider that the Eskimo, or more specifically the ancient Eskaleut, were constituted as a group in the Bering Strait region, with a considerable participation of tribes, migrating from the south, from Kamchatka. It is also highly probable that as a consequence of the constitution of the specific maritime culture of the ancient Eskimo, the cultural links and influences from Asia to America through the Bering Strait, if they did not stop, at least diminished.

However, the ancestors of the Chukchi and Koryak appeared in Chukotka after the Eskimo settled there. The many similarities between the Chukchi, Koryak, and Itelmen on the one hand and American Indians on the other can be explained otherwise. The ancestors of the Indians, migrating from Asia to America, had no reason, so to speak, to leave the Chukchi Peninsula completely empty. On the contrary, only a small portion of them migrated, and the most

significant part would have remained in place. The early neolithic and mesolithic archeological sites of Chukotka probably must be attributed to them. The ancestors of the Itelmen, Chukchi, and Koryak, migrating here from the west, assimilated this local substratum and absorbed many cultural features from them, which explains the striking parallels between Asian and American cultures. Ancient Eskimo were not influenced by this substratum, because they were settled exclusively on the shore.

The overall tendency of ethnic processes in Northeast Asia has been the assimilation of the coastal populations by the interior populations, but not vice versa. The mobility and communicability of the tundra people played an important role in this process, for the maritime settlements were relatively isolated. Although the Chukchi

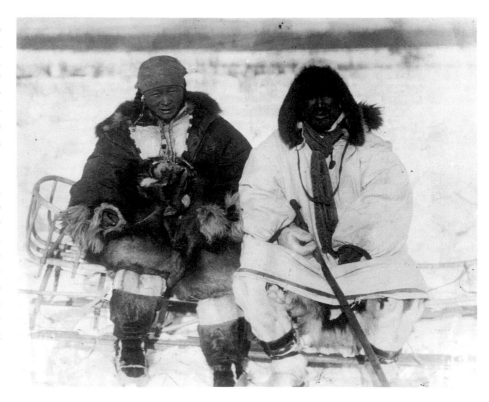

37. Chukchi Travelers

AMNH neg. 11111, Jesup Exp.

Waldemar Bogoras took this photograph of a Chukchi husband and wife relaxing on their reindeer sled on a cold day in Northeastern Siberia. The woman is wearing her warm but bulky one-piece combination suit and fur boots. Scarf, braided pigtails, and beaded earrings and necklace complete her outfit. Her husband is dressed less traditionally, wearing a cloth parka and scarf over fur clothing. He holds a reindeer prod used to guide the animals hitched to his sled.

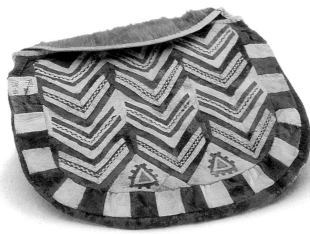

were divided into two distinct groups, culturally and economically, namely the maritime sea hunters and the tundra reindeer herders, these were not isolated from each other. Exchange of products needed by both groups had been in place long ago. These products were first of all reindeer skins for clothing, for the bed curtain (*polog*), and for beds, traded from the Reindeer Chukchi; and blubber, walrus and seal skins, and sealskin thong from the Maritime Chukchi. There was a constant population fluctuation between the two groups by marriage. In some cases, sea hunters shifted to reindeer breeding, but it was more often the herders who had lost their

38. Pouch

Chukchi: MAE 1791-186

This sealskin pouch has a chevron design made of alternating panels of light and dark skin ornamented with strips of appliqué, slit weaving, and spurred triangular motifs, bordered by alternating brown, tan, and green panels. The pouch is typical of work produced by Yukaghir in the Russianized settlements of the Anadyr and Kolyma rivers at which the Reindeer Chukchi trade.

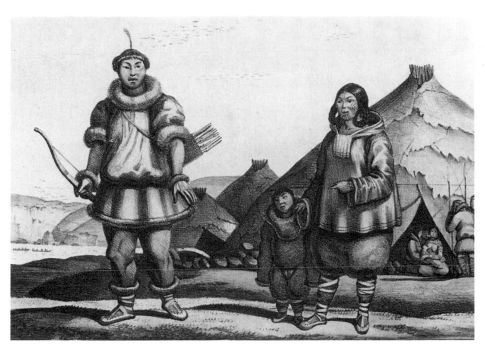

reindeer who became sea hunters. A family, who owned a small herd of about 100 animals or less, practiced sea hunting as an auxiliary means of subsistence. The further to the east, the more significant and developed was the maritime adaptation of the Chukchi, reaching its peak in the Bering Strait region.

Chukchi reindeer herding was the most important in scale, but also the most archaic. Before Soviet jurisdiction was established, with its measures to improve herding, the animals were the responsibility of pedestrian herders. Reindeer sledges were used only as transportation in everyday life. The Maritime Chukchi used dogsleds for hunting trips. Pedestrian herders had to run in the tundra after each reindeer that left the herd. The level of domestication of the Chukchi reindeer was minimal. Even the sled reindeer had to be captured with a lasso, or when attracted by the smell of reindeer urine that every herder carried at his belt in a small pouch. Regardless of the size of their herd, Reindeer Chukchi traded with the Maritime Chukchi, exchanging reindeer hides, primarily, for sea mammal fat, which was used for heating, lighting, and food, and for meat, thong, and sealskins for summer clothing. Without this exchange, Chukchi reindeer herding would have been impossible.

The Maritime Chukchi economy also depended on the reindeer skin trade in the historic period, but before the establishment of the reindeer economy, hides were provided by hunting wild reindeer and polar bear. As far as the preherding ancestors of the Chukchi are concerned, they had little contact with the maritime sea hunters,

but of course, they were fewer than the present-day Reindeer Chukchi, and they did not inhabit the whole tundra but only those areas where wild reindeer were plentiful. Even here, though, judging by legends, they experienced famine sometimes and had to hunt small rodents, such as ground squirrels and lemmings, to survive.

The food of the Reindeer Chukchi consisted mainly of reindeer meat, blood, intestine, and also the contents of the stomach, *rilkéil*, composed of semidigested moss. After the massive slaughter of reindeer in the fall, the large volume of *rilkéil* was prepared for storage, pressed, and frozen. Later it was boiled with blood, fat, and pieces of intestine. The Maritime Chukchi, like the Eskimo, prepared, and still prepare nowadays, fermented walrus meat for the winter, kept in meat caches.

The Reindeer Chukchi lived in *iaranga*s, and the Maritime Chukchi, until the mid-19th century, in semisubterranean houses and later in sedentary *iaranga*s (fig. 258). The main means of transportation was the sled with bentwood suspension runners, pulled by reindeer among the Reindeer Chukchi and by dogs among the Maritime Chukchi. Until the mid-19th century, the dogteam was harnessed in a fan shape, then, under Russian influence, by pairs in a straight long line, numbering between 6 and 12 dogs in a team.

The Chukchi kayak and umiak were similar to the Eskimo's.

The basic hunting and war weapon of the Chukchi, like that of the Koryak and the Even, was a complex bow, reinforced with sinew and

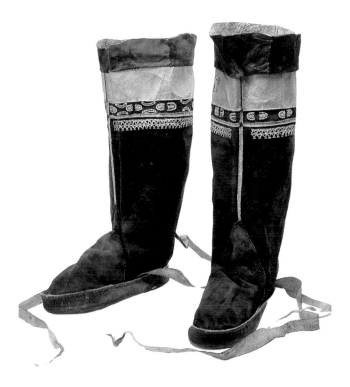

antler strips. Different types of arrowheads were used for hunting wild reindeer, birds, and fur animals and for warfare, the latter having a heavy point that could pierce leather armor from a short distance. Another important weapon was a spear with a thick wooden shaft and a point shaped like a massive knife. This weapon was effective both on the battlefield and when encountering a bear. The taiga hunters, the Even, used it as a machete in the dense forest.

Fishing with hand nets, hooks, and nets on poles had an auxiliary character, as did the gathering of seaweed, shellfish, and wild tundra plants. Bird hunting (partridges, geese, and ducks) and gathering of bird eggs was more important than fishing for the Chukchi people.

The clan type of social organization had become lost among the Chukchi. The Maritime Chukchi social unit was the umiak crew. Men from five or six related families normally formed a crew, the owner of the umiak being usually the helmsman. Sometimes not only relatives but also neighbors of the owner's family were part of the team. Among the Reindeer Chukchi, a similar team was constituted by the members of a nomadic camp, herding the animals together. Patriarchal slavery, the relatively benevolent practice of keeping slaves as auxiliary members of a family group, existed in ancient times among the Chukchi. Slaves usually originated as war prisoners.

Chukchi folklore included myths, tales, life stories, and heroic war legends. The heroes of myths and tales were sea monsters, gigantic predatory worms, human giants, werewolves, six-legged bears, and others. Raven, bear, spider, fox, and wolverine were depicted humorously. The Chukchi had practically no riddles or proverbs but many tongue twisters. The song repertory was not very rich, but the Chukchi knew a large variety of dances and pantomimes and enjoyed mimicry.

Eskimos: Hunters of the Frozen Coasts

William W. Fitzhugh

Alaskan Eskimos are the most numerous and most diverse of all Eskimo populations. Occupying the entire coast of Alaska with the exception of the Aleutian Islands and Southeast Alaska, Eskimos inhabit a wide variety of environments ranging from the North Slope arctic tundras and coasts to the Bering Sea lowlands and the mountainous, forested coasts of South Alaska. Eskimos are known today under a variety of names, "Eskimo" or "Inuit" in Alaska, "Inuit" in Canada, and "Kalaadlit" in Greenland. The geographic extent of their Alaskan territory covers thousands of miles of coastline. To the east, peoples closely related to Alaskan Eskimos occupy the vast expanse of the Canadian Arctic and Greenland, and to the west, across Bering Strait, they inhabited coastal regions of Chukotka (fig. 1). This distribution, more than 6,000 miles (as the raven flies) across the top of the North American continent, made Eskimos the most widespread aboriginal population in the New World.

Throughout this huge region the unity of Eskimo culture is enhanced by their possession of similar languages, similar physical and genetic characteristics, and, to a lesser extent, possession of a common cultural base, the core of which is adaptation to arctic and subarctic maritime environments. Technological, social, and ritual practices surrounding the hunting of arctic marine mammals are the foundation on which most Eskimo cultures rest. For these reasons Eskimo peoples on opposite sides of the North American arctic find more in common with each other than they do with immediately adjacent Indian groups who are their closest inland neighbors.

A set of shared biological features distinguishes Eskimo groups from Indians, Aleuts, and Siberian natives. Genetically, the Eskimo physical type is characterized by a relatively short, muscular body. Facial features are generally thought to be intermediate between those of American Indians and the Asian Mongoloids. Eskimo body type conforms to a general arctic pattern, thought to be an adaptation to cold climate, of flatter faces, shorter appendages, and more compact physique than found among humans in temperate and tropical regions. Genetic studies involving blood types and skeletal and dental morphology tend to confirm an Eskimo biological identity distinct from and intermediate between North American Indians and non-Eskimo Asians, a finding that is consistent with their geographic location between these two population systems (Szathmary 1984).

In actuality, despite similarities, not one but several regionally distinct Eskimo cultures and languages can be identified in the Eskimo ter-

41. Eskimo Dancer

Unlike her more simply dressed Chukchi counterpart, a Bering Sea Eskimo woman took advantage of Alaska's rich supply of furbearers to make this fancy festival parka of ground squirrel, wolf, wolverine, and mink. Imported white Siberian reindeer fur was used for accent. Fur pants, tasseled boots, earrings, and finger masks complete her costume. NMNH: 38451 (maskettes), 38871 (boots), 56070 (earrings), 176105 (parka), T-1611 (pants).

ritories of Siberia and North America. Eskimo languages are part of a larger language system known as Eskimo-Aleut (Woodbury 1984; Krauss, this volume). Eskimo itself is composed of two branches: Inuit, spoken from eastern Norton Sound to Greenland and Labrador; and Yupik, spoken from the shores of Chukotka to Prince William Sound. Although Inuit consists of a single dialect stream, Yupik has five branches, three in Siberia and two in Alaska (fig. 1). The unity of Inuit across the North American Arctic clearly results from the eastward spread of Thule culture from Bering Strait to Greenland about A.D. 1000. This contrasts strongly with the diversity of Eskimo-Aleut languages in the Western Arctic and supports the notion of an Eskaleut linguistic homeland in the Bering Sea region as originally proposed by Sapir (1916). Modern linguists suggest a date of about 4,000 years ago for this Aleut-Eskimo separation (fig. 177).

The contrast between Eastern and Western Arctic languages extends to culture as well. Cultural indicators of the Inuit-Yupik linguistic boundary are evident in many sectors of cultural

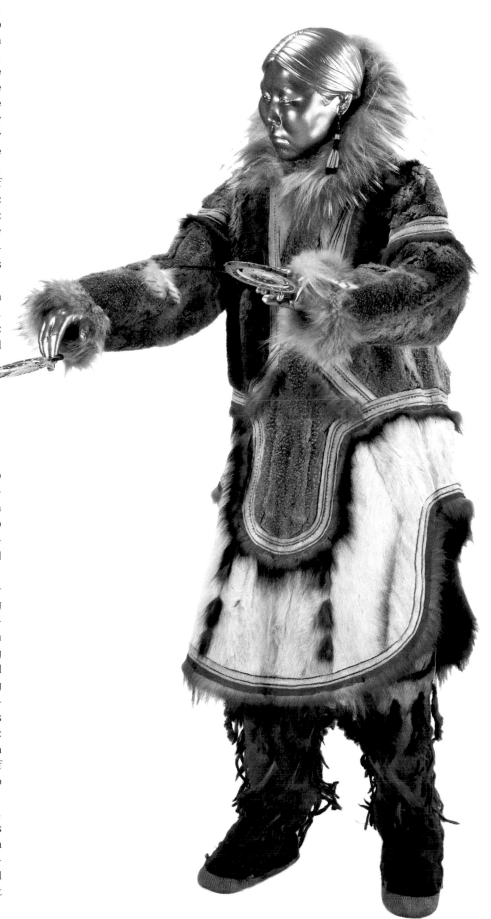

life that in themselves are not closely related to environmental conditions or economic adaptations. Important shifts in mythology occur south of Bering Strait, and many new traits relating to women's and children's culture, like "housewives" (sewing bags), sewing implements, and children's story knives, appear.

This ethnolinguistic boundary located in eastern Norton Sound separated four Inuit-speaking North Alaskan Eskimo groups (North Coast, Interior, Kotzebue, and Bering Strait groups) from three more sharply divergent Yupik-speaking groups south of Bering Strait. The latter included Siberian (including St. Lawrence Island), Bering Sea (including Nunivak Island), and Pacific (including Koniag and Chugach) Eskimo groups occupying these diverse coasts. Hence, linguistic and cultural evidence supports the western homeland hypothesis, contrary to the beliefs of Franz Boas and others who argued for Eskimo origins in Canada.

Given such diversity, any ethnographic sketch, even one limited to Alaskan Eskimo cultures, is bound to be misleading. Therefore, rather than discuss highlights of a composite culture, separate sketches are presented for four regional Alaskan and Siberian groups as they existed at the time of European contact.

North Alaskan Eskimo

The North Alaskan Eskimo (fig. 1) occupied the areas of Alaska north of the forest boundary from Norton Sound to the Canadian border. Living in a variety of arctic and subarctic habitats, the North Alaskan Eskimo were economically diverse. North Coast and Bering Strait groups specialized in hunting whales, walrus, seals, and polar bears. Interior peoples such as the Nunamiut were primarily caribou hunters. Groups around Kotzebue had a more diverse economy utilizing fish, sea mammals, and land game. The largest Eskimo population resided in the Kotzebue area and the smallest on the North Slope interior. However, the largest villages were at the north coast whaling sites where marine mammal, fish, and caribou resources were all available.

North Alaskan Eskimo settlements were concentrated at spits and coastal prominences where marine mammal hunting could be conducted over the ice during winter and by umiak and kayak during the brief open-water season from May to September. Villages consisted of clusters of semisubterranean earth and sod houses (fig. 247) with driftwood or whalebone framing and frequently had populations of several hundred individuals. In addition to dwellings and elevated caches (used to keep food from dogs and marauding wolverines and bears), meat-drying racks, and boat racks, each village had one or more men's houses, known as *karigi*, also used for village ceremonies and festivals. Such men's houses were used by all Eskimo groups in Alaska and to a lesser extent in Canada. They were completely absent, however, in Siberia.

The seasonal round of North Alaskan Eskimo began with the loosening of sea ice in March and the appearance in April and May of waterfowl and anadromous fish. At this time migratory seals, walrus, and whales began moving north along the shore lead, where they fell prey to hunters using darts and harpoons with float gear both from the ice edge and from boats. As in other Eskimo cultures, two types of boats were used, both constructed of sea mammal skins sewn over wooden frames. North Alaskan kayaks were made for single paddlers using double-bladed paddles. Kayaks were suitable for hunting seals and occasionally were used on rivers and lakes for hunting birds and caribou at water crossings. However, because walrus was a more common quarry than seal, large open boats called umiaks were more frequently used by North Alaskan hunters. During the open-water season, umiaks were the dominant form of transport in coastal North Alaska and Bering Strait, used for hunting, trade, warfare, and village movements.

In summer, birds, fish, and sea mammals were the major sources of food, with seal and walrus predominant. Birds were taken with multiple-pronged and blunt-tipped arrows, snares, and bolas. Fish were speared with leisters at stone weirs and were caught with nets and hooks. Harpoon darts were used to catch seals. Fall brought new bird migrations, and a major caribou hunt was conducted to acquire meat and skins for winter food and clothing. Methods for hunting caribou included bow and arrow stalking and communal drives with snares and corrals.

Freeze-up was a quiet period in which people lived off stored food and waited for the sea ice to become firm so that men could move about by foot and dogsled. The early winter months of near total darkness were spent largely indoors, preparing new clothes and holding festivals and ceremonies. As light returned, sealing and polar bear hunting improved, the latter conducted with spears and dogs. In late winter, ice fishing improved, and seals were netted under the ice. Caribou, grizzly bear, and mountain sheep were also hunted, but men had to be careful to wear snow goggles to protect their eyes from snow blindness.

Despite the seemingly large number of resources, life in North Alaska was often unpredictable, and survival could be insured only by successful walrus and whale hunts, with caribou, fish, and birds as important supplements.

Whale meat was especially important for dog food, for without dogs winter hunting, fetching of cached meat, and trade were impossible. Whale meat and blubber also provided the means for early winter festival life when hunting was difficult.

Among northern Eskimos, caribou was the primary material used for winter clothing because the hollow hairs of this animal are one of

42. Baleen Basket
North Alaskan Eskimo: NMNH 372667

The first baleen basket was made at Barrow, Alaska, about 1915 (Lee 1983), after the end of the whaling era. This event resulted from a request by Charles Brower, an American whaler and trader, to Kinguktuk, a local Barrow man, to make a baleen copy of a willowroot basket. The result was so popular that baleen baskets soon became a North Alaskan trademark and a favorite item in the tourist trade. Baleen baskets are made with a single rod core and have ivory finials ornamented, generally, with arctic animals. This basket has a whale tail finial and a fossil ivory starter disc on its bottom.

nature's best insulators. In many areas of Alaska Eskimos wore parkas or frocks made from birdskin, of goose, duck, dovekie, and cormorant, which were nearly as warm as caribou, and far lighter. Summer clothing was made from sealskin, ground squirrel, or muskrat. Foul-weather gear was produced from sea mammal intestines on the coast, and in the interior, from the skins of salmon or other large fish, as in parts of Siberia.

North Alaskan social organization was relatively fluid, with status being determined by hunting skill and ability to provide for community security in terms of obtaining food resources, protecting against outside attack, and maintain-

ing social well-being. Shamans helped interpret signs and performed séances and ceremonies to protect against environmental disasters, disease, and threats from invaders. Status was determined by individual prowess and accomplishment rather than by hereditary or ascribed means. Despite the flexibility of an egalitarian social structure, powerful leaders, known as *umialiks*, emerged from whaling activities, and shamans, who might also be *umialiks*, controlled village spiritual life and had a major impact on community life. In addition, there existed military and trading leaders whose prestige was related to their ability to deal with outsiders, native and European.

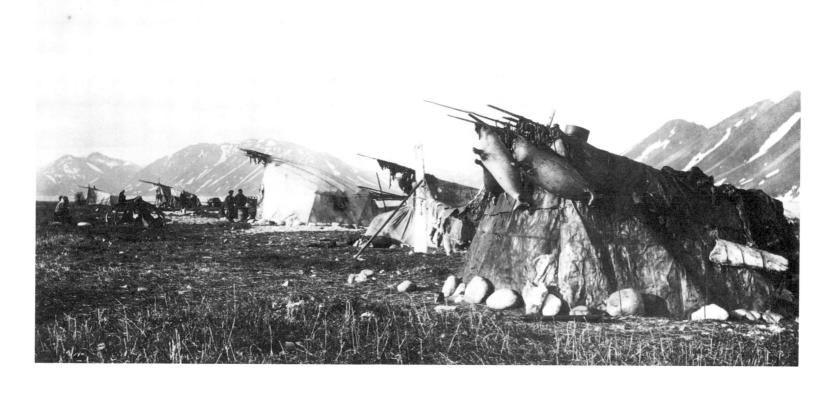

43. Asian Eskimo Village, Plover Bay AMNH neg. 127,519, Jesup Exp. Waldemar Bogoras visited this Eskimo settlement in Plover Bay during his travels around the Chukchi Peninsula in 1901. Skin as well as canvas tents were in use at the time, both being constructed in traditional fashion. Stormy conditions required the use of boulders to hold tent flaps down. Additional security was achieved by hanging cables with weighted ends over the top of the tent. Inflated sealskins used for whaling floats and as food storage containers dry at the tent peak.

Asiatic Eskimos

Asiatic Eskimos occupied the western side of Bering Strait and St. Lawrence Island (Hughes 1984). Formerly numerous, their population was undergoing reduction in the 18th and 19th centuries due to disease and to conflict and amalgamation resulting from Chukchi expansion into the Chukotka Peninsula. Like the North Alaskans, regional economic patterns existed, but as a group Asiatic Eskimos specialized in hunting whales, walrus, and seals.

Asiatic Eskimos lived in large semisedentary clan-based villages along the coast and hunted marine mammals in kayaks and umiaks as did the North Alaskan Eskimos, with whom they shared a similar way of life. Their sites contain large numbers of gray and bowhead whalebones, used both for house and cache construction and apparently also for religious functions. Major sites, such as Whale Alley, indicate the vitality of this whale-hunting tradition and its strong affinities with the traditions of North Alaskan coast Eskimos, with whom they were in contact across Bering Strait.

The economy of all groups of Asiatic Eskimo was similar to that of the North Alaskan Eskimo, except that the absence of significant amounts of land hunting, especially of caribou, gave it a stronger maritime specialization. Even fishing was of lesser importance here than among the North Alaskan Eskimo.

Until the 20th century, the Asiatic Eskimo were divided into three groups with languages that were mutually hardly intelligible: Chaplinski, Sirenikski, and Naukanski (see pp. 146–47). Even more important in Asiatic Eskimo social life than linguistic differences, however, was the division into kin groups, or *nalku*. This feature of Asiatic Eskimo social organization is absent in all Alaskan Eskimo groups. These clans, which were patrilineal (i.e., membership passed through the father's line), controlled rights to resources, residence areas in villages, and even cemetery plots. The oldest, most powerful clans controlled the most convenient locations in a given community and used separate burial grounds from other clans. They controlled access to hunting and fishing areas and determined the composition of whaling crews, war parties, and trade partnerships. Clan politics dominated community decisions, and the ancestral traditions and legends of each clan were maintained separately from those of other clans and were expressed in distinctive rituals and beliefs.

Asiatic Eskimo housing differed from Alaskan houses. Ancient forms were large, round semisubterranean structures occupied by communal families of given clans. In the late 19th century the Chukchi winter tent known as the *iaranga* was adopted. This aboveground structure had stone, sod, and log walls with a domed skin roof. The *iaranga* was divided internally by skin partitions that set off individual family residences known as *polog*s. Another departure from Alaskan Eskimo tradition was the absence of the *kashim*, the men's communal workplace, residence, and community ceremonial center, which for Alaskan groups was a central feature in their social organization.

The Asiatic Eskimo in recent centuries lived in close proximity to the Chukchi and intermarried with them. The population of some settlements, such as Kivak village, was constituted of mixed Eskimo-Chukchi inhabitants. Since they were in close contact with the people of St. Lawrence Island and western Alaska, the Siberian members of the Asiatic Eskimo family often served as intermediaries in the trade between Chukchi and Alaskan Eskimos.

Bering Sea Eskimo

South of Norton Sound lies the vast lowland of the Yukon-Kuskokwim Delta, home of the Bering Sea Eskimo who inhabit its coast, river courses, and tundra to the head of the delta, and south to the Alaska Peninsula. Bering Sea Eskimos speak several Central Alaskan Yupik dialects. They are also culturally diverse, with distinct subgroups located in Norton Sound, Lower Yukon and Kuskokwim rivers, Nunivak Island, and Bristol Bay, home of the little-known and now extinct Aglegmiut Eskimo. Like the North Alaskan Eskimo, Bering Sea Eskimo inhabited both coastal and interior regions, but here the analogy ends. Coastal groups hunted walrus, seal, and beluga but did not engage in the hunting of large whales, which did not visit this coast because of its shallow, muddy waters, which, however, teemed with herring, flounder, and salmon. Interior groups derived their living from fish and bird resources of the Yukon-Kuskokwim Delta and from many land animals, including caribou and grizzly bear, in addition to smaller furbearers whose pelts were highly desired for clothing and were traded north and south, and even across Bering Strait.

One of the most distinctive aspects of Bering Sea Eskimo culture is its complex art and its wide variety of cultural forms. Whether measured in terms of artifact types, design styles, or religious festivals, Bering Sea peoples registered a greater profusion of cultural forms than known historically for other Eskimo groups. In part this resulted from their relatively stable subsistence base and occupation of a large geographic region, including interior regions of the Yukon-Kuskokwim Delta where fish and bird resources, in addition to many types of land game, were available. In some locations along the Lower Yukon and Kuskokwim large permanent villages developed in which semisubterranean winter dwellings and summer plank houses occurred side by side (fig. 249).

Bering Sea Eskimo implements were designed to be pleasing to the animal and natural spirits with which the implements would be associated in use. Hence, ivory harpoon points were or-

44. Retrieval Hook
Bering Sea Eskimo: NMNH 175668
Made to please the spirits of sea mammals, this ivory-pronged boat hook has a spiritual "lifeline" consisting of a broad groove extending down one side on the shaft and up the other. Encircling grooves of this type are common on Bering Sea Eskimo implements and ceremonial items.

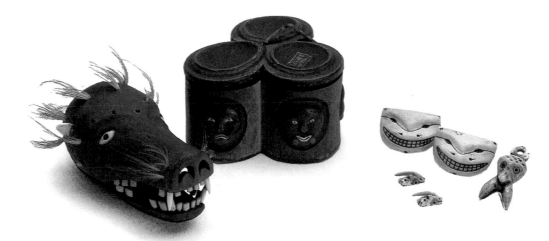

45. Personal Ornamentation

Bering Sea Eskimo: NMNH 176232, 36859, 43720

Bering Sea Eskimos decorated themselves with ivory earrings (seals), pendants (jowly man), and hair clasps (*tunghaks*?).

46. "Beautiful Things"

Bering Sea Eskimo: MAE 571-63 (wolf), 537-4a (box); NMNH 37120 (front spoon), 38635.

Yupik Eskimos of the Bering Sea coast ornamented their belongings to honor the souls, or *inuas*, of animals and objects upon which they depended for survival. These tobacco boxes depict spirits of husband (smile) and wife (frown), and a devilish wolf whose red-painted mouth opens to reveal the storage space. Bone teeth, ivory ears, bristle ornament, and ivory eyes through which blue beads shine complete the masterpiece.

Similar care is given to serving spoons. This set illustrates the mythological transformation between wolf and killer whale.

namented with delicate designs in which the circle-dot motif was usually prominent. Ivory handles for ulus (the curved woman's knife characteristic of Eskimo culture) and pail and bag handles were frequently ornamented with real and beastly animal effigies, and harpoon and dart socket pieces were carved in the form of helping spirits. Many of these carvings and motifs continued artistic traditions rooted in Old Bering Sea and Punuk cultures of the previous 2,000 years. Masking traditions and festival life were equally elaborate. These and other features have led scholars to identify Bering Sea Eskimo cultures as the most artistic of the historic Eskimo groups.

An interesting feature of Bering Sea Eskimo culture is the importance of Raven in their mythological beliefs. Raven stories, many of which are similar to those found among Northwest Coast Indians, have been cited as evidence of contact with Pacific peoples. However, many of the northern Inuit myths are missing along

the Bering Sea coast, especially the central myths of Sedna, the sea goddess, and Loon, seemingly the alternative to Raven as trickster-operative. Traces of Sedna myths exist, however, among Siberian Yupik. Also of note are the many parallels found between Yupik culture of the Lower Yukon and Kuskokwim and Ingalik Indians upriver from them. These Ingalik adopted many features of Yupik culture, including their mythology, festival cycles, masking traditions, houses, and many forms of material culture. Contact between the two groups was frequent and trade well established.

At the time of European contact Bering Sea Eskimos were among the most isolated and most traditional of all Eskimo groups. Because of their occupation of the lowland coasts, which were not frequented by whales or by whalers, their life was being maintained largely as it had been for generations, with limited contact with the outside world. A further feature of their culture was its distribution throughout a wide geo-

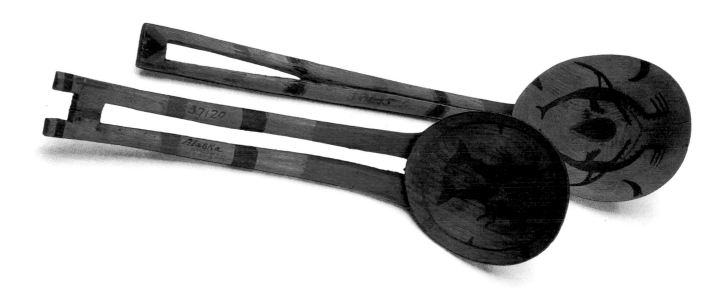

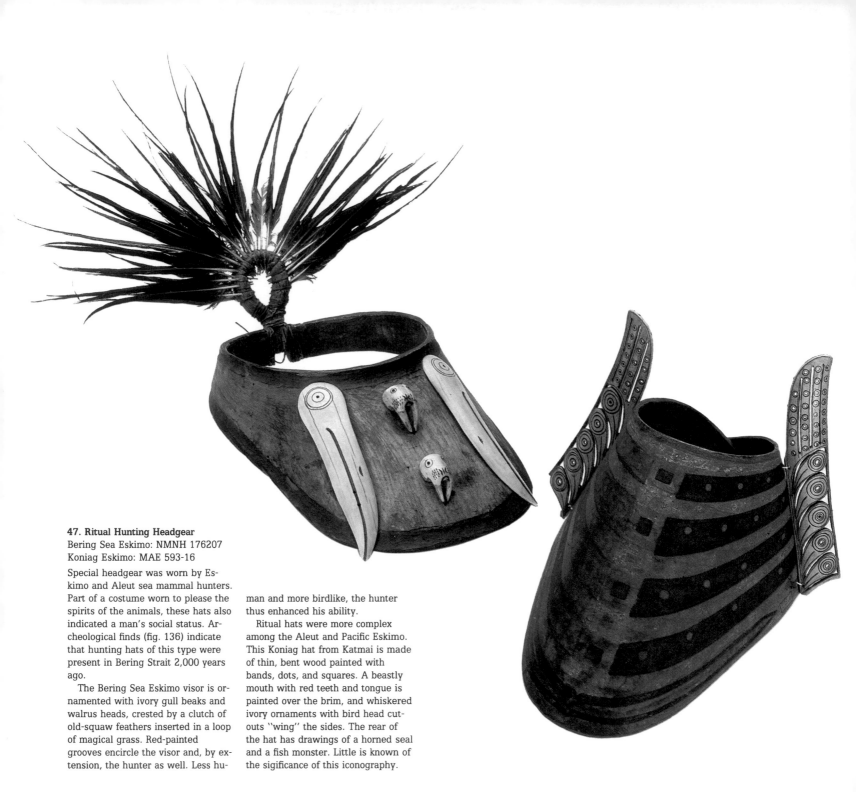

47. Ritual Hunting Headgear
Bering Sea Eskimo: NMNH 176207
Koniag Eskimo: MAE 593-16

Special headgear was worn by Eskimo and Aleut sea mammal hunters. Part of a costume worn to please the spirits of the animals, these hats also indicated a man's social status. Archeological finds (fig. 136) indicate that hunting hats of this type were present in Bering Strait 2,000 years ago.

The Bering Sea Eskimo visor is ornamented with ivory gull beaks and walrus heads, crested by a clutch of old-squaw feathers inserted in a loop of magical grass. Red-painted grooves encircle the visor and, by extension, the hunter as well. Less human and more birdlike, the hunter thus enhanced his ability.

Ritual hats were more complex among the Aleut and Pacific Eskimo. This Koniag hat from Katmai is made of thin, bent wood painted with bands, dots, and squares. A beastly mouth with red teeth and tongue is painted over the brim, and whiskered ivory ornaments with bird head cutouts "wing" the sides. The rear of the hat has drawings of a horned seal and a fish monster. Little is known of the sigificance of this iconography.

graphic region along the coast of southwest Alaska and in the hinterlands of the Yukon-Kuskokwim Delta, where large numbers of Eskimo villages were found along the river courses and the tundra lakes. These conditions provided Bering Sea Eskimos with a population base greater than that of the coastal-dwelling Eskimos and larger and more stable than that of the caribou-hunting Eskimos of the Alaskan North Slope. Although large fish runs, migratory birds, and a wide variety of marine and land mammals provided the means for a secure life, these resources were not particularly suited for intensified resource production, and even contact with Russian fur traders between 1820 and 1867 had relatively little effect in altering Bering Sea Eskimo traditional economy and culture. Serious European epidemics struck during this period, but Bering Sea Eskimos continued to live a rich festival life, using elaborate ceremonial masks and manufacturing artfully designed implements and weapons until the introduction of Christianity began in the 1880s. Even today, traditional Yupik culture remains strong in Southwest Alaska, and language retention is excellent.

Pacific Eskimo

Along the south coast of the Alaska Peninsula, in Cook Inlet, in Prince William Sound, and on Kodiak Island, was found the fourth distinct group, the Pacific Eskimo. Today, these people often prefer to be known as Aleut, and call their language Alutiiq, emphasizing their historically linked ancestry with Aleut peoples with whom they have become associated as a result of Russian colonial enterprises. Anthropologically, Pacific Eskimo culture seems to have been derived from an early establishment of Yupik Eskimo culture in South Alaska with subsequent influence from Aleut and Northwest Coast Indian groups. The South Alaska coast was one of the most productive regions in the North Pacific, with relatively mild climates, prodigious salmon

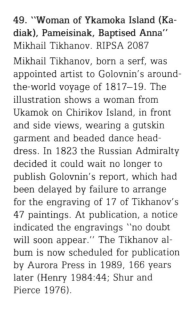

48. Beaded Dance Headdress
Koniag Eskimo: NMNH 90453
This fine beaded headdress was collected from Koniag Eskimo living at Ugashik on the north side of the Alaska Peninsula in 1883. Made of sinew thread and glass beads, it bespeaks of wealth amassed by successful Eskimos in an era when European goods began to flood the North Pacific coasts.

49. "Woman of Ykamoka Island (Kadiak), Pameisinak, Baptised Anna"
Mikhail Tikhanov. RIPSA 2087
Mikhail Tikhanov, born a serf, was appointed artist to Golovnin's around-the-world voyage of 1817–19. The illustration shows a woman from Ukamok on Chirikov Island, in front and side views, wearing a gutskin garment and beaded dance headdress. In 1823 the Russian Admiralty decided it could wait no longer to publish Golovnin's report, which had been delayed by failure to arrange for the engraving of 17 of Tikhanov's 47 paintings. At publication, a notice indicated the engravings "no doubt will soon appear." The Tikhanov album is now scheduled for publication by Aurora Press in 1989, 166 years later (Henry 1984:44; Shur and Pierce 1976).

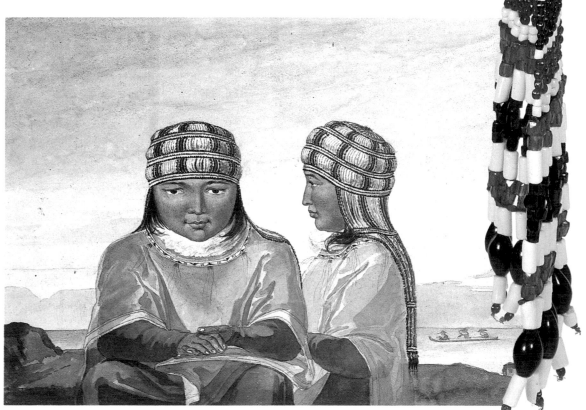

and other fish resources, and large stocks of land game and avifauna.

More is known about the culture and people of Kodiak Island, known as Koniag, and the Chugach of Prince William Sound than about the Eskimo groups of the Alaska Peninsula and Cook Inlet, who shared these territories with Tanaina Indian groups. Kodiak and Chugach groups shared a similar environment. Here, whales, seals, sea lions, sea otters, and fish, including many species of salmon, cod, halibut, and herring, provided the basic sustenance. Land game included grizzly bear, elk, black bear, and caribou, the latter three found only on the mainland. Plant foods were widely used and were even more plentiful than along the Bering Sea coast.

Occupying a mountainous coast with no sea ice cover, Pacific Eskimo groups relied on watercraft almost exclusively for transportation. As in northern Eskimo regions, both kayaks and umiaks were used, but in reversed frequency compared with northern regions. In the Pacific regions, kayaks rather than umiaks were the common mode of water transport, and kayak technology developed to a highly refined art, equivalent to that of the Aleut and the marvel of exploring Europeans. A special adaptation in kayak design was the addition of a second paddler to provide stability and speed needed for sea otter and other types of ocean hunting, war, and use of the bow and arrow.

Pacific Eskimo subsistence combined forms more typical of Bering Sea, Aleut, and Northwest Coast regions. Whaling was conducted in the Aleutian manner, from kayaks, using poisoned spears with long slate points, and seals and sea lions were hunted with both toggling and non-toggling harpoons. Sea otter hunting, the predominant activity during the Russian period, was done with bows and arrow harpoons and with harpoon darts propelled by spear-throwers. Birds were taken with the typical Eskimo tri-pronged bird spear, also thrown with the spear-thrower.

Kodiak Island settlements were among the largest found anywhere in the circumpolar north, rivaling and perhaps exceeding the size of North Alaskan Eskimo villages. Located at prime salmon rivers, or in locations were sea mammal hunting and ocean fishing were productive, these villages consisted of scores of semisubterranean earth and log dwellings occupied by several closely related families. Constructed in the manner of northern Eskimo houses, these houses, known in the historic period as barabaras, had a central common room with a hearth surrounded by a series of two to four small side rooms used by individual families, some of which also contained separate hearths for heat, light, and sweat bath-

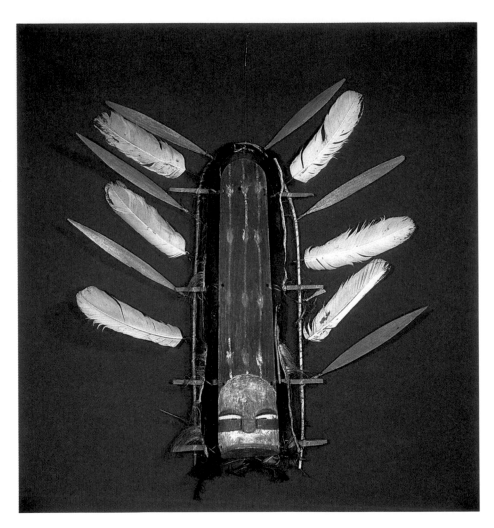

50. "Happy Fellow"
Koniag Eskimo: MAE 571-6

This mask is one of a set used in a "six act mystery" play witnessed by I.G. Voznesenskii on Kodiak Island in 1842, cast as the "happy fellow" (Lipshits 1955). A full rendition of this performance based on Voznesenskii's extensive notes has yet to appear. This mask, like many diverse types used by Koniag people, shares design features with Bering Sea Eskimo masks, including use of hoops and outstretched feathers and bangles, which in northern traditions represented stars and heavens (Nelson 1899:496). Similarities in facial features, use of long-headed plank masks, and bangles also link Koniag masks with those of their Aleut neighbors. Koniag theatrical performances were similar to those performed by Northwest Coast Indians at potlatch feasts.

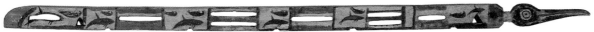

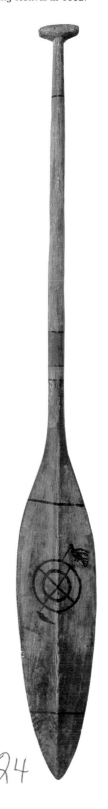

ing. Communal cemeteries were not known, and the dead were frequently buried outside the log walls of the family houses. In addition, most villages had one or more communal houses (*kashim* or *karigi* in northern usage, and *qasgiq* along the Bering Sea coast) in which the men gathered to work and which was used for ceremonies and festival activities. Dwelling structures of the Chugach Eskimo are less well known than those of the Koniags but appear to have been plank structures similar to those of the Tlingit, although of smaller size, a departure from the Eskimo pattern that suggests contact influence.

Pacific Eskimo clothing differed in significant ways from that of Bering Sea and other northern Eskimos, mainly in stylistic features rather than in radical changes of materials. Because of the milder climate, the heavy fur clothing of northern regions was not necessary, and prevailing dress emphasized protection against rain more than cold. *Kamleika*s, full-length frocks made from the intestines of seals, sea lions, and bears, were worn commonly and were often richly ornamented with hair, skin, and feather tassels and colorful embroidery, the latter influenced by Russian styles in the historic period. For more formal occasions, frocks made from cormorant skins, also richly decorated in the characteristic Kodiak colors of red and black, were used. Since this area was out of the heavy frost zone, footgear was rudimentary or nonexistent, as were gloves.

By far the most striking personal equipment was the elaborate headgear used by Kodiak people. This included a variety of red and black painted gutskin caps, ornamented ceremonial headpieces made of beaded weasel skins, womens' beaded dance headdresses (also found among Bering Sea Yupiks), and several types of ritual hunting hats. Among the latter are seal effigy hats used for decoy hunting and elaborate painted and ornamented bentwood hunting hats and visors, which were among a man's most prized possessions. As in the case of clothing and

hunting technology, these hats are closely tied to Aleut traditions. Bentwood hunting hats, however, are not known to have been common in the Chugach area, where men more commonly wore the spruce-root basketry hats typical of Tlingit culture.

Ceremonial life of the Pacific Eskimo was complex, embodying many elements of the Bering Sea Eskimo festival cycle as well as elements of Aleut culture, especially those relating to whaling cults. In 1802, Gavriil I. Davydov observed festivals during his visit to Kodiak, as did I. G. Voznesenskii in the early 1840s; the latter also collected festival masks similar to those traditionally used in Bristol Bay and along the Bering Sea coast (fig. 437). On the other hand, archeological finds dating from relatively recent prehistoric times in the Shumagin Islands suggest contacts with Aleutian whaling ceremony and art.

Thus in many respects Pacific Eskimo societies may be seen as highly developed following a trend of increasing complexity noted in Eskimo cultures from the physically demanding conditions of the Arctic Ocean to the more sociopolitically demanding environment of the Pacific coast. Compared to Bering Sea, Asiatic, and Arctic Eskimo, Pacific Eskimo had higher population densities and more diverse and stable economic resources, and they occupied a culturally diverse region where warfare, slave-taking, social ranking, and role specialization were present to a greater degree than among northern Eskimo groups. In this regard the hierarchically ranked societies of the Pacific Eskimo were an anomaly in the general pattern of Eskimo culture, one which undoubtedly had developed in response to the more advantageous economic conditions of the Pacific coast region. Under these conditions the Pacific Eskimo established a distinctive identity based on age-old traditions blended with Aleut and Northwest Coast attributes at the southern edge of the Eskimo world.

Aleut: Islanders of the North Pacific

Lydia T. Black and R. G. Liapunova

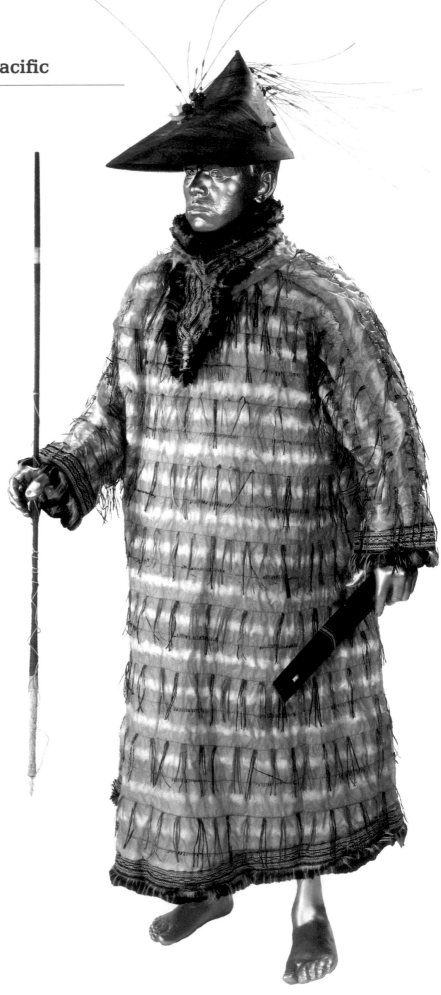

The Aleut, or Unangan, as they call themselves, inhabit the Aleutian archipelago, a 1,300-mile-long volcanic island arc extending from the Alaska Peninsula west nearly to Kamchatka. Traditionally, the Alaska Peninsula to the west of Port Moller was also part of the Unangan territory. In the 19th century, under the auspices of the Russian American Company, Aleuts were settled on the Pribilof Islands (USA) and the Commander Islands (USSR). Today there are 11 Aleut villages in the USA, and a group of Aleuts live on Bering Island in the USSR.

The term "Aleut" originally was a self-designation of the inhabitants of the Near Islands, the westernmost Unangan group, distinct from other Aleuts culturally and linguistically. Today it has become the preferred self-designation of several Alaskan peoples: the Unangan (who speak the Aleut langauge), Alutiiq-speaking Kodiak Islanders (the Koniag), and the Chugach of

Prince William Sound, as well as several Yupik-speaking groups of the eastern Alaska Peninsula. All of these groups came under intensive Russian influence in the 18th century, and in the last 200 years their history followed the same or very similar courses. Members of these groups were considered citizens of the Russian Empire with civil status equivalent to that of free peasants in metropolitan Russia.

In this essay, the focus is on the traditional culture of the Unangan only, island dwellers whose habitat is devoid of trees and, with the exception of the easternmost islands, of terrestrial fauna. For this reason, the Aleut dependence on the sea in the past was total. We shall stress their environmental adaptations and material culture. Readers interested in the Unangan's rich spiritual life should consult specialized publications by Black, Lantis, Laughlin, Liapunova, and Veniaminov in the bibliography.

Aleut settlements were, as a rule, located on bays where there was a good gravel beach for landing skin-covered watercraft. Village locations on necks between two bays were preferred, as such locations provided at least one protected landing or launching site for any given wind direction and served as an escape route in the event of enemy attack. A good supply of fresh water nearby was a necessity, and a good salmon stream was indispensable; other considerations were availability of driftwood and access to stone materials suitable for tool- and weapon-making and mineral paints, sea mammal hauling grounds, and an elevated lookout post from which one could watch for enemies and whales.

Associated with each permanent winter settlement was a fixed territory, trespass upon which could lead to intervillage conflicts. Each local population claimed more than one location suitable for a permanent settlement. Should the resources of one locality become depleted either through overhunting or natural causes, such as earthquake damage, the settlement could then be shifted without conflict with neighbors. The territory of each settlement also included burial grounds.

Though two 19th-century Orthodox clergymen, Father Ioann Veniaminov and Iakov Netsvetov, recorded Aleut traditions and ritual life (Veniaminov 1984), we know little about Aleut beliefs prior to Russian contact. However, their burial practices suggest that they had a complex cosmology, a belief in an afterlife, an elaborate set of notions about death and relation between the body and personal essence or "vital principle," and between the living and the dead. Variation in the mortuary complex existed regionally and over time. Some differences in burial practices were associated with the per-

son's rank and, in some cases, with occupation (particularly in the case of whalers), while others related to the person's manner of death.

Sarcophagus burials (Weyer 1929), both in stone and in wooden double coffinlike structures, are known from the early contact period. The use of double coffins persists to this day and occurs in Orthodox burials. Prehistoric pit burials have also been documented for southwest Umnak Island (Aigner and Veltre 1976). Pit and cave burials associated with whalebones, and corpses placed on or under whale scapulae, have been reported from the Near Islands and from Ship Rock, in Umnak Pass, in the eastern Aleutians. Mummified cave burials, with mummy bundles disposed on platforms or suspended in cradles, have been reported from Kagamil Island in the Four Mountains Islands (Dall 1876; Hrdlicka 1945). Cave burials with corpses placed in rock niches and clefts, reminiscent of cave burials on Kodiak Island, have been found on Unga Island in the Shumagin group (Dall 1876; Pinart 1875). Cave burials associated with kayaks have been reported from the central Aleutians.

In the overwhelming majority of known burials the corpses are buried in flexed position, but extended burials are reported from Kagamil and from Unga. The Aleuts believed that contact with the mummified bodies found in caves granted special powers but that such contact was extremely dangerous. Whalers, however, were expected to engage in such contact and to use substances from corpses on their weapons and kayaks.

Early ethnographic data (Baranov in Khlebnikov 1978; Veniaminov 1984) indicate that slaves were sacrificed at burials of important persons. Dismemberment of enemies and possibly of criminals was also practiced (Laughlin 1980). In protohistoric and early contact times in the eastern Aleutians, members of a community were buried in side chambers of a communal dwelling, and slaves reportedly were buried in rock shelters. The grave goods and the clothing placed with the corpse depended on the rank of the deceased. In a few instances, small bone or ivory masks with no field of vision have been found with burials.

The Aleut, like a majority of the peoples on the shores of the Bering and Okhotsk seas, built semisubterranean dwellings at their permanent winter settlements (fig. 251). These dwellings were entered through the roof by means of notched logs, but their size and floor plans differed from one island to the other. The dwellings of the Aleuts of the Near Islands were small, housing a single household, with the exception of the dwelling of the village leader or chief. His house was larger because it functioned as a

52. Aleut Hunter

Aleut men honored the sea mammal spirits by wearing highly decorated hunting costumes. This high-ranking hunter or chief is dressed in a gut-skin *kamleika* ornamented with colored yarn, appliqué designs, and hair embroidery. The large number of sea lion whiskers on the hat indicates the hunting ability of its owner. Large glass beads, most of Chinese origin, attest to his wealth and successful trading ventures. In his hands are a sea otter dart and throwing board. MAE: 568-1 (throwing board), 593-18 (*kamleika*), 2868-82 (hat). NMNH 175825 (dart)

communal gathering and ritual place, a *kashim,* and also because he accommodated within it some of his supporters. In the eastern Aleutians, sometime before contact, small individual dwellings were replaced by large communal, multifamily dwellings. These longhouses varied in size. In a large settlement there could be up to six large longhouses, from 70 to over 200 feet long and up to 30 feet wide. In ground plan these dwellings were rectangular, oriented on an east-west axis, but at the eastern and western ends sometimes there were extensions running north to south, so that a longhouse could assume a horizontal I shape or look like one leg of a swastika. A large longhouse might have as many as ten rooftop entry hatches, which also served for ventilation and to let in light.

Inside, the longhouse was divided into compartments, occupied by separate households—a head of the family, and his dependents. As Aleuts practiced polygyny, it is assumed that each wife may have had a separate compartment. Each compartment was marked by a post on which was fixed an oil lamp, its rounded bottom fitted into a hollow at the top of the post. Twined grass mats separated one compartment from another.

Aleut society was ranked, with hereditary classes of high nobles, commoners, and slaves. The leaders were recruited from the high nobles or the chiefly elite. This ranking was reflected in allocation of living space within the longhouse and, as mentioned, in burials. The ''east'' and the ''above'' were the sacred dimensions associated with the creator—*Agugux.* At dawn Aleut men emerged on the rooftops of their houses and faced the east to greet the day and ''swallow light.'' The chief and his close kinsmen lived at the east end of the longhouse. The chief's retinue was assigned space within the longhouse by rank along the walls from east to west. A small opening led from each compartment into a side chamber used for storage, as sleeping quarters for children, and for other uses. Occasionally, side chambers had a separate entry hatch. Other side chambers were designed as hiding holes to be used during enemy attack, and some had secret passages to the outside.

Dwellings (fig. 251) were constructed on doubled frames of upright posts that supported crossbeams and rafters. Thin wood poles resting on this framework formed the walls. Thick mats, either of grass or skins, were placed over the wooden framework, followed by a layer of old grass, then a layer of new grass, and finally a layer of sod. From a distance, these houses appeared like grassy hummocks (fig. 16). When available, whalebones were used in house construction.

Food supplies were stored on wooden shelves spread with finely worked mats. Perpendicular to the long walls, at each compartment's boundary, low shelves about 28 inches aboveground served as seats and provided storage space underneath. People slept on these platforms as well as on the floor. Various racks and small shelves held personal belongings. After the appearance of Russians, doors and windows were adopted, but finely worked sea mammal gut remained in use instead of window glass. Wet steam baths, introduced by the Russians, came into widespread use and acquired a ritual purification function.

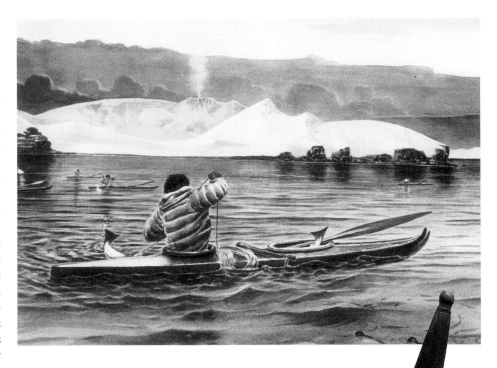

In the 19th century, the use of smaller, individual household dwellings became reestablished. A foreroom was added, and a Russian-type interior stove for heating and cooking. In larger centers, such as Unalaska, Russian-style log and plank houses were used by more-affluent people. By and large, however, the small semi-subterranean dwellings, though modified, continued to be used in many communities until World War II.

Summer dwellings were flimsy, makeshift structures. In the Near Islands, caves provided shelters in summer. When in transit, Aleuts constructed shelter using their watercraft and sea mammal hides.

The watercraft—framework boats covered with sea mammal skins—were the most important items in the Aleut technological inventory. The larger boats, called *baidara*s, resembled the Eskimo umiak. *Baidara*s, especially those from

53. ''Oonalashka Native Codfishing'' H.W. Elliott. SI-NAA 7119-13. SI neg. 73-10975

Aleuts were expert fishermen as well as maritime hunters. This black-and-white watercolor of an Aleut codfisherman is by Henry Wood Elliott, a naturalist who participated in the 1864-66 Western Union Telegraph Survey (p. 91). Elliott was one of the first American scientists to work in Alaska and an early conservationist best known for his efforts to stem the destruction of the Pribilof Island fur seal population (Elliott 1881).

the Andreanof Islands, were 35 to 42 feet long at the keel. This craft was used to transport people over long distances, on visits, to and from summer fishing grounds, or when changing the location of the village. *Baidara*s were also used when chiefs visited their neighbors, on trading voyages, and on military raids. Boat-making was a prestigious skill, and a man aspiring to be a leader was expected to be a master boatmaker and possess at least one large *baidara*.

Every able-bodied adult man had his own *baidarka* (kayak). The village's strength was often expressed in the number of kayaks available. The Aleut kayak was a marvelously engineered craft, and Aleuts were famous for their skill in making and handling it. The early European mariners considered the Aleut kayak the finest of all Alaskan kayaks. Regional differences were expressed in their type and style. In the Near Islands, single-, double-, and triple-hatch kayaks were in use. In the Andreanofs and in the eastern Aleutians, at contact, apparently only single and double kayaks were used. The eastern Aleut kayak was most distinctive of all: narrow and built for speed. Its bifid bow was distinctive, and a flexible three-piece keelson made the craft especially seaworthy (Dyson 1986; Laughlin 1980). The Aleut used double-bladed paddles, but a single-bladed paddle was carried occasionally as a spare. A unique feature was the drip skirt, a device that fitted over the hatch and made the kayak watertight and, together with the *kamleika*, the hunter's gutskin shirt, protected the hunter from getting wet. Sealskin floats for added buoyancy in case of emergency and an ingenious mouth pump (fig. 54) were part of the standard equipment.

In stormy weather, Aleuts joined their kayaks together to ride out storms. It is said that a skilled kayaker could right himself if he overturned. Though no kayaks are made now in the Aleutians, and the skill of kayak-building is believed to have been lost, the Aleut kayak became the prototype for a popular sportscraft now known worldwide.

Aleuts had a strict sexual division of labor. Men worked wood, bone, and metal, while women worked skins and fibers. A man's tool kit included instruments for making *baidara* and *baidarka* frames, among which were straight-edged knives, crooked (sea mammal or beaver tooth) knives, adzes, punching tools, awls, and polishing tools. His weapon inventory was extensive, with each piece suited for specific prey or conditions. The most common weapons were harpoons or darts thrown by means of a throwing board (fig. 193). Harpoons and darts, usually painted red, were constructed with detachable or fixed bone or ivory heads (figs. 76 and 219). Toggling harpoon heads were rare. Blades were of stone, slate, or obsidian. Sea otter darts used drag shaft technology, and harpoons used for larger prey utilized drag floats. Stabbing spears were used to dispatch exhausted animals, and clubs for killing sea mammals, such as sea otters or seals, on shore.

Bird spears and fish spears were multipronged and were similar to Eskimo weapons. In addition, birds were taken by noose, trap, net, and bolas. Fish were taken at weirs constructed in the streams and by spears, arrows, and dip nets. Deep-sea fish were taken by means of gorges and composite hooks. A special hook was used for halibut. Although deep-sea fishing was a province of men, fishing in the streams was often done by young boys and women under supervision of one or two old men. After contact, seining came into wide use and, in the 19th century, gill-netting.

Seal decoys, made of whole inflated sealskins, were used in hunting seals on land. Prior to contact, fur seals were taken pelagically, but after 1786 in the Pribilof and Commander islands, where the North Pacific fur seals haul out to breed, they were harvested on land. Only nonbreeding bachelors were taken after the 1820s.

At sea, Aleut men wore wooden hunting hats. The shape of the headgear indicated a man's rank; a short visor was worn by the young and inexperienced hunters, an elongated visor by the rank-and-file, and open-crown long-visored hats by important mature men. Chiefs, and probably whalehunters, wore the elaborate closed-crown hunting helmet. This helmet was probably

54. Kayak Suction Pump
Aleut: NMNH 168569

The oceanic environment and long crossings between islands required Aleut paddlers to remain at sea for long periods, even for days. Under these conditions removing bilge water through the narrow cockpit hole was impossible. Aleut paddlers developed an ingenious mouth-operated suction pump for this task. Water was sucked into the hollowed out tube and lifted over the side to drain.

55. Aleut Man and Assemblage
Mikhail Levashev. UWL neg. 1771

The first pictorial representation providing ethnographic details of Aleut culture as drawn by Mikhail Levashev at Unalaska in 1768-69. It illustrates a man, his clothing, and a variety of knives, hunting, and war items. Another illustration featured an Aleut woman and her equipment.

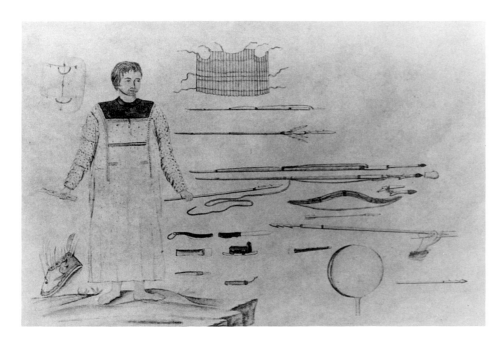

adopted from the Koniag and spread to the eastern Aleutians together with the Kodiak-type whaling complex.

The compound sinew-backed bow was a weapon of war reserved for human prey. Poisoned lances were also used in warfare, as well as war daggers and knives, preferably of metal. Even before the arrival of Russians, Aleuts worked metal, which they obtained from shipwrecks or in trade from the Alaskan mainland, by cold-hammering. The Russians introduced forging techniques to the Aleuts as early as 1772. Slat and rod armor was common (figs. 55, 306), and shields (fig. 75), battle helmets, and special battle *kamleika*s were also used.

Ivory and wood carving were much appreciated skills, and many men possessed ivory carving equipment (fig. 458). Bone and ivory items of religious significance were attached to the kayak, to sealskin floats, to throwing boards, and to hunting hats. It was believed that the sea mammals—but especially sea otters, who were considered to be transformed humans—were attracted by human finery. For this reason men dressed in elegant clothes when hunting sea otter, and carried talismans and decorations.

Items of personal adornment were varied. Labrets were worn by both men and women in the eastern and central Aleutians, but in the Near Islands, only the women wore labrets. Ivory and bone nose pins were worn by men of all groups. Women wore beaded skin bracelets and anklets; men and women wore earrings, mostly of beads; and puffin beaks adorned women's dresses. In the Rat Islands and the central Aleutians, men and women wore feather quills as ear ornaments.

Household utensils were relatively few. Wooden containers, carved and bentwood, were used for water and urine storage and as serving dishes, but because of the scarcity of wood in the archipelago they were not as common or as elaborate as on Kodiak and the Alaskan mainland. Large sea mammal stomachs (''bladders'') had more widespread use as storage containers. Air-dried fish, sea mammal oil, water, edible roots, and berries were stored either in bladders or grass baskets. Bladders were preferred for carrying provisions and water when traveling.

Men's and women's small tools were kept in special containers. At home wooden boxes were used, but when traveling, men carried sea mammal gut pouches that were attached to a cord that passed over the man's shoulder. Women had ''housewives'' of skin and grass that were elaborately decorated with gut-on-gut appliqué and hair embroidery (figs. 88 and 252). Silk, cotton, and wood came into use for decorative embroidery soon after Russian contact.

Aleut men's clothing was made mostly of puffin, murre, and cormorant skins. Cormorant clothing (fig. 268) was especially prestigious. Women's garments were of sea mammal skins—sea otter in the west, sea otter and fur seals in the east. Clothes were worn as a rule skin-side out. The outsides of garments, especially those used on festive and social occasions, were elaborately decorated at neck, cuffs, and hem and along the seams with embroidery of feathers, human hair, and ocher-colored skin strips. After contact, unraveled wool, dyed red or green, was used as seam decoration. Parka yokes were generally colored red. Festive garments, especially lineage clothing worn at the annual winter festival, were decorated with gut-on-gut appliqué and finished with an embroidery overlay of caribou hair. Both men and women wore long, ankle-length, straight shirts with high stand-up collars and raglan-type sleeves. Outer garments of sea mammal intestines, known as *kamleika*s, were worn as protection against the wet.

Women made clothing, bedding, and most of the household utensils, including containers of birch bark, bundles of which were often placed with females at burial. Women made their own sinew thread and multistrand plaited sinew cordage, and men plaited heavy cordage of kelp. Women were highly skilled at needlework, and the waterproof decorated garments they produced were traded by their men to the mainland in exchange for caribou skins, caribou hair, iron, and copper. After contact, these garments were given as gifts or sold to visiting Europeans and important Russian officials. Women made their own needles, mostly from bird bone but also from ivory. Needlecases of bone or ivory were similar to those used in the Eskimo area.

57. Grass Basket
Aleut: NMNH 417767

Attuan women were renowned for their clothlike basketry, producing some of the finest baskets in the world (14-15 stitches/cm). This covered basket is typical of early Attuan work, and features false embroidery (sometimes called overlay) in red, green, blue, and gold hues made from natural dyes. Wild rye beach grass (*Elymus mollis*) was the preferred raw material. Grasswork was an ancient craft in the treeless Aleutian region and was used for many articles, including mats, mitts, socks, and sewing kits. Baskets of this type, however, have not been found in archeological sites and seem to have originated in Attu in the 19th century (Black 1982: 164).

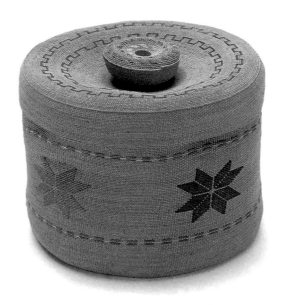

56. Gutskin Cape
Aleut: NMNH 2128

Rainproof gutskin coats were a basic survival item in the wet Aleutian environment. Russian mariners and traders soon discovered the superiority of these lightweight garments and commissioned them from Aleut seamstresses, who altered the style to that of the European greatcoat. When ornamented, these capes were extremely valuable and were used as presentation gifts to visiting captains and dignitaries.

This cape, collected by the U.S. Exploring Expedition under the leadership of Charles Wilkes around 1840, exemplifies the finest of its type. It is constructed of strips of sea lion intestine into which have been sewn tufts of red and green wool and strands of hair. Inserted into the seams in an upward position, the hairs cascade downward like miniature waterfalls. Collar, cuffs, and borders are decorated with bands of dyed membrane strip appliqué couched and embroidered with dazzlingly white caribou hair, and ruffs of iridescent cormorant feathers (fig. 268). Gossimer, waterproof, and regal, such capes were the prize souvenir of high-ranking European visitors to the Aleutian Islands.

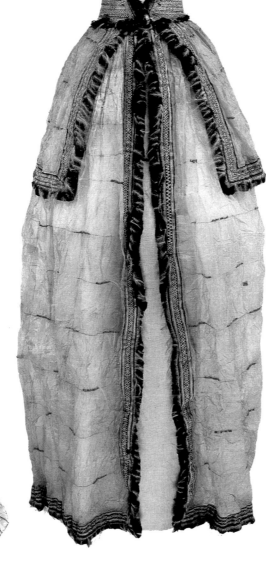

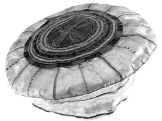

58. Gutskin Hat
Aleut: MAE 571-79

In addition to their bentwood hats, Aleuts wore a great variety of soft hats. Made of gutskin ornamented with tufts of dyed wool, this hat has a complex design of appliqué panels and concentric rings of dyed sea mammal esophagus. As in the decoration on coats, a precise pattern governs the sequence and position of colored panels.

This hat was collected by Voznesenskii in the early 1840s from St. George Island in the Pribilofs, where an Aleut fur seal hunting colony had been established by the Russians.

Ritual clothing was elaborate but is poorly known. Ritual hats and belts were made of sea mammal and bird (eagle and falcon skins, decorated with hair and feathers. Eastern Unangan ritual hats were flat, with a central rosette in gut appliqué on top. Hats from the central Aleutians generally had an elaborate high, protruding frontal piece, which perhaps represented a bird's head and neck. Elaborate costumes and props were used in ritual dances. Dancing shawls of gut are known from the Commander Islands. All festivals were accompanied by drumming, using the hand-held drum of Eskimo type.

Aleut masks differ in style from one region to another and probably by function. The surviving portraitlike masks from Tigal'da were used possibly in winter commemorative feasts in which ancestors were celebrated. Masks from the Shumagin Islands are powerful representations incorporating both anthropomorphic and zoomorphic features and were probably used in whaling ceremonies. These masks were thought by Henry B. Collins to resemble masks of medieval Japan. The complex composite masks from Atka in the central Aleutians remind one of Shang China. Masks from Kagamil Island in the Four Mountains are very different in character and relate more closely to North Alaskan Eskimo masks. Little is known of Aleut mask function or iconography.

Aleut folklore is rich but not well known. Several named classes of narrative and song existed. The eastern Aleuts had several origin stories, some probably historical in nature, others mythological. In one of these, a doglike creature figured as the first ancestor. Raven, widely distributed among other Alaskan groups, appears only in the folklore of western Aleuts, where he is a trickster, not a culture hero. Aleuts believed that spirits were associated with all aspects of their environment. There are indications that the Aleut shared a belief widely distributed among Alaskan Yupik Eskimo in the Thunderbird (fig. 446), a powerful being likened to an eagle who had the power to kill on land and sea.

Illness was believed to be caused by evil spirits, usually set loose by antisocial acts of the sufferers or their kin. The Aleut shamans were primarily healers. In this respect, they had much in common with the Eskimo. The shamans also foretold the future and controlled the weather. The Aleut differed from the Eskimo, however, in that they believed in a universal creator. The creator was associated with the east and the above, as already mentioned, and with the light and life-giving water—a circumstance that made their conversion to Orthodox Christianity acceptable in their own terms of reference. This symbolic overlap explains in part why Orthodoxy today is the basis of Aleut community life and the primary marker of their identity.

As this brief essay shows, the culture of the Aleuts of Alaska was rich and varied and their history complex. In spite of the limitations imposed by their environment, Aleuts developed the technology that enabled them to satisfy their material needs. They also had an elaborate spiritual and ceremonial life and an artistic tradition that included embellishing each and every item they used. In doing so, the Aleut succeeded in creating objects that have a universal aesthetic appeal and are now treasured artistic masterpieces, especially their masks, their carved ivories, and, above all, their splendid ritual bentwood hunting helmets.

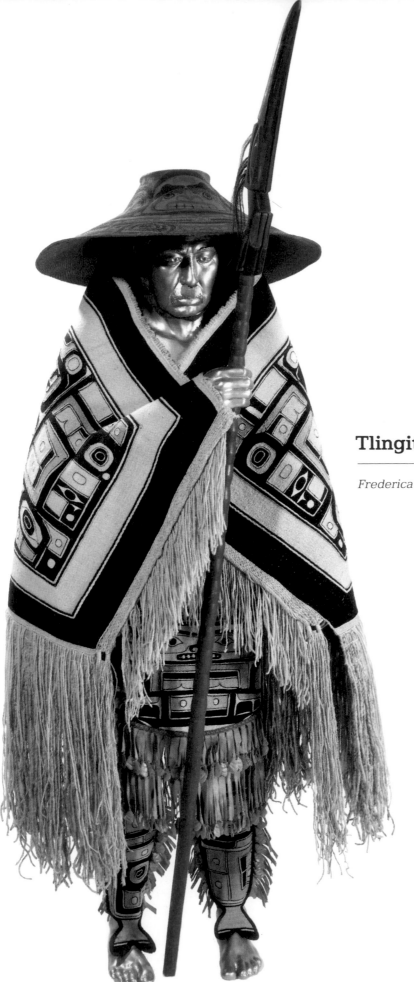

59. Tlingit Chief
Nobility and rank are prominently displayed in the clothing and accoutrements of this Tlingit chief, who is seen with his ceremonial staff as he might look presiding at a potlatch. His robe is a prestigious Chilkat blanket, woven from a combination of cedar bark and mountain goat wool. His apron and leggings are of similar make. His spruce-root hat, like his robe, is ornamented with designs portraying animal totems (''crests''). Outside contacts and trade are indicated by his abalone shell nose ring. NMNH: 20633 (nosering), 88961b (hat), 219504 (robe), 274433 (staff), 341202 (apron), 341202a,b (leggings)

Tlingit: People of the Wolf and Raven

Frederica de Laguna

The Tlingit are the northernmost of the Northwest Coast peoples who lived traditionally by fishing and hunting marine animals and built large plank houses, totem poles, and ocean-going dugout canoes. They were skillful traders and utilized their excess wealth on luxuries given away at splendid feasts (potlatches), which served to honor the dead and to maintain or elevate the rank of the aristocrats. The Tlingit comprised four groups or tribes: Southern, Northern, Gulf Coast, and Inland Tlingit. The latter are not considered here, as their way of life is similar to that of their Athapaskan neighbors in the Yukon Territory.

Tlingit history has been one of movement and mixing of peoples. Archeological evidence indicates an occupation of the islands and mainland of southeastern Alaska for many centuries, even millennia. According to linguists, the Tlingit language may have split from common roots with Athapaskan about 5,000 years ago. Tlingit traditions tell of small family groups venturing in boats or rafts down the rivers under the

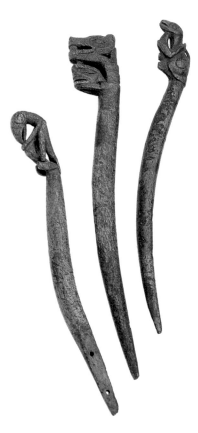

60. Trap Sticks

Tlingit: NMNH 398408-10

Trap sticks functioned as trigger mechanisms in deadfalls used to capture small furbearers. Usually made of whalebone, their figural images were probably intended to lure prey to the trap. The carvings on these sticks include a skeletized bird, a bear or wolf presiding over a corpselike human, and a bird emerging from a fishlike creature. Both hunting magic (p. 151) and crest art (p. 271) are implied by these images.

61. Goathorn Spoons

(Top to bottom) Haida: NMNH 89167. Tlingit: NMNH 9273. Haida: NMNH 88924

The importance of feasting and display motivated Tlingit and Haida artists to produce masterful miniature sculpture—in essence, miniature totem poles—on the handles of spoons and ladles of mountain goat horn.

glaciers that once arched over the waters, suggesting how early migration might have come from the interior, to mix with resident coastal populations. Native history indicates changes in coastal populations as far back as 300 years, when Haida from the Queen Charlotte Islands moved north, displacing Tongas Tlingit, and when Northern Tlingit expanded north across the Gulf of Alaska, intermarrying with Athapaskans and exerting strong Tlingit influence on the Eyak. Through such contacts with other tribes totemic crests and other clan prerogatives have been exchanged and elaborated. The Tlingit seem always to have had an appetite for foreign items such as clothing, songs, names, symbols of rank, secret tricks to be dramatically displayed at feasts, and even foreign supernatural objects to aid the power of their shamans.

The Tlingit life described here was recorded by early explorers of the late 18th and 19th centuries. This period was one of cultural florescence resulting from stimulation by foreign contacts, the fine craftsmanship made possible by steel tools, and the wealth obtained by Tlingits through the European fur trade. This wealth made possible the great Tlingit ceremonies—funerals, house dedications, and memorial potlatches—for which luxury items were made or imported: such things as the great Haida canoes of red cedar; Tsimshian carved rattles, masks, and headdresses; Athapaskan pelts, tanned skins, and beadwork; commercial sheet copper, Hudson's Bay blankets and porcelain dishes; abalone and dentalium shells, and even slaves from southern British Columbia.

The Tlingit live today in a rugged and beautiful country, a land of islands, deep fjords, and steepsided mountains from whose snowfields glaciers descend to the sea. The lower slopes are covered with spruce and hemlock, with red cedar in the south, and an almost impenetrable undergrowth of alders, berry bushes, and thorny devil's club. In the past some tribes with mainland territories hiked up the so-called "grease trails" to exchange fish oil for the furs of their Athapaskan trading partners, but most travel was by canoe. Tlingit even used to paddle hundreds of miles across the open Gulf of Alaska or south to Puget Sound on peaceful trading visits or savage raids. A variety of large and small canoes was used for war, hunting sea mammals, deep-sea fishing, and river travel.

Land mammals, even bears, were usually taken by snares and deadfall traps, although brave hunters with spears (later with guns) "fought" black bears and even the huge brown grizzlies when they emerged from their dens in spring, as if they were human adversaries. Mountain goats, prized for their fat and meat, horns (for spoon handles and the spikes in shamans' crowns), and wool (for Chilkat blankets), were hunted above timberline, but only with the assent of the mountain spirit. Although other furbearers were taken in plain traps, the trigger sticks for marmot traps were decorated, for otherwise, this animal would disdain the trap.

It was on the bounty of the sea, however, that the Tlingit largely depended. Most important were the five species of salmon that every year ascended the rivers and streams. Although rock carvings near the mouths of some of these streams may have been made to attract the fish, it is more likely that they were used to proclaim ownership. Salmon were easily taken by men in weirs and traps or were speared with the harpoon and gaff, but it required the hard work of the women to cut, dry, and store the harvest. So plentiful and reliable were the salmon runs until they were overfished for the cannery industry in the late 19th century that the Tlingit never developed a true First Salmon ceremony like some Northwest Coast nations. Still, care was taken not to offend the fish. Herring and eulachon also appeared in the spring and were caught with fish rakes and dip nets. Spruce boughs were placed in the water for herring to spawn upon, and oil was extracted from eulachon by boiling them in a canoe with hot rocks. Halibut were caught on the open sea with ingeniously fashioned, spiritually active hooks.

In addition to permanently resident birds like eagles, gulls, magpies, crows, and ravens, the Tlingit world is visited each year by myriad flocks of ducks, geese, swans, and songbirds that use the Pacific flyway. Young people fearlessly scaled cliffs to rob nests of their eggs; large birds furnished feathers for decoration and downy skins for warm blankets, as well as meat. Clams, cockles, mussels, sea urchins, crabs, and seaweed were also eaten but were so easy to get that such "beach food" was associated with laziness, and overindulgence was thought to cause poverty and nightmares.

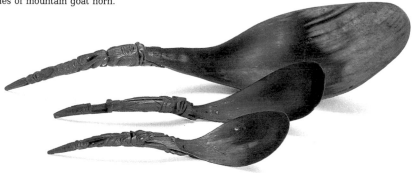

All things—animals, birds, fish, insects, trees, plants, mountains, glaciers, winds, and the sea itself—were thought to possess in-dwelling souls or spirits. Since these were more powerful than human beings, they had to be treated with respect, and there were special rules to be observed in dealing with each species or being: Successful hunting and fishing meant taking a life like that of a person, and could be done only if the creature permitted itself to be killed. The dead animal had to be handled in the proper way. Formerly, it was said, the hunter sang special songs over his prey. Nor was waste permitted; all remains not used for food, dress, tools, or other purposes had to be burned or returned to the water (depending on the species) so that animal spirits could report to their kind on their respectful treatment by humans and could repopulate the species.

Although we may speak of tribes among the Tlingit, these were traditionally only geographic groups, not political units. The Sitkans, or members of a similar group, might consider themselves to be distinguished from the inhabitants of other towns through local customs or manner of speech, but their true allegiances were to their several clans, which were the real units of Tlingit political, social, and ceremonial life. Each tribe or town contained several clans or segments of clans, relationships between which were not always friendly.

Membership in a clan was based on the mother's line. Clans belonged to two sides or moieties, Ravens and Wolves (the latter called Eagles in the north), that were opposites and married and performed ceremonial services for each other. These moieties had no other functions and never met as whole groups. Clans were divided into matrilineal lineages, or houses. A household, as distinguished from a house, was composed of lineage brothers, with married-in wives, their children, and some elders and poor relations. The lineage, like the clan, was a matrilineal descent group.

A clan usually took its name from its supposed place of origin. Such a place, or a landmark encountered in subsequent wanderings, might be taken as a clan crest or emblem. A lineage might also grow and create daughter houses that could eventually become clans in their own right.

The clan owned the most important forms of property: territories for hunting, fishing, collecting wild food, firewood, and even drinking water, and perhaps also exclusive rights to trade routes. Trespassers might be attacked and killed, but anyone claiming relationship to one of the owners was free to use the resource. More precious than these rights in the eyes of the

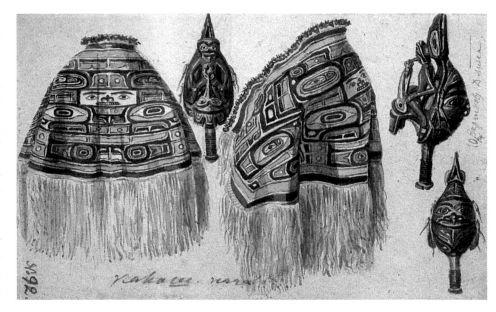

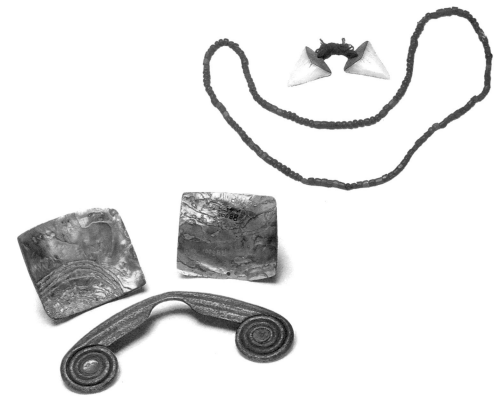

Tlingit were the totemic crests and ceremonial prerogatives vested in the clan and lineage. Rights to these were acknowledged at potlatches when allusion was made to the familiar stories of their acquisition and when guest clan "opposites" accepted payment as witnesses.

The head of a lineage was the "master of the house," and the leader of the most important house was the clan chief or "great man." These men and their immediate families were the aristocrats and were careful to maintain their rank by marrying spouses of equal status, which often required seeking a bride from a distant

62. Personal Ornaments

Tlingit: (Clockwise from top) NMNH 72993, 209550; Haida: NMNH 88900, Tsimshian: NMNH 10313

Abalone shell, shark teeth, glass beads, and iron were highly prized as materials for making body ornaments, and were traded widely. Abalone shell was especially valued, as were shark teeth—two species of which were crests of the Tlingit Wolf phratry. Bead strings and iron ornaments formed into bifurcated scrolls were also popular. The latter motif was popular on Athapaskan knife handles (fig. 304).

tribe, perhaps linking together two chiefly lines through several generations. Nobility, however, depended upon more than birth, since wealth, conduct, and family reputation were also important.

Chiefs were the trustees of common property, with authority to regulate hunting or fishing in clan territories or to mobilize clan wealth for major ceremonies. House heads and other men of rank formed the council of the clan chief. The principal wife of the house chief was the guardian of her husband's treasures and supervised the household work.

Of a lower rank than the aristocrats, who slept in partitioned rooms at the back of the plank house, were the ill-defined commoners, their junior relatives, who slept on the side benches. Lowest of all were the no-accounts who slept with the slaves just inside the door. Slaves were those taken in war, and their descendants. As chattels, slaves were outside Tlingit society, to be bought, sold, killed, or freed at the whim of their masters.

The Tlingit man or woman owed patriotic loyalty to his or her clan, a duty that transcended marital ties. Wars or lawsuits—there was no distinction in Tlingit language—were fought or prosecuted by clans, not by individuals or tribes, although several clans, even from different tribes, might join as allies. Any injury to a person or property of a clan member required compensation, the amount usually having been determined by consultation between the chiefs. In a serious case the whole clan was held responsible for damages if the defendant and his close kin could not make compensation. Most cases were settled by payment of property, but a killing, even if accidental, sometimes led to a feud, which ended only when the losses were evened. The life of a chief was worth so much more than that of a commoner, or even of several ordinary persons, that if a chief was killed, the life of an equal had to be paid. Accounts tell of chiefs and aristocratic men and women who freely gave their own lives to spare their clanmates further bloodshed in cases where the killer was of too low a rank to atone for his own act. Peace was established through the exchange of hostages (deer dancers), who were the foci for magically binding rituals during the eight-day peace ceremonies.

Feuds within a tribe or village were usually settled quickly because relatives on both sides pressed for settlement, but wars between clans in distant villages were savage and sometimes lasted for years, even breaking out again after peace settlements. The Tlingit war party traveled in large war canoes, the chief or his designated nephew directing from the bow and an elderly matron of rank steering. Warriors were equipped with daggers, spears, bows and arrows, and war clubs. The body was protected by armor made of wooden slats or rods, and the neck and head by a wooden collar and heavy helmet, the latter carved to represent his clan crest animal or a ferocious human face. More often, for freedom of movement, the warrior simply tied his hair on top of his head, painted his face, and wore a rawhide tunic painted with a clan crest. Attacks were planned to surprise the enemy in their beds at night. The heads of slain warriors were taken as trophies, and women and children were often enslaved.

Each Tlingit clan was distinguished by its crests, its houses or lineages usually having special versions of these. Crests are symbolic representations of some species of animal, bird, fish, or invertebrate, but also include heavenly bodies, landmarks, and even ancestral heroes and supernatural beings. A clan usually had several crests. Clan history told how ancestors obtained their crests through supernatural encounters. The most important crests of the Raven clans are: Raven, Owl, Whale, Sea Lion, Salmon, Frog, Sleep Bird, Sun, Moon, Big Dipper, and Ocean Waves. On the opposite side are: Eagle, Petrel, Wolf, Bear, Killer Whale, Shark, Halibut, and Thunderbird. Beaver and Golden Eagle (or Fish Hawk) were Wolf-Eagle crests on the Gulf Coast but belonged to Raven clans in southeastern Alaska.

The plank house (fig. 264) and the woven spruce-root hat were the two most important possessions of the clan and its chief on which clan crests were displayed. The rear screen inside the house, the four major house posts, and the facade were carved and painted to illustrate stories about the crests. Crests of clan and lineage also appeared on totem poles (receptacles for ashes of the dead) and grave

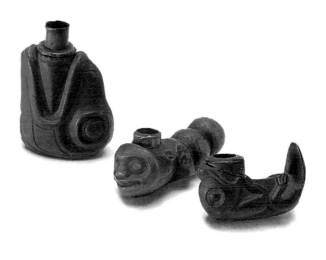

houses; on spoons and ladles, feast dishes, tobacco pipes, speaker's staffs, song leader's poles, drums, and other objects used in ceremonies; on ceremonial garments such as Chilkat blankets, button blankets or beaded shirts, painted aprons, and headdresses with frontlet masks; and on armor, daggers, powder horns, and war canoes.

All crest objects, including the house and grave, were supposedly made by members of the opposite moiety, who were publicly rewarded at a potlatch. The display of any crest required payment to all members of the opposite side who were present, since they were witnesses to the owners' right to that crest. In this way, if the crest was some landmark in the clan's territory, acceptance of the gifts affirmed the clan's territorial rights. Crest objects and other things featured at potlatches were treasured as heirlooms and were safeguarded in the chief's house.

Objects of particular wealth, which were often decorated with crest designs, were the shield-shaped sheets of copper. "Coppers" were appropriate as marriage or potlatch gifts or as the purchase price for land. All Northwest Coast coppers that have been tested are made of European copper, intended for or used as sheathing for ships' bottoms. Although some copper may have been scavenged by the Indians from wrecked ships, most copper was obtained by purchase from European traders. Presumably there was an earlier prototype made of native copper, perhaps like the coppers sketched by Captain Colnett among the Haida in 1787 and described as "their under armour."

The great ceremonies of the Tlingit centered around the dead. The bereaved clan, or hosts, entertained their opposites, the paternal and affinal kin of the deceased, and rewarded them for their funeral services. The giving of gifts—the potlatch proper—benefited and honored the dead while raising or maintaining the prestige of their descendants who bore their names. The rites for men, women, and children were similar, although they were naturally most elaborate for a deceased chief and the installation of his successor.

When such a man died, there were traditionally eight days of mourning, during the first four of which the body lay in state, surrounded by the clan or lineage treasures. Bereaved clan members, wearing old clothes and cut or singed hair, sang the clan mourning songs, and the opposites offered comfort. After four days, the opposites cremated the corpse and put the ashes in the lineage grave house or box. That night the mourners hosted a "smoking feast" at which everyone smoked or took snuff, and tobacco was

put in the fire for all the dead of the clan. The mourning period ended with a feast, at which time the leader called upon all members of the clan, in turn, to introduce a song in memory of a dead relative. Then gifts were given to the guests, those of rank receiving the most. This potlatch was called "feeding the dead." Sometimes a slave was sacrificed.

The mourners were then free to wash and burn their old clothes, except for the widow, who had to leave her face unwashed and remained in the care of her husband's sisters for several months. At this time, a grave monument was erected and the widow distributed all her husband's and her own private property to his heirs, and then married the designated man. The grave was now finished, and the deceased's clan paid for it at a final potlatch.

The great memorial potlatch, known as "setting up the dead," involved all the members of a tribe, either as hosts or as guests, and in addition, a guest clan from another place was invited, making two rival groups of guests who "danced against each other." Only the wealthy could afford to give such a potlatch, although the principal host, who thereby assumed the title and position of his predecessor, was assisted by contributions from all his clanmates. Other houses of his moiety usually helped entertain the guests at this time, so that there were several days of feasting and dancing with dramatic displays of feats of gluttony before the great climax when the property was distributed. Such a major potlatch was planned months, and sometimes years, in advance in order to notify the guests from far away and to accumulate the necessary property and food. It also required the building (or rebuilding) of a new house or houses, or perhaps moving the remains of the clan dead to new grave houses or boxes. The new house would be "danced together" by the host and his clanmates before any guests were entertained, and stood as a memorial to all the dead of the clan or lineage.

Shamanism was an important feature of Tlingit society. In every clan there was at least one shaman, who might be either a man or a woman but was usually male. The shaman's power was greater than a chief's, but sometimes chiefs, or their brothers, were also shamans. Tlingit shamans derived their power from special spirits and from power objects. Shamans were believed able to discover breaches of taboo, control the weather, foretell the future, secure news of distant persons, rescue those captured by Land Otter Men, cure the sick, and identify witches. Shamans could be recognized by their long, tangled locks (to wash or cut which was forbidden) and by their haggard faces and gaunt

65. Raven Rattle
Tlingit: MAE 2448-24

Raven rattles are one of the most characteristic artifact types of Northwest Coast Indian culture. This rattle is of a style dating to the early 19th century. Both the sculpture and the formline detail (p. 287) have a massive angularity often seen in Tlingit art from the early historic period. The rattle differs from most in that there is no sign that the man ever had an extended tongue; there is no frog represented (usually present if the tail bird is reversed); and the figure on the rattle's breast has no recurved beak. There may have once been feathers carved on the bird's tail, but they are no longer present. Some early rattles portray puffins, but this one has the typical raven form.

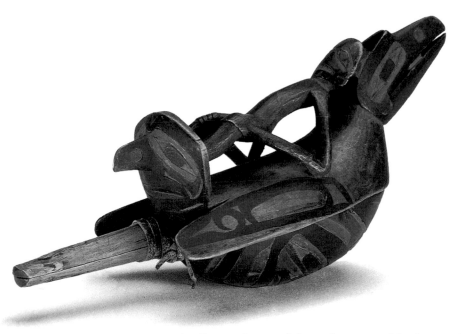

66. Sea Lion Headdress
Tlingit: MAE 5795-12

Crest art was a feature of Northwest Coast art that distinguished it from other North Pacific and Bering Sea cultures. Crests were emblematic insignia (usually animals or mythological creatures) adopted by social groups because of their mythological associations with the group's past. Despite their social affiliation, crest objects could be traded or sold by chiefs. This artistic system differed from the use of animal art in hunting magic, the other major artistic system common to the North Pacific region.

This expertly sculptured headdress in the form of a sea lion probably once had a hide panel attached to the back of the head with a formline design of the animal's body. (Just such a panel is in the collection of the Anthropological Museum of Lomonosov State University in Moscow and may have become separated from its mate.) Long whiskers were inset in holes in the snout, and rows of teeth—probably opercula—lined the mouth. The elegance of the original work is apparent even in its present incomplete state. When worn, it pointed upward, in the normal attitude of the sea lion.

bodies, exhausted from frequent thirsting and fasting. A shaman's powers were acquired on quests in the woods when spirits were encountered, the usual number, accumulated over a period of time, traditionally being eight. Each was represented by the skin or other parts of an animal (talons, beak, jaws) that were put together into a bundle to be worn when practicing, and also by the paintings and carvings on the shaman's paraphernalia: headdresses, masks, rattles, drum, and amulets. The animals most commonly figured on shaman's equipment were the land otter, bear, mountain goat, frog, devilfish, oyster catcher, and even invertebrates. These spirits also appeared to the shaman in human form and probably were ultimately derived from the ghosts of the dead. During performances, each spirit was summoned when the shaman's clanmates sang its song and the assistant beat the drum, while the shaman donned his garb. The spirit then entered the shaman's body and spoke through his or her mouth, usually in a foreign tongue or obscure language.

When someone fell sick of an illness that did not yield to ordinary remedies, and especially if the patient was wealthy and of high rank, witchcraft was suspected. At such a time a shaman of a different clan, and preferably from a different village, was called in to name the one causing the illness and to exact a confession under torture and force the guilty party to undo the harmful spell. The witch or "master of sickness" was often someone, usually a man, inherently evil and consumed by envy of another's good fortune. He was one who possessed or was possessed by a malign spirit or power that made him "crazy" and drove him to frequent graveyards, where he reveled with the dead. It enabled him to change shape, fly through the air, and to kill by black magic. Witches obtained food leavings or scraps of clothing from the intended victim and made them into a doll in the likeness of the latter, placing it in a grave to rot. The evil could be neutralized if the confessed witch removed the doll and plunged with it into the sea. If the victim was cured, the witch might be pardoned, but the evil taint was passed on to all the witch's descendants. Witchcraft was the ultimate treason.

Unlike other members of society, who were cremated at death, a shaman's body was thought not to decay and was placed in a grave house with his dangerous paraphernalia nearby so that a successor in the same clan might soon become inspired.

Despite many years of contact with Europeans, which began in 1741 when Captain Chirikov's vessel *St. Paul* made landfall in the Sitka region, the Tlingit maintained their traditional subsistence and culture for a century, successfully resisting Russian domination and skillfully exploiting European rivalries to their own advantage. However, the first decades after the U.S. purchase in 1867 brought major dislocations to Tlingit society and culture as the territory was flooded by prospectors, adventurers, military and government men, and missionaries. The opening of salmon canneries and the establishment of local businesses and schools resulted in major changes to traditional Tlingit economic and social life. This process was further hastened by the Gold Rush of 1898–99, such that by the end of the century Tlingit acculturation to American society was well advanced.

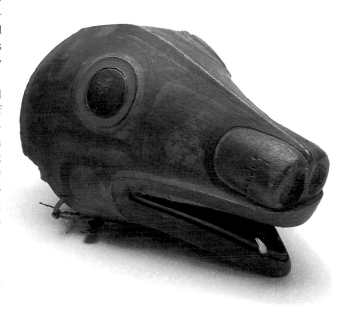

Northern Athapaskans: People of the Deer

James W. VanStone

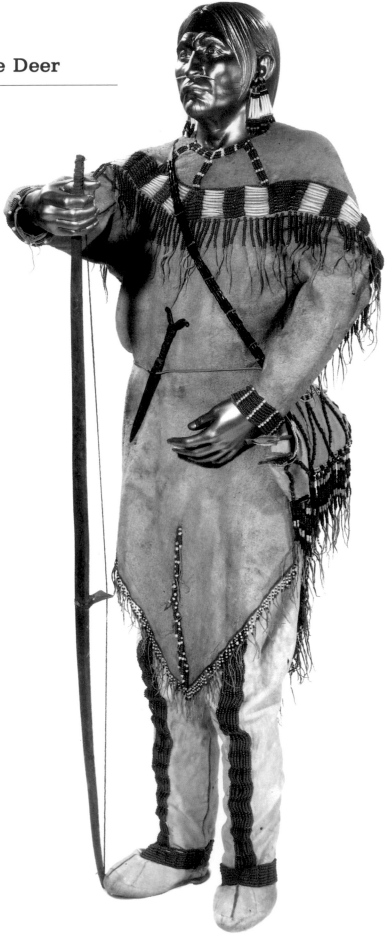

The area occupied by northern Athapaskan Indians lies directly south of the true arctic regions in a belt of coniferous forests broken in places by high mountains and stretches of treeless tundra. Except in the far western portion where the Rocky Mountains occur, much of this area is of relatively slight elevation, and there are numerous low, rolling glaciated hills. The climate of the region is characterized by long, cold winters and short, warm summers. Snowfall is heavier than along the arctic coast, and in general the climate is quite different from the desertlike coastal areas inhabited by Eskimos.

The northern Athapaskans inhabit the western part of this coniferous forest belt, specifically the drainage of the Yukon River and those parts of the Northwest Territories, northern British Columbia, Alberta, Saskatchewan, and Manitoba drained by the Mackenzie River. The total area of Athapaskan occupancy falls naturally into two sections, a Pacific and an arctic drainage area. In spite of the pervasiveness of the northern coniferous forest and its seeming uniformity over vast distances, the mountainous nature of much of the region occupied by northern Athapaskans and its considerable spread—from north to south as well as from east to west—is such that there are few areas of North America within which the environmental contrasts are so great and the natural barriers between native groups so formidable.

The various groups of northern Athapaskans speak languages that belong to the Athapaskan branch of the Na-Dene speech family. In fact, it is primarily language, together with occupation of a common territory, that serves to set off the various Athapaskan groups from one another since, like the Eskimos, they do not have formal tribal organization.

The northern Athapaskan area can be conveniently divided into five contiguous physiographic units that give maximum recognition to the most significant ecological factors that have influenced the lives of the Indians. These are the arctic drainage lowlands, dominated by the basin of the Mackenzie River; the cordilleran, named in recognition of the great mountain chain running in a generally south to north direction through western British Columbia and the Yukon Territory into Alaska; the Yukon and Kuskokwim river basins; the Cook Inlet–Susitna River basin; and the Copper River basin.

The arctic drainage lowlands are occupied only by Canadian Athapaskans, and those groups will not be discussed here. Four Alaskan groups live in the cordilleran region, the Upper Koyukon, Kutchin, Han, and Upper Tanana. All except the Upper Koyukon extend into Canada. The remaining physiographic units are entirely within Alaska. The Ingalik, Koyukon, and Tanana inhabit the Yukon and Kuskokwim river basins; the Tanaina, the only Athapaskan group living on the seacoast, occupy the Cook Inlet–Susitna River basin; and the Ahtna live in the Copper River basin. The most reliable estimates available for the late 19th and early 20th centuries indicate a population of 6,750 for these groups.

The subsistence activities of all northern Athapaskans reflected a changing economic relationship to their environment throughout the year. Athapaskans were exclusively hunters and gatherers, but there were considerable differences in emphasis in the use by specific groups of the natural resources available to them.

Although the arctic drainage lowlands are outside the scope of this account, it can be noted that the people there were primarily hunters, exploiting all the animal resources in their environment, particularly moose and caribou. In the northern part of the cordilleran region occupied by Alaskan groups subsistence also centered around the hunting of large game animals.

However, the Kutchin, extending considerably to the west of the mountain chain, exhibited greater diversity in their subsistence activities. In the east, the Chandalar Kutchin were typically big-game hunters of the high country. Caribou, the most important animal hunted, were taken in surrounds, and when large game was scarce, many small mammals provided an alternative food supply as did a variety of birds, particularly ptarmigan and spruce hens in winter and ducks and geese during the summer months. Unlike other Kutchin, the Chandalar made little use of fish, although they were occasionally taken in winter through the ice.

This lack of emphasis on fishing separated the Chandalar Kutchin from the groups to the west. In the Yukon Flats area, for example, from early July until early September the Indians took salmon with dip nets and basket-shaped traps. When the fishing season was over, the Yukon Flats people hunted moose and caribou until the river was frozen. Although predictable fish runs allowed the Yukon Flats Kutchin to enjoy a certain stability unknown to peoples almost completely dependent on hunting, periods of starvation were known to all the Kutchin and, indeed, to most Athapaskans.

In the Yukon and Kuskokwim river basins fishing was of primary importance and took precedence over all other forms of subsistence. The Ingalik and other inhabitants of this region hunted moose, caribou, bear, and most other subarctic animals, but it was fishing that gave stability to their way of life, a stability not approached in the other physiographic units. In keeping with the importance of fishing and the variety of fish available in the environment, the Ingalik had a highly developed fishing technology. Long-handled dip nets were used for taking salmon in spring and summer, and netlike drags of willows were used in the shallow waters of the innumerable Yukon sloughs. For lake fishing, fish-shaped lure hooks were characteristic and gill nets of various sizes were used in both summer and winter. The most common method of fishing among the Ingalik, however, was the use of basket-shaped traps of varying sizes and shapes for dog salmon, whitefish, losh, blackfish, jackfish, and grayling. They were set in swift water in spring and summer and under the ice in winter. Traps were particularly effective in the muddy waters of the Yukon and its lower tributaries where they could not be seen by the fish. Most fish caught during summer months were dried and stored in caches for dog food as well as human consumption.

For the Tanaina Indians in the Cook Inlet–Susitna River basin, sea mammal hunting was of considerable importance in restricted areas

67. Athapaskan Hunter

The Athapaskans, nomadic hunters and fishermen, did not have an extensive inventory of material culture. Great artistic effort was invested, however, in clothing, jewelry, and weapons. This chiefly hunter's tunic, leggings, and mitts are of tanned caribou or moose skin ornamented with fringes and a bright display of beads and dentalium shells. Dentalium shell earrings, nose pin, and tattoos augment the majesty of his appearance. A quiver, bow, and hunting knife complete the outfit. FM 14937 (quiver), USNM 1857 (tunic, leggings), 43352 (arrows), 153428 (knife), 209941 (bow)

of their territory. The Cook Inlet Tanaina possessed Eskimo-like kayaks from which seals were hunted with bows and arrows or harpoons. Sea otters, whose skins were highly prized in the early period of European contact, were hunted by special parties organized for the purpose. The animals could be killed easily from kayaks with bows and arrows or harpoons in calm weather when they were sleeping on their backs.

The hunting of sea lions was restricted to the Kachemak Bay region. These large animals were usually harpooned, the wounded creature dragging a line with a sealskin float attached until it tired and could be killed by a hunter with a bone-headed spear. Belugas, or white whales, are common in the upper inlet area, where they feed on tomcod. Several hunters were required in taking belugas, which were hunted with the same size of harpoon used for sea lions.

It is clear that in the hunting of sea mammals the Tanaina were heavily influenced by their Eskimo neighbors. Their area was also rich in land animals including black bears, caribou, moose, and, on the eastern edge of the upper inlet country, mountain sheep and goats.

The subsistence patterns of the Ahtna of the Copper River basin have never been described in detail. Although living in a mountainous region rich in game, the Ahtna, like the Yukon and Kuskokwim river basin groups, depended heavily on salmon fishing. In the turbulent Copper River, fishing presented special problems that did not occur often elsewhere in the Athapaskan area. Gill nets and traps were easily swept away by the fast waters, so the Indians depended heavily on dip nets to take the several varieties of salmon as they ascended the river to spawn. Moose and bear were the most important large game animals, but early explorers reported that the Ahtna depended heavily on small game, particularly hares, to carry them through those periods in late winter and early spring when supplies of dried fish were low.

Although the emphasis has been on those activities and techniques that were of particular importance in the major ecological zones of the Athapaskan area, this should not obscure the fact that throughout the region there was considerable uniformity. Every animal in the environment was utilized when the need arose, and many of the methods and techniques used to take them were common throughout the area. Subsistence activities in the western subarctic were highly generalized, at least in comparison to the specialized nature of subsistence in some other areas of North America.

The dwellings of aboriginal northern Athapaskans, reflecting the extreme mobility of most of these groups, were among the simplest constructed by any people in North America. As might be expected, the simplest structures were found among the most mobile groups, and more complex construction was characteristic of the more sedentary peoples. Among every Athapaskan group, the pattern of shelter reflected not only the subsistence activities characteristic of particular times of the year but also climatic variations.

Although the cordilleran region has a considerable north to south range, the dwelling types within this vast region did not exhibit a great deal of variation, and reflected the mobility that characterized the groups that inhabited the region. The Upper Tanana may be considered reasonably typical. The several types of houses utilized by these people can be grouped into two categories: semipermanent and temporary. In the former category was the circular winter house, which consisted of a frame of long, curved poles, the lower ends of which were stuck in the snow; the upper ends did not come together at the top, thus leaving a smoke hole. These poles were reinforced by being lashed to two horizontal poles, the arches of which followed the inner curve of the structure. The typical domed lodge, covered with sewn moose hides, was about 14 feet in diameter, 8 feet high, and required between 18 and 20 hides for its cover.

Summer houses among the Upper Tanana were somewhat more permanent and located near good fishing sites. These dwellings were rectangular in floor plan, with parallel series of poles driven into the ground to make an outside and inside wall. Strips of spruce or birch bark were then laid between them. Sometimes these houses, which were as much as 20 or 30 feet in length and occupied by several families, had flat roofs, but a gabled roof was probably more characteristic. This type of summer dwelling was widely distributed among cordilleran Athapaskans and was also used by the Ahtna of the Copper River basin (fig. 262).

The only temporary shelters used by the Upper Tanana were of simple lean-to construction, covered with bark or boughs. Often two such shelters were built facing each other with a fire between them and each side occupied by a family. This double lean-to construction was typical of many northern Athapaskans in all physiographic units.

It is likely that even the most permanent of the structures just described were not often constructed twice in the same place. In the Yukon and Kuskokwim river basins more sedentary groups like the Ingalik occupied permanent winter villages and summer fish camps usually not far from the winter settlements. The Ingalik live in close proximity to the Eskimo of the lower

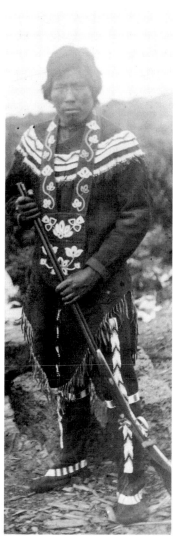

Yukon River, and their culture has been influenced in a number of ways by Eskimos. In few areas is this influence more noticeable than in housing.

The Ingalik erected at least three types of winter houses of varying sizes, all of which resembled to a marked degree the semisubterranean, earth-covered Eskimo house of Southwest Alaska. The smaller structures were about 16 feet long and slightly less wide, but much larger ones were also built. In addition, in their winter villages they constructed a *kashim*, or ceremonial house, which was also semisubterranean and as much as 35 feet by 25 feet in size. It had a cribbed roof, a long entryway that widened to form a separate room, and benches on all four sides. The *kashim*, a characteristic feature of Eskimo villages throughout Southwest Alaska, served as a sleeping room and work room for the men, a place to take sweat baths, and a theater for religious and secular ceremonies.

A number of different dwellings were also constructed in summer villages and fish camps. They were aboveground, rectangular structures with pitched roofs and walls of vertically placed spruce planks, spruce bark, or birch bark strips. The Ingalik also made smokehouses, constructed like the summer houses, for smoking fish.

In the Cook Inlet–Susitna River basin, the Tanaina Indians, who were even more sedentary than the Ingalik, constructed a large log winter house with a gabled roof that could have several rooms and a bathhouse attached. The Tanaina also made semispherical lodges with pole frameworks and bark or grass covering for use on hunting trips during all seasons of the year.

Although northern Athapaskans lacked any concept of group identification beyond that of territory or language, each of the identified groups or tribes was divided into subgroups. It was these subgroups rather than the larger enclaves that had social meaning to the people themselves.

Most aboriginal northern Athapaskans spent at least part of the year in small aggregates or local bands consisting of a few nuclear families, but at certain times of the year the ecology of an area permitted several small units of this type to come together to form a regional band. Summer fishing and fall caribou migrations are good examples of the kinds of situations that permitted local bands to gather as a regional band, usually associated with a particular region, shaped in large measure by the drainage pattern of the land. The regional band exploited the total range of the land as identified by tradition and use. It utilized all the resources within the range and could exist for many generations. The local

band exploited its smaller range and was essentially a grouping of close kinsmen, and since its temporal duration was related to the activities for which it was organized, it might be in existence for only a generation or two.

Both offensive and defensive warfare were known among northern Athapaskans, and this type of activity frequently led to another type of leader: the war leader. These individuals were usually aggressive men who dominated through their physical strength. Generally speaking, war represented retaliation for offenses committed by relative strangers upon members of the group. Since revenge in turn promoted the desire for fresh vengeance on the part of the opposite side, antagonism between groups could be chronic.

The basic unit of social organization among northern Athapaskans was the nuclear family consisting of a man, his wife or wives, and their natural or adopted children. Throughout much of the Athapaskan area, extended kinship was characterized by the presence of matrilineal sib organization, consanguineal kin groups that acknowledged a traditional bond of common descent in the maternal line. These sibs generally were exogamous; that is, a person had to find a mate outside his sib. Sib affiliations played an important part in warfare, marriages, funerals, and potlatches. Matrilineal residence, whereby a newly married couple lives with or near the bride's family, was characteristic throughout much of the area.

An important feature of social organization among many Athapaskans was the potlatch, a ceremony in honor of the dead that is best known as it occurs among Indians of the Northwest Coast. Among Athapaskans, the potlatch was most fully developed among western tribes, a fact that has led to the general belief that the trait diffused from the Northwest Coast into the Athapaskan area. The potlatch was the chief means by which an individual achieved prestige in his own or neighboring bands. If a man aspired to be a leader, he had to give a potlatch whenever possible, and the death of even a distant relative provided an excuse to celebrate and distribute gifts.

If one were to select the single most consistent feature of aboriginal Athapaskan magico-religious belief systems, it would be the significant reciprocal relationship that existed between men and the animals on which they were dependent for their livelihood. Superior-subordinate aspects were largely absent from this relationship, possibly because of a widespread belief in reincarnation in animal form. This belief tended to blur the distinction between animals and men, and to emphasize the fact that the spirits of animals had to be placated if men were to continue their exploitative relationship to the environment.

Another characteristic of the belief system was its individualism. The cultures of hunting peoples must of necessity socialize individuals to a high degree of independence, since survival depends to a large degree on individual skills. From the standpoint of religion, this meant that a great deal of emphasis was placed on individual rituals rather than on community rites.

Personal power was the vital element in religious life and those individuals with the most personal power, the shamans, were the only professional religious practitioners. The shaman and the magico-religious practices he used to control the spirit world were the most important features of northern Athapaskan religion, and were, in most respects, similar to shamanistic practices among the Eskimos and Tlingits. The primary duties of any shaman were to prevent and cure disease. In addition, shamans also brought game to hunters, predicted the weather, and were able to foretell the future.

Although dramatic group ceremonies were not prevalent among the individualistic northern Athapaskans, some did occur, particularly among western groups. The potlatch may be considered such a ceremony, even though its religious elements were of minimal importance. The most elaborate ceremonies were performed by the Ingalik in their village *kashim*s. Many of these were associated with respect for animals, including not only species important for subsistence like salmon but also those that the Indians feared and respected because of their considerable power, such as the wolf and wolverine.

The western subarctic was penetrated from two directions by representatives of European nations. From the east came English fur traders. Having secured their position in eastern Canada, they followed the continental rivers and lakes to the interior of the Canadian northwest, where trading posts were established in the drainage of the Mackenzie River in the late 18th century. From the west came the Russians who, after 1741, explored the coast and ascended the major rivers into the interior. Trading posts had been established among Alaskan Athapaskans by 1840.

It is possible to discern two major phases of contact relations. The early contact period, which lasted approximately between 1700 and 1850, included rivalry between the Hudson's Bay Company and its competitors in the east and the trade monopoly of the Russian American Company in the west. European diseases were introduced, frequently with devastating effects, and the first Christian missionaries entered the region. The stabilized fur trade and mission period, which lasted from about 1850 to 1940, was a time of relatively slow, uninterrupted change, although more rapid in the west after the purchase of Alaska by the United States in 1867. During this second period, Indians had direct access to trade goods and intensive exposure to missionary influence. Mission and later government schools were established, and there was an intrusion of gold miners in some areas, most notably on the upper Yukon River.

Indian life changed in some essential ways as a result of involvement in the fur trade. Aboriginal subsistence activities did not involve extensive trapping, and most of the fur-bearing animals desired by the fur trade were not suitable for food. It was the need to procure food to support life during periods when animals without food value were being hunted that eventually bound the Indians closely to the posts where they traded.

Trapping effectively signaled the end to exploitation of the total environment. Specialized knowledge of animal behavior was still an important adaptive strategy, but its emphasis shifted considerably. Knowledge of the habits of fur-bearing animals and their environments was now of greater importance than a similar knowledge of large game animals and fish. This shift of emphasis and its commercial implications also disturbed the balanced reciprocal relationship between the hunter and his animal spirit helpers, thus undermining a basic aspect of the traditional religious belief system.

Opposite:
"Aleut [of Kodiak Island] in Festival Dress Demonstrating How They Hunt" (Mikhail Tikhanov, 1817, RIPSA 2127)

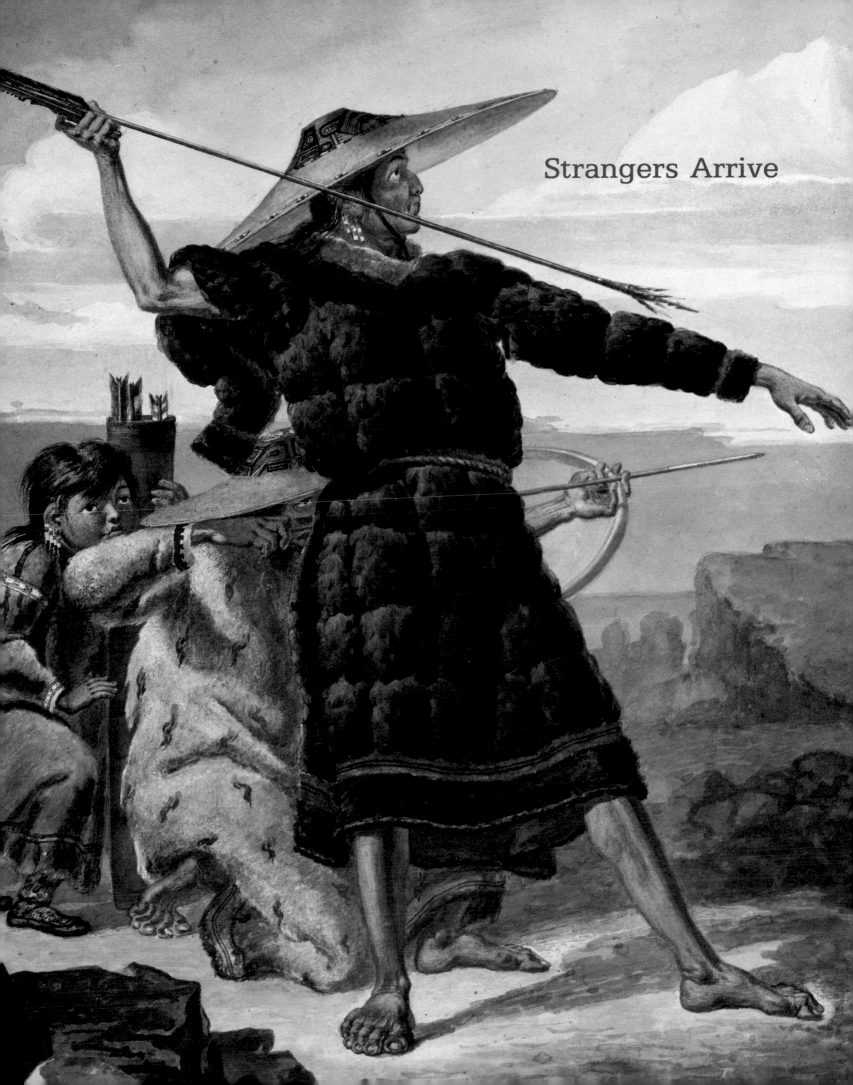

Strangers Arrive

The Story of Russian America

Lydia T. Black

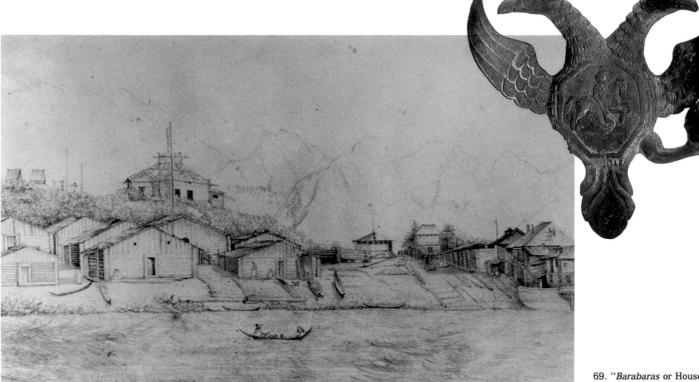

69. "*Barabaras* or Houses of the Koloshi along the Harbor of Novo-Arkhangel'sk"
Pencil drawing by I. G. Voznesenskii, 1843–45. MAE 1142-12

The Russian fort of Novo-Arkhangel'sk ("New Archangel") at Sitka, Alaska, was built in 1804–5 after the Tlingit Indians (called Kolosh by the Russians) overran and destroyed an earlier Sitka fort. Novo-Arkhangel'sk grew into a major trading post and the administrative center of the Russian American Company. The Russians continued to feel threatened by the presence of the Tlingits, who built a large village around the walls of the fort, yet depended on them for fresh food.

70. Russian Double-headed Eagle Crest
NMAH 420307

The double-headed eagle was the imperial emblem of Tsarist Russia, adopted from Byzantine heraldry in the 15th century. Buried plates and brass eagle crests were used to mark Russian claims of American territory, starting with the voyage of explorers Bochorov and Izmailov in 1788. This rare example entered the aboriginal trade network and was excavated in 1934 from a late 18th-century Klikitat Indian grave on an island in the Columbia River, Oregon.

For almost a century and a half, beginning in 1741, Alaska was an integral part of the Russian Empire. Then, overextended in the wake of the defeat in the Crimean War in the 1850s and afraid of British expansion to the North Pacific, the Imperial government in 1867 invited the United States to step in and take over the territory. Two groups of people, more than any others, were responsible for winning, and holding, Alaska for Russia. These were the men of the Russian Navy and, by far the most important, the fur hunters and traders—the seagoing mountainmen of the Russian North. Thus, the story of the Russian expansion onto the American continent begins long before 1741, the year a Russian Navy squadron under Vitus Bering claimed Alaska for Russia. In fact, Russians stood on the Pacific by the beginning of the 17th century, when Salem and Boston and English settlements in Virginia were being founded or were young and struggling. But the story of Russian America really begins on the shores of the Polar Sea, half a millennium earlier.

Pomorie, the coasts of the White and Barents seas, the cradle of Russian polar navigation and home to the ancestors of the men who claimed Alaska, was settled by the Russians between the 5th and 9th centuries. Already between the 9th and the 11th centuries, Russian entrepreneurs were extending their activities to the Ob River in Siberia. Russian fishermen and sea mammal hunters since the 13th century were sailing to Novaia Zemlia for walrus and to Spitsbergen for cod, halibut, walrus, and whales (Belov 1956). By the 15th century, such voyages were a matter of course. Sailings along the shore to the east were also common, but here the mountainmen were but the spearhead. The administrator, the garrison, and the tax collector followed close on their heels. By 1600, by orders of the Tsar, the building of the commercial port of Mangazeia on the Taz River, which empties into the Ob near its mouth, was commenced. This port was second only to the great city of Arkhangel'sk, by then several centuries old. By that year, the Russians also had reached the Yenisei River to the east of the Ob.

Since the 15th century, the idea of a northern, coastal sea route to China and India was current in Russia. Soon, the notion spread to Western Europe. Holland and England, trading through Arkhangel'sk in the 16th century for ships' timber, cordage, beeswax, furs, and other products of the Russian North, entered the search for the Northeast Passage, but through the 17th century there was little success in sailing the long and icebound route along the Polar shores of Eurasia with ships not suited for polar navigation.

In the meantime, Russian fur hunters and traders steadily advanced along the coast, sailing from river mouth to river mouth, penetrating the Siberian interior by going upriver, portaging to the next river drainage to the east, and descending again to the sea. The Lena River was reached early in the 1600s. Between 1633 and 1637, the basins of the Iana and Indigirka rivers were explored. Moskvitin reached the coast of the Okhotsk Sea, 1639–41. Others followed in rapid succession. In 1643, Poiarkov was at the mouth of the Amur River. By 1644 the Kolyma and the Polar shore of the Chukchi Peninsula were reached. The Anadyr River draining into the Bering Sea became known. By the 1680s, the Kamchatka Peninsula was conquered, and in 1711 the Kurile Islands were explored. By this time, the sea route from the Polar to the Bering Sea was well known locally.

In 1647, the expedition organized by Fedot Popov and Aleksei Usov and led by Semeon Dezhnev set out to round the Chukchi Peninsula

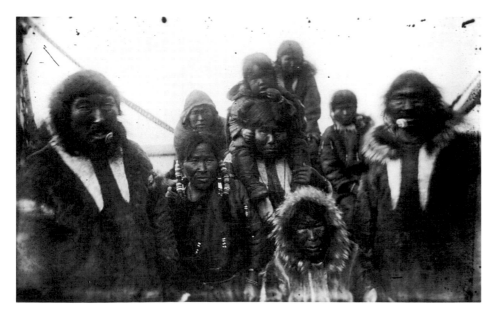

71. North Alaskan Eskimos, Cape Smith
Edward Nelson, 1881. SI neg. 6394
In 1655 Dezhnev reported Chukchi familiarity with the "toothed people"—Eskimos living on the Diomede Islands in Bering Strait. The name referred to the labrets (lip plugs) worn by the Eskimo, and possibly to the walrus tusk gores inset on their parkas.

and reach the Anadyr River by sea. Popov and Usov were men of the White Sea, descendants of a long line of polar merchant-navigators. Dezhnev was a Cossack. The expedition sailed the *koch*, a vessel developed in the Pomorie specifically for sailing in ice-infested polar waters (Belov 1955, 1973). It was derived from the more ancient *lod'ia*, a single-masted barque-type vessel, a variant of the cargo vessels used by the Scandinavian Vikings (Belov 1956). Sev-

eral other expeditions followed the same route within the next 20 years (Orlova 1951). The existence of the "Great Land" to the east of the Chukchi Peninsula and across the "Eastern Sea" was part of local knowledge, and so were the Diomede Islands in the Bering Strait and in all probability St. Lawrence Island.

The navy began to play an active role in the reign of Peter the Great (1682–1725). First under his leadership, then under his successors, the government began consistently to take the lead in exploration of the northern regions and advancement to the American continent. By 1713 the sea route to Kamchatka from the locality that became the port of Okhotsk, the first Russian port and shipbuilding center on the Pacific, was explored. In 1716, the government authorized the Great Kamchatka Command (Bolshoi Kamchatskii Nariad) under El'chin to explore the Siberian northeast. In 1719, Peter sent the first topographers, Evreinov and Luzhin, to survey the Pacific shores. In 1720 they sailed from Okhotsk to Kamchatka, in 1721 to the Kurile Islands. In 1725, following the instructions Peter the Great signed on his deathbed, Bering's first expedition commenced, but Bering, instead of sailing east, went to the north through the strait that now bears his name in 1728 (Fisher 1988). Between 1729 and 1733, an expedition under Shestakov was ordered to explore Kamchatka and Chukchi Peninsula, by land and by sea. As part of this effort, in July 1732, the Navy vessel *Sv. Gavriil* visited the Diomedes and stood off Cape Prince of Wales, reporting the first official contact between the Russian Navy and Alaskan natives.

In the meantime, the government was preparing an enormous exploratory effort in the North, both on the Polar and Pacific shores. This effort, which lasted many years, is known as the Great Northern Expedition. It commenced in 1732 and covered three main areas: the northern arm, comprising several detachments, charted the entire Polar coast of Siberia; the second, under Spanberg, was to chart the Okhotsk Sea and the coasts of Japan; the third, under Bering, was to sail to America, to the Spanish territories in the south, and claim the northwest coast for Russia. Bering's vessels reached the American coast in 1741, establishing Russian sovereignty over Alaska on an international basis. The landfalls made during this voyage determined the boundaries of the territory of Alaska as it is today.

Though the Russian government clearly intended to assert its sovereignty and presence in the newly claimed lands on the American continent, European wars (especially with Turkey and Sweden) as well as internal Russian

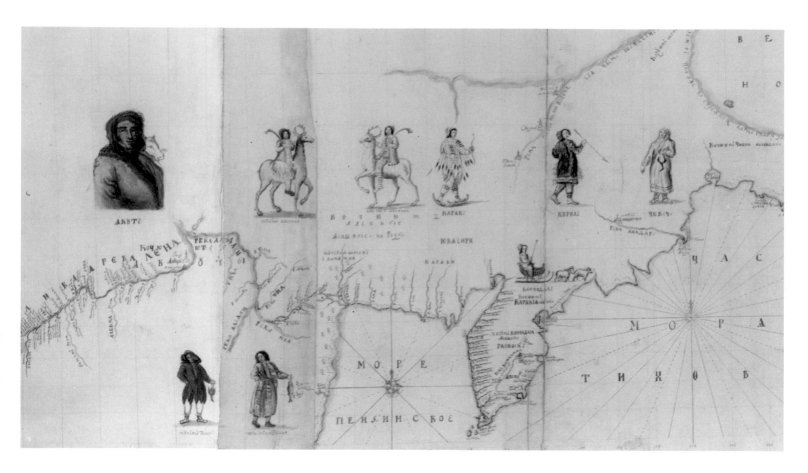

politics intervened. Following Bering's expedition to America until the end of the 18th century the field, once again, fell to the private entrepreneur. The shipowners and builders of Kamchatka and the fur hunters and skippers who sailed in these vessels, built to the ancient northern models, almost to a man were descendants of the sailors and sea mammal hunters and of Cossacks who won eastern Siberia for the crown. The sea held no terrors for them. Beginning in 1745, their advance eastward along the Aleutian Island chain and then along the Pacific coast of Alaska was rapid. Within 20 years, they had a foothold on Prince William Sound and were looking eastward to the Columbia River and northward along the Alaskan coast to Bering Strait.

The early skippers and foremen, sailing with small crews, about half of whom were Kamchatka natives, sought fur seal and sea otter for the Chinese market in Kamchatka and Okhotsk waters and in the Kurile Islands. The move to the Aleutian chain was but an extension of an ongoing enterprise. The environment was familiar, and they could hold their own against the Aleuts. They did not intentionally seek conflict, though sporadic violence occurred. But in

the main, the skippers' object was trade, and they sought to establish trading partnerships with the Aleuts whenever they could. These men were tough, resourceful, and able to endure incredible hardships. Many died on the Alaskan shores; others sailed the Aleutian waters and explored Alaska for several decades.

In the eastern Aleutians, they encountered a formidable people, the Qawalangin of Umnak and Unalaska and the Qigigun of the Krenitzin Islands. Beginning in December 1763, the Aleuts of these two groups, in concert with the people of Unimak Island and the Alaska Peninsula, destroyed four Russian vessels. Of the crews, only 12 men (4 Russians and 8 Itelmen) survived. The Russians, following their original loss, retaliated, and the result was the beginning of the end for Aleut independence.

Other Russian vessels arrived, and prodded by the survivors as well as by considerations of their own safety, one skipper, Ivan Solov'ev, conducted a preventive strike against the Aleuts of Unalaska. By destroying Aleut kayaks, hunting equipment, and war weapons, Solov'ev forced the Umnak/Unalaska alliance to sue for peace. The period of Russian dominance in the eastern Aleutians thus dates to the year of 1766. Spo-

72. Map of Siberia, First Bering Expedition (1725–30)
Royal Library, Stockholm 2:12:17
The first Bering expedition produced the earliest "ethnographic map" of Siberia, with watercolor depictions of Siberian peoples. *Upper row, left to right:* portrait of a Yakut, a mounted Reindeer Evenk man and woman, a Koryak man on snowshoes, an Ainu with harpoon, a Chukchi. *Lower row:* a man with a bird and woman with a fish of the unmounted or "foot" Tungus, an Itelmen with dog sled.

73. Ivory Sea Otter with Pup
Aleut: MAE 2938-6
Special rituals surrounded the hunting of sea otters, viewed by the Aleut as transformed human beings.

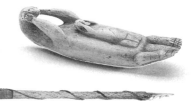

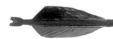

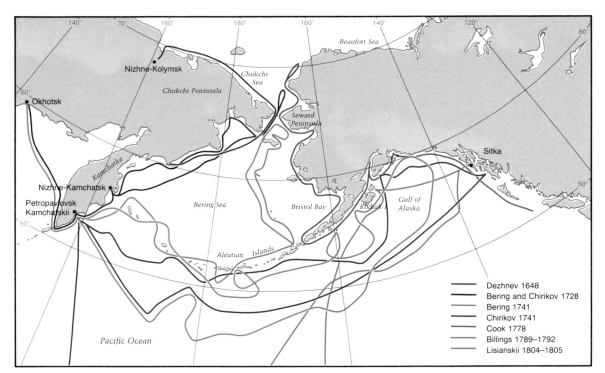

74. Early Voyages of Exploration to Alaska

The 1741 voyages of Vitus Bering and Alexei Chirikov confirmed the existence of Alaska, first reported by the 1648 Dezhnev Expedition. The Billings Expedition and other efforts by Russia to explore Alaska and strengthen its territorial claims were stimulated by competing efforts such as the Alaskan navigations of Great Britain's Capt. James Cook in 1778. Lisianskii's visit to Alaska was part of the first Russian circumnavigation of the globe (1803–1806).

——	Dezhnev 1648
——	Bering and Chirikov 1728
——	Bering 1741
——	Chirikov 1741
——	Cook 1778
——	Billings 1789–1792
——	Lisianskii 1804–1805

75. War Shield

Aleut (Kagamil Island): NMNH 389861

Aleut and Koniag warriors waged successful attacks against the ships and shore parties of early fur trading expeditions. Russian firearms and cannon, as well as the practice of holding native hostages eventually were successful in overcoming resistance.

76. Harpoon Arrow for Sea Otters

Koniag Eskimo: NMNH 16407

Using a technique known as "surround hunting," kayak hunters shot these arrows as they drew an ever-tightening circle around a sea otter in the water. The barbed head buried itself in the otter's flesh, while the shaft detached, unrolled, and dragged behind to retard the animal's escape.

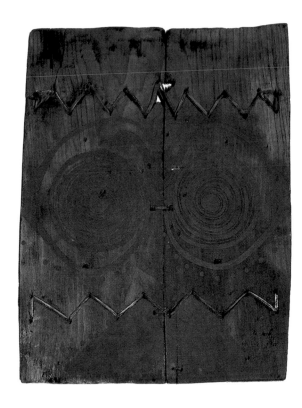

radic resistance to Russian intrusion continued here and there in the Krenitzin Islands and on Unimak, but never again were the Aleuts able to mount a concerted effort of the kind that took place between 1763 and 1766.

In the meantime, with the ascent to the throne of Catherine the Great, in 1762, the Russian government renewed its interest in establishing control in the new lands. Twenty-five years after Bering's voyage of 1741, the navy was once

again to sail to America. The plan was a complex one. The foremost Russian scholar of the age, Mikhail Lomonosov, became interested in the old notion of the sea route to India via the Polar Sea. In 1763, he presented the hypothesis that the sea around the pole, above 80° latitude, should be ice-free because of submarine volcanic action and other factors. He proposed that not only China and India would be much more easily accessible via the cross-polar route but the American continent as well (Lomonosov 1763/ 1952). The project was approved by the admiralty, and in May 1765 a three-ship squadron, commanded by Chichagov, sailed from the Kola Peninsula, past Spitsbergen northward. He reached 80°26' north latitude but was forced to turn back by the pack ice. Next summer, he was ordered by the admiralty to sea again, and again was defeated by the pack ice. In the meantime, the admiralty had dispatched to the Aleutian archipelago a two-ship squadron under the command of Captain Krenitsyn, known as the Levashev-Krenitsyn Expedition. They were to meet Chichagov and exchange officers and crews so that the largest number of sailors would become familiar with the polar route on one hand and with the Kamchatka-America route on the other. The Levashev-Krenitsyn squadron, with most of the experienced local merchant skippers called into service as pilots and navigators, reached Alaska in 1768, departing in 1769. This expedition produced the first navy charts of the Krenitzin Islands, Unimak Island, and the Alaska Peninsula as well as the first ethnographic account of the eastern Aleut people. Invaluable

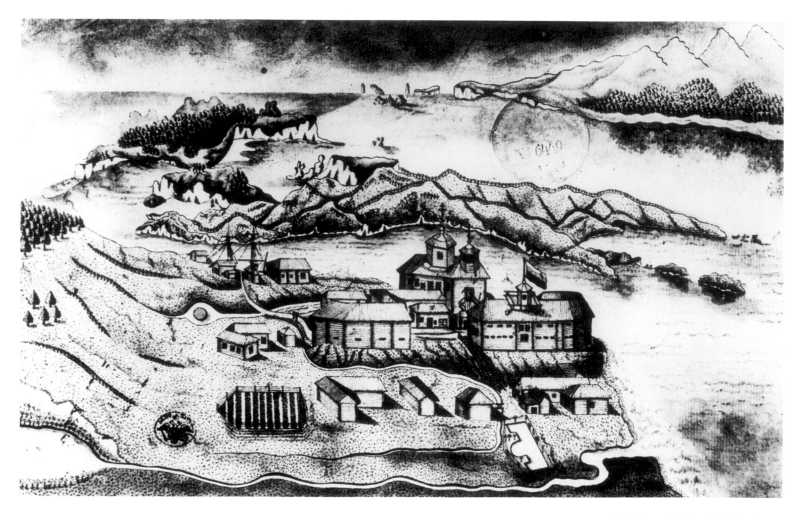

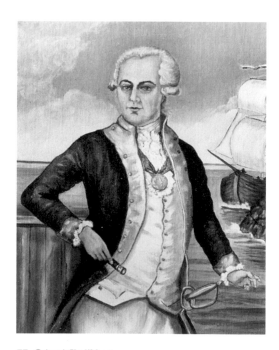

**77. Grigori Shelikhov
(1747–1795)**

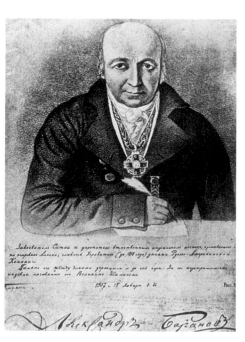

**78. Aleksandr Baranov (ca. 1747–
1819)**

Engraving after a portrait by Mikhail
Tikhanov.

**79. "View of Pavlovskii Harbor from
the North, 1798"**

Attributed to James Shields

In order to take advantage of locally
abundant timber and an excellent
harbor, Aleksandr Baranov moved the
headquarters of Shelikhov's fur trading company to Pavlovskii (St. Paul)
in 1792, at the site of the modern
city of Kodiak, Alaska. Buildings in
the settlement included company
headquarters, Orthodox church, bar-
racks, storehouses, workshops, and
residences.

are Levashev's illustrations. He painted dwellings, costumes, tools, and weapons of the Qawalangin (fig. 55) and produced the first technical sketches of the kayaks and umiaks used there.

This activity of the Russian Navy aroused great interest on the part of Western European powers, and in 1778 Britain dispatched Capt. James Cook to North Pacific waters—a step that could not but alarm the Russian government. In response, Catherine the Great decided to show the Imperial flag in no uncertain terms. Russian discoveries in the Pacific Ocean were for the first time officially proclaimed by the government. Beginning with 1785, a navy expedition to the North Pacific, under Captain Billings, was sailing from Okhotsk, and on December 22, 1786, an Imperial order decreed the sending from Kronstadt of a circumnavigating expedition to the American coast ''for the safeguarding of our land, discovered by Russian navigators.'' The expedition's commander, Mulovskii, had governmental powers, and he was to claim the American coast from Nootka on Vancouver Island in the east to the Near Islands in the west. Ironically, it was the intelligence obtained at Unalaska by Martinez from Potap Zaikov about the coming of this navy squadron that triggered Spanish determination to claim Nootka, where Spain seized the British merchant ships. As a result, the British moved against Spain and gained, by 1790, sovereignty over the coast of what is now British Columbia. But Mulovskii's squadron never sailed. The war with Turkey broke out anew, and in 1787 Sweden and Russia were, also, once again at war. The ships sailed to fight the Swedish Navy.

Consideration of international politics, however, was not the sole motivating power in the plan to establish the governmental presence on the American continent. In 1783, Grigorii Shelikhov equipped three vessels for Alaskan trade and sailed to America. For Shelikhov, trade was not a sole aim. He dreamed of an empire on the American continent, from Prince William Sound to Bering Strait, where settlers would build cities, cathedrals, and schools. He dreamed of a land economically self-supporting, producing its own food, building its own ships, developing industries that would make Alaska an economic center for the world. Thus, Shelikhov differed essentially from the other fur-trading companies operating at that time in Alaska. His goal was not trade with the natives but permanent settlement. For his first base, Shelikhov chose the most populous and hitherto (because of its military strength) largely bypassed island of Kodiak. The conquest was swift and brutal. At one stroke, going in force, Shelikhov gained a foothold that was the key to expansion to the continent. By

1786, he had fortified outposts on Afognak Island and the Kenai Peninsula.

Word of the brutality of the conquest and Aleut complaints about abuses had reached St. Petersburg, and the government was concerned. Billings, whose squadron was to support Mulovskii, received orders to investigate as well as to make the presence of the navy felt by the British. Since 1785 the British had been sending more and more heavily armed and large-capacity merchant vessels to the North Pacific and were flooding the Chinese market with sea otter pelts via Canton. In 1786 alone, nine British vessels were present from Copper Island to Prince William Sound. Billings was to intercept any of the British vessels that were privateers with Swedish letters of marque, especially the brig *Mercury*, which was said to have raided the central Aleut villages. He was also to hold an inquiry into Aleut complaints, particularly about Shelikhov's actions on Kodiak.

Shelikhov was able, however, with support from the governor of Siberia, in whose view Shelikhov's actions were more than justified by reasons of state, to beat the charges. The fact that he was also a builder mattered. Shelikhov established the first school on Kodiak by 1786. He instituted the first agricultural experiments and imported cattle and poultry, and successfully petitioned and financially supported the first ecclesiastical mission to Alaska. The clergy arrived on Kodiak Island in 1794. Here, Aleksandr Baranov, hired by Shelikhov in 1790 to become the manager of the Kodiak District, which encompassed the entire Kodiak archipelago, Cook Inlet, Prince William Sound, the Alaska Peninsula, and the Shumagin Islands, was by this time an absolute ruler. The clergy and Baranov were soon at loggerheads over the issue of Aleut rights. The clergy vigorously protested the economic exploitation of the Kodiak population and social abuses Baranov permitted his men. This stance was one of the major reasons why the Orthodox Church gained strength and adherents so that today it is perceived as a native institution, the primary marker of Aleut identity.

Aleut rights, however, had little importance for Baranov. While Shelikhov issued instructions for expansion to the Bering Strait, using the Pribilof Islands as a platform for the thrust in that direction, Baranov faced more immediate priorities. These priorities were dictated not only by the growing competition of British and American sea otter traders but also by the ever growing need for supplies. In Europe, Napoleon was on the march, and the difficulties of Russian merchants in Alaska were not on the government's urgent list. Baranov had to rely on his own resources. He felt that expansion east and south, to the Columbia River, to California, to Hawaii, was imperative if the colony were to survive.

When Shelikhov died in 1796, Baranov, with the support of Shelikhov's widow, Nataliia, did what he felt to be absolutely necessary: he expanded into the Tlingit territory previously explored and claimed in 1786. In fact, at least one of the bronze crests marking the land as Russian territory had been placed there.

That year Baranov established a settlement at Yakutat and soon thereafter on the island of Sitka (Baranov Island). Both locations were favorite stopping places of the British and Bostonian traders, and the choice was not random. Baranov wanted the Russian presence clearly demonstrated. In this effort, he relied mainly on the native force he recruited, by fair means and foul, of Koniags from the Kodiak archipelago, the Chugach from Prince William Sound, and men of the eastern Alaska Peninsula. The number of Russians was minuscule.

To achieve his aims, Baranov resorted to impressment. Almost all able-bodied Kodiak males were dragooned into service as hunters and warriors, paddling to the Tlingit territory in parties composed of several hundred two-hatch *baidarka*s. At Prince William Sound, these parties were joined by the Chugach, who anticipated revenge on their ancient enemies, the Tlingit. Armed with their traditional weapons, led by their own chiefs, but under overall command of individual Russians, they hunted sea otter for trade and sea mammals for food and, according to Tlingit folklore, raided Tlingit parties and villages. Later, these raids would extend as far south as San Diego and Baja California, when Kodiak and Chugach hunters were hired out by Baranov to American skippers for small salaries and a share of the sea otter take for the Russian American Company.

Back home, the absence of the men condemned the Kodiak villages to untold suffering. Food shortages were severe, skins for clothing and other household needs became almost nonexistent. More and more the population had to rely for relief on Baranov's largess, such as it was. Women worked for meager recompense as fish processors and sewers of clothing needed for Baranov's "army." Old men and young boys were sent out to take bird skins from which the women made parkas issued to their men. Despair reigned in the villages. It was this exploitation that aroused the wrath of the clergy, from Monk German (St. Herman of Alaska) to Archimandrite Ioasaf, Head of Mission, and later of Hiermonk Gideon, sent to Alaska by the Synod of the Orthodox Church. It was this system of impressment that moved navy officers, from Lisianskii

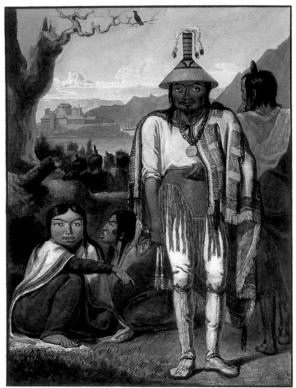

80. "Portrait of Toyon (Chief) Katlian and his Wife"
Mikhail Tikhanov, 1818: RIPSA 2116

Katlian (Kalyáan) was the military leader of the Kiks.ádi clan of the Tlingits in their battles with the Russians in 1802 and 1804. He wears a spruce root crest hat, Russian medal, Athapaskan skin trousers, and a woven ceremonial blanket in the pre-19th century "geometric" style (see fig. 284). In the background are Golovnin's sloop *Kamchatka* and the fortress at Sitka.

in 1804–05 to Golovnin in 1810 and 1817, to denounce Baranov to the government. But in the meantime, Baranov's energy and resourcefulness made possible the establishment of a Russian outpost deep in the Tlingit territory, at first with the consent of Tlingit leadership.

Before long, however, the initially peaceful relations between Baranov and the Tlingit became those of armed confrontation. The reasons were many and complex. Cultural miscommunication was, indubitably, at work. A weir built by Russians on a salmon stream at Yakutat interfered with the salmon run upstream, something that the Tlingit did not foresee when they granted Baranov permission to build a post there. At Sitka, already in 1797 and 1798, parties of Kodiak natives were taking 200 sea otter skins per season, which the Tlingit themselves wanted for trade with the British. The latter were not too pleased, and some leaders objected to the establishment of a permanent Russian base in 1799, when Baranov arrived with three vessels and a fleet of Kodiak Aleuts consisting of 550 *baidarka*s, to found the Redoubt of St. Michael the Archangel (Old Sitka). However, Baranov met with the senior local Tlingit chiefs and concluded an agreement. In return for permission to establish a settlement, he was to trade with them and provide protection against enemies. Unfortunately, the Tlingit did not understand that Baranov would not trade in firearms as the British and Americans were doing, nor that he would not supply any rum.

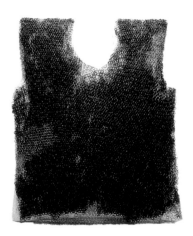

83. Baranov's Chain Mail Shirt
Russian: NMAH 237848

Baranov fought in several bloody engagements with Tlingit war parties in the course of his efforts to expand Russian American Company operations into southeastern Alaska: at Prince William Sound in 1792 and 1799, and at Sitka in 1804. He presented his chain mail shirt to Tlingit chief Naawushkeitl as a gesture of peace, probably in March 1800.

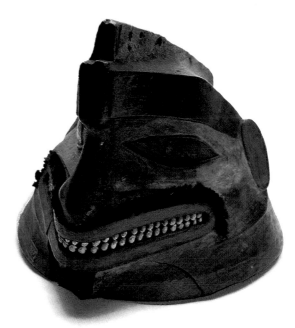

In the fall of 1799, Baranov sent back to Kodiak the Aleut fleet and all vessels but his own small *Olga*, leaving only 60 *baidarkas*—120 men—to provision the post with fish and sea mammals. On the way back, over a hundred Kodiak natives died from shellfish poisoning in Peril Strait. In the wake of this accident, the air was thick with suspicion of witchcraft. The Tlingit expected to be accused of causing the deaths. Indeed, Kodiak natives are said to have killed at least ten important Tlingit men, probably in retaliation for this ''witchcraft-caused'' misfortune. Tension grew. A meeting between Baranov and Tlingit leaders in 1800, when Baranov presented the head of the Kiks.ádi clan with a chain mail shirt, seemed to relieve mutual suspicions. But the respite from tension was short-lived. From the south, via the Haida, British and Americans offered supplies of weapons, firearms and pow-

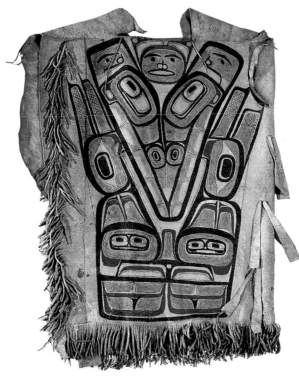

der, even cannon, should the Tlingit mount an effort to oust the Russians. In fact, contemporary Russian sources considered the outbreak of hostilities between the Russians and the Tlingit a direct result of British and American meddling. Whatever the cause, whatever the trigger of the conflict, when it erupted the Tlingit initially had the upper hand.

In spite of the existing tension, Medvednikov, in charge at the post of St. Michael the Archangel at Sitka, felt himself secure. In the spring of 1802, he dispatched most of his men to Frederic Sound to hunt sea otters. Others were sent out to hunt sea lions and seals for food. Only 21 men remained at the unfinished fort, with its palisade not yet completed. On Sunday, June 18, 1802, most of the men were fishing, hunting, or resting. About 12 men were in the main building when the Tlingits attacked in force. Several American sailors are said to have fought on the Tlingit side. Tlingit leader Katlian led the attack. There were few survivors. The fort was burned. The sea otter skins bundled up in the storage loft were taken by the Tlingit, but they did not keep the skins for long. British Captain Barber sailed into the harbor before smoke from the burning buildings had cleared. He threatened to execute the Tlingit leaders who eagerly boarded his ship unless all Russian sea otter skins were surrendered. In the meantime, near Angoon, a party commanded by Urbanov was attacked by the Tlingit and almost wiped out.

Baranov, however, was determined not to give up. In 1804, he, with the aid of the unexpectedly arrived navy vessel *Neva* under Lisianskii, defeated the Sitka Tlingit and reestablished his outpost at a new location, the modern city of Sitka. However, in 1805, perhaps in response, the Tlingit destroyed the Russian outpost at Yakutat. It was never rebuilt. Just the same, the Russian presence in Tlingit territory became an established fact and was never seriously challenged again. Sitka became the center of Russian administration in Alaska and the main port on the North Pacific until the late 19th century.

The establishment of New Sitka, the Novo-Arkhangel'sk, was a turning point in the Russian-Tlingit relations. A kind of symbiosis eventually developed, in which trade played an important part. The Tlingit supplied the settlement with food, fish and game, and after they and the Haida learned vegetable gardening from the

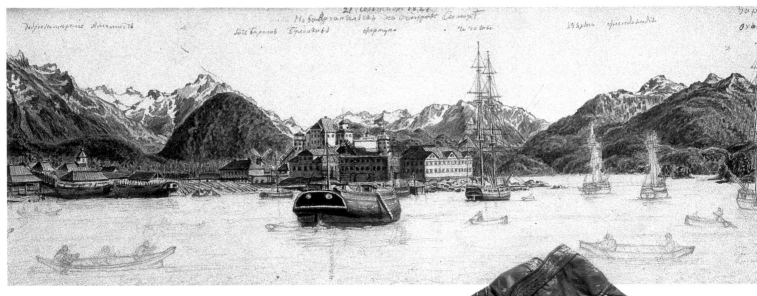

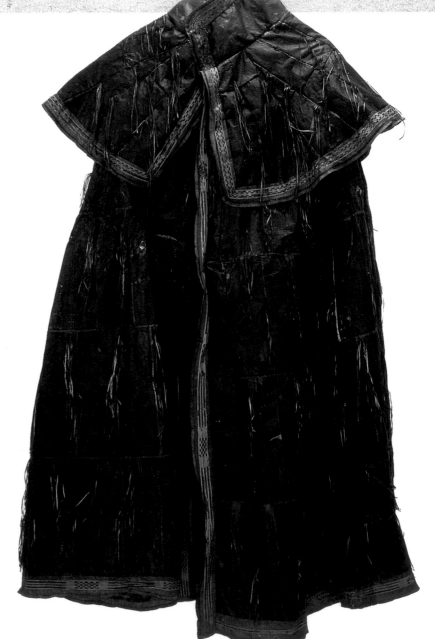

Russians, they even provided a steady source of potatoes to the city. By 1818, almost 1,500 Tlingit occupied their old village site, abandoned in 1804, directly under the palisade of the Russian fort.

Baranov's activities as colonizer were greatly facilitated in 1799 by the granting of a monopoly for exploitation of American possessions to She-likhov's heirs by Emperor Paul I, who reversed his mother's antimonopoly policy. This elimi-nated domestic Russian competition and greatly strengthened Baranov's hand. The Russian American Company, so named in 1799, became the sole economic power and representative of Russian government in the colony. In 1812, Baranov expanded into California, where Fort Ross was founded, again with the aid of Kodiak natives, the Chugach, and the Kenai Peninsula inhabitants; but his attempt to establish a foot-hold in Hawaii failed, largely because of the incompetence of his agent there and the lack of cooperation by the Russian Navy (Barratt 1981).

Beginning with the 1803–06 Krusenstern-Lis-ianskii expedition, Russian naval ships were calling in Alaska with ever-increasing frequency. The end of the Napoleonic Wars in 1814 per-mitted regular sailings from the navy base of Kronstadt around the world to Alaska and the Pacific Ocean, even to Antarctica (Ivashintsov 1980). The commanders had wide-ranging in-structions for inspection of conditions, and their reports of mistreatment of the locals, predomi-nantly eastern Aleutian and Kodiak peoples, eventually resulted in Baranov's removal in 1818. Beginning that year, the governor of Russian America was always a high-ranking navy officer. Serving as a manager for the Russian American Company, he was also responsible for imple-menting state policies in administering the re-

84. Novo-Arkhangel'sk Harbour, September 21, 1827
Unfinished watercolor sketch by Pavel Mikhailov. SRM PM 29010

gion and for relations with foreign powers who claimed interest in Alaskan waters.

The Russian American Company operated under an Imperial charter. When the first monopoly charter granted by Emperor Paul expired, the second charter was negotiated in 1824 for the following 20 years, and then a third. The fourth charter was in the process of being negotiated when the Imperial government began discussion with the United States about transfer of Alaska to U.S. sovereignty. With each charter, the government assigned to the company ever-increasing social service duties in return for the sole right to exploit Alaska's economic resources. The company was obligated to maintain the church, schools, and medical services. Beginning in 1818, smallpox vaccination was attempted. When the 1836–39 pandemic struck Alaska, a massive effort to vaccinate the native population was made. But it was not accepted largely

ing to a fixed price schedule. Those who worked for the company by voluntary agreement were paid wages regulated by an established pay scale (Khlebnikov 1979, 1985).

In any event, under the new managerial practices, the rights of native peoples under direct Russian control in the Aleutian and Kodiak archipelagoes, the Pribilof Islands, Cook Inlet, and Prince William Sound were protected as they were considered Imperial citizens with the civil status equated to that of the free peasants in Russia. Education and social advancement were open to natives and especially to people of mixed ancestry (Huggins 1981). A native middle class, the bulk of whom were creoles (people who could claim Russian ancestry in the male line, no matter how remote), was emerging. A number of natives who occupied positions of responsibility within the Russian establishment were automatically classified as creoles. There are cases when an Alaskan native, educated in Russia and occupying a managerial position, became first a creole, then a "man" (i.e., a Russian of relatively low rank), and some ended as members of the gentry. Such was the case of Kassian Shaiashnikov, who managed the entire Pribilof Island fur sealing operating for the Russian American Company from 1829 to his death in the early 1860s; or of the Kashevarov brothers, some of whom went to Russia in 1867 or earlier, as navy officers and state bureaucrats, while others, those who became clergymen, remained in Alaska.

85. "Inhabitants of the Aleutian Islands"
Louis Choris, 1816-17. AMHA 4.81.68.9
Choris depicts the hunter in traditional garb, while the woman wears Europeanized clothing, braids, and an Orthodox cross.

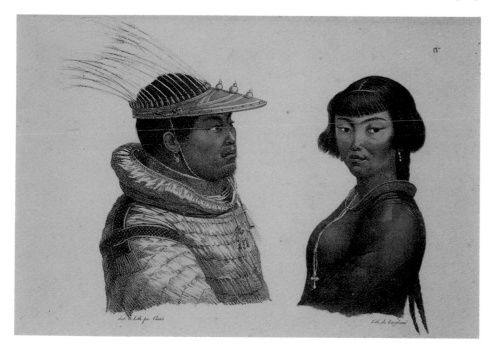

Many Alaskans of native origin explored the Bering Sea coast and Alaskan interior for the Russian American Company from the end of the 18th century to the 1860s. Petr Korsanovskii explored the coasts between the Nushagak and Kuskokwim rivers in 1818 and 1819 and the route from Iliamna Lake to the Mulchatna River. Andrei Ustiugov, an Aleut from Unalaska, in 1819 charted Bristol Bay shores and named Hagemeister Island. Afanasii Klimovskii, in 1819, explored the Copper River. Andrei Glazunov performed the incredible trek from St. Michael via the Unalakleet River to Anvik, from there following the Innoko River to the Kuskokwim, and ascended the Stony River in an attempt to reach Cook Inlet. Semeon and Ivan Lukin, Petr Malakhov, Petr Kolmakov, and others traveled widely in the interior. Aleksandr Kashevarov explored the coast between Pastolik and the Yukon and the Yukon Delta itself in 1834. In 1838, he led an expedition to the Polar coast of Alaska, sailing in a *baidara* (umiak) as far as Point Barrow. Ivan Lukin probably reached the Tanana Valley via the upper Kuskokwim and traded in that direction in the 1840s. In the 1860s, he traveled to Fort Yukon to report on

because the native theories of disease causation were directly opposite to the practice of vaccination or inoculation. The Russians were powerless to prevent the spread of disease, which resulted not only in the great reduction of aboriginal population but also in the belief that Russians deliberately introduced smallpox among the aboriginals.

Furbearer conservation measures were implemented by 1828. Only a strictly limited number of sea otter skins in each district was bought from the Aleuts per year, and the sea otter banks were hunted in rotation (Hooper 1897). Fur sealing was also strictly regulated. The practice of harvesting nonbreeding males and of periodic harvest stoppages was introduced at this time. Aleuts were paid for the skins accord-

86. Gutskin Cape in Russian Style
Aleut or Koniag: MAE 2868-76
This cape, dyed blue-black and cut to approximate the form of a naval greatcoat, was probably made for a Russian officer or merchant captain in the late 18th or early 19th century.

the Hudson's Bay Company's activities there to the governor.

Following the Crimean War and the Opium Wars of the 1850s, which resulted in the virtual collapse of the Chinese market for furs, the Russian American Company made an attempt to diversify the Alaskan economy. Commercial fishing, ice industry, and coal extraction were attempted. None of these enterprises were economically successful, at least not to the degree desired. Fishing, in the absence of canning technology, with salting as the only method of preservation, met with limited success. The coal industry faced the competition of coal from the Vancouver Island area, which was cheaper to transport to the newly developing U.S. ports of San Francisco, Seattle, and Portland.

By this time, the native population of southwestern Alaska, the Aleuts and the Tanaina (Kenaitsy) and Koniags and Yupik-speaking Aleuts from Bristol Bay to Prince William Sound, were participating to some extent in a wage-earning economy, though subsistence activities by aboriginal means continued to predominate. Politically, they were integrated into the Russian Imperial order, retaining, however, local dispute-settlement powers. The Russian American Company administration did not formally intrude in the village life. The Yupik of the Yukon-Kuskokwim drainage, the interior Athapaskans, and the Tlingit systematically participated in the Russian fur trade network while retaining their local autonomy and political independence. A relatively significant segment of the population was exposed to the concepts of education and the availability of public health services, such as smallpox vaccination (the smallpox epidemic of 1863 was checked in Alaska). The clergy devised alphabets for Aleut, Alutiiq, Tlingit, and Yupik languages. Literacy in native languages was developing and native written literature was emerging.

Toward the end of the Russian period, the relationship with the native populations followed an established pattern: since Russia did not desire Russian settlement in the territory, diminution or displacement of the population was not the aim. The successful management of the territory, and the demands of profitable trade, dictated the need for amicable relations. The native peoples were considered citizens of the empire, and those groups who were under Russian dominance since the 18th century formed the backbone of the Russian establishment in Alaska.

The end of the Russian regime, in 1867, came as a shock to the Aleuts, the Koniags, the Tlingits, the Kenai Peninsula Athapaskans, and the Alaska Peninsula Yupik. As one Aleut expressed it in a conversation, "Just as we have learned how to deal with the Russians, when we understood them and they understood us, we had to face a new game with totally different rules. It has taken us almost another century and a half to learn these new rules."

Most of the Russians left Alaska following the transfer of the territory to the USA. Most of the few who remained became paupers (Cracroft 1981): their property rights were not respected by the American settlers, who came to Sitka in

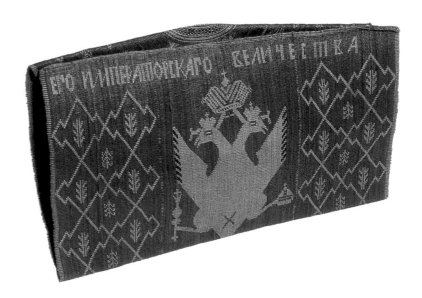

droves, waiting at Sitka aboard ship even before the U.S. commissioner who was to accept the territory had arrived (U.S. Congress 1868). On the very day that the Imperial flag came down, these men staked out every lot in Sitka that had no building on it. Under General Davis, for ten years, the Russian and creole populations were treated as a defeated remnant in a conquered territory. Few were able to obtain even middle-level employment. The creole became the half-breed. Men married to Alaskan women were held in contempt, and eventually they, and their descendants, became absorbed into native communities, as natives. The color bar went up. The Tlingit, who attempted to assert their independence, which they were able to maintain under the Russian regime, were taught submission by the military, culminating in the U.S. Navy bombardment of Wrangell and Angoon.

The sea otter, hunted by private entrepreneurs under the laissez-faire economic policy of the age without any restraint, by the 1880s was on the verge of extinction (Hooper 1897). The canning industry made the territory a commercial fishing paradise. The gold rush brought thousands of seekers for the riches of Eldorado.

87. Othodox Traveling Icon
Even: AMNH 70-5796

The images of the Mother of God and Christ displaying the gospel are of paper, probably clipped from a Russian religious calendar. This Siberian icon is equipped with a belt hook and leather case.

88. Woven Grass Purse
Aleut: MAE 2888-93

The double-headed eagle emblem is here incorporated into the finely woven design of a small Aleut purse, along with the Russian inscription "His Imperial Highness." The emblem and inscription may have been copied from a document.

89. Triptych Icon
Russian from Aleutian Islands: NMAH 25819.130

The central panel of this brass triptych portrays Saints Julitta and Cyricus, to whom prayers are directed for the family and for the health of sick children. Flanking portraits include St. Peter, Michael the Archangel, the Archangel Gabriel, and others. The icon had a cord attached for suspension around the neck.

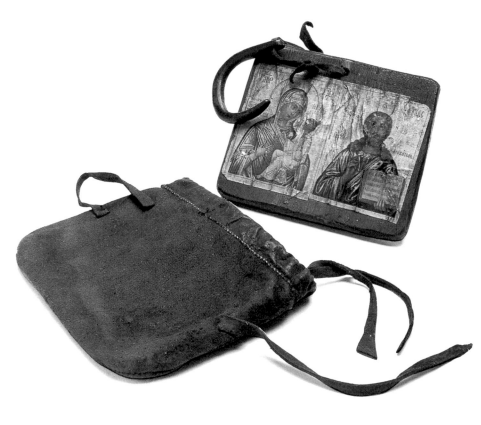

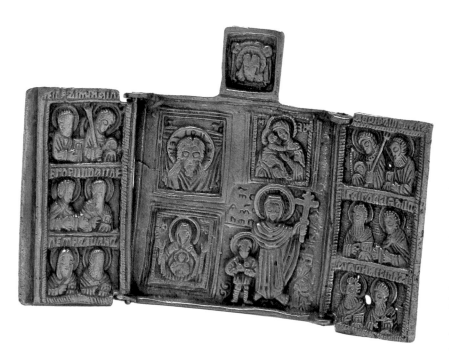

Sitka, the former Imperial capital of Novo-Arkhangel'sk, became a backwater. To the newcomers, for whom Alaska was the last frontier, Russian America was simply irrelevant. For the native peoples of southwestern and southeastern Alaska, on the other hand, the memory of the Russian presence soon came to serve as a model of intercultural communication and integration. This attitude crystallized around the one Russian institution that remained, and grew, while much of the Russian American heritage has disappeared, was suppressed, or was forgotten: the Orthodox Church.

Today, the Orthodox Church in Alaska is perceived by many native peoples, as well as by outsiders, to be a native institution. Aleuts of the Aleutian archipelago and the Pribilof Islands, the people of Kodiak Island, the Alaska Peninsula, Prince William Sound, the Tanaina of the Kenai Peninsula and Lake Iliamna–Lake Clark areas, as well as a majority of the Yupik peoples of the Yukon-Kuskokwim and Nushagak river drainages, constitute the bulk of the Orthodox population of Alaska. A majority of the clergy are Alaskans.

The conversion to Orthodoxy was swift, in spite of the fact that the Orthodox Church does not engage in aggressive proselytizing. In the early period of Russian advance into Alaska, conversions were individual. The faith was spread by laymen, the fur hunters who brought with them aboard their ships the symbols of their faith, built chapels, and regularly conducted prayer services in which any Aleuts present participated. Ties of god-parenthood were established between individual Russian hunters and Aleuts, ties strengthened by name exchanges and name-giving and by the house education provided by some of the godfathers to their new godchildren. Some took their godsons to Kamchatka and Okhotsk, even to Irkutsk, where the young Aleuts lived in their godfathers' households and went to local schools. When these young men returned home to Alaska, they themselves became agents of change, spreading the new faith. The first village chapel in the eastern Aleutians was built by an Aleut leader of Umnak in 1806, as was the first chapel in the Krenitzin Islands in 1844.

The early attempt at systematic mission activity begun in 1794 was short lived. It ended when the Head of Mission, newly consecrated Bishop of Alaska Ioasaf (Bolotov), drowned in the wreck of the *Phoenix* in 1799, together with his entourage and the staff of the seminary that he hoped to establish on Kodiak. However, under his direction the first church in Alaska, the Church of the Holy Resurrection, was built in 1796 at St. Paul (modern Kodiak). After his death, the lay brother Herman, a man of exceptional piety, became the focal point of Orthodoxy in the Kodiak area. After 1808, he built a retreat on Spruce Island where he maintained a school and gave refuge to Aleuts, men and women, who fled to him from oppression by Baranov's henchmen. Loved by the Koniags, he won the admiration and respect of the Russians also, influencing even high-ranking navy officers who met him. He died in 1837, among his people, and after his death his memory was venerated even more than the man was during his lifetime. Already by the turn of the 19th century, he was considered locally to be a saint, and he became acknowledged as a saint by the Orthodox Church in 1970, as St. Herman of Alaska. He is revered today as patron saint of Alaska, as protector of the native peoples, and as the founder of Orthodoxy on the North American continent.

As far as actual mass conversion of the native population to Orthodoxy, the original 1794 mission had little effect, if only numbers are considered. As a model, on the other hand, it is remembered to this day. The monks were expected to convert by example of their lives, not by proselytizing. In fact, they were instructed to ''speak only when asked and to remember at all times that they are guests in somebody else's house.'' But the faith continued to spread by word of mouth, predominantly indirectly through laymen—and that was successful, so much so that by 1819 parish priests were needed in several areas of Alaska. That year, the first parish priest to serve the Orthodox population, Father Sokolov, arrived at Sitka and the Church of St. Michael the Archangel was built there. In 1824, Father Ioann Veniaminov arrived to serve the eastern Aleutian parish and by 1826 built the Church of the Ascension of Christ on Unalaska. Father Frumentii Mordovskii came to serve the parish of Kodiak in 1824. In 1828, Iakov Netsvetov, of Aleut origin, educated at the seminary in Irkutsk, came to serve the western Aleutian parish and built the Church of St. Nicholas on the island of Atka.

True missionary activities commenced only in the 1840s when Ioann Veniaminov returned to Alaska as the first ruling bishop. Clergy from Russia came in increasing numbers during Veniaminov's tenure as bishop, but the native clergy was growing also. After 1867, the majority of the Russian clergy left, and for many years it was the native clergymen who maintained the legacy of the Orthodox faith. Often, these Alaskans held their ground in the face of hostility and even persecution by predominantly Protestant missionaries enjoying U.S. governmental support. Church lands and property were often seized or ''leased'' by commercial interests without due recompense. Even in Sitka the clergy were put under pressure to cede the cathedral lands in the center of town and remove themselves to the outskirts of Sitka, but here this pressure was successfully resisted. Church schools were closed or put under severe pressure. Yet, the clergy persevered.

Today Orthodox churches are maintained or rebuilt in villages where they were destroyed, and in some communities where the dominant religious affiliation is non-Orthodox, Orthodox groups are revived. St. Herman Theological Seminary operates in Kodiak, training clergymen and lay readers not only as church workers but also in community leadership and survival skills, providing education in health aid and crisis intervention. Once thought slated to disappear, following the demise of Russian government support, the Orthodox Church in Alaska remains strong. It is supported solely by the grass roots, by the local Orthodox population. A magnificent Cathedral of St. Innocent of Irkutsk is being built in the city of Anchorage, with all Orthodox Alaskans contributing to the effort. If anything, the number of Orthodox is growing, with a number of Americans of Anglo-European origin joining the church. And through the church, Russian names are perpetuated, as church names and as surnames: Lukin, Malakhov, Chumovitskii, Larionov, are now Alaskan American names.

As Alaska has come of age, as a state of the Union, her people have become concerned with her history. Russian Alaska is an integral part of that history. Interest in the Russian heritage is growing. Architectural monuments of the Russian era are restored; documents of the era are collected, preserved, and translated into English; and the surviving Orthodox Church art and music are respected and admired. Throughout the nation there is the awakening of awareness that Russian America is part not only of Alaskan but also of the nation's history, a heritage to be remembered and treasured.

90. Notched Calendar
Even: MAE 147-4

Several methods were used by Alaskan and Siberian Native converts to Orthodoxy to keep the religious calendar. On this ivory calendar from Siberia each notch represents one day, with feast days marked by special symbols.

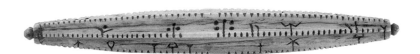

Treasures by the Neva: The Russian Collections

G. I. Dzeniskevich and L. P. Pavlinskaia

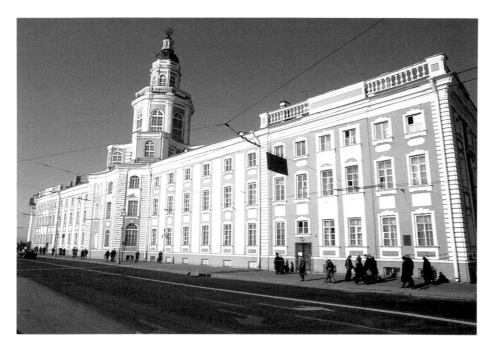

91. Museum of Anthropology and Ethnography

Founded with the personal "Kunstkamera" (art cabinet) of Peter the Great in 1714 in St. Petersburg (Leningrad), the Museum of Anthropology and Ethnography is the oldest museum in the USSR and has been the official repository for the anthropology collections of the Russian Academy of Sciences since 1824 (Stanyukovich 1970).

Originally housed in a small "Chamber of Curiosities," the museum moved to its present location—a site chosen by Peter I on the Neva River—with the completion of a new museum building in 1728. The museum is part of the N.N. Miklukho-Maklai Institute of Ethnography of the Academy of Sciences of the USSR. In addition to holding other famous early collections from expeditions around the world, the museum's American Department houses the Russian America collections utilized in the Crossroads of Continents exhibition.

The Peter the Great Museum of Anthropology and Ethnography, under the Soviet Academy of Sciences, derives from the original Kunstkamera, the first Russian museum, created by Peter the First in St. Petersburg, then the capital of Russia. In 1728 a special building was erected on the banks of the Neva for the new museum, which displayed not only ethnographic collections but also biological curiosities. Like many early museums of the world, it was originally a museum of natural history.

As the first state museum of Russia, the St. Petersburg Kunstkamera played a fundamental role in the development of the natural and social sciences, including ethnology, physical anthropology, and archeology, as well as in national education and museology. The affiliation of the Kunstkamera to the Russian Academy of Sciences in 1724 was a major step: it allowed the Kunstkamera collections to be used for scientific purposes and provided a sounder basis for museum collecting and museum exhibiting methods.

Thanks to the growth of the sciences in Russia, in the 1830s, 100 years after its founding, the museum holdings had increased greatly, so that it became necessary to divide the Kunstkamera into specialized departments for both research and exhibition. In the reorganization that, accordingly, took place in 1831, seven independent academic museums were created, one of them being the museum of ethnography, which was named the Peter the Great Museum of Anthropology and Ethnography (the MAE). The new museum remained in the former St. Petersburg Kunstkamera building.

Towards the end of the 19th century, the MAE became the center of ethnographic work in Russia. Great scientists like A. Sjögren, M. A. Kastren, A. F. Middendorf, L. I. Shrenk, N. N. Miklukho-Maklai, V. V. Radlow, S. F. Oldenburg, D. K. Zelenin, L. Ia. Sternberg, W. G. Bogoras, D. A. Klements, and others worked within its walls.

Since its beginnings, the acquisition of collections at the Kunstkamera has had a governmental character. Systematic collections resulted from special recommendations and instructions given to scientific expeditions or to individual scholars conducting fieldwork. In the 18th and 19th centuries, especially, major scientific expeditions were organized by the Academy of Sciences, aiming for thorough study of the natural history and populations of various parts of the globe. The museum collections from the cultures of Siberia and North America are among the most valuable results of these expeditions.

The MAE owns more than 11,000 artifacts from American Native peoples. This collection was acquired during two centuries, but the most brilliant chapters of the history were the 19th-century collecting activities among the cultures of northwestern North America, Eskimo, Aleut, Alaskan Athapaskan, and Tlingit.

Numerous Russian navigators, travelers, and scholars took part in the collecting of artifacts from the American continent. Newspapers and magazines at the beginning of the 18th century already mentioned American ethnographic pieces in Russia, but the brevity of early museum documentation makes it difficult to identify any of these artifacts that may still survive. Among the early collections, we have reliable documentation only for pieces acquired by the museum after the 1780s. An example is the collection from the 1785–94 expedition of Capt. N. I. Billings and G. A. Sarychev to Northeast Asia, the Bering Strait, the American Northwest Coast, and the Aleutian Islands. All the artifacts from their collection come from the Koniag Eskimo of Kodiak Island. Other accessions from America (e.g., MAE 2520, Tlingit cloaks; and MAE 505), acquired by the MAE from M. K. Boehm, governor of Kamchatka, have been assumed by some to have been given him by Captain Cook's expedition in the 1780s.

The most complete and precious holdings of the American section of the MAE represent the cultures of the Aleut, Alaskan and Koniag Eskimo, Tlingit, Alaskan Athapaskan, and California Indians. These were collected mainly in the first half of the 19th century by members of the Russian American Company and by the Russian navigators around the world.

The first Russian circumnavigation was accomplished by the ships *Neva* and *Nadezhda* (''Hope'') between 1803 and 1806 under the command of I. S. Krusenstern and Iu. F. Lisianskii. Among the 100 ethnographic pieces donated to the museum by Lisianskii after his voyage, a significant number are North American clothing and utensils, means of transportation, craftwork, and religious objects (Tlingit, Athapaskan, and Eskimo from the Kodiak Island area). From this collection, the exhibition displays a Chugach Eskimo bird-shaped wooden bowl (MAE 536-4, fig. 390) and a Koniag Eskimo ivory figurine (MAE 699-1, fig. 92).

Some of the artifacts collected during this expedition were donated to the Museum of the Admiralty Department (later called the Navy Museum), which also acquired many objects from other maritime expeditions and Russian seamen. After 1930 all these were transferred to the MAE, but the collectors and the provenience of the pieces were by then impossible to identify precisely (MAE 4104, 4105, 4270, 5795, 5801, 5803). It is known that accession MAE 633, represented in the exhibition by a Tlingit helmet (MAE 633-8, fig. 81), a Chugach Eskimo spruce-root hat (MAE 633-18, fig. 408), and two Aleut pouches (MAE 633-12, 14, fig. 252), which was originally in the Admiralty Museum, was donated by I. S. Krusenstern after his circumnavigation of the world.

In 1817–18 Capt. V. M. Golovnin completed a voyage around the world on the sloop *Kamchatka*. He visited the Aleutians, Kodiak Island, and Novo-Arkhangel'sk (Sitka), and again the Kunstkamera received a generous donation of objects from North American native cultures.

The exhibit shows a Chugach spruce-root hat (MAE 539-1, fig. 206) from Golovnin's collection.

The next Russian voyage around the world was completed on the sloop *Seniavin* under F. P. Litke (Lütke), resulting in numerous collections that were all put under the management of the Academy of Sciences. The Tlingit collection (woven hats, wooden carved bowls, two daggers, and others) of this series was donated to the Kunstkamera, as well as an Eskimo collection of clothing, utensils, and ornaments.

Most of the collections of the first half of the 19th century were in one way or another related to the Russian American Company. For instance A. F. Kashevarov was from the 1830s to the 1860s in command of various company ships, sailing between Sitka, Kodiak, and Petropavlovsk. Being born himself in Alaska, the son of a Russian teacher and an Aleut woman, he loved Alaskan people and knew and valued the native culture. He gave two collections to the MAE. One of them, from the Alaskan Northwest Coast, includes four Tlingit ceremonial goat-horn spoons, two of which are shown in the exhibit (MAE 518-1a and 1b, fig. 393), and a suit of Athapaskan deerskin clothing.

Another famous navigator, I. Arkhimandritov, also an Alaskan creole (part native, part Russian), was in charge of the general direction of the company. He described the coastline of the Kenai Peninsula, Kodiak Island, and other islands along the North American coast. In 1857 he gave the museum a collection of Aleut masks, one of which can be seen in the exhibit (MAE 538-2, fig. 440).

Among the artifacts donated to the museum by the mining engineer P. P. Doroshin after he conducted geological research in Alaska (he discovered seams of coal on the Kenai Peninsula, among other finds), the exhibition presents a Tlingit wooden bowl (MAE 337-18, fig. 245) and a series of objects from the MAE accession 2448.

Among the collectors of North American artifacts in the MAE, the place of honor is deserved by I. G. Voznesenskii. In 1839 he was sent to America especially to expand the collections of the Academy museums. The Russian Academy of Sciences provided him with careful instructions for collecting ethnographic artifacts together with a list of objects needed by the museum. Voznesenskii spent almost ten years in America, and the results of his work surpassed all expectations. He brought back altogether more than 1,000 North American artifacts. Thanks to his great talents as a collector, his industry, and his honesty, he was able to collect the most precious ethnographic material from the Aleut, Western Eskimo, Koniag, Alaskan coastal Athapaskan, Tlingit, Haida, and Indians of California.

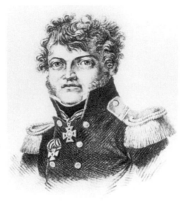

92. Iurii Lisianskii
Koniag Eskimo: MAE 669-1
Bering Sea Eskimo: MAE 2938-2

In 1803–6 the Russian government sent out an expedition under the command of I. S. Krusenstern to explore the feasibility of supplying Russian America by sea rather than by the difficult overland and sea route through Siberia and the North Pacific. Iurii Lisianskii, captain of the second ship, *Neva*, arrived in Alaska just in time to help secure Baranov's reentry into Sitka in 1804 (p. 77). Lisianskii was also instrumental in securing more humane conditions for natives working for the fur traders. His reports contain valuable observations on native life and culture, and he obtained and published ethnographic collections that are among the earliest for the region. They include this carving of a seated high-status Koniag Eskimo with beaded ears, cf. Holmberg (1855–63), and a battle helmet obtained by Baranov after the 1802 Tlingit rebellion (fig. 81; Lisianskii 1814:plate I).

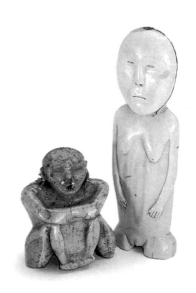

Numerous notes in his diary and his drawings represent important additions to the collection. His collecting methods were unusual for ethnography at the time: Voznesenskii collected objects systematically across functional categories, so that the MAE acquired synoptic series of clothing, canoes, masks, and other artifact types.

Voznesenskii paid attention to every single object, documenting each precisely as to its name, the way it was used, and the materials of which it was made. As a result his collection is particularly valuable for research today.

Voznesenskii's collections, which are well represented in the exhibition, include parts of MAE accession 571, 593, 620, 2448, 2520, 2539, 2667, 2888, and 2938—hunting tools and weapons, clothing, utensils, cult and ceremonial objects, and other material, which not only illustrate but also help reconstruct many elements of the traditional cultures of the Eskimo, Aleut, and Indians.

Under Voznesenskii's influence, L. A. Zagoskin, a lieutenant of the Russian fleet who directed an expedition in Alaska in 1842–44, became an enthusiastic collector. Zagoskin's book (1967) made him the most important ethnographer of his time. In Alaska he made a small but valuable collection, only 43 artifacts altogether, composed of clothing, utensils, religious objects, and others from the Eskimo and Indians of the Yukon basin and the Kuskokwim. The exhibition presents two tobacco boxes collected by Zagoskin (MAE 537-4a, fig. 46, and 537-46, fig. 94).

The Tlingit collection of the MAE is extremely rich, allowing the study of many aspects of this Indian culture. The artifacts related to shamanism are of special interest. Most of these were obtained from the Igumen (Father Superior)

Georgi Chudnovskii, who was sent to Admiralty Island as a missionary in 1891. He spent only half a year there, but this was sufficient for him to build a chapel, baptize almost 500 Indians, establish friendly relationships with the local shamans, and trade with them for numerous cult objects. Of the 96 artifacts collected by Chudnovskii, 67 are of shamanistic nature. In the exhibition a shaman's rattle (MAE 211-2, fig. 371) is displayed.

After the sale of Alaska in 1867, the flow of Native American objects to the MAE somewhat diminished. Except for Chudnovskii's, no more important collections were added. Individual collectors, who either had been to America themselves or had acquired American objects in another way, donated almost all of the new acquisitions. For instance, the vice-president of the Academy of Sciences, L. N. Maikov, bequeathed a collection of Aleut artifacts to the museum in 1878, and Admiral K. N. Pos'et gave two Eskimo statuettes and a pipe. At the beginning of the 20th century, in 1905, as a result of a loan-exchange with a series of great museums of the world, the MAE received a few collections from the American Museum of Natural History in New York, related to the cultures of several Indian groups, including 53 Athapaskan and a few Northwest Coast artifacts. This exchange continued after the Russian Revolution; in 1930 the MAE obtained three significant collections of Pueblo Indian material from the Smithsonian in Washington. A series of collections and objects found their way into the MAE inventory as presents from private individuals.

The first exhibition on the cultures of America opened in the MAE in 1889. In 1948 this exhibition was completely redone. The new exhibition, periodically renewed and reorganized, lasts until this day.

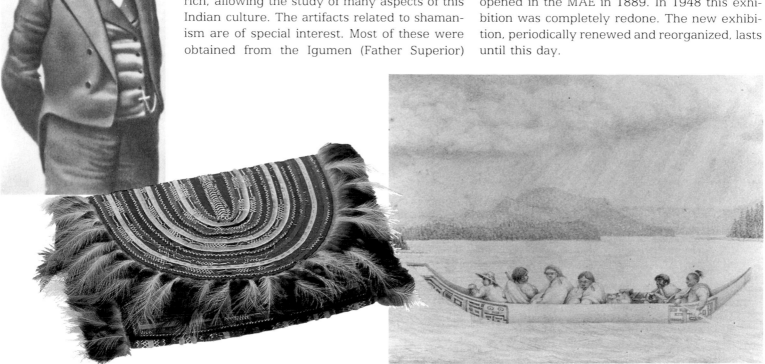

The Siberian collection of the MAE is one of the largest in Russian museums. It consists of more than 36,000 artifacts. The first Siberian objects in the Kunstkamera were collected in the first half of the 18th century by members of the Second Kamchatka Expedition, G. F. Müller, I. G. Gmelin, and S. P. Krasheninnikov. It was then completed by the Academy Expedition of 1768–74 under Academician P. Pallas in Siberia, the Ural region, the Arctic, the Caucasus, and the Volga region. Research and collecting were conducted by V. F. Zuev, S. G. Gmelin (Jr.), N. Ia. Ozeretskovskii, and I. G. Georgi. Despite the loss of their documentation, the few artifacts that survive are of great historical and scientific value. In the museum's catalog they are presently listed as "from the old collection of Kunstkamera." From Northeast Siberia we can mention Asian Eskimo arrow points and harpoons, stone scrapers (MAE 4492, 4495), and a few possibly Chukchi artifacts such as bone engraved plates and miniature statuettes of walrus and mammoth tusks (MAE 4469).

As a result of the ethnographic expeditions of the 18th century, a series of fundamental works was written, which provided the foundation for ethnographic science in Russia. The travels around the world and the research of the Russian navigators of the early 19th century also left their marks on the formation of the Siberian collection, in addition to increasing the American collection of the MAE. Thus for example the MAE collections 666, 668, 752, and 867 were made by Litke, Voznesenskii, and Zagoskin among the Maritime Chukchi and Koryak. They consist of more than 200 objects related to various aspects of the traditional life of these peoples, such as sledges with bone runners, quivers, arrows, bolas, working tools, clothing, utensils, and walrus ivory miniature carvings. Even though these are modest compared with the American collections, they constitute jewels of the MAE Northeastern Siberian collection.

To this we can add a small collection of Evenk clothing from the Okhotsk Sea coast, acquired by the MAE in the first half of the 19th century from K. I. Khlebnikov, the famous explorer of North America and a Russian American Company man (MAE 1, 60).

Nevertheless the bulk of the Northeastern Siberian holdings of the MAE (Chukchi, Koryak, Eskimo, Itelmen, Even) was collected in the late 19th and early 20th centuries. The most important contribution to the MAE collection was the acquisition in 1898 from Nikolai L'vovich Gondatti, who, while scientific secretary of the Anthropological and Ethnographic Society of Moscow University, was in 1893 in charge of the Anadyr district, which included at the time most of the Chukchi Peninsula. Gondatti turned his administrative task to good account by collecting in every corner of the territory he had been assigned to govern. He collected altogether 1,865 artifacts (MAE 395, 407, 408, 422, 434, 441, 442, 443, 444, 445, and 446) representing the cultures of every Northeastern people. These pieces are manufacturing, fishing, hunting, and gathering tools, domestic objects and utensils, clothing, toys, ceremonial objects, and walrus and mammoth ivory carvings (cf. figs. 19, 32, 33, 227; Bogoraz 1901b). The content and the character of these collections show that the collector tried to cover each aspect under every possible form, by presenting not only a unique object but also series of the same object, which form independent collections. Archeological pieces, surface finds, and objects excavated by Gondatti on the Yukaghir Mount on the Anadyr River constitute an independent collection (MAE 872).

In 1898 W. G. Bogoras and W. I. Jochelson, as participants in the Jesup Expedition organized by Franz Boas of the American Museum of Natural History, made an important contribution to the MAE ethnographic collections of Northeastern Asian cultures. In order to study the native cultures of the North Pacific coasts, the link between Asian and American cultures, Boas decided to entrust the study of the Asian part of the project to Russian scientists. In 1898 V. V. Radlov, head of the Russian Imperial Academy of Sciences in St. Petersburg, suggested Bogoras and Jochelson in answer to Boas's request for assistance.

During 1900–01 Bogoras and Jochelson traveled through Kamchatka and Chukotka, collecting data on the language, material culture, social structure, religion, and folklore of the Koryak, Chukchi, Eskimo, and Itelmen as well as ethnographic objects. Some of the artifacts collected during this expedition were given to the MAE (956, 1059), but the largest portion remained at the American Museum. Clothing, ceremonial objects, a complex of funeral objects, toys, various hunting weapons, and craftwork made a unique contribution to the holdings of these museums.

In 1905 Bogoras wrote an invaluable description of the inventory of artifacts brought to the MAE from the Jesup Expedition, which still preserves its scientific relevance. The material collected during the expedition was also the basis for later writings by these two scholars. These works played an important role in the development of Russian and Soviet ethnological sciences. The monographs *The Chukchee* by Bogoras and *The Koryak* by Jochelson, published between 1904 and 1910 by the American Mu-

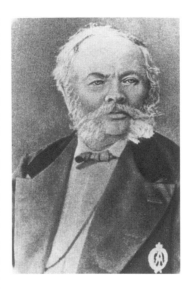

94. L. A. Zagoskin
Bering Sea Eskimo: MAE 537-4b
Voznesenskii convinced Lt. L. A. Zagoskin to collect for the MAE during the latter's explorations in the interior of Alaska (1842–44). Zagoskin's book (1967) is the earliest description of Eskimo and Indian peoples of the Lower Yukon and Kuskokwim rivers. His collections were small but important. This tobacco box is ornamented with effigy figures, a feature that links Bering Sea Eskimo, Pacific Eskimo, and Northwest Coast Indian art.

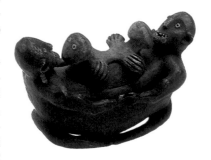

seum, received attention and praise from both Russian and foreign anthropologists.

Bogoras's and Jochelson's activity in Kamchatka and Chukotka incited members of various expeditions in Northeastern Siberia to collect ethnographic objects. In 1901 the MAE received a large collection of Maritime Chukchi material collected along the coast between Provideniia and Kliuchinskaia by A. G. Miagkov, from a gold-digging expedition (MAE 611, 169 artifacts). Soon after, in 1910, the MAE added to its inventory collections made by the Russian geologist I. P. Tolmachev. He collected more than 300 artifacts (MAE 1791) during the first geological survey of the coast of the Arctic Ocean from the mouth of the Kolyma River to East Cape, on the expedition of the Maritime Department of the Ministry of Trade and Industry. Miagkov's and Tolmachev's collections, which include clothing, bows, arrows, smoking pipes, and craftwork, represent quite exhaustively the culture of the maritime hunters of the Arctic coast and complete perfectly Gondatti's, Bogoras's, and Jochelson's collections.

After the Russian Revolution in 1917, collecting of material on the peoples of the USSR became the responsibility of a new generation of ethnographers, educated in several Soviet universities and agencies (Institute of Geography, Institute of the Peoples of the North, Institute of Ethnography of the Academy of Sciences of the USSR), where leading scholars of the MAE, L. Ia. Sternberg, W. G. Bogoras, E. G. Kagarov, D. K. Zelenin, and others, played an active role.

The 1920s and 1930s mark a turn to intensive collecting of material culture from every Siberian group. S. N. Stebnitskii, a member of the Institute of the Peoples of the North, made a particularly interesting collection from the Koryak of the eastern coast of Kamchatka, in 1929. It consists of traditional ceremonial clothing, domestic objects, and children's toys made by Koryak children in the 1920s (MAE 3896). The scholarly description accompanying the collection includes valuable ethnographic information as well.

Simultaneously, his colleague A. S. Forstein conducted some work in the Chukchi Peninsula. Here she made an interesting Eskimo collection, including a ceremonial *kamleika*, ordinary and ceremonial clothing, pouches, and snowshoes (MAE 4210).

The particularity of museum collections from the Soviet period is that they include not only artifacts from the traditional culture but also objects reflecting the development and form of the new cultures of the peoples of the USSR. The most striking example of this is certainly

the large collection of engraved and carved ivory walrus tusks from the famous Uelen workshop, acquired by the MAE in 1951 (MAE 6010; fig. 327). The Uelen workshop was created in 1931 and serves as both an art school and a studio for Chukchi, Koryak, and Eskimo artists, whose ivory and bone carving has gained international renown.

In the 1950s and 1960s, research and collecting among the peoples of Northeastern Siberia were actively conducted by members of the Academy of Sciences of the USSR, namely I. S. Vdovin, I. S. Gurvich, S. A. Arutiunov, V. V. Antropova, and Ch. M. Taksami (MAE 6601, 6355, 6747, 6450, and 6750). These collections fill the gaps in the previous holdings of the MAE. They consist of arrow points, scrapers, woven and fur pouches, oil lamps, toys, ritual masks, and religious objects.

The first Northeastern Asian archeological collections of the MAE were made by Gondatti. The next collections from ancient populations of this area were from the eminent Soviet archeologist S. I. Rudenko, who was responsible for excavation of the famous Pazyryk kurgan tombs from the Scythian period in the Altai region. Being interested in the peopling of the Arctic and the contacts between ethnic groups in this part of Asia, Rudenko conducted fieldwork along the coast of Chukotka from Uelen to Sirenik in 1945, under the Leningrad Institute of History of the Material Culture of the Academy of Sciences of the USSR (now Institute of Archeology) and the (Soviet) Arctic Institute. This first expedition discovered ancient sites near Uelen, Naukan, Dezhnevo, Iandygai, and many other places.

Rudenko's research was continued in the 1950s and 1960s by members of the Institute of Ethnography, M. G. Levin, D. A. Sergeev, and S. A. Arutiunov. The materials excavated from two of the largest sites known to this day, the Old Bering Sea–Okvik–Punuk Uelen and Ekven burial sites, as well as from the ancient settlement of Ekven, constitute one of the most impressive collections in the MAE inventory of ancient cultures of Siberia (MAE 6479, 6493, 6508, 6561, 6588, and 6591). They represent more than 3,000 artifacts covering quite completely the ancient Eskimo culture of the Asian side of the Bering Sea almost 2,000 years ago. Ornate harpoon heads and arrowheads, "winged objects," carvings with the circle-and-dot motif, various domestic objects with engravings, maskoids and combs made of walrus tusk ivory, a wooden mask, and wooden utensils are masterpieces of prehistoric art added to the treasure of world culture (pp. 121–29).

Today the MAE is primarily known as the only

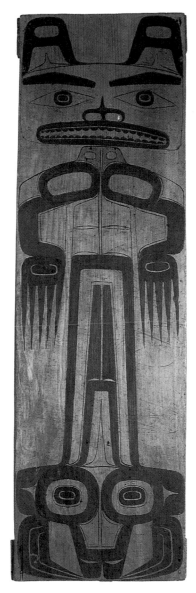

95. Rattle Panel
Tlingit: MAE 2448-30

This panel exhibits some of the finest early Tlingit painting known. Its function is uncertain, but it contains pebbles and may have been a rattle. One side has a highly stylized figure of a bear with an elongated formline body; the opposite illustrates a sea lion. Early style markers include angular formlines, elongated eyelids, and lobed teeth. Although attributed to Voznesenskii, it may have been presented by Grigorii Shelikhov in about 1788.

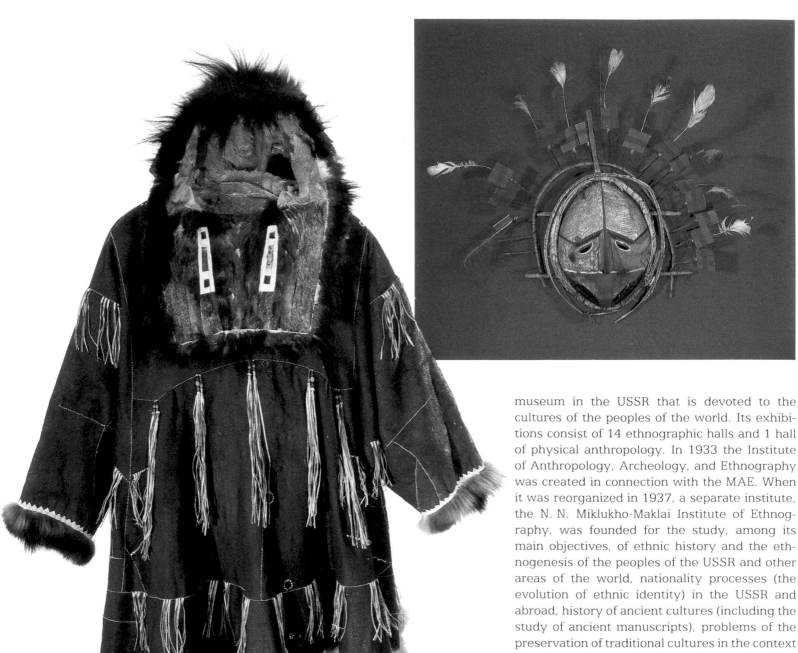

96. "Sand Piper/Woodcock" Mask
Koniag Eskimo: MAE 571-8

A museum preparator by trade rather than an ethnographer, Voznesenskii published little of his Alaskan data, including his notes on a "one act mystery" he witnessed in which this and other masks now in the MAE collection were used. This specimen was too fragile to be loaned for the Crossroads exhibition.

97. Woman's Dance Coat
Koryak: MAE 3896-1

In addition to having many fine Russian America objects, the collections of the Museum of Anthropology and Ethnology hold materials representing cultures of many other areas of the world. This Koryak dance coat was collected in Kamchatka in 1928. It features light, beaded fringes set against dark-tanned reindeer skin and has a chest bib that is common in northeastern Siberian clothing (p. 18). Many of the beads on this coat are of Chinese origin.

museum in the USSR that is devoted to the cultures of the peoples of the world. Its exhibitions consist of 14 ethnographic halls and 1 hall of physical anthropology. In 1933 the Institute of Anthropology, Archeology, and Ethnography was created in connection with the MAE. When it was reorganized in 1937, a separate institute, the N. N. Miklukho-Maklai Institute of Ethnography, was founded for the study, among its main objectives, of ethnic history and the ethnogenesis of the peoples of the USSR and other areas of the world, nationality processes (the evolution of ethnic identity) in the USSR and abroad, history of ancient cultures (including the study of ancient manuscripts), problems of the preservation of traditional cultures in the context of urbanization, and urban ethnography. This research is largely conducted on a multidisciplinary basis that includes ethnolinguistics, ethnopsychology, ethnosociology, demography, and medical ethnology. The intensive program of fieldwork of the institute in all regions of the USSR and abroad adds to the museum's holdings, which at the present time number about a million artifacts: 500,000 archeological objects, 150,000 physical anthropology specimens, and more than 300,000 ethnographic pieces.

During the last 15 years the collections of the MAE have been seen in exhibitions in the USA, Japan, Sweden, Finland, Italy, Bulgaria, and Germany; everywhere they have helped people to realize their own participation in world civilization and to raise their respect for the cultures of other peoples.

Baird's Naturalists: Smithsonian Collectors in Alaska

William W. Fitzhugh

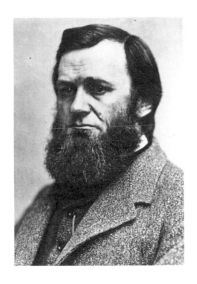

98. Spencer F. Baird
SI neg. 46853

Baird, appointed assistant secretary of the Smithsonian in 1850, arrived with his scientific collection in two railway boxcars. Convinced that Alaska held the key to understanding relationships of animals and peoples across Bering Strait, Baird initiated programs that resulted in the Smithsonian becoming the 19th-century center for North American arctic science.

The transfer of Alaska to the United States in 1867 marked a major turning point in scientific studies of the North Pacific region. The advances of Darwin, Lyell, Agassiz, von Humboldt, and others had changed the ways scientists looked at the world, and these views in turn were being communicated to a public eager for information about exotic peoples, places, and creatures. It was an era in which observation, classification, and interpretation of systematic relationships was replacing classical Eurocentric dogma; an era of science had dawned. It was also a time of optimistic belief in the power of new tools to produce new understandings about the natural world. In the United States, as the frontier expanded west, new fields ripe for scientific study were rapidly uncovered, not the least of which was the natural history of northwestern North America. As knowledge of the natural world, including that of native cultures, expanded across the continent, it was inevitable that Alaska should prove to be a rich source of study. As it happened, the Smithsonian Institution was uniquely positioned to be the primary contributor to the nation's first scientific investigations in Alaska, in the process compiling an unparalleled collection of scientific data.

Early Smithsonian History

When the bequest of English scientist James Smithson was translated by act of Congress in 1846 into creation of the Smithsonian Institution as an "establishment for the increase and diffusion of knowledge among men" there was little consensus about the direction to be taken to pursue this broad mandate. However, with the appointment of Spencer Fullerton Baird as Smithsonian Institution Secretary Joseph Henry's assistant in 1850 the Smithsonian's course in the sciences began to take specific form.

Baird had a notion of the future he saw for the young Smithsonian. At a time when the frontier was expanding westward at a dramatic rate, with Indian cultures and animal distributions in a state of disruption and change, with the threat of extinction mingling with the promise of natural wonders, Baird saw the Smithsonian's role as a dual one: documenting and understanding this new, unfolding, natural world, while at the same time reconstructing its history and preserving its past for future study and edification. Baird saw the Smithsonian as a center for natural history studies that could support field collecting and analysis and could disseminate new findings enriching man's awareness of the natural world widely through publication, lectures, and exhibitions. His most pressing need was to find ways to get bright young naturalists into the field so that they could begin collecting, especially in frontier regions where white man's influence had not drastically changed the natural order.

Partly by design and partly by circumstances, northwestern North America became the testing ground for Baird's vision of a national program of natural history. At mid-century, Russian America south of the Yukon was administratively and economically part of the Old World. These ties were not lost on Baird, who was well acquainted with ideas that the Old and New Worlds must have had early land connections at

Bering Strait to account for the distributions of living and fossil animals. Baird and Henry (who especially promoted linguistic and archeological studies of the Americas) were also aware of controversies about the origin of the American Indians (Haven 1856; also see Fagan 1987; Wauchope 1962). Like Georg Wilhelm Steller and S. P. Krasheninnikov a century earlier, Baird saw possibilities of Asiatic connections across Bering Strait and believed that their historical relationships with New World peoples could be determined by comparative philology and mythology and by studies of skull form, much as comparisons of closely related animals and plants revealed their common history. Baird and Henry saw the unique role of the Smithsonian as serving the needs of government, the scientific establishment, and the public. The fact that northwestern North America in the 1850s and 60s was essentially unknown to American science gave Baird a powerful impetus for advancing his Alaskan program.

In the early 1850s, as Henry and Baird began to articulate this vision, it was lack of means, not of ideas, that was the major obstacle. For a small organization with few staff and facilities, the problems seemed insurmountable. Baird devised an ingenious solution, attaching the Smithsonian to the forces of change themselves to provide means for gathering collections and data from remote regions. Enlisting the support of government boundary survey parties and commercial establishments, Baird created opportunities for scientific collecting among the government and commercial emissaries and agents stationed in outposts in the western and northern parts of North America. Hudson's Bay factors, Indian agents, army and naval officers, medical doctors, land surveyors, boundary commissioners, and other officials were contacted and were supplied with circulars providing instructions on collecting procedures for specimens as varied as bird skins, eggs, plants, fossils,

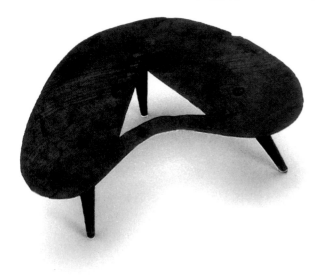

Indian artifacts, and vocabularies. Informed amateur collectors were recruited wherever they could be found—but especially from Chicago, the hotbed of natural history training—spurred to action by Baird's appeal for information and specimens while they still were obtainable.

One of these associates, George Gibbs, had a major impact on the development of ethnographic and linguistic profiles for the Washington Territories. Gibbs's data were obtained in part through use of circulars sent to agents and government representatives, including the governor of Russian America. His goal was to use language distributions and comparisons to reconstruct the Indian history and tribal relationships, a formulation later followed by John Wesley Powell in his linguistic studies. Gibbs's view that Alaskan languages were related to Asian languages, and the growing numbers of scientists who saw American Indian peoples originating from northeastern Asia via Bering Strait, contributed to Baird's belief that ethnological studies in Alaska would provide answers to the problem of relationships between New World and Old World peoples.

Baird's Alaskan program did not materialize overnight (Fitzhugh and Selig 1981). Rather it took form slowly during the 1850s as an outgrowth of the Smithsonian's correspondence with amateur and professional collectors and its requests for donations to the institution's growing collections. During the mid-1850s, while George Gibbs was collecting Indian vocabularies in the Northwest, Baird began to collaborate with a brilliant young naturalist named Robert Kennicott who had been collecting natural history specimens from regions west of the Great Lakes. Earlier Baird had established contact with governors of the Hudson's Bay Company, particularly with Sir George Simpson and his agents managing the company's posts west of Hudson Bay, requesting assistance acquiring collections for the Smithsonian. The Hudson's Bay men were willing but needed training in collection and preservation techniques. What they really needed was someone to provide guidance and coordination. Baird found Kennicott eager for the task and in 1859 sent him north on the Smithsonian's first arctic field expedition.

Kennicott spent the years 1859–63 in the Yukon Territory, arriving back in Washington with his collections to a hero's welcome (Collins 1946; Nute 1943). These included 40 boxes "embracing thousands of skins of birds and mammals, eggs of nearly all the birds nesting in the north, numerous skulls and skeletons of animals, fishes in alcohol and preserved dry, insects, fossils, plants, &c." Baird's report continues:

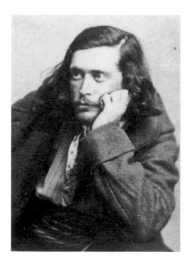

99. Robert Kennicott
Photo: Grove National Historic Landmark

Baird's first arctic enterprise began by sending a gifted young naturalist named Robert Kennicott to northwestern Canada in 1859. Kennicott later went on to lead the first U.S. fieldwork program in Alaska, where he died in 1866. The data collected by Kennicott's team was influential in convincing Congress and the public that Alaska was valuable. Kennicott's ethnological work was the first by Americans in this region and was the foundation for the Smithsonian's arctic program.

100. Sealing Stool
Anderson River Eskimo: NMNH 3978

Baird and Kennicott initiated a collecting program through Hudson's Bay Company officials resident in the Mackenzie District, Canada. This stool used by Eskimos while waiting for seals at their breathing holes was obtained from Anderson River Eskimos by Roderick McFarlane, a local factor. Baird supplied post managers with collecting instructions and funds. Ethnological items were only part of the plan; factors submitted bird skins, eggs, animal pelts, native vocabularies, and other materials. By developing a network of amateur natural historians, Baird built both the Smithsonian's collection and its public and scientific constituency.

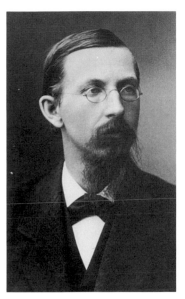

101. William Healy Dall: "Dean" of Alaskan Natural History

SI neg. 1145; SA RU7073 (notebook)

Dall inherited the leadership of Alaskan fieldwork following Kennicott's death in 1866. His book *Alaska and Its Resources* was the first English language treatise on Alaska, and his lifetime scientific contributions were immense. His field notebooks—here illustrating Malemiut Eskimo clothing—are a rich source of primary data.

Not in any way inferior in interest and importance to the natural history collections were those relating to the ethnological peculiarities of the Eskimaux and different tribes of Indians inhabiting the Arctic regions. It is believed that no such series is elsewhere to be found of the dresses, weapons, implements, utensils, instruments of war and of the chase, &c., &c., of the aborigines of Northern America. . . . The materials will serve to fix with precision the relationships of the arctic animals to those of more southern regions, their geographic distribution, their habits and manners, and other particulars of interest, and to extend very largely the admirable records presented by Sir John Richardson relative to arctic zoology (Smithsonian Institution Annual Report 1863:53).

Thus, with B. R. Ross (fig. 67), R. R. MacFarlane (fig. 100), and other Hudson's Bay Company men, Kennicott established the first comprehensive ethnographic collection in North America and, in the view of Henry B. Collins, among the most treasured materials in the U.S. National Museum. Not commented upon was Baird's growing perception of Alaska as a vast but potentially rich wilderness unknown to American science whose secrets could be unlocked if only a means of entry could be found.

The Telegraph Survey and the Purchase of Alaska

While Kennicott was cataloging the arctic collections in Washington in 1865 the opportunity Baird had been waiting for materialized. The Western Union Telegraph Company, with whom Baird had been consulting, had decided to build an overland cable to Europe via Bering Strait to compete with a trans-Atlantic cable plagued by undersea breakage. Kennicott's new information proved invaluable in selecting a route, and at Baird's suggestion, Western Union appointed Kennicott to lead a team to map the route and gave him authority to make collections and observations from this vast interior region, then under tenuous Russian administration.

The operation of the telegraph survey, however, proved more troublesome than either Baird

or Kennicott envisioned. It extended not only from San Francisco to Bering Strait but had a Siberian component as well, and surveys were required in Kamchatka and Chukotka. In the end the results were completely unexpected. It turned out that Kennicott's skills as a field naturalist were not matched by the organizational and leadership abilities needed to manage an unruly group of scientists, each with definite (and different) ideas of their goals and needs. For Kennicott, the outcome was disastrous; he suffered a nervous breakdown, and in May 1866 his body was found on the bank of the Yukon River near Nulato. Kennicott's death, apparently of a heart attack, ended the career of a pioneering American scientist and disrupted the ambitious plans for the telegraph survey. But even as the Scientific Corps regrouped under the leadership of William Healy Dall, completion of the Atlantic cable by a rival company on 27 July, 1866, sealed the fate of the project.

Though the telegraph project failed to complete all its goals, its contributions were invaluable, being the first widespread scientific survey of Alaska, including the Yukon River, Bering Strait, Norton Sound, the Bering Sea coast, and parts of Southeast Alaska. Data were also gathered from Kamchatka and the Siberian shore of Bering Strait. Topographic and geological maps were prepared; observations and collections were made on native cultures, plants, animals, minerals, and climate; and reports were compiled on a wide assortment of other subjects. Although few of these were formally published, the archives of the Smithsonian contain a wealth of primary documentation, much of which contributed to Dall's monograph *Alaska and Its Resources*, the first English-language compendium on Alaska, which was published in 1870.

When members of the Scientific Corps returned to Washington they found the govern-

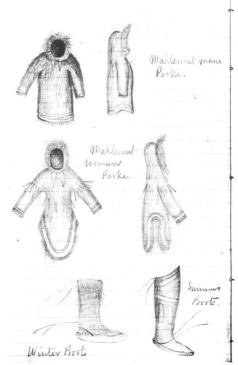

ment deeply involved in debate over the purchase of Alaska. Naturally, Baird was involved, for the Smithsonian was the only government agency with firsthand knowledge of Russian America. Frederick Bischoff, who had spent a year in the vicinity of Sitka studying insects, and Henry Bannister, a paleontologist who knew the Russian literature and who had explored the regions around Norton Sound, south of Bering Strait, testified to the Senate and the Department of State on their observations, while Baird provided information on zoology and minerals. All reported evidence of great promise: a wealth of fur-bearing animals, timber, minerals, fisheries, and whaling, and highly developed native cultures. Quite to the astonishment of Congress and much of the public, Alaska seemed worlds apart from the better known but more impoverished Eastern Arctic regions. This information had a major impact on Senator Charles Sumner of Massachusetts, whose speech ''The Cessation of Russian America,'' of April 9, 1867, to the U.S. Senate presented the most informed view in a debate that was overloaded with rumor and ignorance.

Realizing that the battle for the purchase would not be resolved only in the halls of Congress and government agencies, Baird also spread the word through the Smithsonian's ''telegraph'' network. Mobilizing the institution's information-exchange links, he supplied data on the results of the telegraph survey and copies of Senator Sumner's speech to natural history societies, universities, and Smithsonian correspondents. Partly in response to the Smithsonian's finds, the Department of State concluded the purchase treaty on March 30, 1867, and after a long public debate, Congressional approval was reached on July 27, 1868. Although it remains unclear to what extent the Smithsonian Congressional reports and public information campaign influenced the outcome of the debate, the institution is credited with having played a significant role in this momentous transaction (James 1942; Sherwood 1965).

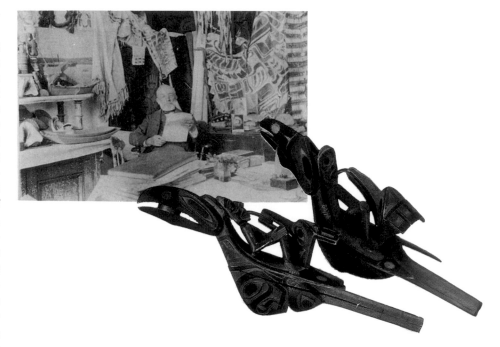

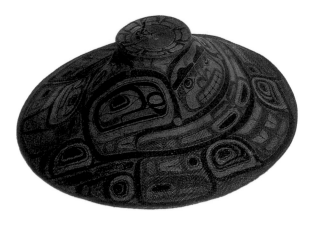

One matter about which there can be little doubt is that the telegraph survey set into motion a Smithsonian program of Alaskan research of unparalleled scope and impact. In addition to the collections and information gathered, and its impact on the purchase of Alaska, some of the major results were crystallization of an Alaskan research program, establishment of contacts with other agencies, and training of scholars, some of whom, like Dall, remained involved in Smithsonian research in Alaska for the remainder of the century, training another generation of researchers. Ornithologist Henry Wood Elliott became a leading conservationist in the fight to save the Pribilof fur seals from extinction by fur hunters.

During the next 30 years the Smithsonian collected from virtually all regions of Alaska, built an immense natural history research collection, and published volumes of basic data, including many volumes on Alaskan ethnology, archeology, and physical anthropology. The fieldworkers involved were largely naturalists with primary training in biological sciences, rather than anthropologists or ethnologists, and as natural scientists they tended to view native peoples and cultures more objectively than many 19th-century scholars. Baird presided over this stream of directed research like a mother hen, coaxing and guiding his naturalists to extend and improve their collections while cajoling the agencies funding them into providing continued support as they collected for the Smithsonian in their spare time.

102. James G. Swan
SI neg. 79-6861; Haida: NMNH 89079, 88795

The Smithsonian's early Northwest Coast collections were obtained primarily by James G. Swan, a correspondent of Baird's living in Port Townsend, Washington (Cole 1985; Doig 1980). Swan's major contribution was in making a large collection of Haida and Tlingit materials for the 1876 Centennial Exhibition. Swan collected these raven rattles in the early 1880s.

103. Crest Hat
Haida: NMNH 88961b

Among the collections the Smithsonian wanted Swan to acquire were spectacular display objects like this large spruce-root hat. Made for noble men, such hats were painted with stylized animal representations and were used as crest regalia by chiefs. The formline design is of an orca, or killer whale, a leading crest of the Raven moiety of the Haida.

Smithsonian Anthropology in Alaska

Following the purchase of Alaska, Baird's groundwork blossomed into a flurry of scientific activity as the government expanded its activities in the territory. Baird secured places for naturalists on many government expeditions and surveys and encouraged officers of Navy and Revenue Service vessels, the forerunner of the Coast Guard, to participate in collection and data gathering. The Smithsonian's *Annual Reports* attest to the success of this effort.

It was clear that scientific research required better documentation than could be obtained through casual collecting efforts. Following the precedents established in the telegraph surveys, Baird turned to his naturalists and, in collaboration with Dall, devised a regional program that took advantage of the many government observation posts that became established throughout coastal Alaska from Sitka to St. Michael. Match-

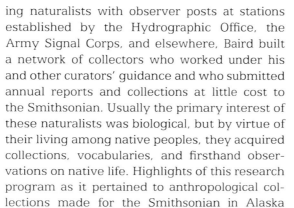

104. Sketch of a Traditional Tlingit House

SI-NAA 129776; SI neg. 45-604-A

Swan's notes include documentation on objects he collected. His comment on this watercolor sketch reads "Form of House of the Indians of Sitka, Alaska copied from a model made by a Sitka Indian, drawn and painted by James G. Swan, Port Townsend, Washington Territory, March 1874." Of a literary but unscientific bent, Swan's documentation did not match that of Baird's northern collectors, many of whom were trained scientific observers.

105. Shaman's Whale Tooth Amulet
Tlingit: NMNH 74990

Taking advantage of the posting of government personnel to the Alaska territories, Baird enlisted men like John J. McLean to collect during the course of other duties. While maintaining weather records for the Army Signal Corps, McLean studied Tlingit life and with funds provided by Baird purchased objects. The images on this shaman's amulet include octopuses, bears, and birds; as is typical of other shamanistic creations, their meaning is unclear.

ing naturalists with observer posts at stations established by the Hydrographic Office, the Army Signal Corps, and elsewhere, Baird built a network of collectors who worked under his and other curators' guidance and who submitted annual reports and collections at little cost to the Smithsonian. Usually the primary interest of these naturalists was biological, but by virtue of their living among native peoples, they acquired collections, vocabularies, and firsthand observations on native life. Highlights of this research program as it pertained to anthropological collections made for the Smithsonian in Alaska between 1867 and 1900 are given below.

Northwest Coast: Swan, McLean, Niblack, and Emmons

The Smithsonian's Northwest Coast research began with the work of George T. Gibbs, who

as noted above is known primarily for his linguistic mapping but who also made contributions to ethnographic collections on the Columbia River Plateau and Puget Sound region. However, it was James G. Swan, another pioneer resident of the Northwest, who became the Smithsonian's primary contributor of early Northwest ethnographic objects. His collections of Makah ethnography (Swan 1869) provided the Smithsonian with a collection from this whaling society at the southern end of the Northwest Coast, with whom Swan lived for many years. Swan became a lifelong correspondent of Baird's and is best known for his collections for the 1876 Centennial Exhibition from the least acculturated northern tribes—Haida and Tlingit—and from central and southern groups, which came at a critical time in the history of these cultures. Carefully documented, these collections included war canoes, memorial poles, a painted house front, masks, ceremonial objects, and many other items. Swan continued collecting for the Smithsonian into the 1880s, but without travel funds, these later collections were less documented (Cole 1985). Swan's collections were partially published by Ens. A. P. Niblack, a U.S. Naval officer who served in Southeast Alaska with the U.S. Coast and Geodetic Survey in 1885–87 and wrote the first monograph on Tlingit culture (Niblack 1890).

Swan's work among the Tlingit was followed by that of John J. McLean in the early 1880s. McLean was posted to Sitka as a member of the U.S. Signal Corps, following in the footsteps of Bischoff, the telegraph survey entomologist. While maintaining weather records for the Signal Corps, McLean documented Tlingit life and culture and made ethnographic collections, especially of shamanic materials. McLean was succeeded in 1884 by Lt. T. Dix Bolles of the U.S. Navy, who also collected shamanic objects, notably a mask whose eyes consist of ritual Chinese temple coins (fig. 442; Bolles 1883). He also compiled the first listing of the Smithsonian's Eskimo collections (Bolles 1889).

By far the most important of the U.S. Navy collectors in Southeast Alaska was Lt. George T. Emmons (Low 1977). Between 1882 and 1900 Emmons developed close relationships with the

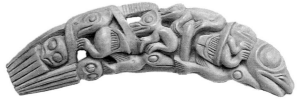

Tlingit and assembled a large collection. Emmons never sold much to the Smithsonian, which already had Swan's impressive Tlingit collection, but he became closely involved with the American Museum of Natural History in the 1890s. This relationship ended, however, after a falling out with Franz Boas, after which Emmons assisted the Smithsonian on various projects. His large collection ultimately went to the Field Museum in Chicago. Emmons spent his life working toward a Tlingit monograph that was to have been published as a volume in Boas's Jesup Expedition series, but he never completed the manuscript, which is only now being published under the editorship of Frederica de Laguna.

Kodiak and the Aleutians: Dall, Turner, Fisher, and Stejneger

The people of Kodiak Island, like those of the eastern Aleutians, came under strong Russian influence in the late 1700s, and by the beginning of the American period much of their traditional culture had disappeared. Nevertheless, William J. Fisher obtained an important collection of several hundred ethnographic specimens from Kodiak while stationed there as a tidal observer for the U.S. Coastal Survey, 1880–85. Fisher's linguistic data, masks, costumes, hunting implements, and other items are among the most important collections from Kodiak in North American collections. He also collected from Bristol Bay, particularly Ugashik (Fisher 1883), and from areas of the Pacific coast of Alaska. After 1885, Smithsonian work on Kodiak ceased

until Ales Hrdlicka began archeological and physical anthropological studies here in the 1930s.

In the Aleutian Islands, similar conditions of Russian acculturation resulted in relatively little traditional material culture surviving, except basketry, after 1867, although important natural history studies were conducted here by W. H. Dall and Lucien Turner between 1868 and 1881. Although a paleontologist with special expertise in snails and other mollusks, Dall made many important contributions to Alaskan anthropology during his long career. He was the first to point out to Baird the rich potential for ethnographic work among the Yupik Eskimo of the Bering Sea coast. His book *Alaska and Its Resources* was for decades the only regionwide compilation. His field notes are full of ethnographic information, and he wrote an early report on the Siberian Chukchi (Dall 1881). He made the first archeological excavations in Alaska, excavated the important whalers' cave at Unga in the Shumagins (fig. 164; Dall 1876), established a cultural chronology in the Aleutians based on stratigraphic relationships (Dall 1873), and wrote an excellent survey of labrets and masks (Dall 1884). Dall, second only to Baird, was responsible for the Smithsonian's continued involvement in Alaskan research in his capacity as the Smithsonian's honorary curator of malacology. Throughout his long career he was employed not by the institution but by the Coast and Geodetic Survey and later by the U.S. Geological Survey.

One of Dall's discoveries was a young naturalist named Lucien Turner. Upon his return from the telegraph survey, Dall recommended

106. E. W. Nelson: ''The Man Who Buys Good-For-Nothing Things''
Portrait, NPG; field photo; SI neg. 6393

Baird's most systematic collector, Edward W. Nelson, began his association with the Smithsonian at age 21. Over a four-year period (1877–81) Nelson assembled the most comprehensive natural history collection (some ''caught by means of my hat'') ever obtained from an arctic region. Nelson's success was due in part to his adoption of Eskimo language, clothing, and travel techniques. His field photos, here of an Eskimo summer camp, were the earliest such record of Alaskan Eskimo life. Nelson's custom of appearing in villages asking for traditional implements earned him the Yupik nickname ''the man who buys good-for-nothing things.''

107. Man's Ground Squirrel Parka
Bering Sea Eskimo: NMNH 176104
Nelson was one of the few naturalists working for Baird who wrote full reports on all aspects of his work. His collections, documentation, and publications on birds, animals, and Western Eskimo culture set scholarly standards for northern science. Even the few specimens he retained in his private collection, including this parka, eventually came to rest in the National Museum of Natural History.

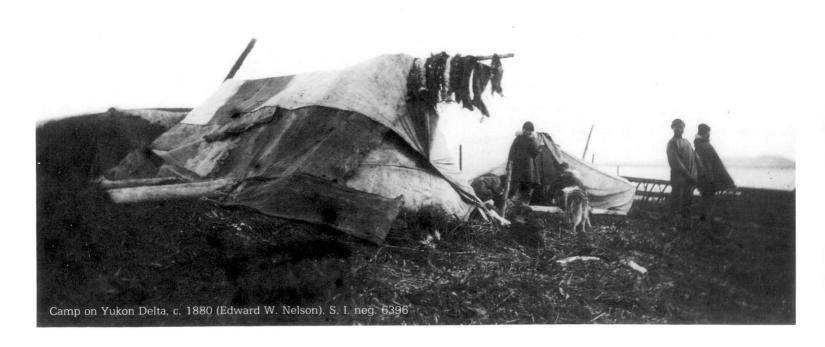

Camp on Yukon Delta, c. 1880 (Edward W. Nelson), S. I. neg. 6396

Turner to Baird for the position of U.S. Army Signal Corps observer at St. Michael, formerly the Russian American Company post at the mouth of the Yukon River. Turner's ethnographic collections from St. Michael were small but spectacular. In 1877 he was transferred to the Aleutians, with similarly excellent results until 1881, and later to northern Quebec (1881–83), where he pioneered Indian and Eskimo ethnographic studies (Turner 1894) about the time Boas first arrived in North America to begin his career on Baffin Island, in 1883.

Leonhard Stejneger, a Smithsonian biologist best known for his work on the northern fur seal and for his biography of Georg Wilhelm Steller (Stejneger 1936), naturalist on Bering's voyage of 1741, followed Dall to the Aleutian Islands. He also worked in Kamchatka and in the early

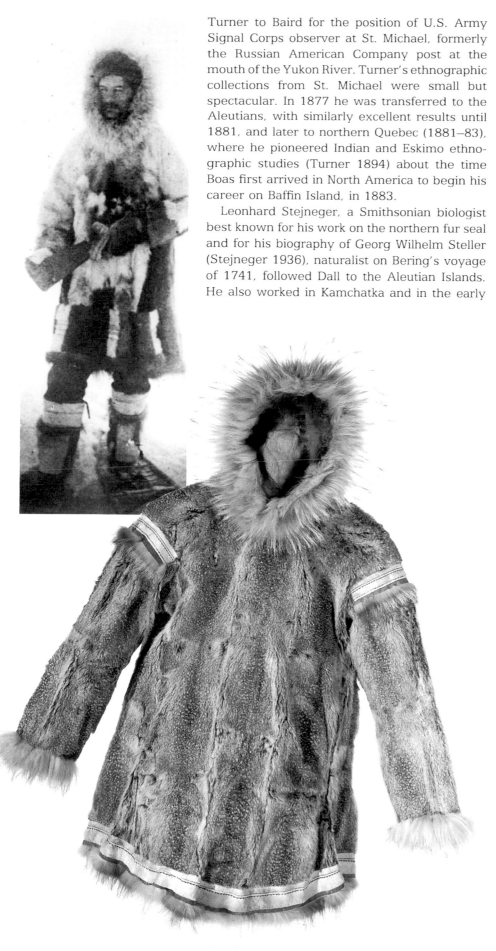

1880s conducted a large biological survey of the Commander Islands. In 1882 Stejneger located and excavated part of Bering's camp on Bering Island where the ship *St. Peter* was beached and where Bering (who perished) and his crew spent the winter of 1741–42. Among Stejneger's records is the following note:

I also visited the place of Bering's death, and the wintering, and spent two days here, digging and surveying. The ruin of the house was measured and described, but my intention of taking a map-sketch and some landscape-sketches of the surroundings was completely frustrated by the never-ceasing rain. The remains found were very scant, small glass beads and sheets of mica, intended for money in the exchange with the Indians, a few iron balls from grape-shot, fragments of a brass plate with Russian armorial ensigns, bolts, and sheaves from the vessel, etc. I have kept these relics, as perhaps the National Museum is interested in receiving only the remains of this unlucky expedition for discovering America from the west (Stejneger manuscript n.d.).

Southwest Alaska: Dall, Turner, Nelson, and MacKay

In 1877, Turner was replaced at St. Michael by Edward W. Nelson, another Chicago naturalist appointed to make weather observations for the Army Signal Corps (Lantis 1954). Nelson remained at St. Michael until 1881, during which time he amassed the most important collection of Eskimo ethnographic materials ever collected from the Arctic. Nelson's work was especially significant in that the Eskimo from this region were almost totally isolated from European contact and had retained much of their traditional culture. Unlike many of the Smithsonian's natural history collectors, Nelson published his collections fully, and his monograph on western Alaskan Eskimo ethnology has become a classic (Nelson 1899, also 1882, 1887). Hundreds of Nelson's Eskimo specimens were exchanged with other museums around the world. Nelson also made more than 100 ethnographic photographs, which, except for those of Alphonse Pinart's of 1871, are the earliest images of Alaskan peoples.

In addition to the Fisher collections from Ugashik (Fisher 1883), important collections were gathered from Bristol Bay by Charles MacKay, Signal Service observer at Nushagak in 1881–83. MacKay drowned in a boating accident while in the field. His collections are important because of the paucity of information on the ethnography of this region, located strategically at the junction of the Aleut, Bering Sea Eskimo, and Pacific Eskimo culture areas. Other collections from western Alaska include those obtained by John Henry Turner along the Yukon in 1889–90 in connection with boundary surveys for the Coast and Geodetic Survey.

Bering Strait: Nelson, Hooper, and Healy

During the early years of the American period, the region around Bering Strait, including Norton Sound, Seward Peninsula, Kotzebue, and the western side of Bering Strait—regions visited heavily by whalers and other vessels—was frequented by Revenue Service vessels and others on official missions. Many of the officers and representatives of government agencies contributed ethnographic collections resulting from these trips. Such collections tended to be poorly documented but were occasionally of great interest because of their exceptional quality. Notable among these collectors were Capt. C. L. Hooper of the Revenue steamer *Thomas Corwin* in 1881 (Hooper 1881, 1884) and Capt. M. A. Healy, who commanded the *Corwin* cruises of 1884–85 (Healy 1887, 1889). Edward Nelson also made collections from Bering Strait while on the *Corwin* in 1881 in company with geologist John Muir.

North Alaska: Ray, Murdoch, and Stoney

Ethnological research was a primary objective of the U.S. International Polar Expedition to Point Barrow in 1881–83. Under the command of Lt. P. H. Ray (Ray 1885), this expedition made important collections from the natives of the Point Barrow region at a time when their culture was under considerable influence from contact with whalers but still retained its traditional character. Much of the data collected was obtained by John Murdoch, who like many others noted above received the post through Baird's recommendation. The collections of this expedition represent the whaling culture of the North Alaskan Eskimo and are especially strong in material culture and technology, less so in social culture, mythology, and other subjects. Murdoch, like Nelson, published the expedition's materials in full, and it, too, has become a classic in arctic ethnography (Murdoch 1892). Murdoch had a long association with the Smithsonian, publishing many articles on Eskimo and other ethnographic subjects, and was Smithsonian librarian from 1887 to 1892. Of all the Smithsonian's Alaskan collectors, Murdoch was the only one who became primarily interested in ethnology, but he never received a curatorial appointment. Ray's and Murdoch's North Alaskan research was extended by the work of Lt. George M. Stoney (Stoney 1890), who explored and mapped the North Alaskan interior between 1884 and 1886 and also made ethnological collections from the Lower Yukon, Kotzebue, and the North Alaskan interior.

Thus, in slightly more than 40 years, between 1859 and 1900, the Smithsonian pioneered the study of Alaskan natural history and anthropology, established one of the world's finest research collections, published large amounts of data, guided the conduct of government science in these new lands, and trained many scientists who were to take up positions in other government agencies as these agencies began to assert their own control over agency research needs. One man in particular was responsible for this remarkable achievement. Spencer Fullerton Baird conceived of the need for Alaskan research at a time when Russia's interest and control over Russian America, which held so many secrets to the understanding of natural history, cultures, and peoples of the New World, was waning. Assisted initially by industry and later by government agencies, Baird, and later Dall, helped recover important ethnological collections at a time when Alaskan cultures were in a state of transition. The importance of these collections, their documentation, and the publications by the scientists who collected them is inestimable.

Yet by themselves, these collections provide only a partial view of Alaskan cultures during the last half of the late 19th century. With Russian collections representing the age of exploration and contact and the Smithsonian documenting the Alaskan cultures in Southwest Alaska and north of the Aleutians in a relatively unacculturated state, Boas turned to the one remaining geographic area for which no Western sources of anthropological materials were available—Northeastern Siberia. In addition to seeking data, Boas also reviewed the questions of Northeast Asia–America connections raised by Gallatin, Morton, Agassiz, Bachman, and others in the early to mid 19th century, and that had energized Henry, Gibbs, and Baird at the Smithsonian in the 1850s, but for which firm answers were still not available. In part this was because the Smithsonian's Alaskan work had been done primarily by biologists and naturalists and not by experts trained in the study of anthropology. Boas was formulating a new scientific discipline and believed a more problem-oriented and rigorous methodology, carried out by specially trained ethnologists, would provide the answers to cultural relationships across Bering Strait. Boas did not foresee that the problems would prove even more durable than he imagined, their solutions seemingly even more remote.

108. Morris K. Jesup
AMNH neg. 2A-5200

A true American success story, Morris K. Jesup (1830–1908) rose from humble origins to become a millionaire in the railroad banking business. He helped found the American Museum of Natural History in 1869 and later became its president and chief financier from 1881 until his death in 1908.

Jesup, a man interested in big problems, was impressed with the scope of the expedition proposed by his young curator, Franz Boas. Jesup's fervent support for the decade-long Jesup North Pacific Expedition—still the largest and most systematic study of Asian-American relationships ever undertaken—earned him a prominent place in the history of anthropological science.

109. Franz Boas
AMNH neg. 2A-5161

When Franz Boas (1858–1942) arrived at the American Museum of Natural History in 1896 he lost no time presenting an idea for a grandiose project on the cultures and history of the North Pacific region. Boas saw the lack of data from Siberian tribes as the major impediment to solving this problem. Between 1897 and 1903 Boas secured funding and fielded research teams, and in subsequent years edited and supervised publications. Initially optimistic about the results, Boas later grew distrustful of his interpretations and never wrote the final report he promised Jesup. Today, the Jesup Expedition's major contributions are in its huge collection of specimens and field data and the detailed publications on a remote and previously unknown region.

The American Museum's Jesup North Pacific Expedition

Stanley A. Freed, Ruth S. Freed, and Laila Williamson

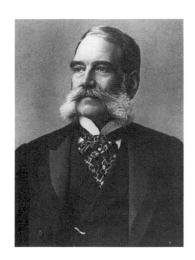

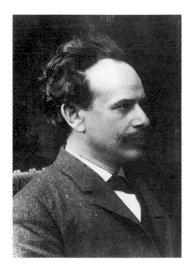

"The biggest of the unsolved anthropological and ethical problems" and one that is "alive with human and historic interest" was how the *New York Times*, in a March 1897 editorial, greeted the announcement that the American Museum of Natural History was about to launch an ambitious investigation of the relationship between the peoples of northeastern Asia and northwestern North America. Named after Morris K. Jesup (1830–1908), then president of the American Museum, the venture involved six years of fieldwork among the principal tribes on both sides of the Bering Strait (fig. 3). Describing the project as "dealing with a subject of great interest . . . the theory that America was originally peopled by migratory tribes from the Asiatic continent," Jesup invited contributions from friends of the American Museum. Apparently finding no takers, Jesup later declared that he would assume the entire expense of the project.

Franz Boas (1858–1942), then assistant curator in the museum's Department of Anthropology and later to become the most distinguished American anthropologist of his time, directed the project. Boas conceived the research to answer three main questions: the origin of the early inhabitants of America, "the relationship between the American race and the Asiatic race, and the relationship between American culture and Asiatic culture" (Boas 1905:92). Although Jesup and the popular press were interested principally in the question of the origin of the Amerindians, Boas seemed little concerned with it, in all likelihood believing that their place of origin was obvious.

Boas moved quickly to set the project in motion. In late May 1897, less than three months after the announcement of the expedition, Boas left New York in the company of Harlan I. Smith of the American Museum and Livingston Farrand of Columbia University for a summer of fieldwork. The three men arrived in Spences Bridge, British Columbia, where they joined James Teit, a Scotsman who had married a Thompson Indian and spoke several Salish dialects fluently. Boas had first met Teit in 1894. "James Teit is a treasure," he wrote to his wife. "He knows a great deal about the tribes. I engaged him right away" (Rohner 1969:139).

Boas, Farrand, and Teit headed north on horseback to investigate the physical characteristics of the Lillooet and Shuswap and the customs and physical traits of the Chilcotin. The party proceeded slowly to the Chilcotin, where Farrand remained for a month while Boas, Teit, and an Indian guide made a difficult journey westward across a wild 3,500-foot plateau north of Tatla Lake and over the Coast Mountains. On July 20, almost seven weeks after leaving Spences Bridge, Boas arrived at the village of Bella Coola, where he met George Hunt, his principal assistant and collaborator. He remained in Bella Coola a bit more than a fortnight working with Hunt on Kwakiutl texts and with Bella Coola informants. On August 5, he left Bella Coola for Numa to catch a steamer for Port Essington on the Skeena River, where he intended to study the Haida and Tsimshian in the company of Harlan I. Smith.

While Boas was awaiting the ship at Numa, another steamer arrived from the north with George Dorsey of Chicago's Columbian Museum (now the Field Museum of Natural History) and some companions aboard. They were on a collecting tour. They disembarked, met Boas, and the group had a brief, very friendly conversation. The next day, Boas wrote to his wife:

This trip of Dorsey's annoys me very much. . . . What makes me so furious is the fact that these Chicago people simply adopt my plans and then try to beat me to it. . . . I don't really think that his trip will interfere with my work, but this treacherous way of acting makes me awfully angry (Rohner 1969:221).

Boas regarded the Northwest Coast as his territory and believed that infringement, without at least the courtesy of consultation, was intolerable. Frederick Ward Putnam sympathized with Boas but from the beginning had pointed out that competition was probably inevitable.

Boas's anger after the chance meeting at Numa was more than a transitory reaction; it reflected

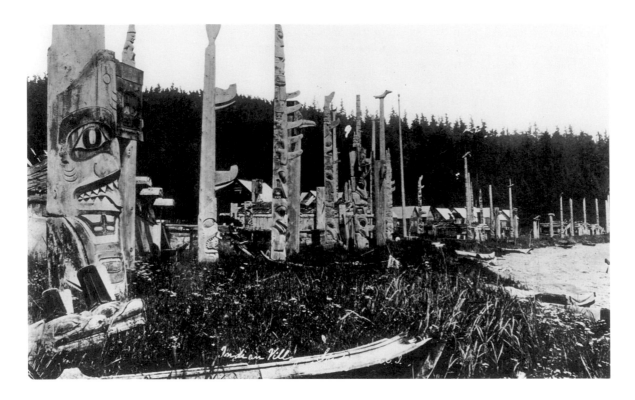

the intense competition, enhanced by personal bitterness, between New York's American Museum and Chicago's Field Museum, which was an undercurrent throughout the years of the Jesup Expedition. Boas had expected to be named as head of anthropology at the new Chicago museum but was passed over. Boas felt that his rejection by the Field Museum was an insult, and Putnam shared his anger. With the financial support of Jesup, Boas and Putnam were in a strong position, and Putnam vowed to best Chicago. Dorsey in Chicago also had strong backing and was as combative as the New Yorkers.

The battle for artifacts was one aspect of the competition, but even more serious from Boas's point of view were Dorsey's efforts to entice George Hunt away from him. At the Numa meeting, the Chicago group asked about Hunt's whereabouts, but Boas wrote, "I was mean enough not to tell them . . . and I have written George Hunt that he should not do anything for them. I have to do this to protect myself" (Rohner 1969:222).

Hunt was the keystone of Boas's personal Northwest Coast research. Hunt's mother was a Tlingit and his father, an English Hudson's Bay Company factor. Raised in Port Rupert as a Kwakiutl, Hunt spoke their language fluently, was literate in English, and was a steady and reliable worker. Boas trained him to transcribe Kwakiutl texts, and much of Boas's Kwakiutl research depended on him (Cannizzo 1983:45, 47–48, 53). Moreover, Hunt was Boas's principal collector, managing to make some remarkable

purchases, such as the Nootka Whalers' Washing House in 1904.

After the summer of 1897, Boas made only one other trip to the Northwest Coast in the course of the Jesup Expedition. In 1900, he visited Spences Bridge for about a week's work in the Nicola Valley. From July 3 to September 9, he was in Alert Bay with George Hunt working with the Kwakiutl. He wrote to his secretary, "The work is interesting, but very unexciting. I am sitting outdoors all day with my interpreters and pump the people."[1]

Boas and his field investigators collected about half of the American Museum's 16,750 Northwest Coast artifacts. From the first, systematic collecting was an important part of Boas's own work on the Northwest Coast and of all the research carried out by the Jesup Expedition. Boas was generally circumspect as a collector of artifacts, carefully establishing a reputation for patience, generosity, and tact. "His heart is pure and kind toward us Indians," said a Kwakiutl chief during a potlatch that Boas gave to pay for the performance of a dance. "My heart is friendly toward him and if he wants anything from us we shall do our best to do what he asks" (Rohner 1969:37).

Most of the formidable body of ethnographic data that Boas and his colleagues collected was published in the *Memoirs of the American Museum of Natural History, Jesup North Pacific Expedition.* Harlan I. Smith, who served at the American Museum until 1911 and eventually became chief archeologist of the National Museum of Canada, established his reputation with

110. Haida Village, Queen Charlotte Islands
AMNH neg. 330387

The Jesup Expedition began work on the southern Northwest Coast in 1897. Boas had already initiated research here with a team interested in combining ethnology, archeology, physical anthropology, and linguistics to solve problems of cultural relationships and development. The British Columbia work served as a testing ground for methods Boas was to apply in his study of Asian-American problems.

This photograph of Skidegate, a Haida village in the Queen Charlottes, was taken in 1900 by John R. Swanton, a Smithsonian anthropologist who collaborated with Boas.

111. Shaman's Apron
Yukaghir: AMNH 70-5620b

This apron was purchased from a Yukaghir shaman whose name was Igor Shamanov. Though part of an entire costume (fig. 326) made for a male shaman, its fur tassels are characteristic of female garments. Sexual ambiguity and transvestism were common features of Siberian shamans. Male shamans often adopted female names, behaved like women, and wore women's clothing.

a series of excavations in British Columbia and Washington. John R. Swanton, who was to produce a prodigious number of publications on the North American Indians, participated in the Jesup Expedition early in his career while a member of the Bureau of American Ethnology, with the bureau and the American Museum dividing both the financing and the information that he collected on the Haida. Livingston Farrand of Columbia University, who went with Boas and Smith in the opening thrust of the expedition into the Northwest in 1897, wrote on the traditions of the Chilcotin and Quinault and on the basketry designs of several Salish groups. Boas's local collaborators, Hunt and James Teit, made substantial contributions. Hunt mainly assisted Boas; his name appears with Boas's on the title pages of Kwakiutl monographs. Teit wrote on the Thompson, Lillooet, and Shuswap. In addition to producing his famous monographs on the Kwakiutl, Boas wrote on the Bella Coola and edited the Jesup series.

The Siberian operations of the expedition, beginning a year later than the American research, covered an area many times as large under much more difficult conditions. Three teams carried out the fieldwork: one in southern and two in northern Siberia. The southern team, composed of ethnologist Berthold Laufer and archeologist Gerard Fowke, was first into the field, operating along the Amur River and on Sakhalin Island in 1898. Laufer continued his fieldwork in 1899. The two northern teams were

headed by Waldemar Bogoras and Waldemar Jochelson.

Born in Germany, Berthold Laufer (1874–1934) took his doctorate from the University of Leipzig in 1897 with a dissertation on a Tibetan text. He decided to make East Asia his specialty and, as part of his preparation, studied no fewer than ten Asian languages. On May 19, 1897, Boas wrote to Laufer that he would receive $500 per year while in the field and his expenses.

Laufer arrived on Sakhalin Island on July 10, 1898, where he remained until March 21, 1899, studying the Nivkhi, Evenk, and Ainu. He began with the Nivkhi and Evenk in northeastern Sakhalin and then headed south to investigate the Evenk and Ainu of central and southern Sakhalin, a departure delayed for $2\frac{1}{2}$ months by influenza and pneumonia contracted among the Nivkhi. The journey by horseback, reindeer sled, and dogsled was difficult and dangerous. Once he broke through the ice and would have drowned had not his guide seen the incident the moment it happened and saved him.

Laufer crossed to the mainland on March 25 and settled in Khabarovsk on the Amur River to study the Nanai (Golde). He estimated his expenses for work on the Amur at 3,000 rubles (about $1,560), explaining, "Nothing is free here except death, which you can have in this country at special bargain rates" (American Museum of Natural History, New York City, Laufer to Boas, March 4, 1899, translated and quoted in Boas to Jesup, May 4, 1899). By the end of May,

112. Bogoras on the Kolyma River
AMNH neg. 22402, Jesup Exp.

Waldemar Bogoras (1865–1936), a populist revolutionary whose ethnological interests developed during exile in Siberia, was hired by Boas to work among the Chukchi. During 18 months (1900–1901) Bogoras traveled extensively in Chukotka while his wife made collections in the vicinity of the Anadyr. Working conditions were terrible; famine and disease were rampant, and Bogoras nearly died of influenza.

Despite harsh conditions, the Bogorases amassed a huge collection: 5,000 artifacts, 450 tales and texts, 75 skulls and archeological samples, 33 plaster face casts, somatological measurements of 860 individuals, and 95 wax cylinder recordings. These collections surpassed Boas's expectations and were eventually published in seven monographs and numerous scholarly papers.

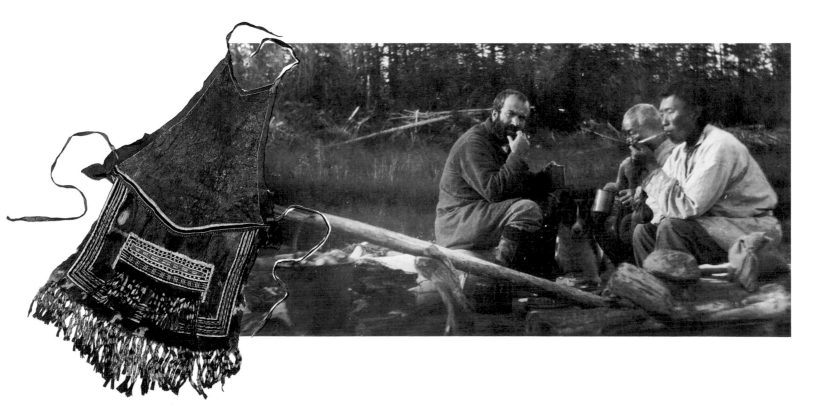

navigation had opened on the Amur, and Laufer descended the river, visiting Nanai and Nivkhi villages on the way. About his work on the Lower Amur, Laufer wrote,

The trip during summer on the lower Amoor was really more trying than the winter campaign on the island of Saghalin. Nobody who has not been there can have an idea of the dreadful horrors one has to undergo on account of the insect-pest, combined with heat and sixteen months' loanly [sic] life in wilderness, which resulted into an extraordinary state of nervousness I never experienced before (Laufer to Boas, November 2, 1899).

Laufer's only publication in the Jesup North Pacific Expedition series is a monograph on the art of the Amur tribes (Laufer 1902). He was especially fascinated by the art of the Nanai and their neighbors and collected many objects that were superb artworks (Kendall 1986:5). After the Jesup Expedition, Laufer lived in the United States for the rest of his life. He was affiliated with the American Museum and Columbia University until he joined the Field Museum of Natural History in 1908, where he spent the rest of his scholarly career.

Boas's plans for fieldwork in northern Siberia were developed with the aid of V. V. Radlov, director of the Museum of Anthropology and Ethnography of the Imperial Academy of Sciences, who recommended Waldemar Bogoras (1865–1936) and Waldemar Jochelson (1855–1937) as best qualified (Radlov to Boas, February 23, 1898). Friends and colleagues, they were Russian intellectuals and revolutionaries who in their youth were exiled to Siberia where they became ethnographers.

In the spring of 1900, Jesup wrote a long letter officially giving Jochelson charge of the work of the expedition in northeastern Asia (Jesup to Jochelson, March 24, 1900). Jochelson and Bogoras would each receive $100 per month. However, Mrs. Jochelson and Mrs. Bogoras, whose "scientific work . . . must be considered as part of the results of the expedition," would receive no separate remuneration.

Arriving at Mariinsky Post at the mouth of the Anadyr River on July 18, 1900, the Bogorases spent their first four months of fieldwork with the Reindeer Chukchi who camped along the seashore during the summer. He laconically described conditions that summer as rather "unfavorable" because of a measles epidemic that in places caused the death of 30 percent of the population (Boas 1903:110).

At the end of October, Bogoras began a journey with a Cossack and a native guide through a territory ranging from Indian Point and St. Lawrence Island on the northeast to Kamchatka on the southwest. Traveling mostly

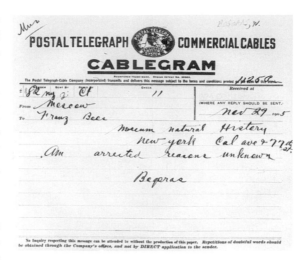

by dogsled, Bogoras was on the move for the rest of his 12½ months in northeastern Asia. He generally remained no more than four weeks in any locality. At times, the journey was an ordeal. Bogoras had influenza on the way back to his base at Mariinsky Post, and his illness became so alarming that his Cossack asked where to deliver his body and official papers in case he died en route. While her husband traveled, Mrs. Bogoras stayed on the Anadyr. She spent her time traveling between Mariinsky Post and Markovo, gathering the greater part of the collections for the American Museum (Boas 1903:110–14; Bogoras to Boas, September 11, 1901).

Back in St. Petersburg in the fall of 1904, Bogoras was settling in for a winter of writing, but political developments were soon to usurp almost all his attention. In 1905 events in Russia were close to a revolution. To Boas, who was trying to extract completed manuscripts from Bogoras and Jochelson, any social disturbance was a threat to the timely completion of the work. He kept gentle pressure on Bogoras in a carefully worded letter, in which he complained of having heard nothing from him for a long time. Bogoras replied from St. Petersburg:

I am afraid that you are right and I feel myself guilty of much neglect to all dear friends in America. But you will understand that an epoch like this happens only once in many centuries for every state and nation and we feel ourselves torn away with the current even against our will (Bogoras to Boas, April 6, 1905).

Boas was upset and immediately wrote to Bogoras, rejecting the idea that exciting social events were a valid excuse for neglecting science. Science was Boas's first priority. However, Bogoras's heart clearly was in politics. He wrote, "You must believe us, that we here do not forget our good friends in America nor indeed anywhere. But the events of the time are so stirring.

113. Bogoras, the Revolutionary
AMNH, Anthropology Archives
Boas received this ominous telegram from Bogoras in November 1905 after Bogoras had returned from the field and was writing up his expedition field notes. Distraught at the incarceration of his collaborator, Boas cabled V. Radlov, director of the Museum of Anthropology and Ethnology: "Bogoras arrested Wednesday Moscow. If wrongly can release be secured for continuing scientific work for Museum."

Bogoras's arrest in Moscow at a Farmers Congress was political; he was a Russian intellectual with membership in revolutionary organizations sharing ideological commitment to peasants and "folk" people. After returning to St. Petersburg from the Jesup Expedition he became swept up in the political ferment of the early stages of the Russian Revolution. Boas, anxious for publication of Bogoras's scientific work, contributed to the successful efforts for his release. In later years, Bogoras went on to publish widely as both ethnographer and novelist, and to head the Institute of the Peoples of the North that established the first Soviet policies for its northern subjects.

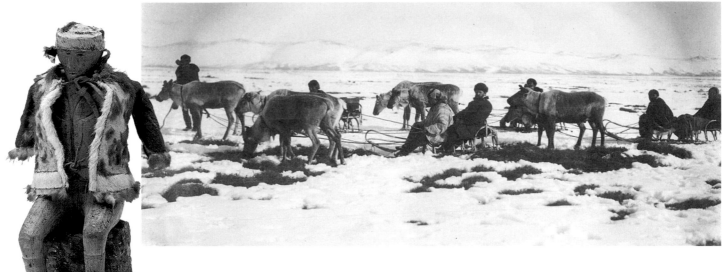

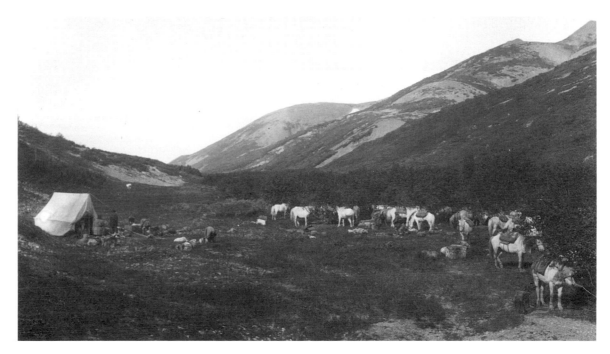

114. Sled Travel in Siberia

AMNH neg. 4155, Jesup Exp.
Koryak: AMNH 70-3040

Jochelson and his wife, Dina Brodsky, shared the danger and exhaustion of Siberian travel: "Bogs, mountain torrents, rocky passes and thick forests combined to hinder our progress. . . A heavy rain . . . caused the provisions to rot." Here Jochelson and Brodsky pause during a spring sled trip with Reindeer Koryaks. Jochelson collected this Koryak doll portraying a Russian traveler in European coat, boots, hat, and buttoned vest. Is it Jochelson?

115. Jochelson Camp in Stanovoi Mountains

AMNH neg. 4199, Jesup Exp.

Waldemar Jochelson (1855–1937) was a colleague of Bogoras's also recommended by Radlov. Jochelson, also a revolutionary whose interest in Siberian ethnography developed during exile, was older and more experienced than Bogoras, and was put in overall charge of the expedition's Siberian work. Working south of Bogoras, Jochelson studied the Koryak, Yukaghir, and Yakut, while Borogas studied the Even, Chukchi, and Asian Eskimo. Jochelson later served as a director of the Museum of Anthropology and Ethnography.

The blood is flowing, the best blood of the country, and no result is to be seen so far'' (Bogoras to Boas, May 13, 1905). In late November, Bogoras wrote to Boas that his only present interest was the Russian situation.

On November 27, Bogoras was arrested in Moscow. Two days later, he dispatched a cablegram to Boas, "Am arrested, reasons unknown''. However, Bogoras was to spend only two weeks in prison before the Literary Artists' Society of Moscow obtained his release by posting bail of 15,000 rubles (Bogoras to Boas, January 10, 1906). After the uprising, Bogoras went to St. Petersburg and from there to Wiborg, Finland. Eventually he returned to Russia and lived the rest of his life engaging in scientific and literary work. After the revolution, he became director of the Institute of the Peoples of the North, an agency concerned with education and develop-

mental work among the northern tribes of Siberia (Krader 1968:117; Boas 1937:314).

Bogoras's work for the Jesup Expedition resulted in seven monographs, most prominently on the Chukchi. He and his wife collected ethnographic data, linguistic notes, 450 tales and texts, 5,000 ethnographic artifacts, skeletal material, 33 plaster casts of faces, 75 skulls and archeological specimens, 95 phonographic records, and somatological measurements of 860 individuals (Boas 1903:115). No modern anthropologist would ever collect such a diversity of data.

Like Bogoras, Jochelson engaged in revolutionary activities as a student. He had to flee Russia in 1875 to avoid arrest. In 1884, trying to enter Russia under an assumed name to continue his revolutionary work, he was recognized at the border and arrested. He served

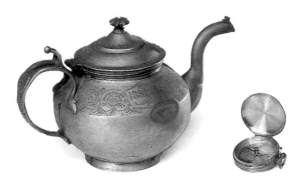

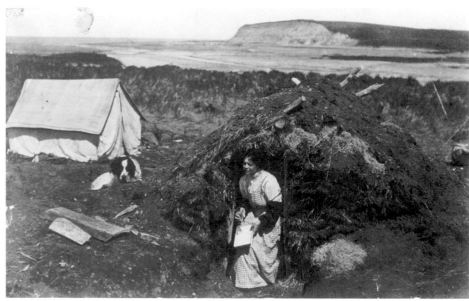

three years in solitary confinement and was then exiled for ten years to Northeastern Siberia. He spent his time in ethnological and linguistic studies of the native tribes, writing articles for various Russian scientific societies.

The Jochelsons were assigned to study the Koryak, Yukaghir, and Yakut for the Jesup Expedition. They arrived in Kushka, a small village at the mouth of the Gizhiga River, on August 16, 1900. During the measles epidemic of the winter of 1899–1900, 179 persons out of a total of 500 had died at Gizhiga, and, contrary to Jochelson's expectations, no Koryak were to be found. The Reindeer Koryak, who usually wintered there, had moved far into the mountains to escape the epidemic. The Jochelsons then went overland to the villages of the Maritime Koryak on Penzhina Bay, living most of the time in native underground dwellings. Jochelson reported to Boas:

It is almost impossible to describe the squalor of these dwellings. The smoke, which fills the hut, makes the eyes smart. It is particularly dense in the upper part of the hut, so that work that has to be done in an upright position becomes almost impossible. Walls, ladder and household utensils are covered with a greasy soot, so that contact with them leaves shining black spots on hands and clothing. The dim light which falls through the smoke-hole is hardly sufficient for writing and reading. The odor of blubber and of refuse is almost intolerable; and the inmates, intoxicated with fly agaric (*Amanita muscaria*), add to the discomfort of the situation. The natives are infested with lice. As long as we remained in these dwellings we could not escape these insects, which we dreaded more than any of the privations of our journey (Boas 1903:104).

The Jochelsons had to make dangerous journeys. Their late-summer trip (August 15 to October 9, 1901) from Kushka to Verkhne-Kolymsk to study the Reindeer Koryak gives an idea of travel in Siberia. Jochelson reported:

This journey was the most difficult one that it was ever my fate to undertake. Bogs, mountain torrents, rocky passes and thick forests combined to hinder our progress. . . . A heavy rain . . . caused the provisions to rot. Therefore we had to cut down our rations from the very beginning. After crossing the [mountain] passes . . . we reached the upper courses of the Korkodon River. by this time our horses were exhausted, and it was necessary to take a long rest (Boas 1903:107).

The temperature was dropping daily, and the Jochelson party knew that they would have to hurry if they were to reach Verkhne-Kolymsk before the river froze. They spent a day building a raft and prepared to float down the Korkodon River to a Yukaghir camp where they could obtain a boat. The descent was made dangerous by numerous rapids, rocky banks, and jams of driftwood. Their guides said that the descent could be made in two days, so they left most of their food with three Yakuts who stayed with the horses and reduced their own allowance to a three-day supply. The journey took nine days; for the last six days, each person received only two cups of flour daily and a little tea without sugar (Boas 1903:107). They spent four days among the Yukaghir of the Korkodon and then set out in a boat for Verkhne-Kolymsk. The river froze when they were 40 miles from Verkhne-Kolymsk, and they had to walk for two days to reach the settlement.

116. Dina Brodsky in Native Hut
AMNH neg. 337626, Jesup Exp. Russian: Uncataloged teapot, compass, Dohmer collection, AMNH

The Jochelsons arived in Gizhiga in August 1900, only to find 179 of 500 Koryaks had died of measles there the previous winter; the remainder had fled into the mountains to escape the epidemic. The Jochelsons attempted to follow, frequently living in underground houses whose squalid conditions, smoke, lack of room, and odor of blubber, they found oppressive. Travel direction was assisted by Jochelson's compass, and camp life was brightened by a brass teapot and glassware. In this photo, Brodsky emerges from a hut with her note pad and drinking glass.

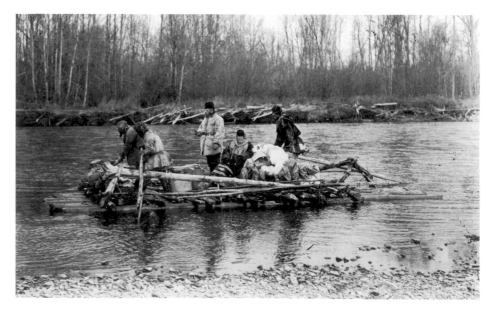

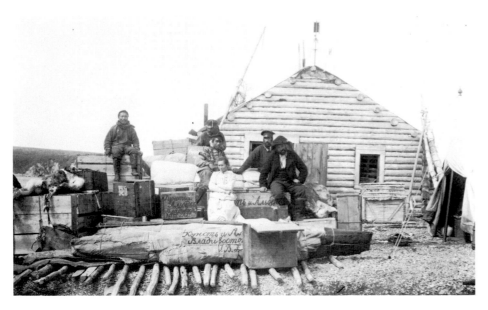

117. Expedition Freight at Marinskii Post
AMNH neg. 1380, Jesup Exp.

Marinskii Post, at the mouth of the Anadyr River, was Bogoras's headquarters and the central location of the Chukchi collecting effort. While Bogoras traveled, his wife collected here and at Markovo Post on the middle Anadyr. In August 1901 the expedition crew and freight (shown here) departed on the annual postal steamer to Vladivostok.

118. Rafting Down the Korkodon
AMNH neg. 4194, Jesup Exp.

Danger was the constant companion of fieldwork in Siberia. Jochelson described the trip from Kushka to Verkhne-Kolymsk as "the most difficult one that it was ever my fate to undertake." Lack of food, freezing conditions, and exhausted horses forced the party to build a raft on which they trusted their luck through rapids and logjams. Even so, freeze-up overtook them, and they had to complete the final 40 miles on foot. Here Jochelson, Brodsky, pet dog, and field party pose in an eddy for a "crew shot" at the beginning of the trip.

The Jochelsons made comprehensive studies of the Koryak and Yukaghir, collected 3,000 ethnographic artifacts, 41 casts of faces, measurements of 900 individuals, 1,200 photographs, 150 tales and texts, phonographic cylinders, skulls and archeological specimens, and a small zoological collection (Boas 1903:109). Jochelson published several monographs on the Koryak, Yukaghir, and Yakut under the auspices of the American Museum. The museum also issued his useful handbook, *Peoples of Asiatic Russia* (1928). Dina Brodsky Jochelson, later to take a degree in medicine, handled all the anthropometric and medical work and most of the photography. She used some of her anthropological measurements for her doctoral dissertation at the University of Zurich, published in *Archiv fur Anthropologie* (1906). She also published a work on the women of Northeastern Siberia, in Russian, in the *Russian Anthropological Journal* (1907).

After the Jesup Expedition, Jochelson led the Aleut-Kamchatka Expedition of the Imperial Russian Geographical Society in 1909–11. From 1912 to 1922, he was division curator of the Museum of Anthropology and Ethnography of the Russian Academy of Sciences in St. Petersburg/Petrograd and collaborator of the Asiatic Museum of the academy. From 1922 until his death in New York, November 1, 1937, Jochelson lived in the United States, where he was associated with the American Museum of Natural History and the Carnegie Institution of Washington (*American Anthropologist* 1930:376, 1938:345).

Based on the results of the Jesup Expedition, Boas discerned a close cultural affiliation between eastern Siberia and the region of southern Alaska and British Columbia; a cultural "break" between the East Siberian tribes and the Eskimo;

and a "fundamental break" between the Northeast Siberian tribes and the Evenk and Yakut. He wrote:

Comparisons of type, language and culture make it at once evident that the Northeast Siberian people are much more closely akin to the Americans than to other Asiatics. . . . The Chukchee, Koryak, Kamchadal, and Yukaghir must be classed with the American race rather than with the Asiatic race (Boas 1905:99).

Boas believed that these Siberian tribes were an offshoot of the American race. According to his theory, Asians first migrated into the New World during a period of reduced glaciation. Advancing ice then separated the Asian and American populations for a long enough time to allow for physical differentiation; when the ice melted, there was a reverse migration of American Indians to Siberia where they came into contact with other Asians moving northward with the retreat of the ice.

Jochelson gave the name "Americanoids" to the people descended from these hypothetical reverse migrants. He was intrigued by Boas's ideas and attempted to support the close affiliation of the Americanoids and Amerindians with evidence from mythology and folklore. Bogoras also emphasized the closeness of the Americanoids and the Amerindians. He wrote:

The mythology and folklore of northeastern Asia are essentially different from the Uralo-Altaic mythology, and point to a group of conceptions and a mode of expression which have little relationship to those of the interior of Siberia; on the contrary, they possess affinities eastward along the shores of Bering sea to the northwestern part of America. From an ethnographical point of view, the line dividing Asia and America lies far southwestward of Bering strait (Bogoras 1902:579).

The Jesup Expedition established the close relationship of the populations of northwestern North America and northeastern Asia and strongly supported the view that the ancestors of the Amerindians came from Asia. The effort of Boas, Jochelson, and Bogoras to go beyond these currently accepted points was not successful. The Americanoid theory never attracted attention and is today largely an historical curiosity. Yet with many aspects of New and Old World relationships currently hotly debated, the ideas of Boas and his colleagues still inspire reflection.

The classic ethnographies and the irreplaceable museum collections, however, are the enduring monument of the Jesup North Pacific Expedition. This accomplishment can never be duplicated. For Boas and his colleagues, their work for the expedition went a long way toward establishing their scientific reputations. Jesup may not have been fully aware of it at his death in 1908, but he did succeed, as was his wish, in attaching his name to scientific work of major importance.

Young Laufer on the Amur

Laurel Kendall

In 1897, Franz Boas wrote to Berthold Laufer of Cologne, a youthful scholar of oriental languages and recent philosophy doctorate of the University of Leipzig. The letter invited Laufer to participate in the Jesup North Pacific Expedition, to lead an expedition to the Amur River in eastern Siberia "for the purpose of investigating the peoples of that region and for making ethnological collections" (AMNH: Boas to Laufer, March 25, 1897).

Laufer arrived on Sakhalin Island on July 10, 1898, set to work, and by September could report, in addition to his progress in Nivkhi (Gilyak) and Tungus languages, "I have taken about [a] hundred measurements and carried on investigations on the physical types and the culture of those tribes, particularly regarding their decorative art, of that I have obtained interesting specimens together with good explanations, daily life, fishing and hunting, social organization, shamanism, medicine and so on; as to their healing methods, I got a very important collection of amulets . . . [for protection] from diseases and representing the figures of various animals." He may not have been enthusiastic about taking head measurements, reporting near frustration in his attempts to apply calipers to the Ainu. "The people were afraid that they would die at once after submitting to this process. Although I had their confidence, I failed . . . even after offering them presents which they considered of great value. I succeeded in measuring a single individual, a man of imposing stature, who, after the measurements had been taken, fell prostrate on the floor, the picture of despair, groaning, 'Now I am going to die tomorrow!' 'Have some brandy and you will be all right.' "

More useful was the recorder, and Laufer reports the taking of songs and tales on wax cylinders when the winter cold did not freeze his equipment to inactivity. He wrote to Boas of the young Nivkhi woman who, after singing into the recording instrument, declared, "It took me so long to learn this song and this thing here learned it at once without making any mistakes. There surely is a man or a devil in this box which imitates me!"

After several months on Sakhalin, he requested "a small instant camera. . . . I am afraid that many interesting things I come across will be lost forever if I can't take a picture" (Laufer to Boas, March 4, 1899). Boas recommended that Laufer hire a professional photographer (fig.

22). With an eye toward future museum exhibits, he also requested images of "one or two of the most characteristic occupations and ceremonials of the people, which we could utilize for arranging a group or two illustrating some of the most salient features of their life."

The scholar of oriental languages did, indeed, have an appetite for fieldwork and offered only the rarest complaint. Almost offhandedly, he mentions his scrapes with highwaymen, influenza, and a near drowning in icy water when his sleigh broke through thin ice. After his difficult first winter in the field, he complains, over a misunderstanding about reimbursement, that tradesmen are better remunerated than "a learned man who puts his health and life at stake" exploring, and at the very end of his Amur trip concedes that the 16 months of hardship and loneliness resulted in an "extraordinary state of nervousness [such as] I [had] never experienced before."

As a collector, Laufer experienced the common frustration that others had been there before him. He appealed to Boas for funds to make a significant collection. "For some time the natives have known the real value of their possessions and what they can get for them. The demand for their things, from Russian amateurs and dealers alike, is very high and so the prices are going up. . . . There is absolutely nothing you could get for free from [the Nivkhi]. They even want payment for trivial communication in money, tobacco, tea, malt spirits etc." Although Laufer fulfilled his mandate to provide a comprehensive selection of artifacts, his collection bears the mark of his own scholarly interests and aesthetic judgments. Ritual life is well represented, and he seems to have been utterly captivated by the rich embroideries and appliqué work of the Nanai and their neighbors.

Laufer's published contribution to the ethnography of Sakhalin Island and the Amur region is disappointingly spare. His major monograph on the Jesup material (Laufer 1902) is not the intended comprehensive ethnography but rather a meticulous study of decorative motifs, lavishly illustrated with collection pieces. Even so, he affirms the value of fieldwork, arguing that "ornaments should not be regarded as enigmas which can be easily puzzled out by the homey fireside. . . . They . . . receive proper explanation from the lips of their creators" (Laufer 1902:1).

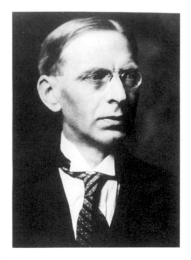

119. Berthold Laufer
AMNH neg. 125308

Berthold Laufer (1874–1934) was the first member of the Siberian team to join the Jesup Expedition. Fresh from his doctorate in Leipzig, he began fieldwork in Sakhalin in 1898. Boas's terms: $500 per year in the field, plus living expenses.

Laufer spent one year on Sakhalin studying Nivkhi (Gilyak), Evenk (Tungus), and Ainu, and a second working with the Nanai (Goldi) and other groups in the Lower Amur. Compared to Bogoras and Jochelson, his achievements were modest. For Laufer, the Jesup Expedition was a learning experience; he later became a productive scholar of Asian culture, holding positions at the American Museum of Natural History and the Field Museum in Chicago.

Opposite:
"Kodiak Island Toyon [Chief] Named Nangquk, Baptised Nikita [from Three Saints Bay]" (Mikhail Tikhanov, 1817, RIPSA 2115)

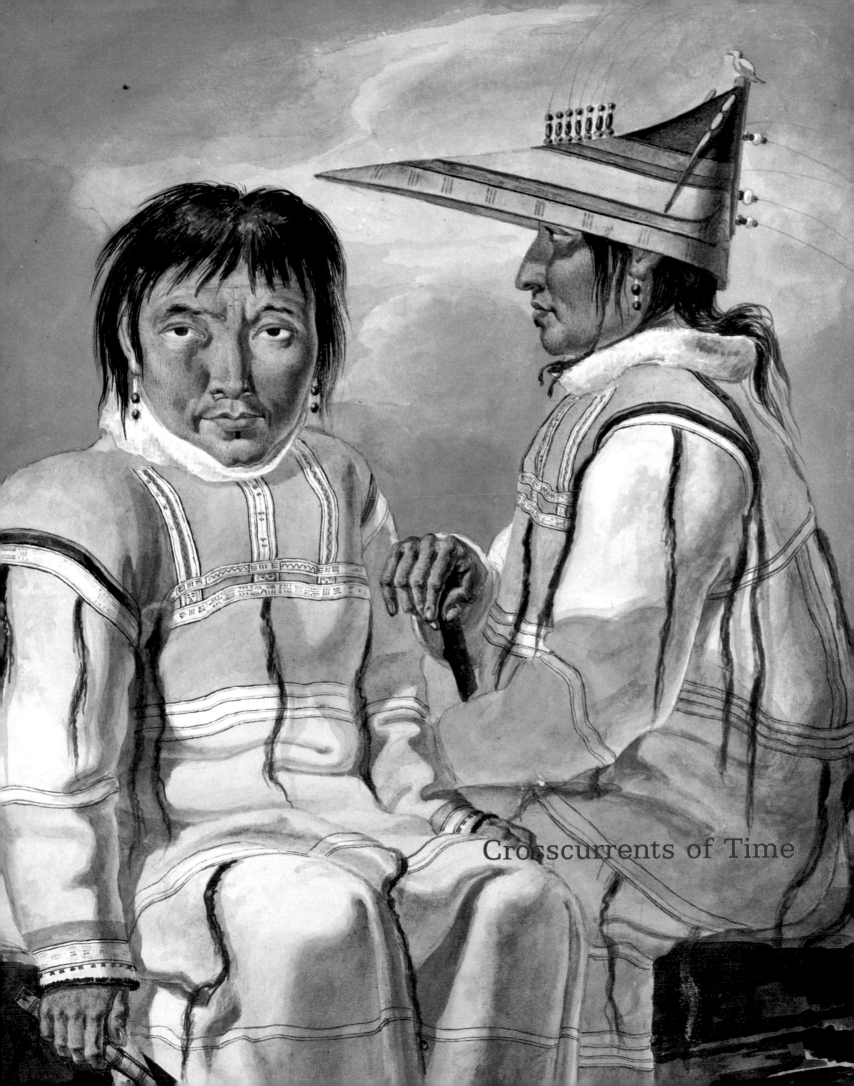

Beringia: An Ice Age View

Steven B. Young

Waves that beat against the shores around Bering Strait often have a troubled, petulant air. They are short, steep, broken into a welter of spray and crosscurrents. They often show a dirty cast of perturbed bottom sediments, and they are mean and tricky to navigate in an open 30-foot umiak. For the past 15,000 years, the waves have been in a winning war with the land. The city of Nome constantly fights for its waterfront, casting thousands of tons of ledge rock against the choppy, bullish breakers.

We often think of sea level as being one of the few fixed, immutable things in this world. We know exactly how tall Mount Denali is, and if the figures were shown to be in error, we would think it was because we had mismeasured the mountain or it had sunk or risen like an immense toy boat floating in a sea of continental rock. Over the long term, though, sea level is about as undependable a geographic feature as can be found. In the course of the last 15,000 years it has risen something like 300 feet, as the last Ice Age glaciers retreated from northern lands and refilled the ocean basins. Even this hasn't been a simple process. The glaciers gave way grudgingly. A few decades of warm summers and the waves lapped inland by a few inches or feet. A siege of cold, snowy winters and the sea stabilized for a time, perhaps even sank back in its bed a few centimeters. Overall, though, the past 15 millennia have been a time of advancing seas, with the greatest rise occurring during the period of perhaps 12,000 to 8,000 years ago. There were corresponding worldwide sea lowerings at various times. An important one occurred between roughly 25,000 and 18,000 years ago, although the seas were apparently a bit lower at the start of that period than they are now.

When we think of the world in the throes of an ice age, we tend to see the northlands disappearing under a mantle of deep ice, such as now covers Greenland. We think of arctic animals—reindeer, woolly mammoths, cave bears—moving southward over the generations as the frost deepens in the ground and the snowbound season lengthens. In truth, though, many of the high-latitude lands never were lost beneath ice. Within hundreds of miles of the Bering Strait, there have never, in the past million years, been more than relatively small, local glaciers. There are bigger glaciers within an hour's drive of Anchorage than ever were found in most of western Alaska during the last ice age.

What we have, then, in many far northern regions, are huge areas of present-day dry land that never were under ice and adjacent areas of shallow sea floor—continental shelf—that emerge as dry land each time the growing ice sheets deplete the seas. We see northern geography as a constantly changing interrelationship between land, ice, and sea, and we see that the land area itself is hardly diminished by advancing glaciers, only relocated, and this largely at the expense of shallow seas.

Nowhere in the world is this situation illustrated better than in the vicinity of the Bering Strait (fig. 121). The shallowly submerged continental shelf extends southward halfway to the Aleutian Islands and northward deep into the Arctic. At a glacial maximum, the exposed sea floor was a subcontinent more than 1000 miles wide. We call this the Bering Land Bridge, but no people crossing it would have known they were on a bridge connecting two continents. Most likely, no one ever really did cross it. Life was probably much better on the old sea floor than on the bleak fells and steppes of what is now Alaska, where howling, frigid winds must have hurled themselves down from the high ice fields and kept the sky a dull mask of blowing grit. Most denizens of Beringia, as we call the ancient land area, probably lived out the generations on the old sea floor and retreated into the stony uplands only as the rising seas threatened.

Winters over much of Beringia would probably have been bitter by even modern Siberian standards. Summers, on the other hand, may have been bright and fairly warm. Although there were probably no forests, there may well have been coppices of cottonwood and thick, dwarf woodlands of scrub willow and perhaps alder. Among the most striking differences between ancient Beringia and the modern world would

120. Vegetation History in Alaska

Pollen produced by vegetation becomes part of the geological record when the grains are deposited in lake sediments or peat bogs. Pollen diagrams produced by counting percentages of pollen types from the bottom to the top of a core taken from these sediments can be used to reconstruct vegetation history through time.

This diagram is a simplified one such as might be derived from a location in central or western Alaska. It represents some 16,000 years and thus extends back to the height of the last glacial advance. Three zones are easily distinguished. Lowest and oldest is an herb zone, dominated by grass, sedge, and sage-brush (*Artemisia*). The later birch zone seems to indicate greater moisture and possible warmth as the Ice Age ended and the Bering Land Bridge was submerged. The top zone, dominated by spruce, documents the spread of typical boreal forest into a previously treeless environment. The few spruce grains in the lower level do not necessarily indicate the local presence of spruce trees. They may have blown long distances in the wind, or been redeposited from older sediments. In an actual diagram, many additional minor pollen types would be represented as well.

have been the animals who lived there. The familiar caribou were around then, as were musk-oxen and moose. But there were many additional, exotic animals, some of immense size and presence. Woolly mammoths, elephants with high-domed skulls, hulking shoulders, enormous tusks, and long, reddish brown hair roamed Beringia at some times. Bison with long, straight horns grazed in mixed herds with small buff-gray horses; probably also included were the saiga antelopes that now occur only in high Asia. Following these herds were an odd array of predators. Lions, cheetahs, and the strange sa-ber-toothed cats lay hidden in hollows and brush patches. A huge, gangly bear, called the short-faced bear, probably was an active pursuer of game rather than a scavenger, fisherman, and opportunist like the modern grizzly. Small mammals and birds would also have been a mixture of the familiar, the exotic, and the extinct. There are also other large animals whose role is more problematical. Mastodons and giant ground sloths were most likely already long extinct by the time of the height of the last glacial age. Beasts such as camels, yaks, and wapiti may have been part of the picture at some time or other. We are still too short on bones and radiocarbon dates to be able to evaluate their significance over time.

We can see that the question "What was it like in Beringia in the past?" is not a simple one. We are dealing with an area the size of a small continent, whose relationship between land and sea altered so rapidly that one might well have seen clear changes over a normal human life-time. Geographical changes would have been accompanied by changes in climate, changes in vegetation, changes in animal populations—probably changes in human society. One of the most important changes has to do with the geographic relationship between Asia and North America. During land bridge times, Beringia was the easternmost extension of Asia. It was more or less completely separated from North America by a broad barrier of ice. Melting ice and rising seas altered the relationship toward the American side, although the minor barrier of the Bering Strait really cuts Beringia more or less in half.

It makes sense to divide the past 20,000 years of Beringian environmental history into three periods. These are closely correlated with events recorded in the sediments of the floors of shallow lakes throughout Beringia, through the deposition of pollen from plants that grew nearby. Changing vegetation results in different kinds and proportions of pollen falling into the lakes, and these changes can be shown graphically (fig. 120). The interpretation of this information

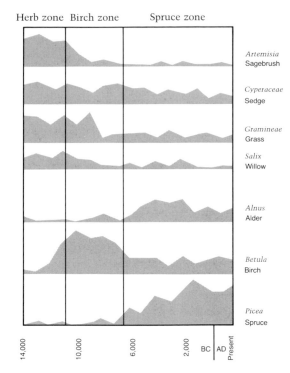

is, as suggested above, as much an art as a science—without intuition the picture is flat and dull, but the embellishments that make it work are almost as much the result of a rich imagination as they are of a scientific approach.

The lowest zone, extending back from roughly 13,000 years ago, is known to palynologists as the herb zone. Its most striking feature is the presence of relatively high amounts of pollen of *Artemisia*, a large group of plants that includes sagebrush as well as familiar garden herbs such as tarragon and dusty miller. Grass and sedge pollen are also common, but trees such as spruce seem to have been rare or absent throughout Beringia. Willow, on the other hand, was abundant. Poplar and aspen, whose pollen is fragile and easily destroyed and which can apparently subsist for millennia reproducing mainly by root shoots, were probably part of the picture.

We see the Bering Land Bridge at this time as a broad, rolling plain. Relief is provided by stabilized sand dunes derived from the emergence of the sea floor thousands of years earlier. Since then, ground ice has built up in the sediments, raising ridges and causing the formation of innumerable shallow thaw ponds. The plain is cut by huge rivers. The Yukon, swollen by summer melt of the great glaciers of the Alaska Range, must traverse 500 miles more land than it does now; it probably has captured other major rivers such as the Kuskokwim. We can imagine thousands of square miles of the land bridge as being a morass of blind channels, sloughs, cutoff lakes, and river bars, the whole covered by a seemingly endless sea of scrub

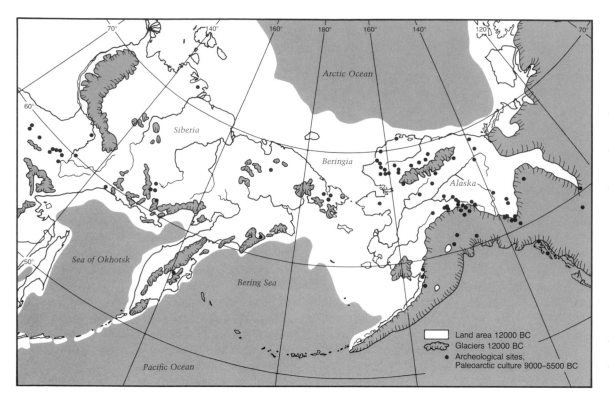

121. The Bering Land Bridge and Sites of the Siberian-American Paleoarctic Culture

This map shows glaciers and coasts as they would have appeared 14,000–15,000 years ago (redrawn from Hamilton *et al.* 1986). At this time the unglaciated lowlands of Alaska were linked to Asia by the broad Bering Land Bridge, while at the same time isolated from the rest of North America by masses of glacial ice. As climate warmed over the next several thousand years, glaciers retreated, sea level rose and cut through the Land Bridge to create Bering Strait, and the land ecosystem underwent major changes, including extinctions of some of the larger Ice Age mammal species. Human populations spread into Alaska from Siberia 11,000–12,000 years ago or slightly earlier, represented by sites of the Paleoarctic culture. The microblades found at these sites link the Paleoarctic people to earlier Siberian Upper Paleolithic groups (fig. 122). (Site distribution from West 1981, fig. 40.)

On the map: 70°, 140°, 160°, 180°, 160°, 140°, 120°, 70°; 60°, 50°. Arctic Ocean, Siberia, Beringia, Alaska, Sea of Okhotsk, Bering Sea, Pacific Ocean.

Legend:
- Land area 12000 BC
- Glaciers 12000 BC
- Archeological sites, Paleoarctic culture 9000–5500 BC

willow brush, swaying in the wind in summer, anchoring drifts of the sparse snow in winter and creating a nucleus for silt deposits during flood times. Back from the rivers the terrain may well have been similar to the steppes of interior Asia. A thin vegetation cover built up of wiry prairie grasses and dwarf sagebrush dominates the ridge tops, while greener sedge meadows lie in hollows and emerge from late-melting snowbeds. Spring comes early after bitter winters, and the steppe undergoes a time of flowering—arctic poppies, anemones, primroses, and dozens of other species—before the endless drying winds of summer raise the glacial dust of the river valleys and gray the landscape.

The picture probably changes quite dramatically along the southern coast of the land bridge. We can imagine hundreds of miles of deeply convoluted coastline: a land-sea of broad estuaries, lagoon and barrier beach systems, salt flats, sedge meadows, and towering dunes. The landfast ice probably built up each winter, and there were probably several months when the offshore seas were dominated by shifting pack ice. But there would also have been many months of open water, a time when seals and beluga

whales abounded in the shallow bays and inlets. Salmon would have invaded every stream, and clouds of waterfowl would have congregated in the lagoons, using them as staging grounds for northward migrations as the rivers and ponds of the interior opened up with the return of summer. This environment, rich as it must have been, must also have been difficult to master for man and other terrestrial mammals. It is hard to imagine a mammal living there who was not an accomplished swimmer or a human who was not a skilled boatman. We can speculate that animals such as horses, bison, and mammoths would have kept mainly to the interior, perhaps wandering down to the grassy coastal dunes during some winters. It needs to be said, too, that this whole question of the nature of the southern coast of the Bering Land Bridge is based on the most tenuous evidence. The alternative, though, is to leave it an empty slate. Although we have no direct data telling us that there were rivers full of fish, it makes no sense to assume, therefore, that the rivers were empty and sterile. But if we do accept the presence of the fish, it is equally absurd to leave out seals, cormorants, brown bears, and mink. Man, as we

122. Composite Knife
Facsimile made by Dennis Stanford
Upper Paleolithic: Kokorevo site, Siberia, ca. 12,000 B.C.

Discoveries of early bone and stone tools strongly suggest that all the native peoples of the Americas can ultimately trace their ancestry to the Upper Paleolithic cultures of northeastern Asia. To make implements for hunting and butchering mammoths, bison, and other large game, Upper Paleolithic hunters glued segments of small stone microblades into a slot along the edge of a bone head, creating a long straight cutting edge. Microblades and the cores from which they were struck occur as early as 20,000 B.C. in Siberian and Japanese sites. Other stone tools from this era include burins (tools for cutting bone and ivory), skin scrapers, and projectile points (fig. 130).

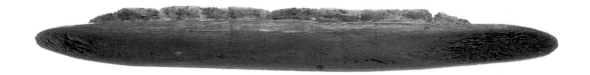

have said, is more problematical, but if he was in Beringia at all, it seems likely that he wandered the sloughs and backwaters of the Bering Sea coast and that he built tents or sod huts—or even mammoth-bone houses such as those found on the Russian steppes—on the low ridgetops.

Having gone this far with our speculations, it is worth asking a few additional questions. For example, what would the possibility have been for coastal, boat-using people from the southern Beringian coast to travel eastward along the glaciated coast of the Gulf of Alaska, perhaps coasting from one ice-free headland to another in search of marine mammals, fish, and seabirds? Similar voyages were made by later Eskimo in northwest Greenland, and they led to new land to the south. Could this have happened on the Pacific shores of North America as the ice began to wane? Another question is whether the hypothetical inhabitants of Beringia might have been two populations, perhaps an inland group that followed the mammoth and bison herds and a coastal group that fished, hunted sea mammals, and trapped migrating waterfowl. How might this situation be reflected in the distribution of language groups or other cultural patterns millennia later? Would traces of these ancient conditions still remain?

Whatever was the situation in southern Beringia, the more marginal environments to the north and east can probably be reconstructed with a bit more confidence, since the possibilities are narrower. The steppe became sparser and increasingly frigid to the north, ending against a permanently ice-locked sea. This sea was probably almost totally barren compared with today's Arctic Ocean. The nearest retreat from the permanent sea ice would have been thousands of miles away in the Atlantic. There would probably have been no walrus, no bowhead whales, possibly a few ringed seals—perhaps an occasional wandering seabird—and no people.

Deep in the interior of what is now Alaska and the Chukchi Peninsula were grim, icebound mountains, silt-covered floodplains, and endless blowing dust. If we can imagine the high plans of interior Asia even colder and more barren, we probably have a good analog. And we can imagine a sparse fauna—a few wild sheep perhaps, small burrowing mammals such as ground squirrels, and marginal populations of predators such as wolves and wolverines.

According to this picture, the heart of Beringia was the land bridge itself. If there were huge herds of game—mammoths, horses, bison, as well as moose and caribou—they would most likely have centered on the bridge, with only stray, marginal groups finding their way into the bleak valleys and high plains of the deep interior. Imagine, then, the rapidly rising seas of 12,000 years or so ago and the profound effects they would have had on animals and man. Equally profound was the effect on the vegetation, and this would, of course, have been transmitted to the other inhabitants.

Picture a time when sea levels may have risen by several feet in the course of a human lifetime. These rises would hardly have been a slow, gentle drowning of beaches and river mouths. Rather, a storm beyond anyone's imagination might have swooped down on a winter day and stripped away the entire line of barrier islands from a lagoon that had been traditional hunting grounds for generations. A decade or two later, the process would have been repeated. Home sites and hunting vantage points would have been undercut by the waves, salt meadows would have become angry shallow seas, and bitter salt and rafts of sea ice would have killed the willow brush and rich sedge meadows of the river deltas. Each generation would have seen new ravages. Finally the seas broke through the remnants of the land barrier and the Arctic Ocean connected with the Bering Sea for the first time in ten millennia or more. No more could a herd of mammoths wander into the summer highlands of Chukotka and back down to the winter grass and willow of the land bridge.

This seems to be the time that the game herds went extinct. Some species survived on the remaining uplands, where they formed the nuclei of our modern caribou and moose herds. Others, like the bison, lasted for millennia but guttered out before historical times, leaving relatives in the great plains to the south. Even more distant are the remnants of the horses and saiga antelopes, deep in Central Asia. And the most magnificent of all, the woolly mammoths, died out everywhere and forever—we shall not see their like again.

We do not know for sure the cause of the extinctions. It is plausible to suggest that the rising seas had much to do with them, but there must have been complex chains of causality involved. They could have involved loss of some necessary food component, loss of a traditional migration route, changes in protection from predation, most of all perhaps changes in human predation. The situation is complicated by lack of good data on the exact time of extinctions. We have relatively few solid dates on the remains of the ancient mammals, and the fact that the latest individual we know of died, say, 15,000 years ago does not prove that their descendants didn't last for a few more millennia. It is interesting to note, in any case, that the mammoths had survived many a rising sea as previous glaciers waxed and waned. Was it a new kind of human culture that made the difference this last time?

The pollen record shows a tremendous, widespread rise in birch pollen throughout Beringia at about 13,000 years ago. We can best interpret this birch zone as being the result of catastrophic invasion of birch scrub over the entire Beringian landscape. If the old steppe vegetation was sparse, it was also widespread and, perhaps most important, diverse and variable. A complex diet would have been available for large herbivores, perhaps changing with the seasons as well as geographically. If, then, the remnants of the lands being lost to the rising seas were overwhelmed by a bitter scrub of resinous birches, the results for bison and mammoth could have been disastrous.

Our mindset as postglacial beings of tropical origin is to see the end of the Ice Age as a return to normal. A long-horned bison or a mammoth probably had a different perspective, as, very likely, did the people who hunted them. We can visualize shrinking, starving bands of the great herd beasts as the seas returned, and we can guess that this had an effect on human population and culture, as it apparently did at the end of the Ice Age in Europe.

In any case, the beginning of postglacial times, which is conventionally placed at 10,000 years ago, occurred at the end of the several-thousand-year period that encompassed the destruction of the land bridge and its unique environment. We see changes occurring at 10,000 years ago and thereafter, but none so radical or widespread as the invasion of the birch scrub. The main

later changes seem to be the spread of spruce into Beringia from some location to the east—perhaps the lower Mackenzie River area—the spread of alder and, presumably, tree birches, probably the expansion of cottonwood and aspen woodlands, and later the spread of peat lands and muskeg. Not too long ago, we tended to view the change from a glacial age to the postglacial as being something of a flip-flop, from full glacial conditions to something similar to the environment of today. We know now that the modern environment is the product of 10,000 years of evolution, building upon pieces of the old land bridge environment, as well as invaders and colonizers from afar. These changes, though, are relatively subtle, and they tend to be localized when compared with the rising tide of birch scrub. Without using an inordinate amount of space, perhaps the best we can say is that the Denbigh Flint people, halfway back to the Ice Age, lived in a land that was recognizable as modern Alaska—a land of spruce forests to the inland; of shorelines near those of the present; of caribou, moose, walrus, and seals and devoid of mammoths, wild horses, and clouds of wind-blown silt. But it was a coastline without the modern beach ridges, and probably a tundra with many subtle differences from that of today. If we were suddenly set down on Cape Denbigh at 2500 B.C., we would probably be faced with a slowly dawning awareness that things were not quite as we were used to. We will be uncovering the exact nature of these differences for decades to come, and the main source of this information will probably be the study of the lives and culture of the people of Beringia.

123. Yukon-Kuskokwim Delta
One of the richest environments of the North Pacific–Bering Sea region is the vast Yukon-Kuskokwim Delta. The delta was the breeding ground for huge flocks of migratory waterfowl, and its rivers, sloughs, and tundra ponds supported large stocks of local and anadromous fish. Although large whales were absent along its coast, beluga were common, as were seals, and walrus could be hunted during their northward migration in spring. Despite the hazards of delta life, which included periodic destruction of low-lying villages in winter and spring floods, the resources of the Yukon-Kuskokwim Delta supported 10,000 Eskimos in the late 19th century, the largest and densest Eskimo population in the world.

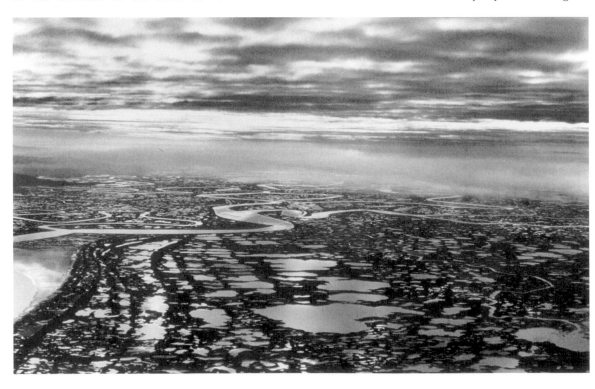

Ancient Peoples of the North Pacific Rim

Christy G. Turner II

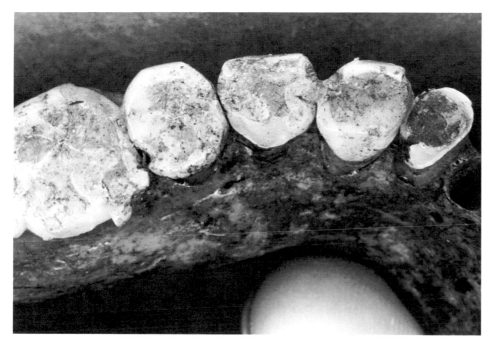

124. Arctic Dentition
McKenzie Eskimo: C.G. Turner neg.
1978:8 ASC 33

Peoples of arctic regions have distinctive dental characteristics that are illustrated in this photograph of a Mackenzie Eskimo male: heavy occlusal wear across the tops of the teeth; flattened outer surface; and chipping of crown surfaces due to crushing bones, use of teeth as tools, and damage from sand and bone in food.

This essay briefly reviews some of the anatomical, genetic, and other biological research that has been carried out on the living and prehistoric inhabitants of Northeastern Siberia and Alaska. The emphasis is on findings that help in understanding where the original homeland of these peoples was located, how they spread into the Americas, and what can be inferred about their later history from intergroup biological variation.

In assessing biological evidence of relationships among human populations, the fact needs to be stressed that evolutionary rates differ between the anthropological trinity of culture, language, and biology. Of these, in the Arctic as elsewhere, culture changes the most rapidly because cultural adaptations (new behavior patterns, inventions) may be rapidly adopted and taught to subsequent generations. At the other extreme, biological adaptation depends on the slow process of natural selection, and advantageous physical characteristics that may randomly appear take many generations to become

established in a population. Language changes at an intermediate rate but generally drifts more slowly than culture because it is not directly affected by adaptive pressures.

Major adaptive problems had to be solved before any humans could inhabit arctic Siberia and North America. The new problems presented by this environment included long periods of intense cold, patchy and highly seasonal food resources, and the lack of extensive support networks of neighbors and kin faced by all pioneers. The cultural solutions to these problems, worked out at least 12,000 years ago, included heat-saving tailored fur clothing and domesticated dogs for hauling bulky fur bedding, skin tents, and other household gear necessary for a nomadic arctic lifeway. Also, at some point in prehistory, dugout or bark-covered frame boats evolved to produce light but durable skin-covered boats for hunting on icy seas or where wood was scarce, as in the Aleutians. Such craft would have increased the resource base following the discovery of the ice-choked Sea of Okhotsk with its millions of sea mammals. Finally, social behavior emphasizing cooperation, sharing, and rapid childhood learning of adult skills would have been recognized early on as critical in an arctic habitat.

Because the late Pleistocene colonizers of the Arctic adapted mainly by cultural rather than by biological means, there has been limited genetic change since then. Modern arctic populations resemble the earliest known arctic inhabitants, as far as can be determined from the shapes of bones and teeth (Debets 1948; Hrdlicka 1945). This relatively simple genetic history, preserved in calcified morphology, allows us to attempt reconstructions of the origins, ancestry, and historical genetic relationships of modern arctic groups with some confidence.

Not all biological qualities are equally useful for origins research, however. Least valuable are those that can be studied only in the living and that are significantly influenced by the environment. Examples of the latter include weight, health, and age. The best features to study are those that are under strong genetic control and that can be examined in both living and deceased people. Teeth, with their many genetically determined crown and root structures, are ideal for this purpose. The hard enamel usually preserves well while buried in the ground, so archeological teeth may be compared with those of living populations. The influences of age, sex, and health are minimal on dental anatomy. Other genetic traits, such as blood types, cannot be studied in ancient skeletal remains. For these and other reasons this essay will focus on the human population history of eastern Siberia and Alaska as presently understood from studies of dental morphology.

Early descriptions of Aleut, Eskimo, and Siberian physical appearances made by Russian fur trappers and explorers noted that these native peoples were of medium stature, robust, moderately dark-skinned, and had dark eyes partially obscured by a skin flap known as the epicanthic fold. They also tended to have small noses, straight black hair, and flat, nearly beardless faces. One of the first published reports on Aleut and Kodiak Island Eskimo crania appeared in an 1859 memoir of the Russian Imperial Academy of Sciences of St. Petersburg, by C. E. de Baer. His measurements showed these crania to be similar to Japanese crania. Craniology dominated the study of the origins and relationships of arctic people for almost a century after de Baer's work, mainly because the face and head were thought to be racially distinctive. The shape of both are determined by the underlying bony structure of the skull, which usually preserves well. Mummified or accidentally frozen bodies, which can provide information on skin, hair, and blood, are rare. Intentional mummification was practiced only in the eastern Aleutians and by the Pacific Eskimo along Alaska's southern coast. Some of these mummies have survived the destructive, wet environment because they were placed in burial caves warmed and dried by underground conduits to hot subterranean volcanic rock.

One of the first Americans to conduct natural history studies in Alaska was William H. Dall (1877). In the 1870s Dall tested old Aleut village sites on several islands and was the first American scientist to interpret his archeological findings by stratigraphic and evolutionary principles. He also described several crania he unearthed, noting that eastern and western Aleuts were very similar, although quite variable, and rather specialized compared with crania belonging to other northern groups he had available for comparison. Without noting it specifically, Dall seems to have recognized the evolutionary significance of the marked geographic isolation that characterizes the Aleutian Islands.

Soon after Dall's pioneering archeology, workers in the newly emerging museum and university field of anthropology turned their attention to western arctic and subarctic populations. The extensive anthropometric surveys carried out by members of the Jesup North Pacific Expedition in Siberia and the Northwest Coast are an invaluable human biological record collected at a time when Russian and American admixture to native populations was less than today. Ales Hrdlicka carried out similar surveys for the Smithsonian Institution on living and skeletal Alaskan Aleuts and Eskimos in the 1930s in his study on the peopling of the Americas, a research objective to which Hrdlicka devoted much of his life (Hrdlicka 1944, 1945). Plaster head casts and measurements made in the field by the Jesup Expedition, by Hrdlicka, and by Riley Moore on St. Lawrence Island in 1912 have been used in creating the mannequins in this exhibition.

While craniological investigation, now strengthened by evolutionary and genetic theory, profitably continues to the present day, other scientific areas of inquiry have emerged. Research into cold adaptation, be it physiological, anatomical, behavioral, or a combination of all three, has developed following World War II. Most of the identifiable cold adaptation by arctic peoples is now seen as being accomplished behaviorally and culturally with clothing and by avoiding sweating, staying indoors in stormy weather, consuming a diet rich in fat and oil for energy, and by other simple but effective means. Despite much research on the flat Asiatic face structure, it still remains uncertain if this trait is an evolutionary adaptation to cold stress.

In the 1940s blood-group genetics were added to the research programs of arctic anthropologists such as William S. Laughlin (1951). Despite the official Soviet ban on genetics at this time, some scientists in the USSR nevertheless managed to conduct blood-group studies on native Siberians. By the 1950s it was evident that Eskimo, Aleut, and native Siberian populations possessed the B gene of the ABO blood system, and American Indians lacked this allele. This, along with the possible linguistic link between Aleut, Eskimo, and Chukchi, as well as craniological similarity (Alexseev 1979), suggested that Aleuts and Eskimos were more closely related to eastern Asians than were American Indians, possibly because they entered the New World later than did the ancestors of Indians. Recently, this view has been reconsidered. Blood-group genetic studies and osteological research by E. Szathmary and N. S. Ossenberg (1978) reveal the distinctiveness of Athapaskan-speaking Indians from all other Indians and their possibly closer relationship to Aleuts and Eskimos. However, Soviet genetic studies on arctic peoples have shown that recent admixture likely has obscured the phylogenetic history hoped for from studies of modern living populations. It has been estimated, for example, that by 1970 as many as 25 percent of all North Alaskan genes were from non-Eskimo sources (Szathmary 1984). Fortunately, prehistoric bones and teeth do not have an admixture problem of this magnitude, so osteological and dental research continues to be important in understanding the origins, relationships, and evolution of the Bering Sea Mongoloids.

As Russian explorers learned more about Siberia and Alaska in the 18th and 19th centuries it became evident that native population density increased from north to south because of the better food supply at lower latitudes. This ecological relationship is also reflected in body size and stature. The far northern peoples are generally shorter than those living to the south. Stature and body build may be an adaptation to northern conditions such as limited calcium and sunlight, which can retard skeletal growth. Facial flatness is possibly a cold adaptation because it, too, decreases from north to south. Early anthropologists gave head shape much taxonomic weight for classifying groups of people, mainly because it was thought to be an evolutionarily neutral feature, but even today the mechanisms responsible for such anatomical change have yet to be identified, and its usefulness for differentiating prehistoric populations remains unclear. Other distinctive features of arctic peoples, such as medium trunk height combined with short arms and legs, may be accentuated by differential growth under the influence of cold stress.

In addition to the probable pressure from natural selective forces, numerically small northern populations are subject to genetic bottlenecking (reduction or limitation of genetic variability) caused by population crashes due to regional starvation, poisoning, disease, or warfare. This and inbreeding probably contributed to some of the known arctic skeletal anomalies, such as T. D. Stewart's (1973) finding that Eskimo groups have frequent occurrences of defective neural arches. Aleuts differ somewhat from their Eskimo linguistic cousins because of random genetic changes that likely occurred in the small founding populations of the isolated Aleutian Islands. The senior scholar of the Aleuts, William S. Laughlin, believes this genetic isolation extends back at least 8,000 years.

Finally, there are many interesting features of Siberian and Alaskan skeletons and teeth that are caused by environmental or cultural factors rather than biological ones. For example, the difficulty of the arctic lifeway shows up in the many fractured and chipped teeth of its prehistoric peoples. This damage occurred when bones were crushed in the mouth to extract all possible nutrient, or when teeth were used as tools when fingers were rendered nearly useless by cold exposure. When Russian explorers and fur hunters first discovered Siberian and Alaskan Eskimos and Aleuts, they found many individuals with facial tattoos, bone pin-pierced nasal septa, and ivory or stone lip plugs (labrets) worn in slits cut through the lower lip or cheek. Years of use eventually wore down the tooth surface in contact with the labret, resulting in archeologically recovered teeth with labret wear facets. This form of facial ornamentation was in vogue among Aleutian Islanders for at least 4,000 years. Another early Aleutian practice, one that was discontinued before historic contact, was extraction of anterior teeth. Intentional removal of teeth is very old in eastern Asia, possibly beginning as early as 17,000 years ago. Because of the small amount of carbohydrate in the arctic diet, no prehistoric Siberians or Alaskans had cavities, although periodontal disease was extremely common and often terribly severe. A condition akin to tennis elbow was sometimes present in adult males, the result of joint stress caused by years of throwing harpoons and spears. Finally, osteoarthritis, present even in young adults, developed from cold exposure and activity-related stress placed on the living skeleton.

Having, to a degree, characterized various aspects of the physical anthropology of the arctic and subarctic peoples of the North Pacific Rim, let us turn to the three fundamental biological questions posed at the outset of this essay: the questions of origins, of the spread of arctic Asian populations into the Americas, and of their subsequent population histories. These problems will be explored using information from my own detailed examinations of thousands of teeth, most of which were obtained from archeological populations by the various investigators mentioned above. The arctic teeth used here were studied by the author in museum skeletal collections in Canada, Denmark, France, Japan, the USA, and the USSR.[1] Table 1 gives frequencies for a few of the more than two dozen dental traits used in this analysis of arctic population history. By comparing the frequencies, one can get a rough idea of the similarities and differences, and therefore the closeness of relationship, between the selected populations. However, a quicker and clearer understanding of affinity and history is gained from the diagrams in figures 125–127.

East Siberian and Native American Origins

The probable biological affinity between the populations studied is shown in figure 125. Any pair linked by a short branch indicates a relatively close relationship, as seen between Egyptians and Europeans. Deep branching, such as between Egyptians and North and South American Indians, indicates a remote relationship. Starting at the trunk of the tree, on the left side, all groups first branch apart into a North Asian–American cluster (Recent Japan, Macro-China, American Arctic, Northeast Siberia–Amur, Greater Northwest Coast, and North and South America) and a non–North Asian–American cluster containing three subclusters. Dental traits thus indicate that all Native Americans are more closely related to northeastern Asians such as Chinese and Japanese than they are to Europeans and that the ancestral origin of East Siberian and Native American populations was likely in eastern Asia. Because Native Americans are more like Japanese and Chinese than like Southeast Asians, the ancestral homeland was probably in Northeast rather than Southeast Asia. Within Northeast Asia the ancestral Native American homeland was more likely in northern China and Mongolia than in Japan. This is because the Jomon people, quite dissimilar to Native Americans, inhabited Japan thousands of years before the large migration of modern Japanese from the mainland began around 300 B.C. The dental analysis also seems to rule out southern Siberia as the ancestral home of Native Americans. It can be concluded that the peoples whose ways of life are illustrated in this exhibition arose from an ancestral stock in North China–Mongolia. According to archeological findings and estimated rates of dental evolution, that stock lived about 20,000 years ago.

Examining the North Asia–American cluster in more detail, the dendrogram shows American arctic people are more like those of Northeast Siberia–Amur than like American Indians. Thus, we can hypothesize that at least two waves or stocks of people—or possibly three—were involved in the initial peopling of the Americas.

How Did the Peopling of the Americas Occur?

Figure 126 is based on the same analytical methods as figure 125, but with territorially smaller groups. Again, the first branching separates a large northern cluster made up of Eskimo, Aleuts, and Northwest Coast Indians. Other analyses of this sort have shown that all North and South American Indians, except those of the Northwest Coast, are closely related, so figure 126 uses only three southern Indian series to demonstrate this basic duality of New World populations. When archeological information is

TABLE 1

Selected Dental Morphology of Beringian and Comparative Groups (%)*

Trait: Tooth:	Shovel UI1	1-root UP1	Carabelli cusp UM1	6-cusp LM1	4-cusp LM2	Protostylid cusp LM1	3-root LM1
N & S America	92	86	38	55	9	38	7
Greater NW Coast	83	93	25	50	4	34	16
American Arctic	69	95	14	50	5	20	31
NE Siberia-Amur	62	93	21	50	6	23	22
Macro-China	96	77	33	36	21	26	28
Recent Japan	66	75	31	43	14	21	24
Jomon	31	75	41	45	20	27	3
South Siberia	37	69	39	20	54	30	2
Macro-early SE Asia	30	57	33	40	32	21	8
Europe	3	58	51	8	71	18	1

* Computer reference: HCLS World 14. Sexes pooled. U denotes upper; L, lower; I, incisor; P, premolar; M, molar. Breakpoints for dichotomized intratrait variation are identified in Turner (1987). Group sample sizes in most instances exceed 100 individuals per trait. Illustrations of these dental traits can be found in Turner (1985).

125. Old World–New World Dental Relationships

This evolutionary tree, or dendrogram, is based on a computer analysis of 25 dental traits in thousands of individuals belonging to the indicated groups. The diagram indicates that Northeast Asians and Native Americans are closely related. Therefore, the ancestral homeland of people who designed and crafted the objects in this exhibition probably originated in North China and Mongolia.

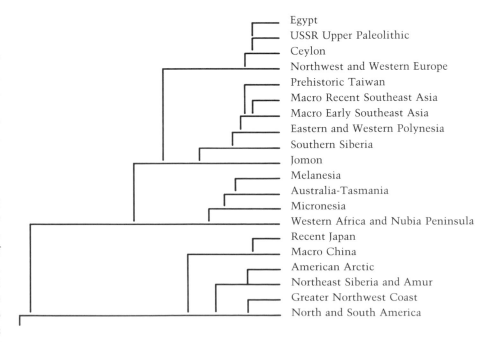

Egypt
USSR Upper Paleolithic
Ceylon
Northwest and Western Europe
Prehistoric Taiwan
Macro Recent Southeast Asia
Macro Early Southeast Asia
Eastern and Western Polynesia
Southern Siberia
Jomon
Melanesia
Australia-Tasmania
Micronesia
Western Africa and Nubia Peninsula
Recent Japan
Macro China
American Arctic
Northeast Siberia and Amur
Greater Northwest Coast
North and South America

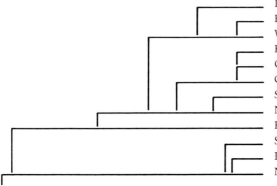

Point Hope
Eastern Aleuts
Western Aleuts
Kodiak
Central Maritime
Gulf of Georgia
St. Lawrence Island
Northern Maritime
Kachemak and Alaska Peninsula
Southern California
Panama
Northern and Central California

126. Western North American Dental Relationships

This dendrogram suggests three migrations were involved in peopling the New World. A basic duality of the Native American population is seen in the deep division between California and Panamanian Natives from those of the Nortwest Coast and Alaska. A second division separates Aleuts and Point Hope Eskimos from Northwest Coast peoples.

127. North Pacific Dental Relationships

This diagram suggests a number of historical relationships between peoples of the North Pacific, Beringia, and the Arctic. Details are discussed in the text.

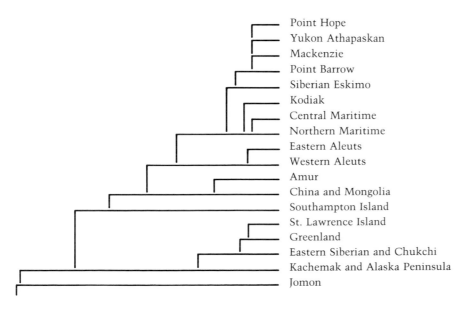

Point Hope
Yukon Athapaskan
Mackenzie
Point Barrow
Siberian Eskimo
Kodiak
Central Maritime
Northern Maritime
Eastern Aleuts
Western Aleuts
Amur
China and Mongolia
Southampton Island
St. Lawrence Island
Greenland
Eastern Siberian and Chukchi
Kachemak and Alaska Peninsula
Jomon

considered it becomes evident that most American Indians are probably descended from the founding population we associate with the mammoth-hunting Paleoindian Clovis culture. This hypothesis is also supported by linguistic and other biological evidence (Greenberg et al. 1986).

The more complex upper cluster can be interpreted several ways. The interpretation favored by the author is that it contains two subclusters. One includes the Point Hope Eskimo and all Aleuts. The second includes all the Northwest Coast Indians from the northern and central Maritime districts (southeastern Alaska and British Columbia) and those of the Gulf of Georgia and Puget Sound. It also includes the St. Lawrence Island Eskimo and the Kodiak Islanders. On cultural grounds Kodiak prehistory has usually been thought of as a product of Eskimo, but Kodiak dental affinity is with the Northwest Coast Indians. Why the St. Lawrence Islanders cluster with Northwest Coast is uncertain. More than likely this is a statistical mismatch resulting from the fact that St. Lawrence Island Eskimo, although Siberian Eskimo by linguistic affiliation, have been joined artificially with the Northwest Coast cluster because no other Siberian group was included in this particular study for them to link up with. As shown in figure 127, given a Siberian choice, St. Lawrence Islanders do link with Siberians rather than Alaskans. A question remains concerning the population history of the two closely related northern clusters. Did they separate in Alaska or, as this author favors for a number of reasons (Turner 1985), in Siberia?

If we follow the latter interpretation of the dental, archeological, and linguistic evidence, the peopling of the New World may be summarized as follows. The first wave of migration was composed of the Paleoindians, who moved through the Beringian region sometime between 14,000 and 12,000 years ago and became established in lower continental North and South America about 12,000 or 11,500 years ago as Clovis and other fluted point cultures. Between 10,000 and 11,000 years ago, sites of the Paleoarctic microblade tradition in the interior of Alaska and eastern Siberia give evidence for the expansion into the New World of the ancestors of the Athapaskan and Northwest Coast Indians. A third wave of New World settlement from Siberia, also thought to date to this early period, is represented by the ancestral Eskimo-Aleuts, who settled along the coasts of mainland Alaska and the Aleutian Island chain. The archeological evidence for this movement has been largely destroyed by rising sea levels, although sites in Japan, the Amur River region, and Anangula (6000 B.C.) in the Eastern Aleutians probably relate to this maritime occupation (Laughlin1980).

Northeast Asian and Northern North America: Biology and History

Figure 127 takes a detailed look at groups on both sides of the Bering Sea. Examining the diagram from left to right as previously, the first branch point separates the prehistoric Jomon people of Japan from all other groups. The Jomon people were not members of the Northeastern Siberian–Alaskan population system. The next branch point separates most of the remaining groups from a cluster made up of Eskimo from St. Lawrence Island and Greenland, East Siberians, and Chukchi, and people of Kachemak Bay and the Alaska Peninsula, usually thought of as Eskimo. With the exception of the Greenland Eskimo, whose recent arrival can be traced back to northern Alaska, this group is characterized as having lived around the shores of the Bering Sea, suggesting a coastal economic, social, and genetic network that did not extend into the Aleutian or Northwest Coast areas. The network may best be related to the expansion of the Eskimo population bearing the Thule culture. The strong separation of this cluster from the other Native Americans suggests much genetic isolation, although it might also indicate a more recent Siberian rather than early Alaskan origin.

As expected on the basis of geographic distance, the Amur and China-Mongolia series are considerably removed from the remaining groups in the upper cluster but are clearly more like Northeast Siberians and Native Americans than were the Jomon people.

The top five groups of the upper cluster (Point Hope, Yukon Athapaskan, Mackenzie Eskimo, Point Barrow Eskimo, and Siberian Eskimo) are all far northern Americans except for the Siberians. However, such American archeologists as Henry Collins long ago pointed out that Siberian Eskimos probably migrated to Siberia from Alaska many generations ago. The anomalous Eskimo affinity of the Yukon Athapaskans in this study seems likely to have resulted from problems of Russian and Eskimo admixture, or both, for in other studies they cluster with Northwest Coast Indians.

The major interpretation to make of this far north American subcluster is that it is not especially similar to the more Siberian cluster containing the Chukchi. This suggests that Eskimos have been genetically separated from Siberian populations for about as long a period of time as have Indians. The case of the Siberian Eskimo indicates that some population movement and genetic exchange has occurred at Bering Strait, however.

The Aleut subcluster is distinctive, supporting the aforementioned view of a long period of genetic isolation. Only minor differences have evolved between eastern and western Aleuts, a fascinating biological finding that matches the relative homogeneity of the prehistoric Aleut culture found throughout the archipelago and other archeological evidence that documents marked cultural stability and isolation through time. Taken together, these facts suggest that the Aleut objects on exhibit, and the early observations of Aleut life made by the Russian priest Ioann Veniaminov and others, might well portray Aleut ways as they were practiced for many millennia.

The final subcluster is the Northwest Coast and Kodiak branch. Apparently, despite their more recent cultural affinity to Eskimos, the prehistoric people of Kodiak Island were genetically more related to Indians than to Eskimos, a possibility hinted at in scraps of ethnographic lore. The Kodiak situation should serve as a useful reminder that cultural history is not predetermined by biological ancestry.

In the final analysis, genetic descent can only be evaluated with the physical remains of people themselves. This is the ultimate reason for the need to preserve human biological collections and conduct skeletal and paleodental research.

Bering Strait is indeed the crossroads of continents. But, not until the Russian discovery of Alaska was it traveled by any people other than the descendants of those first families that moved northward from North China and Mongolia into virgin Northeastern Siberia about 15,000 years ago. This story, which began in very ancient times, can be told because of the genetic history embedded in the coded anatomy of teeth, bones, and many other biological features.

Prehistory of Siberia and the Bering Sea

S. A. Arutiunov and William W. Fitzhugh

128. Cultures and Sites of the North Pacific-Bering Sea Region

For many years it has been supposed that the first people to move into North America passed over the ancient land bridge that joined Siberia and the American continent at the end of the Ice Age. If you were to take the date of the peopling of America as between 25,000 and 14,000 years ago, as some archeologists have claimed, the first inhabitants of North America must have crossed the Bering Land Bridge at a time when large portions of Europe, Siberia, Canada, and the northern United States were covered by great masses of ice. At this time

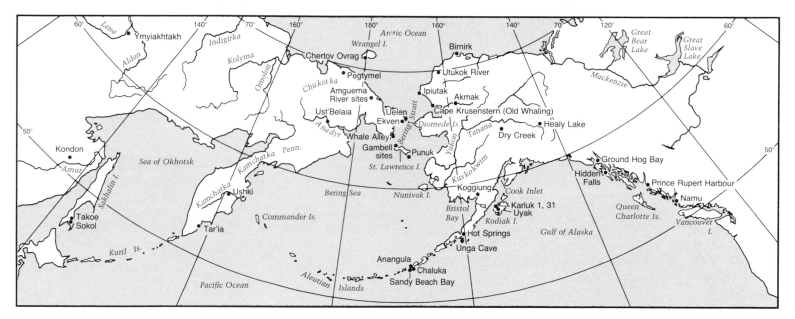

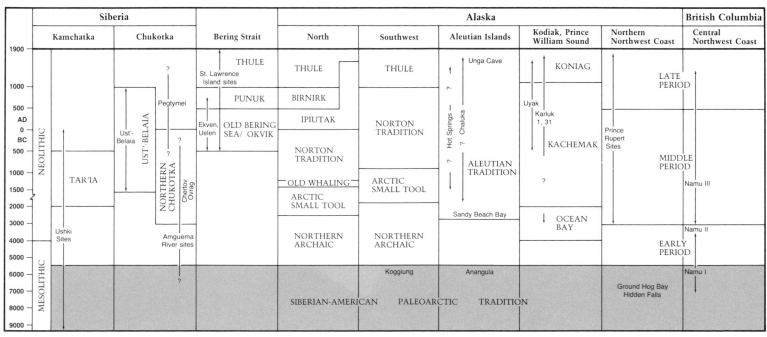

	Siberia			Alaska					British Columbia
	Kamchatka	Chukotka	Bering Strait	North	Southwest	Aleutian Islands	Kodiak, Prince William Sound	Northern Northwest Coast	Central Northwest Coast
1900		?	THULE St. Lawrence Island sites	THULE	THULE	Unga Cave	KONIAG		LATE PERIOD
1000		Pegtymel	PUNUK	BIRNIRK		? Chaluka	Uyak Karluk 1, 31	Prince Rupert Sites	
500		Ust'-Belaia	Ekven, Uelen OLD BERING SEA/ OKVIK	IPIUTAK	NORTON TRADITION	Hot Springs			MIDDLE PERIOD
AD 0 BC	TAR'IA			NORTON TRADITION		?	KACHEMAK		Namu III
500		?				ALEUTIAN TRADITION	?		
1000		NORTHERN CHUKOTKA		OLD WHALING	ARCTIC SMALL TOOL				
1500		Chertov Ovrag	ARCTIC SMALL TOOL					Namu II	
2000					Sandy Beach Bay	OCEAN BAY		
3000	Ushki Sites	Amguema River sites		NORTHERN ARCHAIC	NORTHERN ARCHAIC				Namu II
4000								EARLY PERIOD	
5000									
6000		?		Koggiung	Anangula			Namu I
7000			SIBERIAN-AMERICAN PALEOARCTIC TRADITION				Ground Hog Bay Hidden Falls	
8000								
9000								

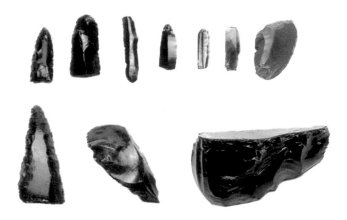

129 Early Man in Siberia
Sakhalin Upper Paleolithic: SKRM (upper) 4072-3, 4072-2, 14, 15, 16, 18, 9; (lower) 4072-4, 7, 1

This assemblage of obsidian tools, from the site of Sokol, dating to 18,000–16,000 B.C., is typical of later Upper Paleolithic cultures of Siberia. Diagnostic tools include wedge-shaped cores (*lower right*) from which blades and microblades were struck for use as knives and composite tools (fig. 122), and as blanks for triangular points whose bases were later thinned for use in slotted hafts. Burins, flake knives, and pointed side-scrapers also occur. Other sites, such as Ushki in Kamchatka, contain bifacial stemmed and leaf-shaped points. Similarities between these complexes and the Diuktai complex of central Yakutia and microblade sites in Japan demonstrate the existence of a widespread Late Paleolithic horizon from which American cultures must have originated.

glacial conditions prevailed throughout the northern hemisphere. At its peak 18,000 years ago, sea level was 100 meters lower than at present, and the lateral extent of the exposed sea floor from the Arctic Ocean to the Pacific would have been nearly 1,000 miles wide. This would hardly have been a land "bridge" at all but rather a huge continental land mass.

However, if you believe, as most cautious archeologists do, that man migrated into the Americas about 13,000 years ago (fig. 121), humans could not have traveled over the surface of this land bridge. By this time the floors of the Bering and Chukchi seas had already been submerged by the rising sea levels resulting from the melting of the Ice Age glaciers, and man must either have entered North America over the frozen sea ice in winter or have crossed the waters of Bering Strait by boat. Archeologists have not solved these questions of the first Beringian migrations largely because no remains

that are unquestionably older than 11,500 years have yet been found either in Chukotka or in Alaska.

Whichever dating one prefers, few sites are known even of the 11,500-year period. Most early coastal sites of early man in the Beringian region were either destroyed initially by rising sea levels at the end of the Pleistocene or by erosion and submergence that has characterized much of this region's geomorphology in the Holocene, the period from the end of the Pleistocene to the present. The sea continues to encroach upon the land even today, and some capes, pebble spits, and shorelines on which the remains of ancient settlements have been studied as recently as the 1950s no longer exist. Nevertheless many archeological remains have been discovered that provide information on the prehistory of the North Pacific and Bering Sea region.

130. Takoie II: Proto-Paleoindian?
Siberian Upper Paleolithic: SKRM (upper) 3670-83, 107, 54, 105, 99, 52, 44; (lower) 795-3764-2, 1; 3670-194, 45, 113

An assemblage excavated in 1973 by Valerii Shubin from the site of Takoie II on Sakhalin Island contains a more highly developed tool inventory dating to 16,000–14,000 B.C. Unifacial core and blade technology continues as the basis for the industry. A variety of microblade cores, microblades, endscrapers, and convergent sidescrapers occur. Most interesting are triangular points of various sizes made on blades, which have carefully thinned bases and partial bifacial flaking. This combination of features begins to resemble a prototype assemblage for American Paleoindian culture.

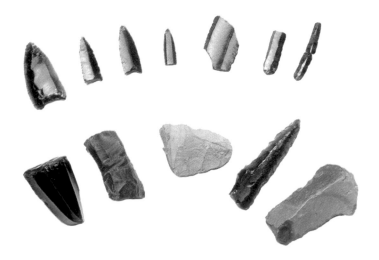

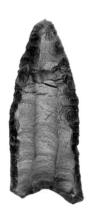

131. Early Man in Alaska
Paleoindian Culture: NMNH 391806

This 11,000-year-old fluted point discovered on the surface near the headwaters of the Utukok River in 1947
(Thompson 1948) was the first firm
evidence of Paleoindian fluted point
culture in Alaska. Typical of Clovis
and Folsom points used by the first
well-documented Indian cultures of
the Americas, such points have no
suitable prototypes in the New
World. The presence of fluted points
in Alaska suggests that Siberia—
poorly known archeologically—may
be their place of origin. In fact, possible prototype technologies containing
concave base unifacial points made
on prismatic blades, like the Takoie II
complex in Sakhalin (fig. 130),
strengthen the case for Siberian
origins.

132. Paleoarctic Tradition
Denali complex: (left to right) UAFM
UA 77-14-3884,-1591; DCr 73-24,
-47,-48,-13,-46; 76-155-4097; 76-
155-3269; 77-44-2659

A large number of sites containing
assemblages with wedge-shaped
cores and microblades, and less frequently with bifacial leaf-shaped bifaces, occur in both Siberia and
Alaska at 9,000–10,000 B.C. These
sites comprise the Siberian-Alaskan
Paleoarctic Tradition, with clear roots
in the Siberian Upper Paleolithic, and
document a major population movement of hunting cultures into the
New World.

Early Man in Siberia and Alaska

Contrary to popular belief, the Beringian region
was not glaciated during the Pleistocene ice age,
and much of Siberia and Alaska was accessible
to human habitation. The dry, cold tundra and
steppe lands, which had little snow, were rich
in grasses and in wildlife that grazed on them.
In southern Chukotka and Kamchatka—where
the grassy steppe was interspersed with stands
of trees—mammoths, bison, and caribou were
plentiful. The climate was severe but was still
suitable for paleolithic hunters. Similar conditions prevailed on the Bering Land Bridge, but
much of modern-day Alaska was extremely
inhospitable.

The most ancient finds from Northeast Asia
were discovered by N. N. Dikov at Ushki alongside a lake in the valley of the Kamchatka River
(fig. 121; Dikov 1965, 1968). Here buried living
floors and stratigraphic levels document cultures
occupying Kamchatka over thousands of years,
beginning about 14,000 years ago. Early Ushki,
the earliest culture found (Level VII), contains
bifacial (chipped on both sides) leaf-shaped knives,
stemmed points, and gravers, as well as a human
burial with stone pendants and beads. In Level
VI, a culture dating to 12,000 or 10,000 years
ago known as Late Ushki was found to use
elongated leaf-shaped bifacial knives, small
wedge-shaped microcores and microblades (fig.
122), gravers, burins, scrapers, and possibly
labrets and fishing-related art. Late Ushki shares
microblades and leaf-shaped bifaces with the
Diuktai Paleolithic culture of central Yakutia and
small microblade sites in Japan, as well as a
variety of Alaskan sites. Among the latter are

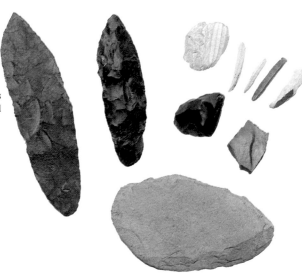

Ground Hog Bay and Hidden Falls on the Northwest Coast; Healy Lake, Dry Creek, Ugashik,
Akmak, and the Denali complex materials (fig.
121).Just how similar the cultures of Siberia and
Alaska were at this time cannot yet be determined, but the presence of a Siberian-American
Paleoarctic tradition immediately following the
submergence of the Beringian Land Bridge appears evident.

The existence of these early Siberian-Alaskan
crossties raises the perplexing problem of American Paleoindian relationships with Siberia. Remains of Paleoindian Clovis (fluted point) cultures have been found throughout most regions
of North America where they date to ca. 9500
B.C. Fluted points also have been found in western Canada and interior Alaska in a trail leading
tantalizingly toward Siberia. Yet, to date, the
search for fluted points in Siberia has been
fruitless, nor have prototype points been found
outside the New World. Hence this first truly
American technology remains anomalous to the
seemingly unrelated Siberian-American Paleoarctic horizon.

The people who left these early sites in Siberia
and Alaska can hardly be considered as direct
ancestors of the people who inhabited these
areas in the historic period. Undoubtedly, many
subsequent movements of peoples and cultural
changes have obscured the historical and ethnic
trails of peoples over the intervening millennia.
Nevertheless, it may turn out, as Dikov has
suggested, that the culture represented in Level
VI at Ushki was the basis for diversification in
Alaska into proto-Eskimo (Denbigh) cultures on
the one hand and proto-Aleut (Anangula) on the
other, although most American specialists prefer
to remain uncommitted on this point.

At the end of the Pleistocene and beginning
of the Holocene about 10,000 years ago, major
changes occurred in the environment of northeastern Asia. Glaciers disappeared, sea levels
rose, and the shoreline took on its present shape
(fig. 121). Climate became more humid and wet,
and swampy tundra appeared in place of the
dry steppe of the Ice Age landscape. Mammoths
and bison died out, and the only remaining large
game animal of the tundra of economic importance to man was the caribou. In coastal regions,
the formation of Bering Strait, connecting the
Arctic and Pacific Oceans, and the general warm-
ing of the seas and reduction of sea ice created
ideal conditions for sea mammals such as seals,
sea lions, walruses, and whales. From this time
on the peoples of Northeast Asia were primarily
fishermen and hunters of caribou or sea mammals.

The Siberian Neolithic

Early Holocene levels at Ushki record the beginning of a new economy. Judging from the large number of burned fish bones, fishing began to play an important role in subsistence at this time. Later, the end of the mid-Holocene climatic optimum coincides with the expansion in Kamchatka of neolithic hunting and fishing cultures dating to the third and second millennium B.C., traces of which have been found by Dikov both at Ushki and at sites on the western shores of Kamchatka. Related cultures have been found in Chukotka in the area of the Amguema River and in the Malta Mesolithic in the Kolyma River basin. Similar changes also occur along the Pacific coast of Alaska and on the Aleutian Islands where settled village life and developed maritime economies are noted in the Sandy Beach and Ocean Bay traditions. It is quite conceivable, even probable, that these parallel developments in Kamchatka and Alaska were historically linked. Further development of neolithic cultures in Kamchatka, including the appearance in the second millennium B.C. of ceramics, ground slate knives, and oil lamps, as well as other elements, led to the formation of the Tar'ia neolithic culture. This culture has some Eskaleut traits (for example, lip ornaments known as labrets) but generally is considered as belonging to cultures of the ancient Itelmen. Houses of the Tar'ia culture, in contrast to the earlier tentlike houses of paleolithic and mesolithic cultures, were large semisubterranean sod and log-walled structures with rooftop smokehole entrances similar to dwellings of the ethnographically known Itelmen and Koryak peoples, and also to house types of prehistoric and historic peoples of western Alaska, the Aleutians, and Kodiak Island. In short, the Tar'ia culture continues the development toward an Eskaleut type of culture begun in the early Neolithic period in Siberia, a way of life that was beginning to be shared widely by peoples throughout the North Pacific coastal region.

Archeological sites of the late Paleolithic and Mesolithic are known to a much lesser extent in Chukotka than in Kamchatka. Those that are known seem related to the Malta Mesolithic from the Kolyma basin and may represent movement of some of the ancestors of the Itelmen from eastern Siberia to Chukotka and Kamchatka.

By the third millennium B.C. in Chukotka, neolithic cultures had developed ceramics decorated with net impressions, and later, by the beginning of the first millennium, with cord-marked impressions. These cultures, designated by Dikov as Northern Chukotka and Ust'-Belaia, have clear parallels with the large suite of Ymyiakhtakh cultures of northern and central Yakutia that date to the same period and must have been important components in the formation of ancient Chukchi and Koryak cultures.

Ust'-Belaia peoples were partially sedentary and were based on hunting the massive herds of caribou that migrated across the tundra (Dikov 1965). Their summer camps were located at the river crossings used by these herds. Fishing provided an important supplementary food source. Burial sites contain skeletal remains of people

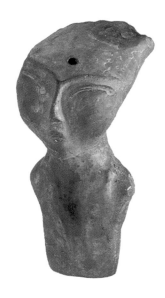

133. "Nefertiti" of the Amur (cast)
Siberian Neolithic: MIHPP Kn-63-48090

Excavations in 1965 in a Neolithic dwelling dating to the 4th-3rd millennium B.C., uncovered a burnished, fired clay female bust. Resembling armless ethnograhic figurines known as *sevons* (spirits of illness and shaman's helpers) and *dzhulins* (female house guardians (fig. 243), such figurines suggest ancient roots for 19th-century art and beliefs.

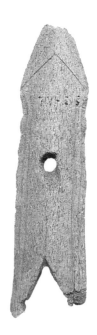
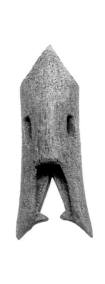
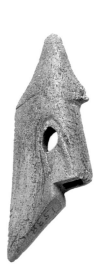
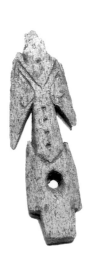

134. Sakhalin Harpoons
Neolithic: SKRM 70-214, 213, 219, 216

A wide variety of harpoon types characterizes the later prehistory of the southern Okhotsk Sea region. Decorated with sculptural and engraved designs, these toggling harpoon styles differ greatly from Eskimo types, indicating isolation from the center of Eskimo development in the Bering Sea. The nontoggling harpoon (*right*), however, is similar to Aleut forms and suggests contacts with the western Aleutians.

135. Boat Model
Old Bering Sea culture
MAE 6479/11-407

Skin-covered watercraft were probably used in the North Pacific as early as 10,000 years ago. This 2,000-year-old ivory model from an Ekven grave has a bifurcated bow and stern similar to those found on modern Eskimo umiaks, and its cockpit face recalls the use of human face plaques in Bering Sea Eskimo kayaks (fig. 198). The face, whale images, and grave find location suggest this model was used in hunting ritual rather than as a toy (pp. 255, fig. 344).

physically intermediate between the modern Chukchi and the continental Mongolids of central Siberia. Grave finds include stone implements and ceramics with check-stamped and hatched decoration typical of Ymyiakhtakh culture. Funeral ceremony included partial cremation. Along with the stone inventory there are also bronze tools originating from neighboring Yakutia and dating to the second millennium B.C. Toggling harpoon heads similar in type to those used by the Dorset Eskimo of the Canadian Arctic have also been found.

The finding of toggling harpoon heads demonstrates that by 1500 B.C. peoples of northeastern Asia had developed efficient methods for hunting sea mammals. Toggling harpoons similar to Ust'-Belaia finds, dating to the same period, have been found at Chertov Ovrag on Wrangel Island and at ancient Eskimo sites around Bering Strait. By this route we arrive at the question of the origin of Eskimo culture and its northern sea mammal hunting adaptation. Here we need to remember that incorporation into a single complex of Eskimo language, culture, and even physical type (which is close to that of the Chukchi) need not imply a single evolutionary development. These strands of historically known Eskimo life may have arisen independently among groups with different backgrounds and physical makeup.

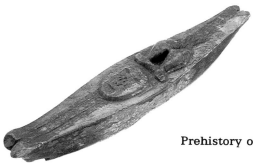

Prehistory of Bering Sea and Bering Strait

136. Hat Ornaments
Old Bering Sea culture
MAE 6587-298, 6587-300

Continuity in hunting ritual between Old Bering Sea and 19th-century Bering Sea Eskimos (fig. 201) is suggested by these hunting hat ornaments from an Old Bering Sea grave. The crest piece on the right has jet eye inlays, sketetized body markings, and holes for hair and wood plug inserts.

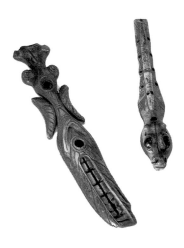

The North Bering and Chukchi seas contain three different ecological regions. The first, western Alaska, has diverse subsistence opportunities based on sea mammals, caribou, birds, and fish. The second region, Bering Strait, is unique for its wealth of sea mammals, especially walrus and whales, and absence or near absence of caribou. The third is the mountainous Chukotka Peninsula, which owing to its limited land fauna supported a relatively impoverished hunting culture before the introduction of reindeer breeding. These three regions figure importantly in the history of Eskimo cultures, a subject that has intrigued scholars since the early 1800s.

Theories of Eskimo origins have variously supported Canadian or Bering Sea theories for more than a century. Finally, in the 1930s the issue was resolved with excavations at St. Lawrence Island by Henry Collins, whose work revealed 2,000 years of Eskimo development in Bering Strait. However, since Collins's oldest sites, representing the Okvik and Old Bering Sea cultures, were fully developed and not rudimentary, the search for Eskimo origins was not finally settled. Soviet archeologists see proto-Eskimo features in neolithic Kamchatkan and Chukotkan prehistory, while American archeologists emphasize early western Alaskan cultures such as

Norton and Choris as the most immediate ancestors of Old Bering Sea, with Palisades, Old Whaling, and earlier cultures of the Arctic Small Tool tradition as the earliest identifiable proto-Eskimo cultures, ca. 4,000 years ago. Beyond this, the trail of Eskimo origins vanishes in the Bering Sea fog.

Until now, considerable attention has been paid to the processes of ethnocultural evolution that took place on the American side of Bering Strait, because only in that location is it possible to follow the gradual development of moderately specialized cultures into specialized proto-Eskimo cultures. We suppose that this process reflects not so much a spontaneous local evolution as an addition to a local American substrate of new characteristics, the infiltration of which took place through the Bering Strait from Asia.

Here it is useful to look at Siberian prehistory. From the end of the third to the end of the second millennium B.C. on the expansive watershed of the Arctic Ocean, from the Olenek River to the Amguema, there existed several variants of the neolithic Ymyiakhtakh culture that have been studied by Iu. A. Mochanov and S. A. Fedoseeva (Mochanov 1969). Its branches in Chukotka were the Northern Chukotka and

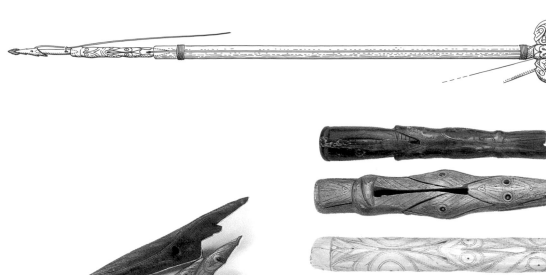

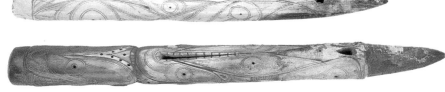

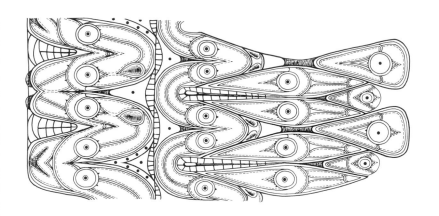

Ust'-Belaia cultures. The latter, at about 1100 B.C., occasionally used bronze instruments for the hunting of both caribou and seals. The economy of this culture is illustrated in part on the Pegtymel petroglyphs dating to the same period (Dikov 1972). Ymyiakhtakh culture, located farther west, was primarily a caribou hunting and fishing culture; however, several of its variants, such as Burulgino in the lower Indigirka River, have stone inventories including burins, knives, and arrowheads whose closest analogies are among the Old Bering Sea Eskimo culture complex in Bering Strait. Late forms of Ymyiakhtakh ceramic technology no doubt influenced Choris and Norton ceramics.

By the second millennium B.C. in northern Kamchatka, cultural developments in the middle period of the Neolithic included elements also found among ancient Eskimo cultures of Bering Strait. On the American side, early Old Bering Sea and Okvik ornament designs such as circle-dot, spurred line, and acute-angle line motifs have not been found in earlier American cultures as they have in the Siberian Burulgino site previously described. This may result, however, from the absence of bone preservation in American sites dating to this period.

The origin of the Eskimo skin-covered kayak, a type of boat known in various forms in many places in the northern hemisphere, is of special interest because of its importance in the Eskaleut adaptation pattern. Undoubtedly, the neolithic inhabitants of Siberia had boats, but no certain evidence of whether these were of bark or skin exists. La Martinier in the 16th century found evidence of skin boats on the shores of the

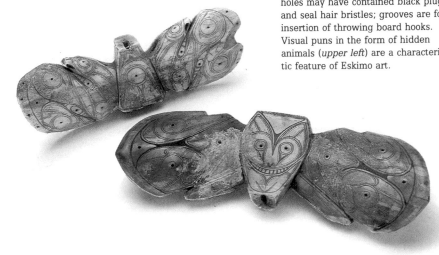

139. Ancient Hunting Magic

Old Bering Sea culture: (top to bottom, left) MAE 6479-269, 6588-72, 6588-139; (top to bottom, right) SI 378054; MAE 6561-126, 6479-17-582, 6479-9-205

Old Bering Sea hunters decorated their harpoons with incised designs and spirit images in the belief that their beauty, which honored the animal spirits, drew game to the hunter. Carvings of spirit helpers and deities further strengthened the power of these weapons. Feathers and wings transformed harpoon heads into swift birds of prey; socketpieces were carved into representations of the hunters' predator-helping spirits; and winged objects were ornamented with images of the powerful controlling spirit, the *tunghak*.

Stylistic diversity and absence of identical designs suggest Old Bering Sea art was produced by individual hunters, rather than by designated craft specialists. Yupik Eskimo hunters of Southwest Alaska continued the traditions of Old Bering Sea hunters into the 20th century.

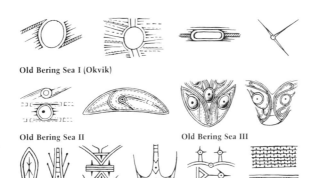

Old Bering Sea I (Okvik)

Old Bering Sea II

Old Bering Sea III

Punuk

Contemporary Alaskan Eskimo

Covarrubias 1954

140. Style Shift in Eskimo Art

Old Bering Sea culture: MAE 6561-329, 6561-256; Punuk culture: SI 356126, 344677, 356128 (top to bottom)

Excavating stratifed house floors at St. Lawrence Island, Alaska, Henry Collins discovered stylistic keys to the 2,500-year development of Eskimo art. The sequence begins with the flat, angular Old Bering Sea I (Okvik) style dating 500 B.C. This was followed by the increasingly ornate, plastic, and curvilinear OBS II and OBS III styles. After A.D. 800, Old Bering Sea art was replaced by simpler designs characteristic of Punuk culture. In addition to changes in ornamentation, wing elements underwent reduction in the Punuk period until only the central post required for throwing board hook insertion remained.

Collins noted the importance of Asian influence in Eskimo art and recognized that Eskimo culture had reached a fully developed stage by 2,500 years ago (Collins 1937).

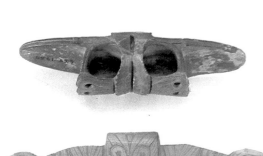

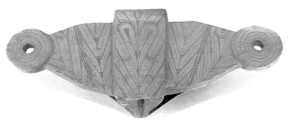

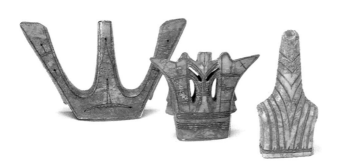

Barents Sea, and during our times Iu. B. Simchenko discovered relics of their existence in Taimyr. Archeologically, kayak models with features similar to umiaks and inland Chukchi kayaks have been found in 2,000-year-old Siberian Old Bering Sea culture sites (fig. 135). Since it would be virtually impossible to live along the shores of the Bering Sea without skin boats, we must assume that they were a necessary element in early arctic maritime adaptation for at least the last 4,000 years.

Like the skin boat, the origin of harpoon technology, which is the basis for hunting sea mammals and for the entire North Bering Sea adaptation, is complex, and many details of its development remain unknown. Harpoon typology suggests two pathways of development corresponding to the two dominant types of harpoons—the barbed nontoggling form and the toggling form (fig. 195). The former probably originated from the old paleolithic fish harpoon that predates man's arrival in Bering Strait by thousands of years and was geographically widespread. The origin of the toggling harpoon, however, is more recent and obscure. Primarily a North Pacific and North American arctic implement, early toggling harpoons have been found in Old Whaling and Wrangel Island Chertov Ovrag sites at 1500 B.C. However, earlier prototypes are known from Maritime Archaic Indian sites in Newfoundland and Labrador as early as 5500 B.C.. Could it be that this early "Eskimo" implement was actually introduced to the Western Arctic by central Arctic Pre-Dorset peoples who we have reason to believe acquired toggling harpoons from Northeastern Indians 4,000 years ago, 500 years before the appearance of toggling harpoons in the Chukchi Sea?

Following the introduction of toggling harpoon technology into the North Pacific, harpoon distribution takes on an interesting pattern. As A. Leroi-Gourhan (1946) and later R. S. Vasilevski (1969, 1971) noted, nontoggling, multibarbed harpoons with lashed stone endblades were used almost exclusively in Kamchatka, Japan, the Kuriles, and the Aleutians; rarely are they found in Bering Strait, where the pattern reverses, toggling harpoons being more common than nontoggling harpoons. In fact, it was noted that the boundary between the two forms closely followed the southern limit of the winter pack ice, nontoggling forms occurring south of the distribution of winter pack ice. From this came the suggestion that toggling harpoons are advantageous in regions where floating ice is abundant because they do not protrude outside of the wound and cannot be broken off when the animal strikes the ice, either accidentally or

123

purposefully, whereas in iceless waters this refinement is unnecessary.

A remarkable feature of the prehistory of the northern Bering Sea is the proliferation of toggling harpoon types and artistic styles and motifs that developed in this region during the first millennium B.C. This complexity cannot be explained simply by functional requirements related to the hunting of different species or seasonal (ice and non-ice) conditions. Rather it seems to result primarily from social and religious changes in which style, as measured by artifact form and artistic elaboration, becomes not only a marker of chronological periods and broad sociocultural identity but also a designation of social subgroups such as clans, families, and even individuals. Whichever explanation one chooses, nonfunctional diversity suggests the growth of populations and creation of social and ethnic diversity from a more undifferentiated culture. By A.D. 0 we may suggest the presence in this region of numerous small groups of people with different ethnic backgrounds and cultural traditions, all of which, however, were adapted to marine mammal hunting and engaged in intergroup contacts across Bering Strait. By this time we find, besides different ethnic groups settled in various regions around Bering Strait, the convergence of an ethnos, a common Eskimo type of lifeway, spreading throughout the region in both Asia and Alaska.

Archeologically, we do not know all aspects or stages of this process. But perhaps we know something of its early development, depicted in the Pegtymel petroglyphs, and of Asian influence in Choris and Norton culture. We also know something of its result: the formation of the brilliant Old Bering Sea complex of cultures—Okvik, Old Bering Sea, and Ipiutak—that were the immediate progenitors of later Eskimo culture history in the Bering Strait region. The relationships between these three cultures have not yet been fully clarified, partly because Okvik and Old Bering Sea cultures are to date known only in this area. In fact, there is reason to believe that each of these cultures, whose typological and radiocarbon dates of about 500 B.C. to A.D. 500 do not allow us to speak of these cultures as dating from different periods, actually may have originated as geographically distinct entities, the Okvik in Southwest Alaska, Old Bering Sea in Chukotka, and Ipiutak in northwestern Alaska. As seen from the perspective of excavations in the Bering Strait, where their distributions seem to intersect, the differences are not easy to perceive, and a single human burial may contain objects decorated in any of the three styles.

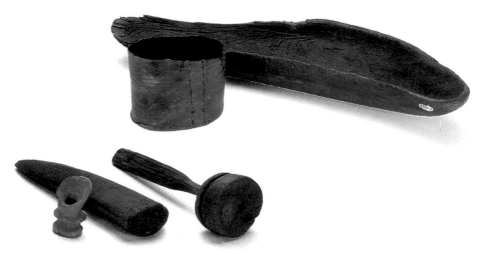

The economic base of the Old Bering Sea complex (including Okvik but not Ipiutak) was the hunting of walrus. Whale hunting was already completely developed but was secondary to walrus hunting in importance. Hunting of other animals had a supplementary character. Harpoons as a rule were thrown with the aid of a throwing board. The rear end of the harpoon shaft was fitted with an ivory "winged object" that acted to counterbalance the heavy ivory socketpiece and harpoon at the front end of the shaft. All of these components were decorated and had both aesthetic and magical qualities; in addition the design may have helped the carver reproduce his implements to a standardized pattern and proportion.

One basic difference between Okvik and Old Bering Sea cultures is seen in their harpoon

141. Containers and Float Gear
Old Bering Sea culture: (upper, l-r) MAE 6588-69, -12; (lower, l-r), -233, -63, -80/61

Wood was available to peoples of Bering Strait only in the form of driftwood. Wood was used for food trays, bucket bottoms, wound plugs, float plugs, and many other items, but is rarely preserved in ancient sites. Often baleen and ivory were more plentiful than wood, and just as serviceable.

142. Women's Work
Old Bering Sea culture: MAE 6588-39, -241; 6561-419, -516; 6588-41, 6508-562; NMNH-372080; MAE 6588-33, -36 (left to right)

Women's work was dominated by the production of warm, tailored skin clothing. Old Bering Sea and Punuk women used beautifully crafted zoomorphic stone-bladed ulus, needlecases, bootcreasers, and sinew twisters. The four-toed ivory foot, an animal reference, functioned as a lice crusher.

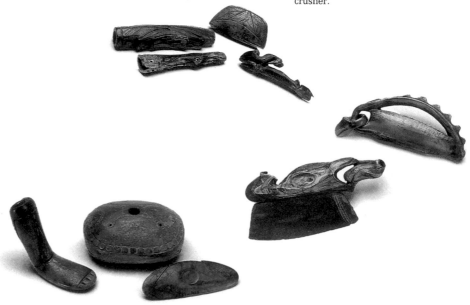

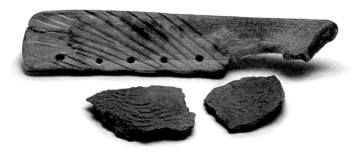

143. Pottery

Old Bering Sea culture: (top to bottom) MAE 6588-74, 6561-1014a,b

Unlike other pottery traditions in the Americas, which developed without external stimulus, pottery spread into Alaska from neolithic cultures of Siberia 4,000 years ago. Used for cooking pots and oil lamps among the relatively sedentary coastal peoples, pottery remained in use in western Alaska until the 20th century. Eskimo pottery was relatively crude and was often undecorated. Ivory paddles with stamp designs were used by Old Bering Sea people to consolidate the wet clay and impart surface decoration.

144. Shaman's Pottery Paddles

Old Bering Sea culture: MAE 6508-547, 6587-564 (bottom)

These ivory pottery paddles show that different stamp designs were used in late Old Bering Sea times. The lower paddle displays the Eskimo penchant for contour-grip handles, skeletal art, and contorted shamanic faces—the latter not visible here but present on the end of the lower handle. Similar faces are found on shaman's drums. The upper paddle illustrates a shaman with outstretched human legs and bear paws transformed into his polar bear spirit helper, in shamanic flight. A bear head is carved at one end, a beast's mouth at the other.

head styles. Old Bering Sea harpoon heads tend to have symmetrical heads with sideblade insets; Okvik harpoon heads tend to be asymmetric and have endblades, but the latter are found in Old Bering Sea as well. Some of the Okvik–Old Bering Sea types cannot be distinguished from harpoon heads found in Ipiutak sites. Walrus ivory artifacts decorated with elegant engraved and sculptural art are common in both of these cultures.

There are, of course, more pronounced differences between Okvik–Old Bering Sea cultures and Ipiutak. The latter did not use oil lamps or knives and points of slate that are characteristic of the former, probably because Ipiutak, like Norton culture, had roots in earlier cultures adapted to coastal life in western Alaska, in which sea mammal hunting was not highly specialized (seals primarily, less often walrus) and which depended to a significant degree on caribou. Whether Ipiutak ever hunted whales is not clear. We must also note that even in Old Bering Sea cultures chipped stone tools do occur, although they are less common than slate points.

Differences in the use of slate and flint tools by Ipiutak and Old Bering Sea cultures may have a rather functional basis relating to their economic conditions. Modern Eskimo people, for example, prefer soft iron for points, knives, and flensing tools rather than hard steel, which is difficult and time-consuming to sharpen. A completely analogous situation exists for the relationship between slate and flint weapons: northern maritime cultures with sea mammal

specializations almost universally adopt slate technology for piercing, flensing, and sea mammal skin processing activities. The preference for ground slate technology at the expense of chipped stone tools through time generally in Alaska is seen also in Bering Strait, where flint or chert tools common in Ipiutak and present in Old Bering Sea are replaced by slate in Punuk times, by ca. A.D. 1000. However, during this time use of iron in Siberia was gaining ascendancy, and slate grinding may have been a suitable, and in many ways a comparable, substitute in areas where metal was scarce and expensive.

Another difference between Old Bering Sea and Ipiutak is seen in the ceramic traditions of Old Bering Sea culture, absent in Ipiutak. Old Bering Sea ceramics were generally of low quality. The types present were usually round bottom cups and bowls with decorations stamped on their surfaces by ivory pottery paddles. Several of these stamp paddles were found at the Ekven site with concentric circle and lined decoration (fig. 144). To some degree this decline in ceramic technology has to be seen against the elevated expression found in the ivory carving arts.

The florescence of the Old Bering Sea complex seems to have been assisted, though only to a limited extent, by the acquisition of metal, particularly of iron, tools. Both linguistic and archeological evidence suggest the Japanese Sea as the source of Old Bering Sea metal. Remains of iron tools have been found at both Ipiutak and Old Bering Sea culture sites. One can therefore suggest that the ornamental art of these cultures developed under the oblique influence of ancient Far Eastern civilization. Especially notable in this regard are early Eskimo sculptures, which are realistic and stylized representations depicting fantastic masks (figs. 138, 147–149). The great number of masks and zoomorphic images in the Old Bering Sea complex seems also to have been related, though through a process not yet understood, to the art of Scytho-Siberian, Shang,

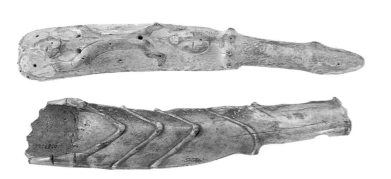

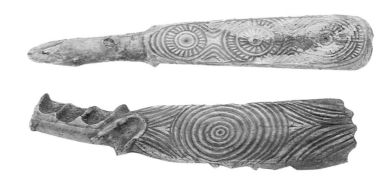

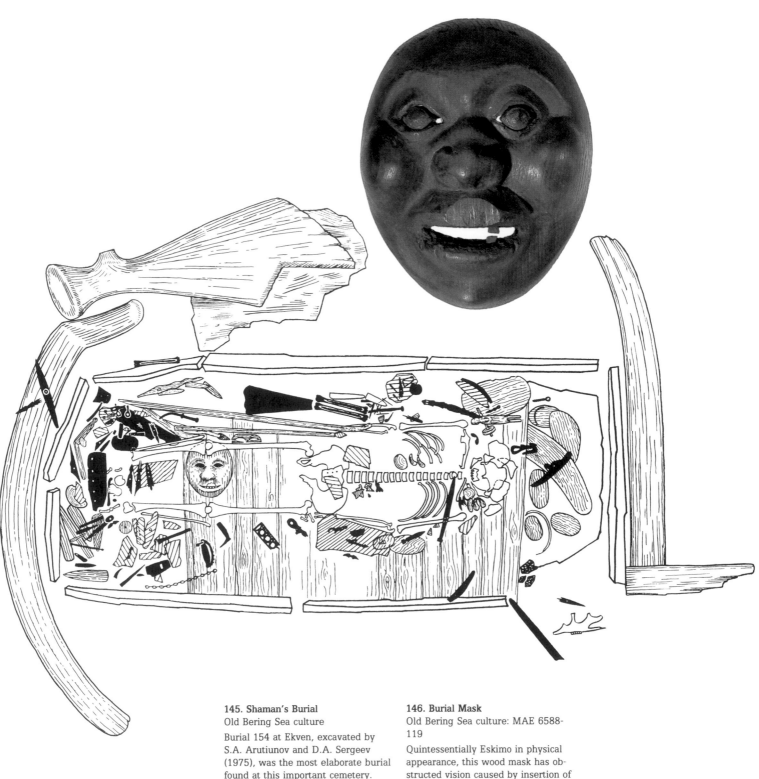

145. Shaman's Burial

Old Bering Sea culture

Burial 154 at Ekven, excavated by
S.A. Arutiunov and D.A. Sergeev
(1975), was the most elaborate burial
found at this important cemetery.
The burial contained the remains of a
woman lying on a wood floor in a
stone-lined grave, surrounded by
many ivory, wood, shell, stone, and
bone tools, including both men's and
women's implements. The large number of finds and presence of drum
handles and masks (including dance
goggles shown above) suggest this
woman was a powerful shaman.

146. Burial Mask

Old Bering Sea culture: MAE 6588-
119

Quintessentially Eskimo in physical
appearance, this wood mask has obstructed vision caused by insertion of
carved bone eyes. Blocked vision is a
feature of Siberian shaman costumes
(figs. 333, 334) and of North Pacific
deathmasks in general. The mask
was probably placed over the deceased's face at the time of her death
to prevent the shaman's spirit from
returning to animate the body, and
was removed to a location between
her knees at burial.

147. Antler Soul Catcher

Ipiutak culture: AMNH 60.1/453

Among the implements found in
Ipiutak graves were sucking tubes,
used by shamans to extract evil spirits from sick people. The assistance
of wolflike helping spirits was required. Compare with fig. 451.

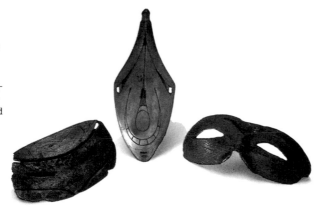

148. Masked Spirits
Old Bering Sea culture: (left to right)
MAE 6561-722, -1000, 6588-118
(left to right)

Mask plaques and a set of dance goggles display a variety of masking traditions and spirits (bird, *tunghak,* and transformed man) known to Old Bering Sea people.

and Eastern Chou peoples on the one hand (figs. 448, 450, 451) and to Northwest Coast Indians on the other (fig. 449). Art, technology, funeral practices, and shamanism somehow seem to be deeply involved in these transfers.

149. Ipiutak Burial Mask
Ipiutak culture: AMNH 60.1-7713
This composite ivory mask was found disassembled at the Ipiutak cemetery at Point Hope, Alaska. Like the Ekven mask, it was probably worn between the time of death and burial. Another composite mask found at Ipiutak was lying disassembled between the knees of the deceased. Stylistic parallels have been noted between these masks and burial masks used by the Eastern Chou Dynasty of China (Collins 1971).

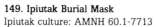

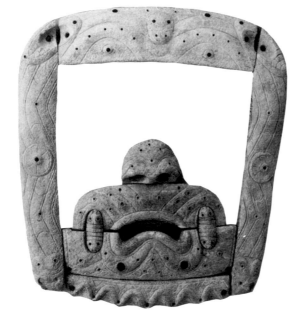

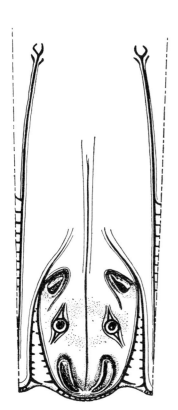

One of the particular characteristics of Old Bering Sea walrus tusk sculpture is its polyiconic nature, the mixing in one space of two or more images that must be seen from different vantage points. Polyiconic art serves as a means for expressing parallelism or connections of "primal incarnation" between people and animals of the land and the sea. Thus a killer whale appears as a sea transformation of the wolf, a shaman turns into a polar bear (figs. 46, 144), the walrus may be transformed into the mountain sheep, or a woman turns into a walrus. These plots

recorded in 2,000-year-old finds are present also in modern Eskimo mythology and folklore and show that the sea orientation of these cultures has been expressed in their ideological structures for thousands of years. Many of the same stories are found among 19th-century Yupik and Inupiat peoples. These traditions are especially strong in the case of the Yupik-speaking Bering Sea Eskimo, whose material and spiritual culture appears derived with little modification from the early Paleoeskimo cultures of Bering Strait.

Attempting to resolve questions of social structure on the basis of archeological material would be quite a thankless task, but there is a reason to suggest that in Old Bering Sea society there existed rather significant social and material differentiation, even perhaps including paternal slavery. Artifacts found in graves suggest the economic status of poor, middle, and rich individuals, a conclusion that is reflected also in the construction techniques and coverings of stone and whale bones found over the graves. Incidents of the finding of particularly rich graves accompanied by graves without artifacts may be explained as the burials of slaves.

Here we should also recall our discussions of stylistic complexity and the fact that the art of Okvik, Old Bering Sea, and Ipiutak cultures seems to reflect more than individual creativeness. Not only are no two implements decorated in the same style; diversity seems to be an end in itself, expressing an individual artisan's identity and, through his works, his respect for the spirits upon whom he and his community depended. This concept, the creation of beautiful works as a sign of respect to the spirits, was deeply rooted in Bering Sea Eskimo life and seems likely to have been a motivating factor in ancient Eskimo production as well. This attitude of individual artistic exuberance, apparently practiced by individual carvers and not simply by master artisans or specialists, contrasts strongly with the replicative, mechanical art of the succeeding Punuk period, a time when corporate social logic and belief in the power of technology itself seems to have gained sway over the spiritual powers and identities of individual hunters and seamstresses. Nowhere is this more obvious than in the shift from individual hunting of sea mammals in the Old Bering Sea cultures to intensified, communal hunting of whales in Punuk.

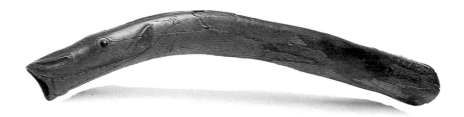

Recent Ancestors

Beginning in the 6th and 7th centuries A.D. in Bering Strait a new type of economy took hold. Especially in the Bering Sea area, Old Bering Sea culture gradually developed into Punuk culture, which spread on the Asian shore from Uelen toward the south to Beringovsk, and also onto St. Lawrence Island, but not, initially, to Alaska, where Norton and Birnirk culture prevailed. As more material is found, the specific characteristics of Punuk culture become clear: massive simple harpoon heads, plate armor for warriors, simplified ornamental forms, winged objects being replaced by three-pronged forms, and other changes that had begun in later stages of Old Bering Sea culture but that were not widespread. The major distinction of the Punuk as compared with earlier cultures was its increased whale hunting specialization. Houses grew larger, as did villages and numbers of sites, all of which reflect population growth. The use of whale bones for house and grave construction increased, and social organization seems to have become more complex. It is also possible to speak about the birth of intertribal cooperation at such sites as "Whale Alley" on Ittygran Island, where ceremonial constructions using skulls and jawbones of more than 100 bowhead whales must have required the cooperative efforts of several villages. By this time also, the growing presence of plate armor indicates that warfare had become as important an element of intergroup social relations as trade and stylistic exchange. Punuk culture continues, with variation, on the Asian side of the strait until A.D. 1500.

Meanwhile, Birnirk culture developed on the shores of the Chukchi Sea. The distribution of this culture extended further south than East Cape on the Asian shore and in the northeast reached Point Barrow. Birnirk culture seems to have developed with influence from Okvik and Ipiutak but with few ties to Old Bering Sea. Birnirk, dating to the 6th through 10th centuries A.D., had considerable Punuk influence in its later stages.

Beginning in the 10th century, Birnirk culture was slowly transformed into Thule culture by the addition of Punuk elements, including whale hunting, which expanded from Bering Strait into North Alaska and the Canadian Arctic at a time when relative climatic warmth facilitated the penetration of large whales into new feeding grounds in the Arctic Ocean. By A.D. 1300 Thule culture was established throughout the North American Arctic from Bering Strait to Greenland. However, with the cooler climates following A.D. 1300, whaling was abandoned throughout much of this region except in Alaska, and a period of readaptation to a life more like the pre-Thule period commenced. Art and material culture styles simplified, and social organization atomized. Canadian Eskimo culture remained in this form until its first contacts with Europeans rekindled social and economic development.

Thus as distinct from the stable, slow pace of cultural development that seems to have occurred in Kamchatka and in the Aleutians, the Bering Sea region, even at high latitudes, demonstrates a different character. Here, adaptation to conditions that were harsh and unstable but at times provided a combination of favorable conditions periodically led to rapid and clear achievements. However, climatic deterioration often resulted in these refinements' being short-lived. Faced with more harsh realities, sea mammal hunting cultures then returned to a simpler level.

The source of the economic-cultural type of the ancestors of the Chukchi and the Koryak originated when peoples whose cultures were based on the early form of caribou hunting and fishing acquired domestic reindeer, which occurred first about the 8th or 10th century (A.D.). True large-scale reindeer herding culture developed here, as everywhere in northern Eurasia, only during the 18th century.

The change from strictly land hunting to a coastal adaptation that included sea mammal hunting among the ancient ancestors of the Chukchi began as early as the middle of the second millennium B.C. However, throughout their development the Maritime Chukchi always remained less specialized sea hunters than the Eskimo, except at the eastern tip of Chukotka.

As far as the Koryak ethnogenesis is concerned, as their ancient development moved further from the ancestors they held in common with the Chukchi, probably in the second millennium B.C., and spread south to the Okhotsk shore in northern Kamchatka, they may have entered into contact with the Eskaleut substrata that occupied these lands previously. After this, ancient Koryak culture of various stages, from the second millennium B.C. to the 15th through 17th centuries A.D. represents a relatively straightforward sequential development. At the

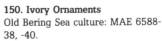

150. Ivory Ornaments
Old Bering Sea culture: MAE 6588-38, -40.

These ivory openwork carvings from Burial 154, the shaman's grave, resemble metal chains and bangles used as power objects on 19th-century Siberian shaman costumes. Ivory copies of exotic west Siberian metal ornaments probably were used for similar purposes by Old Bering Sea shamans on garments and ritual equipment (fig. 212). Nineteenth-century Alaskan Eskimos believed the sounds of chains and rattles pleased sea mammal spirits and helped draw them to the hunter.

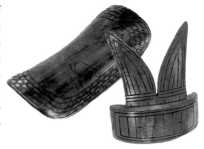

151. Wrist Guards
Punuk culture: NMNH 339833, T-23244

The appearance of Punuk culture after A.D. 800 brought many changes to the smallscale Paleoeskimo societies of Bering Strait. Economic development centered on the hunting of large whales resulted in population growth and increased mobility. Implements of war including armor plate, wrist guards, and bow-and-arrow parts proliferated, and modern trading and raiding patterns became established.

same time, as R. S. Vasilevski notes, Koryak culture development is quite eclectic, with traces of the interior continental culture of the hunters of wild caribou, elements from the south bank of the Lower Amur, and, in terms of its harpoon complex and maritime adaptation, with ancient Eskaleut influences.

On the American side, Eskimo and Aleut prehistory appears to call for relatively stable, progressive development for the past 6,000 years in which distinct regional traditions can be traced forward in South Alaska–Kodiak Island, the Aleutians, and western Alaska. However, major discontinuities occur in each sequence, calling into question ideas of simple population and cultural continuity. For Bering Sea cultures evidence seems to point toward conservatism among the cultures of the Bering Sea coast and interior and a lack of obvious penetration of this coast by Indian groups. But overall, the cultures of western Alaska seem to have responded most dynamically to change in the Bering Strait region, where the potential for intensified resource exploitation was greatest and where the flux of communication with Asian cultures was greatest and novelties more numerous.

Over tens of thousands of years cultural development has taken place along similar paths both in the American and the Asian parts of the Northern Pacific. Upper Paleolithic hunting cultures evolved into taiga and tundra hunters to which Even culture contributed saddle and sled transportation and domesticated reindeer. The coastal adaptation of the Koryaks in many ways is reminiscent of the Aleuts, while the Itelmen, and even more the Nivkhi and Nanai tribes of the Lower Amur, created a fishing culture similar to that of the Northwest Coast Indians. But the homogeneity and common cultural base of these cultures, so widespread in the late Pleistocene and at the beginning of the Holocene, began to weaken by approximately 2000 B.C.. Thus, bronze blades, characteristic of the Ust'-Belaia culture, did not reach America, nor did several new forms of stone implements, reindeer herding, and many other Asian elements. On the other hand, some Asian elements did appear, such as ceramics, iron, art styles, and elements of mor-

tuary ceremonialism and shamanism. It would appear therefore that Bering Strait was never a hindrance to the passage of materials and ideas among local populations living along both its shores. In fact, Bering Strait seems to have operated somewhat as a check-valve, allowing Asian elements to penetrate American territory to a greater extent than American elements did Asia. No doubt a major reason for this directional flow relates to emanations from higher centers of cultural development in Eurasia and to the relative lack of such centers in North America.

The effects of these west to east influences certainly had an impact on the Old Bering Sea culture group and probably also in the formation of Punuk culture and its whaling economy. Thus it seems that over the past 4,000 years at least, Asian influences via Bering Strait may have been most important in North American arctic prehistory, stimulating numerous cultural changes if not population influxes in Arctic Small Tool, Dorset, and Thule periods, while being of less consequence in the Bering Sea and Pacific culture history where American populations were larger, more diverse, and better fed. These areas seem to have resisted northern influence during most periods, and the presence of slat and rod armor, oil lamp types, house types, and other cultural traits speak more strongly for Aleutian rather than Bering Sea links with Asia.

Seen in this light, what is remarkable is that the flow of Asian influence into the Bering Strait region during the past several thousand years seems not to have influenced other cultures of the Americas, perhaps because the Eskimo cultures that lived there were so independent and individual, and so different from the land-based cultures neighboring it, that even though they maintained contacts with the inland tundra-taiga populations, they did not serve as a conduit for culture exchange but rather constituted a relatively impenetrable isolating layer. This fact determined the individual differences in the later direction of the ethnic fate of the populations of the American and Asian subarctic in spite of the almost completely parallel nature of their ecological zones.

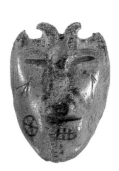

152. Tattooed Maskette
Old Bering Sea/Punuk culture: MAE 6479-522

Naturalistic human faces are rare in Old Bering Sea art, which usually portrays humans as transformed animals. Although found in an Old Bering Sea grave, this maskette has designs common in Punuk and later phases of Eskimo art: rosette, Raven's foot, and spurred line—the latter one appearing later as an identifying mark on hunter's harpoons and arrows. Body tattoos have been used for at least the past 2,500 years in Eskimo prehistory.

153. Pegtymel' Rock Art
Chukotka: Late Neolithic–Early Iron Age, ca. A.D. 0

Rock art from the Pegtymel' River near the Arctic coast of Chukotka provides valuable information not available from other archeological sites (Dikov 1972). The most unusual images are "mushroom people," thought to be spirits of fly agaric, the hallucinogenic mushroom used widely by peoples of Siberia in historic times. Scenes of spearing wild reindeer from kayaks suggest that domestic reindeer herding had not yet been introduced. Images of hunting large whales from umiaks with harpoon equipment may indicate the former presence of Eskimos on the western Chukotkan coast and suggests that Chukchi did not begin their expansion into this area until the middle of the first millenium A.D.

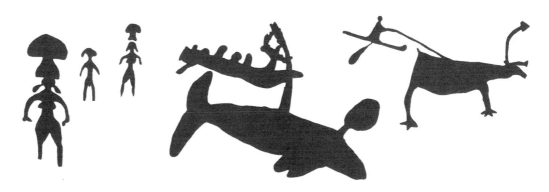

Prehistory of Alaska's Pacific Coast

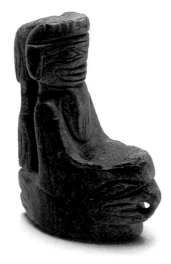

Aron Crowell

The southern coast of Alaska, extending from the Aleutian Island chain to the Coast Range of British Columbia, was home to a group of diverse, complex, and colorful maritime cultures—the Aleut, Koniag, Chugach, Eyak, and Tlingit. Though each was unique in its own right, these cultures were strongly linked to one another by shared ideas and ways of life. This may be seen in numerous aspects of technology, economy and social organization, art, mythology, and ceremonial practices. These similarities imply a high degree of past contact and crosscultural borrowing, a theory whose plausibility is enhanced by the seagoing mobility of South Alaskan groups. This mobility supported the existence of trade networks that linked the whole length of the coast into an extended zone of commerce and interaction. Intersocietal warfare and raiding was also endemic, resulting in the movement of objects and people (slaves and war captives) between groups.

Other similarities may have been the result of parallel development rather than the diffusion of cultural elements between groups. Tlingit culture, for example, is noted for the importance of wealth and status in governing relationships between individuals and clans, and for the system of feasts and counterfeasts that shifted food and wealth between kin groups. It is less well known that similar (if less elaborated) systems of social ranking, which divided society into elites, commoners, and slaves, prevailed among all the cultures of Alaska's southern coast (Town-

send 1980). This was in sharp contrast to the simpler, more egalitarian social systems of more northerly Alaskan and Siberian cultures. This social complexity, rare among the nonagricultural peoples of the world, has been linked by anthropological theorists to the exceptionally rich fish and sea mammal resources available throughout the region, which in turn fostered human population growth, sedentary settlement in large permanent villages, and the emergence of political systems that functioned to control and redistribute food surpluses among different segments of the population (Ames 1981; Price and Brown 1985).

The ethnographic situation thus challenges us to examine the prehistory of the region and to trace the processes by which both shared adaptations and cultural diversity arose. Long archeological sequences at several key sites are available, which provide parallel indexes to prehistoric change in the Aleutians, Kodiak Island, and the northern Northwest Coast, especially for the period after 3000 B.C. The primary sites considered in this essay are Chaluka, on Umnak Island in the eastern Aleutians (Turner, Aigner, and Richard 1974); the Karluk 1 and 31 sites on western Kodiak Island (Jordan and Knecht 1986); and a series of sites at Prince Rupert Harbour, north of the Skeena River in British Columbia (MacDonald 1983). The location and dates of these and other sites mentioned in the text are shown in figure 128.

154. Seated Figure Bowl
Alouette River, B.C.; undated. CMC XII-B-1798
The earliest seated figure bowls are from the lower Fraser River region between 350 B.C. and A.D. 200 (Marpole Phase), but their use may have continued into the historical period among the Shuswap (Borden 1983; Duff 1975). At the end of a girl's puberty ceremony she was sprinkled by a shaman with water and herbs from the bowl, with prayers for the birth of many childern. The iconography is complex—a rattlesnake head lies flat on the figure's breast, while down its back one snake consumes another. Two hawklike faces peer forward and backward from the base of the bowl.

The Earliest Sites: The Paleoarctic Tradition

During the period from 9000 to 5500 B.C., sites of the Siberian-American Paleoarctic tradition, which share a stone tool technology centered on the production of blades for composite hunting weapons, were occupied on the margins of Beringia from Hokkaido, Japan, through Northeastern Siberia, and across Alaska to British Columbia (fig. 121). Although inland site locations and occasionally preserved animal bones indicate the dependence of these early northern people on post-Pleistocene interior fish and game (caribou, bison, elk, mountain sheep, horse), some Paleoarctic coastal sites have been discovered along the seaward flanks of southern Alaskan mountain ranges. The locations of these coastal sites strongly suggest a maritime orientation, despite the lack of faunal remains. They include Anangula (6000 B.C.) in the eastern Aleutians (Laughlin and Reeder 1966; Laughlin 1980), the Koggiung site (6000 B.C.) on the Alaska Peninsula (Dumond 1981), the Ground Hog Bay (Component II, 6800 B.C.) and Hidden Falls (7500 B.C.) sites on the Alexander Archipelago of southeastern Alaska (Ackerman et al. 1979), and the Namu site (Component I, 7100 B.C.) on the mainland coast north of Vancouver Island (Carlson 1979). The earliest of these sites were occupied not long after melting of the coastal glaciers first opened the coast to habi-tation. Johnstone Strait at the north end of Vancouver Island appears to represent the farthest southward penetration of Paleoarctic microblade-using people into North America, although microblades came into use along the southern Northwest Coast and interior Plateau region in later times.

William S. Laughlin (1967) proposed that the Paleoarctic people were ancestral to both Eskimos and Aleuts and developed a maritime way of life while living along the southern margin of the now submerged Bering Land Bridge. There is some difficulty with this idea, since current data indicate that the land bridge was completely submerged by about 12,000 B.C., more than 2,000 years earlier than any firmly dated sites on the coast or in the interior of Alaska. The flooding of the land bridge would not have been an effective barrier to entrance into the New World, however, since Bering Strait is crossable on the ice in winter and by boat in summer. It seems more likely that migration into Alaska from Siberia took place no earlier than about 10,000 B.C., and that maritime settlement first occurred along the Pacific and Bering Sea coasts of Alaska. The earliest shoreline sites would now be flooded by the post–Ice Age rise in sea level, so these very early developments are likely to remain obscure.

Salmon, Seals, and Shell Middens: The Emergence of Large Coastal Settlements

There is a startling difference in visibility between the thin traces of early coastal occupation discussed so far and the massive prehistoric village sites that dot the southern coast of Alaska, the Aleutians, and British Columbia. The village sites are thick mounds of shell, bone, stone, and cultural debris, built up over centuries of continuous occupation. The surfaces of these mounds are often treacherous with the deep pits of collapsed houses, hidden by the luxuriant summer vegetation that thrives in the rainy climate and on the enriched midden soil. On the Northwest Coast, the oldest and lowest shell levels (such as Namu III and the Prince Rupert Harbour sites) have been radiocarbon dated to about 3000 B.C., give or take a few hundred years. This date marks the beginning of the middle period of Northwest Coast prehistory. Farther north and west along the Pacific coast this development occurs slightly later and less dramatically, with transitional examples like Sandy Beach Bay on Umnak Island (2500 B.C.) and Ocean Bay sites in the Kodiak region (4000–2000 B.C.) leading to the establishment of wide-spread and large-scale coastal villages by about 2000 B.C. This date marks the beginning of the Kachemak phase in the Kodiak–Cook Inlet region and the settlement of the Chaluka site on Umnak Island in the eastern Aleutians.

Found in these coastal middens is a whole new variety of tools and weapons needed for the hunting and fishing life of the coast, and the first examples of art and ceremonial objects. Microblades and chipped stone points have been replaced with an emphasis on ground slate implements, and barbed harpoon points for sealing and fishhooks are common. Knut R. Fladmark (1975) has suggested that coastal village sites became common after 3000 B.C. because it was at this time that climatic and geomorphological factors promoted the establishment of massive and dependable runs of salmon in the rivers. Summer salmon fishing produced large food surpluses that supported the permanent occupation of the large coastal villages, as well as the complex ceremonial life that was carried out there during the late fall and winter months.

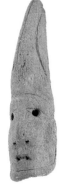

155. Bone Ornament

Hot Springs site, Alaska

1st millennium A.D. NMNH 16089

William Dall collected this ornament from the upper layer of the extensive Hot Springs village site at Port Moller on the Alaska Peninsula (Dall 1877:87). It is completely hollowed out in back and has small lashing holes, as if it had once been sewn on to a hat or clothing, or fitted to the end of some small cylindrical object. The delicately carved face merges with either the arched jaws of a whale or a bird beak, or both—the shape may be intentionally ambiguous.

Social Complexity and Artistic Development in the Kodiak Region

In the intensified maritime focus that emerged after 3000 B.C. we find the beginnings of a remarkable transformation of Pacific hunting, fishing, and gathering societies that led over the course of several hundred generations to the ethnographic complexity and diversity encountered by the first European explorers. These developments included population growth accompanied by increasing numbers of villages, changes in house forms, expanded trade networks, increased warfare, elaboration of ceremonialism, and the development of distinctive regional styles of art and personal adornment. Interwoven with these archeologically observable trends was the emergence of ranked social systems with an emphasis on prestige and wealth.

Intensive surveys and excavations in the Kodiak region have greatly expanded understanding of these complex developments, especially work over the past five years at the Karluk 1 site on Kodiak. The Kodiak sequence offers perhaps the best exemplar of general developments taking place along the Pacific coast, and its description will be followed by comparisons with the data from the Aleutians (the Chaluka site) and the northern Northwest Coast (Prince Rupert Harbour sites).

Ocean Bay Tradition

The Ocean Bay I culture (4000–2500 B.C.) represents an early transitional example of maritime adaptation in the region, predating the general emergence of large sedentary coastal populations by a thousand years or more. This archeological culture is known from more than a dozen sites on Kodiak Island and the Alaska Peninsula, where a local variant is known as the Takli Alder phase (D. W. Clark 1979; G. H. Clark 1977). Preserved food bone from one of the Takli Alder sites indicates that sea otter, seal, sea lion, and porpoise were all being hunted. Barbed bone harpoon heads and stone lamps for burning sea mammal oil also occur in the oldest Ocean Bay levels. A two-phase settlement pattern appears to have already been in place, with small coastal settlements (fall to spring) and summer fishing camps along the banks of salmon rivers.

Judging from the size and number of known sites, and the thinness of occupation levels, the Ocean Bay I population was small, mobile, and thinly scattered. This impression remains, even accounting for the difficulty of locating Ocean Bay sites, since they are more likely to be completely overgrown or buried beneath later cultural deposits. Domestic groups were prob- ably simple nuclear families, judging from the small size and simple rectangular or oval form of the dwellings, which had sunken floors and sod walls. Because organic preservation is rare in sites of this age, we have no indications of what Ocean Bay art or ceremonial practices might have been like.

Ocean Bay I stone tool technology included both microblade manufacture (providing a link to the antecedent Paleoarctic tradition) and the chipping of knives and weapon points from chert. Stone tools made from sawn and ground slate, including long narrow lance blades, were used from the beginning of early Ocean Bay I but became increasingly more common through time and gradually replaced the chipped stone tool kit. This shift to ground slate technology marks the beginning of Ocean Bay II (2500–2000 B.C.) and was paralleled in coastal mound phases all along the Pacific coast. Interestingly, no shift to slate occurs in archeological sequences to the north of the Pacific Eskimo area at this time, nor did Bering Sea developments such as the appearance of the Arctic Small Tool tradition (2500–1000 B.C.) have any visible impact south of the Alaska Peninsula. These data indicate that at this early stage Pacific cultures were developing with a large degree of independence from cultures around the Bering Sea.

Kachemak Tradition

The size and number of sites that date to the succeeding Kachemak tradition (2000 B.C.–A.D. 1100) suggest that both population size and the intensity of resource exploitation greatly increased during this period. Hundreds of house groups and village sites in coastal locations on Kodiak, the Alaska Peninsula, and Cook Inlet are known, situated to maximize proximity to such resources as sea bird rookeries, sea mammal concentrations, salmon streams, and shellfish beds (de Laguna 1975; Heizer 1956; D. W. Clark 1970). Discarded food bone from these sites shows that scores of different species of mammals (including whales), birds, fish, and shellfish were being consumed. Inland sites occur along salmon rivers; the collapsed remains of Kachemak houses occur in great numbers along the 25-mile length of the Karluk River on Kodiak Island, where summer salmon runs of 10 million fish or more were probably once common. Houses are square or rectangular and slightly larger than in Ocean Bay times (averaging about 250 square feet inside), with hearths, storage pits, and small appended storage alcoves. Middens (layered deposits of occupational debris) are often 3 feet thick or more, and the good preservation of bone and shell that is usually present

156. Ornamented Stone Lamp
Uyak site, Kodiak Island, Alaska
Kachemak, ca. 500 B.C.–A.D. 500
NMNH 375349

Massive pecked stone lamps provided with wicks were used to burn sea mammal oil for light and heat inside the house. The bear head in this lamp would have been eerily illuminated by the flame, appearing to float above its pool of oil.

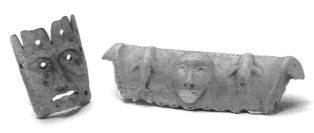

157. Kachemak Carvings
Uyak site, Kodiak Island, Alaska
Kachemak, ca. 500 B.C.–A.D. 500
NMNH 363740, 365592

Bone and ivory carving reached a high state of refinement during the Kachemak phase. The miniature mask (*left*) is crowned with a head-dress and has eye holes like a real mask, suggesting that it may have ceremonially masked a figurine. The imagery on the plaque (*right*) points to its use in whaling ceremonies. The human face is flanked by whales; bird heads adorn the ends of the plaque; and feathers were probably once inserted into the bordering line of small holes. From the back of the plaque projects a lug which served as a hand or mouth grip.

provides a much fuller picture of Kachemak life to the archeologist than is possible for Ocean Bay.

By the late, or developed, Kachemak phases, dating to the first millennium A.D., distinctive technological, artistic, and ceremonial characteristics become evident. The sea mammal hunting and fishing technology is fully developed, including several varieties of barbed bone dart points, toggling harpoon heads, large numbers of net and line weights for fishing, and compound fishhooks. Long, heavy barbed dart heads fitted with barbed slate blades were probably used for poison whaling, as were identical weapons by the historic-period Aleuts. The barbed end-blades known as the Three Saints type probably fit into these dart heads and frequently have inscribed designs that would have functioned as owner's marks, identifying the hunter who had first struck the whale. Ground slate tools predominate over chipped stone and include numerous knives and ulus. All of these tools show careful attention to craftsmanship. Woodworking implements such as hafted planing adzes and wedges remind us of the wooden objects (bowls, masks, carvings, etc.) that are absent or poorly preserved. Oval stone lamps for burning sea mammal oil are often large and ornamented with grooves, bars, female breasts, human and animal forms (fig. 156).

Objects of personal adornment become progressively more varied and common throughout the Kachemak period. Labrets of varied shapes and materials (bone, ivory, jet, amber, marble) are found, along with occasional stone and shell

beads, pendants, earrings, nose rings, combs, and polished stone mirrors. The raw materials used for ornaments and amulets are often from distant sources, implying an expansion of trade contacts throughout the region.

Other objects and practices reveal aspects of ceremonial life, probably concentrated during a winter season of feasts and hunting rituals as in later times. Of particular interest in this regard is an ivory plaque (fig. 157) from the Uyak site on Kodiak island, which depicts a human face flanked by a pair of whales. Zoomorphic bone carvings, figurines, and miniature human masks in bone appear, many of which probably served as amulets. Treatment of the dead, known from the abundant human remains found in village sites, is varied and complex. Multiple types of burials are known, including cremation. Skulls interpreted as trophy heads occur, with features modeled in clay and inset with artificial bone eyes. This use of artificial eye insets parallels practices seen in Old Bering Sea and Ipiutak burial traditions at this time. Dismemberment, cutting and drilling of human bones, and possible cannibalism are indicated by the condition of the human remains and may relate to the treatment of war captives.

Koniag Tradition

The Koniag tradition of Kodiak Island is well documented by excavations in the 1960s (D. W. Clark 1974) and by recently excavated sites at the mouth of the Karluk River, including the Karluk 1 "wet site," where constant groundwater saturation has resulted in excellent preservation of wooden and grass objects, as well as bone, shell, and stone material (Jordan and Knecht 1986). Excavations there have dissected nine levels of superimposed Koniag houses that extend from the contact period (mid-1700s) back to the beginning of the Early Koniag phase (A.D. 1200), and have produced over 20,000 examples of Koniag hunting and fighting equipment (bows, throwing boards, darts, arrows, harpoons, shields, and slat armor), household items (bowls, lamps, grass and split root baskets, knives), boat parts, ceremonial and religious artifacts (masks, figurines, amulets), ornaments, toys, gambling equipment, and numerous other object classes. Strata dating from 3000 B.C. (Ocean Bay I) to ca. A.D. 1000 (Late Kachemak–Koniag) were excavated at the Karluk 31 site on the opposite bank of the river, providing an opportunity to trace the cultural changes that took place during the Kachemak–Koniag transition.

Richard H. Jordan and Richard A. Knecht discount previous theories, which held that this transition at the beginning of the second millen-

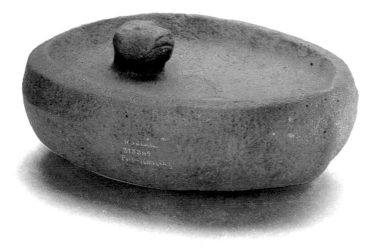

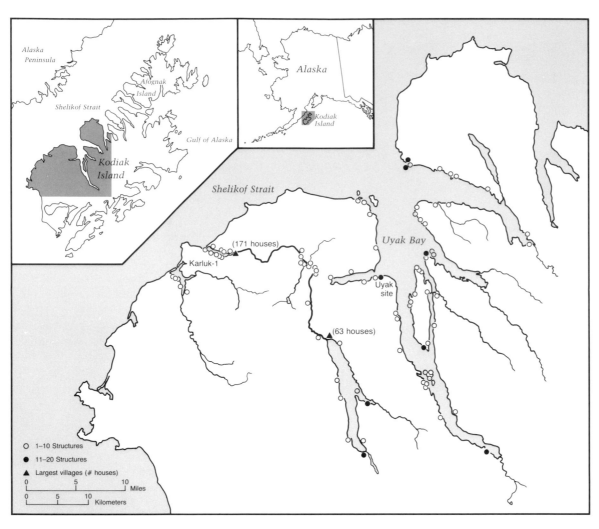

158. Prehistoric Koniag Villages on Northwestern Kodiak Island, Alaska

159. A Prehistoric Koniag Settlement on the Karluk River, Kodiak Island

160. Koniag Masks and Figurines
Karluk 1 site, Kodiak I., Alaska
Koniag, A.D. 1500–1750: Koniag, Inc.
UA85.193.3455, UA85.193.3695, UA85.193.3733, UA85.193.4063, UA84.193.1044

Koniag figurines may have been used for play or in shamanic rituals; some have cut or burn marks, which suggest the latter function. The two figurines on the right wear labrets.

The raised slit eyes and flaring nostrils of the maskette (*left*) are unique, but its pointed head and beaklike mouth are common Koniag mask features. The full-sized mask (*right*) was found lying face down inside a storage box in a collapsed late Koniag house; it is the short-eared owl, frequently depicted in Yupik Eskimo art (fig. 359).

nium A.D. represented an abrupt discontinuity in the archeological record, caused by either the immigration of Asians of a new physical type and culture or by the rapidly spreading influence of the Neoeskimo culture, centered at Bering Strait. North Pacific cultures were far to the south and on the periphery of these events, and continued to develop largely according to their own internal dynamics of change. Between A.D. 900 and 1200, the Karluk sequence does show gradual changes in artifact forms, art styles, and house types that mark the end of Kachemak and the beginning of Koniag culture, but the sudden and broad changes in material culture that would mark an abrupt Neoeskimo influx are absent.

The size and the number of known sites continue to expand during the Koniag period, reflecting population growth that eventually resulted in an estimated 10,000 or more inhabitants of Kodiak Island at the time of Russian contact. Although there are more Koniag sites, the settlement pattern duplicates that established during Kachemak times, so that stratified levels representing both cultures are often present at the same sites. Figure 158, showing the numerous Koniag sites around Uyak Bay and along the Karluk River on Kodiak Island, suggests to the imagination the busy animation of these once populous shores—the smoke and activity of the settlements and the endless coming and going of kayaks and umiaks on the business of hunting, travel, trade, and sometimes war. In coastal locations such as Uyak Bay, large permanent winter villages of up to 20 multifamily houses were interspersed with outlying small settlements and hunting camps that would have been used in spring through fall. The sea mammal, bird, and shellfish resources procurable from coastal settlements were complemented by the tremendous summer concentrations of spawning salmon in rivers like the Karluk. Massive riverbank settlements (fig. 159) most likely represent fishing camps that were reoccupied each year by people drawn from a wide region.

This economic system presents the political problem of gaining access to needed resources in different ecological zones (e.g. coastal versus riverine) in territories settled and controlled by different segments of the population. The abundant food supply permitted Pacific coast popu-

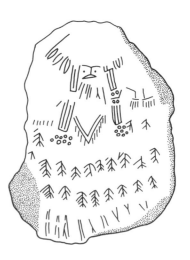

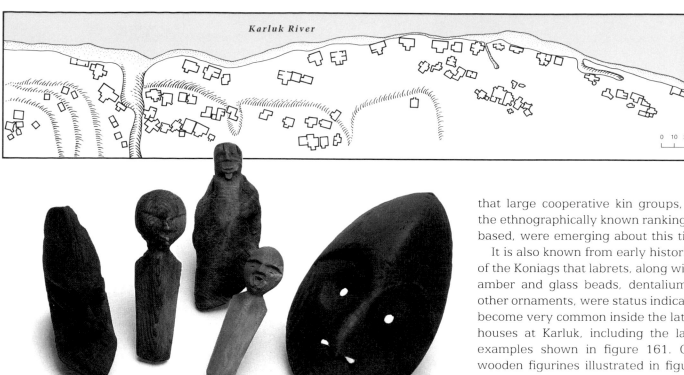

Karluk River

0 10 20 30 40 50 Meters

lations to grow to high levels, a trend that we have traced through several thousand years of Kodiak Island prehistory. We may suppose that with larger populations, unrestricted seasonal movement between prime hunting and fishing locations would have become increasingly difficult. More complex social and political arrangements would have emerged to regulate both direct access to resources and indirect access through trade and redistributive feasts and ceremonies. Local groups controlling important resources, particularly salmon fishing sites, would have been at an advantage in such a system and able to increase their own power and prestige. Hostile access, carried out through warfare and controlled by military alliances, would have also developed. The emergence of political and military leaders and of ranked social systems was the apparent outcome of this process in North Pacific societies.

Several trends that may be indications of increasing social complexity first became evident in the Kachemak tradition and continued and intensified during Koniag times. The great increase in house size is one of those trends. In the 15th century A.D., multiple siderooms began to be added to Koniag houses, and floor areas expanded to 850 square feet or more. Russian observations tell us that extended family groups of 18 to 20 people inhabited the typical Koniag house during the early contact period. The shift in house forms in the early Koniag phase implies

that large cooperative kin groups, upon which the ethnographically known ranking system was based, were emerging about this time.

It is also known from early historical accounts of the Koniags that labrets, along with nose pins, amber and glass beads, dentalium shells, and other ornaments, were status indicators. Labrets become very common inside the late prehistoric houses at Karluk, including the large wooden examples shown in figure 161. Of the three wooden figurines illustrated in figure 160, one wears a hat-shaped labret through the lower lip and another wears large dual cheek labrets. Smaller labrets in unusual shapes and materials (fig. 161) may have had special social meanings or have been nonlocal styles worn by traded or captured slaves.

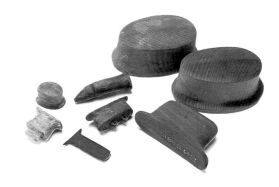

A striking increase in the frequency and variety of ceremonial objects also occurs in the late prehistoric levels at the Karluk 1 site, which seems to indicate a new intensity and variety in ritual observances. Between about A.D. 1350 and 1500 at Karluk and other Koniag sites, large numbers of polished slate pebbles were scratched with the stylized face and clothing of a figure variously adorned with beads, earrings, tattoos, and labrets (fig. 162). The clothing is often detailed in ways that suggest the feathers, seams, and tassels seen on ethnographic examples of Koniag parkas (fig. 268). The significance of this short-lived phenomenon is unknown, but concentrations of these incised pebbles on Koniag

135

house floors at Karluk give the impression that they were rapidly made and discarded as part of a ritual.

After A.D. 1500 a variety of masks and maskettes appear that are identical to forms used by the historic Koniag and Chugach and stylistically related to Bering Sea Eskimo masks. The pointed heads and beaklike mouths of the archeological maskettes in figure 163 may be compared with the 19th-century masks illustrated in figures 368 and 441. Mask hoops and bangles seen on the ethnographic examples become common in Karluk 1 house floor deposits after A.D. 1500, and board masks similar to figure 50 have also been recovered. Hoops surrounding Bering Sea dance masks had multiple symbolic references to transformations between worlds, and similar ideas were probably shared by Koniag mask makers. The pointed heads of the masks may identify them as images of *kalag*s, evil spirits of the woods and caves who were visible only to shamans (Birket-Smith 1953:124). A fascinating cross-Pacific connection is implied here, to the malevolent Siberian spirits, also with pointed heads, of the Koryak (*kala*s) and Chukchi (*kele*s). The beaked mouths are part of a general emphasis on bird imagery in Pacific Eskimo art that apparently developed at this time, including the idea of spiritual transformations between humans and birds. Puffins are carved on Late Koniag bag handles, and a full-sized owl mask from the Karluk site is shown in figure 160. Complex transformation imagery (visual punning) is also seen in a masklike carving from Karluk (p. 105).

Figurines become common in the Late Koniag levels at Karluk (fig. 160), including a remarkable example that is probably a birthing amulet (fig. 165). Some figurines probably represent shamanistic spirit helpers (Birket-Smith 1953:127). Finally, finds of drum handles and rims at Karluk should be added to the inventory of Late Koniag ceremonial objects.

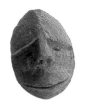

163. Miniature Masks
Karluk 1 site, Kodiak I., Alaska
Koniag, A.D. 1500–1750:
Koniag, Inc.: UA 85.193.4026 (left),
UA 85.193.6311

164. Dance Mask and Attachments
Unga Island, Alaska
Aleut, late prehistoric: NMNH 13002 (mask), 13082R, 13002N, 13082R

The features of this mask, with its massive nose, open nostrils designed to serve as eyeholes, wide mouth, pegged teeth, and incised tattoo-like facial designs, are typical of the masks from the Unga Island burial cave. They have no close parallels in either ethnographic or archeological collections, and remain undated. A bar behind the mouth served as a tooth grip for holding the mask in place. Hundreds of flat decorative pieces, most of them probably attachments for the masks, lay scattered on the floor of the cave. The leftmost example represents a harpoon head.

165. Birthing Amulet
Karluk 1 site, Kodiak I., Alaska
Koniag, A.D. 1500–1750:
Koniag, Inc.: uncataloged

This figurine, with her swollen stomach and supporting hands behind, seems to be very pregnant, perhaps in labor. She may have been a birthing amulet, or symbol of fertility. Her head is decorated with inset human hair.

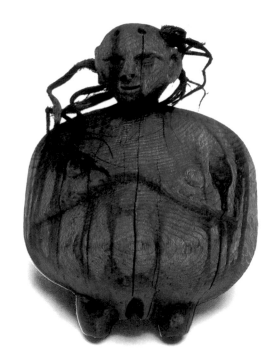

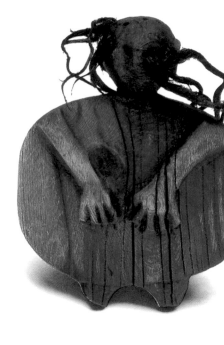

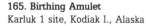

Comparisons West and East: Aleutian and Northwest Coast Developments

The Aleutian Tradition

Interesting parallels to the Kodiak sequence may be traced through the layers of the Chaluka site on Umnak Island in the eastern Aleutians. Aleutian mound sites, the remains of coastal villages that began to be settled after 2500 B.C., contain many artifacts relating to maritime hunting and fishing, including barbed harpoon heads, fishhooks, and spears. Ground slate tools are rare because of a lack of local slate sources, and

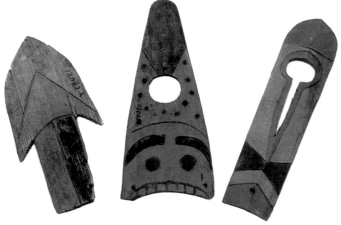

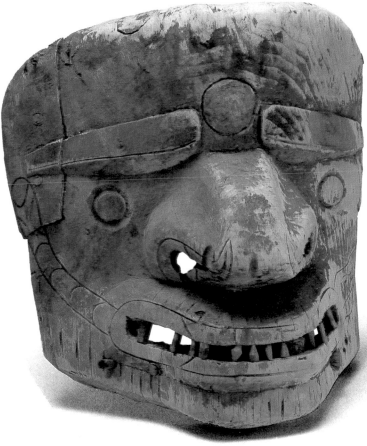

knives, scrapers, and projectile points were chipped from basalt, obsidian, greenstone, and chert. Faunal remains from the midden deposits (over 20 feet thick at Chaluka) include seals, sea lions, whales, sea otters, fish, birds, mollusks, and sea urchins, to which the ancient Aleutians added berries, seaweed, and a few other plant foods. As on Kodiak and the Northwest Coast, salmon was a critical resource.

Parallel to Kodiak developments, a dramatic increase in house size is seen between the small single-family structures of 2500 to 2000 B.C. and the large, multifamily longhouses known from the historic period. The earlier houses were

166. Harpoon Head
Chaluka site, Umnak I.
Prehistoric Aleut, undated: NMNH 395958 (head),
395999 (chipped stone point)
Bilaterally barbed bone harpoon head for sea mammal hunting, excavated by Aleš Hrdlicka in 1938.

domed, sod-covered structures with stone and whalebone wall foundations, probable roof entrances, interior hearths, and stone-lined storage pits (Aigner 1978). In one of these early (2000 B.C.) houses at Chaluka a small stone figure was found of the type termed an "Image of the Diety" by modern Aleuts, which would have been suspended from the rafters as a powerful protecting spirit of the house. The much larger longhouse type (sometimes exceeding 200 feet in length), in which individual family quarters were spatially arranged according to rank, may be less than 500 years old, although its evolution has not been traced archeologically. As on Kodiak Island, multiple-family dwellings must have evolved as populations grew and social organization became structured around large cooperative kin groups under the leadership of high-ranking individuals. Labrets and other ornaments that carry social information about status also increase in number and variety from the lower Chaluka levels (beginning at 2000 B.C.) to the uppermost level (17th century). These changes occurred while most types of hunting weapons and other artifacts remained basically the same, discounting the theory that late prehistoric developments resulted from an influx of a new population and culture into the Aleutians.

Some of the most striking art known from an archeological context in the Aleutians was removed from a burial cave on Unga Island in the late 19th century (Pinart 1875; Dall 1876; fig. 164). Such burial caves were used for the placement of elaborately prepared mummies of men, women, and children, along with offerings and ceremonial equipment of various kinds, including dance masks. The mummies, known as "the dry ones", were thought to carry on all the activities of daily life during the night, including hunting, eating, and dancing.

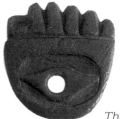

Northwest Coast prehistory may be divided into three periods: Early (8000–3000 B.C.), Middle (3000 B.C.–A.D. 500), and Late (A.D. 500–present) (Carlson 1983). As discussed earlier, it was the settlement of the large coastal winter villages that marks the beginning of the Middle period. The most extensive archeological research carried out on the northern Northwest Coast so far has been at coastal midden sites on the shores of Prince Rupert Harbour, British Columbia, in Tsimshian country. These sites were occupied from about 2500 B.C. into the contact period and provide evidence for the gradual emergence of the complex Northwest Coast social system and of the totemic crest art associated with it. Good information on temporal changes in house size and form is not available, but trade networks, status-related elaboration in ornaments and burial goods, and evidence of shamanism and warfare all appear to increase through time.

Before 1500 B.C. there is no evidence at Prince Rupert for graphic or sculptural art, and perforated tooth pendants are the only items of personal adornment that have been preserved. Beaver tooth knives for carving wood are found, however, cautioning us to remember that without wood preservation most Northwest Coast art of the ethnographic period would have been invisible in an archeological site. By 1000 B.C. labrets and bone pendants appear, and small stone carvings of abstracted animal forms foreshadow future developments in art (fig. 168). It is over the next 1500 years (the remainder of the Middle period) that some of the most dramatic changes occur, however. Along with gradual changes in tool types that will not be discussed here, a new inventory of decorative items develops, often incorporating exotic raw materials that point to the expanded importance of trade: shell, amber, dentalium, and jet beads; copper earrings and bracelets and copper-wrapped tubes that may have been part of rod or slat armor; bent bone bracelets with elaborate incised designs. Bone and stone war clubs appear in graves and caches, and the use of such clubs in war is grimly documented by the occurrence of skulls with crushing indentations. Ribbed amulets are found after 500 B.C., which are probably highly abstracted fish forms used in salmon ceremonies. Organic materials pre-

served at the waterlogged Lachane site demonstrate that boxes, bowls, baskets, and other artifacts made of perishable materials were very similar to those produced by the historic Tsimshian, although still mostly undecorated.

The first real evidence for the development of the abstract formline style of Northwest Coast graphic art is seen in the bone and antler combs that appear at Prince Rupert between A.D. 500 and 1000 (fig. 169). It is quite probable that this style was simultaneously being applied in a wood medium, as seen in ethnographic boxes,

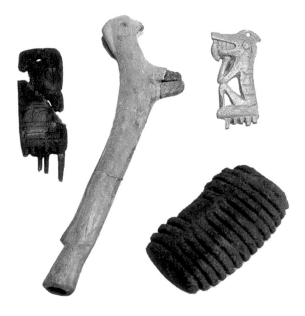

bowls, and other carved items known ethnographically but not preserved in archeological levels of this period. Indeed, with the application of zoomorphic carving to pecked stone artifacts such as mauls, adzes, and bowls between A.D. 1000 and 1500, the essential elements of Tsimshian and other Northwest Coast art styles were in place. We may also speculate that the social meanings behind the art, which were concerned with the totemic animal symbolism of corporate lineages, were developing parallel to, if not driving, the emergence of the new art. Bone pins, zoomorphic labrets, and other new decorative items added in the Late period continue the trend, seen at Prince Rupert as well as all along the northeastern Pacific coast, of elaborating personal adornment, probably linked to the emergence of an elite stratum of society.

167. Eye Amulet
Gitlakdamiks, British Columbia: undated, CMC VII-C-271

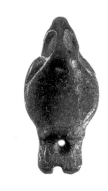

168. Raven Amulet
Boardwalk site, British Columbia
ca. 1000 B.C.
CMC GbTo–31:2178
Raven makes an early appearance in the prehistoric sequence at Prince Rupert Harbor in the form of this carved schist amulet. It is perforated through the tail for suspension, and the hollowed eye sockets may once have held abalone shell inlays.

169. Prehistoric Carvings from Prince Rupert Harbour Sites

Bone Comb (1st millennium A.D., CMC GbTo–34:1805)
This comb shows the use of the eyes, U's, and split-U forms of classic Northwest Coast design.

Miniature War Club (ca. A.D. 100, CMC GbTo–31:211)
A shaman often used ceremonial weapons to fight supernatural battles, which may explain the function of this miniature club.

Bone Comb (ca. A.D. 800, CMC GbTo–23:850)
A wolf is depicted, with an emphasis on its eye, extended tongue, and skeletal ribs.

Segmented Stone (ca. 500 B.C., CMC GbTo–31:X717)
A highly abstracted fish or animal form, this carving shows the ribs and vertebrae only, with head and tail eliminated.

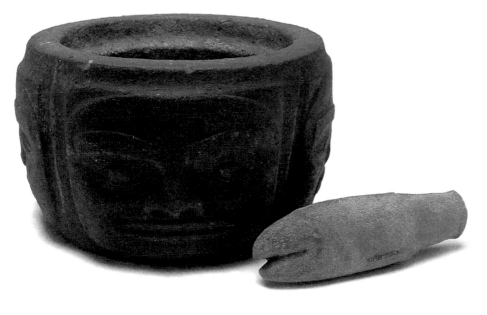

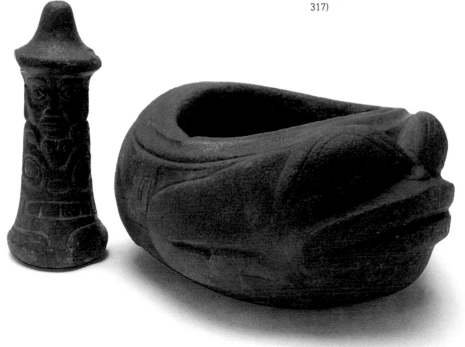

170. Late Prehistoric Northwest Coast Stone Carving
(Clockwise from upper left)

Tobacco Mortar (Skeena River, British Columbia, undated, NMNH 220185)

Stone Club (Fish) (Metlakatla, British Columbia, undated, CMC XII-B-560)

Pestle Queen Charlotte Islands, British Columbia, CMC VII-B-908)

Tobacco Mortar (Frog) (Queen Charlotte Islands, British Columbia, CMC XII-B-317)

Overview

The prehistory of Alaska's Pacific coast peoples is a complicated story for prehistorians to piece together. This was a region that came to support large human populations with diverse and complex cultural traditions, all in a state of constant interaction and change. During the Paleoarctic period a single cultural tradition was present over most of Alaska and eastern Siberia, but from that point on the Pacific coast region of Alaska followed its own course of development, largely independent from the dynamics of the Bering Sea cultural sphere. This must have been largely the result of the contrasting ecologies of the icy Bering Sea and the relatively warm Pacific Ocean, with its more diverse marine fauna and considerably greater resources of fish and shellfish, and the implications of these resources for the growth of more densely packed human populations in the south. If we compare cultures within the Pacific region, some general patterns of similarity and difference emerge that operate on different levels of culture.

At the basic economic level, Aleut, Koniag-Chugach, and northern Northwest Coast cultures had similar adaptations to the environment. This observation includes seasonal patterns of settlement, reliance on watercraft, and dependence on the harvesting and storage of salmon, and extends to many specific tool and implement types; barbed harpoon and dart heads, compound fishhooks and net sinkers, and stone lamps for burning sea mammal oil are only a few examples. It is clear, moreover, that many technical innovations appeared throughout the region at about the same time in prehistory, most notably the replacement of microblades and chipped stone tools by ground slate implements. It is on this cultural level that it is easy to point out parallel developments among Siberian cultures at similar latitudes (large coastal settlements, adoption of ground slate tools, stone oil lamps, large semisubterranean houses without entrance tunnels), which may or may not imply direct contact across the Aleutian chain. A strong candidate for direct diffusion by this route is the practice of poison dart whaling by the Itelmen, Aleuts, Koniag, and Chugach, which appears to have its origins even farther south in the highly developed use of poisons by hunting cultures of the Kurile and Japanese archipelagos (Heizer 1943).

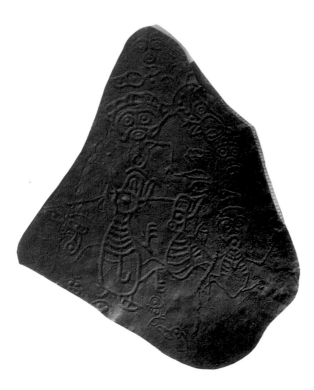

171. Petroglyph (cast)
Tsimshian

Skeletized human figures and bears dance together on this petroglyph from Ringbolt Island in the Skeena River, British Columbia. It probably depicts spiritual communication between shamans and bears, who were animal masters (MacDonald 1983). The location of the panel in a major salmon river suggests that there may be a connection with First Salmon ceremonies.

172. Whale Bone Club
Boardwalk site, Prince Rupert Harbour, B.C., ca. 500 B.C., CMC GbTo–31:522

A warrior's cache excavated at the Boardwalk site contained copper-wrapped armor rods, a stone dagger, copper bracelets, and carved war clubs, including this specimen. The face design is composed of ovoids and U-forms, and is surmounted by an animal image.

The development of complex social structures also presents a remarkable linking theme among Alaskan Pacific cultures and appears to have resulted from a general process of cultural adaptation to both the opportunities of the environment and the stresses of population growth. Increased trade and warfare have been traced as components of this development.

As these complex social systems emerged during the millennia following 3000 B.C., so did a more elaborate and intense ceremonial life and an increased emphasis on artistic expression. It is at this level of culture that diversity becomes increasingly evident throughout the late prehistory of Alaska's Pacific region. At one end of the spectrum of South Alaskan artistic traditions is Aleut art, with its accomplishments in fine grass weaving, decorated clothing, unique mask styles, and the manufacture of painted and highly ornamented hunting hats. Northwest Coast art, with its totemic symbolism and complex graphic style, appears to have started its distinctive course of development around A.D. 500 or earlier. The artistic and ceremonial Koniag inventory that develops through the upper levels at Karluk 1 is equally distinctive yet definitely Eskimo. Painted designs on wooden carvings and bowls are simple and Eskimoid, with no trace of Northwest Coast formline designs. Most masks resemble those of the Bering Sea Eskimo, to whom the Koniag were also related linguistically.

The links between Tlingit and Pacific Eskimo art as known from the contact period are numerous (Holm, this volume) yet have not for the most part been documented archeologically, even from the large and well-preserved Karluk sample. Both twined grass and spruce-root baskets have been found there, but woven hats have not been found in the midden. Frame fragments of a puffin beak rattle, used by the Koniag, Chugach, and Tlingit, have been found in the uppermost Karluk house floor. On the other hand, goat horn spoons have not been found, nor have dentalium shells, a Northwest Coast import and highly valued decorative element on Koniag and Chugach jewelry and hats during the contact period. This largely negative evidence seems to indicate that strong Tlingit influence on Koniag and Chugach art was probably a very late precontact phenomenon and may have been accentuated by the Russian practice of taking large fleets of Koniag, Chugach, and Aleut hunters into Tlingit waters to hunt sea otters.

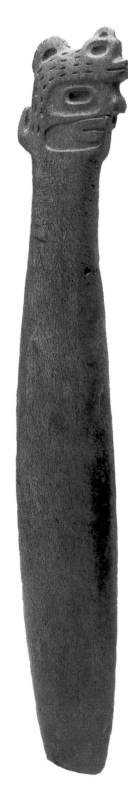

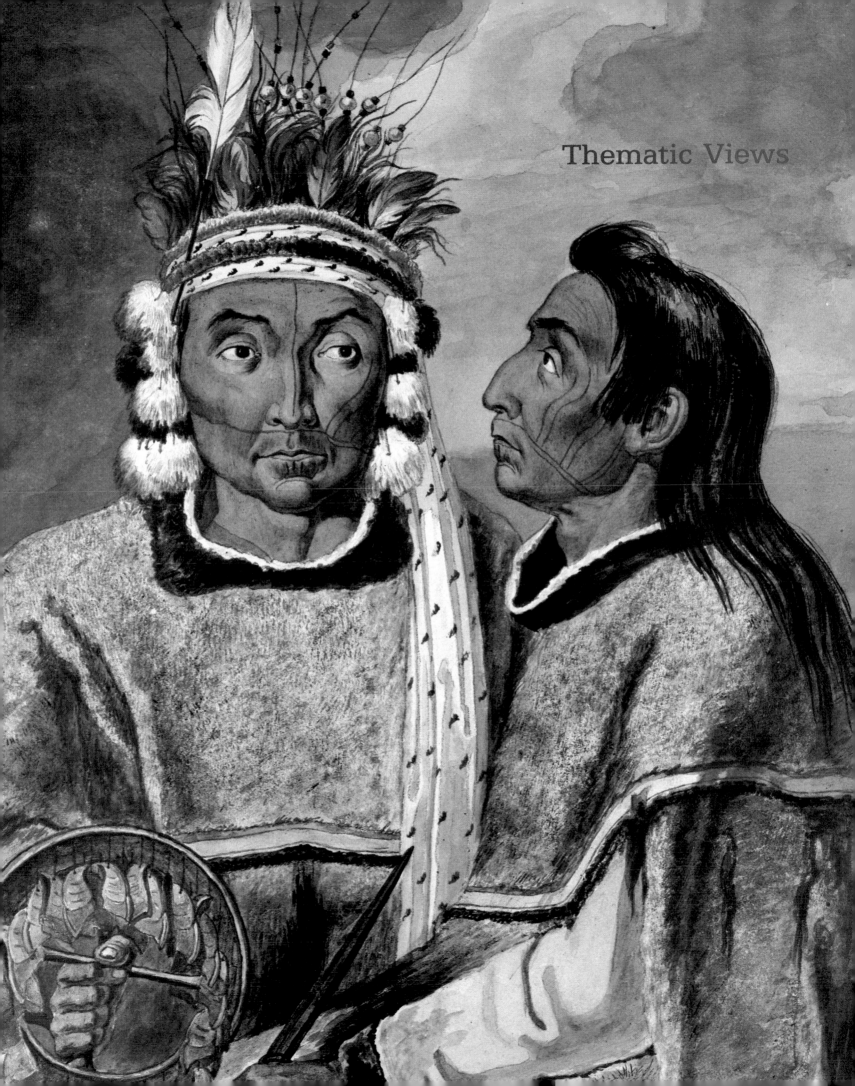

Raven's Creatures

Milton M. R. Freeman

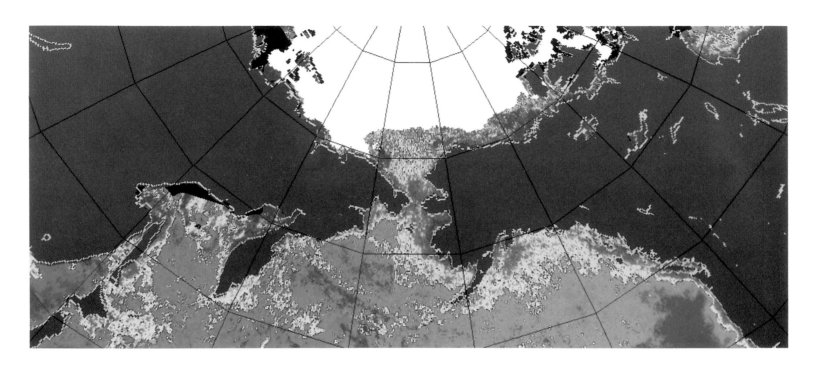

173. Biological Productivity in the North Pacific–Beringian Region
NASA Goddard Space Flight Center
This map shows summer concentrations of phytoplankton (floating microscopic plants) in the surface waters north and south of Bering Strait, composited from satellite imagery for June-September 1979, with the ice margin for mid-August. Phytoplankton concentration is indicative of general marine productivity, which is highest in shallow coastal regions, especially in the Okhotsk Sea, northern Bering Sea, and along the ice-free margins of the Arctic Ocean. The ice-edge margin (ice is shown as white) is particularly productive. The areas of high phytoplankton productivity seen here in red/yellow coincide with the major summer feeding grounds of whales. No data was available from areas shown in black.

The near-shore waters around the margin of the North Pacific are one of the most ecologically productive high latitude environments in the world (fig. 173). High marine productivity is coupled with a biogeography that concentrates resources in rivers and streams, at island passes, and along continental margins, making rich food supplies accessible to native hunters and fishermen. For these reasons almost all societies of the North Pacific Rim had a maritime component in their economies, and even inland peoples depended in part on salmon which spent most of their lives in the sea.

Unlike the land, the northern seas do not experience wide temperature differences between summer and winter; the ocean waters hover at or a few degrees above the freezing point. Since all forms of life inhabiting these low-temperature waters are cold-adapted, nutrient availability rather than temperature is most significant in determining abundance and variety of life. Sunlight, the controlling factor, is nearly absent during the long arctic winter and nearly continuous during summer.

The waters of the greater North Pacific Ocean extend north to the Bering Strait and encompass the Bering Sea and the Okhotsk Sea. North of Bering Strait are the Chukchi and Beaufort seas.

All these seas are cold, being influenced by currents originating in the Arctic Ocean, and have seasonal ice cover. However, along the American coast, including the Aleutian chain, a strong current sweeping across from Japan contributes warmer water, resulting in winters mostly free of sea ice. Absence of sea ice allows the development of rich marine plant and animal communities in intertidal and shallow coastal waters. Production of microscopic and small-sized plant and animal plankton species is essentially a summer phenomenon especially in ice-edge waters (fig. 173).

The result of high plankton productivity is an abundance of animals higher on the food chain that are of direct importance to man. Those easiest to harvest are the edible crabs, molluscs, and sea urchins, species that, in turn, support higher life forms such as fish, birds, and sea mammals that supplied natives with most of the means for survival. More abundant, diverse, and stable than land species, these marine species provided the basis for the larger and more sedentary human populations that inhabit the coastal regions of the North Pacific and Beringian regions.

Of the more than 2,000 species of fish in the region, salmon were of greatest importance to man because their spawning behavior brought them to shores and rivers where they could be caught. Five species of salmon return annually to North American rivers to breed, and six species return to Japanese and Siberian rivers. The richness of cultural development in the North Pacific region owes more to the abundance and security provided by salmon than to any other species. Other fish, like herring, mackerel, cod, and pollack, migrate annually into shallow coastal waters where they can be caught, and they are followed by larger predators such as seals and whales (fig. 207) that, in turn, become available to coastal hunters.

Especially important in arctic marine ecosystems are the large marine mammals, including polar bears (north of Bering Strait), sea lions, several seal species, sea otters, walrus, whales, and the now-extinct Steller sea cow. The gregarious nature of sea otters, walrus, and sea lions facilitated native hunting. Migratory species like whales brought the resource base of the greater Pacific Ocean within reach of northern hunters, whereas resident species like walrus and ice-dwelling seals provided northern hunters with winter sustenance.

Both in North America and Siberia the most important feature of land ecology is the distinction between forest and tundra (fig. 1). Wood was of great importance to man, and its absence in arctic regions delayed human settlement here for thousands of years. In North America the northern boreal forest is dominated by black spruce, whereas on the Siberian side of Bering Strait larch is the dominant northern tree species. However, on both continents, willows, alders, and occasional birch stands extend north into the tundra in protected river valleys, sometimes to the shore of the Arctic Ocean itself, where by default driftwood was the primary source of wood. In these regions the availability of driftwood was important.

Winters in these northern regions are long and cold. Although summers are short, long hours of sunshine result in a surprising abundance of life. For man, the most important land mammals are herbivores: wild caribou in North America and their domesticated relative, reindeer, in Siberia; without their meat, warm fur, sinew, antler, and bone, human survival in the northern interior would not have been possible. Black and brown (grizzly) bears, moose, Dall sheep, mountain goats, otters, and beaver and

other rodents played more minor roles. The carnivores (wolves, wolverines, lynx, mink) were less numerous and less important to man as food, but they contributed skins and furs for garments and other manufactures. Most of these animals were present on both sides of Bering Strait, an exception being the porcupine, which does not occur in Siberia.

The immense birdlife of the North Pacific region, many species of which are also migratory, was also important for human survival. In addition to their food value, bird skins and feathers contributed to clothing, ornamentation, and religious life. Finally, this survey would not be complete without mention of the many edible plant resources available, including the berries, leafy salad plants, and some small tuberous

roots, that add vitamins and tasty treats to the dominant fish, meat, and fat diet.

In the end, biological richness and diversity coupled with the accumulation of human knowledge led to the development of the complex cultures of the North Pacific region. That this knowledge could be distributed rapidly throughout a wide region, as demonstrated by the spread of the aconite poison hunting technique for hunting large whales (p. 172), contributed to producing cultural similarities noted in this vast region.

174. Walrus Herd on the Chukotka Coast

Survival of human populations in Bering Strait and along the coasts of the Arctic ocean would not be possible without the large walrus herds that frequent these regions. Walruses, gregarious creatures, live near the edge of the arctic pack ice, migrating with the seasonal advance and retreat of the pack from its winter margin in the southern Bering Sea to its summer position north of the Arctic Ocean coast. In addition to walrus providing meat for men and dogs, its blubber was a source of fuel for cooking and lighting, its hide was used to cover boat frames, and its ivory tusks and bones provided raw material for innumerable items, from harpoons to ornaments.

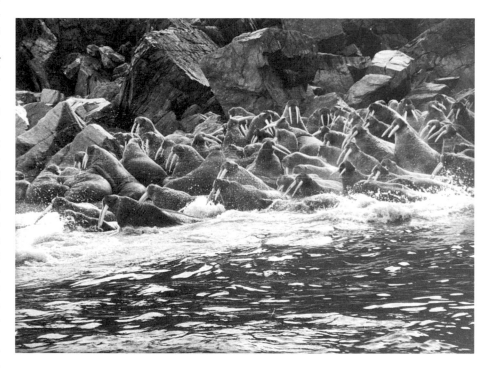

Opposite:
"[Aleut] Inhabitant of Unimak Island Named Umasik, Baptised Vasili" (Mikhail Tikhanov, 1817, RIPSA 2123)

143

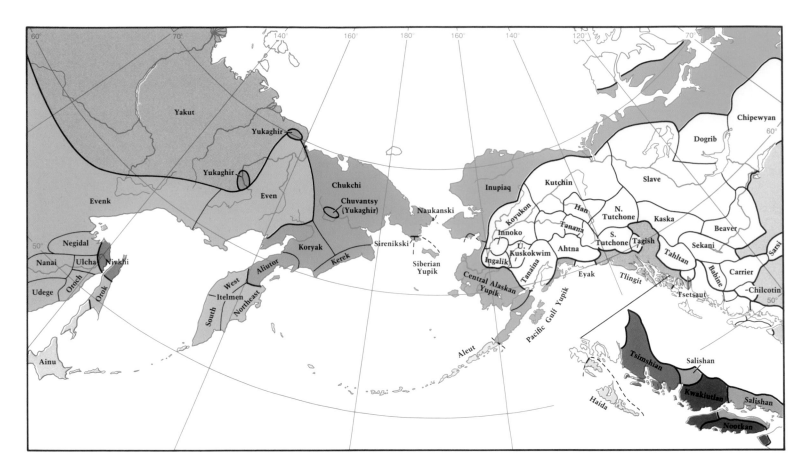

TABLE 2

1980 Populations and Speakers of North Pacific Region Languages

Language Family		Language Name	Population	Speakers
TUNGUSIC		Udege	1,600	500
		Oroch	1,200	490
		Nanai/Goldi (USSR)	10,500	5,860
		* Nanai/Goldi (China)	1,476	300
		Ulcha	2,600	1,010
		* Orok	400	
		Negidal	500	220
		* Solon (China)	19,343	19,000
		Evenk/Tungus (USSR)	28,000	12,070
		* Evenk/Tungus (Mongolia)	2,000	
		* Evenk/Tungus (Oroqen: China)	4,132	4,000
		Even/Lamut	12,000	6,800
NIVKHI/GILYAK		Nivkhi	4,400	1,350
AINU		Ainu	15,000	10
TURKIC		Yakut	328,000	312,000
YUKAGHIR		Yukaghir	800	300
CHUKOTKO- KAMCHATKAN		* Itelmen/Kamchadal	1,400	100
		Koryak and Aliutor	7,900	5,450
		* Aliutor subtotal	2,800	1,930
		Kerek	400	<100
		Chukchi	14,000	10,960
ESKIMO-ALEUT		Inupiaq (Alaska)	12,500	5,000
		Sirenikski		2
		Siberian Yupik	2,000	1,550
		* Chaplinski (USSR) subtotal	900	500
		* St. Lawrence Is. (USA) sub.	1,100	1,050
		* Naukanski	400	200
		Central Alaskan Yupik	18,000	13,000
		Pacific Gulf Yupik	3,100	800
		Aleut (USA)	2,100	700
		* Aleut (USSR)	300	20

Language Family		Language Name	Population	Speakers
ATHAPASKAN- EYAK		Ahtna	500	100
		Tanaina	800	150
		Ingalik	400	80
		Innoko	150	20
		Koyukon	2500	650
		Upper Kuskokwim	150	120
		Tanana	350	70
		Tanacross	200	100
		Upper Tanana	300	200
		Han	260	30
		Kutchin	2,200	1,000
		Eyak	5	2
TLINGIT		Tlingit	10,000	2,000
HAIDA		Haida	1,700	250
TSIMSHIAN		Coast Tsimshian	3,500	200
		Nass-Gitksan	6,000	3,000
WAKASHAN (KWAKIUTLAN)		Haisla	1,000	a few hundred
		Heiltsuk-Oowekyala	1,400	ca.250
		Kwakiutl	3,500	1,000
WAKASHAN (NOOTKAN)		Nootka	4,700	1–2,000
		Nitinat		ca. 60
		Makah	1,000	ca. 25
SALISHAN		Bella Coola	1,300	<1,000

Note: Unless otherwise marked (*), figures for USSR groups are from the USSR 1979 census (with number of speakers converted from percentages) and adapted from Krauss 1982 map of Alaska Native Languages and from *Handbook of North American Indians,* Volumes 5 (Arctic), Volume 6 (Subarctic), and Volume 7 (Northwest Coast, forthcoming).

Many Tongues—Ancient Tales

Michael E. Krauss

175. Languages of the Greater North Pacific Region, A.D. 1900

The native languages shown on the map of the North Pacific area (fig. 175) fall into four main families or groupings, two on the American side of the Bering Strait and two on the Asiatic. From the earliest days of European discovery in this part of the world, linguists have considered possible genetic relationships between American language families and ones in Asia, whence they must have come. Though debate is as lively today as ever before, still no proof of genetic relationship of any native American language family to any Asiatic language family has yet been offered that satisfies even a majority of linguists who have carefully studied such subjects.

So the question remains not whether American languages came from Asia, which most linguists agree must be so, but rather whether any link between specific families has been convincingly demonstrated. At best, such ge-

netic relationships are certainly not obvious, as they are for instance between English and German, or French and Spanish, and even between Germanic and Romance (both being branches of Indo-European). Rather, if they exist, they have been obscured by the passage of time, for establishing convincing links as one approaches 5,000 years of language separation becomes increasingly difficult, and as separations increase toward 10,000 years, it becomes generally impossible. Negative proof, that any two languages are not related, not descended from a common ancestor, is of course impossible. It is therefore possible that all the world's languages might ultimately be related. Thus, as yet, linguistic links between Asia and America remain unproven with the single obvious exception of Eskimo, of which closely related varieties are found on both sides of the Bering Strait.

Language Families

Na-Dene

The dominant Indian language family of northwestern America is called Na-Dene, coined by Edward Sapir (1915) from the Haida and Athapaskan words for "people." This family consists of Haida, Tlingit, Eyak, and Athapaskan, whose relationships are shown in figure 176. Athapaskan is itself a large family of closely related

languages. Centering inland, Athapaskan has spread far beyond its original area of some 2,000 years ago, perhaps in the upper Yukon River region, throughout much of interior Alaska and northwestern Canada, and thence to southern Oregon and northern California, and separately in the Southwest, where it is spoken by Navajo and Apache. The Athapaskan family is a complex of languages and dialects, which consists of some 30 languages, 11 of which are found in Alaska. Today there are over 230,000 Athapaskans; 10,000 are Native Alaskan, 25,000 Canadian, 3,000 Californian and Oregonian, and 195,000 Navajo and Apache.

Coordinate to this vast Athapaskan family is the subbranch Eyak, a single language, which is now nearly extinct. Formerly spoken on the Gulf of Alaska coast from Yakutat Bay to Comptroller

176. Na-Dene Language Group

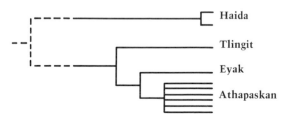

Haida

Tlingit

Eyak

Athapaskan

Bay, where it was being progressively assimilated to Tlingit, its last stronghold at Eyak Lake was discovered by Frederica de Laguna in 1930. Eyak proves to be an important link in showing genetic relationship between Athapaskan and Tlingit.

Of the many languages of the Northwest Coast, Tlingit occupies by far the longest stretch, virtually the whole of the Alaska Panhandle. A single language, Tlingit is easily intelligible throughout its wide distribution because of a relatively recent expansion from the south, judging from the greater dialectical differences within Southern Tlingit. The Tlingit population is approximately 10,000, some of which expanded into the interior of the Yukon Territory in early contact times. The genetic relationship of Tlingit to Athapaskan-Eyak is more distant and somewhat problematical in that although its grammatical structure is very similar to the Athapaskan-Eyak, much of its vocabulary seems to be unrelated and may come from some other unknown population.

Another major Northwest Coast power was the Haida, who inhabit the Queen Charlotte Islands and took over the southern half of Prince of Wales Island from the Tlingit in the early 18th century. After a catastrophic decline from 10,000 to 2,000 in the 19th century, the Southern Haida survivors gathered at Skidegate and the Northern survivors at Masset on the Queen Charlotte side and at Hydaburg in Alaska. Northern and Southern Haida are highly divergent dialects, only partly intelligible to one another. Sapir was the most influential of the linguists who have asserted that Haida in turn is genetically related to Athapaskan-Eyak—Tlingit, and he named the family Na-Dene to reflect this link. Franz Boas remained skeptical about this and about Athapaskan-Tlingit ties, and many modern specialists dispute it.

Eskimo-Aleut

The Eskimo-Aleut family (fig. 177) is best known for its importance in arctic Canada and Greenland, but this represents the recent expansion over the last 1,000 years of but one branch of Eskimo, the Inuit, while the Yupik branch of the family and the Aleut language remain in their ancestral homelands about the Bering Sea.

Though recognized on a sound basis as genetically related to Eskimo in 1818 by Rasmus Rask, the divergence between Aleut and Eskimo is far greater than any divergence within Eskimo, about what might be expected after 4,000 years or more, more than twice the time to which the divergence within Eskimo might be attributed. The sharp linguistic border between Aleut and

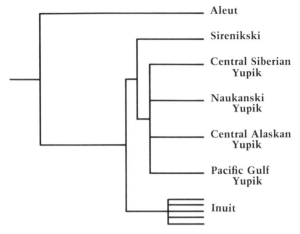

Eskimo is no doubt due not to ancient separation but rather to the complete elimination of prehistoric intermediate languages by Eskimo and Aleut, which now meet on the Alaska Peninsula. Today Aleut is a single language with two main dialects, Western (Attuan and Atkan subdialects) and Eastern. The Aleut population was severely reduced during the 18th century. Also during the Russian period, colonies of Aleuts were established on the Pribilof and Commander islands and remain there to this day.

The Inuit branch of Eskimo (Inupiaq in Alaska, Inuktitut in Canada, Kalaallisut in Greenland) is a continuum of interconnecting dialects, as might be expected from their recent spread. Inuit is practically a national language in Greenland, with 45,000 speakers and an important literature since the 18th century. It is strong, too, in Canada, especially in the East, with 18,000 speakers among a population of 25,000. Inuit seems destined to remain the major native language of the New World Arctic. The dialect (Imaklikskii) spoken by the few Inuit remaining in 1948 on Big Diomede Island in the Soviet Union is now extinct.

The Yupik branch of Eskimo is a broken chain of five languages, which once must have connected from the Alaska mainland to the Chukchi Peninsula via the Seward Peninsula. Pacific Gulf Yupik (also known as Sugpiaq, Alutiiq, Suk, and popularly also known as Aleut because of Russian tradition) consists of two main dialects, Chugach and Koniag. This population was also severely reduced, from about 10,000 to 3,000, during the colonial period.

Central Alaskan Yupik is the largest ethnic group in Alaska and is the language now spoken by the largest number of native persons in both the American and Soviet sides of the North Pacific Rim. It is a single well-defined language with four dialects diverging from the main one: Egegik (Aglegmuit-Tarupiaq); Nunivak; Hooper Bay–Chevak, diverging in the direction of Pacific

Gulf Yupik; and Unaliq in Norton Sound, diverging in the direction of Siberian Yupik or Naukanski in the Soviet Union.

The next link in the Yupik chain is Naukanski, spoken at Naukan on East Cape and since 1958 mainly in St. Lawrence Bay. This language is in several respects intermediate between Central Alaskan Yupik and Siberian Yupik. Siberian Yupik was spoken by the Eskimo along most of the east coast of the Chukchi Peninsula during the 19th century and perhaps also along its Arctic Ocean coast. Siberian Yupik was and still is not only the main Eskimo language of the Soviet Union, where it is known as Chaplinski, but is also virtually identical with the language of St. Lawrence Island, Alaska, where it is now spoken by an even larger number of people, including most children.

Sirenikski is now remembered by only two elderly persons at Sireniki. All but replaced by Chaplinski, Sirenikski is a relic of the Eskimo language earlier spoken more widely on the southern coast of the Chukchi Peninsula. Sirenikski shows evidence of having been so different from Chaplinski that it should perhaps be classed not only as a separate branch of Yupik but also as a coordinate subbranch of Eskimo, with Yupik, as shown in figure 177, or even as a third branch of Eskimo.

It is proposed that the Eskimo languages on the Siberian side represent relatively minor westward movement back to and into the Chukchi Peninsula from Alaska, and that Sirenikski represents the oldest wave of that movement, Siberian Yupik the second, and Naukanski the latest. The Yupik chain was then broken between Asia and America not by the Bering Strait but by progressive Inuit occupation of Seward Peninsula, while on the Asiatic side Chukchi expanded into much of the coastline during the late prehistoric period.

Chukotko-Kamchatkan

On the Soviet side, except for Eskimo and Commander Island Aleut, the easternmost language family or grouping may be called Chukotko-Kamchatkan, consisting of two groups: the Itelmen (Kamchadal) and Chukchi-Koryak. Itelmen was formerly spoken throughout most of Kamchatka in three forms, which may have been separate languages rather than dialects, by a population of perhaps 20,000. Kamchatka was Russianized early, however, and the population was decimated; only Western Itelmen remained long into this century, and that too is now approaching extinction.

The Chukchi-Koryak group, though traditionally considered to consist of two, or more recently four, languages, is perhaps no more diverse than Itelmen was and might yet be considered as a single complex or chain of dialects. The largest and most uniform by far is Chukchi, represented also by the largest population of any of the Soviet native groups on the North Pacific. On the coast between Chukchi and Koryak is Kerek, formerly considered a dialect of Chukchi or of Koryak and now recognized as a separate language, but now also nearing extinction. Within Koryak itself there is significant dialectal diversity; the southern three Koryak subgroups are now considered by some authorities to be a separate language, named Aliutor. The markedly decreasing diversity within Chukotko-Kamchatkan from Kamchatka towards Chukotka may well imply that this family spread in a northeastward direction. Some authorities even propose that Kamchadal is genetically related to Chukchi-Koryak (fig. 178).

Tungusic and Others

Southwest of the Chukotko-Kamchatkan language area is the Tungusic (fig. 179). The major language group of the mainland Okhotsk shore belongs to the northern branch of this Tungusic family. Two languages of this branch, Evenk and Even, have undergone vast expansion. Evenk (or Tungus) is found even past the Yenisey, 2,000 miles to the west, while Even (or Lamut) not only dominates the upper Kolyma region but has also spread to the Arctic Ocean, the Lena River, and Kamchatka. However, the density of Northern Tungusic speakers in the Soviet Union is low, 28,000 Evenk and 12,000 Even, and is mixed with Yakut and others and increasingly with Russian. Negidal is a third variety of Northern Tungusic spoken by a small group on the Lower Amur. Still other varieties of Northern Tungusic are spoken on the Chinese side of the Amur, Orochen and Solon, both probably most similar to Evenk.

The Southern Tungusic languages are a far more compact and diversified branch, subdivided into the Southeastern and Southwestern subbranches. Southwestern Tungusic is Manchu,

178. Chukotko-Kamchatkan Language Group

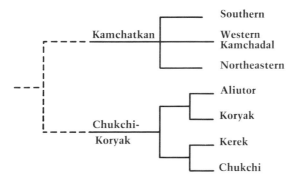

147

now said to be approaching extinction but once the language of the ruling class of China and an empire. Southeastern Tungusic, the dominant language group of the Amur region, is in turn divided into two subgroups, the Nanai-Ulcha-Orok and the Udege-Oroch; the Nanai (or Goldi) are numerically by far the largest group. Here again, the much greater diversity of Tungusic in the south probably implies northward spread.

Another language that has undergone a vast and spectacular spread into Northeastern Siberia, still more recently, during the last few centuries, is Yakut, belonging to the expansive Turkic family, whose origin must lie far to the southwest. Yakuts are by far the most numerous of all Native Siberians, numbering more than 300,000 and occupying much of Siberia to the arctic coast, now even to the Okhotsk shore.

It was, however, the Yukaghir that were formerly spread over the largest part of Northeastern Siberia. As in the case of the Northern Tungusic, Yukaghir population density was very low. They once occupied most of the northern Yakut and Even territory but are now reduced to one of the smallest of Soviet nationalities, in two widely separated and divergent dialect enclaves, the Tundra and Upper Kolyma. The Yukaghir language is not proven to be genetically related to any other.

Another such isolated language is the Nivkhi (or Gilyak) of the Lower Amur and northern Sakhalin, not yet shown to be genetically related

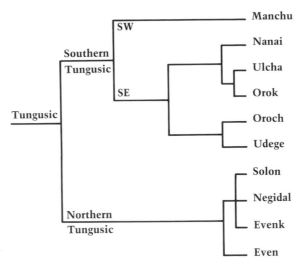

179. Tungusic Language Family

to any other. Ainu, formerly spoken on the Kurile Islands and southern Sakhalin, where it is entirely extinct, and on Hokkaido in northern Japan, where it is nearly extinct, is also not yet proven to be genetically related to any other.

Yukaghir and Nivkhi, and sometimes Ainu, have been classed together with Chukotko-Kamchatkan in a grouping called Paleosiberian or Paleoasiatic. This grouping does not imply any claims of genetic relationship but rather emphasizes that these languages are relics of families much more ancient to the Soviet Far East than the Tungusic and Turkic, which expanded more recently into it from the south and west.

Asian-American Comparisons

The general direction of these movements accords with the obvious eastward trend across the Bering Strait area. Of the movements of languages into America, a most recent theory (Greenberg 1987) is that all but Na-Dene and Eskimo-Aleut belong to a single family called Amerind that came to America 12,000 to 15,000 years ago. Though this theory of the genetic unity of Amerind has not won widespread acceptance, the notion that Na-Dene, as previously noted by Sapir (1916:455), belonged to a different and later wave, and Eskimo to a still later wave, is more widely accepted. Even these much later movements, of approximately 6000–7000 and 4000–5000 years ago according to Greenberg, are old enough that most linguists do not believe Asiatic links for them are proven. Nevertheless Eskimo-Aleut and Na-Dene remain of course the best candidates for such linking.

The most promising candidate for intercontinental linkage would be Eskimo-Aleut, the newest and westernmost American family, with

Chukotko-Kamchatkan an old and easternmost Asiatic one. This possibility was examined in the 1770s by P. Pallas (Coxe 1780:303), who noted that Aleut was remarkably unlike Koryak and Itelmen (and Ainu). Although some typological similarity in sound and grammatical structure exists, studies by linguists over two centuries attempting to link these two families (Swadesh 1962) remain disappointing. At best, they are no more convincing than attempts to link Eskimo-Aleut with other language families of Eurasia. As probably the latest in the long chain of such attempts, one may mention the ideas of one group of Soviet comparativists including S. A. Starostin and others who believe that Eskimo belongs to the so-called Nostratic macrofamily together with Indo-European, Uralo-Altaic, Semito-Khamitic, Dravidian, and others, while Na-Dene belongs to a quite different macrofamily together with Sino-Tibetan, Ket, North Caucasian, Burushaski, and others, called Sino-Dagestanic.

Historical and Modern Development

We shall now consider the historical period, contact of these languages with Russian and English, and their present situation. By 1648 Russian speakers had reached East Cape, and a century later the Aleutians. In 1778 these people heard English for the first time, from members of Capt. James Cook's expedition. Now, in 1988, the vast majority of each of these native populations speaks Russian on the Soviet side and English on the American (and in most cases, on both sides, their children now speak only Russian or English).

However, there are some significant historical twists to this. During the period 1741 to 1867, when Alaska was Russian, Russian was the first contact language for many of the Alaskan groups. The degree and type of this Russian impact can be measured by the number of Russian loan words, usually names for new materials and concepts, in each. These figures can be calculated from our documentation of these languages and because the diffusion from Russian mostly ceased after 1867. Aleut has the most, with about 600; Pacific Gulf Yupik has about 500, Tanaina Athapaskan about 400, Central Alaskan Yupik about 200; Koyukon, Upper Kuskokwim, and Ahtna Athapaskan each have about 80; Ingalik 60, and Innoko 50. One sees the influence fading in the three dialects of the Tanana language as one ascends the Tanana River, from 45 to 35 to 25 such loans, with finally 5 in Tanacross. Upper Tanana, Han, and Kutchin have no loans from Russian, the first contact language in that area being "Slavey" jargon (with French) and English. Eyak has about 30 (mainly via Chugach Yupik). Interestingly, Tlingit has only 9, in spite of the fact that the very capital of Russian Alaska was in their territory, an indication of the cultural resistance of the Tlingit people to Russian domination. In the Bering Strait area, Russian presence was relatively weak. In Inupiaq there are about 15 Russian loan words, and on St. Lawrence Island even fewer, only 10.

In fact, in the Beringian area from about 1850, and on the Asiatic as well as American side of the strait into the 1920s, the dominant contact language was English, first from the Franklin search expeditions and later from American whalers and traders. Thus, ironically, the Alaskan Yupik words for butter, soap, cat, and cow are from Russian: *maslaq, miilaq, kuskaq, kuluvak;* but in Siberian Yupik they are from English: *bara, suupa, kiti,* and *kaakw.* Some of the English loans can also be found in Chukchi and perhaps also in Koryak. This exchange of loan words continues cultural, genetic, and historical exchanges that have characterized the North Pacific region for millennia and is paralleled most especially in the history of ethnological collecting on which this exhibition rests.

Language Policy

During the 1830s and 1840s in Alaska the Russian Orthodox priest Ioann Veniaminov began a remarkable mission school system that included written use of four Alaskan languages: Aleut, Pacific Gulf Yupik, Central Alaskan Yupik, and Tlingit, adapting the Cyrillic alphabet rather well (in the case of the first three) to the sounds of these languages. The first book, an Aleut catechism, was printed in 1834. Vernacular literacy soon became a part of Aleut culture, and to a lesser extent also in Pacific Gulf and Central Alaskan Yupik. Toward the end of the 19th century, American missionary work included some written use of several Alaskan languages, while on the Russian side there was relatively little such activity. During most of the 19th and 20th century, however, American (and Canadian) educational systems excluded and even suppressed the use of these native languages. On the Asian side, in contrast, after the Russian Revolution, Soviet schools began instruction in many of the languages of the northern minority peoples in the early grades, using books in these languages first during the early 1930s printed in the Roman-based "Alphabet of the Peoples of the North" but converted to Cyrillic alphabet in 1936–7. Thus for these schools books were printed in Soviet Eskimo (Chaplinski), Chukchi, Koryak, Itelmen, Nivhki, Even, Evenk, Nanai, and Udege (though not in Oroch, Ulcha, Orok, Negidal, or Yukaghir, because their numbers were so small; not in Kerek, Aliutor, Sirenikski, or Naukanski, because these were not officially recognized as separate languages). A primer was drafted in Commander Island Aleut but was not printed, and for Itelmen and Udege the vernacular programs were short-lived or not implemented. For the others, however, Soviet educational use and cultivation continued into the 1950s. But in the 1960s a policy began to dominate that resembled the American, with vernacular education and publication declining sharply. In the 1970s American educational policy began to favor the use of the native languages of the area, followed soon also by the Soviet. However, on each side, under the cultural pressure of English and Russian, children were no longer learning their ancestral languages from their parents. On the American side most of these languages are spoken now by few or none under the age of 40, with the exception of St. Lawrence Island, where most children still learn the language, as also in a large part of the Central Alaskan Yupik region, and Aleut at Atka. The languages on the Soviet side, with the definite exception of Yakut and possible exception of some Chukchi, are now spoken by few or none under the age of 20. It thus becomes a race against time to document these languages as fully as possible before they are lost, and their revival or survival as living languages in both Asia and America is a question for the coming century.

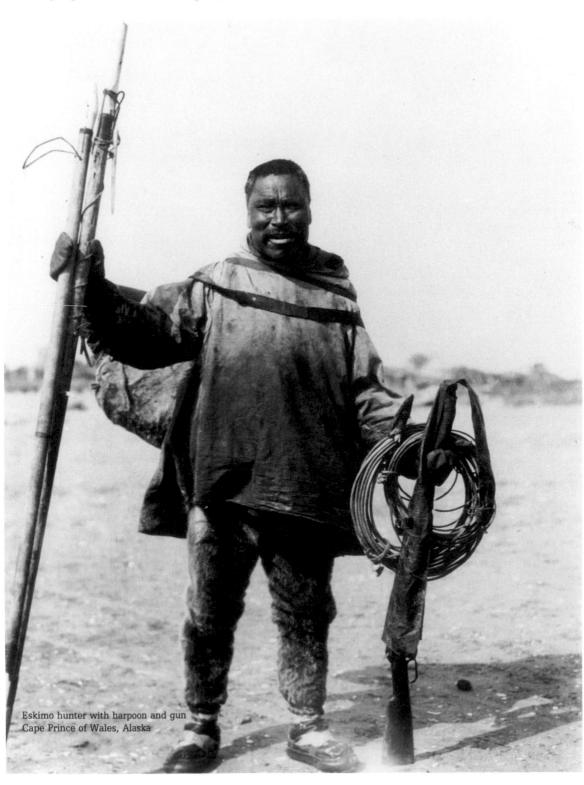

Eskimo hunter with harpoon and gun
Cape Prince of Wales, Alaska

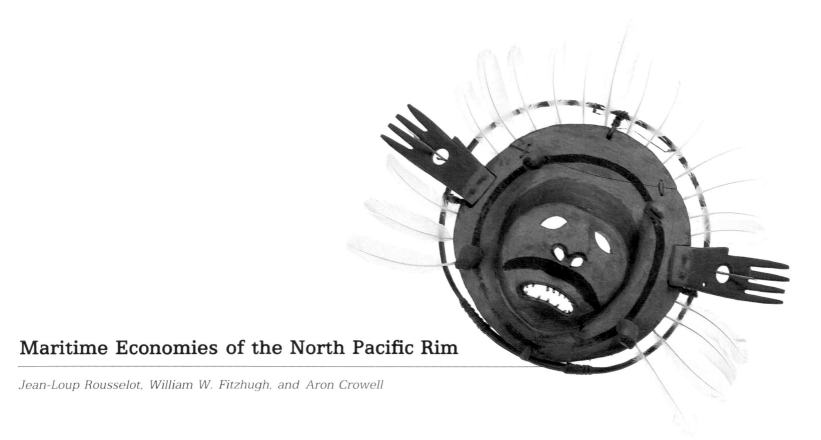

Maritime Economies of the North Pacific Rim

Jean-Loup Rousselot, William W. Fitzhugh, and Aron Crowell

180. *Tunghak*, Keeper of the Game
Bering Sea Eskimo: NMNH 64241

Yupik Eskimos of western Alaska believed that animals were controlled by a master spirit known as *Tunghak*. *Tunghak* lived in the moon, was part animal and part human, was ferocious and powerful, and if displeased could punish man by withhold animals from him. One of the roles of the shaman was to intercede with *Tunghak* on man's behalf.

The hoops and feathers on this mask relate to the *Tunghak*'s residence in the sky. Thumbless hands may refer to impaired grasp. Pierced palms signify the hole in the Sky World which the *Tunghak* controlled and through which animals passed to repopulate the earth.

Most North Pacific and Bering Sea peoples shared the concept of a game master, known variously as *Keretkun* (Chukchi), *Kasak* (Asian Eskimo), *Na'ininen* (Koryak), and *Agudar* (Aleut).

The native peoples of the North Pacific Rim, the great bicontinental arc that circumscribes the northern reaches of the Pacific Ocean, occupy one of the richest maritime environments in the world. Its varied resources include many species of sea mammals, fish, birds, and shellfish, which provide the basis for coastal habitation throughout the year. The ocean exerts a strong unifying influence on the cultures of the region, by providing common adaptational challenges and by facilitating human movement and communication. It was apparent from the earliest era of Russian and European exploration that the seafaring native peoples of the Pacific Rim were linked together in a long intergrading chain by similarities in their ways of life and in physical appearance.

Economic similarities in particular may be traced great distances along the coasts of the North Pacific Rim, while adjoining coastal and inland populations are sharply differentiated in this respect. Typically, coastal groups lived in large villages, occupied permanent winter dwellings on a seasonal or year-round basis, and accumulated large stores of food during the spring and summer for consumption in colder months when food was scarce. Sea mammal hunting and fishing were of primary importance, although considerable regional variation occurred. In northern areas of seasonal sea ice, sea mammal hunting was more important than fishing, whereas in regions south of the Aleutian Islands these conditions were reversed. Hunting

of land animals occurred but was of lesser economic importance. Throughout the region, changing seasonal conditions affected the yearly cycle of economic activity through their effect on animal migration patterns and weather conditions. Some pursuits that had great social and economic importance, such as whaling, could only be practiced for a brief period each year and were highly unpredictable.

Economic activities never exist in a cultural vacuum; they entail social organization, as well as tools and a body of technical knowledge. They require certain kinds of leadership, organization, and investment. They may also be integrated, to a greater or lesser degree, with supporting belief systems that find expression in art, magic, and ritual. In North Pacific cultures the linkage between subsistence practices and religious ideology is particularly strong and is manifested in communal hunting ceremonies, magical and ritual practices connected with hunting, and in the artistry of hunting implements and other manufactured objects. Few culture areas of the world exhibit so close a relationship between the functional and symbolic attributes of material objects.

Magic and artistry are especially evident in the sea mammal hunting technology of the Alaskan Eskimo, Aleuts, and Northwest Coast Indians. Like all North Pacific groups, these peoples believed that hunting success was determined by the willingness of the animal spirits to make themselves available to the hunter, rather than by luck or hunting prowess. Clean and new clothing, the magic power of hunting hats, amulets, and face charm plaques, and the beauty of carefully crafted hunting weapons all served to please and attract the spirits of game animals. Eskimo weapons were sometimes given additional power by being ornamented with the images of predatory animals or beasts, which served the hunter as helping spirits. Bering Sea Eskimo harpoons carried images of wolflike beasts on their socketpieces, and harpoon heads were frequently ornamented with designs of predatory birds like cormorants, gulls, and hawks. Harpoon lines and floats were decorated with ivory rattles that were inset with dark wood or baleen plugs and sprigs of seal hair, float plugs carried spirit face images, and line attachers

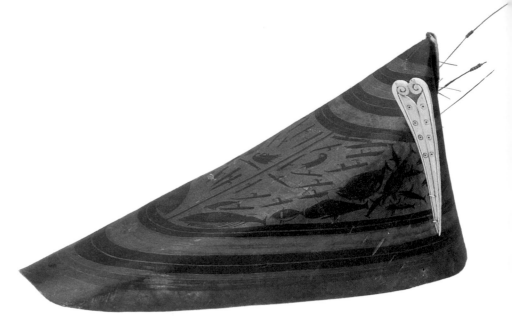

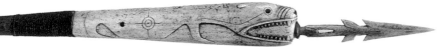

were carved with complex zoomorphic images. In short, the serious sea mammal hunter's equipment was elegantly designed and beautifully maintained as a sign of respect to his prey. These values, as much as functional design, were fundamental to a hunter's success. These practices had ancient origins among early cultures of the North Pacific and are especially noted in the hunting technology and art of the Old Bering Sea culture.

The following description of maritime subsistence systems of the North Pacific Rim portrays ways of life at the time of the first contacts

with Western civilization. However, the millennia that passed before the arrival of Europeans should not be seen as a time of stasis, for it is clear that the aboriginal period saw continual change in artifact design, development of new hunting methods, and flux in the strength and degree of isolation of regional traditions. Although the opening of Alaska and Siberia to new raw materials (metal, glass, cloth) and manufactured implements (nets, rifles, and harpoon guns) changed native cultures, diversified patterns of traditional fishing, sealing, and whaling continue in the late 20th century.

181. Hunting Magic
Aglegmiut Eskimo: NMNH 127766, 127777 (socket piece, point). Aleut: MAE 2868-83 (hat)

To insure hunting success, weapons were decorated with images of powerful predators, and special clothing was worn. This elegant ritual hunting hat shows killer whales attacking large whales and kayak hunters surrounding a sea otter, whose ivory image adorns the peak of the hat.

Fishing

Fish were everywhere important if not preeminent in terms of caloric contribution to the diet, especially in the southern area of our region—Kamchatka, the Aleutians, the southern coast of Alaska, and British Columbia—where fish resources were most abundant. Methods and fishing equipment used in different areas showed relatively minor technical variation but varied in importance according to ecological conditions and the local abundance of various species.

The limited nature and, in some cases, complete lack of rites and ceremonies associated with fishing enterprises is a curious feature of the northernmost Pacific Rim cultures. For instance, among the Bering Sea and North Alaskan Eskimo, little ceremonial or ritual attention was given to fish, even in areas where fish provided the bulk of the diet. Masks representing fish

were rare, whereas those of birds and mammals were common. Perhaps the spiritual elements of sea mammal hunting were more emphasized because it was usually a more dangerous activity than fishing, and because the hunter engaged individual, observable animals rather than an invisible and undifferentiated mass of organisms. Rituals and the invoking of spirit helpers did characterize halibut fishing, but these fish were taken at sea in open boats or kayaks and are large, powerful, and dangerous. Among various Northwest Coast groups the First Salmon ceremony was an important annual renewal rite, reflecting the overriding economic importance of salmon in that region. In this case, however, it was an individual (the first salmon caught) that represented the mass of other fish.

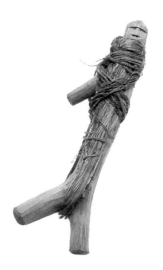

182. Guardian of the Nets
Koryak: AMNH 70-2752

Dressed in magically powerful grass, anthropomorphic amulets (kamak-lo) guarded Koryak nets from the incantations of wicked people and guaranteed a large catch. Periodically these amulets were ritually fed with the blood and blubber of sea mammals.

152

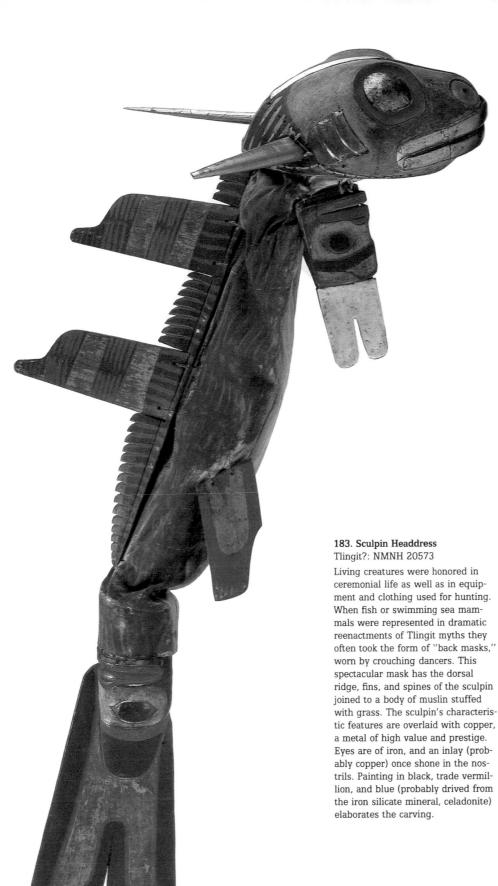

183. Sculpin Headdress
Tlingit?: NMNH 20573

Living creatures were honored in ceremonial life as well as in equipment and clothing used for hunting. When fish or swimming sea mammals were represented in dramatic reenactments of Tlingit myths they often took the form of "back masks," worn by crouching dancers. This spectacular mask has the dorsal ridge, fins, and spines of the sculpin joined to a body of muslin stuffed with grass. The sculpin's characteristic features are overlaid with copper, a metal of high value and prestige. Eyes are of iron, and an inlay (probably copper) once shone in the nostrils. Painting in black, trade vermillion, and blue (probably drived from the iron silicate mineral, celadonite) elaborates the carving.

Net and Weir Fishing

Some fishing methods were designed for mass harvesting, especially of salmon and other fish that spawn in rivers. Salmon were the most important fish resource of the North Pacific and were taken by all groups as far north as Bering Strait. Not only were salmon a major summer food but they were also preserved for fall and winter use and provided the economic basis for fall and winter festival life. Five species were available, each of which had different characteristics in terms of the timing of runs, preservability, taste, and nutritional value. In mid-June, when the first salmon runs begin, they were caught by fishermen wearing waterproof clothing who pulled seines and gill nets through the shallows. The Tlingit and Pacific Eskimo took salmon concentrated at V-shaped river weirs using harpoons with small barbed or toggling heads, and the Tlingit also used funnel-shaped basket traps. In the Eskimo region, salmon were netted or taken with three-pronged leisters after being channeled into ponds using stone or wooden weirs. Salmon fishing ended in September or October with the conclusion of the spawning runs.

Herring were also an extremely important resource for many North Pacific peoples. Herring were caught in early summer when they swarmed into shallow shore waters, attaching their spawn to seaweed and rocks. In some areas spawn was so thick that it could be gathered with pole-mounted rakes set with dozens of bone splinter teeth, and with cedar-bark seines. Gill nets were also widely used in the streams and along shore for herring, sea-run trout, and other fish.

Halibut Fishing

Open-water fishing from watercraft was important for the Northwest Coast Indians, Pacific Eskimo, and eastern Aleuts. Of all the various fishing techniques, halibut fishing was the most highly developed and required the greatest ritual attention. These huge bottom-feeding creatures were caught at depths down to 150 fathoms and attained weights up to 600 pounds, although most fish caught were in the 20-to-100-pound range. Ens. A. P. Niblack, who observed Tlingit halibut fishing, commented: "A primitive halibut fishing outfit consists of kelp-lines, wooden floats, stone sinkers, an anchor line, a wooden club, and wooden fish hooks. It is impossible with our most modern appliances to compete with the [Tlingit] Indians in halibut fishing. With their crude implements they meet with the most surprising success" (Niblack 1890:299).

On the Northwest Coast, halibut fishing was conducted in dugout canoes from spring to fall

153

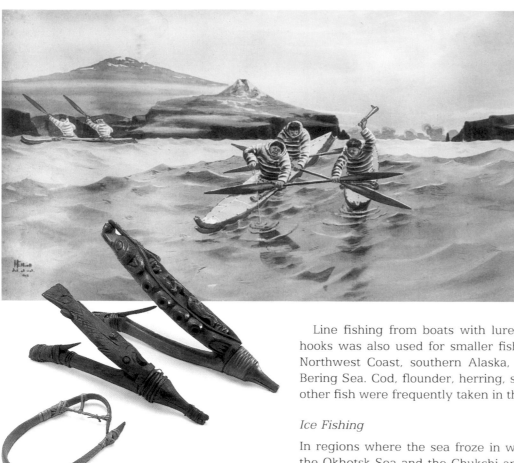

184. Ocean Fishing
Henry W. Elliott, 1872: SI-NAA 7119-7, SI neg. 73-10872. Tlingit hooks (top to bottom): MAE 2539-3; NMNH-46349, T-717

Although sea mammal hunting engendered more ritual and artistic elaboration, halibut fishing ritual was also highly developed south of the Bering Sea. Tlingit halibut fishing was done from wooden dugouts while Pacific Eskimo and Aleut fishermen used kayaks, as shown in this painting. Group fishing and special paddle bracing was needed to kill and land a large fish.

Many Northwest Coast halibut hooks were crudely carved, probably by individual fishermen, like the hook (*center*) depicting a salmon with a hooked snout, as it appears during spawning. Others were powerful works of master carvers, combining animals and humans in incongruous composites. The hook at the upper right is shaped like a canoe and shows a sea lion-like creature with its long tongue curved back over his head, rows of octopus suckers along its sides, and flippers. In the "canoe" a fisherman hauls in a halibut, from under whose tail emerges a human face. These enigmatic parts cannot be interpreted, except to say that they relate to the power the hook was expected to exert on the fish.

Equally ingenious hooks were used to catch black cod. A long slip of hardwood, usually split from the branchroot in a partially rotted log, was steamed and bent into an elongated hoop, one end of which became the hook, the other the shank. In use the ends were spread apart with a thin stick that dislodged when the cod took the hook, allowing the ends to spring closed and set the point. A brace reinforced the curve of the hook from the pull of the fish.

using hooks embellished with representations of mythological creatures. These hooks were baited with octopus and were anchored by stone sinkers about two feet off the sea floor. Sections of bull kelp, knotted together, provided flexible and nearly unbreakable lines up to 150 fathoms in length. Bird-shaped floats were attached to the tops of the lines. When a fish was hooked its weight pulled the bird float upright, signaling a catch. The fisherman then gingerly drew the halibut to the surface and dispatched it with a blow from a club.

The northern Northwest Coast halibut hook (fig. 184) was V-shaped and was made of two pieces of wood, a smaller shank joined to a thicker body fitted with a bone barb. The thicker body section was more buoyant and held the hook in the proper orientation in the water. The body was carved with representations of helping spirits: individual or composite groups of birds, bears, seals, humans, and mythological monsters. Ingenious inventions, suited exactly for the behavior and anatomy of halibut, these hooks were designed so that it was impossible to catch a halibut larger than a man could haul into his boat; a larger fish could not get its mouth into the V opening far enough to become hooked on the barb.

Line fishing from boats with lures or baited hooks was also used for smaller fish along the Northwest Coast, southern Alaska, and in the Bering Sea. Cod, flounder, herring, sculpin, and other fish were frequently taken in this manner.

Ice Fishing

In regions where the sea froze in winter, as in the Okhotsk Sea and the Chukchi and northern Bering Sea (fig. 185), and in interior lakes and rivers, lures, baited hooks, and jigs were used. Ice fishing was often done by old people, women, and children in late winter and early spring when food was scarce and hunters were occupied elsewhere looking for larger prey.

Among the Chukchi and Eskimo, ice fishing began with the chopping of a hole through the ice with an antler or ivory chisel or pick. Floating pieces of ice were then removed with a scoop or with a baleen strainer. This type of ice fishing was conducted with short fishing rods 12–18 inches long that doubled as line reels. Eskimo and Chukchi rods were single pieces of wood with notched ends that served as line reels when not in use. Koryak rods were longer and more elaborate, having pistol-grip handles and ivory line guides (fig. 185). The line consisted of kelp, sinew, or, in northern regions, strips of baleen or bird quill, both of which maintain flexibility and do not become knotted or brittle when frozen. The lines were fitted with ivory or stone weights and small lures. Western Eskimo groups produced beautiful composite lures of colorful ground stone and ivory ornamented with orange crested auklet bill fragments and glass beads (fig. 186). Sometimes lures were used in combination with leisters to spear fish that would not strike the lure itself. In another technique, known as jigging, fish were attracted to a mov-

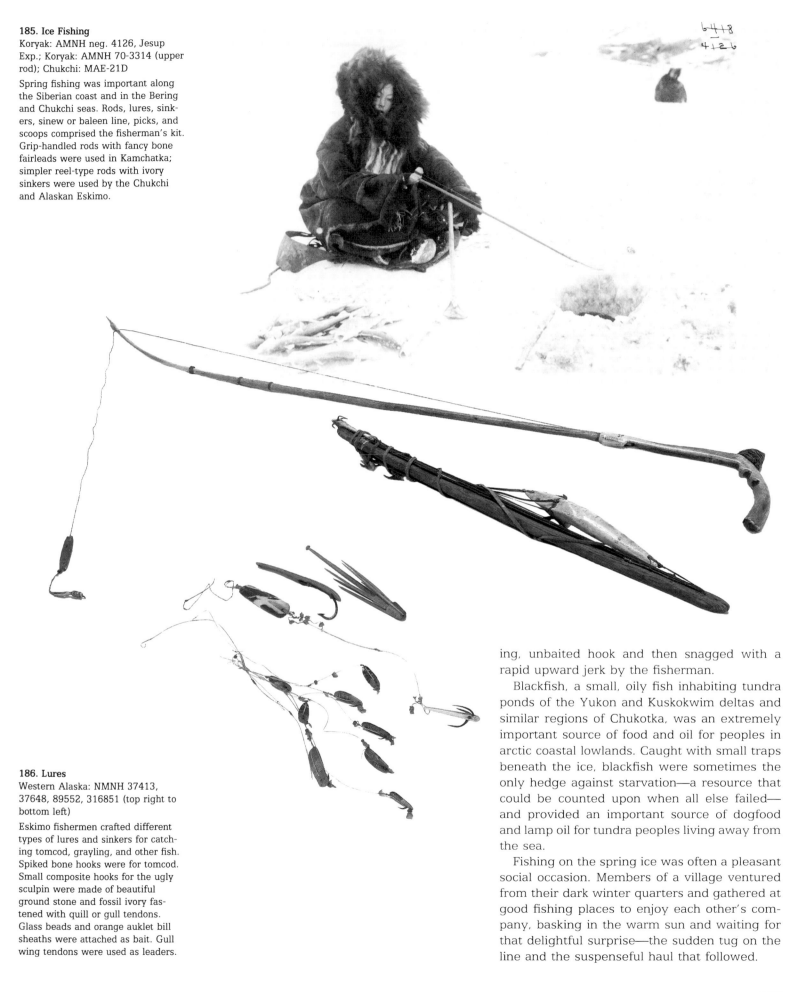

185. Ice Fishing
Koryak: AMNH neg. 4126, Jesup Exp.; Koryak: AMNH 70-3314 (upper rod); Chukchi: MAE-21D

Spring fishing was important along the Siberian coast and in the Bering and Chukchi seas. Rods, lures, sinkers, sinew or baleen line, picks, and scoops comprised the fisherman's kit. Grip-handled rods with fancy bone fairleads were used in Kamchatka; simpler reel-type rods with ivory sinkers were used by the Chukchi and Alaskan Eskimo.

186. Lures
Western Alaska: NMNH 37413, 37648, 89552, 316851 (top right to bottom left)

Eskimo fishermen crafted different types of lures and sinkers for catching tomcod, grayling, and other fish. Spiked bone hooks were for tomcod. Small composite hooks for the ugly sculpin were made of beautiful ground stone and fossil ivory fastened with quill or gull tendons. Glass beads and orange auklet bill sheaths were attached as bait. Gull wing tendons were used as leaders.

ing, unbaited hook and then snagged with a rapid upward jerk by the fisherman.

Blackfish, a small, oily fish inhabiting tundra ponds of the Yukon and Kuskokwim deltas and similar regions of Chukotka, was an extremely important source of food and oil for peoples in arctic coastal lowlands. Caught with small traps beneath the ice, blackfish were sometimes the only hedge against starvation—a resource that could be counted upon when all else failed—and provided an important source of dogfood and lamp oil for tundra peoples living away from the sea.

Fishing on the spring ice was often a pleasant social occasion. Members of a village ventured from their dark winter quarters and gathered at good fishing places to enjoy each other's company, basking in the warm sun and waiting for that delightful surprise—the sudden tug on the line and the suspenseful haul that followed.

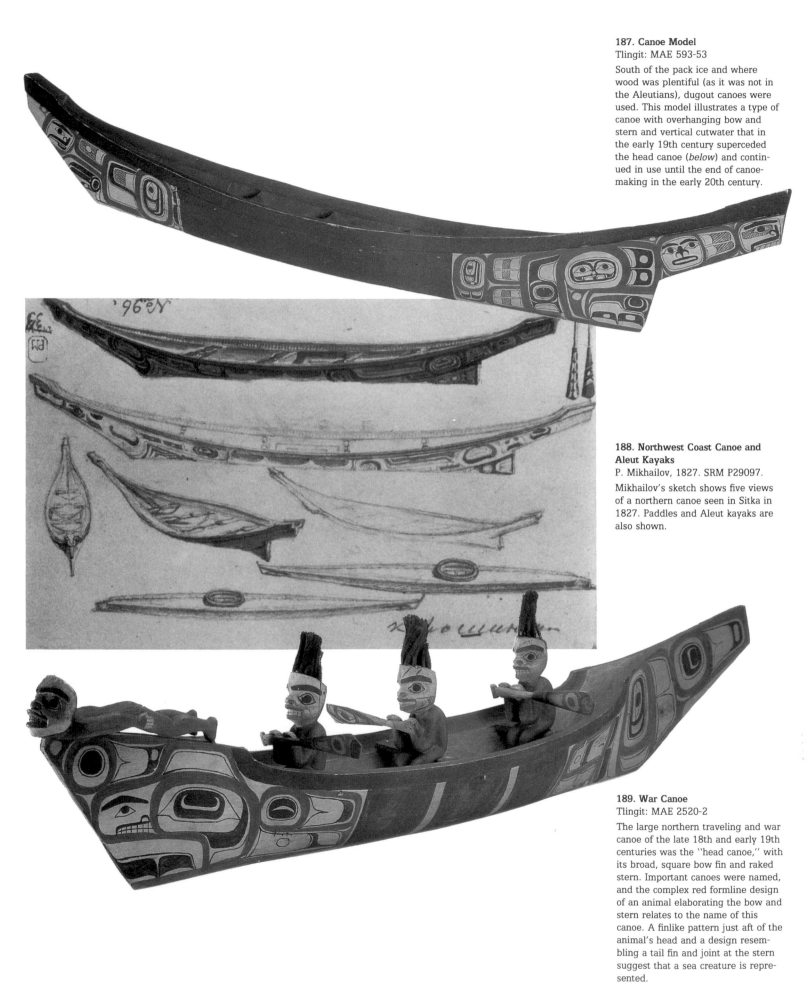

187. Canoe Model

Tlingit: MAE 593-53

South of the pack ice and where wood was plentiful (as it was not in the Aleutians), dugout canoes were used. This model illustrates a type of canoe with overhanging bow and stern and vertical cutwater that in the early 19th century superceded the head canoe (*below*) and continued in use until the end of canoe-making in the early 20th century.

188. Northwest Coast Canoe and Aleut Kayaks

P. Mikhailov, 1827. SRM P29097.

Mikhailov's sketch shows five views of a northern canoe seen in Sitka in 1827. Paddles and Aleut kayaks are also shown.

189. War Canoe

Tlingit: MAE 2520-2

The large northern traveling and war canoe of the late 18th and early 19th centuries was the "head canoe," with its broad, square bow fin and raked stern. Important canoes were named, and the complex red formline design of an animal elaborating the bow and stern relates to the name of this canoe. A finlike pattern just aft of the animal's head and a design resembling a tail fin and joint at the stern suggest that a sea creature is represented.

156

Northwest Coast Canoes

The art of dugout canoe making reached a high state of development on the Northwest Coast of America, with more than a dozen distinctly different types of canoes known during the historic period. Some of these were confined to very specific areas of the region, while others had wide distribution.

The classic northern canoe was a graceful craft with upswept and overhanging bow and stern, elegant sheer, and a distinctive square cutwater under the bow. It was made in sizes ranging from tiny one- or two-person boats to great seagoing traveling canoes said to be as much as 70 feet in length with a beam of 10 feet. They were excellent sea boats and were probably perfected by the Queen Charlotte Haida, who carried on a brisk trade in canoes.

The most spectacular of the early historic period canoes was the "head" canoe with its large, roughly rectangular fin extending from the bow and a similarly large, but tapered fin at the stern (fig. 189). Head canoes did not survive the early contact period. Models and drawings are the only record we have of this important canoe type.

North of the distribution of red cedar, a small to moderately large canoe was made of spruce (de Laguna 1972:337). This "Sitka canoe" (or "spruce canoe") had the typically northern feature of thin fins extending from the bow and stern. Closely related to the spruce canoe in form was the cottonwood canoe typical of Klukwan and other villages of the rivers (de Laguna 1972:336). Of all Northwest Coast canoes, Tlingit cottonwood canoes exemplify the technique of producing, by steaming and spreading, a vessel wider than the log from which it was carved.

All of these and other canoes were propelled by single-bladed paddles, while canoes used in rivers were commonly driven by poling. Everywhere on the coast they were sailed before the wind using sails of matting or thin planks. After European types of fore-and-aft sails of canvas were introduced in the late 18th century, Indians very successfully sailed their keelless canoes on points up to a beam reach, close to a right angle to the wind. Thereafter most canoes of any size were equipped to step masts. Later in the contact period many canoes were fitted with rowlocks and oars.

Bill Holm

190. Steering Paddle
Haida: NMNH 73544
Long, broad-bladed paddles were used by the steersman of large traveling canoes. Crew paddles were shorter and more pointed. Designs on paddles related to the design on the canoe, this one being an octopus with long, sucker-lined tentacles. The paddle is made of tough yellow cedar.

Sea Mammal Hunting

Sea mammal hunting was of paramount importance to peoples of the North Pacific region. Sea mammals provided them with their most important animal resource, considering the value of these animals not only as food but also as providers of oil, skins, ivory, and other products without which life in this environment could not have been sustained. The importance of this activity is seen in the development of sophisticated hunting equipment and also of costumes, ornament, and ritual, which, taken as a complex, is perhaps the most striking and elaborated feature of North Pacific maritime societies.

Techniques for hunting North Pacific sea mammals—including pinnipeds (seals, sea lions, and walrus), sea otters, and small and large whales—were extremely varied but conformed to two basic systems: harpooning with float or drag gear, and the use of poisoned projectiles. The latter method was used only for large whales and was practiced exclusively by Itelmen, Aleut, and Pacific Eskimo hunters; variations on the former were used for all sea mammals from sea otters to huge whales. The following discussion treats the hunting of the small- and medium-size sea mammals separately from large whale hunting, which, despite its similar technology and principles, was attended by a separate

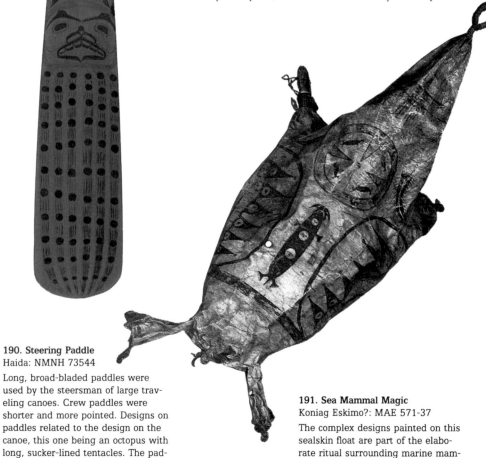

191. Sea Mammal Magic
Koniag Eskimo?: MAE 571-37
The complex designs painted on this sealskin float are part of the elaborate ritual surrounding marine mammal hunting.

ceremonial complex and had different implications for social and economic organization.

Seasonal availability of the smaller sea mammals varied, but the most important hunt was carried on during spring and summer when the weather was calm and the animals had a heavy layer of fat and when their skins and pelts were in prime condition.

Differences in equipment and hunting techniques were correlated with differing habits and environments of the animals. In the north, hunting from the ice edge or at breathing holes was more important than open-water hunting from boats, whereas in the southern Bering Sea and in Pacific waters most hunting was done from boats. Some techniques required cooperative hunting parties, either in large boats or in fleets of kayaks, while others were conducted by single hunters, the specific method being determined by the numbers, size, aggressiveness, and alertness of the prey.

Most important, the pinnipeds and small whales supplied the hunter's family (and dogs) with food. But they also provided a number of other products. Sea mammal blubber, in addition to being a dietary staple, was rendered into oil for use in lamps for heat and light; skins were used for clothing, thongs, and boat covers; and ivory teeth and tusks were used in a variety of functional and decorative industries and were important trade items. Of all the sea mammals, the sea otter was the least used in prehistoric times but was the dominant quarry during the Russian period because of its importance in the fur trade.

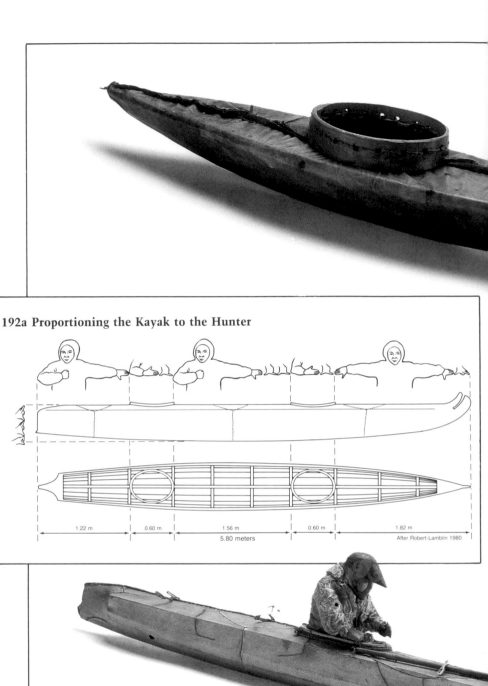

192a Proportioning the Kayak to the Hunter

1.22 m 0.60 m 1.56 m 0.60 m 1.82 m
5.80 meters
After Robert-Lamblin 1980

Open Water and Ice Edge Hunting of Seals, Walrus, and Sea Otters

Weapons used in the hunting of sea mammals in the Arctic and Subarctic exhibited a great deal of technical variation. They may be classified into arrows, darts, harpoons, and lances on the basis of shaft diameter and mode of propulsion. Arrows, shot from bows, are short with thin shafts; darts are longer but still lightweight weapons that may be hand-cast but are usually propelled with throwing boards; harpoons have longer and heavier shafts and may be thrown or used as thrusting weapons; lances (or spears) are variable in length with heavy shafts, and may also be thrown or thrust. Lances were used primarily to administer killing wounds to animals that had already been secured with darts or harpoons. A basic distinction that cuts across these categories is whether the point or head of the weapon is detachable or nondetachable. Darts and harpoons were the most important weapons for hunting sea mammals in open water

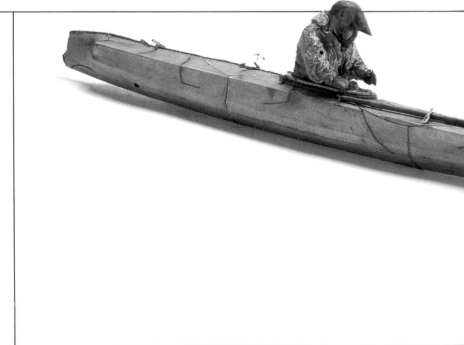

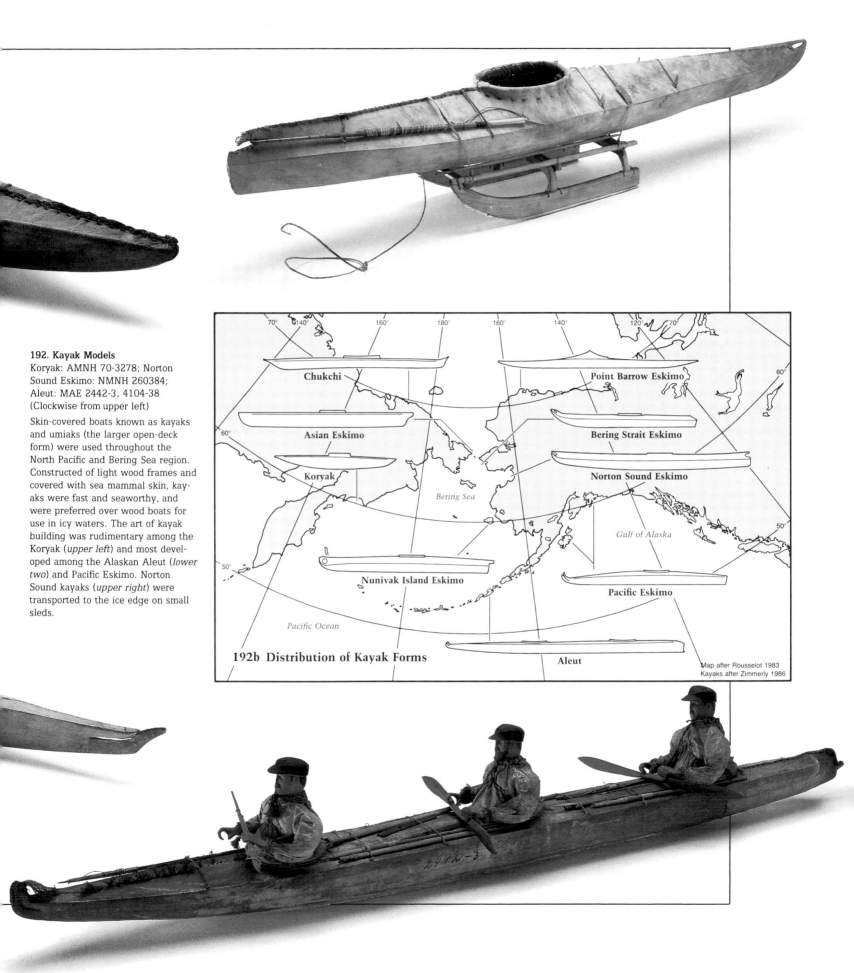

192. Kayak Models

Koryak: AMNH 70-3278; Norton Sound Eskimo: NMNH 260384; Aleut: MAE 2442-3, 4104-38 (Clockwise from upper left)

Skin-covered boats known as kayaks and umiaks (the larger open-deck form) were used throughout the North Pacific and Bering Sea region. Constructed of light wood frames and covered with sea mammal skin, kayaks were fast and seaworthy, and were preferred over wood boats for use in icy waters. The art of kayak building was rudimentary among the Koryak (*upper left*) and most developed among the Alaskan Aleut (*lower two*) and Pacific Eskimo. Norton Sound kayaks (*upper right*) were transported to the ice edge on small sleds.

192b Distribution of Kayak Forms

Chukchi

Point Barrow Eskimo

Asian Eskimo

Bering Strait Eskimo

Koryak

Norton Sound Eskimo

Bering Sea

Nunivak Island Eskimo

Gulf of Alaska

Pacific Eskimo

Pacific Ocean

Aleut

Map after Rousselot 1983
Kayaks after Zimmerly 1986

and always had detachable points that remained in the body of the animal after impact. Dart and harpoon heads conformed to two basic designs of different origin and different utility according to ice conditions.

The barbed, or male, harpoon head was the most ancient form, dating back to paleolithic times. It consisted of a bone, antler, or ivory point with a row of barbs along one or both sides, and a base that had a hole or flange to which a line was tied (fig. 195). The butt end of the head fit into a socket at the front end of the weapon shaft. It detached and remained in the animal after impact, while the shaft floated free. The other end of the line remained attached to the shaft, boat, or some type of float.

The barbed form was the dominant type used throughout the North Pacific south of the sea-ice zone. In ice-infested waters, this type was replaced by the Eskimo, or toggling, harpoon head (fig. 195), a female-socketed implement that was designed to be implanted beneath the skin and blubber with the aid of a slender foreshaft connecting the head to the shaft. The foreshaft allowed the toggling head to penetrate deeply into the animal so that when the shaft detached, the head twisted sideways beneath the animal's skin and could not be pulled out. The worldwide distribution of these two types, barbed forms occurring along open-water coasts and toggling forms in regions of seasonal ice cover, clearly demonstrates the superior efficiency of the toggling form for use in icy regions where breakage, either accidental or purposeful, of the protruding butt element against ice permitted the animal's escape. Such losses could be substantially reduced, and holding power increased, by use of the toggling principle.

Whether using a barbed or toggle-headed dart or harpoon, the basic hunting method was similar. Typically, the hunter silently approached the seal in his skin-covered kayak and when within range hurled his weapon. The animal was restrained by the drag created by a float or float board attached to the end of the harpoon line. Alternatively, the line would be attached to the dart or harpoon shaft, which dragged behind and impeded the animal's escape. The actual killing of the harpooned animal was done with a lance or club. Specially designed repeating

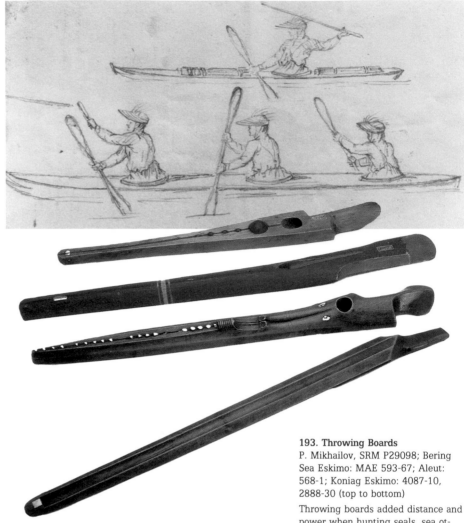

193. Throwing Boards
P. Mikhailov, SRM P29098; Bering Sea Eskimo: MAE 593-67; Aleut: 568-1; Koniag Eskimo: 4087-10, 2888-30 (top to bottom)

Throwing boards added distance and power when hunting seals, sea otters, and whales with darts. Like kayaks, styles varied regionally. Known historically from Bering Strait to Southeast Alaska (fig. 388), they had almost disappeared in Siberia before the historic period. Beaded designs (*top*), black and red paint, and sea otter teeth and sculptural figures (*lower two*) were favored by Bering Sea Eskimo, Aleut, and Koniag hunters.

194. Throwing Darts
Aleut: NMNH 175825; Bering Sea Eskimo: NMNH 43746, 33956 (top to bottom)

Darts, a kind of heavy-duty arrow, were launched with throwing boards at small to medium sized sea mammals. Aleut sea otter darts (*top*) were shorter and lighter than Bering Sea seal darts (*bottom*) because the quarry was smaller, but they worked the same way. When the animal was struck, the shaft disengaged and dragged sideways behind the animal, hindering its escape. Bird darts (*middle*) with multiple prongs were also launched with throwing boards.

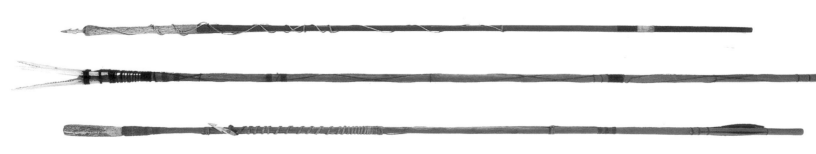

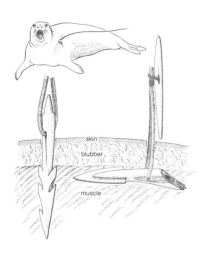

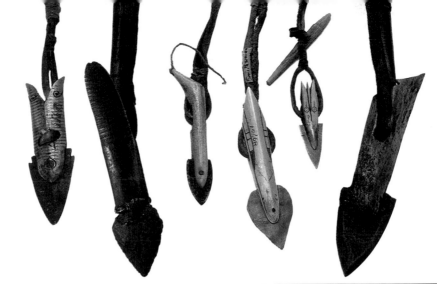

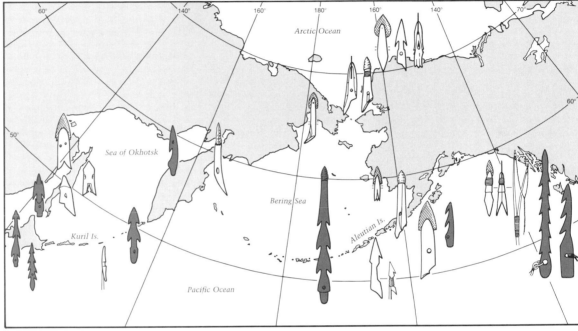

195. Harpoon Technology
MAE 656-42, 5031-1, 434-17/2, NMNH 89761, 37571, 168625 (left to right)

Two types of harpoon technology are used in the North Pacific. The simplest, distributed mostly in ice-free waters, is the nontoggling or 'male' harpoon point that holds an animal by its barbs. The second and more complex form is the toggling harpoon point, historically a later development associated with sea mammal hunting in arctic waters. Toggling beneath the skin and blubber where it cannot be broken off by ice, it holds heavier quarry like walrus and whales. The toggling forms shown here are from the Orochi, Koryak, Chukchi, and the North Alaskan, Kuskokwim, and Bristol Bay Eskimo.

196. Lances
NMNH 153731, 36058, 382259 (top to bottom)

When an animal was exhausted by struggling against the harpoon, it was approached and killed with a lance. Two types of lance are used in western Alaska, the northern fixed point lance (*above*, with chert blade) that could only be used from an umiak, and, south of Bering Strait, the repeating lance. The latter could be rearmed for multiple thrusts.

lances (fig. 196), with successively inserted detachable heads, were employed by Bering Sea Eskimo in killing harpooned white whales (beluga). This technique permitted a large number of killing thrusts to be made in a short time, because the hunter did not have to struggle to withdraw the lance after each thrust.

The size of the prey was a determining factor in selecting the right weapon. Light darts with toggling or barbed heads propelled with throwing boards were used for small seals (fig. 193), while larger seals and sea lions required heavier equipment. Some darts were especially designed for taking seabirds on the surface of the water (fig. 194). For hunting sea otters, which were hard to approach, very light darts propelled with

throwing boards and ''harpoon'' arrows (arrows with detachable barbed or toggling heads) were used (fig. 76). The use of light equipment permitted Pacific Eskimo and Aleuts to carry more weapons and to launch them from great distances, a technique that permitted a single boat to capture many animals at one time. In addition, the surround technique, in which fleets of kayaks encircled whole groups of sea otters, corralling them in the center until the hunters had expended all their weapons, was highly effective for hunting these gregarious animals.

The use of harpoon arrows required two-man kayaks in which the stern paddler stabilized the boat while the bowman shot. This method, used by the Pacific Eskimo, may have been adopted

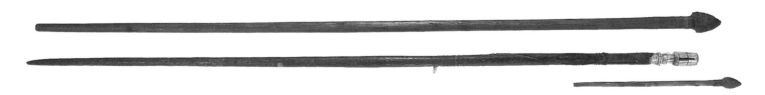

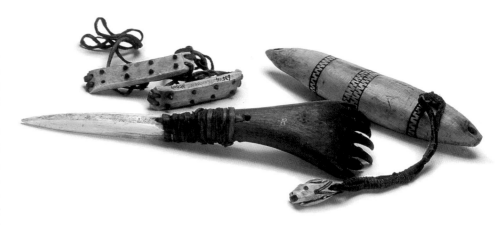

from Northwest Coast Indians. Tlingit hunters, who hunted from more stable dugout boats, used the bow for hunting small sea mammals and large barbed harpoons for hunting larger game.

In May and June, seals and beluga whales approached the shore to feed on fish and often entered estuaries and rivers. In such situations, groups of hunters drove them into shallow water, where they were speared. In some cases, hunters erected scaffolds for shoreside hunting or simply hid among the rocks at good hunting spots, wearing seal helmet disguises.

Walrus, a pagophilous or ice-loving creature, was hunted throughout its distribution from the southern Bering Sea into the Arctic Ocean with heavy harpoon equipment and spears. Because walrus tend to occur in large herds and frequently defend themselves, they were usually hunted from open skin boats carrying four to eight hunters. Walrus harpoons had long foreshafts, permitting the harpoon head to be forced deeply into the animal, and were attached to long lines made from sealskin thong and to sealskin floats, often richly decorated with ornaments and rattles. The successful walrus hunter required strength, courage, and skill, and he had to have the means to maintain his equipment, crew, and boat. For these reasons, walrus hunting had greater social ramifications than sea otter or seal hunting. Walrus were also hunted with the aid of a baleen clapper, which was slapped on the water to drive the walrus to shore, where they were speared by waiting hunters. Shore hunting also occurred at rookeries and haul-out places by men using harpoons and lances.

By the end of the 19th century, many of the traditional methods of sea mammal hunting had disappeared. However, firearms did not replace harpoons, which remained as auxiliary weapons. Gaining the advantage of distance, hunters shot to wound rather than kill, and then hurried to attach harpoons to the animal before it was killed with the rifle. In this way the sinking and loss of the dead animal was prevented.

Winter Sealing

In early winter and in spring seals were caught in large mesh nets made of strips of seal-hide thong stretched beneath the ice. Lying nearby, the hunter would scratch the surface of the ice with a scratcher made in the shape of a seal's flipper, to which seal claws were attached. Seals, sociable and curious animals, were attracted by the sound and became enmeshed. At this time of year hunters also stalked basking seals with harpoons. Wearing white intestine clothing, the

hunter approached on his belly, sometimes behind a white shield. Keeping a sharp watch, the hunter crawled forward while the seal napped, and "froze" when it woke every few minutes to check for danger. The hunt climaxed with the hunter's final dash and throw; he had only a single chance. At a time of food scarcity, survival depended upon success, and a single error had grave consequences for hunter and family.

Winter and spring were also the time for sealing at the breathing holes that some seal species keep open through the sea ice. Waiting patiently over the breathing hole, sometimes for hours, required concentration and stamina equivalent to that required to stalk basking seals. A single sound could alert the approaching seal. Use of a harpoon with a long foreshaft enabled the hunter to thrust his weapon deeply into the seal, attempting to kill it. If not, the hunter faced an unpleasant predicament, trying to hold a harpoon line with several hundred pounds of fighting seal in one hand while attempting to dispatch it with a spear through a small hole in the ice with the other.

Breathing-hole sealing was considered unpleasant work and was practiced only under conditions of scarcity. The technique could only be used in areas of firm ice cover, and for this reason was rarely practiced in the southern sea ice regions. In open-water regions winter sea mammal hunting was conducted with nets and harpoons that had floats attached to their shafts.

197. Hunting on the Ice
NMNH 63514, 63876; MAE 668-2; SI 38754; FM 53453

Special equipment was developed by Eskimos living in the icy regions of Bering Strait. Among these were heavy ivory seal net weights; ice scratchers to calm the nerves of suspicious seals being stalked by hunters over the ice; drag handles and small sleds to haul animals home; and ice creepers to give one's boots traction. The sled below is made from oak scavenged from wrecked whaling ships.

198. "Wife" and "Husband" Charms
Bering Sea Eskimo: NMNH 340373a

Face charms were attached inside the cockpits of some Eskimo kayaks to protect the hunter from harmful spirits. Similar to charms representing "the wife" (frown) and "the husband" (smile) used for protecting the home, this pair protected the ocean traveler.

199. Walrus and Sealing Harpoons
NMNH 45475, 153727

Walrus harpoons were heavier than sealing harpoons and had larger heads. Seal hide was used as line. Ice picks at the butt end balanced the shaft and were used for testing ice thickness.

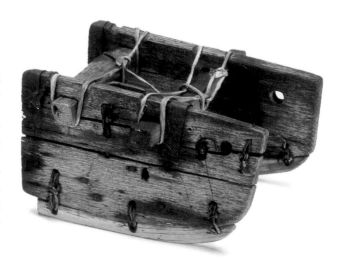

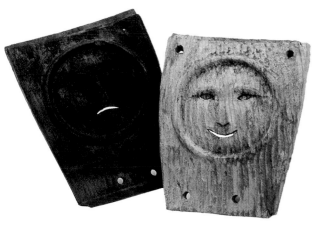

Hunting Ritual

Practices to insure the success of the hunt, and to mollify the spirit of the animal caught, were widespread in the North Pacific. Hunters carried amulets to protect them from evil spirits and charms to make their presence acceptable to the prey. Ivory sea otters were attached inside the kayaks of Bristol Bay and Aleutian Island hunters; Bering Sea Eskimo carried smiling and frowning male-female face plaques lashed inside their kayak cockpits; and other types of charms and fetishes were used by other groups. In addition to boat charms, hunters carried personal charms and amulets made of ivory, feathers, bird beaks, and pieces of skin in bags at their belts or sewn into their clothing.

Sea mammal hunting was supported by a wide variety of ritual and ceremonial activity beyond the practice of the hunt itself. Boat manufacture was accompanied by the performance of rituals intended to protect the hunter, and the annual calendar of ceremonial life included harvest festivals honoring the spirits of sea mammals upon which the community depended. During these festivals hunters reenacted symbolic hunts and returned the bones, bladders, or other parts of the animals captured to the sea as a gesture of respect meant to replenish the supply of game.

Throughout the North Pacific region, hunters had strict procedures that governed the ownership and sharing of sea mammal game, beginning with correct attribution of hunter and prey. Hunting marks on harpoons insured that the identity of the hunter who harpooned the game was known. The primary division of the meat and skin and the symbolic spirit of the animal were awarded to the hunter making the first firm strike. Rights to portions of the catch depended on the size of the animal and the role of the secondary hunters. The larger the animal, the more elaborate the sharing ritual. For large animals such as walrus and bearded seals caught from umiaks, meat was shared evenly among the members of the boat crew and those present at the division. Skins went to the owner of the boat, as did the head and tusks when a walrus was caught.

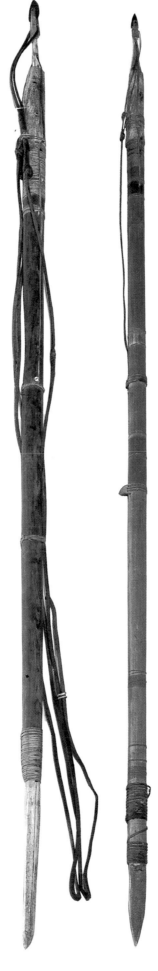

Whaling

Aboriginal whaling in the North Pacific, Bering Sea, and Chukchi Sea reached a high degree of development long before the arrival of Europeans in this region. In fact, techniques used by Siberian and Alaskan whalers of the Punuk and Thule cultures in the 7th through 13th centuries were the most advanced in the world at that time. It was not until Europeans learned how to use toggling harpoons by contacts with Eskimos in the Eastern Arctic in the 17th century that this gap closed and European whalers began to reap huge gains by adopting this efficient technology. Only then did the combination of new hunting technology and seagoing vessels allow European whalers to extend their reach into North Atlantic waters and, later, into the Pacific.

The exact origin of whaling among North Pacific Rim peoples remains unknown, but in the Bering Strait the first large whaling harpoons occur in 2,000-year-old archeological sites of the Old Bering Sea culture. Prior to this, North Pacific peoples probably utilized whale products like bone, teeth, blubber, and meat by scavenging the carcasses of dead whales. Although the beginnings of whaling seem indicated in Old Bering Sea times, several centuries elapsed before whaling began to play a dominant role in the life of Punuk culture (A.D. 600–1200) and in subsequent cultural phases of the Bering Sea and North American Arctic. Most of what we know about the origins of whaling comes from these arctic regions. At present, relatively little is known archeologically about whale hunting by the peoples of northeastern Asia, southern Alaska, and the Northwest Coast. As discussed below, the whaling techniques of the Kurile Island Ainu, Itelmen, Aleut, and Pacific Eskimo were based on the use of poisoned darts or arrows and thus differed radically from the harpoon and float whaling practiced in the Bering Sea and southern Northwest Coast. Poison whaling is of uncertain age (Heizer 1943).

A significant feature of the distribution of North Pacific Rim whaling in the historical period is that it was not uniform but rather occurred in some regions and not in others. This resulted, in part, from variations in the migratory patterns of the several species of whales most important in native subsistence: the gray, bowhead, fin, and humpback whales (fig. 207).

Bowhead and gray whales were the focus of Bering Sea and Chukchi Sea umiak whaling, because they are slow swimming and relatively docile, making approach by paddling or sailing boat crews possible. Gray whales winter in lagoons off Baja California and Mexico and travel north along the coast of western North America

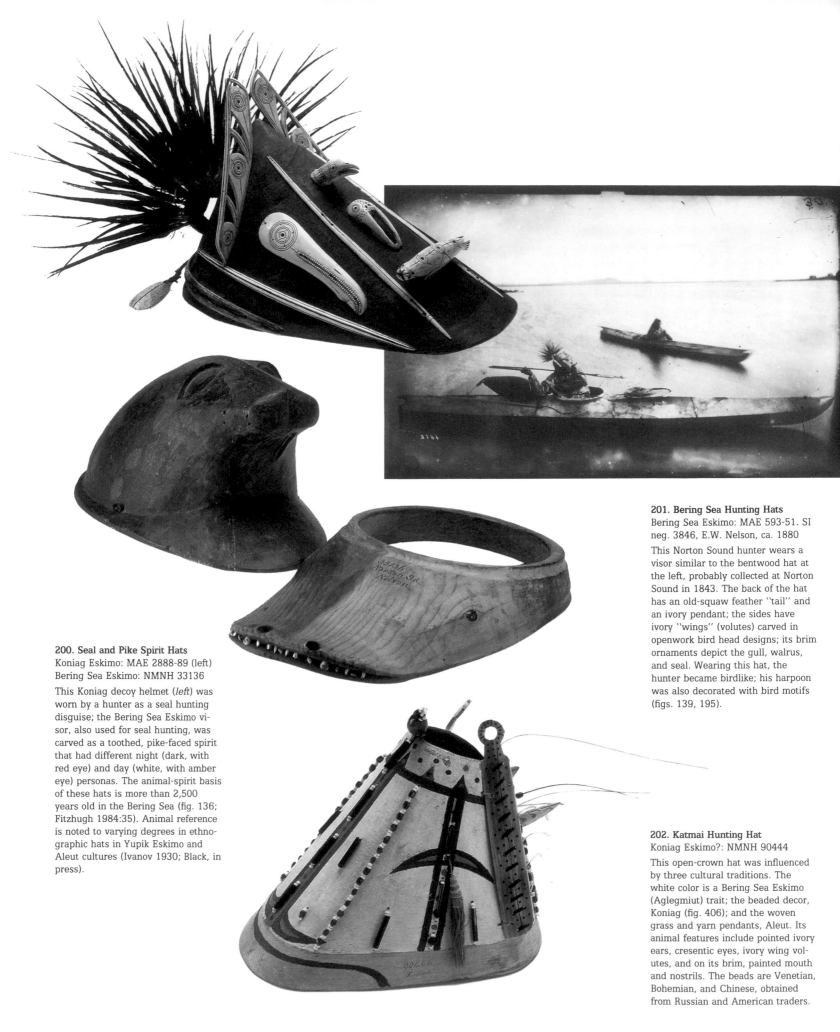

201. Bering Sea Hunting Hats
Bering Sea Eskimo: MAE 593-51. SI neg. 3846, E.W. Nelson, ca. 1880

This Norton Sound hunter wears a visor similar to the bentwood hat at the left, probably collected at Norton Sound in 1843. The back of the hat has an old-squaw feather "tail" and an ivory pendant; the sides have ivory "wings" (volutes) carved in openwork bird head designs; its brim ornaments depict the gull, walrus, and seal. Wearing this hat, the hunter became birdlike; his harpoon was also decorated with bird motifs (figs. 139, 195).

200. Seal and Pike Spirit Hats
Koniag Eskimo: MAE 2888-89 (left)
Bering Sea Eskimo: NMNH 33136

This Koniag decoy helmet (*left*) was worn by a hunter as a seal hunting disguise; the Bering Sea Eskimo visor, also used for seal hunting, was carved as a toothed, pike-faced spirit that had different night (dark, with red eye) and day (white, with amber eye) personas. The animal-spirit basis of these hats is more than 2,500 years old in the Bering Sea (fig. 136; Fitzhugh 1984:35). Animal reference is noted to varying degrees in ethnographic hats in Yupik Eskimo and Aleut cultures (Ivanov 1930; Black, in press).

202. Katmai Hunting Hat
Koniag Eskimo?: NMNH 90444

This open-crown hat was influenced by three cultural traditions. The white color is a Bering Sea Eskimo (Aglegmiut) trait; the beaded decor, Koniag (fig. 406); and the woven grass and yarn pendants, Aleut. Its animal features include pointed ivory ears, cresentic eyes, ivory wing volutes, and on its brim, painted mouth and nostrils. The beads are Venetian, Bohemian, and Chinese, obtained from Russian and American traders.

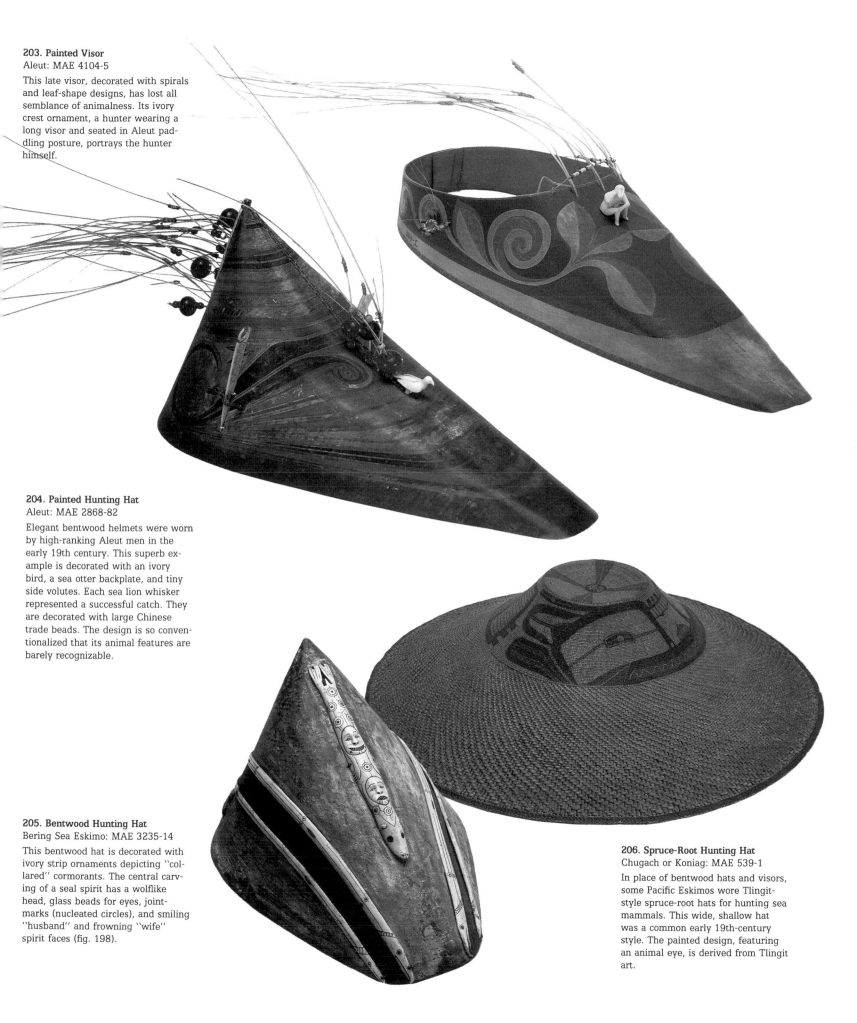

203. Painted Visor
Aleut: MAE 4104-5

This late visor, decorated with spirals and leaf-shape designs, has lost all semblance of animalness. Its ivory crest ornament, a hunter wearing a long visor and seated in Aleut paddling posture, portrays the hunter himself.

204. Painted Hunting Hat
Aleut: MAE 2868-82

Elegant bentwood helmets were worn by high-ranking Aleut men in the early 19th century. This superb example is decorated with an ivory bird, a sea otter backplate, and tiny side volutes. Each sea lion whisker represented a successful catch. They are decorated with large Chinese trade beads. The design is so conventionalized that its animal features are barely recognizable.

205. Bentwood Hunting Hat
Bering Sea Eskimo: MAE 3235-14

This bentwood hat is decorated with ivory strip ornaments depicting "collared" cormorants. The central carving of a seal spirit has a wolflike head, glass beads for eyes, jointmarks (nucleated circles), and smiling "husband" and frowning "wife" spirit faces (fig. 198).

206. Spruce-Root Hunting Hat
Chugach or Koniag: MAE 539-1

In place of bentwood hats and visors, some Pacific Eskimos wore Tlingit-style spruce-root hats for hunting sea mammals. This wide, shallow hat was a common early 19th-century style. The painted design, featuring an animal eye, is derived from Tlingit art.

in the spring. Their route takes them through Unimak Pass at the eastern end of the Aleutian chain and into the rich feeding grounds of the Bering and Chukchi seas. With the advance of summer they turn south, following the shores of Chukotka into the Pacific. Bowhead whales are more oceanic and were not hunted except in the narrow leads through the sea ice that they follow north, and which bring them close to shore at points of land and offshore islands. Like the grays, bowheads followed the ice leads north into Bering Strait and the Arctic Ocean until their progress was blocked by ice, at which point they turned south and followed the Siberian coast to the Pacific.

Migrating gray and humpback whales were hunted on the Northwest Coast, but only by the Nootka of Vancouver Island and the Makah, Quileute, and Quinault of the Olympic Peninsula. The absence of whaling in historic times by more northerly groups of Northwest Coast Indians was a cultural phenomenon and not related to lack of available prey. Pacific Eskimo and Aleut whaling was undertaken in open water from kayaks and focused primarily on humpbacks and fin whales. Fin whales are concentrated during summer in the Gulf of Alaska and along the Aleutians, while humpbacks range farther north but stay in open water south of the pack ice; neither species was therefore likely to be taken by Bering Sea whale hunters. Whaling was not reported in the western Aleutians by the earliest Russian observers, possibly because migration patterns concentrate whale populations close to the Alaskan mainland. The Pacific Eskimo and Aleut whaling method was apparently not suited for the taking of gray whales.

Whaling was important for a variety of reasons but primarily for the immense food value of these huge creatures. A successful hunt produced mountains of meat that could be dried and stored for future use during leaner seasons, and it also insured a festive ceremonial season. Dogs as well as people shared in this wealth. Important as meat was, however, whale blubber and oil were perhaps of even greater economic importance.

Umiak Whaling in Arctic Regions

The onset of European whaling in the late 19th century resulted in decimation of the stocks of large whales hunted in the Bering Strait before documentation was gathered on the practice of aboriginal whaling by Siberian natives. That this activity was widespread and exceptionally productive is evident from the oral traditions of the Koryak, Chukchi, and Siberian Eskimo, and from

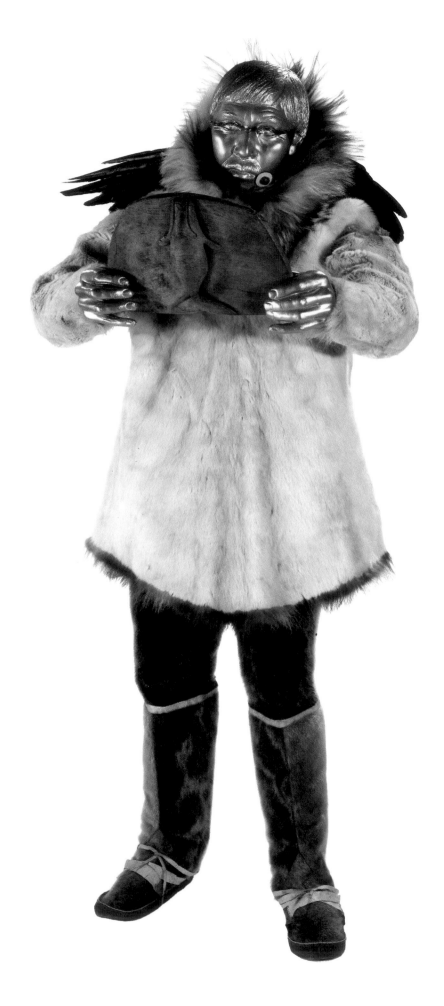

207. Spring-Summer Ranges of Whale Species in the North Pacific, Bering, and Chukchi Seas

The whale species shown here—bowhead (*Balaena mysticus*), gray (*Eschrichtius robustus*), fin (*Balaenoptera physalus*), humpback (*Megaptera novaeangliae*), and beluga (*Delphinapterus leucas*)—were the principle species hunted by Siberian and Alaskan native whalers. Bowheads are still hunted today by Eskimos on St. Lawrence Island and along Alaska's northern coast. Both traditional hunting methods and the relative importance of different whale species varied greatly between different groups of coastal hunters.

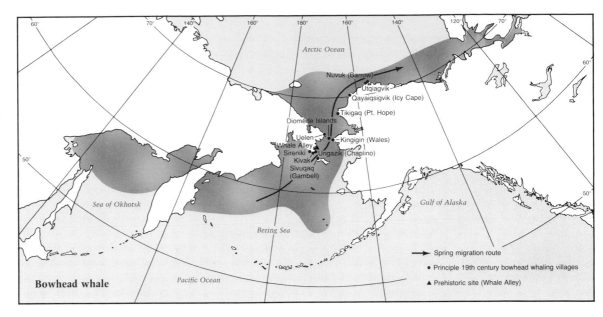

Bowhead whale

→ Spring migration route
● Principle 19th century bowhead whaling villages
▲ Prehistoric site (Whale Alley)

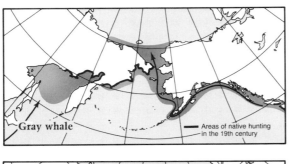

Gray whale

Areas of native hunting in the 19th century

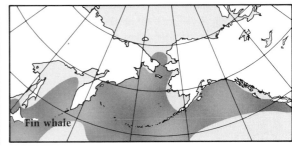

Fin whale

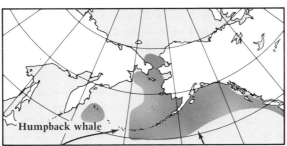

Humpback whale

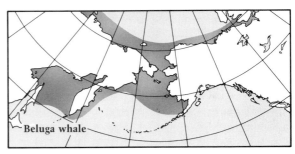

Beluga whale

208. The *Umialik*: North Alaskan Eskimo Whale Boat Captain
NMNH 153734 (parka), 280111 (pants), 203720 (boots), 37663 (labret); FM 53423 (whale plaque)

The *umialik*—captain and owner of a North Alaskan Eskimo whaling boat—stands ready, ritually prepared for the difficult and dangerous task of leading his crew in the capture of a bowhead whale that may weigh 75 tons or more. The raven skin he wears is a powerful amulet and badge of office; the soot marks on his face are a tally of previous kills; and the whale charm plaque he holds will be hung in the bow of the umiak to magically compel whales to draw near. The *umialik* is dressed in a hooded reindeer parka with gores representing walrus tusks, waterproof sealskin pants and boots, and a single labret with a large blue Chinese bead.

the many archeological sites found along the coast of Chukotka, which contain large amounts of whalebone. Skulls, jaws, and ribs of bowhead and gray whales had been used at these sites for construction of houses and elevated storage racks and for ritual purposes. Some of the larger Siberian sites, such as Whale Alley (Arutiunov et al. 1982; Chlenov and Krupnik 1984), contain thousands of whalebones, many of which still stand like sentinels over the landscape, testimony to the hunting success of ancient hunters and to the role of whales in their ceremonial observances.

Aboriginal whaling along the northwest coast of Alaska has been studied more extensively (Spencer 1959). Here, whaling began with the opening of spring leads near the major capes, such as at Wales, Point Hope, and Point Barrow. For the North Alaskan Eskimos an annual period

of renewal began in early March, when umiaks received new covers, people made new clothing, and whaling implements, lines, and floats were refurbished. Attention to whaling magic, sexual abstinence, and solemnity marked these preparations, with the *umialik*s—the whaling captains—assuming almost priestly roles, overseeing all community activities in advance of the hunt, including rituals intended to greet the oncoming whales and the business of seeing that each crew was well taken care of and prepared. Whaling crews were close-knit groups of kinsmen that functioned as cooperative social and economic units throughout the year under the leadership of the *umialik*.

As the time for the appearance of the whales neared, umiaks and whaling gear, including ritual equipment, were moved out to the ice leads by dogsled, and hunting camps were

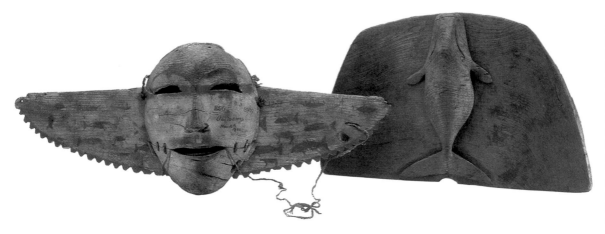

209. Ceremony and Magic: The
North Alaskan Eskimo Whale Cult
North Alaskan Eskimo: NMNH 89817
(left); FM 53423

To summon the village to feast on
whale meat in the *karigi* and to celebrate the end of the whaling season,
whalers danced house to house wearing masks and breast gorgets (collected as a matched set, *left*). Pride
and status are signified by the
"whaleman's mark"—the black band
across the eyes of the mask, here
complemented by lip and chin daubs.
Painted on the gorget are umiaks,
whales, bears, and (beneath the
mask, in red) a giant grasping a
whale in each hand (cf. fig. 444). A
plaque for suspension in the umiak's
bow (*right*) charmed whales to the
boat, its magic aided by a quartz
crystal inset on the obverse side.

established. Here the hunters remained, sometimes for days or even weeks, their gear maintained in ready condition, always poised for an
instantaneous launch should the lookout report
signs of an approaching whale. The slightest
sound or deviation from prescribed ritual was
thought sufficient to spoil the hunt. Meanwhile,
the women and children, who were forbidden
to be present on the ice, had to obey strict rules
of behavior, remaining silent and not engaging
in otherwise routine activities, such as sewing.
The *umialik*'s wife was especially important in
her role representing the whale during the hunt;
she had to remain docile to insure the whale's
similar behavior, and her dignified silence in-
duced the whale to come willingly to the hunters.

When a whale was sighted, the whaling crew,
composed of 7 to 10 men, ran the umiak into
the water, made their approach, and struck. If
more than one umiak crew was present each
vied for the honor of the first strike, as this
guaranteed both prestige and the choicest share
of the distribution. Umiaks making secondary
strikes were also important in securing the catch
and received shares commensurate with the
order of their strike. Meanwhile the whale sounded
and struggled against the lines and floats, later
to be subdued and lanced. It was then towed to
the ice edge where the *umialik*'s wife, dressed
in finery, greeted it ceremonially with songs and
gave it a drink of fresh water. The whale was
then hauled up on the ice or, if too large, was
butchered into segments for hauling out. Crews
and villages gathered for shares in the division
of meat, blubber, baleen, and other products.
The head and the largest share of meat and
blubber went to the *umialik* who first struck the
whale, with secondary shares for his crew. Other
crews received appropriate shares, and from
these fixed portions the kill was shared with
other members of the community. A successful
hunt meant food for an entire community for
several months and was often followed by ceremony and feasting, to which neighboring villages would be invited.

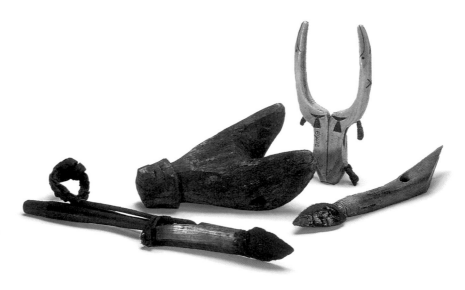

210. Koryak and Eskimo Whaling
Koryak: AMNH 70-3240, 70-2737;
North Alaskan Eskimo: NMNH
89418, 398238

The harpoon head and anthropomorphic bow line guide (*left*), which
was also a charm called the "Manager of the Boat," were used in Koryak whaling umiaks. The Eskimo
harpoon rest was also magic, with its
whaletails and carved whale prongs.
An "X" marks the whale's first vertebra, the location of its soul.

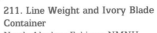

211. Line Weight and Ivory Blade
Container
North Alaskan Eskimo: NMNH
48384; FM 53420

The graphite weight aided in securing a line around the flukes of a dead
whale; the box held harpoon blades
symbolically inside the intended prey.
A blue bead marks the first vertebra.

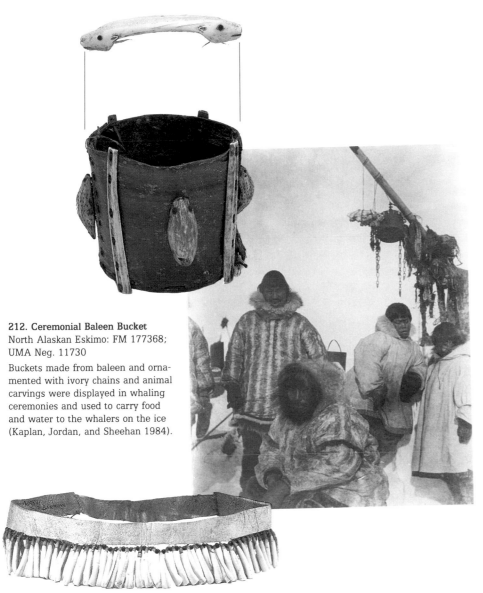

212. Ceremonial Baleen Bucket

North Alaskan Eskimo: FM 177368;
UMA Neg. 11730

Buckets made from baleen and ornamented with ivory chains and animal
carvings were displayed in whaling
ceremonies and used to carry food
and water to the whalers on the ice
(Kaplan, Jordan, and Sheehan 1984).

213. *Umialik's* Headband

North Alaskan Eskimo: NMNH
209841

The *umialik* and his wife were focal
points of the ritual complex that surrounded North Alaskan Eskimo whaling. Their actions were subject to numerous taboos and restrictions meant
to avoid offense to the spirit of the
whale. The *umialik* ritually curated
an assortment of whaling charms that
he inherited or was given by his shamanic advisors. These might include
pebbles, teeth, insects, ivory or baleen carvings, and stuffed birds. His
headband, worn on the hunt, was
hung with beads and the teeth of the
mountain sheep.

214. Whaling Charms

North Alaskan Eskimo: NMNH 56703
(top), 381859, 89577

Chipped-stone whaling charms were
made in the shapes of whales, humans, bears, birds, seals, and other
creatures. The were kept in charm
boxes, or worn on the clothing and
headbands of the *umialik* and harpooner.

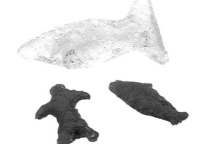

Even though whaling was frequently unsuccessful, hunters would often take walrus and
seals that were discovered during their vigil,
sharing ivory, meat, and skin as described.

Whaling ceremony and ritual practices were
intended to honor the spirits of whales so that
they would allow themselves to be captured.
These practices insured that no offense might
be taken, and in the case of whaling, with its
vast underpinnings in the economic, social, and
technological aspects of life, attention to hunting
magic and associated ceremony was considered
critical to community survival. Failure to catch
a single whale might threaten starvation or
dispersion of the community.

Many ritual items were carried in the umiak
itself or on the persons of the *umialik* and his
crew. Charm boxes contained amulets prepared
by the *umialik* or a shaman to insure hunting
success and safety, including such items as
chipped stone effigy whales and pieces of quartz
crystal, a potent vision-inducing material (Kaplan, Jordan, and Sheehan 1984). The umiak
was also fitted with ornamented harpoon rests
and plaques bearing the images of whales,
reminiscent in concept of face plaques and sea
otter charms used in Bering Sea and Aleut
kayaks. Harpoon blades were kept in special
whale-shaped boxes, and ritual wooden freshwater containers were kept at the whaling camp
for use in the greeting ceremonies.

The mass extermination of whales by American whalers in the late 19th century resulted
in a major decline of native whaling in arctic
regions of Alaska and Siberia. This native hunt
was strictly a coastal hunt, usually conducted
near the shore or at the ice edge, while European
whaling occurred both in coastal and deep-sea
areas. The success of the American whalers in
the open sea drastically reduced the numbers
of whales available to native hunters along shore,
placing them at great disadvantage competitively in addition to undercutting a focal point
of native life. With the rise of alternative means
of subsistence in the 20th century, reliance on
whales as a food source diminished, but the
importance of whaling in economic and cultural
terms never disappeared. Although Alaskan Natives no longer observe most of the religious
rituals connected with the hunt, they continue
to share the meat and blubber in traditional
patterns that reaffirm social ties and provide a
strong sense of ethnic identity. Recently, with
the rise of the international whale conservation
movement, some native groups, such as those
in Siberia, have been banned from practicing
aboriginal whaling, but Alaskans, who never
interrupted their whaling tradition, have been
successful in maintaining an annual quota.

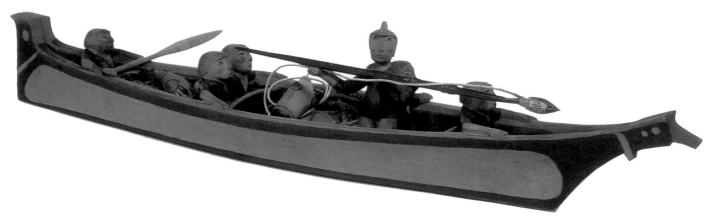

Northwest Coast Whaling

Vancouver Island and the Olympic Peninsula of Washington were home to the Nootka, Makah, Quileute, and Quinault Indians, who were the great seafaring whalers of the Northwest Coast (Frachtenberg 1921; Olson 1936; Drucker 1951). Although whale meat was not their primary food, whale hunting was the ultimate challenge for men in these societies, and, as in the Arctic, whaling took a central cultural role.

Whales were present here from the beginning of May through the end of June. They were pursued in dugouts carrying a crew of eight: six paddlers, a steersman, and a harpooner who also served as boat captain. Traditionally, the crew members wore nothing but their basketry hats, which provided protection from sun and rain.

The search might last for days. When a whale was sighted, the crew had to paddle hard but silently to approach the prey, always from the left side. The harpooner delivered his blow with a direct thrust, as a throw would not have embedded the harpoon head deeply enough to hold. Accuracy was crucial; the harpoon had to be placed close behind the whale's left flipper. After a successful strike the remaining canoes in the flotilla joined chase, striking with other harpoons each time the animal surfaced. Throughout, sacred hunting songs were sung to help drive the whale toward shore to reduce the towing distance after the kill. The chase ended with the whale lying exhausted from exertion and blood loss. The lead canoe then approached and the harpooner severed the tail tendons with a chisellike blade mounted on a long pole, to prevent the whale from sounding again, and then delivered a mortal blow with an elk-horn lance. Floats were then attached to the carcass, its mouth was tied shut, and the boats began the hard task of towing the whale to shore.

A complete whaling harpoon consisted of a shaft, a foreshaft, a harpoon head, a harpoon line, and three or four inflated sealskin floats.

The shaft was of heavy yew with tapered ends, measuring 14 to 20 feet in length. Harpoon heads were made of thick-shelled mussel blades encased in two elk-horn valves coated with spruce gum. The harpoon line was of tough twisted cedar root, 40 fathoms long, with three or four inflated hair seal floats. In Nootkan whaling, as in northern Eskimo whaling, the line and floats were cast free from the boat to be dragged behind the whale, impeding its escape while avoiding the dangerous ''Nantucket sleigh-ride'' characteristic of the European whaling tradition.

The origin of Nootka whaling is not known. However, whaling was important in the life and culture of Makah people who lived at the Ozette site south of Cape Flattery. Whaling gear from this well-preserved archeological site dating to about A.D. 1400 is nearly identical to that from the ethnographic period. A rich complex of whale-related ceremonialism was also recovered from this remarkable village, destroyed by a mud slide. The many similarities between this southern Northwest Coast whaling tradition and those of Asia and the Arctic have stimulated speculation, but no certain conclusions have been reached with archeological data. The most peculiar similarities are those between Nootka

215. Whaling Canoe Model
Makah: NMNH 72936

Famed as expert canoe-makers and seamen, the Makah and their neighbors were the only Northwest Coast Indian peoples to hunt whales in historic times. Whaling was a dangerous and prestigious pursuit, undertaken with the aid of ritual observances and a highly developed technology. The whaling canoe was fast and seaworthy. In this model the harpooner stands with his heavy yew wood harpoon, fitted with a mussel shell-bladed head, line, and attached sealskin floats. His crew is prepared to back from the whale at the instant the harpoon strikes.

216. Whaling Float
Makah: NMNH 23387

Inflated sealskin floats attached to the harpoon line slowed the whale and shortened his dive. Makah and Nootka floats were typically painted with red and black circles around the four closed holes in the skin, one of which was fitted with a stoppered nozzle for inflating. The arrangement of the colored circles and diamond-shaped feather designs was the property mark of the whaler.

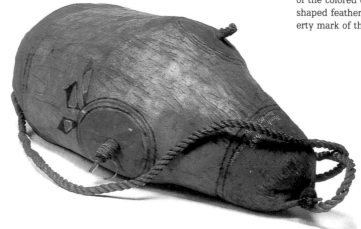

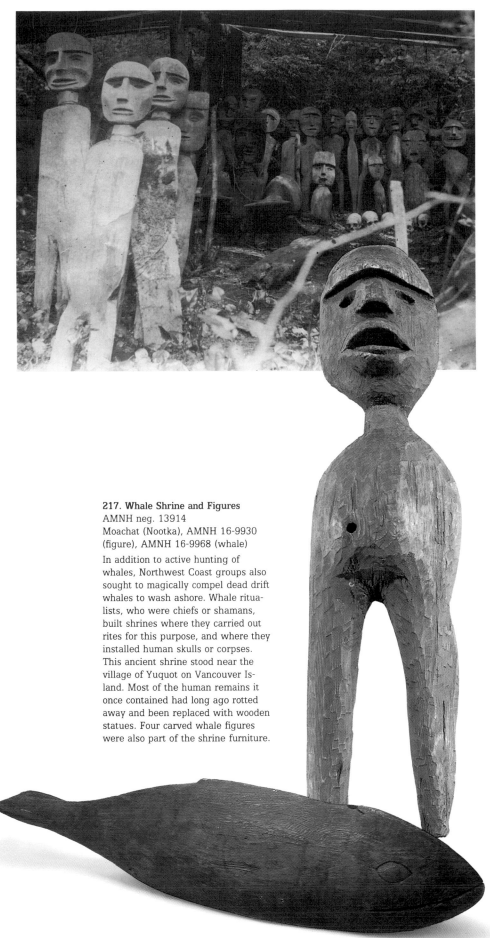

217. Whale Shrine and Figures
AMNH neg. 13914
Moachat (Nootka), AMNH 16-9930 (figure), AMNH 16-9968 (whale)

In addition to active hunting of whales, Northwest Coast groups also sought to magically compel dead drift whales to wash ashore. Whale ritualists, who were chiefs or shamans, built shrines where they carried out rites for this purpose, and where they installed human skulls or corpses. This ancient shrine stood near the village of Yuquot on Vancouver Island. Most of the human remains it once contained had long ago rotted away and been replaced with wooden statues. Four carved whale figures were also part of the shrine furniture.

dugout canoes and Alaskan Eskimo umiaks (Duff 1964, 1981a). These similarities even include details like the zigzag designs that run the length of Nootka dugouts beneath the inside gunwales, a pattern that seems to mimic the lacing of skin covers in Eskimo umiaks (Holm 1983:92).

Correspondences with Bering Strait whaling also occurred in Nootka ceremonial practices. Nootka tradition required the whaler's wife to lie in the whaler's sleeping place under a new cedar-bark blanket when the hunt began and to remain there, immobile and without food or water, for the duration of the hunt. As in North Alaska, the Nootka whaler's wife embodied the whale; her activities were transmitted to it and vice versa. If she made sudden movements, the whale would also. When the whalers returned, she went to the shore to greet the whale, commenting on its great thirst, after years in the sea, and pouring a drink of fresh water into its mouth. She then sang and danced her greeting.

Societies involved with whaling all had special ceremonial festivals, in addition to rituals that took place during the actual time of the hunt. One of the best known is the Eskimo festival called the Messenger Feast. This feast took place after a successful hunt and was announced when an *umialik* would send a messenger to neighboring villages inviting them to feast with him. The feast helped create social solidarity and spread the recently acquired wealth beyond the *umialik*'s village. Presentation of lavish feasts built the reputation of the *umialik* beyond that of a family and village provider and established him as a man of power, generosity, and esteem. The Messenger Feast was the most important social event of the year, bringing renewal and rebirth and reaffirming the social values supporting the whaling complex. In this manner, the accumulation and distribution of wealth and the advancement of individual and community status in North Alaska correspond to the potlatch system on the Northwest Coast, where circumstances provided use of more durable goods in these exchanges.

These similarities between Siberian, Alaskan, and Northwest Coast whaling methods, material culture, and customs have been noted for many years (Lantis 1938). It seems unlikely that whaling developed separately in each separate geographic region, but the timing and nature of the supposed cultural connections are not yet understood.

Kayak Whaling

Whaling methods of the Aleut and Pacific Eskimo contrasted sharply with the umiak whaling of Bering Sea cultures and more closely resembled whaling methods employed by the Ainu of the Kurile Islands and the Itelmen of the southern Kamchatka Peninsula in Siberia. The Aleut and Pacific Eskimo technique differed from the northern method in three major ways: use of kayaks rather than umiaks or dugouts; use of poisoned darts cast with throwing boards, rather than harpoons; and utilization of whales after they died and drifted ashore, rather than capturing them directly. The Itelmen shot whales with poisoned arrows from wooden dugout boats, and a similar variation was apparently used by the northern Ainu.

The crucial element in this method was the use of an aconite poison made from the root of the monkshood plant (*Aconitum* sp.). Aleutian and Pacific Eskimo whalers regarded human fat derived from the bodies of deceased whalers or ''rich persons'' as an essential and magically potent ingredient, which was added to the poison. Although less efficient than harpoon hunting, which provided a firm attachment to the animal, use of poison and collection of dead whales allowed the hunters to recover 10 to 50 percent of the whales struck.

Kayak hunting was conducted during the summer months on the open ocean, sea ice never being present in these regions. Hunters would embark in one or more two-holed kayaks with the main paddler in the stern and the hunter, who also paddled, in the bow, where he had access to the whale darts laid out before him on the deck. The search for whales was aided when calm seas permitted spouting whales to be seen at great distances, but the whaler also relied on medicine songs to bring him into contact with his prey. These songs were considered central to whaling success and were passed down from ancient whalers; in other cases, whalers who could not gain access to songs, or who needed new ones, created them anew. Once sighted, the whale was approached silently, again from the left side, and the spear was hurled at a spot behind the flipper. The wooden shaft detached from the thin, poisoned slate blade and floated free, to be retrieved, as the whale sounded. In the Aleutians, a barbed, stone-tipped head was used that detached from the dart after penetrating the whale's skin.

The hunters then returned to shore to await the effects of the poison, exacerbated by the working of the point in the wound. The stricken

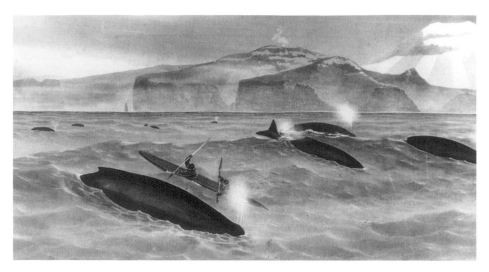

whale, killed by the poison or drowned because of poison-induced paralysis in the flipper nearest the wound, was generally dead within three days. During this time the hunters sat, singing songs to the whale, in front of a sacred cave containing the mummified bodies of the great whaling ancestors. If all the complex rituals leading up to the whaling venture had been strictly observed, not only by the hunters themselves but also by the community as a whole, the whale would die and float into the cove in front of the village. As this rarely occurred, more practical steps were also taken, including keeping a careful watch of the whale's movements, if visible, or if not, estimating the effects of wind and tide so that a successful search for the carcass might be made in due course. In some cases, kayakers were able to drive a dying whale toward the village. The hunter who had struck the whale could be determined by examining his owner's mark scratched on the blade embedded in the carcass.

Use of the poison hunting technique allowed a small group of hunters, in small boats, to strike as many whales as they could successfully approach. This avoided a large investment in expensive equipment and could be carried out without large boat crews. Although less efficient than harpoon whaling, the method produced adequate results. In this technique, elaboration occurred not in technology but in the development of arcane knowledge surrounding poison production and ritual, including the elevation of the whaler's social position and postmortem status. Disposal of deceased whalers in sacred caves was vital to the conduct of ongoing whaling practices and insured prominence of whaling ancestors in the ritual and mythological life of Aleut and Pacific Eskimo peoples.

218. ''Aleutians striking humpback whales: off Akootan Island, Bering Sea''
Henry W. Elliott. SI-NAA 7119-9, SI neg. 84-1816

Kayak whaling using poison-tipped darts was practiced from the eastern Aleutians to Prince William Sound, but this method may have been a contact period introduction from Kamchatka (Heizer 1943). The rituals surrounding the hunt and the preparation of whaling poison, including the use of the mummified bodies of dead whalers, were elaborate and suggest ancient roots, however. Aleut, Koniag, and Chugach whalers were feared for their supernatural powers. Elliott's painting captures the drama of an Aleut hunt off Akutan Island, but is less than accurate in some details. Most imporantly, whale darts were cast with the aid of a throwing board, not thrust directly into the whale.

219. Whale Dart
Aleut: MAE 4270-44

Aleut whale darts had barbed bone heads with chipped-stone endblades. The head was coated with enough aconite poison to paralyze one flipper of the whale and cause it to drown. With luck, the dead whale would be found floating or washed up on shore. Koniag whale darts had long, poison-coated slate blades that broke off in the wound.

Hunters, Herders, Trappers, and Fishermen

James W. VanStone

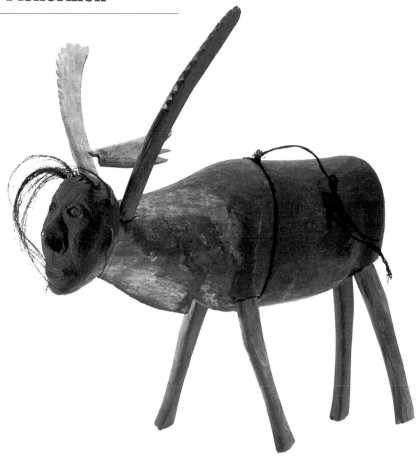

220. Caribou Spirit
Bering Sea Eskimo: NMNH 56026
In the Bering Sea Eskimo conception of the world the caribou, like all other animals, possessed a soul (*yua*) in human form that sometimes revealed itself and was capable of human speech. The function of this Bristol Bay caribou-human carving is unknown, but the cord around its middle suggests that it was suspended, possibly from the ceiling during the Bladder Festival. During that hunting ceremony it is known that caribou skin strips and bladders were hung up along with sea mammal bladders, wooden bird carvings, and miniature paddles.

Although most Pacific Rim peoples practiced a subsistence emphasis oriented primarily toward the marine ecosystem, rivers and river mouths have always been economically important to all of them, and many groups, particularly those without direct access to the seacoast, were heavily dependent on inland game animals. Peoples of the Pacific Rim, from the coast of British Columbia to the mouth of the Amur River, have traditionally exploited all aspects of their environment even while emphasizing one particular ecosystem.

Large game animals of primary subsistence importance on the North American side of the Bering Sea were the woodland caribou, barren ground caribou, and moose. On the Asiatic side, several groups relied heavily on a domesticated relative of the caribou, the reindeer. In alpine areas of northwestern North America the mountain goat and Dall sheep have been important resources, but always in addition to moose and woodland caribou. Black bears are widely distributed on both continents but were never a major food resource, although they were of ritual importance to some peoples. Of the small mam-

mals, hares were widely exploited and were often a source of midwinter food when large game was scarce.

All arctic and subarctic mammals larger than voles, lemmings, and shrews were included in the fur trade economy. European fur fashions, which changed frequently, greatly influenced the income and activities of native trappers. In addition to the many fur-bearing animals that were basic to the trade, large game was also included for the hides and the meat that was supplied to workers in the fur trade.

Along all the streams that have major salmon runs, native peoples depended heavily on the seasonal catch of several species of these fish. Even in areas where there were no salmon, the availability of fish in most lakes and streams made them an important seasonal resource. With the increase in the size of dog teams during the historic period, large quantities of fish were required for dog food. Migrating waterfowl, particularly numerous species of ducks, were an important source of food for brief periods, especially in the spring.

River Fishing

The several species of salmon were the most important fish economically throughout the Pacific Rim area. Salmon fishing depends on the behavior of the fish at spawning time. Salmon live in salt water but spawn in freshwater rivers, streams, and, in the case of one species, lakes. When the young fish hatch, they live in fresh water for only a short time and then make their way to the ocean. Two, three, or four years after spawning, depending on the species, the mature fish school in bays and inlets before making their way up rivers to spawn. It is these periodic runs that offer the best opportunity for intensive fishing.

For the Indians of the Northwest Coast, salmon fishing was vital for subsistence and a major influence on their lifestyle. Several kinds of harpoons, nets, and traps were used. Weirs were constructed that permitted the flow of water but directed the fish in such a manner that they could easily be trapped, netted, or harpooned. For fish as large as salmon, harpoons were preferred to spears because the fish could not tear loose as easily as they could from a weapon

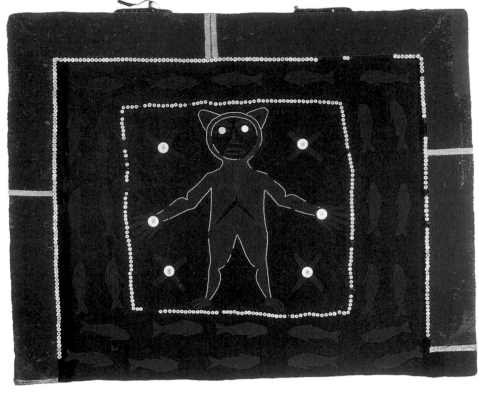

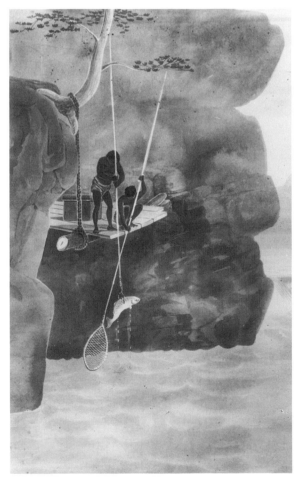

with a fixed point. Salmon were netted with dip nets manipulated from scaffoldings erected over streams, from canoes, and from catwalks erected on large weirs. Cylindrical traps with funneled entries were placed on the bottoms of streams and the fish directed toward them with weirs.

In addition to the predictable abundance of salmon, these fish were important on the Northwest Coast and elsewhere throughout the Pacific Rim area because they are easily preserved. Smoke dried, the flesh would last a considerable time even under humid coastal conditions. In a few days a family could catch and preserve sufficient salmon to last them for several months, thus providing leisure time for other activities. The peoples of the Northwest Coast were the only sedentary hunter-gatherers in North America, and their rich culture was primarily the result of the abundance of salmon.

Other varieties of fish also occur in annual runs. Herring and smelt spawn along beaches, and eulachon run in the lower courses of rivers north of the Fraser. Although not as important as salmon, they were taken in large quantities with dip nets and eaten fresh or dried. Eulachon, however, are so oil-rich that they cannot be dried, but they were preserved for the oil, which was a luxury for the Indians. The runs of these species occurred in spring and summer, when the previous fall's supply of dried salmon was

221. Button Blanket
Tsimshian: NMNH 274676

As described in the Tsimshian myth of "The Prince Who Was Taken Away by the Spring Salmon" (Boas 1916:192), each species of salmon has its own chief and village beneath the sea. When the cottonwood leaves fall into the Skeena River, it is a signal for the salmon to leave their villages to head upstream, led by their chief, the First Salmon. It is not known what myth is illustrated by this flannel-appliquéd button blanket, but its humanoid central figure may represent a salmon chief. Alternatively, it may be the submarine monster Nagunaks, whose crest helmet is shown in figure 383.

222. "Interior or 'Stick' Indians spearing in the canyon of the Fraser River"
Henry W. Elliott, 1891. SI-NAA 7119-6, SI neg. 84-1808

Many methods were used on the Northwest Coast for catching salmon during their annual spawning runs, including dip-netting and spearing from platforms suspended over the water.

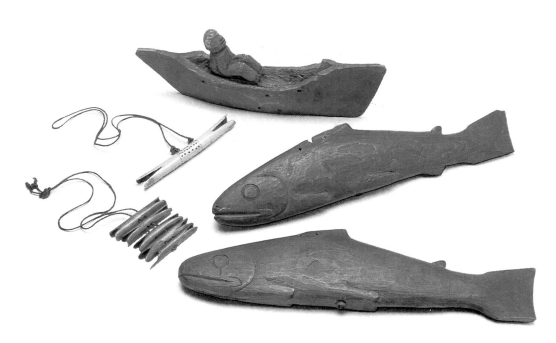

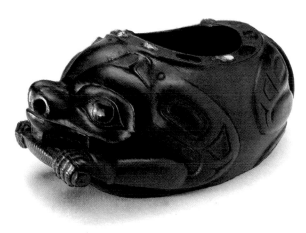

low. Fishing with hook and line was reserved
for large species such as cod and halibut.

Indicative of the importance of salmon to the
Indians of the Northwest Coast was the importance associated with the arrival of the first
salmon each year. Salmon were believed to
voluntarily sacrifice themselves for the benefit
of people, and thus it was necessary that they
be treated respectfully. The first fish taken each
year was conveyed by a priest to an altar in the
presence of the assembled group and positioned
with its head facing upstream so that the rest
of the salmon run would not head back to sea.
Throughout the rite, during which the fish was
treated as an honored guest of high rank, constant reference was made to the continuation of
the run. A speech of welcome was made, songs
and chants were sung, and the fish was cooked
and served to those present. The First Salmon
rite was typical of the placation-of-game ceremonies prevalent throughout the Pacific Rim
area.

Among Alaskan Eskimo, the greatest dependence on fish occurred among various coastal and
riverine groups, especially those on the central
and lower Kobuk River, the Noatak River, and
the Lower Yukon, as well as coastal groups in
the Norton Sound, Kuskokwim Bay, and Bristol
Bay areas. These people, together with Eskimo
on Kodiak Island and the Kenai Peninsula, had
access to five species of salmon entering the
rivers to spawn as well as several other species
of freshwater fish. Salmon were caught in gill
nets or in traps set in association with weirs.
Individual fish were taken with harpoon darts.
The most important freshwater species, whitefish, was trapped and netted.

In central Kamchatka, as well as on the Northwest Coast and in the Amur-Sakhalin area, a
seasonally rich environment enabled the people
to lead a sedentary life of comparative leisure
during half the year. Among the Itelmen, life
revolved around fishing, particularly the taking
of the local species of salmon, which, as elsewhere, had to be exploited to the fullest extent
during the relatively brief period in which they
were available to each community. At those
times, everyone worked, the men catching the
fish and the women hanging them to dry. Most
salmon were taken in weirs fitted with basket
traps, but nets of several types, made of nettle
fibers, were also used. Fish were also speared
from riverbanks and dugout canoes.

Next in importance to fishing in the Itelmen
economy was the gathering of wild vegetable
products, which was more important here than
elsewhere in the Pacific Rim area. The local flora
was exploited to the fullest extent by women,
who were the gatherers. All edible plants were
utilized, and others were collected for household
or medicinal use. The nettle was an extremely
important plant, being the source of fiber cor-

dage and thread and thus the essential raw material for the manufacture of fishnets.

Fish were also of primary importance in the diet of the Nivkhi of Sakhalin Island and the lower Amur River, and their life was regulated by the seasonal runs of salmon and sturgeon. Seines and nets of various sizes, mesh, and construction made of nettle fiber were used. Nets were set out from shore and erected serially, primarily for night fishing. The heaviest nets were used for sturgeon. Elaborate fish traps were constructed in conjunction with weirs, and large bag nets were employed for fishing from boats and also for winter ice fishing. Fish were also taken with rods, gaffs, hooks, and a variety of harpoons and hand nets. For navigation of shallow waters and narrow creeks the Nivkhi used a dugout made of a single poplar trunk; birchbark canoes were also used. The choice of settlement location was determined to a large extent by dependence on large-scale fishing. River settlements were often occupied year-round.

Land Hunting

Land game was abundant on the Northwest Coast, especially deer, elk, black and grizzly bear, and wolf. Furbearers included beaver, mink, land otter, fisher, and marten. Flights of waterfowl followed the Pacific flyway in their seasonal migrations to and from their arctic and subarctic nesting grounds.

Land animals were hunted and trapped in a variety of ways depending on the habits of the various species and the nature of the terrain. Individual stalking, group drives, surrounds, spring pole and simple snares, pitfalls, and bows and arrows were all utilized. Nevertheless, land hunting was of relatively minor importance because of the emphasis on exploitation of sea and river products. Among the Indian groups living along the coast, there were a few villages situated at the head of tidewaters or on rivers. Sea mammals were less accessible in these areas, and consequently land game was more important.

Although land hunting was important to all Alaskan Eskimo, even to those where the mar-

itime emphasis was strongest, the environment of the Brooks Range in northwest Alaska where the Nunamiut live offered perhaps the least potential for a balanced economy. Among these Eskimo the annual subsistence cycle focused on the hunting of caribou. Although accessible throughout the year in small numbers, caribou were most abundant during early summer when the herds moved north and in the fall as they moved south. The most successful method of taking migrating animals was through the cooperative efforts of a number of hunters and families. Two converging lines of cairns made of rocks or sod were erected at a place where the caribou were likely to concentrate. These cairns looked like men to the animals. Near the converging point earthen mounds were constructed to hide the hunters, and snares were set in circles beyond the mounds. As the caribou approached the cairns, women and children appeared behind the herd and frightened the animals toward the hunters, who shot them with bows and arrows. Those not killed were caught in the snares and speared. Cairns were also used to guide the caribou toward lakes where they could be killed easily by hunters in kayaks. Caribou meat was eatable at any time, but the skins were best when taken from animals in the summer and early fall. The meat and skins from cooperative hunts were divided equally among the hunters.

Many species of land animals as diverse in size as ground squirrels, wolves, and Dall sheep were also taken in snares. Bears were also snared and wolverines taken in rock deadfalls. Moose, which were numerous in the willows along rivers and streams, were shot with bows and arrows. Migrating ducks and geese were also available seasonally. The Nunamiut shared a caribou-hunting emphasis with Eskimo of the upper

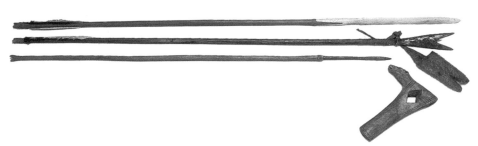

225. Arrows and Shaft Straightener
Chukchi: AMNH 70-6980b,e,d;
North Alaskan Eskimo: NMNH 383300

Bow and arrows served the Chukchi in both war and in the hunting of wild caribou, small game, and birds. Arrows of many types, some with skin sheaths to protect their sharp points, were made for different game. The ability to split a blade of grass with the point of an arrow was proof of the greatest skill in archery. The Eskimo arrow shaft straightener was used as a wrench to true arrows in the process of manufacture.

226. Bows
Koniag Eskimo (Alaska Peninsula): MAE 593-64 (top); Chugach Eskimo: MAE 2913-20

Painted images of caribou, sea otter, and beaver reflect the fact that the Koniag and Chugach hunted on both land and sea using bows. Visible on the upper bow of this pair is the sinew cable backing typical of Eskimo bows; an ivory plate at midlength adds even more strength and elasticity. The inner side of the longer bow is shown, with the bowstring removed. The use of red and black paint to decorate weapons is similar to Aleut practice, as is the decorative use of fine hairs and strands of yarn on the Alaska Peninsula bow.

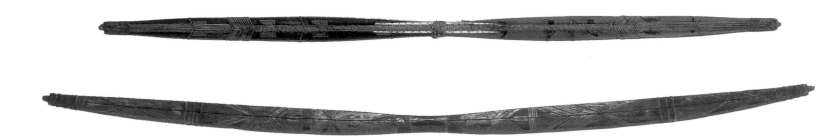

Noatak and Kobuk rivers, but caribou were also important to people living along the Bering Sea coast, where the animals moved in summer to avoid insects.

Among Athapaskans, big-game hunting tended to be most important to those people living at the headwaters of the major rivers and their tributaries and to those whose territories encompassed the divide between the Pacific and arctic drainages. Like the Nunamiut, Athapaskan hunters made their greatest harvest when the animals were massed together and thus especially vulnerable. Caribou massed for migrations were taken either in surrounds placed in mountain passes or from boats when the herds were crossing rivers. Athapaskan hunters used a kayak-form canoe covered with birch bark and decked at both ends. It also served for fishing and visiting fish traps and nets.

Migrating waterfowl were exploited when they massed in breeding areas and were molting. Moose were hunted from canoes when swim-ming in rivers, and thus helpless, or run down in the deep, crusted snow of late winter, which supports the weight of a hunter on showshoes but breaks and retards the movement of a much heavier moose. In large areas of the Athapaskan region there were few game animals, and changes in annual populations, such as caribou migration routes, frequently caused starvation among native populations.

Among the Nivkhi hunting was of secondary importance to fishing as a means of subsistence, but it was nevertheless significant as a source of wealth and prestige. Forest animals were hunted primarily for their pelts, which, during the contact period, provided the currency for acquiring prestigious trade goods.

The Nivkhi utilized hereditary winter hunting territories based on lineage affiliation. A man hunted alone within his section of a territory and inspected his traps every three or four days. Sables, the most important fur-bearing animals, were taken in noose and deadfall traps designed so as not to injure the animal's pelt. A typical trap was constructed within a tree hollow with the bait just inside the hollow. The animal, in reaching for the bait, was strangled by a falling stick. Another form of trap involved a trigger mechanism that released an arrow or, in the case of big game, a spear. The Nivkhi did not hunt with dogs.

Bears were hunted cooperatively by groups of kinsmen, the objective being to capture the animal alive, chain and lash it to a platform made of several sleds, and return it to the village, where it played an important role in lineage rituals. The best hunters sometimes hunted bears alone to kill them. The animal was located in its winter lair, the entrance partially blocked, and the bear roused to be killed with a multi-pronged pike or spear as it attempted to escape.

Animals hunted for other than ceremonial reasons included deer, moose, wolves, and lynx. Hares were killed for food and for ritual purposes. The fur, especially the head and ears, was believed to offer protection from evil spirits. The ownership of lynx pelts conveyed high prestige. A variety of birds, especially waterfowl, were killed with small arrows and, during the molting season, clubbed with sticks; ptarmigan, grouse, and partridges were taken in snares. Weapons employed in hunting, principally the compound bow, spear, lance, and pike, were also used in war.

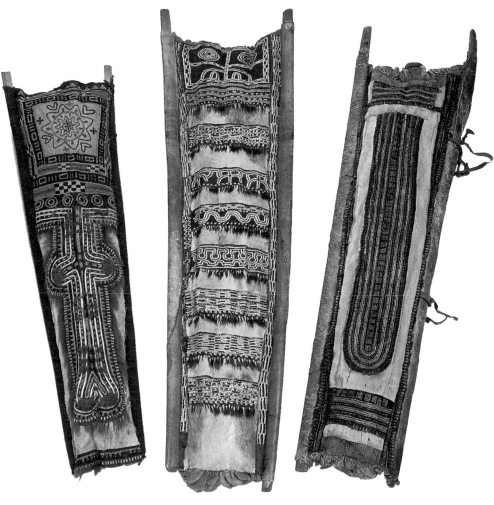

227. Siberian Quivers
Koryak: MAE 956-87; Chukchi: AMNH 70-6980a; Chukchi: MAE 408-71 (left to right)

The meanings of the ancient designs and symbols embroidered on Koryak and Chukchi quivers were no longer known by the time these examples were collected 85-90 years ago. The silk-embroidered funeral quiver on the left was meant to be burned with the hunter on his pyre; an anthropo-morphic design fills its lower panel. Decorated quivers contrast with the generally plain aspect of Chukchi craftwork.

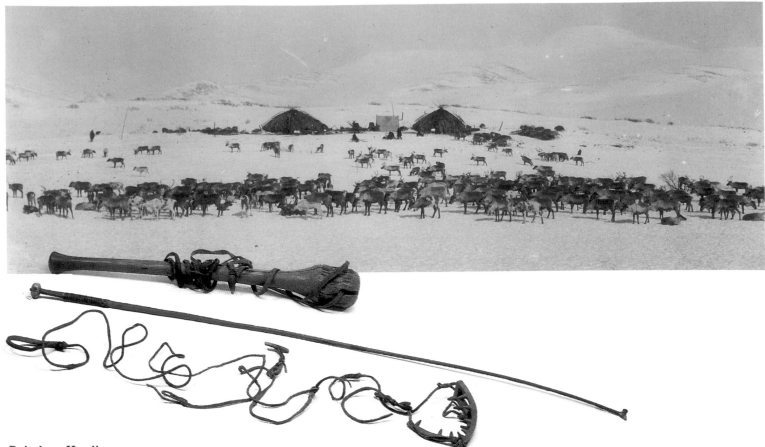

Reindeer Herding

In Northeastern Siberia live the only people along the Pacific Rim whose subsistence depended primarily on a domestic animal. Among the Koryak of the upper Kamchatka Peninsula and the east coast of the Okhotsk Sea, there were maritime hunters on the coast as well as reindeer herders in the interior and some groups that had a mixed economy. The Chukchi, neighbors of the Koryak to the north, were also divided into maritime and reindeer groups.

For the reindeer-breeding Koryak, these animals provided the principal item of the diet as well as the basic material for clothing, skins to cover dwellings, and sinew for thread. The Koryak kept large herds, often exceeding 100 animals, in contrast to most Eurasian reindeer-breeding groups, which followed a pattern of intensive breeding using small herds exploited for dairy products and transportation but seldom slaughtered. Both the Koryak and the Chukchi employed reindeer for drawing sleds but did not ride them.

Among the Koryak a reindeer herd grazed near the encampment in winter. As soon as this pasture was exhausted, a search was undertaken for another. When one was selected the entire camp, consisting of double tents of skin, moved to the new site, and herdsmen moved the herd. These migrations took place four or five times during the winter. In spring, before calving,

females were separated from the rest of the herd. Calving time was a difficult period for the reindeer breeders since the newborn calves had to be protected from predators and also kept from freezing. At this time the herdsmen were assisted by members of their families, and even old people and children helped in guarding the herds.

Following the calving season, the herds were driven into the mountains for the summer. Choice of a summer pasture was of utmost importance and determined the welfare of the herd for the entire year. Summer herding required considerable skill and experience as well as knowledge of the reindeer's requirements and conditions of the tundra. During this period the Koryak encampment was moved to a summer site, usually on a riverbank where the meat diet could be supplemented with fish. In the fall the herdsmen brought the herd to the camp, and this annual occasion was one of the major holidays of the Koryak and the time of important ceremonies and rituals.

Reindeer herding among the Chukchi and Koryak was accomplished without the assistance of dogs. A good herder required agility, good eyes, and considerable skill with a leather lasso if he was to protect the herd from wolves and snowstorms in winter, foxes and ravens in spring during the calving season, and from insects in

228. Reindeer Herders of Siberia
AMNH neg. 4169, Jesup Exp.; Chukchi: 70-6979a, 70-7684, 0-239

Koryak reindeer herders, here in a spring encampment (Jochelson's tent in center), led a nomadic life, constantly moving on as the herd required new pasture. Reindeer supplied food, skins, and draught power. Chukchi reindeer sled driving equipment included the training club (*top*), used for violently jerking the reins while breaking in a new animal to the sled; an ivory-tipped driving whip, and a harness trace with a spiked bone bit that dug into the animal's neck when pulled by the driver.

spring and summer. It was necessary for the herders to remain with the herd at all times.

Chukchi herdsmen were brought to Northwest Alaska with reindeer herds in 1891–92 for a herding program instituted by the U.S. Bureau of Education at the suggestion of Dr. Sheldon Jackson, a Presbyterian missionary. The intention was to provide Alaskan Eskimos with a new source of food to offset the decline in sea mammals caused by unrestricted killing of whales, walrus, and seals by commercial interests during the second half of the 19th century. There was a small market for the meat and skins, and it was hoped that the Eskimos could derive a cash income from their sale and that reindeer would replace dogs for local transportation.

The reindeer herds were, at first, frequently owned by non-Eskimos, especially individuals at the missions. In the early years of the project Lapps from northern Norway replaced the Chukchi, and a system of apprenticeships for Eskimos was established. As they became experienced in herding through working with the Lapp herders, Eskimos became individual owners of deer. After 1918, the reindeer industry gradually became dominated by companies, such as the Loman Brothers in Nome, who owned trading posts and transport as well as stock. Their monopoly continued until the Reindeer Act of 1937, which restricted the ownership of reindeer to natives, but by this time the industry was in a considerable decline.

Involvement of Alaskan Eskimos in the reindeer-herding program can be understood by examining the participation of people from one village. In 1894 two men from Point Hope were sent to the reindeer station at Teller on Seward Peninsula to learn herding practices, and one of

them brought part of his herd and some government deer back to the village in 1908. At first the reindeer did well at Point Hope. Most of the animals were individually owned and identified by special marks on the ears. However, this proved to be an unsatisfactory arrangement because the herds were hard to separate on the basis of individual marks. In 1926 all deer were counted into one herd, numbering 4,100 animals, owned by a joint stock company of Eskimos. Six years later there were 6,000 deer. The herd seems to have maintained its size until 1938, when the first sizable decrease was noted, and by 1945 there were only 500 animals. In 1947 the herd was returned to the government because it was too small to pay its way. A herder was hired, but when, in 1948, he left the herd to get supplies, the remaining 250 animals disappeared.

The attempt to make reindeer herders out of the Alaskan Eskimos was unsuccessful for a variety of reasons. The deer themselves were subject to various parasites and were killed in large numbers by wolves. If not carefully watched by the herdsmen, they tended to wander off with the caribou; certain areas were overgrazed through careless herding. Most significant of all, perhaps, was the fact that the coastal Eskimos of Northwest Alaska were a sedentary people who followed a definite cycle of hunting and fishing quite foreign to the nomadic routine of close herding practiced by Siberian reindeer herders. At Point Hope, for example, even the most dedicated herdsmen desired to return to the village for the spring whaling activities, and it was at this time that large numbers of deer wandered away and were lost.

229. Alaskan Reindeer Herders
Glenbow-Alberta Institute neg. NC-1-890

In this Lomen Brothers photograph Alaskan Eskimos pose with their sled reindeer near the Kuzitrin River on the Seward Peninsula (1920s). The experimental grafting of reindeer herding, a Siberian economic pattern, onto Alaskan Eskimo culture enjoyed only brief and limited success.

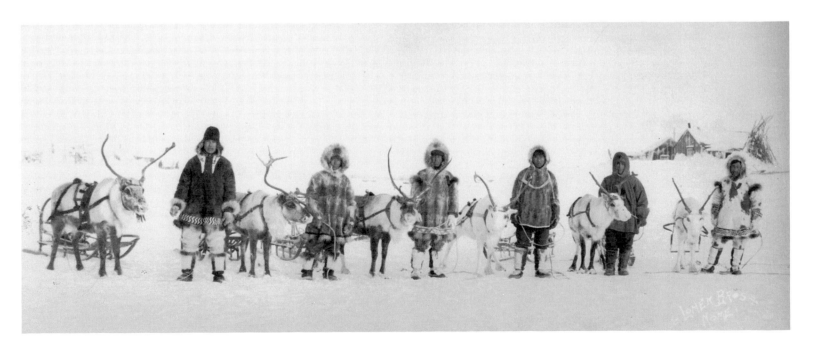

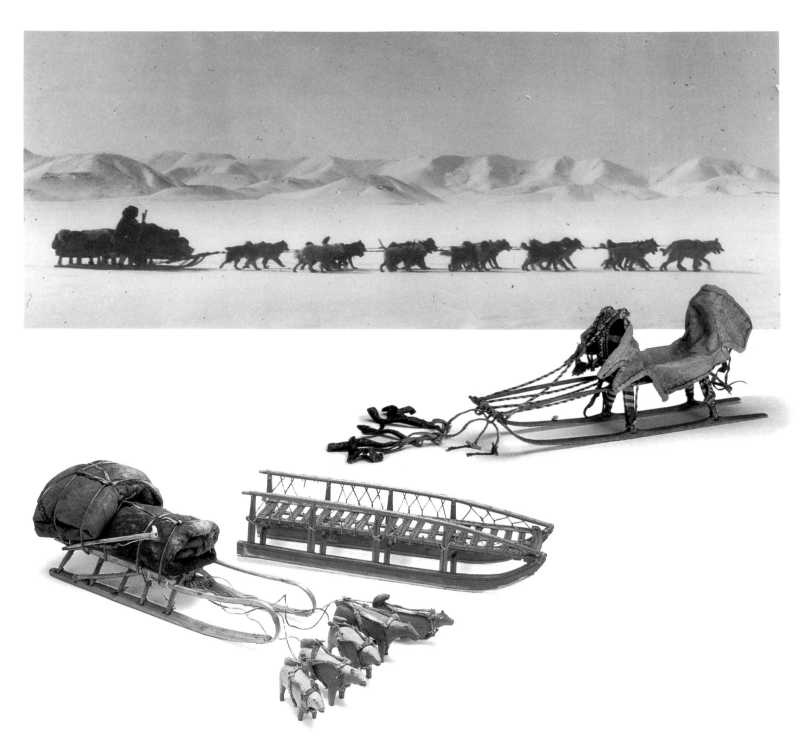

Transportation

For the Alaskan Eskimo and Athapaskans, land travel with dogs and sleds was important for hunting caribou and fur trapping, as well as for setting fish traps through the ice. Eskimos required such transportation for hunting sea mammals at the edge of the ice, and both peoples visited trading posts and distant relatives in other villages or where special festivals were being held. Several different forms of sleds were used throughout western Alaska, varieties developed in response to ice and snow conditions and the type of activity for which the sled was required. Small hand-drawn sleds were used to haul meat and transport kayaks to the edge of the ice. Traditionally Eskimo dog teams were small, seldom more than three to five animals hitched in tandem to a central tow line with a single leader. Larger teams and lighter sleds were introduced by Euro-Americans in the fur trapping era, and both Eskimo and Athapaskans were thus required to process large quantities of dried fish for dog food.

During the aboriginal period, all winter hunting by most northern Athapaskans was carried out on foot since dogs were not yet used for pulling sleds or toboggans. Therefore, snow-

230. Dog Sledding

AMNH neg. 2420, Jesup Exp.
Sled Models (left to right) Chukchi: AMNH 70-7888; Bering Sea Eskimo: NMNH 260531; Itelmen: MAE 864-1

Dog sledding was primarily the practice of coastal and riverine groups. The old harnessing method, practiced by both Siberians and the Alaskan Eskimo, was a fan arrangement in which each dog was tied directly to the sled (models.). The Russian tandem method (photo) allowed faster speeds.

shoes were important items of material culture, and many groups made two types. The first, called hunting snowshoes, were long and rounded in front and were used for walking over fresh snow. The second type, travel snowshoes, were shorter with a pointed and sharply upturned front end. These smaller snowshoes allowed the wearer to sink more deeply into the snow and were used for walking on a previously broken trail or, in later times, to break a trail for a dog team. Eskimos in Southwest Alaska used snowshoes similar to the travel type for traversing land where protected conditions resulted in the accumulation of soft, deep snow. In Northwest Alaska Eskimo used crude, short snowshoes for travel over sea ice. Their primary purpose was to distribute the weight over a wider area when crossing new or weak ice.

The Itelmen were dog breeders, but unlike the Alaskan Eskimo, dogs played only a minor role in their economic life. The Itelmen sled, with its saddlelike superstructure, could carry no load and was a unique form with no obvious parallel elsewhere in the Arctic or Subarctic. There is no evidence to indicate another style of sled for transporting freight, but the Russians did introduce such a sled that became an integral part of post-contact Itelmen culture. Dogs were tied up and fed on fish in winter but turned loose to fend for themselves in summer.

The principal means of transportation for the reindeer-breeding Chukchi and Koryak were reindeer, and the maritime groups traveled by dogsled. Reindeer sleds were of two types, a light traveling vehicle and a heavier one for hauling freight. The traveling sled was made of slender poles held together with hide lashing, curved antler stanchions, and narrow runners curved in front. A pair of reindeer were harnessed not on the front but slightly to the left so that the driver could see everything in front of him. As a rule, only one man rode on the sled, sitting astride it and balancing with his feet. The reindeer were managed with the aid

of long reins and a whip with a bone tip. Freight sleds were heavier and pulled by a single reindeer. They were used primarily during seasonal movements for transporting household belongings, women, and small children. Travel by dog team among the maritime Chukchi and Koryak underwent substantial changes after the middle of the 19th century. The fanlike method of harnessing dogs and the sled of the reindeer type were replaced by the so-called eastern Siberian sled and tandem hitch.

The Even of east-central Siberia were also reindeer breeders, the deer being ridden and employed as pack animals during the long journeys involved in hunting furs and meat and on summer trips to rivers for fishing. Thus the reindeer differed from the Chukchi and Koryak breed, being larger and having greater strength and endurance ("Lamut reindeer"). Harnessing to sleds was practiced only in northern Kamchatka and other areas bordering the territory of the Chukchi and Koryak where the reindeer-harnessing complex was borrowed in its entirety.

On the Lower Amur River dogs served as draft animals and also provided fur for clothing and meat for food. The traditional Nivkhi sled was long and narrow, and the driver straddled it, his feet on short skis. Although light and fast, these sleds could transport considerable weight. The dogs were harnessed to a tow line alternately rather than in pairs. By the middle of the 19th century, this sled had been replaced by a heavier Russian form.

Nivkhi hunters used long and relatively wide skis made of larch or birch. One form was unlined and worn on trips to fishing sites, for wood cutting trips, and for visits to neighboring villages. This type of ski was particularly well suited for travel over deep, soft snow. For hunting, when speed and silence were required, skis lined on the bottoms with several layers of seal, moose, or deer skin were preferred (fig. 231).

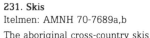

231. Skis
Itelmen: AMNH 70-7689a,b
The aboriginal cross-country skis used by many Siberian groups were covered on the bottom with slick reindeer-leg skins or sealskin (the latter, in this case), with the hair turning backward to assist in ascending hills, yet smooth enough to glide down. In touting the efficiency of these skis, Bogoras noted that Even skiiers running alongside his dogsled could easily keep up without visible strain for miles.

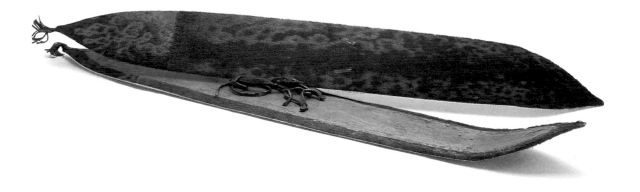

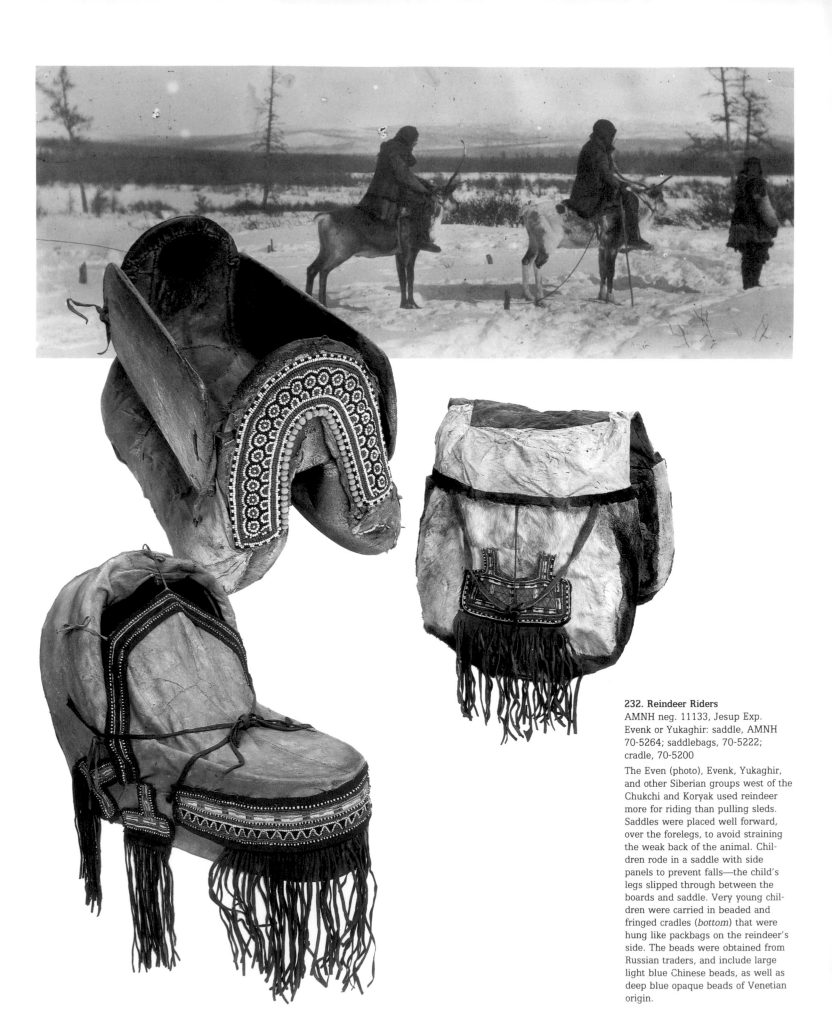

232. Reindeer Riders

AMNH neg. 11133, Jesup Exp.
Evenk or Yukaghir: saddle, AMNH
70-5264; saddlebags, 70-5222;
cradle, 70-5200

The Even (photo), Evenk, Yukaghir,
and other Siberian groups west of the
Chukchi and Koryak used reindeer
more for riding than pulling sleds.
Saddles were placed well forward,
over the forelegs, to avoid straining
the weak back of the animal. Children rode in a saddle with side
panels to prevent falls—the child's
legs slipped through between the
boards and saddle. Very young children were carried in beaded and
fringed cradles (*bottom*) that were
hung like packbags on the reindeer's
side. The beads were obtained from
Russian traders, and include large
light blue Chinese beads, as well as
deep blue opaque beads of Venetian
origin.

Economic Patterns in Northeastern Siberia

I. I. Krupnik

The local and ethnic variants of traditional subsistence systems known in northeastern Asia and Alaska in the late 19th and early 20th century can be divided into six basic types: settled maritime hunting (type 1); seminomadic hunting and herding (type 2); seminomadic hunting and fishing (type 3); intensive fishing (type 4); intensive reindeer herding (type 5); and the creole-introduced economy of Russified or Americanized settlers (type 6). This essay discusses the five types that occur in Siberia. Type 3, confined to Alaska during this period, is discussed in a subsequent essay (p. 193). The first three of these economic systems have ancient origins in neolithic cultures of Northeastern Siberia. Intensive reindeer nomadism and Russified mixed economy, on the other hand, emerged only in the 17th and 18th centuries. This essay describes the cultural, geographic, seasonal, and historical aspects of these eco-

233. Economic Systems of Siberia and Alaska (Late 19th Century)

Both contrasts and similarities are apparent in this comparison of traditional Siberian and Alaskan economic patterns. Maritime hunters, who subsisted mainly on sea mammals and lived in large, stable communities, occupied most coastal areas on both sides of Bering Strait. Intensive salmon fishing dominated the Northwest Coast and overlapped sea mammal hunting in Southwest Alaska, but also occurred on Siberia's Kamchatka Peninsula. The strongest intercontinental contrast was between the intensive reindeer herders of northeastern Siberia and the caribou hunters of interior Alaska; only the former were food producers. In many areas of Russian influence a Creole or mixed economy had developed since contact, which combined cash and subsistence sources of income.

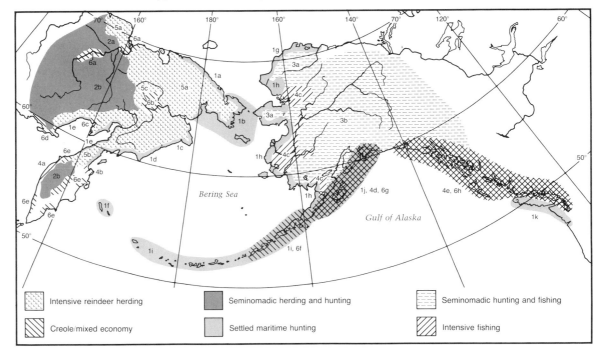

Intensive reindeer herding   Seminomadic herding and hunting   Seminomadic hunting and fishing

Creole/mixed economy   Settled maritime hunting   Intensive fishing

nomic types as they relate to the traditional, pre-1900 populations of this region.

The distribution of traditional economies of Northeast Siberia fall into three geographic regions that follow major environmental zones (fig. 233). The coastal zone, following the shores of the Arctic and the Pacific oceans, was inhabited by the sea mammal hunters and, on the extreme south, by sedentary fishermen. The second zone, which included the maritime lowlands and mountainous areas of the Chukotkan and Koryakan plateau, the Anadyr plateau, and the surrounding mountain range, was the territory of nomadic reindeer herders. Finally, the third inner zone of continental mountain ranges and plateaus was occupied by the seminomadic hunter–reindeer herders. The Russian Siberians (or Russian settlers, Starozhili) and creole (mixed Russian-native) population, who practiced a mixed economy, inhabited peripheral regions and pockets within the larger three zones.

Economic Systems in Siberia and Alaska

Siberia	Alaska
1. Settled Maritime Hunting	
a. Arctic Chukotka	g. North Alaska Coast
b. Bering Strait	
c. Kerek	h. West Alaska Coast
d. EasternKoryak	i. Aleut
e. Western Koryak	j. Pacific Eskimo
f. Commander Is.	k. Nootka-Makah
2. Seminomadic Herding and Hunting	**3. Seminomadic Hunting and Fishing**
a. Arctic	a. Arctic
b. Subarctic (taiga)	b. Subarctic
4. Intensive Fishing	
a. Itelmen	c. West Alaska Riverine
b. South Koryak	d. Gulf of Alaska
	e. Northwest Coast
5. Intensive Reindeer Herding	
a. Chukchi	
b. Koryak	
c. Chuvantsy	
6. Creole/Introduced Economy	
a. Kolyma	f. Eastern Aleut
b. Anadyr	g. Kodiak
c. Gizhiga	h. Northwest Coast
d. Kamchadal	Mixed
e. Russian Settler	

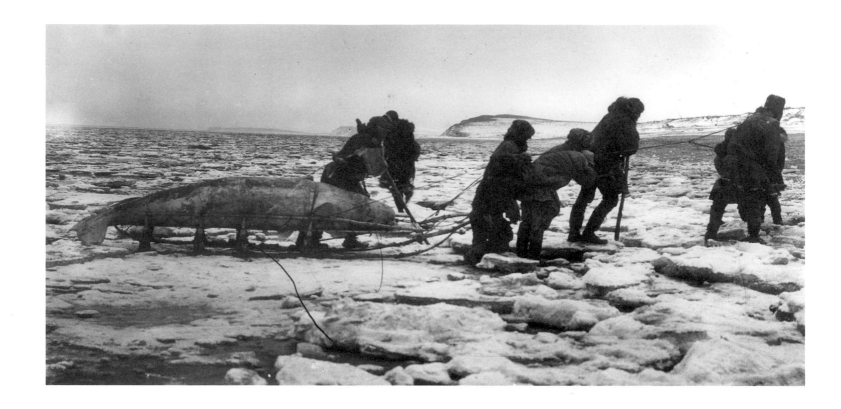

Ancient Hunting and Fishing Economies

Settled Maritime Hunting

Settled maritime hunting (type 1) was the prevailing form of subsistence on the maritime coastal area from Cape Billings to the western and eastern shores of the Kamchatka Peninsula, on the mainland coast of the Okhotsk Sea at the mouth of the Taui River in the 17th and 18th centuries, and at the mouth of the Siglan River in the 19th century. At the end of the 19th century, more than 7,000 sea hunters including Asian Eskimo, Aleut, Maritime Chukchi, Maritime Koryak, and Kerek lived a sedentary life in permanent settlements in this territory. Here, in various places, they hunted small sea mammals such as seals, sea otters, and sea lions, as well as larger species like bowhead and gray whales, walrus, and beluga with bark and wood-frame boats and skin-covered kayaks and umiaks, using toggling harpoons, spears, nets, and traps. Fishing, bird hunting, and gathering of plants, berries, and seafood supplemented the sea mammal diet throughout the territory. Dog-sled transportation played an important role in this economy. In general, the hunting of land animals was of minor importance in this coastal region.

The annual cycle of these sedentary hunters consisted of a succession of seasonal movements with one or two peak periods of intensive activity, usually in the summer or spring and in the fall during the annual sea mammal or fish migrations. At this time the population secured fresh food for people and dogs and prepared large amounts of food for winter consumption. Throughout the year the staple food was fresh, frozen, or fermented meat and sea mammal fat, preserved in caches dug into the frozen ground, and fresh or dried fish. In winter, sea mammals caught at the ice edge and in pockets of open water at the time of freeze-up and ice fishing occasionally provided fresh food.

The sedentary sea hunters lived in large settlements numbering from several dozen to a few hundred people. They occupied a territory with precisely fixed coastal boundaries. Within the boundaries of such a territory each community had usually one or two central settlements, containing both summer and winter houses, and a few summer camps or hunting stations. As a rule, the annual migration on dog sledges or in umiaks within the limits of the territory did not exceed a few dozen miles.

At the end of the 19th century, sedentary sea hunting as a group's major subsistence activity was represented in northeastern Asia with a few local or ethnic variations. These variations were, from north to south (fig. 233), the Arctic Chukotka type (1a), which existed from Cape Billings to Cape Serdtse-Kamen' on the Arctic coast, was practiced by the Maritime Chukchi, and included the hunting of seal and polar bear by individual

234. Koryak Bringing Home a Beluga Whale
AMNH neg. 1423, Jesup Exp.

The Maritime Koryak were formerly great whalers, but 19th-century commercial hunting by American whaling ships in the Sea of Okhotsk nearly destroyed this source of livelihood. By the time they were studied by Jochelson, the Koryak took only an occasional small whale, such as this beluga (white whale). The complex ceremonies surrounding whaling were still carried out, however.

hunters; the Bering Strait type (1b) in the eastern, southern, and partly northern coasts of the Chukotkan Peninsula, in which Asian Eskimo and Maritime Chukchi practiced collective hunting of whale and walrus; the Kerek type (1c) on the southern coast of the Anadyr Bay and the coast of the Koryak plateau, as far as the Gulf of Nataliia, where a subgroup of the Koryak practiced seal and walrus hunting, mainly without harpoons, and hunted birds in bird colonies; an Eastern Koryak type (1d) along the cliff shores of the Koryak plateau and the eastern coast of Kamchatka to the mouth of the Uka River, where sedentary Koryak-Aleuts on the Karaga and Uka rivers fished, hunted summer seals and small whales with nets, and speared walrus at haulouts; a Western Koryak type (1e) from the western coast of Kamchatka to the mouth of the Uka River, were sedentary Koryak from the Palana, Kamen', Paren', Itka villages, and mixed Koryak-Even groups engaged in fishing, seal hunting with nets and harpoons at haul-outs, and collective whale hunts in umiaks; and a

Commander type (1f) in the Bering Sea and Mednii Islands, where Aleuts and creoles were involved in commercial hunting of seal and sea otter at haul-outs, an economy that began in the early 19th century when the Russian American Company established itself in the Commander Islands.

Unlike the maritime hunters of northern Alaska, the sedentary hunters of northeastern Asia did not have to leave the coast to hunt wild caribou in remote regions of the tundra every summer. The products they needed—meat and skins— were obtained from the nomadic reindeer herders in exchange for maritime products. As a result, long-term partnerships between coastal and tundra inhabitants—both individual families and whole communities—allowed mutual relationships to develop. In years or periods of starvation on the seacoast, the sedentary population moved in masses to the tundra to join the nomadic groups; correspondingly, during difficult periods on the interior, reindeer herders would move to the coast.

235. Chukchi Duck Hunters at Cape Wankarem

SI neg. 6924, E.W. Nelson, 1881

Sea birds and migratory fowl were an important supplement to the diets of maritime hunters. Flying birds were captured using bolas (fig. 13), here worn around the head where they would be instantly available to hurl at passing flocks. Bolas were given up after shotguns came into use and made the birds too wary to pass within bolas range.

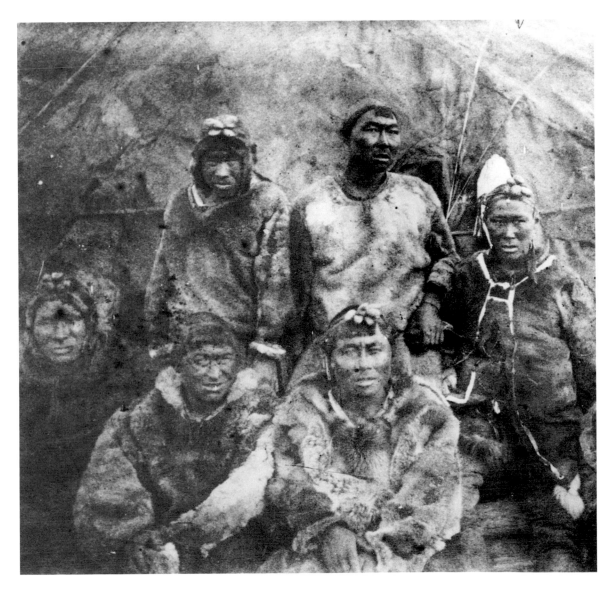

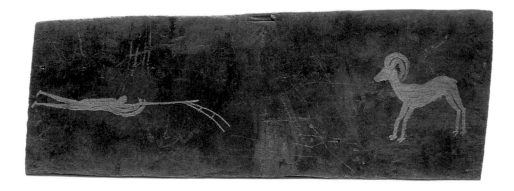

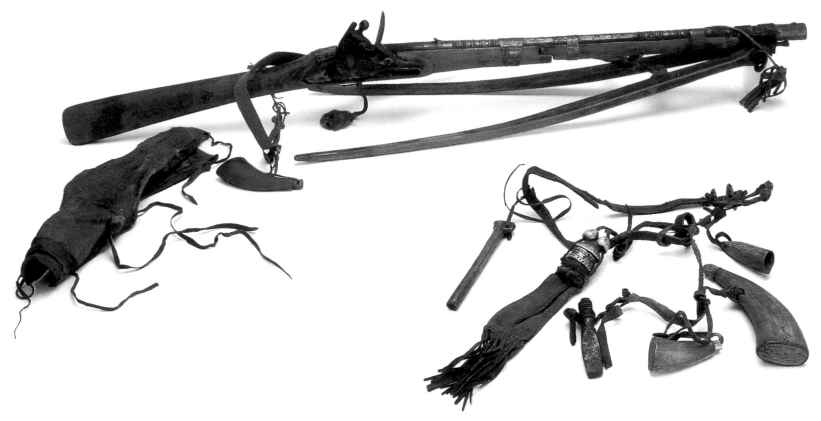

Seminomadic Hunting and Herding

The hunting-herding economy (type 2) in Northeast Siberia was characteristic of the Even people of the basin of the Kolyma, Anadyr, and Penzhina rivers and the inland parts of Kamchatka, as well as of the Tundra Yukaghir of the lower Kolyma, representing approximately 3,000 people. This form of subsistence was in the process of development before the arrival of the Russians but underwent major transformations during the 17th and 18th centuries. The custom of raising reindeer for transportation was brought by the Even to the Northeast during their eastward spread in northern Siberia, as was the special breed of strong saddle reindeer, so-called Lamut reindeer. Reindeer were used exclusively for transportation and were consumed as food only in case of starvation. The number of reindeer ran from a few head per family up to two or three dozen. The basic form of subsistence

before contact consisted of large game hunting, like wild reindeer, elk, bear, snow sheep. Fishing played a lesser, although significant role. Gathering was relatively unimportant. The nomadic hunters did not practice sea hunting.

In the vast, mountainous, and almost impenetrable inland regions of northeastern Asia, the Even settled in stable groups of a few dozen families. Each group had its own territory, although the limits of the hunting territory were, of necessity, flexible. The nomadic hunters did not have permanent settlements. With the Russian penetration of the Northeast, the Even became involved in trapping and hunting of furbearers, which, until then, had had a subsidiary character only. At first fur had been a means to pay taxes, but later fur trade became a commercial enterprise. Originally the demand was for mink; then squirrel, ermine, and marten

236. Russian Firearms

Koryak: AMNH 70-3543 (board)
Chukchi, AMNH 70-5695 (gun),
70-5698 (gun kit)

The guns available to Siberian hunters and herders at the turn of the 20th century were for the most part Russian flintlocks, fitted out with homemade stands and gun kits. This gun kit was worn as a belt and includes a ramrod, bullet bag, powder horns, and powder measure. The gun barrel and firing mechanism were covered with a skin bag or cloth to protect them from moisture. A hunter (*top*) takes aim at a mountain goat on a Koryak cutting board drawing.

in the taiga and the arctic fox and wolverine in arctic regions took its place. In the 19th century the fur trade provided the hunter-herders with up to 90 percent of their cash income.

The traditional method of hunting wild reindeer and elk was to follow individual prey on saddle reindeer or on skis, often with the help of hunting dogs. The Even used firearms before any other group of Northeastern Siberia, by the middle and end of the 18th century. They were considered excellent marksmen. The intensification of the hunting economy and the introduction of firearms allowed the Even to enlarge their territory considerably in the 18th and 19th centuries, by taking over central Kamchatka and the basin of the eastern confluents of the Kolyma, such as the Omolon and the Aniui, which had been inhabited earlier by Yukaghir hunters on foot.

At the end of the 19th century, with the depletion of wild reindeer, the Lamut hunters of central Kamchatka and of the Okhotsk Sea began to shift towards production herding of reindeer for meat and hides.

In the traditional annual cycle, at the beginning of fall, seminomadic hunter-herders set the reindeer free in open pasture in the taiga and engaged in fishing. At the first snow the reindeer were gathered, and the group moved to distant hunting grounds, sometimes as far as several hundred kilometers away. Here, until the beginning of spring, the hunters and herders practiced intensive fur trapping and hunting of wild reindeer and elk. After the birth of the calves, they moved back to the summer camps again.

237. Fox Trap
Chukchi: AMNH 70-6453

The traditional Siberian fox trap had a long striking arm held under tension by twisted sinew cables inside a wood or whalebone body. The trap shown here is half-cocked; when set the arm was held back by a trigger attached to a cord, and the whole device was buried in the snow. At the other end of the cord was the bait, usually a fish head; the first pull on the bait released the arm and the fox was struck on the head.

In the 19th century, under the influence of contact and commercial fur trade, hunter-herder subsistence underwent a specific change. Commercial nets made of horsehair or hemp became widespread, increasing fishing productivity. Trade food items such as flour, tea, and sugar, and also tobacco, cloth clothing, and manufactured utensils became available in everyday life. The greater availability of trade goods made the fur trade all the more important in subsistence, and hunters had to look further and further for new hunting grounds. Two regional variations of seminomadic and trade economy developed: the arctic type (2a) in the tundra, where hunting molting birds, massive hunts of wild reindeer at river crossings, and other activities learned from the local Tundra Yukaghir played a notably important role; and the initial subarctic type (2b) in the taiga and broken forest.

Intensive Fishing

Intensive fishing (type 4) still existed at the end of the 19th century as a basic subsistence form only among the native population of Kamchatka, the Itelmen, and partly among their neighbors, the most southern groups of sedentary Koryak from the Uka, Karaga, and Palana villages. For these last groups, representing a total of approximately 1,500 people, intensive fishing was a complement to sea hunting.

Despite abundant resources of salmon and other fish species migrating every year to the coasts of Northeastern Siberia, the area of specialized sedentary fishing economy was significantly less here than on the Northwest Coast of North America. Nothing comparable to such developed forms of social organization and art, characteristic of sedentary fishing societies of the American continent like the Tlingit, Haida, Kwakiutl, and others, existed in Siberia.

One can reconstruct the form of subsistence of the sedentary fishermen of Kamchatka from descriptions written in the first half of the 18th century. Fishing of migratory species of salmon (pink, sockeye, coho, chum, chinook) swimming up the rivers of the peninsula every year to spawn constituted the basic form of subsistence. The most efficient technology was weir fishing. Nets made of nettle fiber and various kinds of hooks and fish spears were also used. Gathering of wild plants played an important role, and hunting birds and land game such as bear and fox played a subsidiary role.

The economic cycle of the sedentary fishermen included one peak season only, the summer migration period of the fish. As fish was the staple food throughout the year, huge stocks were prepared in the summer for winter use:

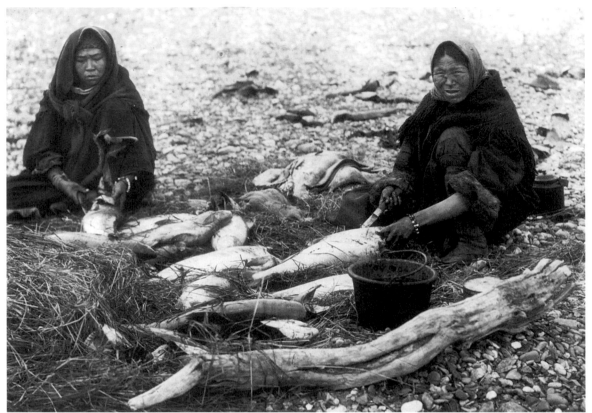

238. Koryak Women Cleaning Fish
AMNH neg. 1656, Jesup Exp.

The salmon are being cleaned and split in preparation for drying. Dried and/or lightly smoked salmon was an important food among coastal groups, even those not having an intensive fishing adaptation, because it could be stored for winter consumption.

sun-dried fish, called *iukola*, fish meal, and fish fermented in pits. Fish was also the staple food for sled dogs.

The most striking feature of the subsistence of the Itelmen fishermen was their relatively weak use of sea and coastal resources. Meat from sea mammals was appreciated, but the fishermen took little part in hunting them; game was caught only along the shore because their dugout canoes were not serviceable on the open sea.

The population of the sedentary fishermen consisted of closed kinship and economic groups of a few hundred people. Each group inhabited a river valley or the basin of a few confluent rivers, in a few settlements of 50 to 100 people. Each of these settlements had one to three communal semisubterranean winter houses and a few dozen family houses for use in the summer. Near the permanent winter settlements, established at some distance from the seashore, were also temporary summer camps close to the mouth of the river where most of the fishing took place. The yearly move of fishermen within their territory covered no more than a few miles.

With the arrival of the Russians in Kamchatka in the 18th century, the subsistence system of the sedentary fishermen underwent drastic changes. With the attempt to intensify the fur trade, the most valuable fur animals were rapidly depleted. Following the example of the Russian settlers and under the pressure of the Russian administration, the natives took up garden agriculture, mainly growing of beets and potatoes, and later began to raise milk animals and horses. The breeding of sled dogs also became important because of the needs of the Russian administration and the lack of other means of transportation.

By the end of the 19th century, the sedentary fishermen had adopted numerous features of the Russian culture. They lived in log cabins, wore trade clothing, and used trade utensils. They had garden vegetables and livestock, for which they had to store hay for the winter. New ways to prepare fish—salted, smoked—came into practice, and new ways to consume it too, by baking homemade breads of fish meal, or bread of wild plants mixed with fish or fish eggs. As far as their way of life and economy were concerned, the sedentary fishermen resembled the Russian Siberian and creole population.

Introduced Economies

Intensive Reindeer Herding

This type of economy (type 5) was the only form of arctic subsistence based entirely on food production, with an organized resource of large herds and regular consumption of the products of the slaughter of domestic reindeer. Since the late 18th century and early 19th century, this became the basic mode of subsistence of three ethnic groups of tundra nomads—the Reindeer Chukchi, Koryak, and Chuvantsy—sustaining 11,000 to 12,000 people. Having evolved from a mixed reindeer economy, the large-scale nomadic reindeer herding went through several stages. The period of accumulation of large herds among the Koryak took place in the late 17th and early 18th centuries, and among the Chukchi and Chuvantsy in the second half of the 18th century.

The daily social and working life of the nomadic herders was organized around a stable settlement, the nomadic camp, composed of three to four families who collectively looked after the family herds of reindeer. Such nomadic camps of 15 to 20 people, with a joint herd averaging between 800 and 1,500 reindeer in all, made regular migrations within a delimited territory and were part of a larger social group of 150 to 200 people. The limits of the communal pastures, the itinerary of the nomadic community, and the nomadic camp were fixed by customary law of the herders but might vary slightly with yearly conditions. In some areas a larger nomadic community, known as the territorial group, occupying the basin of a large river or some other precisely delimited zone, existed.

The yearly cycle of the reindeer herders consisted of regular trips around their territory with successive use of seasonal types of pasture. The annual itinerary usually covered 50 to 100 miles, or up to 250 miles at the most.

Most herders moved towards the seacoast or the lowlands near the sea during the summer months, where men hunted seals and fished. Among the inland nomads, the nomadic camp split in the summer. Women, older people, and children remained in the settled summer camps in a river valley, where they fished, while men herders, carrying minimal equipment, led the reindeer to their summer pastures in the highlands, returning a few months later. These nomads lived year-round in a transportable framed dwelling covered with reindeer hides, called an *iaranga*. They traveled on foot in the summer and on reindeer sledges in the winter.

Practically all the products they needed were available within their own territory. Exchanges of surplus reindeer hides and meat gave the nomads access to sea mammal meat and fat, thongs, skins, and trade goods. The owners of large herds frequently subsisted entirely on herding and exchange. The middle-income and poorer herders, owning less than 300 to 500 reindeer per family, had to rely more heavily on maritime hunting, fishing, fur trade, and bird hunting. All nomadic groups consumed a large amount of wild plants. Hunting large land animals, such as wild reindeer, elk, snow sheep, and bear, continued to play an important role in the subsistence of reindeer herders in the 17th and 18th centuries. But, in the 19th century,

239. Home of a Rich Reindeer Koryak

AMNH neg. 4157, Jesup Exp.

A reindeer herder's wealth was measured by the size of his herd. The chief of the Taigonos Koryak had 5,000 reindeer, twelve herdsmen with their families, three tents, and more than 150 sleds. In this photograph, supply sleds are drawn up around the tent of a rich herder; some are used to hold down the reindeer skin tent cover. Rich men were also central figures in the operation of the Koryak and Chukchi trade networks.

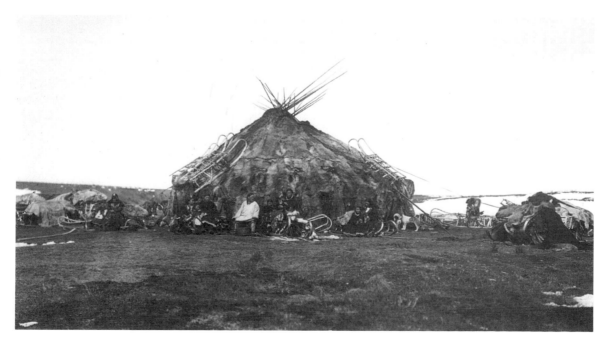

hunting lost its significance, because of over-hunting. Consumption of trade goods like flour, tea, and sugar was minimal up to the mid-20th century. Dogsled transportation was practically nonexistent among the reindeer herders.

The difference between the three ethnic variations of large-scale reindeer herding among the Chukchi (5a), the Koryak (5b), and the Chuvantsy (5c) were minimal. All nomadic groups of northeastern Asia had similar material cultures and very similar uses of natural resources, although hunting had a greater significance among the Reindeer Chukchi, primarily in the arctic regions, and fishing among the Reindeer Koryak. There was a category of active tradesmen among the wealthy and middle-income herders who exchanged with their poorer countrymen furs for trade goods and live reindeer and benefited by selling fur at a high price.

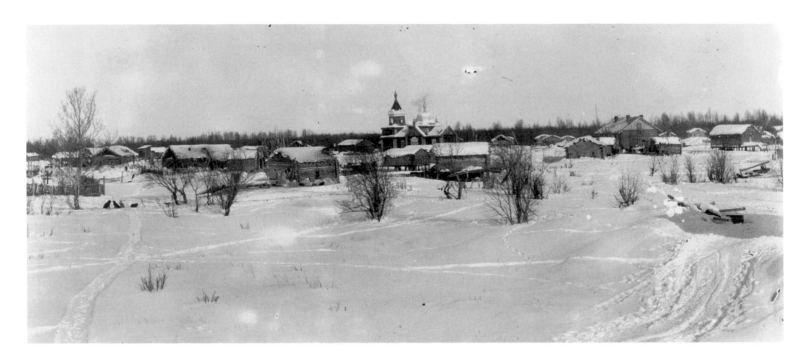

Russian Settlers and Creole Mixed Economy

The mixed trade economy of the Russian settlers (Starozhili) and creole populations (type 6) emerged in the 17th and 18th centuries with the arrival and the constitution of a permanent Russian population in Northeast Siberia.

At the end of the 19th century, the Russian and creole (mixed native-Russian) population was made up of the following groups: the Kolyma River people (6a), consisting of two groups on the lower Kolyma and on the middle Kolyma, each of 500 to 600 people; the Anadyr River or Markovo people (6b), numbering about 300 to 400 individuals; the Gizhiga River people (6c), about 500, on the mouth of the river by the Okhotsk coast; the Kamchadal (6d) of the Okhotsk coast, being a Russianized Koryak-Even-Yakut population of 800 living at the mouth of the Taui River; and the Russian settlers (6e), also called Russian Siberians or Starozhili, about 2,000 people in the valley of the Kamchatka River and the eastern and western coasts of the Kamchatka Peninsula.

Practically all these groups lived in the same villages with the native population: the Kolyma and Anadyr people with the Yukaghir, Chuvantsy, and Even; the Gizhiga people and Kamchadal of the Okhotsk coast with the Koryak and the Even; the Russian settlers with the Itelmen-Kamchadal.

The Russian Siberian form of subsistence became more complex at the end of the 17th century and 18th century, under the strong influence of the economics of the native population, but adapted to specific Russian economic traditions. With the decline of fur trade at the end of the 17th century, and the lesser significance of Russian garrisons and Cossack fortresses in the area in the 18th century, the Russian settlers of the Siberian Northeast had to find a local means of existence. They started to practice intensive river fishing, hunting (primarily of wild reindeer and birds), and, in the 19th century, garden agriculture.

The Russian Siberians and creole people lived in relatively large sedentary settlements of a few hundred inhabitants, as a rule. They were grouped in village communities with an elected direction. The land was nominally owned by the

240. Markovo
AMNH neg. 1327, Jesup Exp.

Markovo, on the middle Anadyr River, was typical of Russian towns in the administratively remote regions of eastern Siberia. Bogoras wrote scathingly of the abuses of Russian colonial officials, here concerning the collection of taxes from the Chukchi: "I know also of cases where the chief of the district would lose at card-playing the whole amount of the taxes of some community, and then would make the accounts so complicated that they had to pay it again the next year as arrears." (1904–09:715)

community. During the year, episodic or seasonal trips were made from the central settlement, which was composed of log *izbas*—traditional Russian houses—to the family plots where people lived in cabins or semisubterranean houses.

The territory used by the Russian Siberians was relatively extended and presented a system of seasonal use of the various types of land divided in family or individual plots. Annual moves took place usually within a few dozen kilometers, a hundred at the most, from the main settlement. The type of subsistence of the Russian Siberians was more mobile than that of the sedentary native population.

The economic year of the Russian Siberians included a few peaks of economic activity, when the necessary amount of products was gathered and huge quantities of food for people and dogs were stocked for the winter. The basic economic activity of all these groups was summer fishing of migratory fish caught with nets or seines or by native methods using weirs and traps. In addition, fish was prepared with recipes borrowed from the native population: *iukola*, fermentation, and others. The northern groups, the Kolyma and Anadyr people, hunted wild reindeer at river crossings during spring or summer migration, as well. The Kolyma and Gizhiga people and the Kamchadal of the Okhotsk shore practiced seal hunting to a certain extent, and in the 18th century and early 19th century the Gizhiga people and Kamchadal even joined the sedentary Koryak on whaling trips. All groups without exception actively hunted bird and land animals—bear and fox—and gathered plants and berries.

To a greater degree than the natives, the Russian settlers relied not only on production of consumption goods but also on imported goods, obtained as periodic state subsidies or by the Cossacks as payment for their services. All the Russian settlers were greatly involved in fur trade, trapping and hunting arctic fox, wolverine, and wolf in the north, and squirrel, sable, fox, and marten in the south.

The northern groups on the Kolyma and Anadyr rivers were involved in trade with the Reindeer Chukchi, exchanging imported goods for fur and reindeer meat and hides. In all these activities, dogsled transportation, borrowed from the natives and improved by the Russian settlers, was an important feature in the settlers' economy. Nevertheless, diversification of settler subsistence types did not guarantee their long-term stability, and all Russian Siberian and creole populations suffered periodic famine, massive loss of dogs, and epidemics. The combination of all these features produced the specific type of economy of the Russian settlers and creole population by merging the native forms of subsistence with a trade-oriented market economy.

It is as a result of the settlers' population that a form of production economy spread in the Siberian Northeast in the late 18th and early 19th centuries that included garden agriculture, animal milking (which implied a regular harvest of hay), and use of horses, which was adopted later by the natives as well.

Economic Patterns in Alaska

William W. Fitzhugh

Many of the economies utilized by Siberian peoples were also practiced by native peoples of Alaska through the end of the 19th century. The greatest correspondences in economic patterns between the two regions are found in the settled maritime and intensive fishing economies. These patterns also account for many of the similarities noted among the cultures of the North Pacific–Bering Sea region. The greatest differences between Siberia and Alaska are found in the land economies and those related to acculturative influences. The absence in northern North America of any form of native domestic animal production (excepting dogs and various relatively unsuccessful post-1890s reindeer and musk-ox experiments) resulted in the persistence among Alaskan and British Columbian interior peoples of a form of seminomadic hunting-and-fishing economy that had disappeared even in remotest northeastern Asia after the introduction of domestic reindeer in the 17th century.

Extending the previous discussion (fig. 233), we may note the presence of the following economic types in northwestern North America: settled maritime hunting (type 1), seminomadic hunting and fishing (type 3), intensive fishing (type 4), and introduced economies (type 6).

Settled Maritime Hunting

As in coastal Siberia, the populations of coastal Alaska and the Northwest Coast derived much, if not all (in the case of some Aleut groups), of their food from marine resources. As has been discussed in the preceding chapters on prehistory, maritime economies have ancient roots here, and they continued to be the mainstay of coastal peoples into the 20th century. Comparing economic types in Alaska and Siberia, some maritime economy variants are shared by both regions, while others are not. Along the arctic coast of Alaska east of Point Hope is found a North Alaska Coast subtype (1g) that combines elements of the Arctic Chukotka (1a) and Bering Strait (1b) subtypes, differing only in the relatively greater emphasis given to caribou hunting as an important supplement to the annual whale and walrus hunts that were (and continue to be) the primary focus of North Alaskan Eskimo life. Approaching Bering Strait, and especially at Cape Prince of Wales and on St. Lawrence Island, this economy merged with the Asian Bering Strait subtype (1b), with its emphasis on whale and walrus hunting, caribou being absent. In these regions, as in the eastern Aleutians and Kodiak, furs had to be supplied by trade, and bird-skin clothing often replaced the warm caribou fur parkas prevalent elsewhere in these arctic regions. As in northeastern Asia, settled maritime life depended, in part, on exchange with interior populations for materials needed but unavailable in the most specialized maritime environments. The roots of this specialized maritime tradition extend back nearly 2,000 years to the Old Bering Sea cultures.

A West Alaska Coast economic subtype (1h) existed into the 20th century from Kotzebue to the Alaska Peninsula, excepting in Bering Strait. In these regions of relatively shallow seas and seasonal pack ice, Inupiat and Yupik Eskimo hunted seals, walrus, and beluga; fished; hunted birds and collected bird eggs; and, to a lesser degree, hunted land animals. Large whales did not frequent these regions, so the intensive whaling economy that had developed in Bering Strait and North Alaska was only weakly expressed in much of western Alaska.

The maritime economy of the Aleut subtype (1i), also present in some areas of Kodiak Island, was essentially an ice-free variant of the Bering Strait economy, with the hunting of whales, sea lions, fur seals, and birds; fishing; and collecting of shellfish and seaweed being the major subsistence activities. Land mammals were few, and caribou were absent. After Russian contact, commercial sea otter hunting greatly altered the traditional Aleut economy, settlement patterns, and population structure.

The Pacific Eskimo subtype (1j) characterized the economies of Kodiak, the southern Alaska Peninsula, and other regions of Cook Inlet and Prince William Sound. Sharing many resources with the Aleutians, peoples of this region had in addition large seasonal salmon runs and, except on Kodiak Island, significant amounts of large land game. Variability, for instance between regions rich in salmon and others rich in sea mammals, resulted in local groups' specializing in different resources, resulting in regional economic diversity as an important feature of the Kodiak economy, to a greater extent, even, than in Siberia. In the late prehistoric and early historic period, whale hunting with aconite poison was locally important.

For reasons that are not understood, the economies of northern Northwest Coast cultures did not include whaling, even though whales were important in their mythology and art. And although smaller varieties of sea mammals were hunted on an annual basis where available, with the exception of a major post-contact emphasis on commercial sea otter hunting, the Tlingit economy was far less dependent on maritime hunting than on fishing. However, large sea mammal hunting, especially the hunting of large whales, was an important activity in the southern reaches of the Northwest Coast, among the

241. "Eskimo whaling and walrus camp, Icy Point, Arctic Ocean, Alaska. Lookout created of drift logs."
Henry W. Elliott, 1891 SI-NAA 7119-5, SI neg. 84-1817

The lookout has probably sighted one of the herds of walrus that appear in midsummer as the sea ice breaks up and the floes move northward into the Chukchi Sea. Walrus were important quarry for northern maritime hunters, providing meat, ivory, and thick, tough skins that were split and used for umiak and tent coverings. In a good season, a single community might take more than 100 walrus. Teepee-like skin tents were used as summer dwellings.

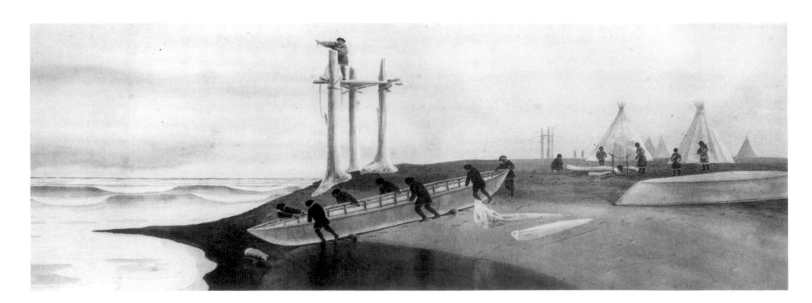

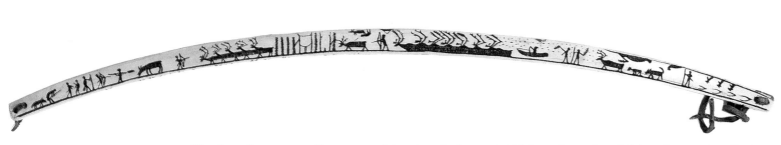

242. Ivory Drill Bow
Alaskan Eskimo: MAE 571-52

The scene depicted here is a caribou drive, a method of communal hunting practiced by the interior North Alaskan Eskimo. Long converging lines of poles or rock piles set up on the tundra funneled a caribou herd toward a large corral, usually placed on the other side of a stream or pond. Hunters closed in behind the herd, waving pieces of clothing (*right*). The caribou could be speared in the water from kayaks, shot with arrows in the corral (*center*), caught in snares at the corral exits, or killed with spears (*left*).

Nootka of western Vancouver Island and the Makah, Quileute, and Quinault tribes of the Olympic Peninsula in Washington (subtype 1k).

Seminomadic Hunting and Fishing

Most of the interior groups, including the Nunamiut Eskimo of the Alaskan North Slope and various Athapaskans, relied to one extent or another on caribou, mountain goat and sheep, moose, and elk and a variety of other land animals. Fishing also played an important role in the life of interior peoples, being most important on the Lower Yukon but everywhere serving as a supplement to land game. Great variation existed in the types of hunting techniques utilized, which ranged from communal drives at water crossings or topographic constrictions, with corral and fence systems in regions where caribou were plentiful, to individual stalking and snaring. Pitfall hunting, such as was practiced by wild reindeer hunters in northwestern Russia and northern Scandinavia, was not used, although snaring was; nor were rights to hunting locations or drive systems owned by individuals or corporate groups. Rather they were the communal property of the regional group. The North American type of seminomadic hunting probably once was widespread in Siberia before domestic reindeer were introduced into that region. In the absence of domestic animals the American economic type is radically different from the Siberian seminomadic herding and hunting economy (type 2), enough so to be assigned a separate status (type 3) with Arctic (e.g., Nunamiut and Seward Peninsula, subtype 3a) and Subarctic (subtype 3b) variants. The latter subsumes essentially all of the Indian culture economies of interior Alaska.

Intensive Fishing

As in parts of Siberia, fishing assumed great importance for many peoples of coastal Alaska and the Northwest Coast. Second only to settled maritime economies, fishing was the most widespread economic pattern in the North Pacific region. In fact, this pattern takes its most characteristic form from the Northwest Coast (4e), where annual salmon and other fish runs in the rivers, as well as productive ocean fishing, provided the economic base for the world's most complex hunting and gathering cultures.

Intensive fishing, however, is not restricted to the Northwest Coast, where it was linked with

shellfish and marine fishing. It was locally important also in the Gulf of Alaska economies (4d) of Kodiak, Cook Inlet, and Prince William Sound and also in the West Alaska Riverine economies (4c) among Yupiks along the rivers flowing into the Bering Sea, the Ingalik Indians of the Lower Yukon and Kuskokwim rivers, and the Inupiat of the Noatak and Kobuk river regions.

Introduced Economies

Beginning with the Russian expansion into the Aleutians, and later into other regions of Alaska and points south, new forms of economy took root among native cultures of the region. These economic elements varied according to patterns of Russian involvement, which were minimal in interior Alaska but had major impacts on native groups in such areas as the Aleutians (6f), Kodiak (6g), and parts of the Northwest Coast (6h), especially in Sitka. In addition to the fur trade, in which sea otter was dominant, Russian contact resulted in such changes as wage employment, introduction of agriculture and domestic animals in some areas, and even total incorporation of privileged Natives into Russian society. At the height of the sea otter trade in the early 19th century, the impressment of Aleut and Kodiak natives severely disrupted native subsistence activities, as did also the introduction of infectious diseases and hostilities of various kinds. Despite these changes, however, most native peoples continued to rely on natural resources for their sustenance and used native hunting techniques. It was not until the American period that major economic changes, such as commercial fishing, cannery operations, the gold rush, and massive white infiltration, began to affect native economic life radically, beginning in Pacific Alaska and spreading gradually into the Bering Sea and Alaskan interior.

Attempts were made to install a domestic reindeer economy in the Seward Peninsula in the 1890s to compensate for the reduction in marine mammal stocks resulting from intensive commercial whaling and walrus hunting, but they failed to have more than a local impact. It seems unlikely that anything short of Chukchi colonization of Alaska would have created conditions for success of a practice so alien to Alaskan tradition and belief.

Dwellings, Settlements, and Domestic Life

Aron Crowell

The houses of the native peoples of Alaska and Northeastern Siberia may be viewed simply as technological support systems—life-sustaining shells enclosing a microenvironment of heat, light, food, and protection from the elements. Many successful designs were developed under the constraints of locally available materials, weather conditions, and functional requirements (portability, permanence, size). Yet aboriginal houses had many functions and cultural dimensions—they were homes, workshops, social environments, sanctuaries from evil spirits, theaters for religious ceremonies. Charms and ritual practices protected and sanctified the home. On a social plane, living arrangements mirrored the structure of society, so that kinship and marriage, social schisms and alliances, and differences in age, sex, and status were all expressed in who lived together under the same roof or as neighbors in a village, and in the protocols of sleeping and seating. This spatial metaphor applied even to the ancestors, whose continuing importance to the community was expressed by the proximity of their graves and memorials to the living village. Social divisions and status relationships dictated the spatial arrangement of the dead, reflecting the continuity of the social order.

Some of the symbolic functions of houses in communal ceremonies and shamanistic performances are detailed elsewhere in this book (de Laguna p. 61; Fienup-Riordan p. 264; Serov p. 254.) In ceremonies the house or, in the case of the Eskimo, the ceremonial house (*karigi, qasgiq*) became a nexus between the secular and sacred worlds. In hunting festivals such as the Eskimo Bladder Festival, the Chukchi *Keretkun* ceremony, and the Koryak whale ceremony, animal spirits were entertained in the house as honored guests. Passage through house orifices (entrance tunnels, doorways, smoke holes, the holed Tlingit house screen) by the celebrants symbolized passage between worlds and between different states of being. The Yupik Eskimo shaman rose through the skylight of the *qasgiq* or descended into the entrance passage to enter the undersea world of the seal spirits. The house could also become in effect a representation of the cosmos, as when a hooped and feathered model of the sky world was suspended from the ceiling in the Yupik Eskimo Doll Festival (Yugiyhik) (Nelson 1899:496).

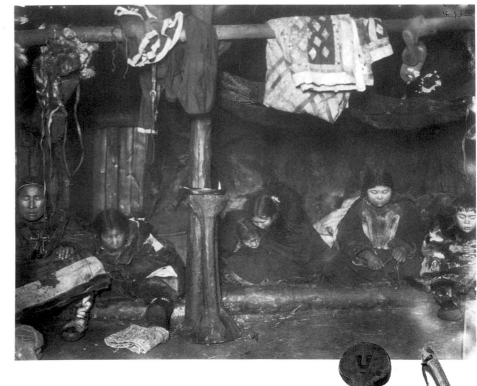

In this essay a selection of both winter and summer homes, as well as of interior and coastal types, is discussed to give an idea of the diversity of dwellings occupied by the native peoples of the Crossroads area. Included are examples of the earth or sod-covered semisubterranean houses of maritime peoples on both sides of Bering Strait, Asiatic and Alaskan skin tents, and the aboveground wooden houses of the Nivkhi, Athapaskan Indians, and Tlingit. Although snow houses were the main type of winter dwelling among the Central Eskimo of Canada, they were seldom used in Alaska. Rectangular snow houses were occasionally built as temporary structures by the North Alaskan Eskimo.

North Pacific peoples dependent on hunting almost always lived in several different locations and in several different types of houses over the course of a year. Seasonal shifts in settlement were integrated with the annual appearance of fish and game in specific locations. The Tlingit Indians, for example, occupied their elaborate plank houses only during the late fall and winter months, when stores of dried salmon, oil, and berries permitted them to congregate in the village and to curtail their subsistence activities during the ceremonial season. In spring and

243. The Koryak Home and Its Guardians: The Sacred Fireboard
AMNH neg. 4135, Jesup Exp.;
AMNH 70-2859 (fireboard),
70-2860a,b,c, (spindle, bow)
Bundled in furs, Maritime Koryak women and children sit in the light of the blubber lamp inside their winter house. The home was protected against evil spirits by many charms, including the anthropomorphic fireboard. Fire was made by the friction of the spindle whirling on the board.

244. Northern Simplicity: Whale Bone Bucket
Asian Eskimo: MAE 668-17

This well-made bucket of whale bone, bent and riveted together and fitted with a wooden bottom, reflects both the scarcity of wood in the Bering Strait region and the generally simple style of household implements made by northern cultures such as the Chukchi, Asian Eskimo, and North Alaskan Eskimo.

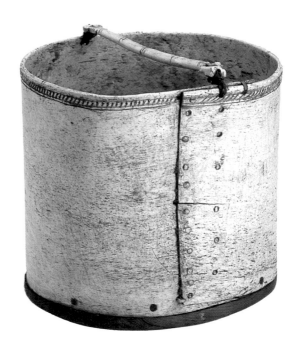

summer, the families of the village were dispersed at many hunting and fishing sites, living in simple shacks covered with split boards or bark. This pattern of winter aggregation and summer dispersal, associated with shifts in dwelling type, prevailed among most other groups. Exceptions occurred where both winter and summer needs could be met at one location or covered by storage of surplus food, although even then a change in dwelling type was typical (e.g., the North Alaskan Eskimo, below). In situations where the need for mobility was more nearly continuous (Siberian reindeer herders, interior Eskimo, and some Alaskan Indians) year-round residence in skin tents was typical.

Certain broad trends in house design followed the arctic-to-subarctic environmental gradient. The climate control elements of house construction (earth insulation, double tent walls, entrance passages, inner sleeping chambers) became less critical or were absent in southern structures, and at the same time wood and grass were more abundant as materials for constructing and appointing the house. Heating methods switched from arctic oil heat (sea mammal or reindeer fat melted and burned in stone or clay lamps) to subarctic wood-burning hearths, although oil lamps continued to be used for lighting.

A north-to-south trend of increasing house size is also evident, connected to the environmental gradient in both direct and indirect ways. Large houses were easier to build and heat in the south, because of the greater availability of wood and warmer temperatures. Yet the social environment was also critical—larger houses were occupied by larger households, an expression of social complexity that was tied indirectly to the richer environment and higher population densities among southern groups.

Lineage-based social organization (division into clans based on male or female bloodlines) was predominant south of the Bering Sea, occurring in the Crossroads area among the Even, Nivkhi,

245. Northwest Coast Elaborations
Tlingit: MAE 337-18 (bowl)
Haida: NMNH 89022 (stone dish)
Tlingit: MAE 2448-26, 2448-28 (paint brushes)

The art of woodcarving and painting reached a high state of development among southern Alaskan peoples, including the Northwest Coast Indians. This bent-corner beaver bowl was apparently new when collected in the mid-19th century, its paint and abalone shell inlays still bright and unworn. The joined corner and red cedar bottom are fastened with spruce-root lacing, and opercula decorate the rim. Ground mineral paints were mixed in the stone dish: graphite and magnetite for black, celadonite for blue, and hematite for red, mixed in a medium of chewed salmon eggs. The two paint brushes have bristles of porcupine guard hairs, and handles carved to represent a killer whale and an emaciated, corpselike figure, perhaps of a shaman.

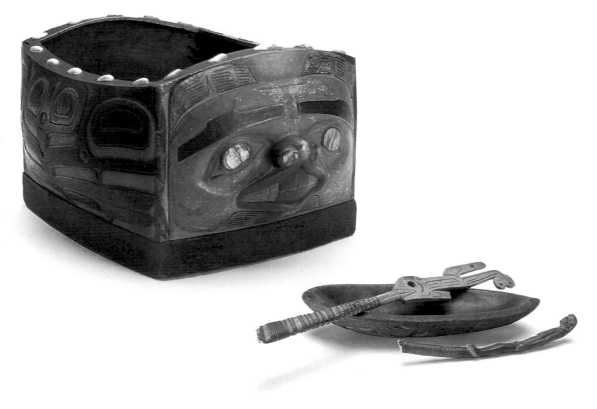

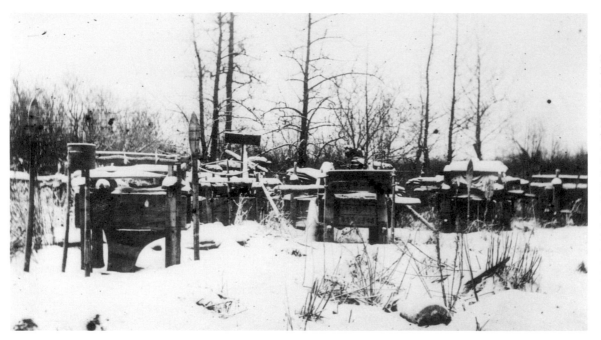

Nanai, Itelmen, Aleut, Pacific Eskimo, Athapaskan tribes, Eyak, and Tlingit. Lineage organization was the foundation upon which formalized cooperative relationships between large numbers of kinsmen were institutionalized. Exclusive claims to hunting and fishing territories, and to the predictable and large food surpluses that they produced, were held by the lineages. The cohesiveness and corporate nature of the lineage were often expressed by the coresidence of its members. Thus 50 or more members of a Nivkhi patrilineage and their in-laws might occupy a single underground house (Black 1973), and the large households of Aleut and Tlingit houses were composed of many cooperating families related by matrilineal kinship. Status hierarchies among individuals and lineages in these groups were also the primary organizing factor in village life and in the arrangement of houses in the settlement.

This organizational complexity stands in contrast to the more flexible, egalitarian, and small-scale organization of northern groups such as the North Alaskan Eskimo, Chukchi, and Koryak. Here the basic economic unit was the family group, usually consisting of several nuclear families linked by patrilineal kinship, which lived and hunted or herded together. Clan organization was nonexistent, and households were comparatively small. Cooperative relationships between households were centered around trading partnerships and subsistence pursuits requiring group effort, such as whaling among coastal groups and management of the reindeer herd among the Reindeer Chukchi and Koryak. Bering Sea Eskimo social organization was similar to this pattern except in the striking residential division between men and women (see below). There were in addition suggestions of the operation of patrilineal clan principles among the Bering Sea Eskimo in the inherited totemic marks (symbolizing the wolf, gyrfalcon, raven, etc.) used on hunting weapons and other possessions (Nelson 1899:322; Lantis 1984b:218). Totemic marks were also placed on grave boxes in the cemetery that adjoined the village, to identify the patrilineage of the deceased. Bering Sea Eskimo lineages seem to have functioned primarily in the inheritance of particular forms of hunting magic and were not ranked or significant in the economic organization of the village.

The patrilineal clans that were well developed among the Asiatic Eskimo (including St. Lawrence Island) present an exception to both the general pattern of Eskimo social organization and to the latitudinal pattern of organizational complexity under discussion. Asiatic Eskimo clans were named, exogamous (requiring marriage outside the clan), and under the leadership of a senior male of the line. Clan membership determined the composition of whaleboat crews, hunting rights in certain territories, and residence location, with segments of the clan living under the same roof and clan houses being grouped together in the village. Each clan also had its own burial area.

Semisubterranean Houses of Alaska and Siberia

North Alaskan Eskimo (Inupiat)

The winter house of the coastal Inupiat (fig. 247) was similar to houses used all the way across the North American Arctic from northern Alaska to Greenland. It was a solid, permanent construction, reflecting the settled life of North Alaska's whaling villages. Each house even had a name: "All wet around it," "The people who face the sun," and "People with lots of mice" were names in use at the old village of Utqiagvik, at Point Barrow (Spencer 1959). The rectangular house was constructed of driftwood and whalebones, with the plank floor several feet below ground level. A thick insulating layer of sod blocks covered the house, except for a membrane-covered skylight. The house (*iglu*) was entered through a long underground entrance tunnel, which trapped cold air below the level of the house floor, preventing it from entering the inner room of the dwelling. Much activity took place in the entrance passage and its side

chambers, which included storerooms (also used as sleeping areas), a frozen meat locker, and a kitchen area where food was cooked and eaten. Inside the upper chamber were several oil lamps for heat and light, a fur-covered sleeping bench, and drying racks for clothes and boots. In the heated inner chamber few clothes were worn. Household furnishings were sparse; there was no furniture, and utensils such as tubs, bowls, dippers, and stone-headed mauls for crushing bone were simple in design and undecorated.

The household was an independent economic unit, in which the hunting and manufacturing activities of the men were complemented by the female activities of sewing clothes, boots, and boat covers, preparing food and skins, and raising the children. Household membership was quite flexible but typically included 8 to 12 people of several generations who were closely related by blood and marriage. Status differ-

247. North Alaskan Eskimo Winter House
Bancroft Library neg. 12511
The long entrance tunnel and wood-lined inner chamber heated with oil lamps were characteristic of the North Alaskan Eskimo winter house. The exterior view was taken at Point Hope in 1886, showing the tunnel entrance (*left*) and meat rack.

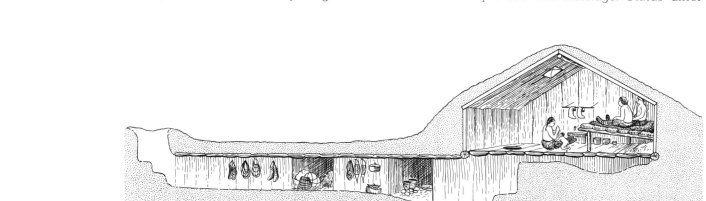

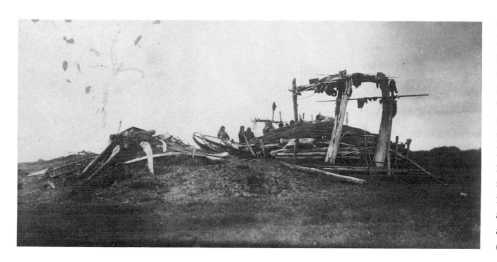

ences in North Alaskan Eskimo society were based primarily on age and sex and were reflected in domestic behavior such as sleeping arrangements. The house owner and his honored male relatives slept on the elevated bench, while women, younger men, and children slept underneath or were "inhabitants of the entrance passage." Whaling, with its requirements for large amounts of cooperative labor and joint ritual effort, was an integrating force in the social system. *Umialik*s (whaleboat owners) were important men in the village, and the *umialik* and members of his crew lived near each other and resided in the same large ceremonial house (*karigi*) during the whaling season.

Bering Sea Eskimo

The semisubterranean winter houses used by Alaskan Eskimo from Bering Strait south showed much local variation, but some basic structural differences from the North Alaskan house are apparent in all varieties. As shown in the Nunivak Island example (fig. 249), houses of the Bering Sea Eskimo were larger, the main room measuring about 15 feet square, and were entered through a large wood-roofed entrance passage at almost ground level. Houses often had an additional underground entrance tunnel, used in winter only, which acted as a cold trap. Wide sleeping benches were built around three sides of the main room, in contrast to the single platform in the northern house type. The roof differed from the central ridgepole construction of the North Alaskan Eskimo house; it was gabled, with four interior support posts. On the barren northern shores of Alaska wood was scarce and seldom used for cooking or heating, but among the Bering Sea groups a central fireplace heated the house, placed below a square smoke hole in the ceiling. Clay oil lamps mounted on stands pushed the darkness back into the corners of the room. Grass was used for matting on house benches and walls, as well as for kayak mats, baskets, socks, rope, and many other applications.

One of the most outstanding features of Bering Sea Eskimo social organization was the high degree to which gender roles were formalized and ritually differentiated (see Fienup-Riordan, this volume). As might be expected, this principle was reflected in housing arrangements.

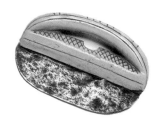

248. Ulu (Woman's Knife)
Bering Sea Eskimo: NMNH 36316

A girl started at a very young age to help her mother and learn the many skills involved in food preparation and the manufacture of clothing. Her most useful tool was the ulu, like this small one with walrus ivory handle and blade of trade iron.

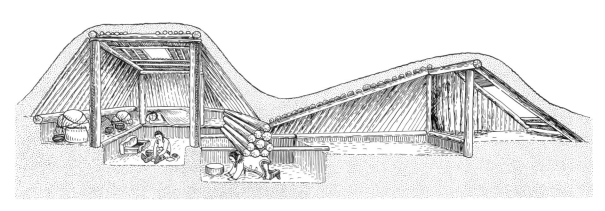

249. Bering Sea Eskimo Winter House
The large winter houses built by Bering Sea Eskimos had gabled roof supports, sleeping platforms on three sides, and a central fireplace with a smoke hole overhead. They were usually occupied only by women and children; the main residence of the adult men was the *qasgiq*, or ceremonial house.

250. Toys for Learning
AMNH neg. 1520, Jesup Exp.; Alaskan Eskimo: NMNH 153659 (bow), 45524 (arrow), 260441 (harpoon), (56045) top, (89800) whizzing stick

A future Koryak hunter takes aim. Many Eskimo toys (*right*) helped children learn adult skills; others were purely for fun.

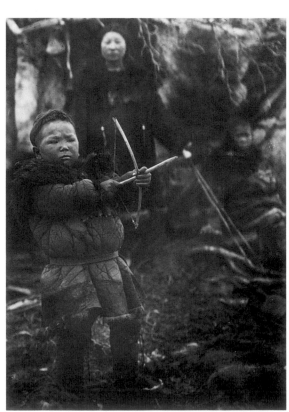

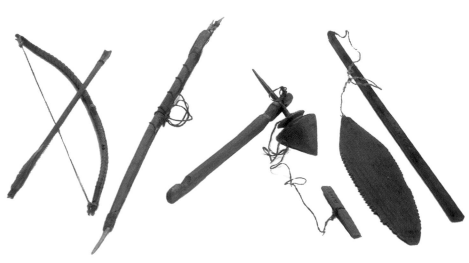

The large central ceremonial house or *qasgiq* was also the primary domicile for the men and boys of age five and older during the winter season when the family groups congregated in the main villages. Here the men ate, slept, worked, smoked tobacco, played games, and took sweat baths, and here the boys absorbed the knowledge and oral traditions that would serve them in their role as adult hunters. It was in the spiritual environment of the *qasgiq* that hunting implements were fashioned and imbued with their magic, and where cosmological beliefs and craftsmanship were combined in the pro-duction of decorated bentwood bowls, carved boxes, ivory fittings and amulets, and ceremonial masks. Women did much of their work in the home, processing and distributing the products of the hunt, teaching and caring for children, sewing carefully tailored garments, boat covers, and boots, weaving basketry, and carrying out their roles in the spiritual life of the community. Girls also began at a young age to absorb the knowledge they would need as adults and played with dolls, story knives, and miniature versions of their mother's tools.

Koniag and Chugach

The Koniag and Chugach (Pacific Eskimo) of southern Alaska also lived in Eskimo-type semi-subterranean houses, which differed from Bering Sea houses primarily in the complete lack of entrance tunnels (the entrance was through a ground level doorway), lack of sleeping benches in the main room, and the addition of multiple side rooms used as sleeping chambers, store-rooms, sweat-bathing lodges, and sometimes as burial chambers. Although *qasgiq*s were used for ceremonies, they were not used as male residences as among the Inupiat and the Bering Sea Eskimo. Koniag households were large (18 to 20 persons), and membership was apparently based on lineage affiliation.

Aleut

The construction and social aspects of the Aleut winter longhouse (fig. 251) are discussed in detail by Lydia Black in this book (p. 53). Eastern Aleut houses were the largest semisubterranean houses in the region, ranging from 70 to over 200 feet in length. Aleut houses lacked entrance passages, which were not necessary in the relatively mild climate of the region. Extensive use of grass was made in covering the house and furnishing it with fine and coarse mats and baskets. The treeless insular environment some-times led to the substitution of whale ribs for scarce timber in the framing of the house roof.

Entrance into the house was through the ventilation holes in the roof, via notched log ladders, a trait also seen in the semisubterranean houses of the Maritime Koryak, Itelmen, coastal Even, and Nanai. Among the Nanai, entry by this manner was made only during the Bear Festival but is suspected to have been in general use in fairly recent prehistoric times (Jochelson 1907). Ladder entry through the roof has been considered a significant trait linking southern Siberian cultures with the Aleutians and even with prehistoric Northwest Coast houses, a dis-tribution implying direct cultural connections across the Aleutians (Collins 1937).

Estimates by early Russian observers of the number of people living in the average longhouse are variable and reflect the rapid decline in

251. Aleut Winter House

The eastern Aleut winter house (fig. 16) was the largest type of semisub-terranean dwelling in the North Pa-cific region, occupied by many related families, each with its own lamp and living compartment. Living spaces were assigned according to rank by the lineage leader, who occupied the most prestigious location at the east-ern end of the house. As in the Ko-ryak house (fig. 253), entrance was gained by way of one or several roof holes equipped with notched ladders.

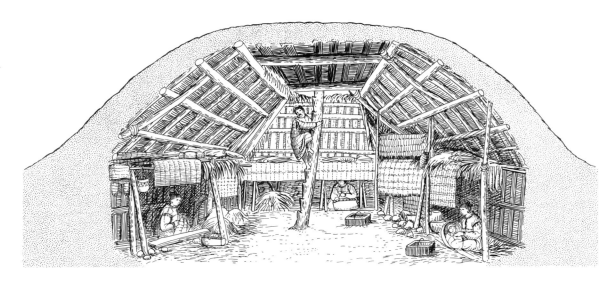

population suffered by the Aleut people after contact; by the late 18th century households averaged between 20 and 30 people (Lantis 1970:174). Household membership was determined by matrilineal clan affiliation, and the interior arrangement of families was strictly ordered by rank.

Koryak

In the Maritime Koryak house (fig. 254), a mixture of Eskimo-like house features and distinctly Asian ones is apparent. The house was partially underground and constructed on an octagonal plan, with double walls: an outer layer of logs and inner paneling of heavy planks, with grass stuffed between for insulation. Driftwood was plentiful in this region, and house timbers were also floated down rivers to the coast from the interior by the Koryak. The interior dimensions of the main room might be as large as 40 by 50 feet. The vaulted roof was supported by four interior posts, as in the southern Eskimo house. A single wooden sleeping platform for house guests was another Eskimo feature, although the resident families of the house slept along the side walls in sleeping tents reminiscent of the inner sleeping rooms (*pologs*) of Chukchi and Koryak reindeer herders' tents. A unique storm roof in the form of an inverted funnel was designed to break up the flow of wind and keep the top of the house from being buried in snow in the howling fury of Siberian blizzards. The top of the house was reached by an exterior ladder, shown in the drawing.

Most houses were occupied year-round, and different entrances were used according to the season. The rooftop entrance hole was used in winter only and also served as a smoke hole for the wood-burning hearth. The floor below was reached by a 15-foot-long ladder with cut-out footholes (fig. 253). The Russian ethnographer Waldemar Jochelson had a difficult time using these ladders when living with the Koryak during the winter of 1899–1900. Rising smoke from the fire blinded his eyes, his boot-clad feet were too large for the footholes, and the edges of the ladders were smooth and slippery with a mixture of grease and soot from the fire. He dryly advised that when falling into the house "one should by no means let go of the ladder, or he will land in the house on his back." The summer entrance was an aboveground wooden passageway, similar to the summer entrance of a Bering Sea Eskimo house. A second winter entrance was a covered porthole in the top of the summer passage, which also served as a draft regulator for the fire. Men considered it beneath their dignity to go through this entrance, but women,

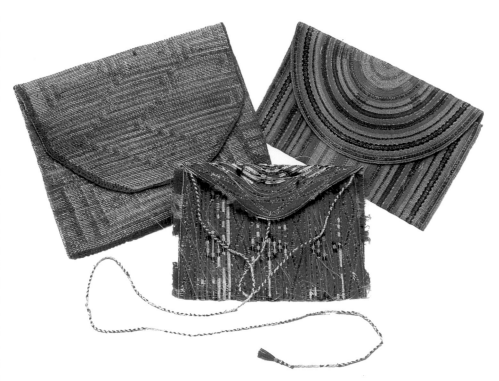

children, and sexually "transformed" men employed it.

The household consisted of a patriarchal family group, numbering from 6 to as many as 40 persons. A concern with spiritual protection of the home and family against *kalas* (evil spirits who brought disease and death) was a prominent feature of both Chukchi and Koryak domestic life. The Koryak house was a sanctuary from the *kalas*, who came from the darkness to attack the settlement, attempting to enter the house from underground through the hearth fire or by creeping down the ladder. The house ladder itself was therefore an important guardian charm and was carved with a small face on its upper end. The family fire was also a sacred and powerful family protector. Other guardians of family and hearth were kept in a shrine by the door and included the sacred fireboard (fig. 243), the family drum, the sacred arrow, and wooden figurines wrapped in grass. The fireboard was "dressed" in sacrificial sedge grass and "fed" by smearing fat on its mouth during ceremonies. Also kept in the shrine were various small wooden figures made from forked willow branches, which functioned in the hunting ceremonies that took place in the house and, along with the fireboard, served to protect and increase the family's livelihood. The Sun Worm charm (fig. 338) was hung in the sleeping chamber to protect women during pregnancy and prevent sterility. The entire village was guarded by a charm post, where offerings and sacrifices were made of grass, dogs, and the blood and fat of animals killed in the hunt.

252. Aleut Grass Pouches
(Clockwise from upper left) MAE 4104-26, 633-12, 633-14

These Aleut pouches were probably made for sale to early 19th-century travelers. Those on the upper left and upper right are skillfully woven from finely split grass, both dyed and in natural shades. The bottom pouch is blue-painted linen, overlaid with thin strips of painted skin, gutskin thread and dyed hair embroidery, yarn fringes, and long fine hair.

253. Koryak Winter House Interior
AMNH neg. 4131, Jesup Exp.

This photograph shows details of Koryak house construction and post-contact domestic life. The sacred ladder descends from the soot-encrusted ceiling to the hearth below, where two women sit with a Russian copper trade kettle. A metal washtub, packing crates, and other trade goods are also visible, while fur clothing and boots hang from a drying rack.

254. Maritime Koryak Winter House

The houses of the coastal Koryak were substantial log structures entered via the rooftop smoke hole in winter and through an above-ground entrance passage in summer. The entrance passage faced the sea and was kept open during the summer to allow free access to the visiting spirits of sea mammals. The top of the house was surrounded by a funnel-shaped construction that kept it from being drifted over during blizzards.

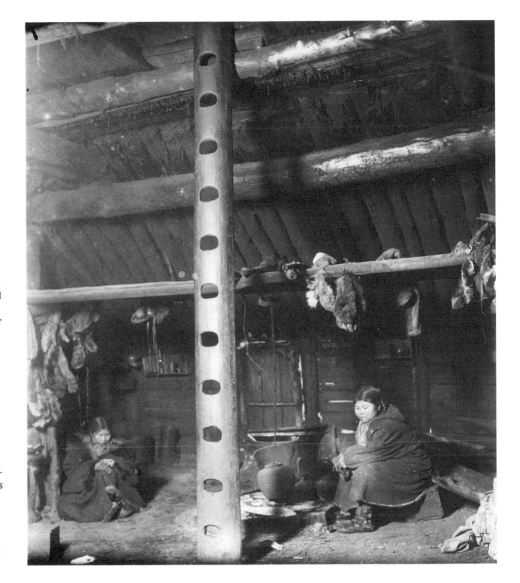

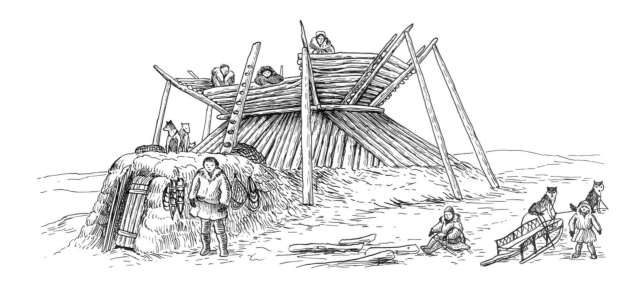

Asian and Alaskan Skin Tents

Skin tents provided a versatile architectural solution to the problem of staying warm yet mobile. Skin tents were used year-round by Asian reindeer-herding groups in the Crossroads area, and their use extended far to the west in Siberia. In Alaska, skin tents were used by the caribou hunters of North Alaska throughout the year. Skin-covered, domed lodges were used as winter houses by the Kutchin and other Athapaskan groups. Conical skin tents were used on hunting trips and as summer residences among the Bering Sea Eskimo and coastal Inupiat.

255. Summer Camp at Cape Lisburne
SI neg. 3855, E.W. Nelson, 1881
Light tents were used for summer travel and hunting along the coast; seals and an umiak are shown spread out on the beach.

256. North Alaskan Eskimo Skin Tent

North Alaskan summer tents were covered with reindeer skins or sealskins until the 1850s, when replaced by canvas sailcloth obtained from American whalers through trade and shipwrecks.

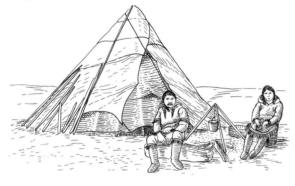

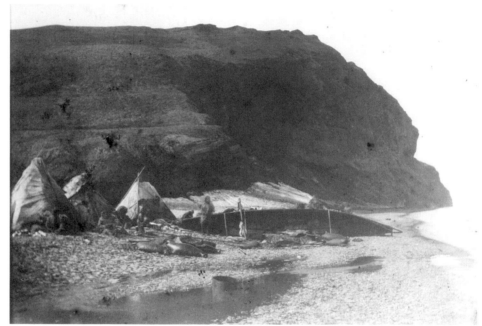

Even

Sergei A. Arutiunov (p. 38) considers the *chorama-diu* skin tent of the nomadic hunting and herding Even (fig. 257) to be a transitional form between the simple conical tent (a North Alaskan example is shown in fig. 256) and the *iaranga* tent of the Reindeer Koryak and Chukchi. The *chorama-diu* framework had a lower portion that formed a vertical wall, giving it a distinctive shape. The covering of the tent was made alternatively of reindeer suede, fish skin, or larch bark, depending on the season and location of the group. Although such a tent had the advantages of portability on the Evens' pack reindeer and ease of erection, it would not have been adequate for the severe arctic conditions to which the Koryak and especially the Chukchi *iaranga* was subjected.

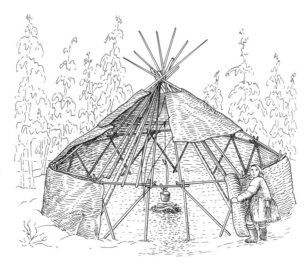

257. The Even Tent
The Even required portable shelter year-round to carry out their nomadic herding, hunting, and fishing way of life. The skin tent covering could be easily removed and packed on the backs of reindeer when camp was moved.

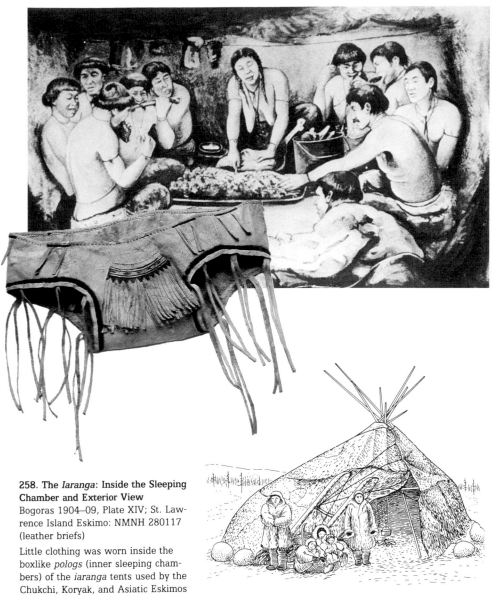

Chukchi and Koryak

The *iaranga* used by Chukchi and Koryak reindeer-herding groups was an adaptation of the Even-type skin tent to conditions of high winds and severe winter cold (fig. 258). It was used, however, in all seasons. An *iaranga* stood 10 to 15 feet high and was between 15 and 25 feet in diameter. The poles were lashed together in a strong but elastic framework, and the entire structure was secured against strong winds by taut lashings tied to large rocks and loaded sledges. The cover might also be deliberately frozen to the ground by pouring water around its base. The distinguishing feature of the *iaranga* was the construction of boxlike inner sleeping chambers (called *polog*s). Only one *polog* was used in Chukchi tents and was placed against the back wall. Two or three sleeping chambers were typically required by the larger Koryak household, placed around the sides and back of the tent. The main room of the tent remained unheated and was used mainly for storage and cooking over a wood fire. (By way of comparison, the principle of heating only a small inner room to save fuel was not employed by Alaskan Eskimo caribou hunters, who instead used a double tent cover during the winter. The dead air space between the covers increased the thermal efficiency of the house.) The close confines of the *polog* were easily heated to a high temperature by a single oil-burning pottery lamp and the body heat of the occupants, who often removed most of their clothes for comfort. Waldemar Bogoras commented on the close quarters of Chukchi tent life:

258. The *Iaranga*: Inside the Sleeping Chamber and Exterior View
Bogoras 1904–09, Plate XIV; St. Lawrence Island Eskimo: NMNH 280117 (leather briefs)

Little clothing was worn inside the boxlike *polog*s (inner sleeping chambers) of the *iaranga* tents used by the Chukchi, Koryak, and Asiatic Eskimos of the Chukchi Peninsula and St. Lawrence Island; they could become sweleringly hot from the heat of a single oil lamp. Both men and women would strip down to tasseled leather briefs like this men's pair.

259. Toys
Chukchi: MAE 434-83 (ball);
Tlingit: NMNH 209567; Chukchi:
MAE 434-80d (dolls)

Chukchi kick ball games were played by both children and adults. A Chukchi girl kept her dolls after marriage to hasten conception. Tlingit dolls with marble heads were made by Tlingit mothers for their daughters.

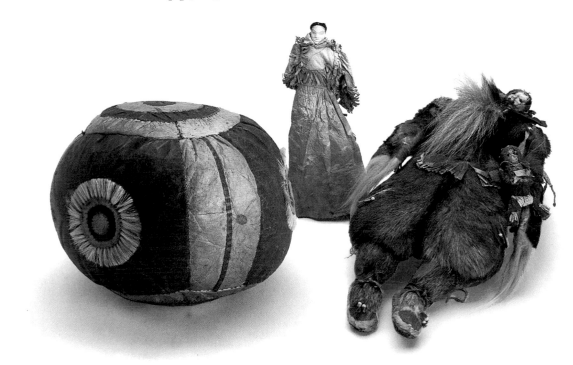

The Chukchee sleeping-room . . . affords little room for the stranger. A few extra men crowd it considerably, and are compelled to sit crouching in the strangest positions while eating or conversing. When there are a number of guests, they can only thrust their heads in, and must keep the rest of their bodies outside of the room, lying flat on their stomachs, and raising themselves up, like so many seals, from under the tent-cover, which is fastened around their shoulders (Bogoras 1975:173).

The Chukchi tent and camp could be read as a social map upon which were delineated simple status distinctions based on age, sex, and wealth (in reindeer). Within the sleeping chamber, the senior male of the Chukchi household and his wife slept on the lefthand side (the "master's place"), while younger members of the household, guests, and strangers slept on the right. Each Chukchi nuclear family had its own tent, and a camp rarely contained more than three tents of related families, usually headed by brothers, cousins, or a father and his grown sons; the total population of a camp rarely exceeded 15 people. The owner of the herd, or the majority of it, was the Master of the Camp, whose family tent was always larger and always sited at the northeast end of the line of tents in a tundra camp. The Master of the Camp exerted his decision-making authority in matters of management of the herd and in deciding appropriate times for sacrifices and ceremonies. Koryak camp organization was similar but with larger herds and camp populations.

The central focus of economic and ceremonial concern among reindeer herders was the welfare of their animals. The Reindeer Koryak sacred fireboard (fig. 260) was the deity of the family fire, protecting home and hearth against evil spirits. It was also the Master of the Herd, who along with his charm assistants kept away the wolves, prevented sickness, and prevented the animals from straying. Fire was thought to have been the progenitor of the first reindeer (Jochelson 1975:87), and in the ceremony welcoming the return of the herd from summer pastures a new fire was started with the fireboard, and burning brands from it were thrown at the approaching herd to greet them.

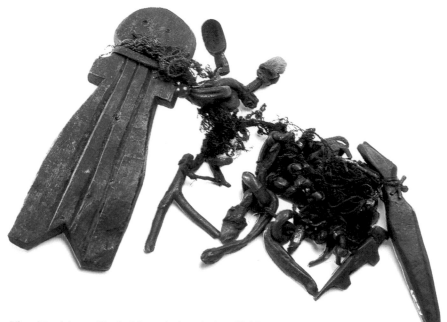

The Maritime Chukchi and the Asian Eskimo used a variant of the *iaranga*. Whalebones were often substituted for wooden poles in the lower part of the tent framework, a wall of sod was added around the bottom of the tent (reflecting greater permanence of the house location and the less nomadic lifestyle of coastal inhabitants), and walrus skins were used as flooring. The tent cover was made of reindeer skins traded from the Reindeer Chukchi. Coastal *iaranga* households were several times larger than the households of the Reindeer Chukchi. As among the North Alaskan Eskimo, the organization of Maritime Chukchi villages was based on the economic cooperation and spatial proximity of boat crew members and the Boat Master (equivalent to the North Alaskan *umialik*). There was no equivalent, however, of the Eskimo *karigi* (ceremonial house). In the summer, walrus skin—covered tents were pitched nearby in the same settlement. Archeological evidence indicates that the Asian Eskimo formerly used wood and whalebone-framed underground houses like those of the Inupiat Eskimo of Alaska prior to adopting the *iaranga* from the Chukchi at the end of the 19th century.

260. Master of the Herd
Reindeer Koryak: MAE 6750-16a

In addition to its sacred role as source of the hearth fire and spiritual guardian of the family against evil spirits, the fireboard also protected the economic welfare of the household. Thus the Maritime Koryak fireboard was thought to help in the hunt for sea mammals, while the Reindeer Koryak fireboard, known as the Master of the Herd, protected the reindeer from disease and predators. The charms tied to this fireboard with sinew and thongs include little forked figures representing "boys" or "herdsmen," a wooden spoon used in sacrifices, a small wooden image of a watchdog, beads, and a divining stone with a hole through it. A larger legless animal image (*right*) is the wolf, which is thus kept near the guardian figure and away from the herd. The fireboard was kept with other charms in the family shrine, and periodically "clothed" in a grass collar, and "fed" by rubbing grease on its mouth.

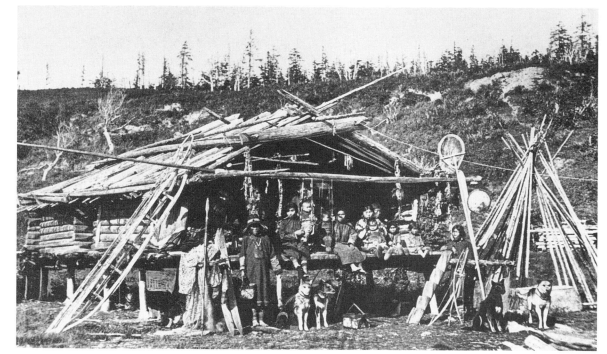

261. Nivkhi Summer House on the Amur River
Photo: AMNH, Jesup Exp.

The Nivkhi occupied large subterranean winter houses, shifting residence in the summer to log structures built on piles at good fishing and sea mammal hunting locations. The social and religious symbolism connected with Nivkhi houses was highly elaborate (Black 1973). In building a new house, shamanisitic divination was important for choosing a spiritually propitious location.

262. Athapaskan Indian House

Pole-framed structures covered with spruce or birch bark and insulated with moss were built as multi-family communal houses by many Athapaskan groups, including the Tanana and Ahtna. These were the most permanent dwellings constructed by these seminomadic hunters and fishermen.

263. Gambling Sticks
Tlingit: NMNH 75423

Gambling was universally popular on the Northwest Coast. In one game, rods such as this set in polished hardwood with abalone shell insets were shuffled under a loose bundle of shredded cedar bark, and the bundle then divided. The players then had to bet on which bundle contained a specific marked rod.

Wooden Houses

Several varieties of aboveground wooden houses were used by native peoples in the southern part of the Crossroads area. Some Bering Sea Eskimo erected log houses for summer use, with front and rear walls made from vertical upright planks; many Athapaskan Indian groups built rectangular pole structures for winter and summer use covered with strips of birch bark (fig. 262); and several basic types of wooden structures used in Siberia included the Nivkhi summer plank house raised on stilts (fig. 261).

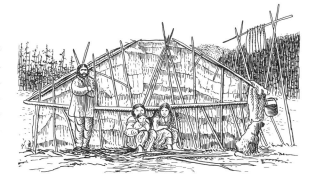

The most substantial and decoratively elaborate wooden structures were the large winter plank houses of the Northwest Coast. Northwest Coast houses and villages provide an especially complex example of the spatial expression of social structure. Figure 264 depicts the Whale House of the Tlingit Ganaxtedi Clan at the village of Klukwan in southeastern Alaska (Emmons 1916), and the discussion that follows addresses the houses and villages of the Tlingit (Shotridge and Shotridge 1913; De Laguna 1972).

The matrilineal clan system of the Tlingit is described in this volume by Frederica de Laguna (p. 60). There were four nested organizational levels. At the highest level was the division of society into halves (moieties), the Ravens and the Wolves. Each moiety was in turn divided into named clans, each clan was made up of several lineages (local divisions of the clan, usually spread out between several neighboring villages), and each lineage was composed of a number of large communal households. Status

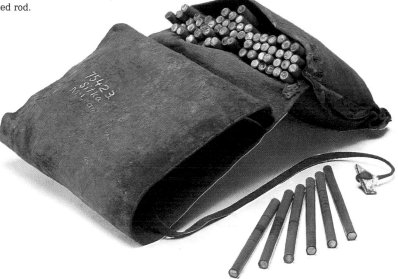

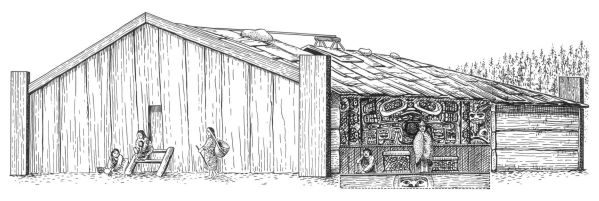

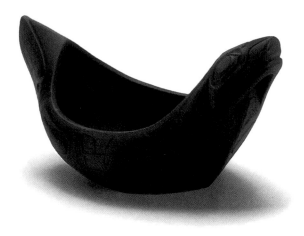

265. Grease Bowl
Haida: NMNH 23409

The social and ceremonial elaboration of the Northwest Coast was supported by abundant food resources. Animal oils—of eulachon fish, salmon, sea lion, and whale—were easily stored and a basic foodstuff. One of the principle sources of oil was the harbor seal, which was also the most commonly used theme for carved bowls used to contain oil. Here the fat creature is poised with back arched as if stretching on the beach or on an ice floe.

latent spiritual power, occupied a separate area hidden among the trees, reflecting the separation of the shaman from the rest of society in both life and death.

The house was a large wooden structure sometimes over 50 feet square, with a single frontal entrance facing the water. It was framed in spruce and planked with easily split hemlock; the houses of wealthy clans were finished inside with red cedar. Four major house posts held up the roof, carved and painted to represent the totemic crest animals of the clan and to represent significant events in the oral tradition of the lineage. Similar themes were sometimes depicted on house front paintings. Above the central hearth was a large square hole that admitted light and allowed smoke to exit, usually fitted with a movable wind screen used to adjust the ventilation of the house. As shown in figure 264, the interior floor was excavated to create two rising tiers that surrounded the sunken hearth area. The wood-planked upper tier was

distinctions were drawn at all levels, so that every Tlingit individual had a rank within the household, each house was ranked within the clan, and each clan ranked within the moiety. This organizational system was mirrored in the layout of a Tlingit village. The houses were arranged in a long line along the shore of a protected cove or riverbank, the houses of each clan clustered together, and the house clusters of the most prestigious clans located at the center of the village.

All of the subsidiary structures of the village reflected the same organization. In southern Tlingit villages totem poles stood before each house, portraying the crest animals and history of the lineage. Along the beach were the canoe shelters, fish-drying racks, and smokehouses owned by each house; behind the houses were caches where provisions were kept, in addition to bathhouses, and huts where women were confined at childbirth. The grave houses, which held the ashes of the dead, ran along behind the village or stood at one end, arranged by the same principles of status and affiliation as the houses of the living. These arrangements expressed the whole generational cycle of birth and death and the integration within the household of all aspects of production and reproduction. The grave houses of shamans, guarded by tall carved guardian figures and charged with

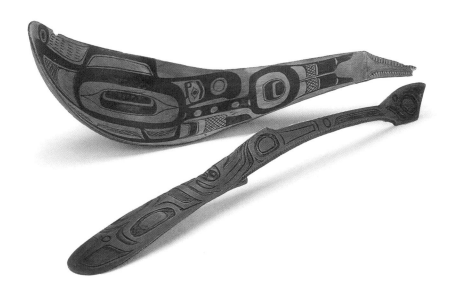

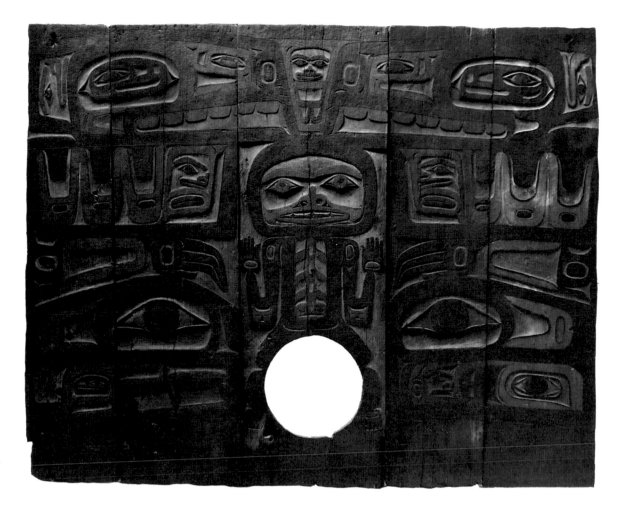

266. House Screen
Haida: CMC VII-B-1527

This cedar plank partition is carved
and painted with a crest of the Haida
Eagle House at Howkan, in Southeast
Alaska. It would have screened off
the chief's apartment at the end of
the house. Exit through the belly of
the screen's central figure symbolized
rebirth.

267. Spoons
Tlingit: NMNH 60144, 60147

Tlingit spoons included large painted
ladles (*upper*) as well as carved soapberry spoons (*lower*). The ladle is
painted with black formlines in the
image of a killer whale, identifiable
by the large, perforated dorsal fin
sweeping back from the head. The
soapberry, native to the dryer parts
of the coast and interior plateau, can
be whipped in water to a stiff pink
froth, considered a delicacy and
prized for feasts. The carved design
on this paddlelike spoon for eating
the froth represents a fish, probably a
salmon. A tiny human face on the
back of the head may be Salmon Boy,
who was taken away by the salmon
and who returned to teach humans
how to properly treat the fish so that
they would return each year to benefit mankind.

divided into family apartments by walls, small
decorated screens, or stacks of piled belongings,
and the lower tier was primarily a sitting bench.

Tlingit households ranged in size from about
25 to 50 people, including male members of the
same clan (related to each other as brothers,
maternal uncles, nephews, or cousins), their
wives (always from a clan of the opposite moiety),
unmarried women and girls, and young children.
A certain number of slaves would also be resident, depending on the wealth of the household.
This large group of people functioned as the
basic social and economic unit of Tlingit society.
Most property was held communally; fishing,
hunting, berry picking, and trading were joint
activities of the household; and food was cooked
and eaten commensally.

As we have seen, the division of house inte-
riors into socially distinct spaces on the basis of

status was a cultural universal among Northeastern Siberian and Alaskan cultures. The place
of honor was always the location farthest from
the door. Among the Tlingit the end apartment
belonged to the house chief (*yitsati*), families of
lower rank ranged along the sides of the house,
and slaves were "dwellers by the door," on call
to fetch water or wood or to carry out other
tasks at the command of the true "house people." An elaborately carved screen separated
the apartment of the *yitsati,* an inner sanctum
in which were kept the valuable crest objects of
the house. Entrance into the apartment was
through a hole in the belly of the crest animal
depicted on the screen, so that the *yitsati* symbolically went into the womb of the crest animal
and was unified with it until he reemerged or
was "reborn" into society again (Jonaitis
1986:133).

This survey demonstrates some of the ways in which houses, as well as their contents and their arrangement into villages, reflect environment, economy, and social structure. From an archeological perspective, houses in the North Pacific–Bering Sea region show a long history of development reflecting general processes of social and economic change. The earliest houses were the tents of Ice Age big-game hunters, known from west of our area at sites such as the 15,000-year-old Malta site on the Belaya River (Gerasimov 1964). Malta houses were constructed with the products of the hunt; over excavated foundations rose a mammoth tusk and caribou antler framework, covered with skins. The interior contained the separate hearths of up to three families, probably representing a cooperative family group comparable to the Chukchi, Koryak, or Alaskan Eskimo household. Tool patterning on the Malta house floors suggests that male and female work areas were on opposite sides of the hearths.

The Paleoarctic hunting groups that spread into Northeastern Siberia and Alaska at the end of the Ice Age (after 9500 B.C.) occupied skin-covered structures that had a shallow excavated floor and a single central hearth. A rectangular house with a short entryway was excavated in Level VI at the Ushki site on the Kamchatka Peninsula and may have been either skin or sod covered (Dikov 1977). Variations on the skin-covered tent remained in use into historic times throughout Alaska and Siberia by interior hunters and herders, whose nomadic way of life required an easily moved dwelling suitable for small households and year-round occupation. Small conical tents were used as summer dwellings or portable hunting shelters by coastal groups.

The process of adaptation to coastal environments, which intensified over the last 6,000 years in both Siberia and Alaska, led to the development of larger and more permanent dwellings that were ancestral to the winter houses discussed above. On the southern coast of Alaska, small semisubterranean earth-covered structures without entrance passages were in use by 4000 B.C.. Aleut houses at 2000 B.C. were domed underground structures that probably had roof entrances and eventually developed into the large communal longhouses known from the historic period. Between 2500 B.C. and A.D. 0 the coastal semisubterranean house with a central hearth, interior support posts, and shallow entrance passage evolved along the western coast of Alaska and in Northeast Siberia (Ackerman 1982), ancestral to the Bering Sea Eskimo winter house. This house type was used by people of the Denbigh and Norton culture phases. Other archeologically known coastal house designs from the second millennium B.C. did not continue into the historic period. These include the large multiroomed houses of the Old Whaling culture (1400 B.C.), which had side rooms and shallow entrance passages, and the large oval houses of the Choris phase (1600–500 B.C.). The North Alaskan Eskimo house, with its long, deep entrance tunnel and absence of a hearth, clearly had its roots in the early Eskimo cultures of Bering Strait after A.D. 0: Old Bering Sea, Birnirk, Punuk, and Thule. Ipiutak houses (A.D. 0–900) were more clearly related to the Bering Sea Eskimo type; they lacked entrance passages but had sleeping platforms around three sides.

These house types represented a large labor investment and were permanent dwellings designed to be used for many years. They were thus suitable to a more sedentary way of life based on the abundant and stable food resources of the coast. This stability is reflected in long-term trends of increasing population density and house size among the coastal populations of Alaska and Siberia. A well-documented case is St. Lawrence Island (Collins 1937), where the dramatic increase in house size from the Old Bering Sea to the Punuk phase is thought to be based on the high productivity and new organizational requirements of large-scale whaling. Dramatic increases in house size over time also occurred among the southern cultures of the Beringian region (Aleut, Koniag, Chugach, Tlingit) as the productivity of the coastal environment came to be fully exploited through new technologies and the emergence of complex forms of social organization.

Needles and Animals: Women's Magic

Valérie Chaussonnet

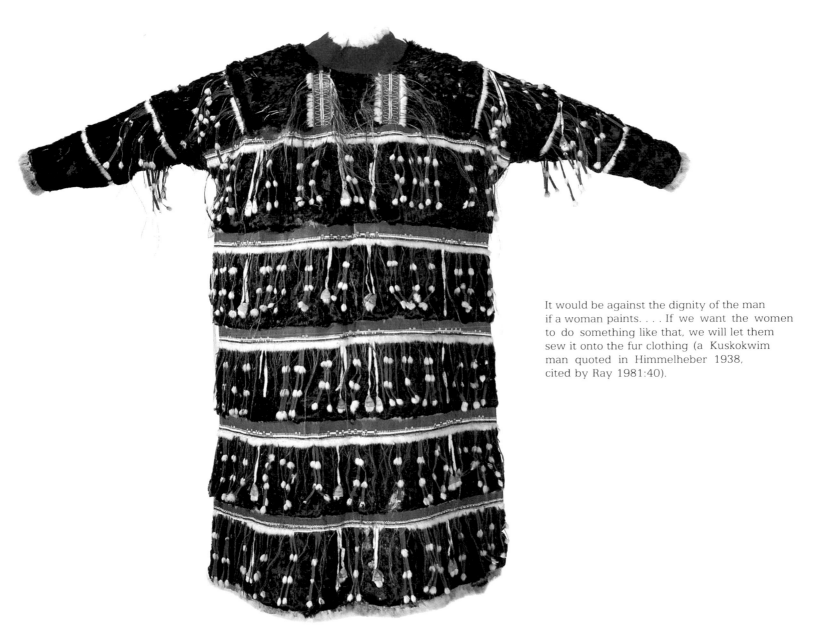

It would be against the dignity of the man if a woman paints. . . . If we want the women to do something like that, we will let them sew it onto the fur clothing (a Kuskokwim man quoted in Himmelheber 1938, cited by Ray 1981:40).

268. Koniag Birdskin Coat
Koniag Eskimo: MAE 2888-84
Hundreds of iridescent neck skins of the pelagic cormorant were used to fabricate this spectacular ceremonial garment (cf. fig. 2). Its beauty is enhanced by red-and-white tufted tassels of dyed skin and gut, long fine hairs and strands of yarn worked into seams, delicate white cormorant flank feathers, tiny embroidered seam designs, a trade cloth collar, and white fur trim.

Today, the traditional native clothing of the North Pacific has been totally or partially replaced by manufactured European-style clothes. Sewing traditions, however, are still alive, and the elaborate garments that impressed the early traveler and that served to visually differentiate one group from the other (fig. 72) are still worn on occasion. In the modern context of rapidly diminishing ethnic distinctiveness, clothing is worn and exhibited as a flag, a marker of ethnic identity. But even before the adoption of European-style clothing and the consequent trans- formation of clothing into ethnic costume, women as seamstresses played an extremely important role in the expression of cultural values and meaning. While appropriating some stylistic and technical elements from neighboring peoples, the women of each group cut and embroidered clothing according to distinctive cultural aesthetics, recognizable throughout their material culture. Apart from their role as the guardians of sewing traditions, seamstresses expressed through clothing the magical beliefs and the symbolic values of the group. Social positions within the group were expressed by characteristics of clothing that marked gender, age, and status.

The link between clothing and identity can be understood in reference to the ideology of spiritual transformation. In Northeastern Siberia and northwestern North America, people, animals, and spirits were subject to metamorphosis. No being had a single, invariable shape. Garments, like masks, could effect or make reference to spiritual transformation. Cosmological links between humans and the animal world were also

Style and Function

The strength of stylistic tradition and its relationship to group identity were apparent in examples of garments poorly adapted to the physical environment and climate. The Even, recent immigrants to the North, made Chukchi- or Koryak-style parkas for long sledge journeys but retained their traditional thin, tight, and open garments for everyday wear. Moreover, the Yukaghir, under Even influence, adopted this style of clothing, even though it was much more suitable for the warmer climate of the southern taiga than for the severe climate of the northern tundra (Jochelson 1908:388).

Although Chukchi and Koryak male clothing was functionally outstanding, typical female clothing demonstrated some strongly nonfunctional attributes. The combination suit, or *khonba* (figs. 36 and 271), typical of Chukchi, Asiatic Eskimo (including St. Lawrence Island), Koryak, and, in the past, Itelmen women, was cumbersome and impractical. Waldemar Bogoras (1904–09:245) reported that young women complained about its shortcomings. He described the *khonba* sleeves as "very full, and so long that they interfere with the work of the woman." Normal tasks often required that one or both arms be removed from the sleeves. The sleeves often slipped down by themselves, because of the deep neck opening. Neck and shoulders were thus exposed to the cold, especially among Chukchi and Eskimo women, who, unlike Koryak women, did not wear a parka over the combination suit. In winter, however, the *khonba* was worn in two layers, with the fur of the inner garment against the body.

As a whole, though, seamstresses in Alaska and Northeastern Siberia were remarkably ingenious in using local resources to create garments appropriate to the local climate and way of life. White people often took advantage of indigenous clothing, especially in the most rigorous regions of the North Pacific and Bering Sea. Bogoras (1904–09:234) noted that "the style of clothes used by Chukchee and Koryak

evident in the requirement that the clothing be carefully and beautifully made to please the spirits of the animals upon whom the group depended for survival.

Social and spiritual elements were thus combined with technological requirements in the design and manufacture of a piece of clothing. The effectiveness of a garment must be partially gauged in social, magical, and aesthetic terms, which in some cases outweighed the practical function of the clothing.

men in winter is admirably adapted to its purpose. It therefore prevails among most of the tribes of northeastern Asia, including the Russians." Murdoch (1892:109) recalled that after one season of wearing ready-made shirts and coats obtained from ships' crews, the Point Barrow Eskimo packed these away and rarely wore them again, and then only in summer, since their own clothing was better suited to the environment. Waldemar Jochelson (1908:588) observed that "excepting those entirely Russianized, very few Koryak wear chintz or calico shirts under the fur clothing."

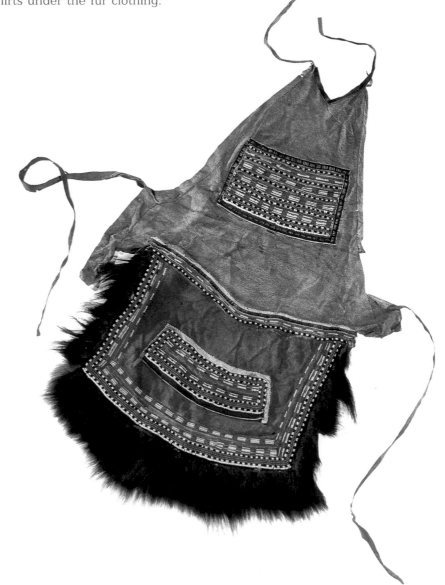

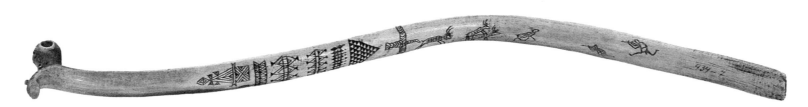

Most clothing from the northern parts of the North Pacific region was made from reindeer fur, which was warmer than any other because of the insulating nature of its hollow hair. Insulation and preservation of body heat, especially during the winter months, were increased by wearing two layers of fur garments of the same cut. This practice applied not only to Koryak and Chukchi clothes but also to the Northern Alaskan and Bering Sea Eskimo parka and pants. Reindeer, killed in the summer (rather than in the fall, when their fur was too thick for clothing), provided a soft and much lighter skin than mountain sheep or bear. Mountain sheep, however, was often used in the past instead of

271. Reindeer Koryak Mother and Children in Fur Clothing
AMNH neg. 1528, Jesup Exp.

Koryak women wore the *khonba*, a one-piece combination suit with wide sleeves, similar to the child's fur suit except for its open neck and lack of hood. Layers of clothing were usually doubled in winter. The mother here wears an outer hoodless parka over her *khonba*. Her parka and that of the children have a front "bib" flap (p. 19). The little boy at left is wearing his parka hair-side-in.

272. Infant's Combination Suit
Chukchi: MAE 395-11

This tiny combination suit has a flap between the legs for changing the infant's moss or soft hair diaper. Suits made for toddlers and older children had hand and foot openings and were worn with separate boots.

reindeer for the inner layer of the *khonba* (Prytkova 1976:40, citing Merck). It was also used by the North Alaskan Eskimo for parkas and by the Yukaghir for a rough type of winter coat. During the summer months the tattered remains of winter clothing, the fur of which had been damaged by spring rains, were worn. For this reason, the appearance of Northeastern Siberians in summer was, in Bogoras's words, "exceedingly shabby" (1904–09:248). The Even made summer coats by shaving the remaining fur off worn-out winter coats.

Dehaired sealskin was used everywhere for boot soles. For this reason, and since reindeer fur was much warmer than sealskin for winter clothing, maritime peoples exchanged sea mammal products and reindeer fur with interior peoples. Maritime groups used sealskin to make summer pants. Sealskin was not warm, but it was waterproof, whereas reindeer fur had to be protected from water to retain its insulating qualities (fig. 208). Alaskan, Aleut, and, to a certain extent, Chukotkan peoples made a remarkable type of waterproof garment from sea mammal or bear intestine (gutskin), which they wore by itself or over fur clothing. Interior groups, especially the Even and Yukaghir, made waterproof garments for the warmer seasons from the hide of that part of the tent that had been cured in the smoke of the hearth. As seen in the exhibition, the skin of a great number of other animal species, including fish and birds, was also used. Their importance varied locally.

It is in the cut and design, rather than in the material, that tradition might conflict with functional requirements. The wide sleeves of the *khonba* are only one example of this. In another, Donald W. Clark (1984:194) noted for the Koniag and Chugach Eskimo that "to work while wearing a parka, people inserted their arms through slits at the side rather than through the virtually nonfunctional [very narrow] sleeves."

The diffusion of such traditions, as evidence of past cultural connections between the Old and the New Worlds, was what Gudmund Hatt, whose work was contemporary to the Jesup Expedition, had in mind when he established a typology of northern clothing. Hatt's typology (1969) was based on the clothing patterns and the development from simple original forms into more elaborate types. He divided northern clothing into two complexes: the moccasin-snowshoe-cloak complex, and the sandal-boot-poncho complex. The former, designated an inland culture, was typical of Even, Nanai, Yukaghir, and Athapaskan types of clothing. The latter, considered the earlier of the two, was typical although not limited to the coast-culture area, including the American and Asian Eskimo, Koryak, and Chukchi.

The *khonba*, according to Hatt, was developed as a garment for Koryak, Chukchi, and Asiatic Eskimo women from a common northern children's garment of the same cut as the *khonba*, but provided with a hood. For him, one-piece clothing such as the *khonba* originated as an animal costume, similar in conception to the way a bearskin, for example, might have been "put on, as far as possible, in the manner in which the animal had worn it," i.e., with the back on the back, and the front legs as the sleeves (Hatt 1969:95, 97). In fact, the legs of the *khonba* were often made from reindeer leg skin. This allowed Koryak seamstresses, in particular, to combine aesthetic and symbolic elements by alternating dark and light vertical bands of skin (fig. 346). The pieces in the exhibition show that the shape of the original animal skin had a great influence on the cut and design of clothing.

Animals, Seamstresses, and Hunters

Animal skin, transformed into a second skin for humans by the work of the seamstresses, still maintained its animal identity. From the killing of an animal through the tanning, cutting, and sewing of its skin into a piece of clothing, the qualities and characteristics attributed to it in life were maintained and passed on to the wearer of the finished garment. This important spiritual principle linked animals, hunters, and seamstresses together in an intricate and circular set of relationships. The continuity of animal identity is made explicit in Bogoras's comment, for example, that in Chukchi beliefs "skins ready for sale have a 'master' of their own. In the nighttime they turn into reindeer and walk to and fro." In Siberia and Alaska, amulets made from animal skin were believed to turn into the original animal when needed. Properties of other animal parts could demonstrate this principle as well. Baleen used in making the wooden hunting hat of the Nunivak Island kayaker, for example, allowed him to pass safely through the currents like a whale, just as the wood of the hat or a grass attachment, as land elements, guaranteed his safe return to the shore (Lydia Black, personal communication).

A direct consequence of the continuum between live animals and animal products for clothing was that women had to observe certain rules in their art and show respect for the material, as did the hunters of the game. Eskimo women were forbidden to sew while men were hunting important game, for fear this work might offend the animals. In addition, the clothing they produced had to be beautiful, with regular and perfect stitches (see Fienup-Riordan essay on p. 263 in this volume) so that the hunter wearing the garment would please the game. North Alaskan men therefore dressed in fine new clothing for whaling. Seamstresses of the North Pacific dressed not only hunters but also their

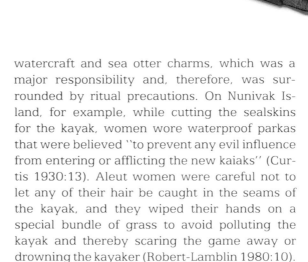

watercraft and sea otter charms, which was a major responsibility and, therefore, was surrounded by ritual precautions. On Nunivak Island, for example, while cutting the sealskins for the kayak, women wore waterproof parkas that were believed "to prevent any evil influence from entering or afflicting the new kaiaks" (Curtis 1930:13). Aleut women were careful not to let any of their hair be caught in the seams of the kayak, and they wiped their hands on a special bundle of grass to avoid polluting the kayak and thereby scaring the game away or drowning the kayaker (Robert-Lamblin 1980:10).

Concern with female pollution of the hunting material explains why the manufacture of thong among the Chugach Eskimo "was the only kind of skin working in which the men took part" (Birket-Smith 1953:74). This same fact was recorded by Jochelson (1908:629) among the Ko-

273. Needlecases

(Clockwise from upper left) North Alaskan Eskimo: NMNH 33700. Chukchi: MAE 688-6. Oroch: 138-42. Bering Sea Eskimo: NMNH 176229. Chukchi: MAE 666-15b

Two types of needlecases were used—tubes with stoppered ends (Oroch and Bering Sea Eskimo shown here) and open-ended tubes into which needles enclosed in leather strips were pulled (fig. 274, above; Chukchi and North Alaskan Eskimo examples here). There were marked cultural variations in shape and decoration, however, as this small assortment demonstrates.

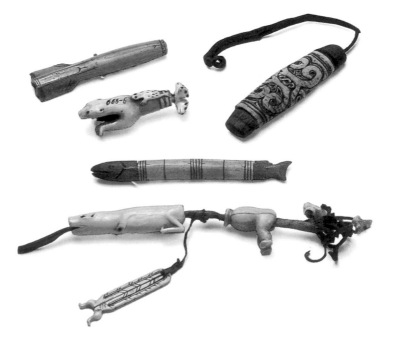

274. Tools of the Seamstress
(Clockwise from top) Bering Sea Eskimo: NMNH 30764. North Alaskan Eskimo: NMNH 398246, 24436

The beautifully crafted wooden box with ivory fittings once held a woman's sewing equipment: a needlecase or two, sinew thread, buttons, useful scraps. Such boxes were made by men for their wives. The handle of the stone-bladed skin scraper (*center*) was carefully shaped to fit the contours of a woman's palm and fingers, easing the fatigue of scraping and thinning hides to prepare them for clothing. The needlecase (*bottom*) is a tube of sheet copper into which was pulled a sealskin strip holding bone and/or steel needles for safe storage. The ends of the strip are fringed and decorated with outgrown children's ''starter'' labrets.

ryak. A Tlingit informant told Frederica de Laguna (1972:422) that in Dry Bay ''men, not women, skinned the seals. . . . This [was] in contrast to the practice at Yakutat, where 'the women don't want the men to touch it after they get the seal', and where the flenzing [was] women's work.'' This explanation demonstrates the problematic and shifting boundary between the animal as hunted game and as sewing material.

The seamstress helped reconcile humans and animals, not only by indirectly participating in hunting but also by reinforcing the transformational relationship between them in the clothing that she made. The iconographically oriented western mind has tended to focus on numerous fine examples of woven or appliquéd animal representations on garments such as the Northwest Coast blankets. Seamstresses of the North Pacific region, however, by taking advantage of the animal qualities of the raw material, also used a more direct means to signify the human-animal symbiosis. A striking example was noted by Birket-Smith (1953:65), who stated that ''for rainy weather the [Chugach Eskimo] men had a sort of combination suit made of black-bear skin. The skin of the head formed a hood, and the skin of the legs, which was cut open along the sides, served as sleeves and mittens, respectively as trousers and boots.'' Such an impressive animal costume made of the whole animal was quite rare and recalls the belief held in both Northeastern Siberia and Alaska that the black bear was a man who could peel off his skin. But the use of tailored animal parts to cover the corresponding parts of the human body was extremely common. Although visually less noticeable, this practice served the same transformational function as the Chugach bear suit. The use of animal leg skin, in particular of caribou-reindeer legs, to make leggings and boots was universal in Alaska and Siberia. The Chukchi made leggings with bear leg skin and sewed

bear leg skin on the elbows of their seal hunting parkas (Bogoras 1904–09:239). In Siberia and Alaska mittens were often made of reindeer leg skin or bear paw, and hoods were usually made from the skin of the head of a caribou, fox, dog, or wolf, on which the ears were often preserved. North Alaskan Eskimo men and boys wore a headband made from the skin of a dog or fox head, with the nose in the middle of the forehead, which seemed extremely valuable to them (Murdoch 1892:142). Headbands of the same type were collected among the Bering Strait Eskimo by Edward W. Nelson (1899:33), who also observed a type of headdress made of a whole arctic fox ''sewed that the head of the fox rests on the crown of the wearer with the body and tail hanging down over the back. These caps are very picturesque and give the wearer a remarkably dignified appearance.''

Animal tails were universally incorporated into the garments, either as the actual tail, like in some Even coats, or as an inspiration for the large U-shaped flap, as in Eskimo women's parkas (fig. 276). According to John Murdoch (1892:138) the Point Barrow Eskimo wore ''attached to the belt various amulets and at the back always the tail of an animal, usually a wolverine's. Very seldom a wolf's tail [was] worn, but nearly all, even the boys, ha[d] wolverine tails, which [were] always saved for this purpose and used for no other.'' The tail as part of the garment was an ancient feature of Northeastern Siberian clothing; in the 19th century it

275. Beaded boots and Leggings
Koryak: AMNH 70-5260a,b; 70-5185a,b

Made from shiny dark reindeer-leg skins, these man's boots and leggings display geometric beadwork patterns heavily influenced by Yukaghir and Even decorative styles. The red flannel trade cloth with which the boots are trimmed was a popular and highly valued commodity in both Siberia and Alaska.

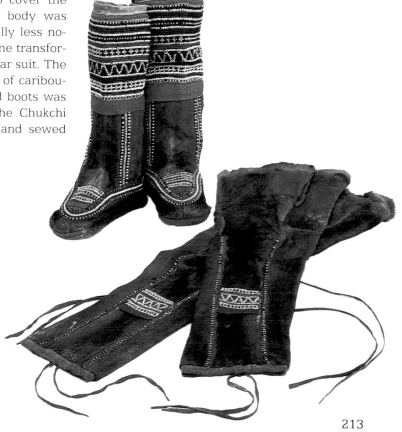

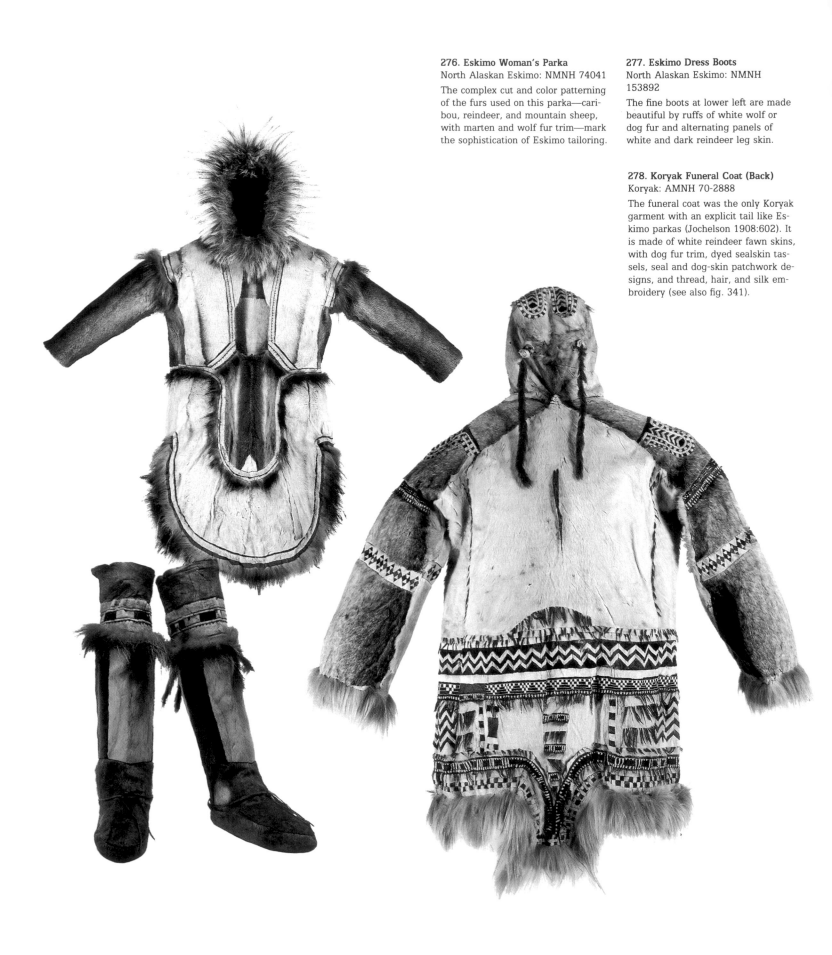

276. Eskimo Woman's Parka
North Alaskan Eskimo: NMNH 74041

The complex cut and color patterning of the furs used on this parka—caribou, reindeer, and mountain sheep, with marten and wolf fur trim—mark the sophistication of Eskimo tailoring.

277. Eskimo Dress Boots
North Alaskan Eskimo: NMNH 153892

The fine boots at lower left are made beautiful by ruffs of white wolf or dog fur and alternating panels of white and dark reindeer leg skin.

278. Koryak Funeral Coat (Back)
Koryak: AMNH 70-2888

The funeral coat was the only Koryak garment with an explicit tail like Eskimo parkas (Jochelson 1908:602). It is made of white reindeer fawn skins, with dog fur trim, dyed sealskin tassels, seal and dog-skin patchwork designs, and thread, hair, and silk embroidery (see also fig. 341).

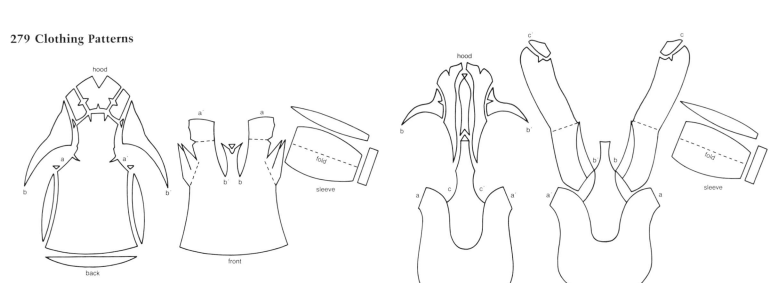

a. North Alaskan Eskimo male parka pattern

b. North Alaskan Eskimo female parka pattern

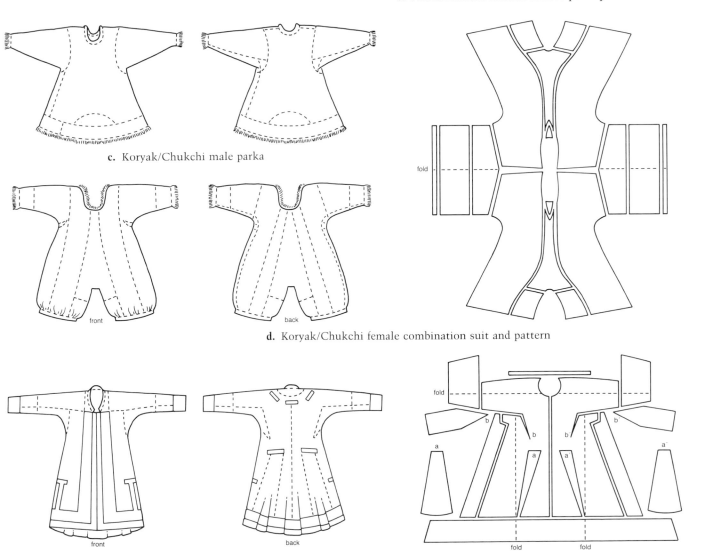

c. Koryak/Chukchi male parka

d. Koryak/Chukchi female combination suit and pattern

e. Even male and female coat and pattern

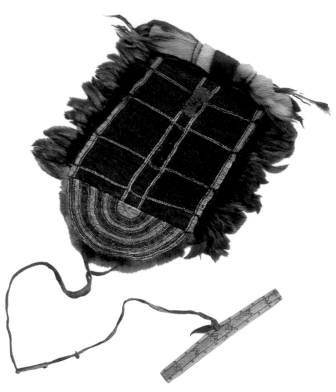

was lost in Koryak and Chukchi coats, except for one type of Chukchi female hooded coat (Prytkova 1976:44) and in the Koryak funeral costume. The tail design was preserved in most Yukaghir and Even coat patterns and was accentuated by fur trim and beadwork.

In addition to animal symbolism, the tail motif was further used to mark the division between men and women. The complex relationship to animals and the importance of division of labor in relation to the game was reflected in every aspect of the life of the group, including in the clothing. One of the main markers of gender was the flap of the coat, although the meaning of particular flap shapes was not consistent among different groups. The elegant rounded U-shaped flap typical of North Alaskan female clothing was an important sexual marker, similar to the U-shaped flap of the sewing bag or "housewife," and to the outline of the female knife or ulu. The male parka of the North Alaskan Eskimo was provided with a slightly rounded bottom piece added in the back (fig. 279), recalling the flap found on male parkas of Eastern Eskimo groups. The Athapaskan buckskin shirt was provided with flaps as well (at the back and front for male, and at the back only for female shirts), but of a pointed rather than rounded shape. Among the Even, the lower hem of the male apron was rounded, whereas that of women tended to be cut straight.

Far from limiting the seamstresses' possibilities, the fact that the raw material was preshaped and charged with animal identity stimulated her creativity and guided her work towards a distinctive cut, according to which particular char-

acter of the animal she wished to emphasize. Practically all garments were manufactured with skins or hair from several different species, the arrangement of which—each with its own plastic characteristics—made her work an exercise of virtuosity and probably of great enjoyment. The pattern of a garment such as the Northern Eskimo female parka, inspired by the shape of a large caribou skin, reveals how complex and elaborate a design could be obtained by piecing together the different skins according to shapes, colors, and type and length of hair. The result was the reconstitution of an animal creature as monstrous as it was beautiful. Such a design, fixed as a cultural style, was a pattern for other skin parkas, such as the ground squirrel parka (fig. 41), and was reproduced with no relationship to the shape of the original "square" small pelts.

The various and contrasting shades of the skins were used aesthetically and symbolically to underline the cut and joints of the garment. In Alaska an impressive effect was obtained by the gores, wedgelike inserts, of both male and female Eskimo parkas, which imitated walrus tusks. Labrets, which both men and women wore under their lower lips, reinforced the walrus image. A parka such as the sumptuous white reindeer-skin parka with dark "tusks" (fig. 208) synthesized the two principles used by the North Pacific seamstresses to signify the dynamic (transformational) relationship between humans and animals. The juxtaposition of the reindeer's body, neck, and head skins onto the person's (the metonymic process) was combined with the (metaphorical) representation of the walrus, whose qualities were acquired not through the skin that once belonged to him but through an image.

280. Eskimo Sewing Bag
Bering Sea Eskimo: NMNH 127353

Small sewing articles were rolled up inside sewing bags (also called "housewives") that had U-shaped flaps like the female parka. The cord could then be wrapped around the rolled up bag, and held in place by tucking the ivory crosspiece under the cord. The bag is made from caribou ear skins.

281. Chilkat Blanket
Tlingit: NMNH 219504

The most prestigious robe of Northwest Coast Indian nobility in the 19th century was the Chilkat blanket. Highly stylized designs in dyed mountain goat wool were woven into the textile, the warp of which was wool with a cedar bark core. Here the central panel represents the killer whale. The creature's head is at the bottom, the tail at the top, and the two sides of the dorsal fin extend outward from the central face, which represents the blowhole. The bottom fringes of the blanket are nearly as long as the height of the woven panel.

282. "Indian of Mulgrave"
Tomas de Suria, 1791

Tlingit everyday clothing before contact included the simple heavy skin cloak, worn here with a woven spruce-root hat. The iron dagger may identify this Indian as one who figured in a threatening encounter with a member of the Spanish Malaspina Expedition in 1791 (Vaughan et al. 1977).

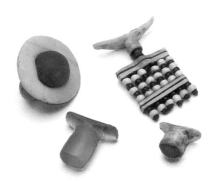

283. Eskimo Labrets
(Clockwise from upper left) North Alaskan Eskimo: NMNH 37663. Bering Sea Eskimo: NMNH 16204, 38800, 44906

Labrets were ornaments that projected through slits in the lower lip (at one or both corners of the mouth for men, above the center of the chin for women; see fig. 71) and were held in the mouth by a flared retainer piece in back. Lips were pierced for a child's first labret at puberty. Design and materials varied widely: (clockwise from upper left) limestone with a split Chinese wound bead; ivory with seed beads; ivory with wound bead; bottle glass.

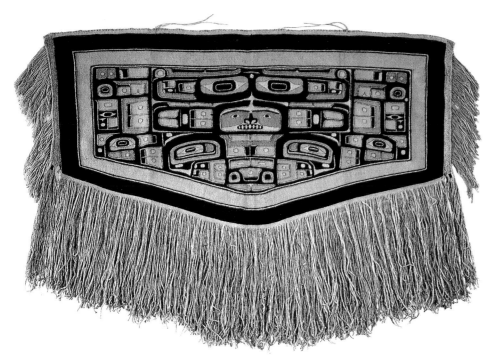

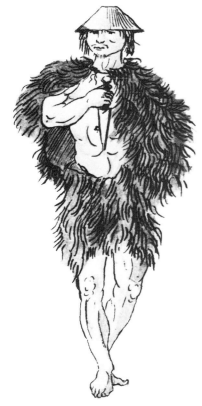

284. Geometric Woven Blanket
Tlingit: MAE 2520-6

Robes of this type date to the early historic period on the Northwest Coast (cf fig. 80); few exist today. They were twined of finely spun white mountain goat wool yarn, with designs in dyed yellow and dark brown yarn.

Totems and Tattoos

Other examples of North Pacific clothing demonstrated principles of zoomorphic representation that were different from those discussed so far. On this clothing, the representation of animals was not related to the cut of the clothing or to the correspondence of body parts between the animal and its wearer, but was an often complex and abstract surface representation. The most striking and famous example was the animal imagery of Northwest Coast blankets.

The form of animal iconography in Northwest Coast art is discussed by Bill Holm in this volume (pp. 281–93). Blankets bearing this rich iconography were worn and displayed for special occasions, but in everyday life the Northwest Coast Indians wore untailored fur capes (fig. 282), plain woven blankets, and buckskin pants and shirts mostly traded from the interior (Athapaskan) Indians. A rare type of geometric woven blanket was inspired by basketry (fig. 284). The highly decorated blankets were "robes of nobility," and most displayed realistic or conventionally coded crest animals (Holm 1983:57). In the Northwest Coast context, the social and political content of these "totem poles on cloth" (Jensen and Sargent 1986) differed from an animal image—the walrus, for example—on Eskimo parkas. The numerous motifs of Tlingit face painting, worn at potlatches, were also representations of crest animals (Swanton 1908:plates 48–54). Among the Tlingit, when parts of animals were used, these were prestigious animals that were incorporated in ceremonial clothing

as a sign of wealth and status. Whole ermines on a headdress or bear ears, for example, served the same purpose as a copper (fig. 380), and small coppers were sometimes inserted in the bear ears, while ermine pelts were associated with the valuable abalone shell (fig. 379; Jonaitis 1986:103, 20). The relationship with animals and the use of animal motifs in clothing were thus very different from the personification observed among the Eskimo.

The art of the Northwest Coast seamstress-weaver was iconographic and two dimensional, in contrast to that of Eskimo seamstresses, who created and decorated garments as three-dimensional, volumetric forms. Technically speaking, Chilkat woven blankets were exact copies of designs painted on pattern boards. The decoration on Tlingit button blankets (the material for which usually came from Hudson's Bay Company blankets) consisted of appliquéd flannel cloth and mother-of-pearl buttons, and the hide of the armor shirt (fig. 82) was crudely cut and used as a canvas for the application of painted designs. The same motifs were applied to boxes, house fronts, and other objects, and the symbolism of the blankets and shirts did not derive any specific character from the fact that it covered or wrapped the human body. As a matter of fact, the ceremonial leggings and apron worn by the Tlingit figure in the exhibition were not woven as such but were cut from a blanket. Not all women were weavers. The Northwest Coast weaver was a professional artist, just as a male painter was. She dressed the blanket, as it were, and thus, indirectly, dressed people. The hierarchically organized motifs worked into the blanket were a statement of the wearer's status. The blanket served as both a physical and a symbolic barrier between the nobility and the common people (Jonaitis 1986:99).

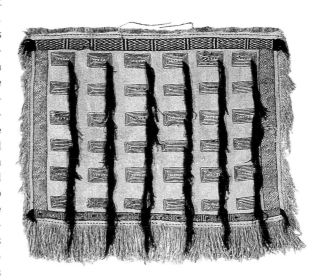

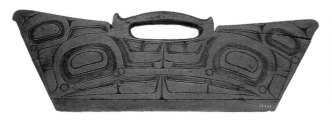

Amur River fishskin coats (fig. 414) were another example of garments used as surfaces for the presentation of a formal iconography. The lower hem, the collar, and the front opening—on the right side for ordinary clothing and in the middle for a ceremonial coat—were bordered with colored beads, which served as a frame for the elaborate ornamental composition covering the surface of the garment. According to Berthold Laufer (1902:5),

the animals which appear in the designs of the Amur natives are just like those who play an important part in Chinese art and mythology. It is indeed most remarkable that animals, such as the bear, the sable, the otter, and many others which predominate in the household economy, and are favorite subjects in the traditions as well as in daily conversation, do not appear in art, whereas the ornaments are filled with Chinese mythological monsters which are but imperfectly understood.

Moreover, the highly stylized motifs were ''read'' by very few and were believed to have only a decorative purpose by most. Seamstresses, however, knew a variety of complex motifs by heart and took pride in reproducing them exactly. Because of their proximity to the Chinese, Nanai women, in particular, were extremely skilled in embroidery, including silk embroidery. As among

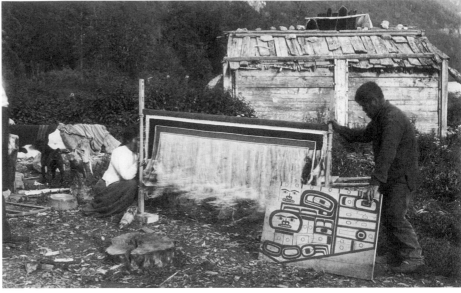

the Tlingit, the same motifs found on clothing also covered the surfaces of wooden tools, boxes, bowls, and many other objects of everyday life. The use of patterns for clothing was similar to the use of painted boards as design guides by the Chilkat blanket weavers. Fish skins were sewn together with invisible seams, and the large surface obtained was treated as a piece of whole cloth. Fake side seams might be embroidered as on a silk or cotton coat. Like the motifs, the elegant shape of the coat was borrowed from the Chinese.

The emphasis on motifs superimposed on the garments with a possible symbolic value—geo-

285. Bark Shredder
Tlingit: FM 13747

To prepare it for use in making blankets, clothing, and basketry, cedar bark was shredded to a soft flexible state with an ulu-like shredding tool.

286. Tlingit Blanket Weaving from Pattern Board at Kluckwan
AMNH neg. 46173, Harlan Smith

Painting of pattern boards was a male specialty, while reproducing the half-design as a full Chilkat blanket was a female profession.

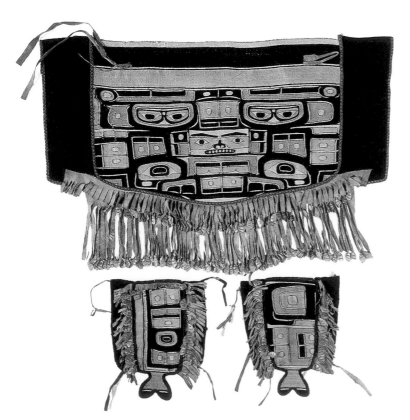

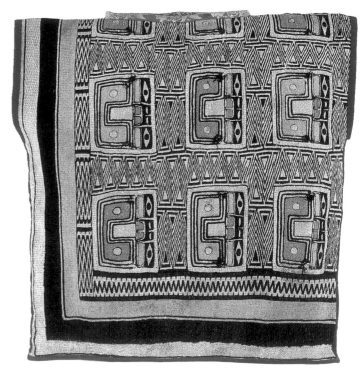

287. Paper Appliqué Pattern
Nivkhi: AMNH 70-1936b

Patterns painted on paper and birch-bark stencils were used as design guides by seamstresses in Amur River cultures when decorating fish-skin coats and other garments. Spiral designs representing fish and cocks flank a grinning beast face.

288. Amur River Fishskin Coat
Nanai: AMNH 70-628

Chinese inspiration is evident in both the cut and ornamentation of this embroidered salmonskin coat, shown here in back view. The ornamental figures that are arranged symmetrically over the surface of the garment are stitched-on appliqués of dyed salmon skin. The figures are highly stylized representations of animals drawn from Chinese mythology. The only real seams in the garment are between individual fish skins, but false seam designs extend up its sides.

289. Tunic
Tlingit: CMC VII-A-360

This woven mountain goat wool tunic, made from part of a blanket that had been cut up and distributed at a potlatch, is stylistically intermediate between early geometric blanket designs (fig. 284) and the later formline designs of Chilkat blankets (figs. 281, 290). Its rectangular figures once had pendant yarn tassels, as in the geometric style. Like later Chilkat blankets it has solid black-and-yellow borders, but has no cedar bark in the warp.

290. Dance Apron and Leggings
Tlingit: NMNH 341202, 2a, 2b

A wraparound apron and decorated leggings were often worn by the nobility along with a Chilkat blanket on ceremonial occasions. The woven pieces of this set were originally part of a single blanket depicting a diving killer whale, which was probably cut up and distributed to guests during a great memorial potlatch. The woven pieces have been extended with trade blanket material and bordered with skin fringes. Puffin beaks attached to the fringes rattled together with the movements of the dancer.

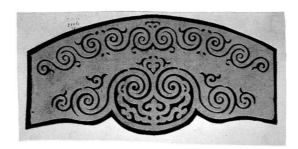

metric rather than representative, and decorative, possibly magical, rather than totemic—could be seen in the clothing styles of the Aleut, southern Alaskan Eskimo, Koryak, Athapaskan, and Even. Since the seamstresses of these cultures exploited the aesthetic more than the symbolic qualities of the material from which the garment was cut, and added ornamental elements onto it, their work is related to that of the Tlingit weaver and the Amur seamstress.

The skins traditionally used by Aleut and southern Alaskan Eskimo seamstresses—small mammal pelts, bird skins, and especially gut skin—were plastically neutral when sewn together, and the composite material could be cut in any pattern, like a piece of cloth. Garment patterns used in areas relying on small skins for clothing manifested a different aesthetic orientation from patterns based on the use of large hides. In southern Alaskan Eskimo and Aleut

garments, the skins were sewn together in straight horizontal bands, with the usual addition of a square breast piece. The parkas had straight bottoms without side slits. Parkas of this type did not show a gender differentiation. Except for the collar, the back and the front of the garment were similar.

Although the cut appeared rather simple and straight, the ornamentation, by contrast, was extremely elaborate. Decoration of this type of garment tended towards rhythmic repetition, which answered at a smaller scale the repetitive patterns of the composite material itself: the rows of dozens of spotted ground squirrel pelts, scale-patterned fish skin, or iridescent cormorant skins. Gutskin might be partly bleached to produce an alternating pattern of gold and white strips. The tails of small animals were often worked into the design, along with tassels of various other materials. They were inserted into the seams to underline the horizontal band effect, a decorative use that stood in contrast to the representational use of tails on Eskimo zoomorphic parkas.

The aesthetic of the horizontal in clothing is well represented in the exhibition. On the Kodiak cormorant parka (fig. 268) the vertical seams between the bird skins were made invisible, while the horizontal seams were enhanced by

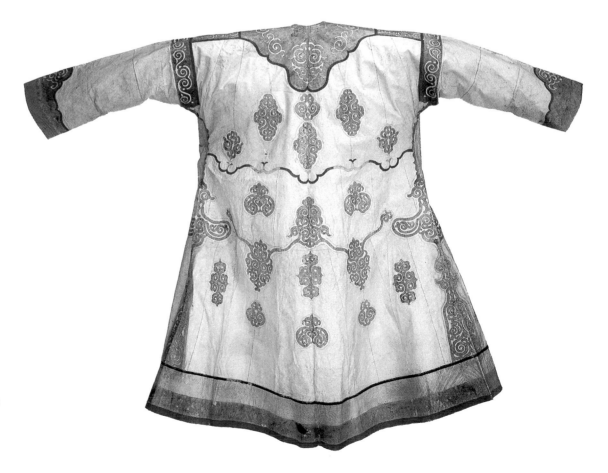

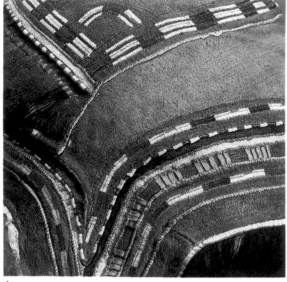

A

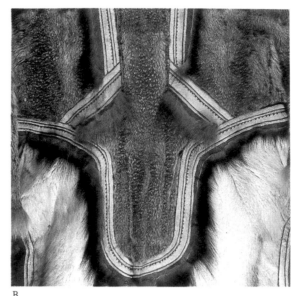

B

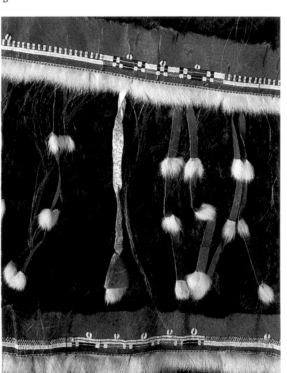

D

C

291. A Close Look at Decorative Techniques

(Clockwise from upper left)

A. Even

(earflap of woman's cap, AMNH 70-5601e, cf. fig. 31)

Tanned reindeer skin, with embroidery of dyed moose or reindeer hair; alder-dyed seal pup fringe

B. Bering Sea Eskimo

(front of woman's parka, NMNH 176105, cf. fig. 41)

The white fur in the lower panels and welted border strips is imported reindeer skin. The spotted skins are Arctic ground squirrel, and the trimming is wolverine.

C. Koniag Eskimo

(front of cormorant skin coat, MAE 2888-84, cf. fig. 268)

The broad horizontal bands are neck and upper breast skins of the pelagic cormorant; intermediate bands are red-colored skin embroidered with white and dyed sinew thread and red-, green-, and blue-dyed yarn or hair, and edged with white fur. There are also narrow horizontal strips of skin painted a sparkling black with paint containing specular hematite. Attached are tassels of red leather and white gut skin, tufted with white fur, some ending in beaks of the tufted puffin.

D. Aleut

(neckline and amulet of gutskin parka, MAE 593-18, cf. fig. 52)

The neckline is bordered with embroidery of colored skin strips and sinew thread, and feathers of cormorant breast (dark) and flank (white). Ornamenting seams between the gutskin strips are dyed gutskin fringes and yarn. The amulet is woven grass.

strips of white and red dyed reindeer skin, embroidered patterns, and fringes (fig. 291, close-up). The fringes in the seams were a feature commonly found on gutskin parkas (figs. 52, 56, 86, and 292). One practical explanation is that the fringes served as a protection against rain, which could flow along them rather than wetting the seams—although this would not apply to fur parkas of the same design. The ornamental aspect of fringes, however, was probably more important. The extraordinary care with which the Aleut seamstress joined the strips of gutskin together using tiny ornamental stitches and hair embroidery (fig. 56) seems to indicate a particular concern with emphasizing the horizontal element of the design. The stylized

anthropomorphic amulet hidden in the collar of an Aleut parka (fig. 291) also featured woven horizontal bands on its head and body, which may schematically represent the parallel lines painted on hunting hats and the horizontal banding of the actual parka to which the amulet was attached. The horizontal stylization of the anthropomorphic amulet dispels any doubt about the visual intention of the gutskin parka design.

Gutskin parkas among Eskimo and Aleut were not only practical but had also a religious function (fig. 350). According to Dorothy Jean Ray (1981:56), "almost all shamans [in South Alaska] wore one when curing as well as when performing miracles under the sea and in other secret places." Gutskin parkas were worn for dancing

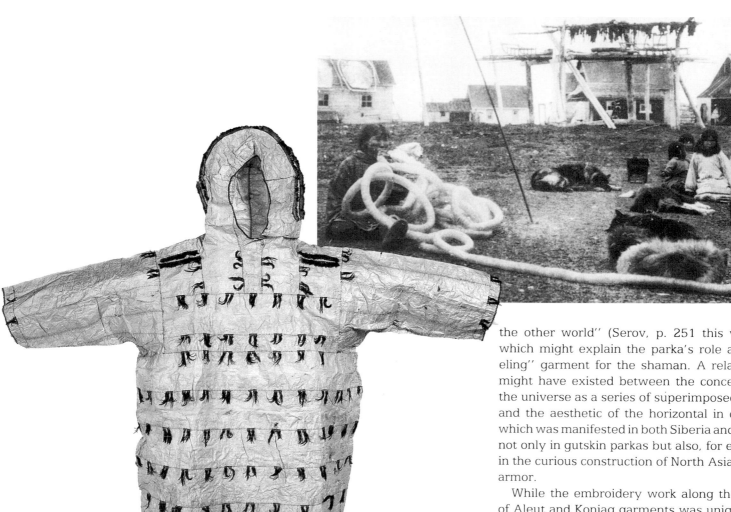

292. From Guts to Garment
St. Lawrence Island Eskimo: NMNH T-1676. SI neg. 82-8286, Henry Collins, 1930 (Gambell village, St. Lawrence Island)

Cleaning and inflating yards of walrus intestine were the first steps in creating beautiful, waterproof gutskin garments like the dress parka shown here. The inflated intestine was hung up to dry; if in winter, it would be bleached white by the wind and cold. The seamstress sewed strips of split, dried intestine together with sinew thread to create a parka, working tiny auklet beaks and feathers into the seams for decorative effect. Fine St. Lawrence Island gut parkas were traded to the Maritime Chukchi, who wore them in ceremonies honoring *Keretkun*, walrus-god and Master of the Sea.

ceremonies too. Their protective power against female pollution has been noted earlier. In the North too, among the Maritime Chukchi and Asian Eskimo, gutskin parkas were worn as ceremonial garments for the *Keretkun* ceremony and other festivals (Bogoras 1904–09:393). For this particular occasion, the Chukchi obtained beautifully worked light gutskin parkas from St. Lawrence Island seamstresses.

But it remains unclear what important quality of the garment endowed the wearer with power and created a boundary around his or her person. Was there a particular power attached to gutskin as a material? Was there a relationship between the waterproof quality of the garment and protection from spirits, in which case the seams, as joints in the material, would be particularly important? A connection might also have been present between the intestines from which the garment was made and the bladders that served such an important role in the hunting ceremonies of the Yupik Eskimo. In Siberia the loops made by intestines symbolized the "crooked path to

the other world" (Serov, p. 251 this volume), which might explain the parka's role as "traveling" garment for the shaman. A relationship might have existed between the conception of the universe as a series of superimposed worlds and the aesthetic of the horizontal in clothing, which was manifested in both Siberia and Alaska, not only in gutskin parkas but also, for example, in the curious construction of North Asiatic hoop armor.

While the embroidery work along the seams of Aleut and Koniag garments was unique in its delicacy, in Northeastern Siberia the manufacture of fur mosaics, slit embroidery, and hair embroidery on the *opuvan*, the large strip sewn as lower hem of the coats (fig. 421), gave Koryak seamstresses the reputation of being fine embroiderers. The beautiful *opuvan* of the Koryak dancing coat is a good example of the geometric patterns used by the Koryak. Even when not ornamented, the lower hem of the Koryak and Chukchi coat was always added as a separate strip to the body of the coat (fig. 329).

Athapaskan tunics, on which the lower hem was cut into pointed flaps with modest ornamentation and fringes, displayed a large and elaborate band of beads, dentalium shells, or quillwork on the chest and the sleeves, encircling the body, and a red line often underlined the seams and the ornate bands. In Siberia and North America quillwork and hair embroidery were replaced by or combined with beadwork, as soon as colored glass beads became available through trade. As for the red lines, they are reminiscent of the Eskimo lifeline that bordered objects, and they are found on Naskapi Indian coats from Labrador as well. Both men and women wore dentalium shells and beads in the form of head bands, earrings, and bracelets. Their faces were tattooed with lines on the chin,

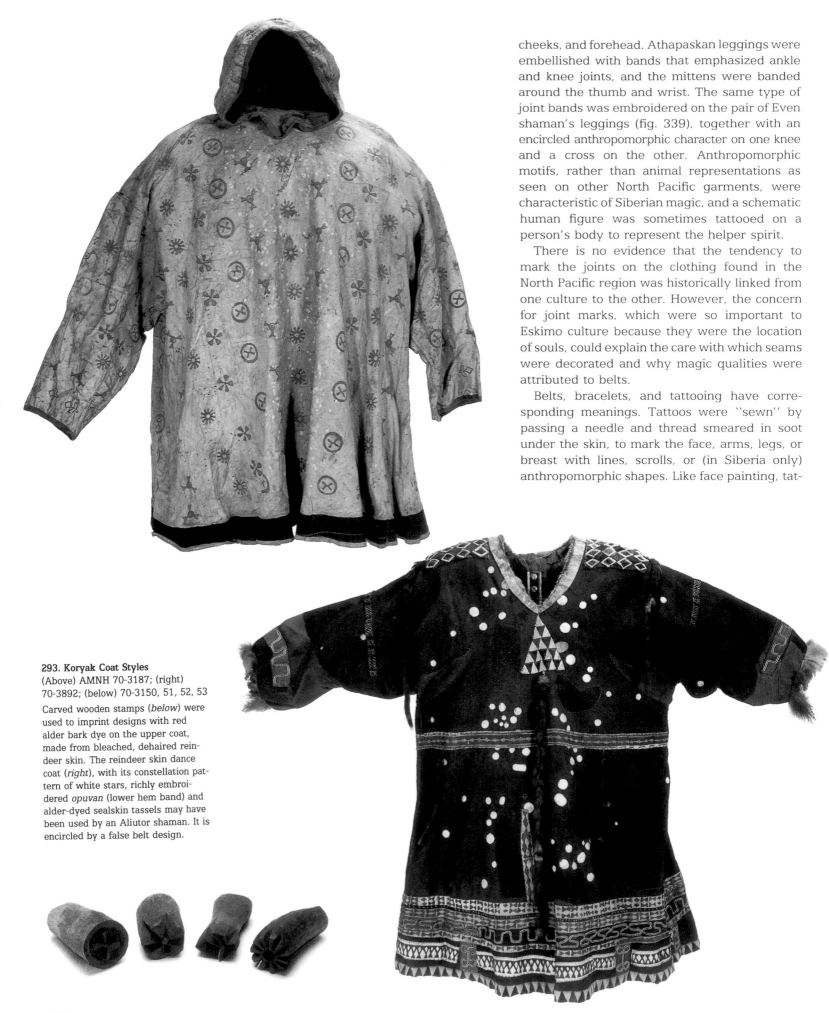

cheeks, and forehead. Athapaskan leggings were embellished with bands that emphasized ankle and knee joints, and the mittens were banded around the thumb and wrist. The same type of joint bands was embroidered on the pair of Even shaman's leggings (fig. 339), together with an encircled anthropomorphic character on one knee and a cross on the other. Anthropomorphic motifs, rather than animal representations as seen on other North Pacific garments, were characteristic of Siberian magic, and a schematic human figure was sometimes tattooed on a person's body to represent the helper spirit.

There is no evidence that the tendency to mark the joints on the clothing found in the North Pacific region was historically linked from one culture to the other. However, the concern for joint marks, which were so important to Eskimo culture because they were the location of souls, could explain the care with which seams were decorated and why magic qualities were attributed to belts.

Belts, bracelets, and tattooing have corresponding meanings. Tattoos were "sewn" by passing a needle and thread smeared in soot under the skin, to mark the face, arms, legs, or breast with lines, scrolls, or (in Siberia only) anthropomorphic shapes. Like face painting, tat-

293. Koryak Coat Styles
(Above) AMNH 70-3187; (right)
70-3892; (below) 70-3150, 51, 52, 53
Carved wooden stamps (*below*) were used to imprint designs with red alder bark dye on the upper coat, made from bleached, dehaired reindeer skin. The reindeer skin dance coat (*right*), with its constellation pattern of white stars, richly embroidered *opuvan* (lower hem band) and alder-dyed sealskin tassels may have been used by an Aliutor shaman. It is encircled by a false belt design.

222

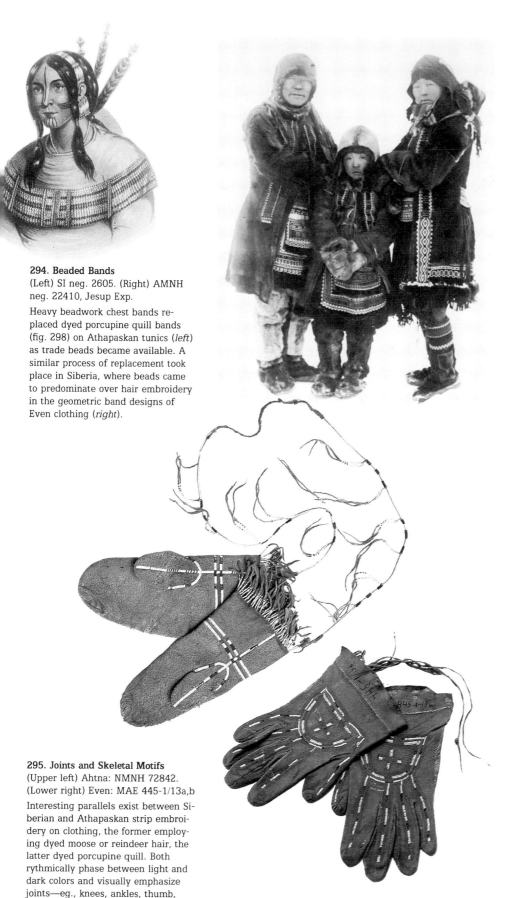

294. Beaded Bands

(Left) SI neg. 2605. (Right) AMNH neg. 22410, Jesup Exp.

Heavy beadwork chest bands replaced dyed porcupine quill bands (fig. 298) on Athapaskan tunics (*left*) as trade beads became available. A similar process of replacement took place in Siberia, where beads came to predominate over hair embroidery in the geometric band designs of Even clothing (*right*).

295. Joints and Skeletal Motifs

(Upper left) Ahtna: NMNH 72842. (Lower right) Even: MAE 445-1/13a,b

Interesting parallels exist between Siberian and Athapaskan strip embroidery on clothing, the former employing dyed moose or reindeer hair, the latter dyed porcupine quill. Both rythmically phase between light and dark colors and visually emphasize joints—eg., knees, ankles, thumb, wrist—or skeletal features of the wearer. On the Athapaskan mittens, where only the thumb may move separately, this joint is marked, while on the Even gloves the joints and bones of each finger are traced.

tooing served a decorative or prestigious function, or else served the same purpose as an amulet. Koryak and Chukchi women were tattooed, as were Eskimo women, among whom the most common motif was a series of lines on the chin, which was intended as a fertility charm. These were applied after puberty and marked the passage to womanly status. Other magic lines and motifs were tattooed as a measure against disease. They were inscribed on the painful area as a protective device against the evil spirits responsible for the affliction. As seen in early illustrations, tattoos used to be much more complex and widespread, among both women and men. Nineteenth-century enthnographers reported that this tradition was being lost, along with the wearing of labrets. The meaning of most of the motifs was also forgotten. Other lines were drawn on the body by means of bracelets, arm bands, and breast bands, which encircled the limbs and bodies of the Eskimo and Chukchi and to which beads and other ornaments were sometimes attached. These attachments were considered as amulets, at least among the Chukchi (Bogoras 1904–09:258, 346). Belts represented a major line of demarcation, physically, on the clothing, as well as symbolically, on the person. Eskimo women's caribou teeth belts served as curing amulets (fig. 296), and Chukchi and Eskimo men's belts carried animal tails, ancient harpoons, and other amulets. John Murdoch described (1892:136) such a belt whose edges were dyed in red, as a lifeline would have been. According to Father Ioann Veniaminov (1984:222), the Unalaska Aleut wore "a belt plaited of sinew or grass spoken over [with an incantation] and with mysterious knots . . . on the naked body as certain protective means against death during attacks upon enemies and strong wild animals." Eskimo belts were precious and passed from father to son or from mother to daughter.

In the various regions of the North Pacific, lines were tattooed on people and drawn, beaded, and embroidered on the clothing that wrapped them. These lines, as lifelines, as a sign of passage (from childhood to adulthood), or as protection against spirits, were ornamentally or stylistically more prominent in certain areas, whereas other groups reserved them as a magic or shamanistic rather than artistic motif.

223

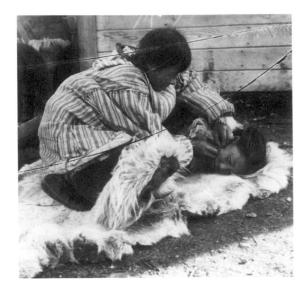

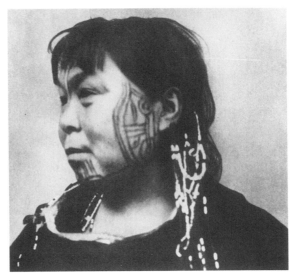

Fringes, Tassels, and Passages

One dimension of clothing that an exhibition or a photograph cannot convey is the effect produced by a garment when it is worn in motion. Moving fringes and tassels accentuated and animated ornamental bands, seams, and hems.

Chilkat blankets were called "fringes around the body" (Emmons 1907). During a potlatch, unworn blankets were displayed flat against a wall, allowing a full view of each complex composition. Others were worn, and, as Bill Holm (1975:152) remarked, their perfect symmetry was therefore broken at the shoulders, and the message of the design lost. During the dances, however, the long and heavy fringes gave life to the blanket. Holm commented that "the constant flow of movement, broken at rhythmic intervals by rather sudden . . . changes of motion-direction characterizes both the dance and art of the Northwest Coast" (1965:92–93). This suggests that the movements of both dance and art were, in the Northwest Coast context, metaphors for spiritual transformation (Carpenter 1973:284). The metamorphosis represented in the fringed blankets was thus more abstract than the animal personification or transformation symbolized in the Chukchi *khonba* or in the Eskimo "tusked" parka, for example, and it was, among the Tlingit, enacted during rituals only.

Similarly, the fine goat-hair fringes on Aleut gutskin parkas or the fur tassels on South Alaskan and Bering Sea Eskimo parkas might have served both visually and symbolically as a dynamic element of clothing. Clothing served as a protective yet spiritually permeable interface be-

tween a person and the world, in which the seams played an important role. Fringes and tassels, inserted in the seams, were conduits through which magic could operate: ermine tails or puffin and auklet beaks, for example, were often parts of the fringe work, as colorful ornaments and as amulets (figs. 268 and 290). In this sense, fringes were reminiscent of the attachments found around the lifelines that encircled masks, bowls, and many other objects.

In Siberia, where the color red symbolized life, red tassels of dyed seal pup skin were common ornaments. These were traded, first as skin from the maritime groups to the Even, then as red tassels from the Even, who were excellent dyers, back to the Chukchi and Koryak. They were sewn onto dancing garments (fig. 293), onto shamanistic garments and hats (figs. 332 and 333), and onto Chukchi sealskin "wrestler's trousers" as a mark of bravery and fierce temperament (Bogoras 1904–09:237). The same type of tassel was attached to armor, together with an anthropomorphic (helper-spirit) figure (fig. 302). Other fringes, tassels, and bead strings were sewn onto clothing to produce movement and beauty (fig. 97). They also added an audible component to shamanistic performances.

North Pacific clothing invites those who have the chance to view it to be attentive to the subtle dancing magic that seamstresses imprisoned in their seams.

Jewelry from the North Pacific region was made of ivory, metal, and trade beads. Examples include the small representative carvings of

296. Caribou Teeth Belt

Bering Sea Eskimo: MNMH 358255

Hunters removed the lower front teeth of the caribou they killed, which were used to decorate women's belts. The hundreds of caribou represented by the teeth on this belt, along with the lavish use of very old blue Chinese trade beads, indicated the prosperity of the wearer and her family. Flagellation with caribou teeth belts was a curing method.

297. Tattoos of Womanhood

(Left) Asiatic Eskimo, AMNH neg. 22323, Jesup Expedition. (Right) St. Lawrence Island, UM neg. 723725, Charles Hughes, 1954–55

Eskimo tattooing of the chin, nose, cheeks, legs, and arms was performed at puberty, and an ability to stoically endure the pain of the procedure was proof of a woman's readiness to bear children. The chin marks were a charm for fertility, but no explicit meanings were known for the elaborate and varied cheek patterns of the Asiatic Eskimo, beyond their esthetic value.

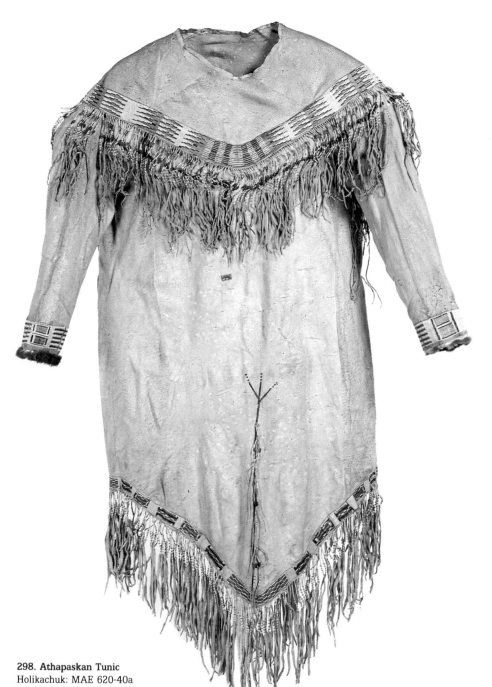

298. Athapaskan Tunic
Holikachuk: MAE 620-40a

This man's shirt in soft, tanned caribou or moose skin is ornamented with porcupine quill band designs, fringes of skin strips decorated with quills, and beaver fur cuffs. Painted red lines extending up front and back end in Raven footlike symbols. This old and beautiful example of Athapaskan quillwork was collected on the upper Innoko River, Alaska, by Voznesenskii in the 1840s.

Eskimo jewelry and ornaments (fig. 263), decorative geometric bands (fig. 324), fringes (fig. 299), and red tassels (fig. 325). Jewelry therefore paralleled design styles seen in clothing and may have served similar symbolic functions.

Both men and women wore jewelry, although the styles were not necessarily identical. Bogoras (1904–09:259) noted that many Chukchi men wore women's earrings, generally by the order of a shaman. By direction of the shaman, Chukchi men also wore women's-style boots on occasion. This transvestism was a ploy to hide and protect the person from evil spirits, in the same way that sick people had their faces blackened so that the evil spirit would not recognize them as human (Serov, p. 245 this volume). Transvestism in the shaman's garments represented his or her position between the male and female worlds. The shaman's position between the human and the spiritual worlds was symbolized by the use of contrasting colors: black and red, or dark and light (fig. 334). The passage between gender identities and other passages throughout the lives and deaths of Siberian people were marked

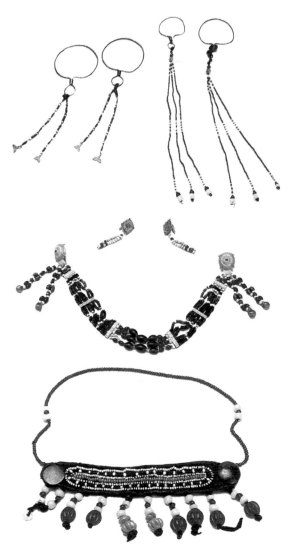

299. Koryak and Eskimo Ornaments
(Top left, pair) Koryak: AMNH 70-3753a,b. (Top right, pair) Koryak: AMNH 70-3216a,b. (Center, pair) Bearing Sea Eskimo: NMNH 127473. (Center) Nunivak Island Eskimo: NMNH 340332. (Bottom) Koryak: AMNH 70-3590

Earrings and necklaces framed the face in bright colors and motion. Koryak copper wire ear ornaments (*top*) are hung with long dangling strands of beads, ending in brass whaletails and large beads. Very little metal was used in Alaskan jewelry (*center*), but delicate ivory elements were often used to accent the deep colors of glass beads. Chinese "vase-melon" beads hang from a Koryak hair band (*bottom*).

on clothing with the same care that the Alaskan Eskimo represented the transformational relationship with the animal world (fig. 341).

Clothing was an interface between each person and the surrounding world. It both imbued the wearer with power and identity and protected him or her from evil spirits. Iconographic motifs, colors, and ornaments were added to clothing to serve these functions. The material and the cut of the clothing, as this essay has tried to emphasize, also conveyed cosmological meanings.

In northern Alaska, the Eskimo parka was a representational three-dimensional piece of art adapted to the human body and was charged with the meaning contained in the various pieces of fur and in its symbolic cut. A man-walrus, man-reindeer, or man-bear would illustrate, as would a visual pun on an Eskimo carving, the transformational quality of the inhabitants of the world.

Animal parts and fur were used as amulets by Tlingit shamans. However, the representation of crest animals on blankets was a sign of secular status, rather than of the relationship between people and animal spirits. It was the movement of the fringes of the Chilkat blanket or the shimmering of the lines of mother-of-pearl buttons on button blankets that served as a metaphor for metamorphosis.

Linear beadwork or quillwork, tattooed lines, belts, fringes, and bracelets among other groups marked not only the physical and spiritual limits of the body but also openings and passages that were conduits for communication and transformation.

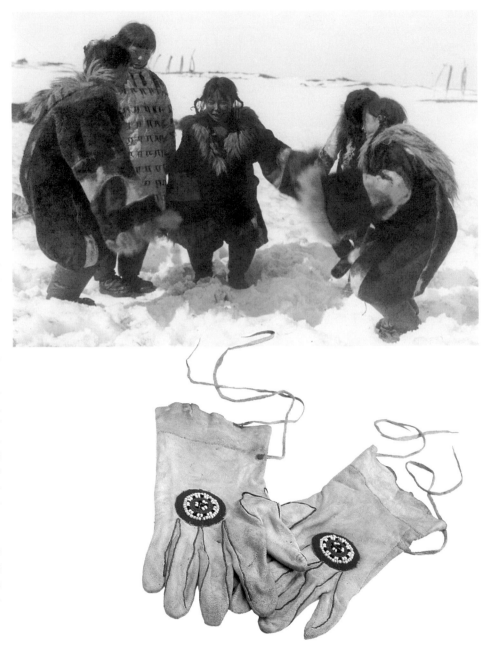

300. Dress Gloves
Even: AMNH 70-5601g,h

Even women were highly skilled at tanning and sewing reindeer skin, as seen in these soft, supple gloves with accented seams. Trade bead medallions decorate the backs of the gloves.

301. Girls Dancing
AMNH neg. 1344, Jesup Exp.

These Maritime Chukchi girls dancing for fun in the snow wear reindeer fur combination suits with their typical long, wide sleeves and open necks with fur ruffs. One girl at left wears a fancy gutskin parka, probably made by St. Lawrence Island Eskimos (cf fig. 292). In the background are whale rib tent frames.

War and Trade

Ernest S. Burch, Jr.

Similar cultural developments on both sides of Bering Strait suggest that people have been moving back and forth across it for thousands of years. Indeed, human migration and inter-action between Chukotka and Alaska probably have been more or less continuous ever since the strait was most recently formed, some 14,000 years ago. Unfortunately, the specific nature of human relations across Bering Strait remains obscure until very recent times.

The first recorded reference to intercontinental relations did not come until the mid-17th century. Semeon Dezhnev, sailing eastward from the mouth of the Kolyma River, passed south through the strait and eventually ended up at the Anadyr River. He reported that on two islands located to the east of the easternmost tip of Asia, lived the ''Tooth People.'' They were called that because they wore ''tooth ornaments made of ivory which protrude through holes which they pierce through their lips'' (Dmytryshyn et al. 1985:332). Although Dezhnev characterized the Tooth People as Chukchi, their use of labrets indicates clearly that they were Alaskan Eskimo; the islands must have been the Big and Little Diomede islands, which are located in the middle of Bering Strait.

Information about contacts across Bering Strait remained spotty for a long time after Dezhnev's voyage. We are fortunate that the North Alaskans wore labrets, for it is only through occasional rumors about the Tooth People passed on by Chukchi to Russians on the Kolyma River that we know that some kind of intercontinental relations must have been taking place. But we really know nothing substantive about those relations until the end of the 18th century, when a series of Russian (and later English) exploring expeditions began to visit the region.

Our information for the 19th and 20th centuries is reasonably good, although naturally less complete than one would like. For this period, trade and warfare were really the only two kinds of relations that took place to any significant extent across Bering Strait. In this paper I attempt to summarize what was involved in these activities over the past 200 years.

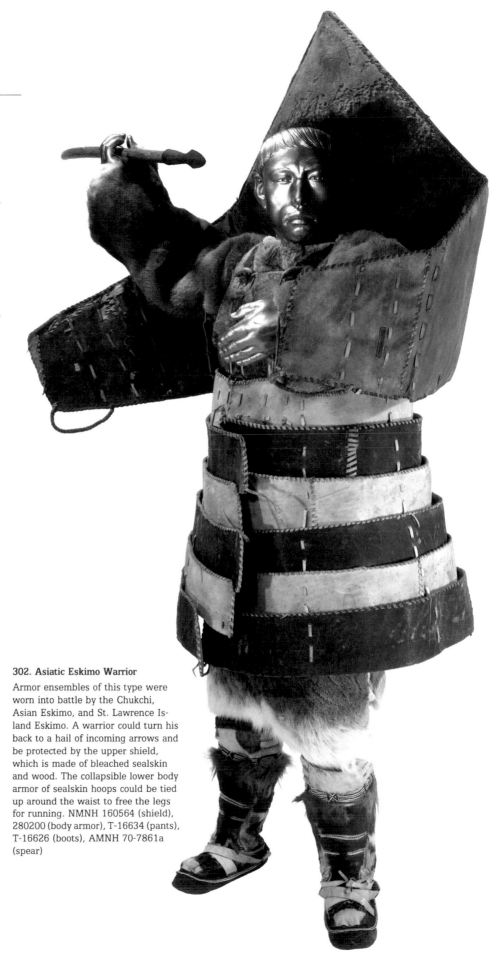

302. Asiatic Eskimo Warrior

Armor ensembles of this type were worn into battle by the Chukchi, Asian Eskimo, and St. Lawrence Island Eskimo. A warrior could turn his back to a hail of incoming arrows and be protected by the upper shield, which is made of bleached sealskin and wood. The collapsible lower body armor of sealskin hoops could be tied up around the waist to free the legs for running. NMNH 160564 (shield), 280200 (body armor), T-16634 (pants), T-16626 (boots), AMNH 70-7861a (spear)

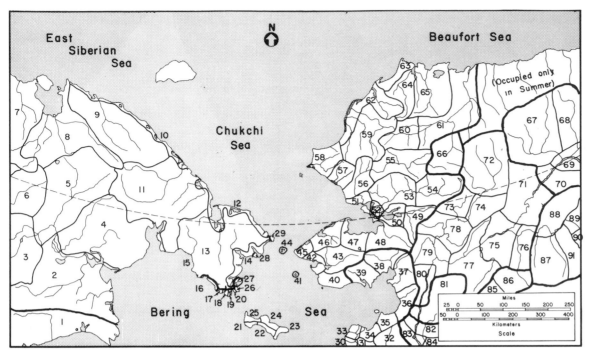

303. Provisional Political Map of the Bering Strait Region (ca. 1800–1825)

The thin lines indicate boundaries between native societies (or nations); the heavy lines delineate major language boundaries.

TABLE 3

Provisional List of Nations in Northern Beringia, Ca. 1800–1825

Koryak Area
1. Kerek

Chukchi Area
2. Viluneilet
3. Taelkapelet
4. Unmelet
5. Kuuluusilet
6. Ettelet
7. Dry Anyuy
8. Saalet
9. Petiymel
10. Errilet
11. Umvaamelet
12. Kuulukelet
13. Chukchi Peninsula
14. Bering Strait Coast
15. Aivalet

Sirenikskii Yupik Area
16. Sirinegmiut

Chaplinskii Yupik Area
17. Imtugmiit
18. Avatmiit
19. Qiighwaaghmiit
20. Tashighmiit
21. Pauvuilagmiit
22. Sikuuvugmiit
23. Kialigagmiit
24. Kukuligmiit
25. Sivugarmiit
26. Uŋazighmiit
27. Napakutaghmiit

Naukanskii Yupik Area
28. Nunatmiit
29. Nuvuqaghmiit

Central Alaskan Yupik Area
30. Kuigluarmiut
31. Kuigpagmiut
32. Iqurmiut
33. Qaerauranermiut
34. Pastulirmiut
35. Taprarmiut
36. Unalirmiut
37. Caxtulirmiut
38. Kuuyugmiut [?]
39. Kaɬuarmiut [?]

North Alaskan Inuit Area
40. Ayaasariarmiut
41. Ukiuvuŋmiut
42. Sinrarmiut
43. Qaviazarmiut
44. Imaqɬiit
45. Kiŋikmiut
46. Tapqarmiut
47. Pittarmiut
48. Kaŋigmiut
49. Siilvium Kaŋianigmiut
50. Kiitaarmiut
51. Qikiqtarzuŋmiut
52. Kuuŋmiut
53. Akunirmiut
54. Kuuvaum Kaŋianirmiut
55. Nuatarmiut
56. Napaaqturmiut
57. Kivalliñirmiut
58. Tikirarmiut
59. Utuqqarmiut
60. Kaŋianirmiut
61. Kuukpigmiut
62. Silaliñirmiut
63. Kakligmiut

64. Kuulugzuarmiut
65. Ikpikpaŋmiut

Kutchin Area
66. Diʔ hai Gwičin
67. Neečit Gwičin
68. Van Tat Gwičin
69. Gwičyaa Gwičin
70. Tsətet'aičin

Koyukon Area
71. Stevens Village-Tanana
72. Nikhto Hot'ana
73. Hogatza
74. Qunutna Xotanə
75. Tanana-Nowitna
76. Kantishna
77. Nogi Xotanə
78. Huslia-Dalbi
79. Kodilqaq Xotanə
80. Yudoʔ Xotanə

Holikachuk Area
81. Holikachuk

Deg Hit'an Area
82. Anvik
83. Bonasilla
84. Georgetown

Kolchan Area
85. East Fork
86. Telida-Minchumina

Tanana Area
87. Nenana-Toklat
88. Minto
89. Chena
90. Salcha
91. Wood River

When we first come to know about the region, both Alaska and Chukotka were inhabited by several different cultural groups. On Chukotka these were the Chukchi and the Sirenikski, Chaplinski, and Naukanski Yupik Eskimo. In western and central Alaska, they were the North Alaskan Inupiat and the Central Alaskan Yupik Eskimo, and the Kutchin and Koyukon Athapaskan Indians. Each of these large entities was subdivided into linguistic subgroups of various kinds, but the only ones relevant to the present discussion are what Dorothy Jean Ray (1967) has termed tribes and which I have called societies (Burch 1984).

Informants of mine who were born in the early 1880s, while these societies were still operating in northern Alaska, referred to them in English as "nations." I adopt that term here to make the point that they performed the same basic functions for their members that modern nation-states do for us today. These functions were of course performed in very different ways, because these societies were both tiny (a few hundred to perhaps two thousand people) and organized along different lines than modern nations are. All of them were segmental, in that they comprised a number of families and clans, but completely lacking in any government or other type of organization with a nationwide span of control. Nevertheless, the citizens of each one perceived of themselves as being ideologically, politically, and territorially distinct from their neighbors and were willing to fight to maintain that status.

A map of the nations occupying northern Beringia ca. A.D. 1800–1825 is presented in figure 303. The map is keyed to Table 3, which lists each nation by its native name, if known, and by a descriptive label, if not. This map is highly speculative and is presented as a first approximation rather than as a fully documented set of conclusions. The details have been most fully worked out for the North Alaskan Inupiat area (Burch 1980; Ray 1975) and least adequately resolved for the Chukotka coast. Hopefully, further research will permit the substantial refinement that this map and list require to be considered truly accurate. However, for the present purposes precise accuracy is not necessary; the map does present an accurate model of what the real situation evidently was like at the time, even if many of the details may be wrong.

The importance of these traditional nations to the present discussion inheres in the fact that war and trade took place between them and not between the more general cultural groups, such as the Chukchi and the North Alaskan Inupiat, as the general literature would suggest. There was at least as much fighting going on between nations *within* the North Alaskan Inupiat realm, for example, as there was between North Alaskan Inupiat nations and, say, Koyukon or Kutchin nations (Burch and Correll 1972).

304. Athapaskan Indian Weaponry
Prob. Kutchin: NMNH 2024. Ahtna: MAE 2667-14

Long knives with flaring, voluted handles were used for both hunting and fighting. They were originally made from copper obtained through the native trade system; later examples like this one collected in the 1860s are made of trade steel. Lashed to wooden poles, they were used by especially daring hunters to kill bears. Heavy caribou antler clubs were carried by Ahtna warriors for hand-to-hand combat. This highly ornamented example has a hide-wrapped, fringed handle, ornamented with beads and hair embroidery. Red ocher has been rubbed into the patterns engraved on the club.

War

As the Bering Strait region emerged from the mists of prehistory in the 18th century, hostility seems to have prevailed over trade as the dominant theme of international affairs. This was true both within and between language areas. The Chukchi and Eskimo in particular were aggressive people by disposition and effective as fighters. Their men constantly prepared for combat through vigorous physical exercise, weaponry training and drill, and prac-

tice in dodging missiles. It is not surprising that the peoples of Chukotka were the only native people in all of the empire who were not subjected by the Russians by force of arms. The Russians tried to defeat them during the 18th century but abandoned the effort in 1774.

Warfare could begin for a number of reasons, such as revenge for past grudges, intrusion into one another's territory, and murder. In such small nations personal animosities and the family and clan loyalties of ordinary people had a significant impact on international affairs. Since these peoples had been in contact with one another for centuries, there was always a backlog of unavenged offenses to help turn a seemingly trivial incident into a *casus belli*.

Since there were no governments or positions of national leadership in these tiny countries, the first problem was to muster an attacking force. If an offense was serious enough, this was an easy matter because many men would vol-

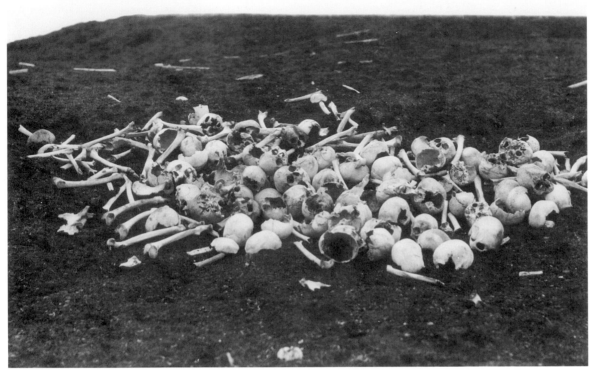

305. "Battlefield Near Point Barrow"
Neg. 120809, National Museum of Denmark. Leo Hansen, 1924
A pile of broken skulls and bones marks an old Eskimo battlefield on the tundra of northern Alaska, photographed by the Danish Fifth Thule Expedition (Rasmussen 1927).

unteer. If it was not so severe, the incident might simply be added to the growing fund of grievances and left for future action. To be effective, a military force had to number at least several dozen men. In extreme cases all of the healthy adult men in the entire country could be involved. Another possibility was to form an alliance with people in other nations and combine forces for a major attack on an especially troublesome country. In one such case in Alaska the members of three or four nations formed an alliance against the Tikirarmiut nation, of Point Hope. They defeated the Point Hopers in open battle, killing perhaps as many as 200 men in the process (Burch 1981:14). The Chukchi and the Asiatic Eskimo no doubt formed similar alliances to deal with the Russians.

Weapons consisted of bows and arrows, lances and knives. Other accoutrements of war in Alaska were slat armor made from pieces of bone or ivory and protective vests made of furs (Nelson 1899:Pl. XCII). On Chukotka both Eskimo and Chukchi warriors sometimes wore heavy protective body armor and cuirasses (VanStone

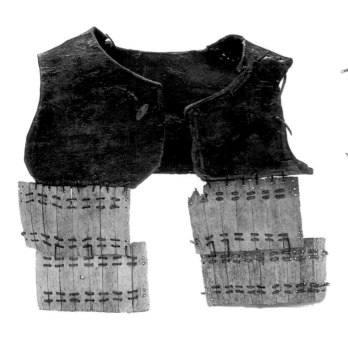

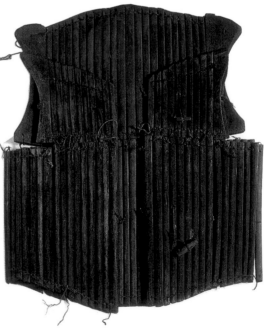

306. Plate and Rod Armor
North Alaskan Eskimo: NMNH T-1886. Aleut: NMNH 17249
Armor made with overlapping rows of small plates was in use all the way from Japan to Bering Strait. As far north as Koryak territory the plates were made of iron, replaced by bone and ivory plates among the Chukchi and Eskimo. This Eskimo example from Bering Strait (*left*) has bone plates and an upper section of thick hide. The rod armor (*right*), from a prehistoric Aleutian Island burial cave, is the only complete example of Aleut armor in existence. Its cedar rods are lashed together with finely plaited sinew cord.

230

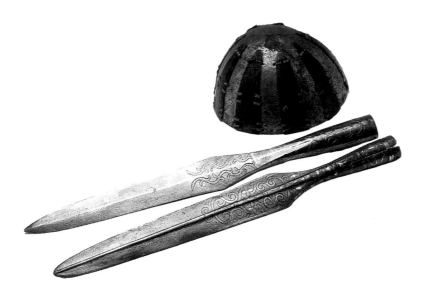

Alaskan Eskimos also knew how to form and maneuver battle lines in an open confrontation. They understood interval spacing, the principle of mass, and the importance of terrain and wind conditions. Open battle began with a firefight with bows and arrows and eventually proceeded to shock encounters with spears, clubs, and knives. Apparently the Koyukon and Athapaskan Indians used the same tactics, since accounts of Eskimo-Indian wars recounted by Eskimos indicate that both sides were operating by the same basic procedures. The Chukchi, presumably, were at least as skillful in such matters.

In Alaska the sole objective of war seems to have been to kill the enemy: men, women, and children. However, attackers deliberately tried to let one person escape to spread the word to compatriots never to offend the attacking nation again. Women were sometimes taken prisoner, but usually this was for only a brief period; eventually they were tortured—often horribly—before being put to death. Warriors on the Asiatic side seem to have been more interested in keeping women captives as slaves.

At least some hostilities occurred across Bering Strait and also between people living on the Asiatic mainland and St. Lawrence Island. In one instance, a party of Naukan and Uelen people raided the former village of Kauwerak, on the Seward Peninsula. In another, a party of Siberians was annihilated on the Alaskan shore of the Chukchi Sea a short distance north of Cape Krusenstern; the event is memorialized in the name of a nearby lagoon, Kotlik Lagoon, which is based on the generic Alaskan Inupiaq term for a Siberian, namely, "qutliq." On the other

307. The Art of the Armorer
Koryak: AMNH 70-3822 (helmet).
Koryak: MAE 956-92. Nivkhi: MAE 202-102 (spear points)

The forging and inlaying of iron was an art that spread to the Koryak perhaps via the Evenk but ultimately from the Chinese or Japanese. Koryak iron weapons and armor reflect these southern influences. The shape and decorative patterns of the Koryak spearpoint (*upper*) imitate the more elaborate Nivkhi example (*lower*) from near the Chinese border.

1983). People maintained themselves on the alert and in constant readiness to repel attack, and virtually all of the early explorers commented on the "good order" in which weapons were kept.

The tactics of native war have been described in detail only for Alaskan Eskimo (Burch 1974). The favored procedure was to mount a sneak nighttime attack on an enemy village, either catching the inhabitants asleep or else all gathered together in the community hall for a festival. If the defenders got trapped inside the hall they might be doomed. However, men were always armed, and many community halls had secret escape tunnels for just such an eventuality. Even successfully launched sneak attacks could sometimes be repulsed.

308. Tlingit Armor
MAE 2454-8 (left); NMNH 60241 (right)

For body protection the Tlingit wore slat armor, hide armor, or both in combination. The slat armor cuirass (*left*) is made of tough hardwood slats wrapped with hundreds of feet of two-ply sinew cord. Sections are joined with heavy skin laces and panels, and the overall shape was carefully fitted to the torso to protect vital organs. The painted hide armor tunic (*right*) is ornamented with carved bone "sharks' teeth" and Chinese coins. Chinese coins were widely traded on the Northwest Coast, not surprising given that the traders' principal market for their furs was China.

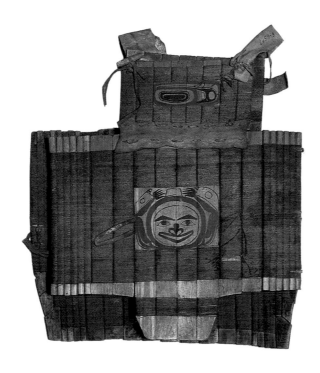

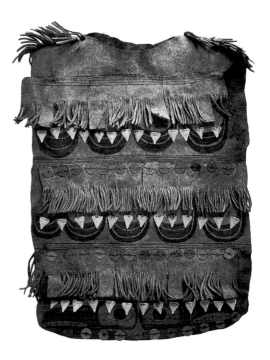

231

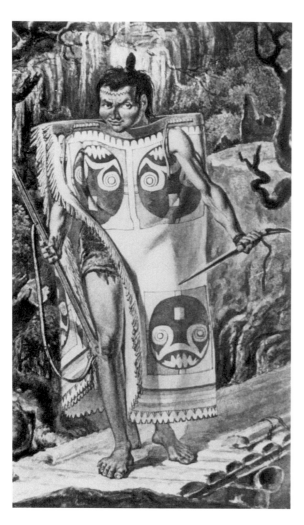

side of the strait the members of the Billings Expedition in 1791 were offered access to some captive women who had been taken in some kind of an encounter with Alaskans (Sauer 1802:252) Unfortunately, almost nothing is known about the details or the extent of warfare between the peoples of Chukotka and Alaska.

The same general pattern of warfare that existed in the Bering Strait area extended for a considerable distance southward around the North Pacific Rim along both its eastern and western margins. Warfare was clearly a widespread phenomenon among the peoples of this part of the world during the late prehistoric–early historic period. In general, both the objectives of war and the means of making it were pretty much the same everywhere, although, the farther south one got, the more important booty and the capture and enslavement of enemies became as strategic goals. In all areas, the incidence of warfare declined as a result of depopulation following the introduction of European epidemic diseases (and the often attendant famines), the breakdown of traditional native political boundaries, and the self-conscious interference by Europeans in native affairs. By the end of the 19th century—several decades earlier toward the south—warfare had essentially ceased as a dominant theme of interregional relations among different native groups.

309. "A Kolosh Warrior from Baranov Island"
Mikhail Tikhanov, 1818, RIPSA 2114

The warrior is wearing painted hide armor and carrying a dagger and flintlock rifle.

310. Tlingit Helmets and Visor
Clockwise from upper left: NMNH 168157, MAE 571-17, MAE 2454-17 (helmets); MAE 5795-9 (visor)

Battles were transformed by the fantastic helmets worn atop the heads of Tlingit fighters into clashes of towering supernatural beings. The helmet on the upper left is a scowling warrior's face, once bristling with bear fur whiskers and thick shocks of human hair. His pierced hands stretch across the front rim of the helmet, joined to a stylized body painted over the back. To the right is a black-faced helmet with abalone shell eyes and teeth, similar to the spirit faces portrayed on shamans' masks. The bottom helmet is probably a bear in part human form, with both bear's and man's ears, although a tail or finlike flap of painted leather on the back of the helmet suggests another creature may have been intended. A visor (*bottom left*) was worn below a helmet and covered the warrior's face to the level of his eyes; shallow notches in the upper edge allowed fuller vision. It was held in place by biting a loop of heavy spruce-root pegged to the inside. Ornamented battle helmets, some with animal crests, were also worn by early Japanese and Chinese warriors.

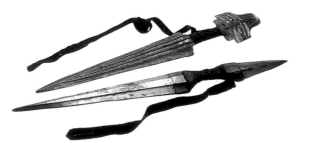

311. Tlingit Daggers
NMNH 221184 (top); 9288 (bottom)

The sculptured pommel of the upper weapon is a split profile image of a sea-grizzly, inlaid with abalone shell. The double-bladed lower dagger could be thrust both up and down without regripping, making it especially deadly in close combat.

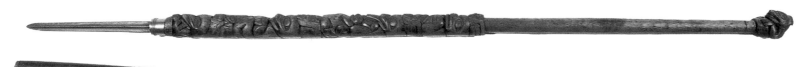

312. Spear
Tlingit: NMNH 75419

Carved like a totem pole with interlocked crest and mythical figures, this spear also served as a ceremonial staff.

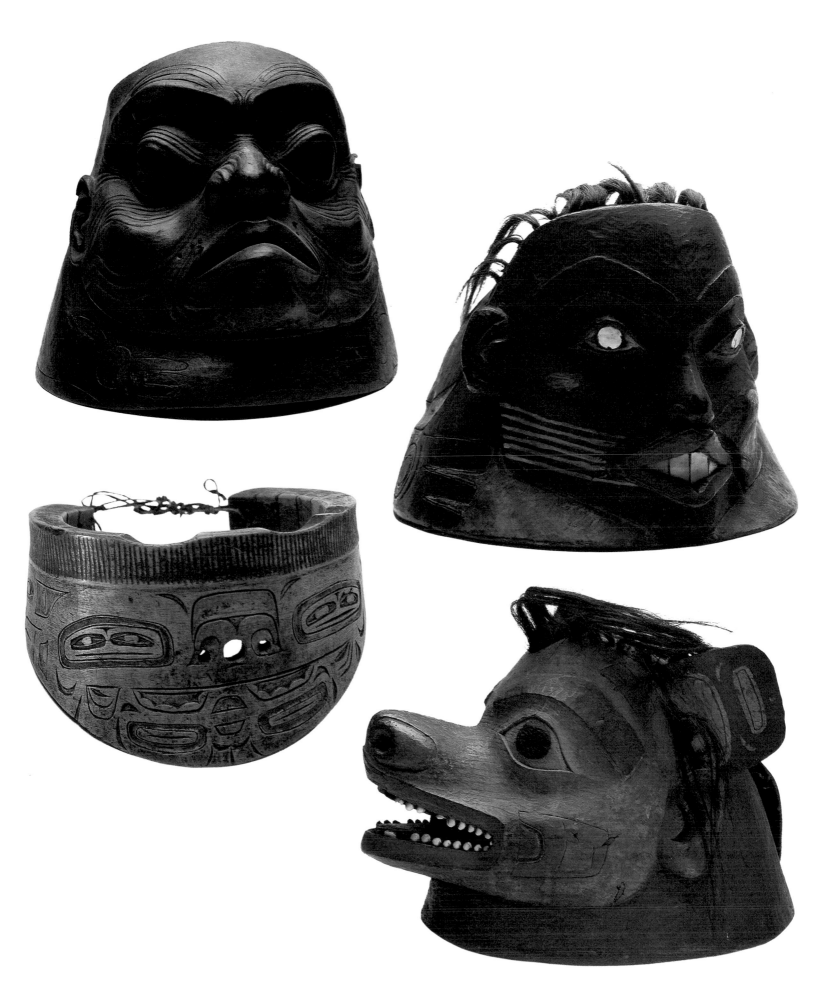

233

Trade

The origins of international trade in the Bering Strait region are lost in the distant past. We may suppose that it went on to at least a limited extent for centuries prior to the period of particular interest here, but there simply is no information about it. What evidence does exist suggests that in the 17th and 18th centuries, hostility must have been the dominant theme in international affairs, but in subsequent decades it was eclipsed in importance by trade.

The first step in setting up trade relations between two nations within the general Bering Strait area was to show that the individuals involved had peaceful rather than hostile intentions. This was accomplished through an open approach by the representatives of one nation to those of another, ideally on neutral ground, otherwise at some distance from a settlement. As the two groups of strangers converged, but while still at a distance, various signals were given—waving empty hands, conspicuously setting aside weapons, holding aloft furs or other goods—all to suggest that trade, not war, was what the visitors had in mind. The presence of women in the visiting party also was a sign of peaceful intentions. For example, when the Beechey Expedition approached St. Lawrence Island for the first time in July of 1826,

the natives . . . launched four baidars [open boats], of which each contained eight persons, males and females. They paddled towards the ship with great quickness, until they were within speaking distance, when an old man who steered the foremost boat stood erect and held up in succession nets, walrus teeth, skin shirts, harpoons, bows and arrows, and small birds; he then extended his arms, rubbed and patted his breast, and came fearlessly alongside (Beechey 1831,I:331).

The second step was probably what has come to be known as silent trade. As demonstrated to Otto von Kotzebue by a North Alaska Inupiat, the process was as follows:

The stranger first comes, and lays some goods on the shore, and then retires; the American [Inupiat] comes, looks at the things, puts as many skins near them as he thinks proper to give, and then also goes away. Upon this the stranger approaches, and examines what is offered him; if he is satisfied with it, he takes the skins, and leaves his goods instead; but if not, then he lets all the things lie, retires a second time, and expects an addition from the buyer. In this manner the dealing seems to me to continue without speaking, and there is no doubt but the Tschukutskoi [Chukchi] obtain here the skins for the Russian trade (Kotzebue 1821,I:228).

A similar pattern of trade was also used by unacquainted Koyukon Indians and North Alaskan Inupiat (Anderson 1974–75:68). No doubt,

especially in the beginning, such transactions must have been undertaken in an atmosphere of considerable tension, since the common pattern was to attack and try to kill total strangers if they were inferior in numbers or weaponry, or to flee from them otherwise.

Silent trade was also used between unfriendly nations in Chukotka. However, they had also developed a pattern of closer, if no less hostile contact.

In very ancient times there was a kind of fair in [Naukan] or in [Uelen] which was held outside of the village, on the flat seashore, for fear of hostilities. . . . The people came to trade fully armed, and offered their wares to each other on their spearpoints; or else they would hold a bundle of skins with one hand, and with the other a bared knife, in readiness to raise a fight upon the slightest provocation (Bogoras 1904–09:53).

Between at least some nations, however, trade—or some other kind of positive relations—must have been established early enough for fairly effective international and interlinguistic communication to have developed by the late 18th century. For example, in 1791, the men of the Billings Expedition met at Cape Rodney, on the Seward Peninsula, North Alaskan Inupiat who understood the ''Chukchi'' language—it actually may have been Naukanski Yupik (Merck 1980:186; Sauer 1802:245). Also of interest is the fact that Chukchi or Yupik-speaking people on Chukotka knew the Inupiat names for many places on the Alaskan coast, both at the time of the Billings Expedition and earlier. By the second half of the 19th century, at least the leading native traders in many areas probably were bilingual or multilingual, and in areas such as the Chukotka coast, where Chukchis and Yupik Eskimos were in close contact, virtually the entire population of some villages may have been bilingual (Menovshchikov 1964:836).

A major event in the development of intercontinental trade in the Bering Strait region was the establishment in 1789 of an annual market at the juncture of the Aniui and Kolyma rivers, some 800 miles west of Bering Strait. The Aniui fair vastly increased the supply of European goods available to the Chukchis, at the same time creating an enormous demand for furs that the Chukchi alone could not satisfy. To meet this demand, they expanded their contacts with people in Alaska, and a complex intercontinental trade network quickly developed.

During the first half of the 19th century, trade between Chukotka and Alaska probably reached a peak, with the Chukchi acting as middlemen

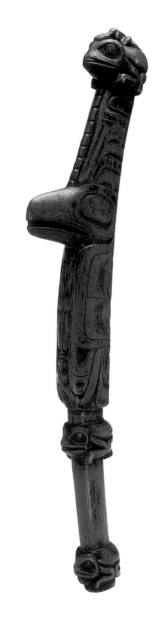

313. War Club
Tsimshian?: NMNH 20610
Few weapons rival the elegance of this fine wooden club, with the raven's beak for a striking point. The form was probably derived from the antler club of the Athapaskans (fig. 304). Two frogs crouch flanking the grip and another, topped with a reclining human figure, caps the club. Between his folded wings, the raven grasps another, inverted human. Abalone shell once glittered in the wing feathers. Such clubs were once true weapons, and later were used as emblems of chiefly rank. It is said they were sometimes used to kill slaves on ceremonial occasions.

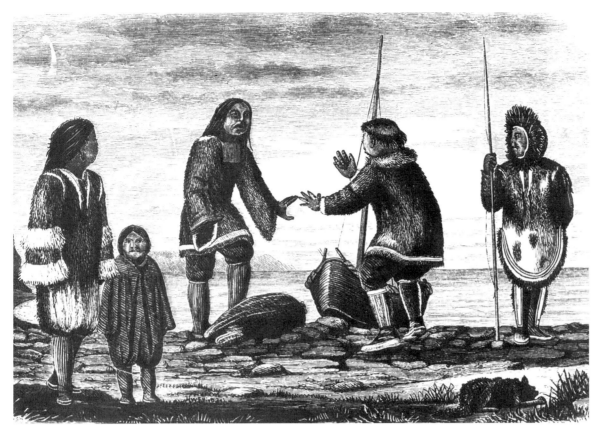

between the Alaskans, on the one hand, and the Russians, on the other. The primary nodes of the trade network at the beginning of the century consisted of several native fairs in Alaska and a number of government-organized winter Russian-native fairs in Asia. The locations of these fairs are shown in figure 316. In the early years the goods that entered this system from the Russian end were glass beads, iron, metal buttons, articles of adornment, needles, pots, kettles, knives, spears, bells, scissors, and axes; tobacco, a minor item in the early years, had become perhaps the single most important one by 1810. In return, the Russians received furs: marten, beaver, red fox, white fox, muskrat, river otter, lynx, and wolverine. Other trade items received by the Russians were walrus tusks, baleen (whalebone), seal and walrus skins, bearskins, and a miscellaneous assortment of manufactured goods. Strictly native elements in the intercontinental trade were domesticated Chukchi reindeer skins, for which there was a growing demand in Alaska, and wood (for bows, arrows, and other objects), which was in short supply on Chukotka. Also involved in the primarily native trade was a diverse array of manufactured goods, such as articles of clothing, figurines, bowls, masks, and pipes, of which a sample is illustrated on these pages. These items traveled both east and west and depended more on the fancy of individual buyers than on a

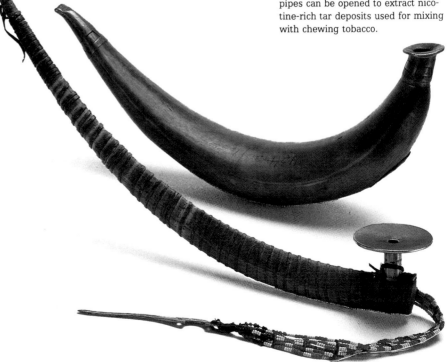

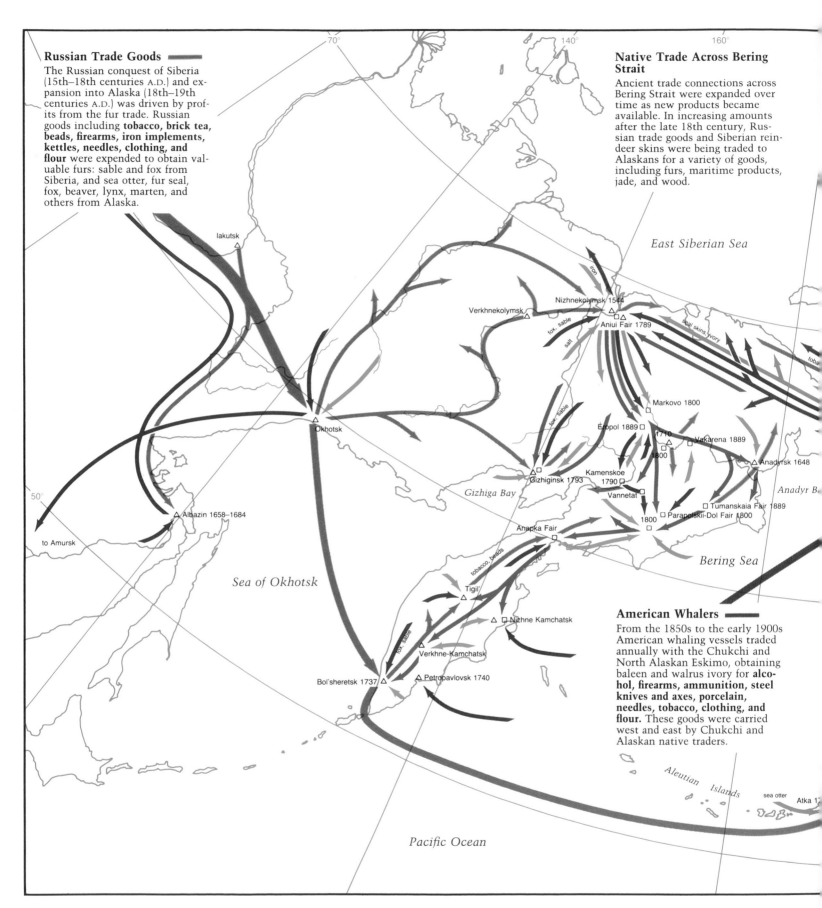

Russian Trade Goods ━━━━

The Russian conquest of Siberia (15th–18th centuries A.D.) and expansion into Alaska (18th–19th centuries A.D.) was driven by profits from the fur trade. Russian goods including **tobacco, brick tea, beads, firearms, iron implements, kettles, needles, clothing, and flour** were expended to obtain valuable furs: sable and fox from Siberia, and sea otter, fur seal, fox, beaver, lynx, marten, and others from Alaska.

Native Trade Across Bering Strait

Ancient trade connections across Bering Strait were expanded over time as new products became available. In increasing amounts after the late 18th century, Russian trade goods and Siberian reindeer skins were being traded to Alaskans for a variety of goods, including furs, maritime products, jade, and wood.

East Siberian Sea

Iakutsk

Verkhnekolymsk

Nizhnekolymsk 1544

Aniui Fair 1789

fox, sable

salt

Seal skins, ivory

iron

Okhotsk

Markovo 1800

fox, sable

Eropol 1889

1710

Vakarena 1889

1800

Anadyrsk 1648

Anadyr B

to Amursk

Albazin 1658–1684

Gizhiginsk 1793

Kamenskoe 1790

Vannetat

1800

Parapolskii-Dol Fair 1800

Tumanskaia Fair 1889

Gizhiga Bay

Anapka Fair

tobacco, beads

Bering Sea

Sea of Okhotsk

Tigil'

Nizhne Kamchatsk

American Whalers ━━━━

From the 1850s to the early 1900s American whaling vessels traded annually with the Chukchi and North Alaskan Eskimo, obtaining baleen and walrus ivory for **alcohol, firearms, ammunition, steel knives and axes, porcelain, needles, tobacco, clothing, and flour.** These goods were carried west and east by Chukchi and Alaskan native traders.

fox, sable

Verkhne-Kamchatsk

Bol'sheretsk 1737

Petropavlovsk 1740

Aleutian Islands

sea otter

Atka 1

Pacific Ocean

316. North Pacific Trade Systems (ca. 1775-1900)

Trade fairs and extensive native exchange networks existed long before Russian contact. The colored arrows show generalized movements of native products, with some local specialities highlighted. The dates of Russian posts, sometimes built at the same locations as ancient fairs, trace the expansion of the Russian fur trade across Siberia and southern Alaska. New native fairs sprang up as the volume of trade increased in the 19th century. The movements of Hudson's Bay Company and American whaler goods are also shown. Chinese and Japanese products, including tea, tobacco, pipes, beads, and armor also entered the North Pacific exchange network, primarily via Russian traders but also by way of shipwrecks on American shores and direct Japanese contacts in Kam-

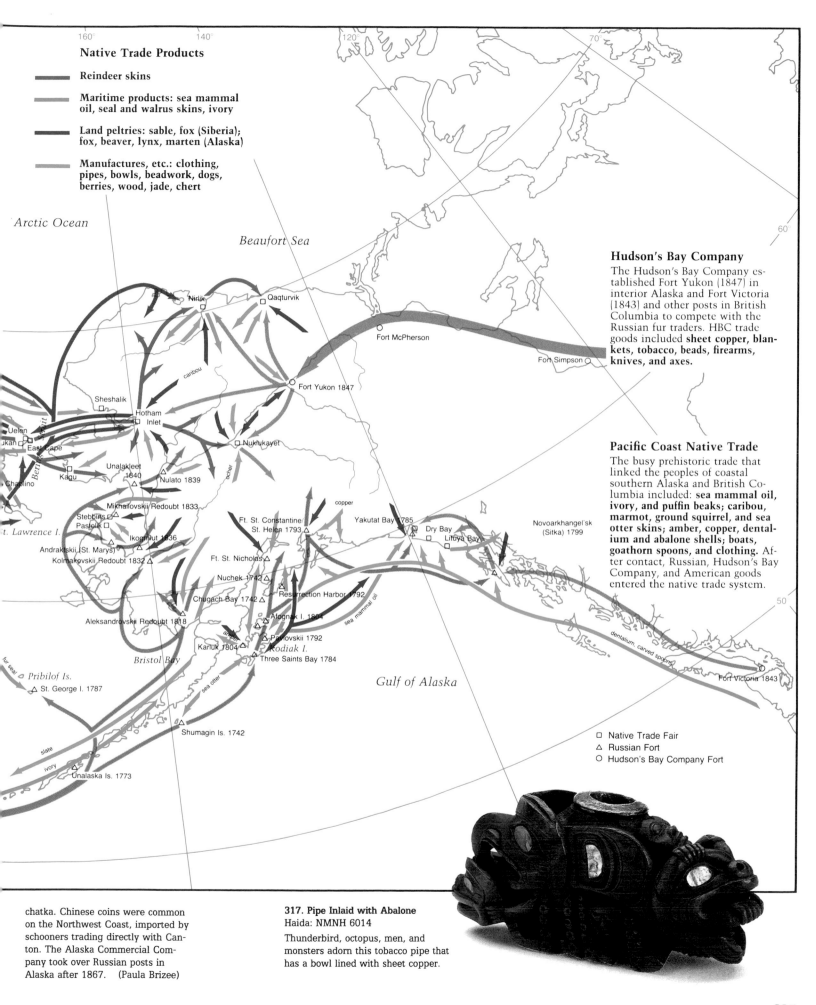

Native Trade Products

— Reindeer skins

— Maritime products: sea mammal oil, seal and walrus skins, ivory

— Land peltries: sable, fox (Siberia); fox, beaver, lynx, marten (Alaska)

— Manufactures, etc.: clothing, pipes, bowls, beadwork, dogs, berries, wood, jade, chert

Arctic Ocean

Beaufort Sea

Nirlik
Qaqturvik
Fort McPherson
Fort Simpson
Fort Yukon 1847
caribou
Sheshalik
Hotham Inlet
Uelen
East Cape
Chaplino
Nuklukayet
Kagu
Unalakleet 1840
Nulato 1839
ocher
copper
Mikhailovskii Redoubt 1833
Ft. St. Constantine
St. Helen 1793
Yakutat Bay 1785
Dry Bay
Lituya Bay
Novoarkhangel'sk (Sitka) 1799
t. Lawrence I.
Stebbins
Pastolik
Ikogmiut 1836
Andraktskii (St. Marys)
Kolmakovskii Redoubt 1832
Ft. St. Nicholas
Nuchek 1742
Resurrection Harbor 1792
Chugach Bay 1742
sea mammal oil
Aleksandrovskii Redoubt 1818
amber
Karluk 1804
Afognak I. 1804
Pavlovskii 1792
Kodiak I.
Three Saints Bay 1784
Bristol Bay
sea otter
Gulf of Alaska
dentalium, carved spoons
Fort Victoria 1843
fur seal
Pribilof Is.
St. George I. 1787
slate
ivory
Unalaska Is. 1773
Shumagin Is. 1742

□ Native Trade Fair
△ Russian Fort
○ Hudson's Bay Company Fort

Hudson's Bay Company

The Hudson's Bay Company established Fort Yukon (1847) in interior Alaska and Fort Victoria (1843) and other posts in British Columbia to compete with the Russian fur traders. HBC trade goods included **sheet copper, blankets, tobacco, beads, firearms, knives, and axes.**

Pacific Coast Native Trade

The busy prehistoric trade that linked the peoples of coastal southern Alaska and British Columbia included: **sea mammal oil, ivory, and puffin beaks; caribou, marmot, ground squirrel, and sea otter skins; amber, copper, dentalium and abalone shells; boats, goathorn spoons, and clothing.** After contact, Russian, Hudson's Bay Company, and American goods entered the native trade system.

chatka. Chinese coins were common on the Northwest Coast, imported by schooners trading directly with Canton. The Alaska Commercial Company took over Russian posts in Alaska after 1867. (Paula Brizee)

317. Pipe Inlaid with Abalone
Haida: NMNH 6014

Thunderbird, octopus, men, and monsters adorn this tobacco pipe that has a bowl lined with sheet copper.

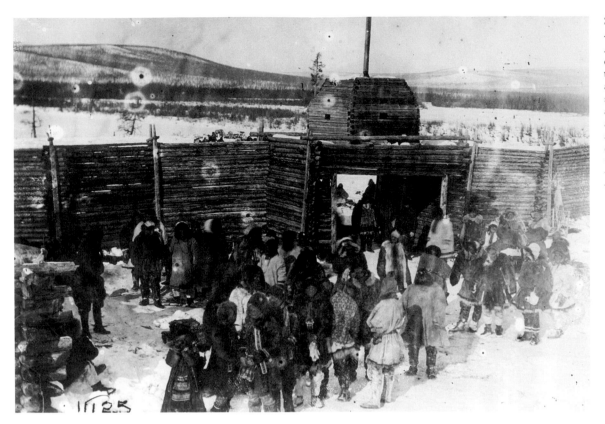

318. Aniui Trade Fair
AMNH neg. 11125, Jesup Exp.

A crowd of Chukchi and Even gathers inside the gate of Fort Aniuisk in the Kolyma River district during the annual spring trade fair. Here Russian traders bartered tobacco, knives, and copper kettles for Siberian fox and reindeer skins and Alaskan furs and ivory obtained by Chukchi traders from the Eskimos at Bering Strait. One *pud* (36 lbs.) of tobacco was worth ten red fox skins or 40 walrus tusks.

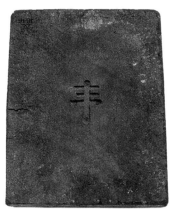

widespread demand for the products concerned.

The major nodes in the trade network were supplemented by a large number of smaller ones. Indeed, for all practical purposes, every Eskimo, Indian, and Chukchi settlement was a trading center, and the normal routes by which people traveled about the country were also trade routes. The region encompassed by the network that contributed directly to the intercontinental trade extended the whole way from the middle Yukon River, in Alaska, to the Kolyma River, in Siberia. This system, in turn, was connected to others that spanned most of northern North America and northern and eastern Eurasia.

The original Bering Strait trade network began to be disrupted in the second decade of the 19th century by European explorers. These men came by ship, which enabled them to bring along a good supply of trade goods and also to carry home a substantial number of furs and native artifacts. They were followed a decade or two later by Russian traders based in southern Alaska, who began to establish permanent posts along the southern margin of the region of present interest in the 1830s. The Hudson's Bay Company, based in London, England, entered the competition in 1847 with a post at Fort Yukon. The locations of these posts are shown in figure 316. Both the explorers and the Alaska-based traders acted to draw the Alaskan trade away from the Chukchi, hence from the Russians.

The system changed again in 1848, when American whalers discovered the rich whaling grounds north of Bering Strait (Bockstoce 1986). The whalers were followed or accompanied by a number of small trading vessels, many of which were based in the Hawaiian Islands and therefore not subject to U.S. or Russian regulations at their home port. While the whalers generally stayed out to sea during the early years, the traders were in frequent contact with natives on both the Asiatic and American coasts. It was primarily through their efforts that firearms and whiskey, in addition to the more traditional trade goods, arrived in native hands. Later on, as whale stocks declined, the whalers turned to taking walrus; when they had nearly exterminated the walrus population, they turned to trading. They also hired natives from both Alaska and Chukotka to work for them, occa-

319. Tea Brick
AMNH 70-3846

Powdered Chinese tea, mixed with sheep or ox blood as a binder and compressed into bricks, was also an important commodity in Russian-Native trade. Tea was consumed in prodigious quantities to ward off the Siberian cold.

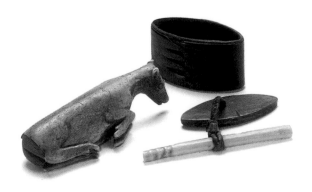

320. Tobacco and Snuff Boxes
North Alaskan Eskimo: NMNH 56512. Bering Sea Eskimo: NMNH 33013

On the left is a beautifully rendered carving in antler of a foetal caribou, which held the owner's precious supply of tobacco or snuff. Snuff taking spread to Alaska along with the rest of the Asian tobacco complex, and many Alaskan snuff boxes are Asian in design like the oval, baleen-covered leather example on the right, from Norton Sound. Its shape and interlaced seam are derived from birchbark snuff boxes made by the Chukchi, Koryak, and other Siberian groups. A birdbone snorting tube is attached to the lid.

321. Koryak Tobacco Paraphernalia

AMNH 70-5123 (pipe); MAE
956-65a,b (box and beaded pouch)

This leather box covered with embossed birchbark and encased in a beaded pouch was used by a Koryak tobacco chewer to safeguard his or her tobacco and half-chewed quids. It has two compartments, each with its own hinged lid. Chewing tobacco was blended with ashes in both Siberia and Alaska. The brass pipe decorated with floral patterns and blue cloissoné is Chinese in origin. The iron pipe cleaners attached with chains are another detail copied on some pipes of native manufacture (fig. 315).

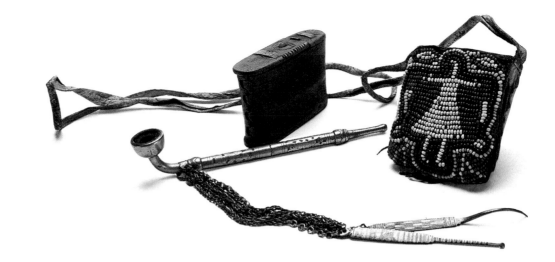

322. American Whalers

"A Northern Whaling Scene,"
Charles Scammon, 1874. Bomb gun
(Cunningham and Cogan, 1874),
NMAH 56334a

United States whaling vessels in the Bering, Chukchi, and Okhotsk seas after 1848 were a new source of external contacts, trade, and social change among coastal native peoples. Bowhead whales were hunted from open boats as in this illustration (Scammon 1874) and the blubber was rendered down aboard the whaling ship. The "bomb lance," an explosive shell, was fired into a whale after harpooning to kill the animal before it could escape under the ice. The bomb was shot from a massive breech-loaded gun whose recoil often floored or injured the gunner.

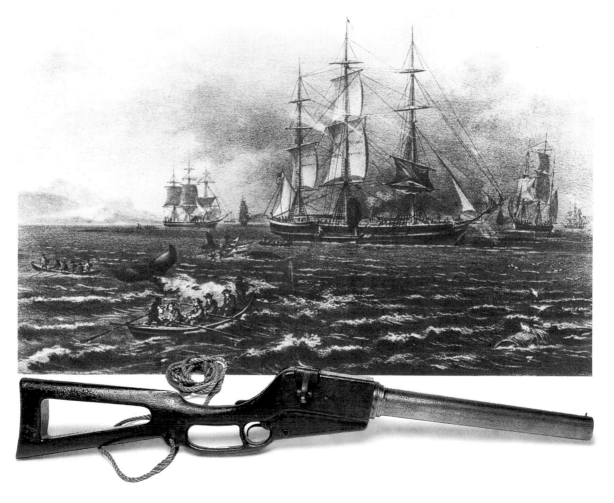

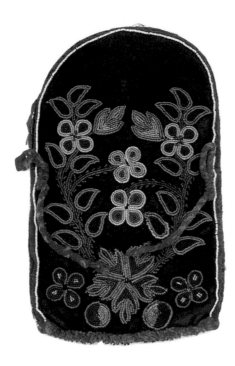

traders with permanent establishments on shore. More important, the Russian and particularly the United States governments began to keep officials permanently based in the region. For the first time, Great Power politics became an important factor in native relations across Bering Strait.

By 1900 disease, famine, and outside cultural influences had so thoroughly disrupted life on both sides of Bering Strait that the traditional native nations had ceased to exist as viable social units, and warfare—which had been on the decline anyway—ceased along with them. Interregional trade continued to take place, however, although at a reduced level, and intercontinental trade specifically was still taking place as late as the mid-1920s (Jenness 1929:78; Rasmussen 1927:357). But, as the new Soviet government extended its control to the Far East, the US-USSR border—which runs between Big and Little Diomede islands—gradually closed. Native contacts across Bering Strait continued at a greatly reduced rate but, for the most part, became limited to social visits between relatives and friends who had become dispersed over the previous two decades. In the late 1940s, even those contacts were brought to an end.

sionally carrying them eastward along the Arctic coast to or beyond the Mackenzie River delta (Nuligak 1966:36). Eventually, whalers took over most of the coastal trade, as the supply of whales became exhausted and the price of whale products dropped dramatically. Together, these forces cut the extensive east-west trade right at its geographic center. For most of the second half of the 19th century, Bering Strait continued to be the focus of trade flowing westward from Alaska, but it also drew the Chukchi trade eastward, away from the Russians.

The early years of the 20th century saw a continuation of the trends initiated in the last quarter of the 19th. The whaling industry continued to decline and pretty well disappeared by about 1914. A few ship-borne traders continued to travel the coasts of Chukotka and Alaska, but they were increasingly replaced by

323. A 2,000 Mile Journey
Northen Ojibwa: AMNH 70-5873

Details of the beaded floral designs on this cloth pouch identify its probable place of origin as the Lake Winnipeg region in Manitoba, Canada—nearly 2,000 miles east of the Chukchi Peninsula where it was collected (Kate Duncan, pers. comm.). Other Northern Ojibwa Indian objects are also known to have made their way to Alaska and British Columbia via native trade networks, another reminder of the long distance contacts and influences that helped shape North Pacific cultures.

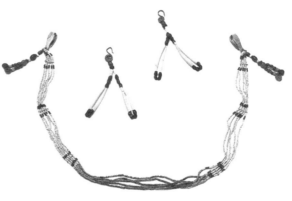

324. Alaskan Bead and Dentalium Shell Jewelry
Bering Sea Eskimo: NMNH 56070 (pair), NMNH 340331

Tubelike dentalium shells, illustrated here on a pair of earrings from Bristol Bay, were rare and costly items in the Pacific Coast trade network (cf. fig. 316). Earrings and necklace are combined in a single piece of jewelry purchased on Nunivak Island in 1927 (*below*). Beads were saved and reused for generations, so that this piece includes a few early 19th-century "wound" beads (dark blue-green oblates) along with a variety of newer tube and seed beads.

325. Chukchi Beads
Clockwise from lower left: AMNH 70-7455; 70-7267a,b; 70-7435; 70-7781a,b; 70-6620

A great variety of trade beads from European and Chinese production centers ended up in Siberia. Chukchi bead jewelry was often accented by bright bits of metal, like the brass navy buttons on the center necklace and the cartridge ends on the earrings. The uppermost strands of beads in this grouping were for intertwining with the hair of a woman's braids.

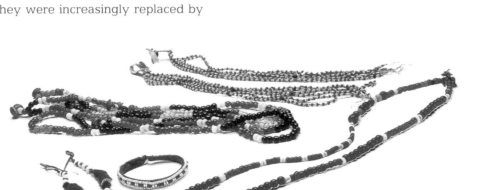

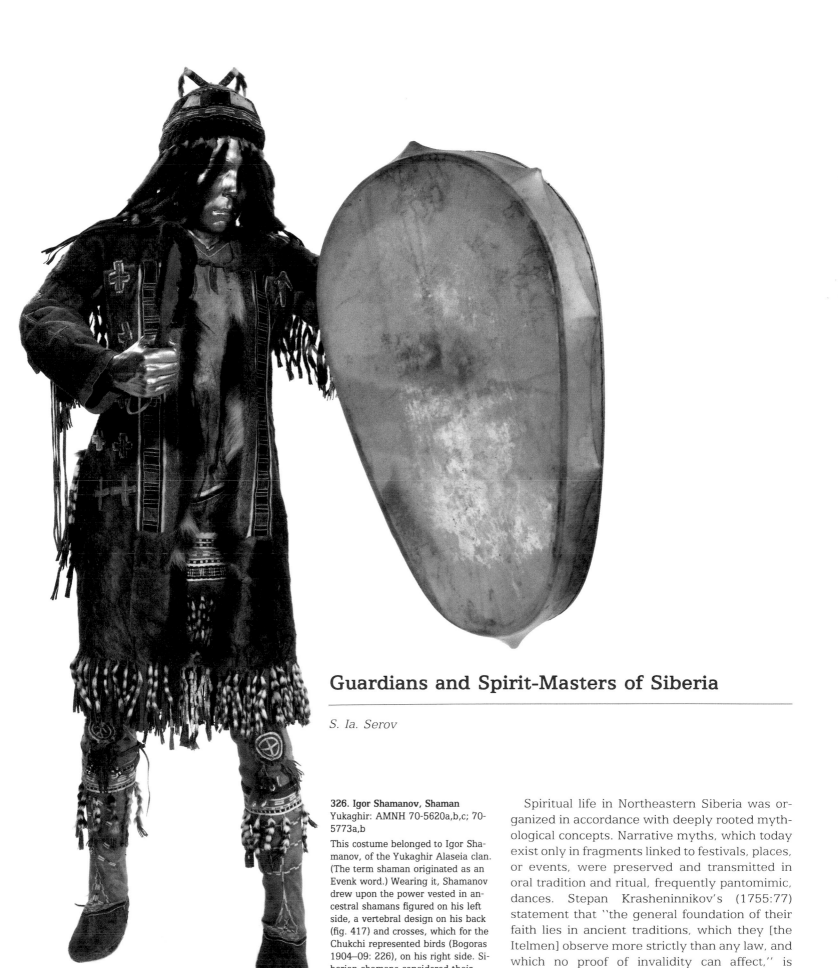

Guardians and Spirit-Masters of Siberia

S. Ia. Serov

326. Igor Shamanov, Shaman
Yukaghir: AMNH 70-5620a,b,c; 70-5773a,b

This costume belonged to Igor Shamanov, of the Yukaghir Alaseia clan. (The term shaman originated as an Evenk word.) Wearing it, Shamanov drew upon the power vested in ancestral shamans figured on his left side, a vertebral design on his back (fig. 417) and crosses, which for the Chukchi represented birds (Bogoras 1904–09: 226), on his right side. Siberian shamans considered their coats to be bird skins, which enabled them to achieve shamanic flight.

Spiritual life in Northeastern Siberia was organized in accordance with deeply rooted mythological concepts. Narrative myths, which today exist only in fragments linked to festivals, places, or events, were preserved and transmitted in oral tradition and ritual, frequently pantomimic, dances. Stepan Krasheninnikov's (1755:77) statement that "the general foundation of their faith lies in ancient traditions, which they [the Itelmen] observe more strictly than any law, and which no proof of invalidity can affect," is applicable to every ethnic group of Northeastern Siberia.

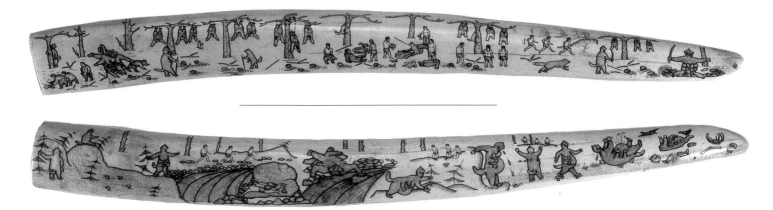

Folklore and Cosmology

The folklore of the Chukchi, Siberian Eskimo, Even, Koryak, and Itelmen is syncretic and includes more than one style or folkloristic genre. Thus, the Siberian Eskimo designate as "tales" a series of creation myths, accounts of magical events, and animal stories, whereas life stories and heroic tales belong to a different genre. The most remarkable examples of origin myths are found among the Chukchi and Siberian Eskimo.

The cosmos itself was conceived by the Northeast Siberian peoples as a series of five, seven, or nine vertically superposed worlds, "our world" being the central layer. The sum of what was considered material wealth (sea mammals, fish, reindeer, and other animals and things), as well as the number of people in the totality of the worlds, was constant, so that one killed on earth would add one to the population of another world and vice versa. The Chukchi believed that those who died on earth went to the sky world; they were then reincarnated in their descendants on earth and eventually went to the underground world after their second death. According to Krasheninnikov (1755:77), the Koryak and the Itelmen believed "that the earth is flat and that underneath it there is a sky similar to ours, with another world below, whose inhabitants have winter when we have summer, and summer when we have winter."

There were numerous concepts concerning the people of the upper world. According to some, here lived the powerful protector of human beings; according to others it was peopled with the dead, who lived lives like people on earth. The smoke of the funeral pyre was the

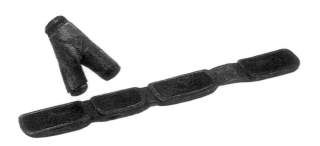

route to the sky for the deceased. The heros in tales and myths, or the shamans during their performance, traveled to the sky world through holes made near the stars, or along a rainbow or a sun ray, or on an eagle or a thunderbird. In a Chukchi myth, light was given to man by Raven, who with the help of a ptarmigan perforated the membrane between two worlds with his beak (Bogoraz 1939:40–43). The membrane between worlds was believed to be so thin that when the first tractor was introduced in the village of Paren', an old woman feared it might crush the inhabitants of the lower world (Gurvich 1987:84).

Scholars have pointed out that folkloristic themes in the North Pacific region form two blocks of material. On the one hand there is a group of Koryak and Itelmen themes, and on the other a group of Chukchi and Eskimo themes. These relationships exist despite the lack of linguistic ties within the folkloristic groups themselves. Koryak and Itelmen are not linguistically close, nor are Chukchi and Yupik Eskimo. Yet Chukchi and Koryak, folkloristically separate, are linguistically related. For example, the folklore of the Aliutor is similar to the Koryak-Itelmen block, whereas their language is related to Chukchi (Meletinskii 1979).

Among the central mythological figures of northeastern Asia was Raven, named *Kurkyl'* by the Chukchi, *Koshkli* by the Siberian Eskimo, *Kuikynniaku* by the Koryak, and *Kutkh* by the Itelmen. For the Chukchi and the Eskimo, Raven was first of all the primeval figure whose major exploit was obtaining light for the people. In the majority of the texts Raven does not take part in the creation of man. This was the task of a creator whose image was amorphous. In other versions, people emerged spontaneously from various objects. Two major variants in the "bringing of light" theme exist. In the Chukchi variant, Raven pierces the membrane between our world and an unlocalized world of spirits that is sometimes good, sometimes evil, according to different versions, and dawn rises. In the

327. *Kelet* Myth
Chukchi: MAE 6010-38

This walrus tusk, carved at the Uelen artist workshop in the 1940s (p. 317), illustrates a *kelet*, or evil spirit legend. The *kelet*, a monster with eight limbs and pointed head, captures three women and hangs them in a tree. When he returns to eat them he finds they have escaped across a river. "How did you cross?" he asks. "We drank it dry," they reply. The *kelet* tries to drink the river, but realizes he has been tricked. He swims across and gives chase, but his swollen belly bursts. The women escape and vultures gather.

328. Ancestor Guardian and Sacrificial Bowl
Chukchi: MAE 422-77; AMNH 70-6690

Among many Siberian groups "guardians" were worn to protect the wearer from evil spirits. Most guardians were made of wood and were carved in simple human form, with faces, torsos, and limbs, or simply as Y-shaped crotches. This guardian was an ancestor spirit that protected a family's material goods.

Sacrificial slaughtering of dogs and reindeer also was used to influence spirits. More common were the ritual sacrifices offered in place of live animals. This segmented bowl was used to offer blood and tallow to the four "directions": dawn, zenith, evening, and nadir.

329. The Koryak Raven Game
AMNH neg. 4150, Jesup Exp.

This photograph shows the beginning of the Raven game in which Raven (*left*) seeks to capture the young ravens holding coattails behind Mother Raven, opposite him, beginning with the last in line.

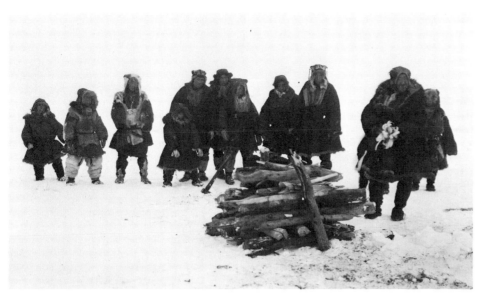

330. Koryak Child's Cremation
AMNH neg. 6468-4129, Jesup Exp.

While Jochelson was working among the Koryak, a young girl died. After being dressed in funeral clothes (fig. 341), she was carried to the cremation place and laid on the pyre. Her possessions were buried in a small hole so that she would not return home for them, and a set of women's tools was placed on the pyre, together with a bag of gifts intended for those who had died the previous year. Then the fire was lit. When the body was consumed, alder and willow bushes were strewn around the pyre, and rituals were performed to keep her spirit from following the funeral party home.

other, entering the lighted world, Raven steals from a little girl, the daughter of an evil spirit (*kele*), her balls containing the celestial bodies. By breaking the balls Raven frees and puts into the sky Sun, Moon, and the stars. This second variant was widespread in Chukotka and among Alaskan Natives and even occurs in South America.

For Koryak and Itelmen, Raven was primarily an ancestor figure. He was called Creator in shamanistic incantations but not in myths. The celestial bodies existed before the earth, so that in local Koryak-Itelmen myths (but also in some Chukchi myths), Raven created only the earth. People were born from an incestuous marriage, repeated in the next generation, between Raven's son and daughter. Among the Chukchi, the incestuous brother and sister were not connected with the Raven cycle.

Raven as a cultural hero, however, was a common motif for both the Koryak-Itelmen and

Chukchi-Eskimo blocks. In Georg W. Steller's and Krasheninnikov's accounts, natives of Kamchatka believed that *Kutkh* taught people how to sew clothing from leaves and hides, to weave fishnets, to build canoes, and to beat the drum. The departure of Raven from earth after fulfilling his duty is characteristic of Kamchatka myths. There is no promise from Raven that he will return. His departure is linked to the creation of mountains and hills, which were formed under Raven's skis. *Kutkh*'s anthropomorphism as he departed was so strongly expressed that neither Steller nor Krasheninnikov suspected his identity as Raven.

Another image of Raven, clearly demonstrated in Koryak-Itelmen myths, is that of the trickster. Raven's erotic adventures are well known and were probably responsible for Krasheninnikov's remark that Itelmen (Kamchadal) tell of *Kutkh* "such obscenities that it would be too indecent to write them down" (1755:73). The Chukchi, unlike the Kamchatka natives, distinguished the personalities of Raven in different genres: he is a creator and cultural hero in the myths and a trickster in the tales. The Siberian Eskimo borrowed Raven stories from Chukchi folklore. The Raven theme is hardly developed in Yukaghir and Even mythology.

The myth of the girl who did not want to marry was known in the Chukchi and Eskimo region. This myth culminates in her creation of people and sea animals, and she becomes Mistress of the Sea. Known as *Sedna* among the Canadian Inuit (Eskimo), she was usually called *Samna* or *Sana* (she "who lives below") by Asiatic Eskimo. The Reindeer Chukchi, having borrowed this theme from the Eskimo, created a version in which the woman did not end up in the sea but went to the tundra, where she created people, reindeer, and sea animals.

Raven's deeds were still being told in the 20th century but only in reference to the creation of the world. The belief in spiritual animism of places and things survives today. In the 1940s, Siberian Eskimo texts about the Master of the Upper World, called *Kiiagnyk*, were recorded. A similar deity, the Chukchi god *Tynagyrgyn* ("Dawn"), was also present in the Eskimo pantheon alongside other deities. The Eskimo Mistress of the Sea is *Samna*; for the Chukchi, this role was taken by a male character, *Keretkun*. He and his wife were the masters of all sea animals. The name of the master or spirit of each forest, river, hill, was not always known, but their existence was not doubted, and a lucky hunt or a safe camp had to be guaranteed by a sacrifice, often symbolic, to the master of the place.

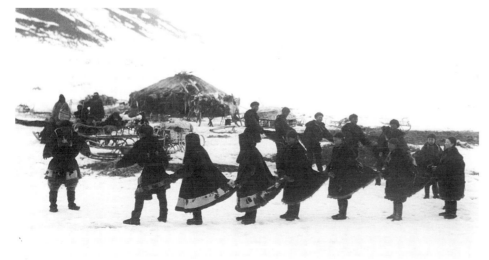

243

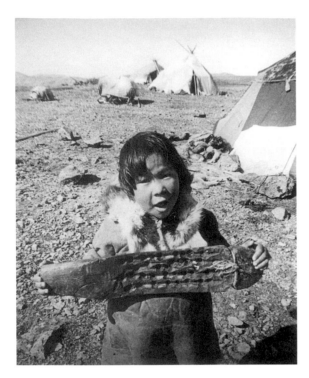

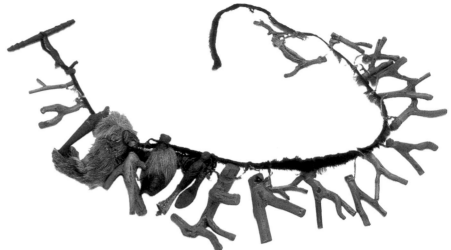

"All that exists lives. The lamp walks around. The walls of the house have voices of their own. Even the chamber-vessel has a separate land and house. The skins sleeping in the bags talk at night. The antlers lying on the tombs arise at night and walk in procession around the mounds, while the deceased get up and visit the living."
(Chukchi shaman quoted in Bogoras 1904–09:281)

Spirits and Souls

According to Bogoras, the Chukchi believed that every object had "a voice" (master-soul), lived a life like that of people, and could express its will. A person's soul was like the soul of an object, an animal, or a plant, although the soul of a plant was small and weak. A person, besides his main soul (which governed the whole body), also had souls in different organs. When a limp developed or an inner organ was sick or wounded, it was believed that the soul of this part of the body had been lost. Even human waste was thought to be capable of animation. In similar fashion, Northeast Asians viewed most phenomena of the natural world in anthropomorphic terms, and some species were thought to live in communities similar to men's. For example, there were polar bear people, mouse people, wolf people, and spider people, but there were no wild reindeer people or seabird people (Krushanov 1987:89).

Beliefs in metamorphosis and animation of objects were closely connected. For the Koryak, as for the Eskimo (fig. 45), killer whales turned into wolves in winter when the sea was frozen and hunted reindeer on land like they hunted whales in the sea. As in many areas of the northern hemisphere, the black bear was thought to be a human in a bear skin.

People could turn into animals, and vice versa, although this belief was not formulated as such. But in myths and tales, it was obvious that when a human and an animal met, the animal, although retaining his name, had a human shape. The

principles of zoomorphism and anthropomorphism were sometimes more concrete. In tales of the Greenlandic, American, and Siberian Eskimo, the soul of a deceased person reincarnated successively into a dog, a bear, a wolf, a fox, and a bird. In another Eskimo tale, known under many variations as "the woman who delivered a whale," a whale used to meet his lover, not in the form of a whale but as a man coming out of the nose of the whale and who is the whale's soul. The husband of the woman struck the whale lying on the beach with his spear, but the whale did not die until the "man," leaving the woman, entered the whale's nostril again (Menovshchikov 1987:16–26). It seems that the whale's soul, returning to the body, received the same wound, and only then did the actual death of the body occur.

The idea of metamorphosis was represented in Old Bering Sea art through polyiconic forms (visual puns). An amulet from Ekven (Arutiunov and Sergeev 1975:plate 80.18) combines features of five different animals. Heads of a killer whale and a wolf, transformationally related, were carved on opposite ends of the amulet. Such links between animal species, including man, continue to be reflected in the art of the Chukotka-Alaska region.

Spirits of the home (guardians) and the personal amulets were often anthropomorphic. The wooden fireboards (figs. 243, 260, 331) used to light the ritual fire in the home were always carved in human form. Guardian spirits were

331. Chukchi Guardians
Andres Slapinsh photo, 1983.
Chukchi: AMNH 70-7810

Among many guardians, one of the most important was the sacred fireboard (fig. 243) which was used with a firedrill to light the family fire. Koryak and Chukchi fireboards were given simple human form.

Because the world was full of spirits, many of which could cause misfortune, a thoughtful person carried a charm string in a leather pouch around one's neck. Each charm, or *okamak*, represented a particular guardian and had a designated name. This string includes a large number of male charms, and a special furwrapped female charm known as "the wooden woman" or "the mistress." Charms made of animal parts are also seen on this string.

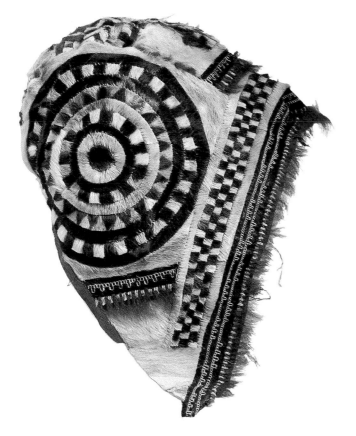

332. Man's Funeral Cap
Koryak: MAE 956-82

Koryak funeral ritual involved the preparation of elaborate funerary costumes. This man's funeral cap, like other parts of the costume, was made of white reindeer fawn fur onto which were stitched geometric piecework designs, embroidered bands, dyed wool tassels, and ruffs of the downy hair of young seals.

often represented by a forked branch looking like a body with legs (figs. 182, 210, 338, 345). Personal guardian spirits made of wood or animal hide were sewn to the clothing, worn at the belt, or hung around the neck. When sick, the Chukchi tattooed their hands and faces with humanlike figures to chase away the spirits of disease. A Chukchi might tattoo on his shoulders a representation of the soul of someone he had killed, to turn the soul into his helper.

There were cases when the relationship between a person and his or her guardian spirit was expressed in marital terms. Among the Chukchi, these partners were called Ritual Wife or Ritual Husband. It is probably these supernatural ''members of the family'' that Krasheninnikov observed among the sedentary Koryak in the person of two stones, the larger one being the ''wife'' and the smaller the ''son'' of a Koryak man. According to Krasheninnikov (1755:164), these stones were ''dressed with clothing, put to bed with [the Koryak], and occasionally joked and played with.'' The same type of spirit was contained in leather fertility dolls that were passed down for generations from mother to daughter.

Spirits were sometimes considered neutral, or even benevolent, but most of the time were aggressive and offensive. Even souls of dead relatives might, as among the Asian Eskimo, become dangerous after a few years when they began to long for company and tried to capture the souls of their kinfolk. Evil spirits were those of dead people who had led evil lives. To protect against them, the earth or snow around the dwelling was sprinkled with human urine or with old lamp oil. Besides family and personal amulets, firearms and weapons, and especially drums, were most effective for protecting against evil spirits because these spirits did not like loud noises.

Evil spirits (*kelet*s) lived, according to Chukchi belief, in the upper world or underground, but not in the sea. Otherwise, they inhabited a wild world, symmetrical to man's, on the other side of a vertical separation. The *kelet*s had various appearances, but they were, as a rule, much larger or smaller than humans and had ugly pointed heads. Evil spirits were associated with the color black and are shown in drawings with black faces. *Keretkun*, Master of the Sea Animals, was represented as a tall, mean-looking man with a black face. The faces of sick people were commonly painted with black graphite among Siberian Eskimo and Maritime and Reindeer Chukchi to deceive the spirits of sickness into believing that the sick man was not a human whose soul could be stolen but another spirit. The image of a helping spirit bringing to his shaman master a red or a black garment represented, in Bogoras's analysis, the choice given to the shaman to become a benevolent or an evil shaman. Even though one must be cautious with too specific an interpretation, one cannot help noting in the color symbolism of the people of Northeast Asia that black was the color of the other world and of death, while red was the color of life. Face and hand painting with red ocher or the blood of a sacrificed animal was an important element in Chukchi wedding and funeral rituals. Ceremonial and shamanistic garments were ornamented with red tassels of twisted wool or fur.

Red and black were conflicting colors, whereas white played a neutral role. Among the Siberian Eskimo, an aging shaman's loss of strength was symbolized by his wearing of white clothing, which was also the color of funeral garments. A combination of all three colors was used on divination sticks of Eskimo weather-tellers. This color symbolism was applied to the sacred realm only; in everyday life, white garments were thought to be the most beautiful.

The cult of ancestors existed among all peoples of Chukotka and Kamchatka. The Koryak sacrificial places near the settlements were called Grandfather or Grandmother.

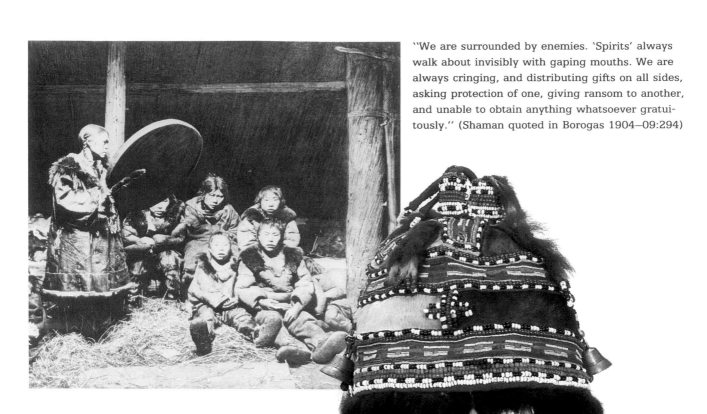

Shamanism

Shamans in Chukotka and Kamchatka could be either men or women. Among these maritime groups, there was no sharp distinction between professional shamans and others, as found elsewhere in Siberia. As a matter of fact, individual and familial shamanism prevailed. For instance, a hunter might, when required, attempt to foresee the future, heal the sick, and fight evil spirits with shamanistic weapons; and a community shaman who was economically supported by his kin helped his family first of all.

I. S. Vdovin distinguishes two forms of shamanistic performance among the Chukchi. One is a mass performance based on general religious concepts and oriented towards the ancestors and personified forces. The other is the individual performance. The view that shamanism is a form of religion, common in 1930s ethnography in the USSR, is not shared by Vdovin, A. P. Okladnikov, and other scholars who define shamanistic faith as belief in the connection between the shaman and evil spirits and see the shaman's role as defending people against these evil forces.

The lack of a separate category of professional shaman is consistent with the lack of a shamanistic costume. The Maritime Chukchi and Eskimo shaman's robe was decorated only with tassels and pendants of seal pup fur. There was no special headdress among the maritime people, although Reindeer Chukchi shamans grew their hair long and braided it. An exception among the Eskimo was the special white clothing worn when foretelling the weather during the whale

333. Tasseled Shaman's Hat
AMNH neg. 337173, Jesup Exp.
Yukaghir: AMNH 70-387
Household shamans like this Koryak woman performed routine rituals and wore no special clothing. Professional shamans, who could also be women, had elaborate costumes. This Yukaghir shaman's hat is made from the short white-and- brown fur taken from the legs of reindeer and has the long fur tassels that were also characteristic of Even shaman's hats. The color division, white on the wearer's right side, dark on his left, signified the shaman's dual role, participating in the world of men (light) and the world of shades and spirits (darkness). Beads, dyed moosehair embroidery, and brass bells and rings (not visible, but see cover illustration) complete the ornamentation.

Yakut and Evenk shamans festooned their coats with metal chains, spirit figures, and ornaments. These jingling attachments aided in attracting friendly spirits.

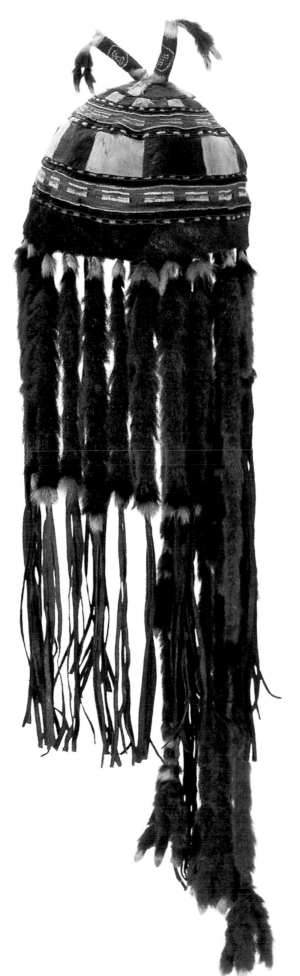

334. Hat of a "Transformed" Shaman
Yukaghir: AMNH 70-5620

The small leather cylinders seen on the top of Shamanov's hat (*right*) are symbolic antlers, equivalent to the iron antlers on Evenk shaman hats (fig. 335). Faces of *wolmadono* representing shades of deceased shamans are stitched into each prong.

In addition to his tasseled hat, Shamanov wore a tasseled, fringed apron (fig. 326), a woman's garment style. Men's aprons did not have fringes. In addition to adopting women's clothing, sexually 'transformed" Siberian shamans adopted female language and behavior.

Tassels were made from the soft fur of the young spotted seal, dyed red with an infusion of the inner bark of larch and alder. Emblematic of Siberian spirit life, they were used both as insignia and as lively swinging ornamanets on costumes and amulets.

335. Antlered Shaman's Hat
Evenk: AMNH 70-5772d

Evenk shamans' hats, like the one at the far right, are often decorated with iron antlers representing the wild reindeer, whose spirit (*ge'lken*) was the special protector of this shaman. Another class of spirit, probably representing ancestral shamans, as in fig. 334, float across the brow, and appear as tasseled stick figures with beaded circular heads along the sides.

ceremony. Bogoras (1939:136) saw the lack of a shamanistic outfit among the Maritime Chukchi as a result of their performances' taking place mainly in the bed chamber (*polog*), which was so hot when everyone was gathered inside that elaborate garments could not be worn. Narrow white fringes on the sleeves and appliqué designs were borrowed from Tungus-speaking neighbors, but these coats were worn only when performances were held outside or in the cold part of the dwelling (Prokof'eva 1971:56, 48–50).

The Yukaghir shaman's coat was originally a plain female coat. By the end of the 19th century it had been exchanged for a coat characteristic of the Tungus-speaking groups symbolizing a bird, eagle, or stork (figs. 326, 417). The apron and boots remained those of a woman. The Even shaman's outfit was similar to the Evenk's. The left part of the coat was made of dark suede and the right part of light suede, a sign of the shaman's belonging to two worlds (cf. fig. 333). The apron, similar to a woman's, and the pendants on the back were embroidered with rep-

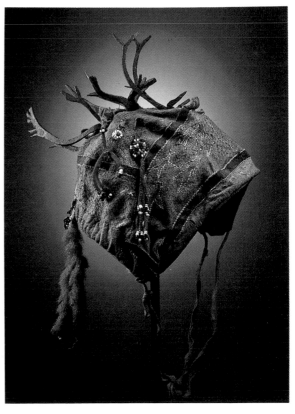

resentations of spirits. The headdress had iron antlers, and on the gloves were tufts of bear fur to symbolize the shaman's designated helping spirit, or protector.

Eighteenth-century travelers in Kamchatka noticed the plain look of male and female shamans. The only exception seems to have been among the Kerek, whose shamans were dressed

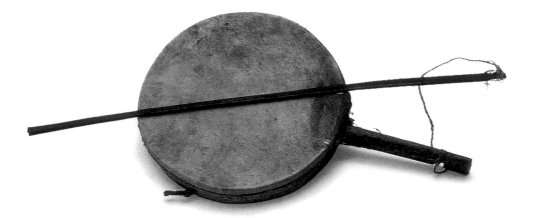

336. Toy Drum
Chukchi: AMNH 70-6548

Chukchi drums, made of walrus
stomach tissue stretched on a bentwood hoop, are similar to the drums
used by Asiatic and Alaskan Eskimo,
and different from those used by
other Siberian groups. This toy drum
is played with a baleen stick.

337. Magic Surgery
Chukchi: AMNH 70-6793, 70-6792

Scratching-Woman, a transvestite
shaman, told Bogoras he operated on
sick people with these tools. Tied to
the iron knife is a huge glass bead
obtained by his grandather from the
*kelet*s. The ivory "knife" (an old armor plate) was a present from the
Milky Way. Its leather images include
a *kelet* from the direction of darkness, with arms longer than its legs
(*left*); the *kelet* Iumetun (*center*),
with one arm and one leg and vertical eyes; and on the right, a crawling
kelet sent by an enemy to attack him,
but which he subdued and tamed.

in long, open embroidered robes trimmed with
dog fur, and fur caps with tassels (cf. fig. 293).
The Chukchi and Koryak considered Kerek shamans to be the most powerful of all (Leont'ev
1983:60).

One usually became a shaman after a reve-
lation. The shamanistic call could result from
apparitions of spirits in dreams or during sickness, or from a voice heard while hunting. But
few shamans were strong enough to subordinate
the spirits, who were not always willing to come
when called. If angry for some reason, the spirit
might leave the shaman or punish him. For the
Chukchi, the spirits were far from being friendly
to one another. When called by the shaman,
they quarreled, and only the shaman's persua-
sive entreaties and threats could pacify them.

The performance (*kamlanie*) was the most
important activity of the shaman. It varied between ethnic groups, within a single group, and
even within one settlement according to the
strength and reputation of the shaman. Both in
Chukotka and in Kamchatka, fly agaric, the
mushroom *Amanita muscaria*, was consumed,
by men only, before the *kamlanie*. Krasheninnikov noted that the Itelmen "affirm that whatever madness they may display is, invisibly,
ordered by the fly-agaric" (1755:109–10). The
Cossack Efrem Purgin, who spent 30 years
among the Koryak in the 18th century, noted
that to strengthen the power of the intoxicating
mushroom the participants, after eating the
mushroom, "pour their urine into a bowl or a
cup and drink it again" (Kos'ven 1962:280).

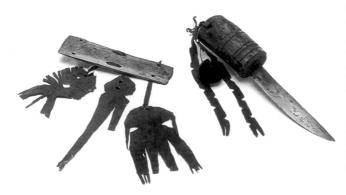

According to the Chukchi, fly agaric took people
by the hand and led them along a crooked path
into the land of the dead (Bogoraz 1939:5).
During the *kamlanie*, hallucinations were often
provoked by self-hypnosis through singing and
drum beating (cf. fig. 153).

Chukchi drums were similar to drums used
by the American and Siberian Eskimo—circular,
with an outside wooden handle; the membrane
was made of walrus stomach. Drumsticks were
of two kinds: a small baleen stick for performances inside the *polog* and a longer wooden one
for outside. Drums of the Yukaghir, Even, Koryak, and Itelmen were oval and were held by
a handle inside the drum frame. Except among
the Eskimo and Chukchi, ritual drums were
different from dancing drums. Ritual drums had
bells and metal rings inside and sometimes grass
or rag dolls and beads. When a shaman died,
his drum was broken and was laid on his grave
so that its spirit could become a new drum in
the otherworld. The drumstick remained in the
family to be used for divination.

For the *kamlanie* in the *polog*, the shaman
undressed to the waist, doused the lamp, and
asked the participants to be seated and to remain
silent, since otherwise the spirits might not
come. Then the shaman started to sing rapidly,
beating his drum. Lesser shamans, using incantations, received some information from the
spirits during this simple performance. Powerful
shamans, however, sang themselves into a trance,
during which their soul traveled on the "boat"
(the drum) to the lower world to divine the
future or retrieve the soul of a sick person. In
contrast to North America, masks were not worn
by Asian shamans. The language the shaman
used with spirits was not intelligible to ordinary
people; sometimes it was another real dialect or
just sounds without content.

Women were considered better shamans than
men, as in most ecstatic cults. The phenomenon
of change of sex, noticed among the Koryak and
Itelmen, may have been related to this. A male
shaman not only dressed as a woman but also

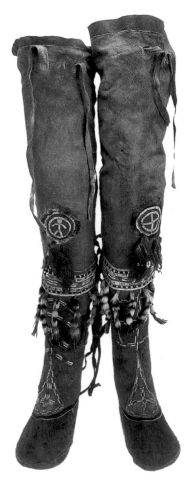

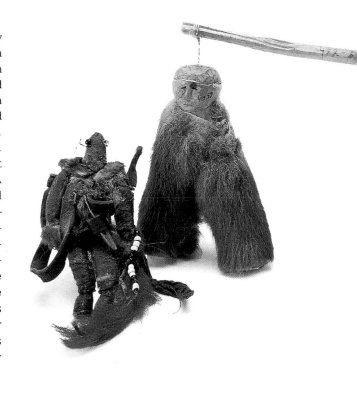

338. Sun-Worm and Divining Guardian
Koryak: AMNH 70-3594
Chukchi: MAE 422-59

This Sun-Worm doll, a guardian of women, has fur clothing, beady eyes, a fur tail, and a hexagonal nut strung on a lanyard. The body contains a worm, "the vivifying one," that falls from the sky into a woman's root basket and protects her from sterility.

The suspended guardian is used for divining. The soothsayer holds the guardian in the air and asks it questions. If the answer is "yes," the guardian swings; if "no," it remains motionless.

339. Shaman's Leggings
Even: 70-5773a,b

Tassels and embroidered spirit figures and other designs were embroidered onto this set of shaman leggings. Though they were collected from the Even, the style indicates Evenk (Tungus) influence.

340. Divining Pouch
Chukchi: AMNH 70-6691

Appended to this divining pouch made of reindeer skin is a polished chunk of graphite. When in use the bag probably held soothsayer's bones.

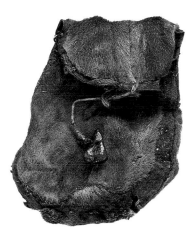

adopted women's manners and work. Many cases of men turning into women and vice versa were known among the Chukchi and Siberian Eskimo. This was apparent in transvestism and in changes of hairstyle, voice, and manners. In such cases, men spoke the female dialect and women the male dialect. Among the Koryak, where no specifically shamanistic outfit existed, the shaman sometimes wore one female boot and one male boot during the *kamlanie*. A transformed shaman kept his or her original male or female name. Complete change of sex—both in attitude, behavior, and physical features—was present in Northeast Siberian folkloric texts. A transformed woman did not participate in male activities, but a "soft," womanlike man did women's work. In the context of the belief in metamorphosis and change of sex, this phenomenon is difficult to separate from a larger tradition of homosexuality, especially since, as Bogoras noticed, homosexuality occurred mainly during youth.

Divination and Family Ritual

Besides curing, the basic duty of a shaman was the divination of weather and of movements of sea animals and other game. Such information could be obtained during a *kamlanie* but in general was sought before the first hunt of the year with the help of a drumstick tied to the head of the *umialik*, the whaleboat captain. Speaking the right answer, the *umialik* felt his head becoming light. The Itelmen practiced levitation with the leg, which the shaman tried to lift with a red string at each question.

Seal scapulae (shoulder blades) or, among the Reindeer Chukchi and Even, reindeer scapulae were used for divination. Coastal groups also divined with whale scapulae in the whale ceremony. In the latter case, the shaman applied burning charcoal to the scapula and interpreted the cracks that appeared. The information sought was the location and movements of whales and the paths their spirits took in returning to the sea after the ceremonies.

The most common method of divination was to suspend a stone, wooden amulet, or animal skull, which would swing when the correct answer to a question was given. The name of a newborn baby was chosen this way. Since it was believed that an ancestor had been reincarnated as the baby, the names of deceased relatives were pronounced by women while observing a stone amulet (anthropomorphic among the Koryak) suspended from a tripod or bipod made of sticks, which swung at the name of the reincarnated relative. The Even announced the birth of a baby boy by saying, "Father is back!" or for a baby girl, "Father returned, but

he wanted to be a woman." The name of an Even baby (i.e., of a reincarnated relative) was guessed when the baby was old enough to speak by interpreting his or her responses to questions posed when held in the arms of the paternal grandmother. For the Kerek, a little boy was the reincarnation of his maternal grandfather, and if the latter was still alive, the great-grandfather. A little girl was the reincarnation of her maternal grandmother or great-grandmother. The name was given accordingly.

To avoid being found by evil spirits, for example after a serious illness, one could change one's name during life, but only with great danger. The new name was often insulting or ugly-sounding. In the Eskimo tale "The boy from Chaplino," the boy takes the name of his deceased brother, thinking that the "upper people," believing him dead, would not take him with them. Taking a new name was equivalent to killing the bearer of the old name and being born again.

Numerous rules and taboos surrounded the periods before, during, and after delivery. As soon as a Chukchi woman knew she was pregnant, she had to look with her husband, at dawn, toward the rising sun, the dwelling place of benevolent spirits. Similarly, a Koryak woman had to go to the community shrine to ask protection, burn pieces of fat, meat, and hare fur, and sacrifice strings of colored beads. A pregnant Even woman was accompanied by an experienced woman who made sure she observed rules that, like postnatal rules, had both hygienic and symbolic aspects. A pregnant woman was forbidden to visit or receive guests at her home, to see other pregnant women, to touch fishnets and other tools, to go out at night, or to eat fatty foods.

At the delivery the Even usually called a midwife to massage the stomach of the pregnant woman and deliver the baby. In the *iaranga* (skin tent) all curtain ties had to be untied, and all lids were left off the pots to facilitate the baby's exit. The midwife cut a boy's umbilical cord with his father's knife and a girl's with her mother's. Then the baby was wiped with soft wood shavings, placed on a board, and wrapped in skins. The Chukchi cut the umbilical cord with a stone knife, then wiped the baby with a bunch of grass soaked in the mother's urine, and then burned the grass. The Itelmen laid the baby in soft grass. The Even buried the placenta, but the sedentary Chukchi and Koryak placed it outside the dwelling, under a symbolic shelter. Krasheninnikov thought the placenta was thrown away to be eaten by dogs, who in Kamchatka and Chukotka were enemies of evil spirits (fig. 342). For the first days after a birth, a Chukchi man could enter the bed chamber only after being purified by a neighbor's household deity or by holding a puppy against his body.

After delivery, the mother's abdomen was bound with straps for three days; she then put on new clothing, or if old clothing was worn, it had to be purified in the smoke from the ritual hearth. On the fifth day the mother, the newborn, the family amulets, and three of the six poles of the dwelling were painted with reindeer blood. Only then was the baby given a name (Bogoraz 1939:175–76; Popova 1981:158–63).

Marriage among the people of Chukotka and Kamchatka was an individual ceremony, although certain forms of group marriage were preserved. Associated with marriage was the custom of bride work. The conditions and length of the groom's obligation to the parents of the bride were discussed in advance. At the end of the period of bride work among the Koryak and Itelmen, the groom had to catch the bride outside her house and touch her genitals as a ritual of possession. This was not easy because as soon as the bride's parents assented, the bride bundled herself up in several combination suits over which she strapped belts and nets. If she herself did not resist, at least her female friends and kin harassed the groom to hinder his efforts. If thwarted, he might try again later, but should he fail decisively, he forfeited compensation for his bride work.

Usually, the young couple lived at the husband's parents' house. The wedding ceremony per se included a sacrifice to the household deity, painting the spouses' faces, and a feast. Krasheninnikov remarked that in an Itelmen wedding in 1739, people on the way to the groom's house recited incantations to a dry fish head, which was later placed at the foot of the entry ladder for all to step on, before being burned in the ritual hearth.

Funeral Practice

Among the natives of Kamchatka and Chukotka, concepts about the organization of the world and the relationship between humans and supernatural beings were clearly defined in the funeral rites. Four means of transferring the dead from this world to the next coexisted in this region: fire (cremation), earth (subsurface burial), air (surface burial), and water (disposal at sea). However, cremation and surface burial prevailed.

In instances of voluntary death, known among Chukchi and Koryak, an individual requested death by spear or strangulation at the hands of a friend or relative and was burned together with his or her belongings. In cases of natural death, more elaborate rituals were conducted that began with wiping the body with a bundle of grass to signify that the person departing from this world was being born in another. The corpse was then dressed in fine white funeral clothing (figs. 278, 332, 341). The Koryak put the deceased's right glove on the left hand and harnessed the reindeer drawing the corpse in reversed order. The Koryak sacrificed a grown dog to take the place of the dead in the house during the funeral rites, and the Chukchi sacrificed a dog pup.

The deceased was then taken from the house, not through the regular door but through a special hole cut in the wall. Later, this hole was carefully mended so that the soul of the deceased could not find its way back into the house to take souls of the living. For the same reason the Koryak of the Okhotsk Sea coast left the funeral location three times, two of them being false departures in which the mourners covered their tracks by placing a stone or drawing a line across the path to prevent the spirit of the deceased from following the funeral party back to the village. Once the body had been laid at the chosen place, cuts were made on the stomach and the throat to free the soul. The sled and weapons left near the corpse were then broken

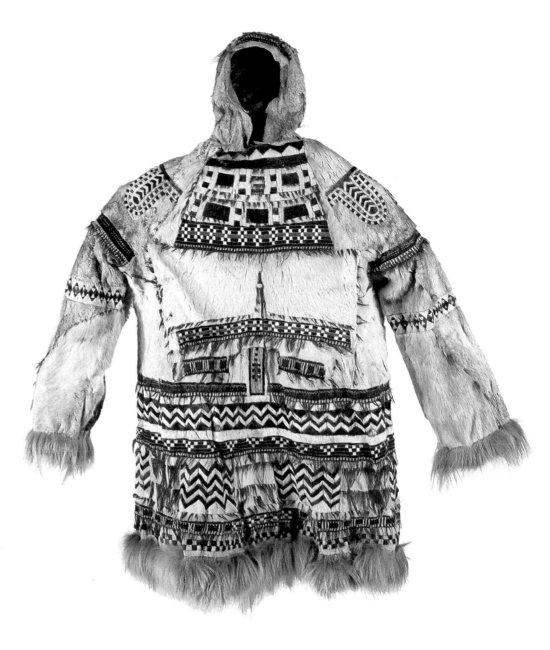

341. Man's Cremation Costume
Koryak: AMNH 70-2888, 70-2887a,b,
70-3234a,b

A Koryak funeral costume included a
parka, leggings, boots, hat, and
quiver (fig. 227), all made from the
white fur of reindeer fawns. Months
in the making, costumes had to be
worked on at night, secretly; if the
garments were seen, or work was
completed in advance, death would
soon follow. As a result, the days between death and cremation were
ones of feverish, sleepless work.
While the women sewed, the men
passed the time playing cards upon
the deceased, whose body was displayed in the house.

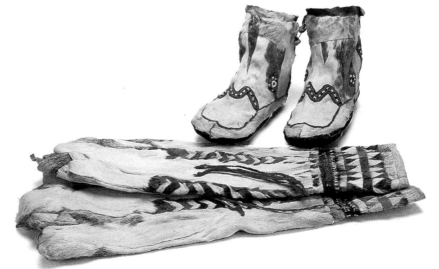

to serve the dead in the other world. Reindeer (among the Reindeer Chukchi and Koryak) and dogs (among the maritime peoples) were sacrificed at the funeral place. A sacrificed dog was left on the grave, his entrails exposed in loops. These loops represented the crooked path taken by the deceased's spirit to the otherworld. To facilitate this travel the Chukchi left two *iaranga* poles, termed legs, at the grave site; the Koryak cut the soles of the funeral boots. The body was then either left on the ground to be eaten by dogs and wild animals or, more often, cremated on a log pyre, its soul rising to the sky world in the column of smoke (fig. 330).

Subsurface burial as a funeral rite was known but was not common in the area. Another funeral custom found among the Maritime Koryak and Kerek was disposal of dead in the sea, after having pierced the side of the corpse with a knife to insure "drowning." The Even laid their dead both on the ground or on a platform in a tree. The Itelmen buried babies in hollow trees.

After the funeral, the participants had to be purified. In the Koryak purification ritual (Gurvich 1980:174–75, 202–22, 239), those returning to the village were met by the women and girls who had not participated in the funeral, who whipped the men with branches or fumigated them with burning sticks and sometimes sprinkled water on them. The Itelmen ritual involved crawling through hoops of green twigs. Similar rituals were common among many Eurasian peoples, who performed them to cure disease and during festivals. The hoops of green branches represented life-giving natural forces. By passing through the hoops one symbolically passed from an old or bad period of life into a new one, reborn and purified. For a sick person, the Itelmen made a "door" with the entrails of a dog between two vertical poles and walked through it with the sick person.

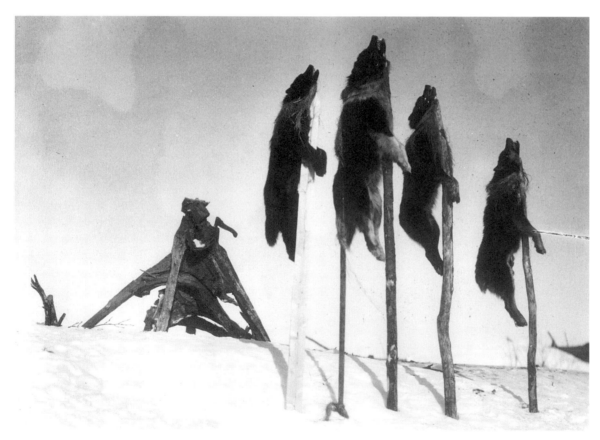

342. Koryak Dog Sacrifice
AMNH neg. 1562, Jesup Exp.

Among the Koryak the sacrifice of live animals included only dogs, while among the Reindeer Koryak and Even, it also included reindeer. Associated with the eastern spread of reindeer breeding, live sacrifice was present among the Reindeer Chukchi, but not among Maritime Chukchi, Asian Eskimo, or peoples of northwestern North America.

To guard against evil spirits Koryak dogs were stabbed in the heart and were displayed wearing grass collars on poles around the village.

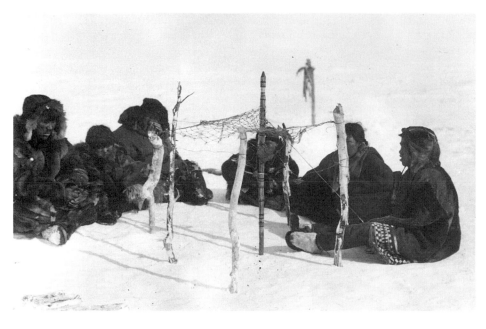

Festival Cycles

A yearly cycle of seasonal festivals, including hunting (harvest) festivals and celebrations of an occasional nature, were held throughout Northeastern Siberia. The latter were organized if someone was instructed to do so in a dream or for rites of passage, such as a young man's hunting initiation, or for other special events. Annual celebrations did not take place on fixed days but were held within specific seasons. They lasted from one to two days to several weeks.

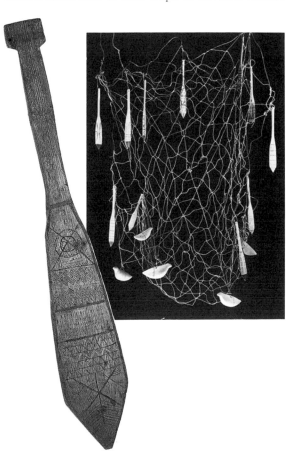

There was no difference in the way individual, family, or community festivals were organized. Tradition held that the festivals were open to strangers and members of other ethnic groups, but in reality visitors were rarely invited.

The purpose of the hunting festivals was to honor the souls of the animals killed during the previous season and to insure their regeneration so that the number of animals on earth remained plentiful and constant. In Koryak and Itelmen ritual, regeneration of individual animals was given more emphasis than among the Chukchi and the Eskimo, for whom game was sent to man by a master: *Keretkun* for the Chukchi, or *Samna* or her male equivalent, *Kasak*, for the Eskimo. In both cases the animals were treated as guests visiting the humans, and certain rules had to be observed. Among them were "treating the guests" and "seeing off the guests." The latter was accomplished by returning parts of the game, usually bones or pieces of meat, to the elements. Continuance of the relationship between animals and human society was assured by saving a portion of the body of the animal or by ritual eating of its meat by the whole community.

Most scholars consider the fall-winter festivals as the beginning of the yearly cycle. Krasheninnikov (1755:84) noted, "At the end of summer and fall activities, no work could be started before the festival, and people were not visiting friends." For Bogoras, the first celebration of the annual cycle was the "sacrifice to the sea," which was, like the "sacrifice to the dead," organized at the end of the summer, before the move to the winter settlement. This was more a ritual than a festival. In its simplest form, it consisted of the hunter's displaying his harpoon and other weapons to the Master of the Sea, asking for good luck, while the hunter's wife brought an offering of reindeer meat and blood, or a dog might be sacrificed. The first community festival after the busy summer and fall season was the Itelmen purification festival at the end of the fall. The Chukchi equivalent was a harvest ceremony, taking place several times a year, after a good hunt. A regular observance was held every year in late fall or early winter. The function of both Itelmen and Chukchi festivals was to mark the boundary between years. There are few descriptions of these ceremonies. It is known that the Koryak burned stuffed seals or seal effigies made of alder twigs at the fall festival so that the seals would return.

The "putting away of the umiaks," corresponding in time with the refurbishment of winter dwellings, was also an end-of-season Koryak festival. After the skin boat cover was removed from the umiak frame, a fire was lit nearby with the fireboard and drill. Then the ashes from the summer hearth were carried to the communal shrine, where a new hearth was lit from the live fire. The summer side entrance to the semisubterranean house was closed, and the ladder was installed in the roof entrance of the house. The representations of the spirit at the upper and lower ends of the ladder were "fed" with fat and offered incantations. The ceremony concluded with symbolic launching of the frame of the umiak, carrying the fireboard ("the father") wrapped in fur clothing to which a model harpoon was attached.

The main Chukchi festival at the end of the fall was the *Keretkun* festival. The corresponding Eskimo celebration was *Kasak* (or *Saiak*). *Keretkun*, Master of the Sea, was, as we have noted, a tall anthropomorphic character with a black face and a bad temper. He lived at the bottom of the sea with his wife. The equivalent Eskimo figure, *Kasak*, is not so well defined. Both Chukchi and Eskimo believed the Master of the Sea attended the ceremony and then went back to the sea. The Maritime Chukchi probably borrowed the idea of this deity from the Eskimo. The Chukchi actually were closer to the Aleut in their use of *Keretkun* masks for pantomimic dances, whereas masks in general were used by Koryak, Eskimo, and Chukchi in winter ceremonies only. The anthropomorphic masks were made of skin among the Eskimo and the Chukchi and of wood and grass among the Koryak (figs. 346, 424). By 1900, the different masks seem to have lost whatever identity they may once have had.

The *Keretkun* festival was a family celebration to which guests were invited. It took place inside the house. The important element of the setting for the Eskimo was the central pole of the *iaranga*. For the Chukchi a special pole was passed through the top of the smoke hole, from which the power of the ceremony was derived and to which the sinew *Keretkun* net was attached, its edges being fastened to the walls. Painted models of birds and paddles were hung from the net. For the Eskimo, the ceremony began by pouring sea water down the pole, thereby bringing the Master of the Sea into the house with the water. Later, a dance was staged in which *Kasak* was impersonated with the aid of a mask that had been empowered from contact with the pole. The model paddles, and actual paddles and umiak seats painted with hunting scenes, were also used for magical purposes. The spirit of the umiak was thought to live in these objects, which were offered for food. All such objects had to be tied by sinew lines to the pole or otherwise were placed in the center of the *iaranga*. In some settlements the painted

boards and paddles were burned at the end of the festival, and in others they were kept for the next year, in which case the drawings were erased and were repainted. The representation of *Keretkun* was burned, and the remains of sacrificial food were thrown into the sea.

Many elements of the *Keretkun-Kasak* festival are found in the whale festival that also occurred in October or November. In this festival, drawings, masks, and figurines were used. Chukchi and Eskimo painted whale tails at the corners of their mouths or whole whales, vertically, on their mouths and noses. The Chukchi and Eskimo hunters, led by the *umialik* who had harpooned the whale, danced around the body of the whale on the shore. The women offered a drink of fresh water to the whale, considered to be visiting as a guest, and, among the Koryak, fed it alder twigs. Then the women cut pieces from the nose, lips, eyes, flippers, and flukes of the whale. Before flensing, a hood of grass was put on the whale's head as a funeral ritual. This was equivalent to the Alaskan Eskimo ritual of slitting a seal's eyes before the butchering so that his soul would not see the bloody procedure. The festival itself started shortly after the whale was flensed. During the feast the whale was fed again, and pantomimic dances were executed. The women danced first, in the same number as the hunters of the umiak, and then the hunters danced with them. Eventually all the participants danced, sometimes in masks.

Besides the feast, other entertainment at the whale festival included contests of wrestling, jumping, and running. Gifts were invariably exchanged. Since the presents had no material value, they were merely a way to reaffirm community bonds. In most cases these gifts

345. Whale Festival Altar Objects
Koryak: AMNH 70-3246,-2992,-2856

For Koryak people the Whale Festival was an important ceremonial event. Similar to the Chukchi *Keretkun* and the Bering Sea Eskimo Bladder Festival, the Whale Festival was to honor the spirits of whales caught and insure their return to the sea so that the species would be renewed.

During the festival a carving of a whale and a ritual whale-shaped dish containing an offering of a drink of fresh water for the whale spirits was placed on the household shrine along with other guardians normally maintained there. This shrine consisted of a grass mat upon which were placed the anthropomorphic family guardians (dressed in grass "neckties"), the sacred fireboard (fig. 243), the Master of Nets (fig. 182), and the house guardian.

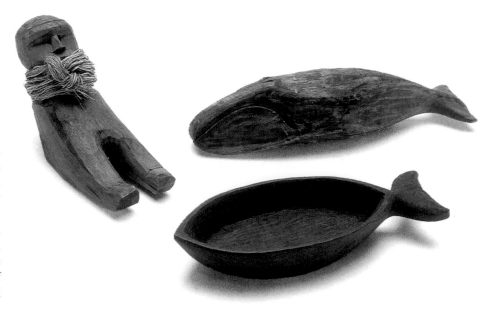

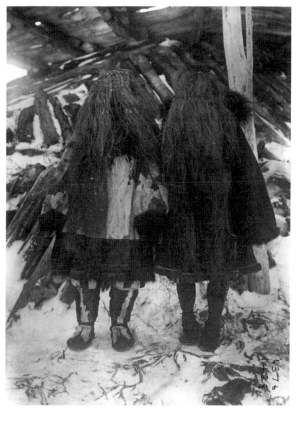

346. Masked Koryak Women
AMNH neg. 1428, Jesup Exp.

Jochelson took a unique series of photographs during various stages of a whale festival that he witnessed among the Maritime Koryak. This photograph shows women dressed in grass masks, worn during the crucial stage in the festival when an entreaty was made for the return of the whale's soul to the sea. A similar type of grass mask was placed over the head of the whale when it was being butchered, so that it would not see the bloody procedure.

Among northeastern Siberian groups masking was relatively uncommon at the time of the Jesup Expedition and was present primarily among the Koryak, who, in addition to using grass masks, wore simple wood masks in the Seal Festival, and on other occasions.

were exchanged indirectly. In the Koryak seal festival in the fall, for example, the guests arrived at the festival house disguised in masks. The hosts tried to pull off the masks. If they succeeded, they offered their guests tea and food. If not, the masked guests were not served but silently showed the hosts a model of the gift they wished to receive, and only after receiving it did they take off their masks. The hosts could ask for gifts too. In these exchanges, refusal was not an option. Among the Chukchi the children served as mediators and were sent by the parents to ask for a present or to make a return one. Sometimes the exchange was performed without the givers' and receivers' seeing each other, by passing presents under the *polog* curtain.

Among the peoples of Chukotka and Kamchatka, ritual games were conducted with the whale spirit as part of the whale ceremony. The Chukchi whale ceremony ended with a pantomime of a hunt (cf. fig. 343). Inside the *polog* a wooden whale figure was suspended by four thongs, to each of which was attached a wooden model of an umiak with hunters. After ritual pantomimic dances, someone blew a cloud of white powder or graphite from the spout of the hollowed-out whale effigy, at which point it was suddenly lowered, causing the umiaks to slide down the thongs and strike it in imitation of a successful whaling hunt. In their private ceremonies the Eskimo also hung a whale figurine at the ceremonial pole or at the crossing of the *iaranga* poles and occasionally fed it with fat. To protect against disease, members of the household swung or threw the effigy to each other. The Koryak placed the actual head of a whale, dressed in its hood of grass, on a crossbeam of the dwelling. At the end of the ceremony two women in grass masks sang incantations to the whale's spirit. Then the men carried the head together with two seals into the forest. The return of the guest was guaranteed by offering part of the whale to the elements, as in a person's funeral. Krasheninnikov remarked on an Itelmen ceremony performed with a whale figurine made of grass and fish meal (*iukola*). A woman with a whale representation on her back crawled into the house and two people hit the whale with entrails while making calls like ravens. The ritual was completed when the whale effigy was torn into pieces and eaten, a widespread type of eucharistic ritual.

The spring umiak festival was also important in the annual cycle. It took place when the sea was free of ice. Members of the umiak team, led by the *umialik,* made a sacrifice to the Master of the Sea and then took the umiak frame down from its whalebone platform and recited incantations over it. The next day, the umiak was carried to the shore and put on a wooden platform, and sacrifices to the sea or to the Master of the Sea were made. The Koryak recalled that in former times a dog was sacrificed and the fire and the umiak were fed.

Another festival, the head festival, took place in early summer. Heads of walrus and bearded seals were taken from the caches and were set in a circle where they were fed by the elders. Then the umiak team tied a line to the largest walrus head and dragged it across the ground, as they did after a successful walrus hunt. There followed a feast of head meat, after which the remains were burned.

In recent decades these festivals have died out or become attenuated. When observed, they have usually been reduced to minimal form, including, sometimes, dances.

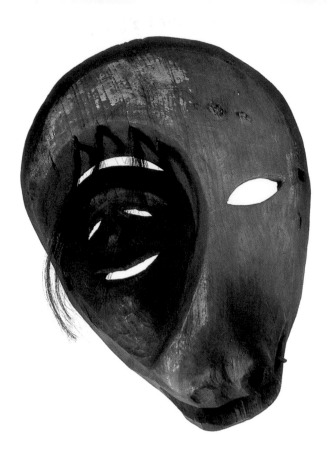

Eye of the Dance:
Spiritual Life of the Bering Sea Eskimo

Ann Fienup-Riordan

Much of what has been written concerning arctic peoples emphasizes their ability to survive in a frigid and inhospitable environment. Relatively little has been said about the values that make such survival culturally meaningful (but see Briggs 1970). On the contrary, a close look at the value systems of the peoples of the Far North reveals less environmental determinism than cultural imagination. The following is an attempt to represent the system of symbols and meanings that continue to guide the daily lives and ritual activities of the contemporary Yupik people of western Alaska. The representations in this essay are derived in part from late-19th- and early-20th-century reporters (e.g., Nelson 1899; Lantis 1947) but mostly from the author's own field observations from the present day, along with recent work on ceremonialism by Morrow (1984) and Mather (1985).

The loss of spiritual traditions in Siberia and some regions of Alaska by the time their cultures came to be recorded makes understanding of the rich, continuing culture and language of the Central Yupik peoples all the more important as a model for visualizing traditional belief systems and ideologies that were once more widely distributed in the North Pacific–Bering Sea region.

The Relationship Between Humans and Animals

Unlike the coastal Eskimo to the north, the Yupik Eskimo relied on neither the bowhead whale nor the walrus for their sustenance. Although the shallow coastline precludes the presence of either of these larger sea mammals, the coastal waters of the Bering Sea abound with a variety of seals as well as beluga whales, occasional walrus, and sea lions. The daily lives of the men and women of the Bering Sea coast were centered on the conquest of these sea mammals, as well as of an impressive variety of fish, land mammals, and waterfowl. In their dealings with these animals, the Yupik Eskimo did not view themselves as dominant over dumb, mute beasts that served them. Neither did they see themselves as dependent on or subordinate to the animals. On the contrary, they viewed the relationship between men and animals as collaborative reciprocity by which the animals gave themselves to the hunter in response to the hunter's respectful treatment of them as nonhuman persons.

According to the worldview of the Yupik Eskimo, human and nonhuman persons shared a number of characteristics. First and foremost, the perishable flesh of both humans and animals belied the immortality of their souls (''*yuas*''). All living things participated in an endless cycle of birth and rebirth of which the souls of animals and men were a part, contingent on right thought and action by others as well as self. For both men and animals, the soul was identified as the principle that sustained life. For sea mammals, the soul had an anatomical locus (the bladder). For human and nonhuman persons, the soul

347. Black Bear Inua Mask
Bering Sea Eskimo: NMNH 48986

Alaskan native peoples, like Siberians, believed that animals and objects possessed souls that could change into human and other forms. This concept is seen most clearly in inua masks made by Bering Sea Eskimos. This mask represents a black bear with its semihuman inua appearing in its right eye, partly obscured by human hair. Hunters often told of seeing inuas in the fur, feathers, or eyes of animals they were hunting. An encircling red-painted groove gave the mask spiritual life. One of a pair of two similar masks, perhaps used in a paired dance performance, this mask has lost its original white paint, its tongue, and its arcing array of white feathers.

remained in the vicinity of the body for a specified time after death before going to an extraterrestrial realm to await rebirth. For humans, an essential aspect of the person was reborn in the next generation. The newborn child regularly received both the name and with it the soul of a recently deceased relative in the ascending generation. Finally, inanimate objects were also believed to possess souls. Thus hunting implements were decorated not only to please or attract animals but also to impart life into and please the objects themselves.

Side by side with this belief in an essential spiritual continuity bridging the gap between the past and the future, the Yupik people allowed that men and animals alike possessed awareness. According to Joe Friday of Chevak:

We felt that all things were like us people, to the small animals like the mouse and the things like wood we liken to people as having a sense of awareness. The wood it is glad to the person who is using it and the person using it is grateful to the wood for being there to be used (Friday 1985).

As they gradually grew to maturity and gained awareness, both humans and animals were the recipients of a multitude of prescriptions (''*alerquutet*'') and proscriptions (''*inerquutet*'') for the culturally appropriate living of life. Three related ideas, however, may be seen to underlie this elaborate detail: the power of a person's thought, the importance of thoughtful action in order not to injure another's mind, and, conversely, the danger inherent in ''following one's own mind'' (Fienup-Riordan 1987:8ff).

As to the first point, the power of a person's thought, the clear message was that a person's attitude was as significant as his action. Thus young men were admonished to ''keep the thought of the seals'' foremost in their minds as they performed daily duties. In all these acts, by the power of their mind they were said to be ''making a way for the seals'' whom they would someday hunt. In the same way, a pregnant woman must keep the thought of her unborn child first in her mind to assure its well-being.

348. Grizzly Bear Spirit Realm
Bering Sea Eskimo: NMNH 38734
This mask represents the masked face (note mask bars on eyes) of a grizzly bear spirit confronting his traditional food, a salmon. His whiskers are made of quills, and three old-squaw feathers are set into his brow. In addition to an encircling painted ring, bentwood hoops called *ellanguat* (lit. pretend cosmos or universe) fitted with swan feathers surround his head. Similarly decorated hoops used in the Doll Festival were represented to Edward Nelson (1899:496) as being symbolic of the universe, with feathers and downy plumes being stars and snowflakes.

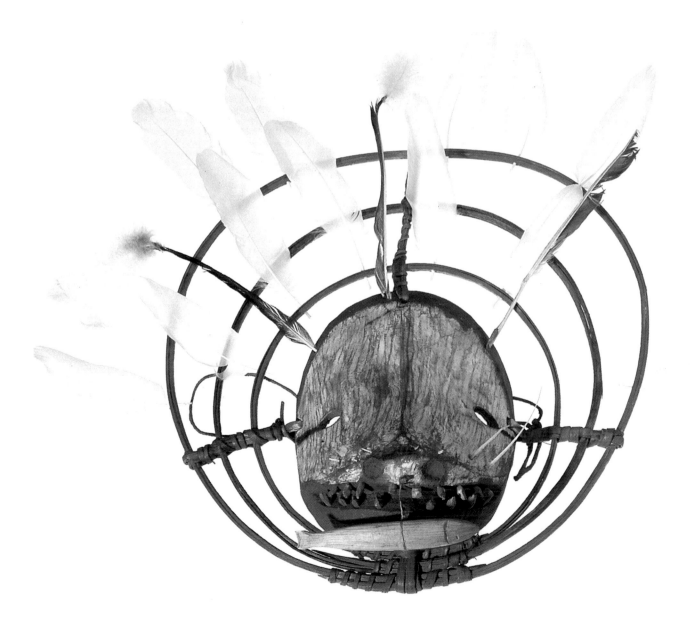

Animals were also subject to this stricture. For example, oral tradition describes how young seals were admonished by their elders to "stay awake" to the rules, both literally and figuratively, so that their immortal souls might survive the hunter's blow. If they were asleep when they were hit they would "die dead, forever" (Fienup-Riordan 1983:179).

In all tasks undertaken, the appropriate attitude was considered as important as the action. Conversely, for humans and animals the "power of the mind of the elders" to affect their future was cited as reason both to give help to an individual elder and to avoid their displeasure. One contemporary account admonished that young people be careful to perform these charitable tasks at night, so that no person would see them:

Only at night he clears the path.
If he does it during the day,
letting the people see him,
already then,
through the people he has his reward.

But if he does that with no one watching him
and nobody is aware of him,
only the one watching him,
the ocean or the land, . . .
the *ellam yua* [person or spirit of the universe] will give him his reward.

Second, as proper thought could effect success in the domain of human and animal interaction, so careful thought must reign over thoughtless action in order not to injure the mind of the other person. Ideally, smoothness and agreeableness should mask a person's emotions. This rule was as important in animal-human as in intrahuman interaction. For example, it was out of consideration or respect for the animal's mind that the hunter was admonished never to brag about either his projected accomplishments or past success. This same consideration also motivated his verbal apology when dispatching his prey.

Last of all, a number of traditional tales recalled the consequences of a person's following his own mind as opposed to following the advice of his elders. The results were usually disastrous, with retribution often experienced by the wrongdoer as well as his companions. In the oral tradition, some animals are identified as descended from human beings who were transformed as a consequence of willfully disregarding the rules.

In the end, human and nonhuman persons can be seen to share two fundamental characteristics: an immortal soul and mind or awareness. This essential similarity in turn creates the common ground on which their interaction is played out. Just as human hunters are capable of conscious decisions as to what and where to hunt, animals are likewise capable of conscious decisions that affect the success of individual hunters (e.g., the decision of a seal not to approach a hunter who appears to him as careless in either thought or action (Fienup-Riordan 1983:180).

As a result of the qualities of personhood shared alike by humans and animals, the basis for a mutual and necessary respect is established. One such instance of respectful action is the care given to animal bones. For example, great effort was made to remove every scrap of meat from seal bones. If this was not done, the seals would perceive the bones as loudly singing, warning them not to give themselves to those careless people. Traditionally bones were either buried, burned, or submerged. It was felt to be essential that bones not be left to lie around for fear they would be stepped on by men or chewed on by dogs. Moreover, the bones of food given away must be returned to the donor. The respect shown to animal bones was motivated by the desire that the animals be able to "cover their bones" in the future, that is, to return as edible game.

Although human-nonhuman interaction is made possible by the common possession of an immortal soul and a mind meriting respect, men and animals are also clearly differentiated. Within the oral tradition, these differences are least evident in the traditional tales of time out of mind. Moreover, the reality of the mythical

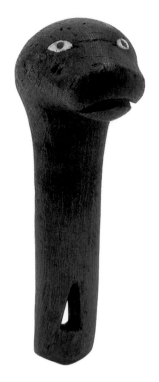

349. Fish Club
North Alaskan Eskimo: NMNH 64218
This club (cf. fig. 184) takes the form of a fish predator, the seal. Its ivory eyes are inlaid with dark wood plugs, and its whiskers and lashes are shown by finely incised lines and remnant stubs of fur. The scratch between the eyes indicates it is a masked spirit.

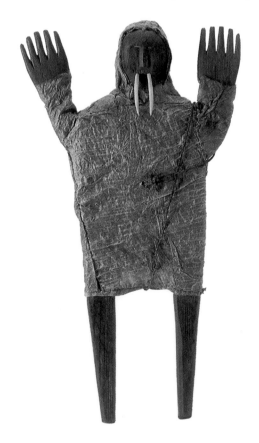

350. Walrus-Man
North Alaskan Eskimo: NMNH 89827
This powerful figure, made from a board, has (restored) tusks and ivory eyes, and wears a gutskin parka. A sinew line, probably for suspension, passes through a hole in the stomach.

Its identity and function are not known, but the pose suggests *Kikamigo*, the giant figure seen on Barrow gorgets standing amidst hunters and sea mammals with his arms upraised (fig. 444; Murdoch 1892:371, 394; Ray 1977:87). As a walrus-man in gutskin clothing it also resembles *Keretkun*, the Chukchi Master of the Sea, who had a special connection with walrus, lived at the bottom of the sea, wore gutskin clothes, and was represented in the *Keretkun* ceremony in the form of a figurine (Bogoras 1904-1909:316, 392; Serov, p. 254; see also Ray 1981: fig. 37).

258

351. Transformation Mask
Bering Sea Eskimo: NMNH 393152

A blood-stained *tunghak* is seen in
the face of this bird mask, which
combines stylistic features of Eskimo
and Indian art. Inua and *tunghak*
masks are common in Bering Sea Eskimo culture, but the use of fur,
painted hair, and cylindrical ear ornaments are typical of Ingalik Indian
masks. The mask was collected in
Norton Sound, but seems likely to
have originated among Eskimo-like
Ingalik Indians who lived upstream
on the Yukon River.

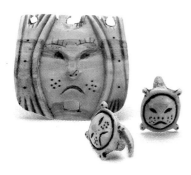

352. Seal Inua Ornaments
Bering Sea Eskimo: NMNH 37763,
43727 (pair)

Preoccupation with seals, a dominant
feature of Yupik Eskimo economic
and religious life in southwestern
Alaska, is seen in these earrings and
in a beltbuckle showing a seal inua
bounded by flipper designs.

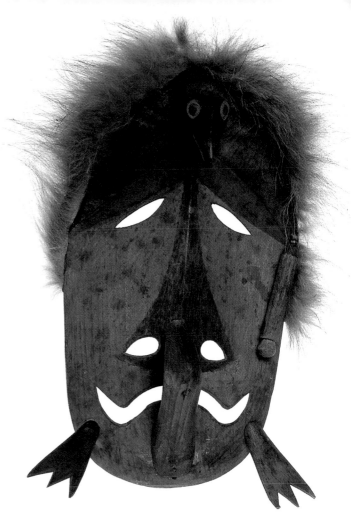

space-time they describe is still believed to be
present, although largely invisible. In these tales,
animals are often encountered who lift up their
beaks or muzzles, transforming themselves into
human form (e.g., Nelson 1899:394, 453). In the
tale of Ayugutaar, a Nelson Island hunter who
was visited by a wolf, the hunter's initial encounter with the wolf is described as follows:

After doing something around its head
and doing something to its mouth
when it faced him,
it became this way
taking its hood off.

In the same way, gaining awareness (''*ellange-*'')
is sometimes equated with peeling back the skin
of an animal, as when the puppies born to a
Nelson Island woman who had married a dog
peeled back their fur and revealed themselves
to their mother in human form. Nineteenth-
century transformation masks are a vivid portrayal of this perception of reality (fig. 435;
Fitzhugh and Kaplan 1982:215).

Along with the depiction of animal-human
transformations, the oral tradition also recalls
the subsequent process of differentiation by
which the physical and behavioral contrasts
between humans and animals occurred. For
example, the origin of the wolverine with its
vicious personality is attributed to the frustration
and subsequent transformation of a man following his desertion by his spirit wife (Tennant and
Bitar 1981:263). In these tales, contemporary
animal species are identified as descended from
transformed human beings.

Perhaps the most vivid accounts of animal-
human interaction, and those that best portray
both the similarities and the differences between
animal and human society, are tales that describe
humans visiting animal society and animals living within human society. An example of the
first is the story of the boy who went to live
with the seals (Fienup-Riordan 1983:177ff). On
arriving in the seals' underwater home, the boy
perceives his hosts as humans of differing sizes
and shapes, depending on their species identity.
Conversely, animals can enter human society,
as in the case of the wolf who takes human form
and comes to dwell with the hunter Ayugutaar.
However, the animal nature of the former is
always apparent, as in Ayugutaar's guest's pro-
pensity to crunch bones when he eats.

Although these tales depict animals as humans
and describe their social interaction, they also
serve to underline the differences between them.
For example, in the story of the boy who went
to live with the seals, emphasis is placed on
contrasting perceptions by describing the seals'
experience with humans from the seals' point
of view. From the seals' perspective, humans

who failed to live by the rules would appear
distorted in one way or another:

People would be walking
and one of the men on shore
would be seen as
having a necklace of many things
such as old mukluks.
Some men were encumbered as such.

It is said that
those are the ones
who continually walk
under everything that is hanging.

In the same way, after drinking from a bowl or
dipper, a person was required to make a stylized
removal motion, in which the right hand was
passed back and forth across his face to clear
his vision. If a man failed to perform this removal
motion, he would not be able to see game even
though it was well within his view. At the same
time, the animals would see him as having the
bowl stuck in the front of his face. Thus, the oral
tradition represents the perceptible differences
between humans and animals as overt and
perhaps illusory appearances that mask underlying resemblances between them. This hidden
world in which animals look like humans, speak
Yupik, wear clothes, and eat *akutaq* (a mixture
of berries, fat, seal oil, boned fish, sugar, and
other ingredients, sometimes called Eskimo ice
cream) figures in the stories as more real than

the conventional human experience of animals as speechless and differently formed.

In the end, the view persists that animals were once closer to humans, used human clothing and speech, but were gradually differentiated from their human counterparts. Their possession of mind as well as their rebirth after being killed and eaten by humans are described as essential aspects of their personhood, real yet unavailable to conventional observation. The ritual treatment given animals by Yupik people in western Alaska today presupposes these same shared aspects of personhood. To this day, animals are believed by some people to observe what is done to their carcasses, communicate with others of their kind, and experience rebirth after death. These aspects of the animal as a nonhuman person underlie and set the stage for everyday experience.

The Relationship Between Men and Women

Just as differences exist between humans and animals, there are also differences between men and women. This distinction traditionally framed, and continues to frame today, activities in everyday life. At the same time, the domains of hunting and procreation are ultimately joined and together are viewed as essential to assuring the reproduction of life.

To begin with, a well-documented sexual division of labor traditionally circumscribed daily activity in western Alaska. Men hunted while their mothers, wives, and daughters processed their catch. Men were largely, although not wholly, responsible for the provision of raw materials, while women worked in the house to produce food and clothing. The moment the hunter reached home, he lost jurisdiction over his catch. Along with processing the kill, women were also largely responsible for its distribution.

Into the 1940s, this division of tasks was replicated in a significant residential division. Men lived together communally in a large central dwelling (*qasgiq*) in which they worked, ate, slept, instructed male children, entertained visitors, took sweat baths, and held elaborate celebrations. Women and children, on the other hand, lived and worked in smaller sod houses (*enet*).

The residential division of the sexes that characterized village life had important ritual as well as social significance. In a variety of contexts, the women's house was comparable to a womb in which biological, social, and spiritual production were accomplished. It was in this house that women worked to transform the raw materials supplied by their men into food and clothing for the people. When a woman was pregnant, her activity within and exit from the house were likened to that of the fetus within her own body. For instance, upon waking each morning a pregnant woman must quickly rise and exit from the house, before she does anything else, so that her child's exit from the womb will be a speedy one (Fienup-Riordan 1983:184, 218).

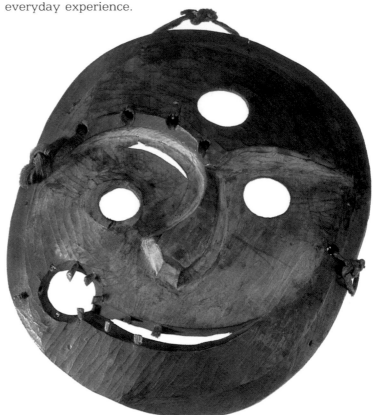

353. Lunar *Tunghak*
Bering Sea Eskimo: NMNH 38645
Bering Sea Eskimos believed the supreme diety that controlled animals, the *tunghak,* lived in the moon. It was to him they sent their shamans to plead for game and other favors. In addition to their ferocious, blood-stained mein, *tunghak* masks reflect lunar themes. This mask displays toothed orbs and crescents, and portrays the twisted-face ''old man in the moon.'' The right eye originally was masked by drooping hair, and feathers were mounted around the rim.

Furthermore, both the women's house and her womb were, under certain circumstances, equated with the moon, the home of *tunghaks*, the spirit keepers of the land animals. Spring itself was marked by the cutting of a door in the side of the women's sod house to permit ready egress. A similar opening in the moon was necessary to release the land animals for the new harvest season. As part of their effort to insure success in the coming year, shamans would journey to the moon (also sometimes a euphemism for sexual intercourse), where they were said to use their power to induce land animals to visit the earth.

Not only was the women's house viewed in certain contexts as a symbolic womb, productive of animals as well as men. Women's activity and inactivity were also directly tied to a man's ability to succeed in the hunt. First and foremost, contact with women was carefully circumscribed so that a man could retain his power to pursue game. Traditionally, men and women had distinctive eating utensils reserved for their exclu-

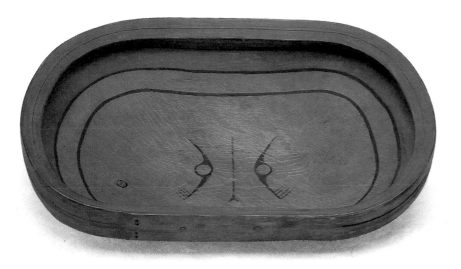

354. Conventionalized Animal Face
Bering Sea Eskimo: NMNH 33060

Two nucleated circles are the basis for this simple rendition of an animal's face, showing eyes, nose, whiskers, and markings. Nucleated circles (also known as the circle and dot) have been used for thousands of years in Eskimo art. In the Central Yupik language, they are called *ellam iinga*, meaning "eye of awareness." These and other symbols were used by Bering Sea Eskimo to support their complex transformational view of the spirit-world.

Many different kinds of illustrations were used on the inside of bentwood food bowls, including animals, legendary beings, and hunting scenes. No doubt, people learned (and told) stories from these designs while eating. Bowls with bentwood rims were used by women; unrimmed bowls by men. Although collected from an Eskimo village this bowl was attributed to Ingalik Indian manufacture (Fitzhugh and Kaplan 1982:238).

sive use. Women's bentwood bowls were made with a rim, and men's bowls were blunt-edged. In bed with his own wife, a man was warned never to sleep facing her, lest the braid of her hair appear hanging in front of his face and subsequently block his vision.

Women's air was also considered polluting to young hunters and dulled their senses. According to Paul John of Toksook Bay, a man's breath soul (*anerneq*) was particularly vulnerable to contamination from such contacts. That such proscriptions affected a man's ability to hunt is attested to in a description of a shaman's visit to the underwater home of the seals occurring during the celebration of the Bladder Festival at the coastal village of Chevak. When peeking in the skylight, the shaman overheard the conversation of the "bladder people":

Some of them will say they had a good host and will go back to the same host. Some of them will say they had a bad host because the host always made him smell female odor and would say he is not going back to his former host (Friday 1984).

At the same time that female odor repelled animals, the smell of the land was believed to attract them. For this reason, hunters fumigated themselves with the smoke of wild celery, Labrador tea, and blackberry bushes, among other things, to prepare for the hunt.

355. Ornamented Sewing Gear
(Top to bottom) Bering Sea Eskimo: NMNH 176142, 43661, 16140, 43535; Aleut: 316777

These women's sewing implements include a thread spool, a bootcreaser (to crimp and gather the soles), a seal-shaped fastener for a woman's "housewife," or workbag, an awl, and a birdbone needle blank. In ivory graphic arts, an Eskimo specialty, nucleated circles served variously as eyes, as jointmarks, and simply as decorative elements.

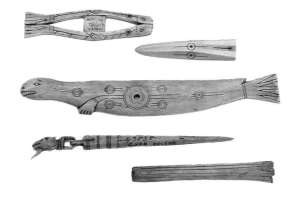

At the same time that a hunter had to protect himself from the depleting effects of unclean air, socially restricted sight was necessary to procure powerful supernatural vision. Likewise, young women were admonished from direct eye contact with hunters.

In all social as well as ritual situations direct eye contact was, and continues to be, considered rude for young people, male or female, whereas downcast eyes signify humility and respect. Sight is the prerogative of age, of knowledge, and of power. For example, the powerful man in the moon has a bright face, and people fear to look at him and must look downwards. The powerful shades of the dead were traditionally said to hear and see nothing at first. However, by the time they reached the grave, they had attained clairvoyance (Nelson 1899:425). Finally, powerful images and hunting fetishes were supposed to watch for game and, by clairvoyant powers, sight it at a great distance (Nelson 1899:436).

A material manifestation of vision imagery is seen in the nucleated circle that appears as decoration on many hunting charms as well as objects of everyday use (figs. 181, 195, 355, 357). The circle-dot motif, so common in Eskimo iconography, is specifically designated *ellam iinga* (literally, "the eye of awareness") in the Central Yupik language. The nucleated circle has, in the literature, been designated as a joint mark and, as such, part of a skeletal motif. Alternately, it has been labeled a stylized woman's breast that might then be substituted for a woman's face (Ray 1981:25; Himmelheber 1953:62). The sexual and skeletal motifs may well have been part of its significance. However, it was not merely that the nucleated circle marked joints but rather that joints were marked with circular eyes (Fienup-Riordan 1986, 1987a). Here William Thalbitzer's (1908:447ff) observation on the Greenlandic Eskimo is particularly significant: "According to Eskimo notions, in every part of the human body (particularly in every joint, as for instance, in every finger joint) there resides a little soul."

Throughout the Arctic, joint marking was associated with social transformation in various contexts. For example, in western Alaska the wrists of young men and women were tattooed with dots on the occasion of their first kill or first menstruation, respectively. Ritual scarification has also been observed among the Siberian Yupik Eskimo (Bogoras 1904:408), and Waldemar Bogoras records that among the Maritime Chukchi of Northeast Siberia tattooed joint marks once served as a tally of homicides. When these tattooing customs are considered in the context of the custom of applying eye-shaped markings

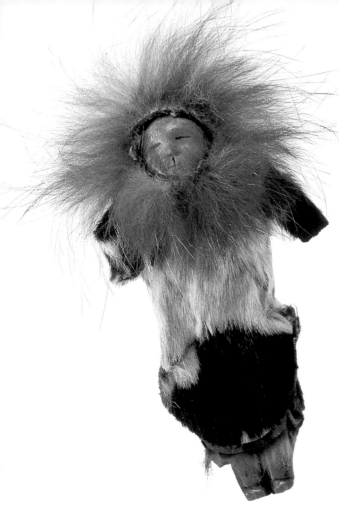

to the joints, it strongly suggests that the tattooed joint mark is itself the rudiment of the eye motif (Schuster 1951:18).

As in the circle-dot motif as applied to material objects, the puberty tattoo denoted enhanced vision. In fact in the oral tradition, one mark of a transformed character is the appearance of black circles around the eyes. Dark circles also appear as goggles on Bering Sea Eskimo 19th-century objects (figs. 45, 358, 362, 435, 437, 438). These goggles identify beings as supernatural, are puns for masking, and refer to their state of transformation. One contemporary Central Yupik hunter recalled his mother circling his eyes with soot when, at age nine, he returned to the village after killing his first bearded seal (Fienup-Riordan 1987a:43).

Not only were joints marked with eyes as a sign of social transformation. Actually cutting an animal or human on the joints was also associated with spiritual transformation, as when the joints of dangerous animals were cut to prevent the animal's spirit from reanimating its body. In the same way, the shaman might be ritually dismembered prior to his journey to the spirit world. Traveling out through the smoke hole or down through a hole in the ice, he would visit the *yuas* (souls) of the fish and game to entreat them to return the coming year. The nucleated circle, both an eye and a hole, thus recalls the ability to pass from one world to another, as well as the ability to see into another world.

An example of the relationship between socially restricted sight and powerful supernatural vision is contained in the traditional tale of the boy who lived and traveled with the seals for one year to gain extraordinary hunting knowledge and power:

And his host [the bearded seal] said to him,
"Watch him [the good hunter], watch his eyes, see what good vision he has.
When his eyes see us, see how strong his vision is.
When he sights us, our whole being will quake,
and this is from his powerful gaze.
When you go back to your village, the women,
some will see them, not looking sideways, but looking directly at their eyes.
The ones who live like that, looking like that,
looking at the eye of women,
their vision will become less strong.
When you look at women your vision will lose its power.
Your sight gets weakened.
But the ones that don't look at people, at the center of the face,
the ones who use their sight sparingly,
as when you have little food, and use it little by little.
So, too, your vision, you must be stingy with your vision,
using it little by little, conserving it always.
These, then, when they start to go hunting,
and use their eyes only for looking at their quarry,
their eyes truly then are strong.

In the above the finite nature of human sight is especially significant. A hunter's vision, like his thought and breath, must not be squandered. Significantly, a man's ability to harvest animals as an infinitely renewable resource was contingent on his careful use of his own finite personal human resources. Moreover, a hunter's ability to succeed in the hunt was not only tied to his care of the animals but also to his relationship with women.

Not only did a woman's actions impact the power of the hunter to attract and overcome game but also, in specific contexts, a woman's actions were believed to affect directly the actions of the fish and game the hunter sought. For instance, when her husband went in search of certain land animals at fall camp, a woman was required to remain at rest within the house, sometimes called her "den," neither working nor coming outside. In some instances, she was equated with the hunter's prey, her inactivity directly related to the inactivity (and subsequent

356. Child's Doll
Bering Sea Eskimo: NMNH 129236

This doll is typical of those owned by every young Bering Sea Eskimo girl. The dolls were armless so their clothing could be removed easily for seasonal changes of fashion. Girls were not allowed to play with dolls inside the house or during winter. They had to await the coming of spring, signaled by the arrival of geese. If they cheated, the geese would fly past without stopping and winter would pass without summer directly into winter.

357. Storyknife
Bering Sea Eskimo: NMNH 127403

For a Yupik Eskimo girl, an ivory storyknife was her most treasured plaything besides her dolls. Made by her uncle, the storyknife was used to draw pictures and shorthand symbols in the sand, illustrating stories she made up or heard. This storyknife, like most, has an image of a bird—probably a puffin—on the hilt, in addition to a collar motif, three nucleated circles, and a skeletized spine. No certain information exists on the symbolism of storyknife decoration, but it appears to represent stylized birds.

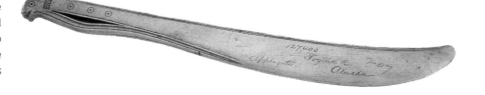

huntability) of the animals her husband sought as described elsewhere with regard to the whaling ritual (p. 168). In other cases, the care with which she worked was felt to impact directly the willingness of animals to give themselves to her husband. For instance, if a man's wife was a sloppy seamstress, her irregular stitchery would cause animals to run away. Finally, in the case of sea mammals, a woman was felt to attract or draw the animals by virtue of the fresh water she gave their thirsty souls immediately following their successful capture. While performing this action, the woman would talk to the seal, saying, "See our water here is tasty, very inviting."

At different stages in her life, a woman affected men differently. For a young woman, the most important event in her maturation was celebrated following her first menstruation. At this time, a girl was sequestered, her condition comparable to that of the fetus in her social invisibility, restriction of movement, and the prohibition against both childhood and adult activities:

Then in the spring time,
when they became aware that she had become a woman,
they let her sit down.
They put a grass mat in front of her,
and then behind her they made a door.
They didn't let her go out through the regular doorway.
Only through the back door . . .
And those girls who had become women,
they let them wear old clothes,
and their mittens had no thumbs.
And when they went to the bathroom they put their hood on
without looking around,
and their head bowed really low.
They go to the area where trash was taken.
They would urinate in the dumping place.
These are some of the things for those who had sat down.

Here a number of elements evoke the power of the menstruating woman to impact the harvest. These include the image of the thumbless hand (figs. 180, 436) simultaneously signifying the idea of impaired grasp and its relation to game productivity (Nelson 1899:395), as well as the restricted sight and use of a hood described above as prerequisite for male hunting power.

On the occasion of her "standing up" after this period of isolation, the girl was required to give away her childhood playthings, including small dolls and their clothing, to other prepubescent females (fig. 356). The restrictions surrounding the use of these dolls are particularly meaningful. Young girls were forbidden from using their dolls during the winter or inside the house, their use being restricted to the outside after the return of the geese. Their dormancy

in the interior of the house during the winter and their emergence in the summer replicates both the transformation of their owners through puberty restrictions into women capable of giving birth and the birth process itself (Fienup Riordan 1983:218). It was believed that if a young girl was to play with a doll outside the house before the arrival of spring, the birds would pass by and winter would move into winter with no intervening season. Here again inappropriate female activity was directly tied to cosmological upset and subsequent human disaster.

Not surprisingly, one of the first women to impact a hunter's relationship with animals was his mother. While she carried the fetus, a woman's actions were not only believed to influence the immediate well-being of her child but also its future abilities as a hunter.

And it was an *inerquun* that never,
through the window,
was she to try to see what was going on.
She was only to check by going through the door.

When she's curious about something,
she is to go outside and find out about it.

And if she does that,
when her son grows up
and goes hunting,
when the animals hear him and become curious,
they would show themselves to him and be caught.

All those things that she is doing
to that baby of hers, if it's a boy,
towards the times when he will be trying to do things,
the things she does or doesn't do while pregnant affect them.

His mother then,
like the one who makes his catch available,
like the one who makes his catch visible,
she will give to the one she is carrying.

A number of rules continue to tie the actions of the mother and child (male or female) throughout its growing up. For instance, a woman was traditionally admonished never to breast-feed her child while lying down but rather to sit up and unabashedly bare her breast for him to make him tough and strong. Were she to be lazy, her careless attitude and action would directly undermine her child's future hunting ability. As he grew, a mother constantly taught her son the rules by which he would live. Significantly, her advice focused on the distance he must keep from women:

A child,
if it is a boy,
he is never to go near a female.
He is not to look at a female squarely in the face.
And on the lee side of a female he was to pass,
and never was he to be stepped over by a woman.

Then, finally, at the age of five or six he was ready to leave her: "Leaving his mother, moving out of his mother to those men, he joins them."

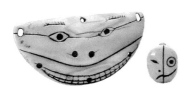

358. Reality, Masked
Bering Sea Eskimo: NMNH 37745, 43670

Concepts of transformation and masking, so pervasive in Bering Sea Eskimo belief, were illustrated on women's jewelery. A masked semihuman *tunghak* decorates this hair ornament, and a seal-person transformation appears on an earring. Belief in the mutability of the physical and the spiritual, of multiple worlds and realities in constant transformation, was the basis for highly creative Bering Sea Eskimo art.

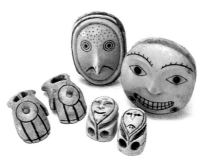

359. Ivory Kayak Ornaments
Bering Sea Eskimo (clockwise from top): NMNH 43509, 176145, 44709, 37063, 43538

The large float plugs are decorated with a human face with beaded eyes and labrets and a short-eared owl with red mineral eyes. The line fasteners (*lower right*) illustrate gender iconography: smiles (corner labrets) are male; frowns (center labrets) are female. Spearguards are decorated with performated hands, a common *tunghak* motif.

The Window Between the Worlds: Houses, Holes, Eyes, and Passages

When young boys came to live in the men's house (*qasgiq*), they entered the social and ceremonial center of the Yupik world. It was in the men's house that they would receive technical training as well as careful instruction in the rules that they must follow to become successful hunters. Under the tutelage of their fathers and uncles, even very young boys were expected to rise early and work diligently in the performance of a number of manual tasks. It was the boys' job to keep the communal water bucket continually filled, as well as to keep the entryway and skylight of the men's house cleared of snow.

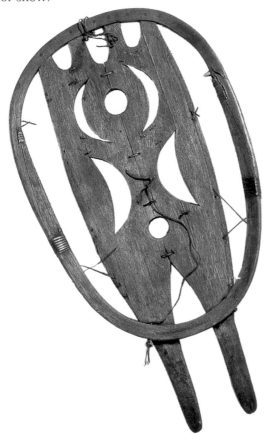

As in a woman's work, the performance of these tasks had both practical and ritual implications. For instance, the water bucket must be kept full at all times to attract the seals, who were always thirsty for fresh water. Likewise, boys were required to keep the water hole constantly free of ice and to take care to drink from it only in a prone position to please "the old woman of the hole," who would subsequently send them good luck in hunting. Here the water hole was explicitly designated the window of the world below.

In stories such as "The Boy Who Went to Live With the Seals," the male seal spirits were depicted as living in an underwater men's house

from within which they could view the attention of would-be hunters by watching the condition of the central smoke hole in their underwater abode. If hunters were giving them proper thought and care, the smoke hole would appear clear. If not, the hole would be covered with snow and nothing would be visible. When their visibility was obstructed in this way the seals would not emerge from their underwater world or allow themselves to be hunted. It was this vision that young men sought to maintain as they carefully cleared ice from skylights and water holes (Fienup-Riordan 1983:178).

The performance of a number of important ceremonies in the men's house dramatically reinforced the notion of the ice hole and smoke hole alike as passageways between the human and nonhuman worlds. For instance, one of the most important traditional ceremonies was the Bladder Festival, held annually to insure the rebirth of the *yuas*, or spirits of the seals, which were said to be located in their bladders. During the closing performances of the Bladder Festival, the shaman would climb out through the skylight to enter the sea, visit the seal spirits, and request their return. Likewise the inflated bladders were removed through the *qasgiq* smoke hole at the end of the festival and taken to the ice hole. There they were deflated and sent back to their underwater *qasgiq* with the request that they return the following year (fig. 366).

In addition to serving as a passage permitting movement and communication between the world of the hunter and the hunted, the central *qasgiq* smoke hole was also a passageway between the world of the living and the dead. For example, in the event of a human death, the body of the deceased was pulled through the smoke hole, after first being placed in each of its four corners. By this action the deceased, on the way from the world of the living to the dead, gradually exchanged the mortal sight that it lost at death for the supernatural clairvoyance of the spirit world (Nelson 1899:425). Although both the smoke hole and the ice hole were rectangular rather than round, this does not undercut their significance as spiritual eyes. One variant of the circle-dot motif is, in fact, a rectangle with four small projections, one at each corner, within which was carved a dot surrounded by concentric circles (fig. 299). In fact, the numbers four and five figure prominently in Central Yupik ritual, representing among other things the number of steps leading to the underworld land of the dead. The Bladder Festival rituals use four corners and four sets of hunting and boating gear. At one stage in its performance, the

360. Floatboard and Paddles
Eskimo: MAE 11-167
Bering Sea Eskimo: NMNH 36057
Yupik cosmology is represented in this unique but undocumented kayak floatboard, whose cutouts can be read either as lunar phases or a human figure. In addition, animal regeneration may be indicated by the round holes, since the souls of new animals (particularly seals) are brought into the world through the sky-hole, and leave it by being sunk through the ice hole at the end of the Bladder Festival (fig. 366).

The paddles are decorated with a female sexual emblem seen when the blades are conjoined, and have *tunghak* faces cut into their handles.

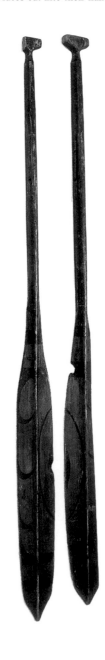

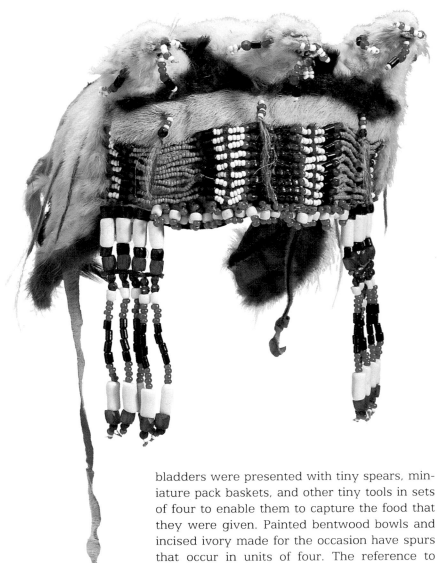

361. Beaded Ermine Skin Dance Headdress

Koniag Eskimo: NMNH 90451

This headdress collected on the Alaskan Peninsula in 1884 combines spiritually powerful land and sea predators—ermine and pelagic cormorant—in a ceremonial headdress. Three ermines with beads attached to their jaws, nostrils, and ears project from the brim over an elaborate beaded brow panel. The ermine skins are quilted into a base of cormorant skins, and red wool and grey (human?) hair tassels hang from the sides of the headdress. Beaded pendants ''obstruct'' the dancer's vision, a necessary requirement for certain dances. Obstructed vision is also a characteristic of Siberian Shaman hats (fig. 333).

362. Dance Fans

Bering Sea Eskimo: 38855a,b

Whereas men wore gloves, women danced with delicately carved fans, also called finger masks, in each hand.

bladders were presented with tiny spears, miniature pack baskets, and other tiny tools in sets of four to enable them to capture the food that they were given. Painted bentwood bowls and incised ivory made for the occasion have spurs that occur in units of four. The reference to square or rectangular holes and the quadrangle functioning like a circle and dot may form a logical symbolic complex with this added sacred dimension.

Not only did the motif of the ringed center connote spiritual vision and movement between worlds but the act of encircling was also performed in various contexts to produce enhanced spiritual vision or as protection from spiritual invasion. For example, during the Bladder Festival, young men ran counter clockwise around the village before entering the men's house bearing bunches of wild celery needed to purify the bladders and ''let them see'' the gifts of the people. Likewise, when a man hunted sea mammals at certain times of the year, he had to circle his kill in the direction of the sun's course before retrieval. The boat itself was also ritually circled before launching in the spring, both in Alaska and in Siberia (Usugan 1984; Moore 1923:369; Bogoras 1904:404ff). Similarly, on the third or fifth day after the birth of a child in western Alaska, the new mother traditionally emerged from her confinement, marking her return to social visibility by circling the house, again in the direction of the sun's course. Finally,

on the fifth day after a human death, the grave was circled in the direction of the sun's circuit by the bereaved to send away the spirit of the deceased. All of these ritual acts recall the magic circle reported by Knud Rasmussen (1927:129, 1931:60) from the Netsilik region, whereby people walked in a circle around strangers who approached their camp so that their footprints would contain any evil spirits that might have accompanied the newcomers.

The performance of a marriage dance (*ingulaq*) during the Bladder Festival on Nelson Island continues the image of the ringed center with the connotation of vision as well as movement between worlds. This was a slow, stylized dance by a young bride who appeared with lowered eyes and bedecked in the furs and finery produced for her by her newly acquired mate. This dance often depicted a particularly successful harvesting episode. The marriage dance performed on this occasion provided a strong image of the complementarity between the production of game and the reproduction of life. While literally dancing the successful hunt, the bride held her skirt below the waist and rhythmically ''fluffed it up to ward off old age and to let her have children.'' This expansive gesture by a sexually mature woman was in sharp contrast to the rule requiring young unmarried girls to hold their skirts tightly down around their legs when entering or exiting the *qasgiq*. If they failed to do so, it was said that the old men would grab at their vaginal areas ''to teach them respect.''

When a woman performed the marriage dance, she appeared before the audience with studiously down-cast eyes. On this occasion, as in other dance performances, her head was encircled with a beaded wolverine crown (cf. figs. 361, 365). The effect of this head ornament was simultaneously to restrict her view as well as to protect her from supernatural powers. It is possible that the grass masks used by some Kamchatkan peoples as well as similar grass head coverings occasionally used in western

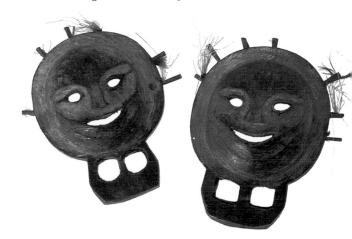

265

Alaska also functioned to restrict human sight and protect the dancer from the effects of powerful supernatural vision (fig. 346).

The grass and beaded headdresses were far from the only paraphernalia used in Central Yupik Eskimo ceremonials. A major focus among Bering Sea Eskimo was masked dancing. Following the Bladder Festival a ceremony designated *Kelek* occurred, during which shamanic visions of the spirit world were translated into carved masks, which were used in elaborate dramatic performances. Ritually powerful masks were created representing both the spirits of the game (*yuas*) as well as the *tunghaks*, or shaman's spirit helpers (figs. 180, 348, 436). These large hooped masks are in the oral tradition directly equated with the circle-dot motif described above, and their powerful supernatural gaze directly contrasted to the restricted sight of the other performers.

Like the circle-dot motif, the large hooped masks functioned as eyes into a world beyond the mundane. First of all, the mask was structurally a ringed center. The face of the mask was often framed in multiple wooden rings called *ellanguat* (literally, "pretend cosmos" or "universe"). These concentric rings represent the different levels of the universe, which was traditionally said to contain five upper worlds and the earth (Ray 1967:66). This same heavenly symbolism was repeated in ceremonial activity in which the masked dancer was a key participant. For example, multiple rings, also called *ellanguat* and decorated with bits of down and feathers, were lowered and raised from the inside of the men's house roof during the traditional Doll Festival and were said to represent the retreat and approach of the heavens, complete with snow and stars (Nelson 1899:496; Ray 1967).

The image of the encircling ring can also be seen in the rounded dance fans, fringed in both

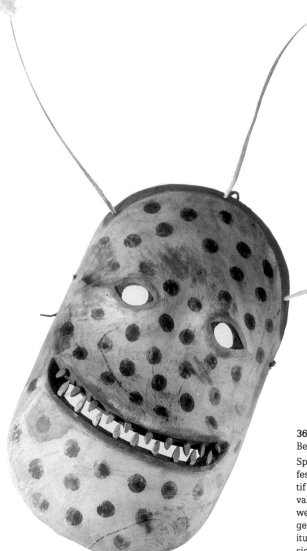

363. Spotted Mask
Bering Sea Eskimo: NMNH 153627
Spots were important in a number of festivals, but the meaning of this motif is not clear. In the Bladder Festival the bladders hung in the *qasgiq* were painted white with colored fingerspots (possibly equivalent to spiritual eyes?) to promote spiritual vision of the seal inuas. In other festivals, men's and boy's bodies were painted and spotted when they paraded from house to house.

fur and feathers, held in the hands of the dancers. These fans are reminiscent of the mask worn by the central dancer, often having animal or human faces. With their eyes respectfully downcast during the performance, women even now speak of the fan's eye as seeing for them while they dance.

Finally, the open-work design of the fans held by Yupik Eskimo dancers is to this day explicitly compared to the pierced hand found as an appendage on many traditional masks. The hole in the hand's center, like the opening in the dance fan, is by some accounts a symbolic passage through which the spirits of fish and game come to view their treatment by men and, if they find it acceptable, repopulate the world. Thus the dancers, both male and female, holding dance fans and arms extended in the motions of the dance, are like gigantic transformation masks, complete with animal-spirit faces to which the wooden pierced hands are appended.

Given this perspective, one may reasonably contrast the efficacy of the mask's supernatural sight to the lowered gaze of the human perform-

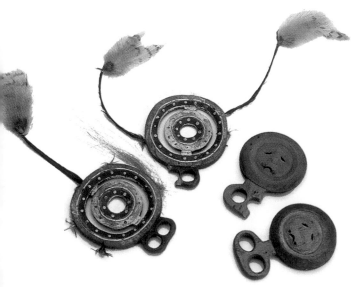

364. Nucleated and Walrus-Face Dance Fans
Bering Sea Eskimo: NMNH 38451 (pair), 37127, 38649
These dance fans illustrate two common varieties used in the Yukon-Kuskokwim Delta region. Both sets originally had caribou fur trim. The pair on the left also has old-squaw feathers trimmed with down, and its hoops, spots, and ringed centers probably relate to spiritual vision. The other pair depict walrus spirits, possibly walrus-men.

ers who dance so that they truly ''see,'' and that the spirits see them. According to one contemporary Yupik elder, the traditional application of a white clay base and colored finger spots to the bladders inflated for the Bladder Festival was likewise an attempt to promote spiritual vision on the part of the souls of the seals. The painting of the wooden masks, as well as the painting of the body of the dancer, had a similar effect, allowing the dancer to become visible to the spirit world and in fact to embody the spirit at the same time that his human identity was hidden from the world of men.

In sum, the Yupik universe was traditionally depicted as subject to constant alteration yet ultimate unity in the repetition of reproductive and productive cycles. It is, ultimately, both the alterations and unity that the hooped mask and the performance of masked dances embody. The use of the hooped mask provides a vivid image for the system of cosmological reproduction through which the Yupik Eskimo traditionally viewed, and to some extent continue to view, the universe. The same image of supernatural sight that dominates the hooped mask can also be seen in the rounded lamp and the ringed bowl, the hole in the kayak float board and the decorative geometry of traditional ivory earrings, the central gut skylight opening from the men's house and the decorative celestial rings suspended from its ceiling for a dance performance. The world was bound, the circle closed. Yet within it was the passageway leading from the human to the spirit world. Rimmed by the *ellanguat* and transformed by paint and feathers, the eyes of the mask, themselves often ringed, looked beyond this world into another.

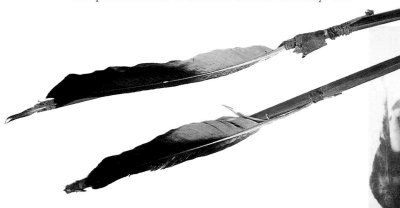

365. Festival Dress
SI neg. 6370, E.W. Nelson, 1881
Bering Sea Eskimo: NMNH 49060, 49061

In some festivals Eskimo women danced with large eagle feather wands made of golden eagle wing feathers tied to slender rods. Plumes of eagle down were attached to the tips of the feathers, and tufts of wolf or Siberian reindeer fur to the base. These wands have lost their attachments, shown in the accompanying photograph taken at a festival in Andraevsky on the Lower Yukon River. The women wear ermine skin dance fillets whose hanging portions restrict sight and relate to the concept of spiritual vision. The use of ermine and sight-restricting panels also occurs on Koniag dance headdresses (fig. 361). The ermine, a powerful spirit ally, was respected for its quickness and courage, exemplary in such a small creature.

The Traditional Yupik Ceremonial Cycle

After freeze-up in November Yupik Eskimo gathered in their winter villages, where they enjoyed a number of public celebrations that marked winter as the ceremonial season. Five major ceremonies were performed during this period, three of which focused on the creative reformation of the relationship between the human community and the spirit world on which they relied. In all three of these ceremonies (the Bladder Festival, the Feast for the Dead, and the masked dances known as *Kelek*) members of the spirit world were invited into the community, formally hosted, and finally sent back out of the human domain. This ritual movement effectively recreated the relationship between the human and spirit worlds and placed each in the proper position to begin the year again.

The Bladder Festival

The celebration of the Bladder Festival (*Nakaciuq*) marked the opening of the winter ceremonial season. At the time of the winter solstice, the bladders of seals killed that year were inflated and brought into the men's house. These bladders were believed to contain the animals' souls, and during their stay in the men's house they were treated as honored guests. The bladders were hung across the back wall, a position comparable to the position of honor in the men's house occupied by the elders, who were likewise nearing the time of their departure from this world.

The primary function of the Bladder Festival was to reverse the separation of body and soul effected at the time of the seal's death. The Bladder Festival proper was preceded by a ceremony known as *Qaariitaaq* in many areas. During *Qaariitaaq*, the village boys had their bodies painted and were led from house to house each night, where they were given food by the women. Through this ritual circuit, the children opened the community to the seal spirits.

Aaniq (literally, ''to provide a mother'') was held directly after *Qaariitaaq* and introduced the Bladder Festival proper. During *Aaniq*, two older

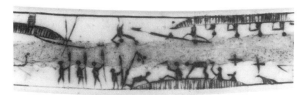

men, dressed in gutskin parkas and referred to as mothers, led a group of boys who were termed their dogs around the village. The men collected newly made bowls filled with *akutaq* (a mixture of berries, seal oil, boned fish, and tallow) from the women, a reversal of the usual pattern of women bringing cooked meat to their men in the men's house. In many areas *Qaari-itaaq* and the Bladder Festival each lasted for five days, a number that corresponded with the five steps that separated the world of the living and the dead.

During the Bladder Festival, the men's house and its residents were ritually purified by sweat baths as well as by the smoke from wild celery plants. Routine activities were set aside, and the days were devoted to athletic competitions between married and unmarried men, instruction in and performance of commemorative songs, and the presentation of special feast foods. All of these activities were performed with the intent to draw out the souls of the seals, residing in the bladders hung along the wall of the men's house.

On the last night of the Bladder Festival, the entire village as well as invited guests from nearby villages gathered in the men's house. Gifts were given by parents to celebrate their children's accomplishments. The wooden dolls of the young girls who had come of age were distributed. Finally, a huge villagewide distribution took place, in which large amounts of frozen and dried fish, and sealskin pokes full of seal oil were given away. When giving these gifts, each donor was particular to say that everything had been given to him. Giving gifts in someone else's name, particularly that of a deceased kinsman, was a feature of a number of ceremonial distributions. To this day in western Alaska, social ties between the living are both created and maintained through the relationship between the living and the dead.

Finally, at the close of the Bladder Festival, pairs of young men took the inflated bladders along with bunches of wild celery out through the central smoke hole and down to a hole in the ice. There the bladders would be deflated and returned to their underwater home, where they would boast of their good treatment and subsequently allow themselves to be taken by the villagers the following season.

The Feast for the Dead

The annual Feast for the Dead (known in some areas as *Merr'aq*, from a word meaning water) was the public occasion on which the spirits of the human dead were invited into the human community to receive the food and clothing they required. It was initiated when men placed stakes at the graveside, effectively opening the village and inviting the spirits to enter as in the ceremonies prior to the Bladder Festival. As in the Bladder Festival, the village was ritually cleansed in preparation for the arrival of the spirits. Moreover, great care was taken during the ceremonial period to limit any human activity (such as sewing or chopping wood) that might injure or cut the souls as they entered the village.

The Great Feast for the Dead, *Elriq*, was a much more complex and elaborate event. It attracted hundreds of people from the far corners of the Yukon and Kuskokwim Delta and continued for four to six days. *Elriq* was sequentially hosted by different villages within a single subregion. Within each village, the feast was hosted primarily by a single individual, aided by his relatives. The major distributions took place on the fourth and fifth days of the ceremony, when first the women and then the men ritually clothed the living namesake according to the sex of the deceased relative. Gifts were brought into the men's house through the gut skylight, the reverse route used to remove the human body at death.

The Gift Festival

Another important winter ceremony was the "commercial play" known as *Petugtaq*. This event is usually described as an exchange of gifts between the men and women of one village. Normally the gifts given were relatively small. The men might begin the play by making tiny replicas of things that they desired, such as grass socks, bird-skin caps, or fish-skin mittens. These replicas would be hung from a wand or stick and taken to the women of the village. Each woman then chose one of the images and prepared the item requested. When all was ready, the women brought their gifts to the men's house, where they presented them to the men, who were duty-bound to provide a suitable return.

In some areas at least, enjoyment derived from the pairing of both biologically and socially unlikely couples in the exchange, because no one knew who had made a specific request until the actual distribution. In this context the pairing of cross cousins was considered particularly delightful. In Yupik the terms used to refer to cross-sex cross cousins were *nuliacungaq* ("dear little wife") and *uicungaq* ("dear little husband").

366. The Bladder Festival
Norton Sound Eskimo: NMNH 44399

This pictographic panel from an engraved ivory drillbow collected at Cape Nome illustrates the culmination of the Bladder Festival, held in December at the winter solstice. After several days of ceremonial activity, the bladders, in which resided the souls of all the sea mammals killed during the previous year, were taken out of the *qasgiq* and sunk through a hole in the ice, releasing the spirits to be reborn as new animals next year. In this panel a procession of men bearing four ritual paddles and a staff of bladders surround the ice hole, while men with knives stab the bladders, one by one, and sink them.

The Bladder Festival is one of a group of harvest renewal festivals, such as the Chukchi *Keretkun* and Koryak Whale Festival, found in the North Pacific-Bering Sea region. Some details of the ceremonies are nearly identical, suggesting cross-cultural contacts.

367. Festival Masks

Norton Sound Eskimo: NMNH 33106, 153623

Masks played an important role in the festival life of Yupik Eskimo peoples. Yupik ceremony included a great variety of mask types, including huge *tunghak* masks that were suspended from the roof of the *qasgiq*, to be danced behind; plaque masks such as the one on the left, which were worn but not danced with; and smaller face masks (*right*), worn by active dancers. Most of the masks used in ceremonial performances had special transformational qualities relating to legend or religious belief, presented in iconographic forms not well understood today. Even so, as works of art, they stand as major achievements. Following their use in ceremonies, most masks were thrown away or burned, their spiritual essence rising to the heavens in smoke.

On the left is a probable black bear mask combined with bird (Raven?) imagery, and on the right a half-face transformation mask (cf. fig. 358), possibly a *tunghak*, with "toothed" crescent mouths and eye.

Marriage between cross cousins was not traditionally prescribed. However, teasing complete with sexual innuendo characterized the relationship between cross cousins, as distinct from the much more serious and respectful relationship between siblings and parallel cousins, and the proper day-to-day relationship between husband and wife.

The Messenger Feast

Another major ceremony held during the winter season was *Kevgiq*, from the name for the two messengers sent to invite the guest village to the festival. *Kevgiq* was characterized by a mutual hosting between villages, whereby one village would go to another to dance and receive gifts. It was initiated when a host village presented its guests with a long list of wants, and the guests subsequently reciprocated with a list of their own. Besides collecting the articles to be given, each village composed songs describing the desired articles and naming the individual from whom the object was requested.

There was considerable rivalry as to the quality and the quantity of the gifts given during *Kevgiq*, and in some areas the guests were designated *curukat*, or attackers. *Kevgiq* was circumscribed by a calculated ambiguity, as the line between friend and foe was a fine one.

Although *Kevgiq* shared common features with the other ceremonial distributions, it stands out as a particularly elaborate display and distribution of the bounty of the harvest, providing a clear statement of respect to the spirits of the fish and game. Two important functions of *Kevgiq* were the redistribution of wealth within and between villages and the expression and maintenance of status distinctions.

The Masquerade Festival

The final major annual winter ceremony was *Kelek*, or *Itruka'ar*, sometimes referred to as the Masquerade. The complex ritual event involved the singing of songs of supplication to the spirits of the game (*yuas*), accompanied by the performance of masked dances under the direction of the shaman. Ritually powerful masks were created especially for the event and represented the spirits of the game as well as the *tunghaks*, the shaman's spirit helpers. In the preparations for *Kelek*, it was the shaman who directed the construction of the masks through which the spirits were revealed as at once dangerous and helpful. Their use, in enactments of past spiritual encounters, had the power to evoke them in the future. As in the Bladder Festival, songs were written and performed by the men of the community to draw the spirit world.

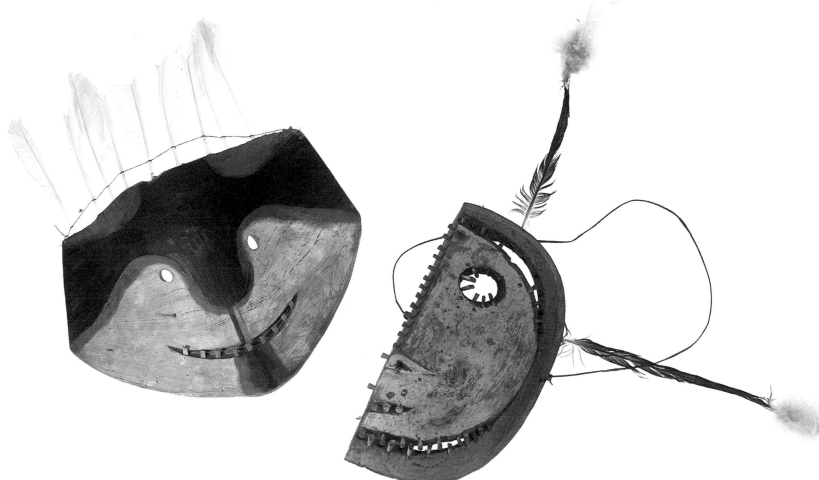

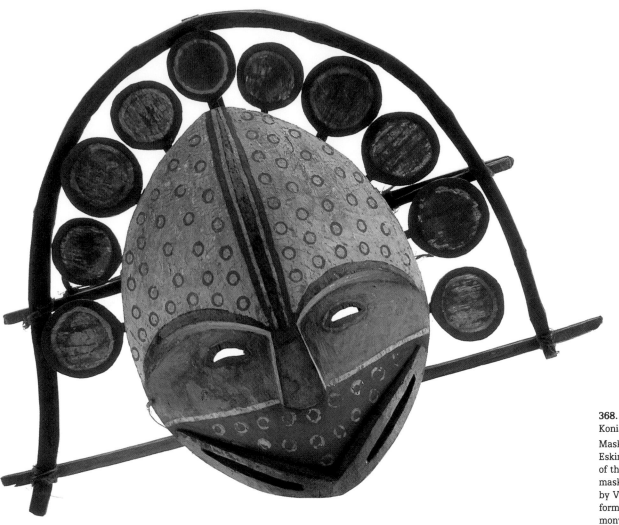

368. Bird Mask
Koniag Eskimo: MAE 571-12
Masking traditions of the Pacific Eskimo were as developed as those of their northern Yupik relatives. This mask may be one of the set obtained by Voznesenskii in 1842 from a performance of a Kodiak Island ceremony. Its feathers missing, the mask depicts a bird-man spirit. Three-quarter hoops and circular appendages are typical Koniag traits, as is circle decoration, which may be equivalent to spots used on masks from the Bering Sea coast.

369. Dance Rattle
Koniag Eskimo: NMNH 90438
Puffin beak dance rattles had special significance for the Koniag, occurring in their art as well as in actual ceremony. This dance rattle is made of two hoops to which dozens of cast-off beak sheaths of the tufted puffin have been attached with sinew ties. An illustration of this type of rattle was noted on a Koniag ceremonial paddle (fig. 51). Although widespread in the historical period, only one of these rattles has been found in a prehistoric Koniag site, dating to the early 18th century. These rattles may have been a recent introduction from the Northwest Coast, where they also occur. Perhaps the resemblance of rattles, hoop, and crossbar grip to the structure of Siberian shaman drums is coincidental.

Summary

In sum, at least five major events made up the annual ceremonial cycle in western Alaska. Individually these ceremonies served to emphasize different aspects of the relationship between humans, animals, and the spirit world. The Bladder Festival along with related ceremonies insured the rebirth and return of the animals in the coming harvest season. In the Feast for the Dead living namesakes were ritually fed and elaborately clothed to provision and honor the souls of the human dead. The Great Feast of the Dead (*Elriq*) served the same function within human society as the Bladder Festival within animal society, expressing and insuring continuity between the living and the dead. The intravillage *Petugtaq* and the intervillage Messenger Feast (*Kevgiq*) played on, exaggerated, and reversed normal social relationships between husband and wife and between host and guest. *Kevgiq* also served important social functions, including the display of status, social control, and the redistribution of wealth. At the same time it provided a clear statement to the spirits of the game that the hunters were once again ready to receive them anew. Finally, the Masquerade (*Keleq*) involved masked dances that dramatically recreated past spiritual encounters to elicit their participation in the future. Together the ceremonies comprised a cyclical view of the universe whereby right action in the past and present reproduced abundance in the future.

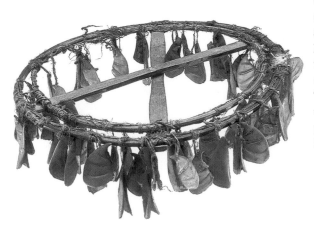

Potlatch Ceremonialism on the Northwest Coast

Frederica de Laguna

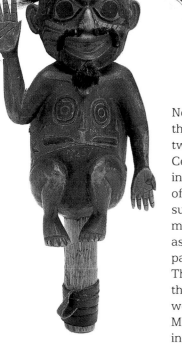

370. Shaman's Rattle
Tlingit: NMNH 9257

This rattle may represent the shaman himself or one of his spirits. His collarbones and vertebrae are sculpted in relief. The grinning face and animated posture of his detailed hands give vitality to the figure. Human hair forms his moustache, beard, and hair, which is long and disheveled in the manner of Tlingit shamans. Asymmetrical paint designs on the face are also typical of shamans.

371. Tlingit Curing Ceremony
AMNH neg. 335775; MAE 211-2

Tlingit curing shamans wore masks, robes, amulets, and rattles. Black oyster catcher rattles were unique to shamans and were used to cure illness caused by witchcraft. The bird is shown with neck arched as in its bouncing, chattering courtship dance. On its back the torture of a suspected sorcerer is seen, surrounded by halibut fins and octopus tentacles.

Northwest Coast ceremonialism was founded on the religious belief in personal encounters between men and supernatural spirits or beings. Ceremonies involved the elaborate display, by individuals, by kin groups, or by secret societies, of the powers or privileges obtained through such supernatural encounters. Display privileges might include names, titles, crests (emblems), as well as songs, dances, costumes, ceremonial paraphernalia, ritual acts, and magical feats. These were sanctioned or explained by tales of their supernatural origins, and the rights to them were validated by gifts to the invited audience. Much of representative art in carving and painting had ceremonial functions, drawing its inspiration and themes from the same supernatural experiences.

The shaman was one who had received powers from personal encounters with supernaturals. Although the spirits that had served a dead shaman were sometimes believed to return more readily to a close relative than to another, each novice shaman had to seek the power for himself

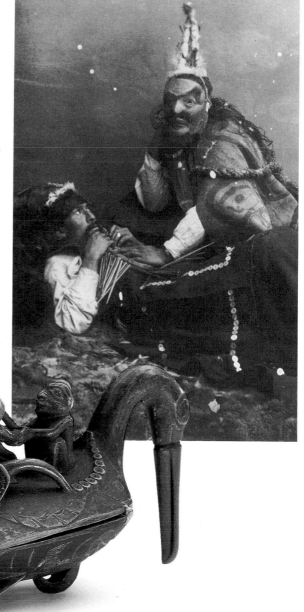

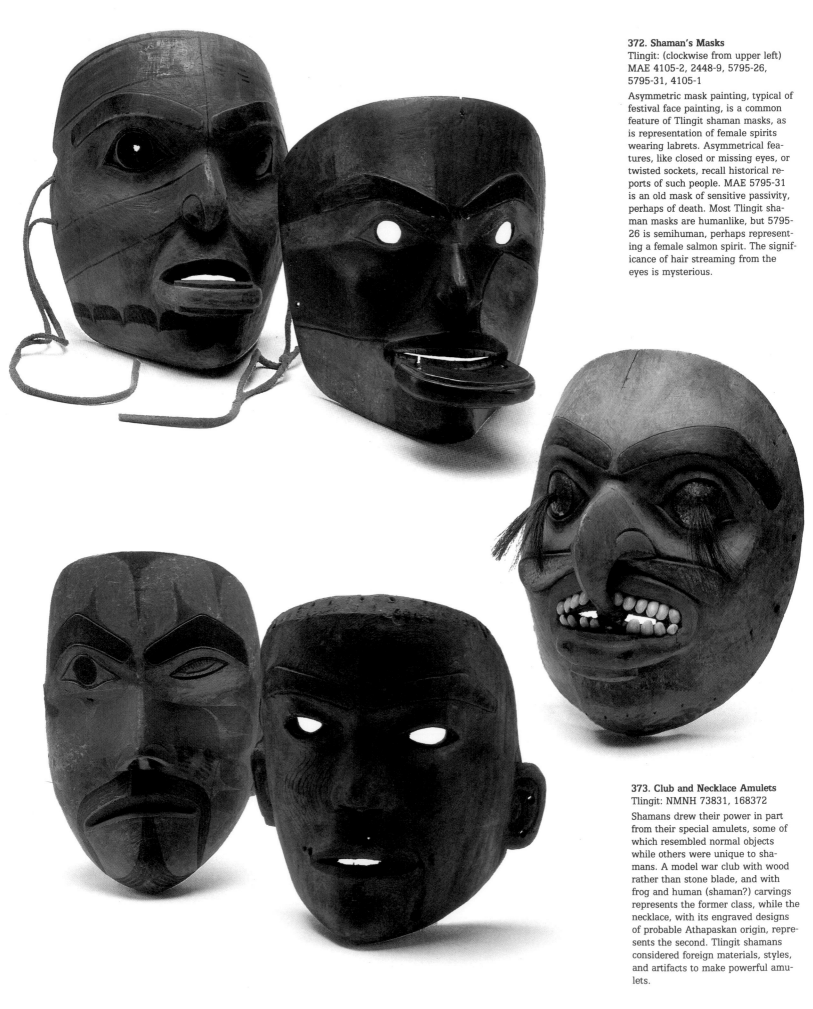

372. Shaman's Masks
Tlingit: (clockwise from upper left)
MAE 4105-2, 2448-9, 5795-26,
5795-31, 4105-1
Asymmetric mask painting, typical of
festival face painting, is a common
feature of Tlingit shaman masks, as
is representation of female spirits
wearing labrets. Asymmetrical features, like closed or missing eyes, or
twisted sockets, recall historical reports of such people. MAE 5795-31
is an old mask of sensitive passivity,
perhaps of death. Most Tlingit shaman masks are humanlike, but 5795-
26 is semihuman, perhaps representing a female salmon spirit. The significance of hair streaming from the
eyes is mysterious.

373. Club and Necklace Amulets
Tlingit: NMNH 73831, 168372
Shamans drew their power in part
from their special amulets, some of
which resembled normal objects
while others were unique to shamans. A model war club with wood
rather than stone blade, and with
frog and human (shaman?) carvings
represents the former class, while the
necklace, with its engraved designs
of probable Athapaskan origin, represents the second. Tlingit shamans
considered foreign materials, styles,
and artifacts to make powerful amulets.

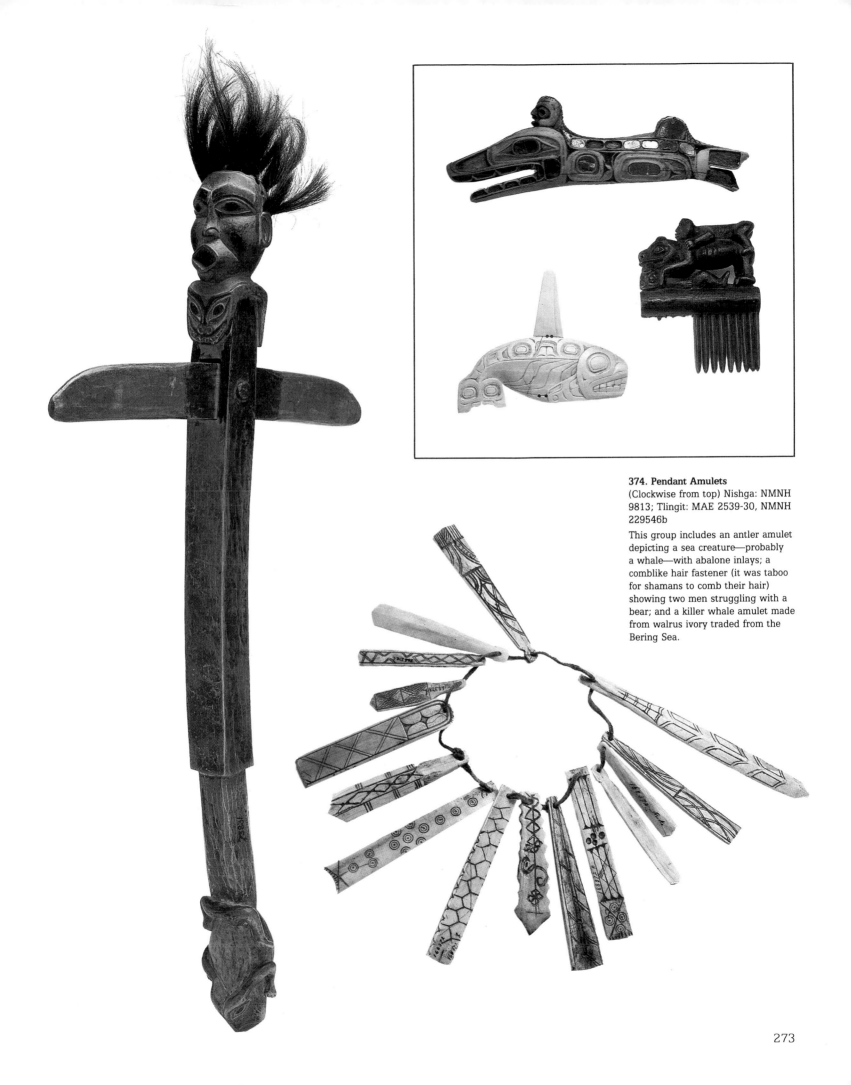

374. Pendant Amulets
(Clockwise from top) Nishga: NMNH 9813; Tlingit: MAE 2539-30, NMNH 229546b

This group includes an antler amulet depicting a sea creature—probably a whale—with abalone inlays; a comblike hair fastener (it was taboo for shamans to comb their hair) showing two men struggling with a bear; and a killer whale amulet made from walrus ivory traded from the Bering Sea.

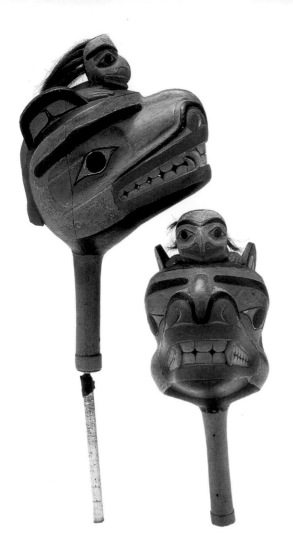

or herself after receiving the call. The supernatural was most often met in its animal guise, but this was only the outer shape, or garment, which the supernatural could doff to show its "real" humanlike form. This transformation was symbolized by the elaborate animal and bird masks of the central Northwest Coast, which opened to reveal the human face inside.

The shaman often kept a piece of the supernatural animal or used its likeness as a powerful charm. The totemic animal crest, however, was the secular memento of a similar supernatural encounter, inherited as the emblem of a kin group. The totem poles of the southern Tlingit, Haida, and Tsimshian remind us, in fact, of the representations of the Siberian shaman's guardian spirit in the form of a bird, perching on a pole in front of the tent. The system of crests, associated titles, and their ceremonial display was most highly developed among the Tsimshian and was especially characteristic of the other peoples with matrilineal descent, the Tlingit and the Haida.

Among the Tsimshian, Kwakiutl speakers, Bella Coola, and Nootka, there existed winter ceremonials in which the spirits were invoked to inspire the novices being initiated into the secret societies. Like family or clan crests and secular titles, the rights to sacred names, songs, dances, and ritual acts were inherited in family lines. Use of these prerogatives, however, required initiation into the secrets involved, a rite of passage that paralleled the spirit quest of the shaman. The chief or family head, as the religious leader, controlled the initiations and determined which roles the initiates should play, just as the chief controlled the display of secular crests. The most dramatic secret society performances originated among the Bella Bella (northern Kwakiutl) and from there spread in attenuated form to the Haida and Tlingit and also southward as far as the Columbia River.

All ceremonies involved the sharing and giving of food and the giving and receiving of property. Such feasting and transfer of wealth, carried out formally on a large scale and preferably to guests from outside the village, is the potlatch, to call it by the widely known word from Chinook jargon. Feasting and gift-giving were necessary after every display of ceremonial rights, and full-scale potlatches were normally given in the

375. Bear and Duck Rattles
Tsimshian: CMC VII C339, 340
Tlingit: NMNH 20828

Great diversity of rattle types existed among Northwest Coast groups. These Tsimshian rattles take the form of bears with humanoid figures peering between their ears. They were probably carved as dance rattles for a chief. Tufted puffin beaks were used as tinklers on Tlingit aprons and leggings, on circular frame rattles, and on baton rattles such as the one below, carved as an abstract duck. Wings, tail, and head are detailed with formlines; the long neck forms the handle. Such rattles were used in sets by shamans and dancers.

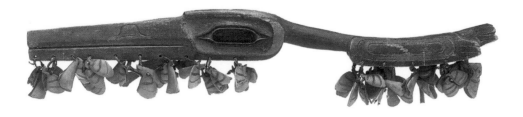

376. Shaman's Bow
Tlingit: NMNH 324930

Wands, batons, spears, daggers, and other items were used for display, carried in the hands by Tlingit chiefs and shamans on state occasions like potlatches and festivals. This oversized bow has a carved human head at each end, one singing and one talking. Similar paired faces were carved on shaman's headrests used during fasting (Wardwell 1978:87). Ceremonial bows were often made with matching arrows, and were sometimes used in curing ceremonies.

377. "Kolosh Indians from Sitka Island, 1842"
Il'ia Voznesenskii. MAE 1142-32

Voznesenskii's painting appears to depict the dance of a Tlingit initiate into a secret society known as the "Dog Eaters." This ceremony spread over the northern coast in the late precontact period, probably originating among the Bella Bella or Heiltsuq. The initiate, with red-painted face, is possessed by the motivating spirit and is hungry to eat raw flesh. He wears cedarbark rings over his shoulders and eagle down in his hair. He acts wild, and attendants, whose faces are painted and also wear eagle down, restrain him. In the Kwakiutl version, "Hamatsa" which is still performed, rattles are used to calm the new dancer, as shown at the right. Drumming and singing are also part of the performance.

378. Shaman's Rattle
Haida: NMNH 89052

Globular rattles were used by shamans all over the northern coast to combat evil spirits. Both sides of this rattle portray crouching figures, the center one with a beaklike nose, surrounded by others with long U-shaped fins stretching from their heads. The meaning of these figures, like most shamanic art, is derived from supernatural experiences and cannot be deciphered without information from the owner, who in this case was Tsilwax, a shaman from New Gold Harbor in the Queen Charlotte Islands.

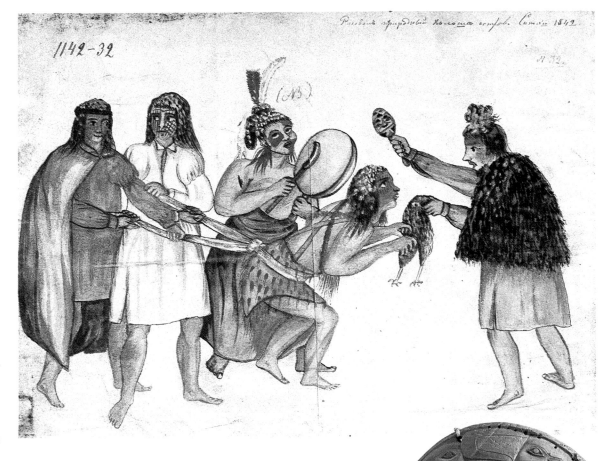

winter season, when the summer's work had assured ample supplies to feast the guests. This season of dark skies was also the time when supernatural forces were most strongly felt, as the spirits drew near the village. Potlatching and sacred dances were combined into elaborate ceremonial sequences, never two alike, during which houses might be built and dedicated, totem poles raised, marriages made or ceremonially unmade, valuable names and titles given or assumed, the deceased memorialized and their heirs formally installed, novices initiated into the secret dance groups, ceremonial debts discharged and new ones imposed.

The piling up of blankets to be given away, the Midas gleam of valuable "coppers" illuminated by grease-fed flames that threaten the roof planks, the serving of enormous portions of rich foods in crest-carved boxes and bowls, the processions of singers and performers behind the dance paddles of their leaders, the splendor of eagle down floating from the headdresses of blanket-clad dancers, the thuds of bare feet on the hardened earth, the thwack of pounding batons on resounding planks, the rumble of box drum or skin-covered tambourine that seems to penetrate the very body of the listener, the eerie whistles ("voices of the spirits") crying from the woods, the elaborate dramas performed with masks and artifices to simulate bloody killing and other fearful acts, the terrifying evocation

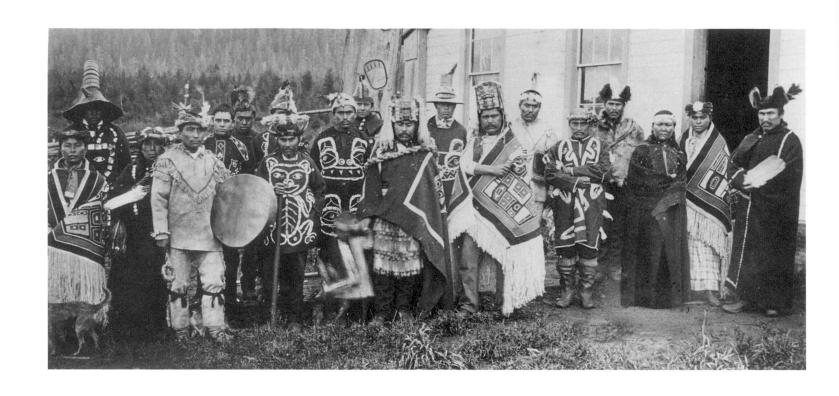

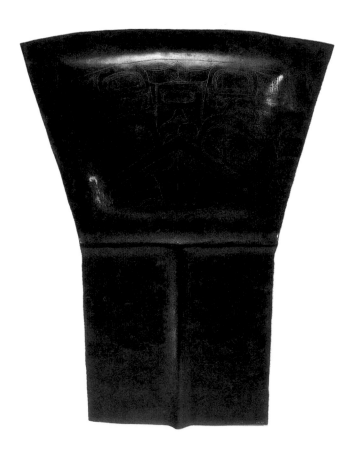 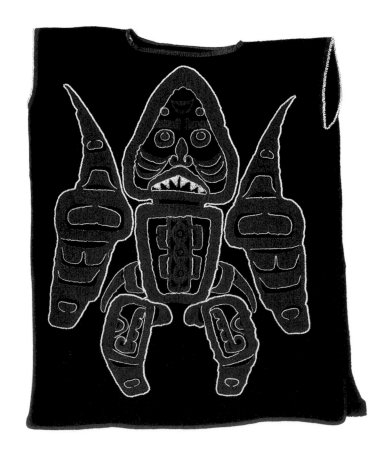

379 Potlatch Gathering
BCPM neg. PN 11880, G.T. Emmons, 1885

Emmons took this photograph of a group of Tlingit of the Nanyaayi clan posed in ceremonial dance costume in front of Chief Shakes' house, known as the "Dogfish" house, in Wrangel in 1885. Chief Shakes stands in the center, dressed in a Chilkat blanket.

380. Copper
Tlingit: FM 19022

From Vancouver Island northward, Northwest Coast chiefs prized plaques of copper, which represented wealth and prestige. Their peculiar and distinctive shape, flaring at the top and embossed with a T-shaped ridge on the lower half, has never been satisfactorily explained, although there is some evidence that it refers metaphorically to a human body. Valuable coppers had names, and often a painted or engraved representation of the appropriate creature on the top, or face, of the copper. This one shows a beaver, identifiable by his large incisors, high, rounded nose, and the two halves of his tail in the upper corners. Coppers were displayed at important ceremonial occasions, where they attested to the high rank and wealth of the owner. They were sometimes given away, whole or cut in pieces, at a potlatch or placed on the grave of a chief.

381. Appliqué Tunic
Haida: NMNH 89194

A dogfish covers the front of this dancing tunic, appliquéd in red flannel and outlined with white beads. It is presented in "split" form, with pectoral fins and halves of the dorsal fin at the sides, and the sides of the second fin and the tail below. The high forehead (the dogfish's nose), gill slits, and sharp teeth are further recognition features. On the back is a sea wolf, a mythical being with a wolf's head, paws, and tail, and the killer whale's dorsal fin and flukes. Sea wolf and dogfish are both crests of the Haida Eagle moiety.

of his spirit familiars by the shaman running around the fire with rattle and clash of bone necklace until he falls exhausted in a trance, the dignified recital of the legend authenticating the crests and displays of a chief—all these are elements characteristic of Northwest Coast ceremonials.

Through intermarriage, trade, and the appropriation of rights to ritual privileges from other groups by capturing or even killing the owner, such displays were spread up and down the coast, and ceremonies were elaborated by the addition of foreign features or the invention of new ones.

No matter how varied in form or stated purpose, these occasions were alike in dramatizing the power, privilege, and wealth of those who gave or sponsored them. Such displays were made with pride, for it was only the wealthy chief, of a wealthy group, with the additional support of his wife and her relatives, who could afford to give a ceremony of any importance. A woman chief, holding her position in default of a suitable male, could also sponsor ceremonies, similarly assisted by her husband and his people. Lesser chiefs in the group might either contribute to the resources of their superior or host smaller affairs of their own, but everyone shared in the glory, since the contributions of each were publicly recognized.

Guests, the necessary witnesses to the prerogatives claimed, were also honored and "paid for their trouble," those of rank and wealth receiving extra, and would remember the generosity of the gift when they in turn became hosts. So binding was the obligation to pay witnesses that when potlatch guests danced in their crest regalia to thank their hosts, the guests had to pay the hosts. Although the Tlingit shaman required payment before attempting a cure, the shaman and his relatives would distribute gifts to their opposites when he first exhibited his powers. This validated his professional name, that of his principal spirit.

"Chiefs fight with property," the Kwakiutl have said, and there was certainly a warlike aspect to much of Northwest Coast ceremonialism. Rivalry tended to follow traditional lines, often between two groups of invited guests; the local group or those first to arrive and the out-of-town later arrivals. The latter would approach in a line of canoes abreast, and though they might dance and sing onboard to show peaceful intentions, the formation was that of an armed landing party, ready to storm the beach. At a Salish potlatch they might indeed engage in a violent and often bloody shoving match with prior arrivals. Among other tribes, the potlatch host might don warrior's garb to show that he

was not afraid to sacrifice property, which in the past might include slaves (war captives) given to the guests to kill. (The method most often employed by the Tlingit was by strangulation with a pole across the neck, in the way that the sacred bear was killed by Asiatic tribes of the North Pacific.) Pride and arrogance, especially among the Kwakiutl, might pit one chief against another, and the way to silence a rival was to overwhelm him with gifts that he could not return or ruin him in a competition of property destruction. Usually, however, the host chief was punctiliously polite in receiving his guests, as was the guest chief in offering the comfort of his crests (symbolically) to the bereaved host of a funeral potlatch. All offerings were received with profuse thanks. Even the touchy Kwakiutl chiefs claiming the highest privileges would reassure each other that their "word was true" and express thankfulness that the other was indeed "still walking in the road given to our grandfathers by the Winter Ceremonial Spirit" and obeying "the laws laid down by the ancestors at the beginning of the world." The authorized joking and buffoonery that enlivened even the most serious ceremonial occasions undoubtedly relieved the tension and anxiety and were particularly relished when they mocked the prerogatives of the chiefs.

Status and privilege, both secular and religious, were inherent in the names or titles borne by aristocratic men and women, "Real People," as the Tsimshian called them. Increasingly important names would be assumed by one who had inherited or received the rights to them. Securing such status for one's self and passing it on to a successor was a dominant concern and often the real reason for the ceremony. Some songs, dances, and performances connected with sacred names were exhibited only when they were being given to an heir or to a son-in-law for his children. Thus, the most important ceremony among the Haida was the house-building potlatch given by a chief and his wife to the husband's clan on behalf of their children, the father's "opposites," for only children so honored could become chiefs, while those whose parents gave lesser ceremonies had lower status, and the no-accounts were the children of parents who had never potlatched. There were few without status, since a potlatching couple would sponsor the children of relatives and adopt orphans.

The principal reason for a Nootka potlatch was to transfer a chief's prerogatives to his children (names, dances, territorial rights), and a potlatch invariably ended the Shamans' Dance (or Wolf Dance) initiation, which also transferred privileges. The Nootka loved giving these ceremonies

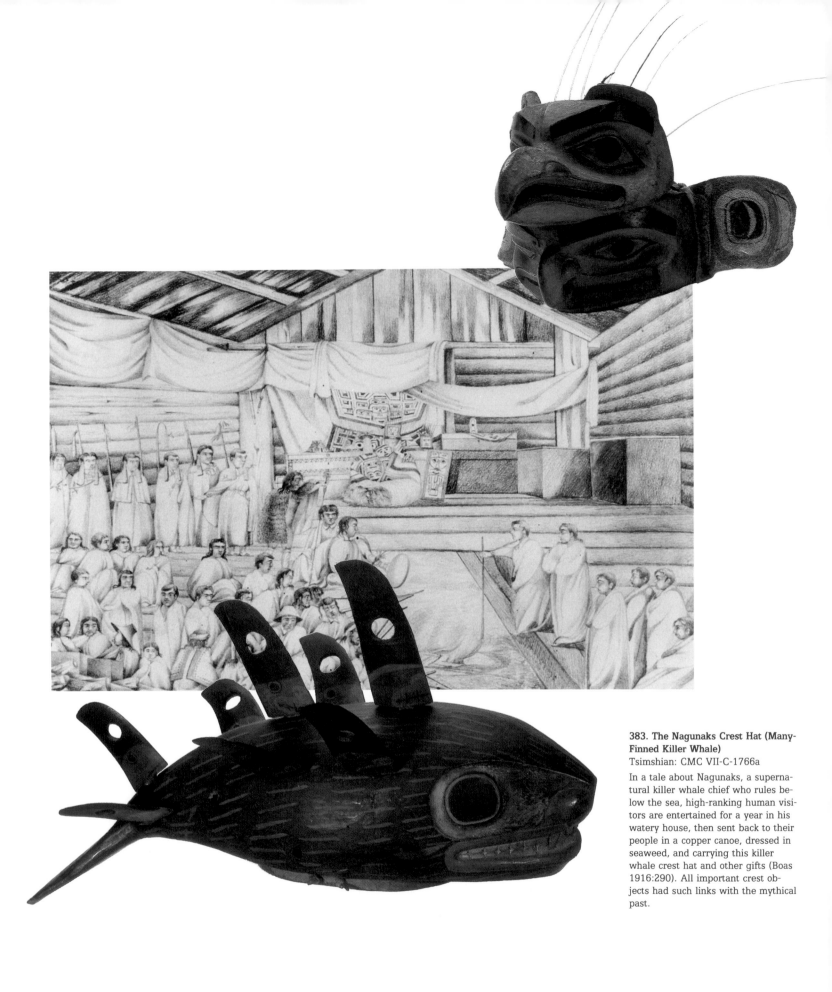

383. The Nagunaks Crest Hat (Many-Finned Killer Whale)
Tsimshian: CMC VII-C-1766a

In a tale about Nagunaks, a supernatural killer whale chief who rules below the sea, high-ranking human visitors are entertained for a year in his watery house, then sent back to their people in a copper canoe, dressed in seaweed, and carrying this killer whale crest hat and other gifts (Boas 1916:290). All important crest objects had such links with the mythical past.

382. Crest Headdress
Tlingit: MAE 571-19

Raven's head protrudes from the
forehead of a hook-beaked creature in
this double crest headdress. Painted
hide flaps extend from the sides of
the lower head, suggesting the identity of a sea-being. At one time,
many more sea lion whiskers and a
fringe of baleen strips radiated from
the top. Headdresses like this one
were worn in potlatches and on festival occasions, and were displayed
along with family emblems and heirlooms at the memorial for a deceased
chief.

**384. "The Funeral of the One-Armed
Kolosh Chieftain (Kukhantan)"**
Il'ia Voznesenskii. MAE 1142-28

Voznesenskii sketched this drawing
from observation of a Tlingit Chief's
funeral in Sitka in 1844. Providing
excellent ethnographic detail, it
shows the dead chief in state,
dressed in a Chilkat blanket and frontlet headdress decorated with sea lion
whiskers and surrounded by other
Chilkat blankets, a copper, a painted
conical crest hat, and chests of valua-
bles. Mourners, perhaps chiefs, wearing ear or hair ornaments line the left
wall, against which ceremonial staffs
are propped. A large gathering of
men and women, some wearing labrets, button blankets, and painted
spruce-root hats, sits before the fire,
around which the visiting chiefs' ceremonial spears have been laid. A
drummer, probably a shaman, sings;
and behind him a figure, possibly
someone representing the deceased,
stands with painted or darkened face,
fur cape, and staff. To the right,
cloaked figures, probably orators, one
with a chief's staff, pay respects.

The name of the deceased indicates he was of the Wolf moiety, so
many of the mourners assembled
would have been their "opposites,"
the Raven moiety. The close kin of
the deceased would have been
dressed in mourning rags, their faces
smeared with soot. After two to four
days of mourning, a hole was broken
through a side wall of the house,
through which the deceased and his
possessions were carried to his funeral pyre. After cremation, women
gathered the remains and deposited
them in a special burial house.
(Pierce 1975:15).

so much that it was the children and youths who
held the high titles, while their elders, the
"retired" chiefs, directed affairs from backstage.
Secure in their prestige, these former chiefs no
longer had to worry about the protocol of their
own seating or the order in which they received
gifts, in contrast to their Kwakiutl neighbors,
who squabbled over such matters. The Nootka
had no use for coppers, and did not kill slaves
at ceremonies; rather, they often initiated slaves
to add more drama to the event. Since everyone
was initiated, there were no secrets about the
supernatural wolves and how they were impersonated. It was all a well-staged drama, with
excitement, fun, and gorgeous display.

Of much more importance to the Nootka was
the knowledge of magic formulas and sacred
rituals, originally obtained from encounters with
the supernatural and inherited as closely held
family secrets. The ceremonies involved were
never public. Most potent of such powers was
that of the Nootka chief who owned the ritual
for calling dead whales to drift ashore on his
beach. One such rite involved a sacred shrine
with human corpses stolen from their graves
and rigged like puppets so that they could be
made to imitate the harpooning of a whale (cf.
fig. 217). Another chief owned the ritual of
calling whales through a human skull used as a
trumpet. Only ceremonial bathing to the point
of numbness, repeated many days, purified and
prepared the chief for such awesome rites.

The theme of death, and ambivalent feelings
toward the dead, ran through many ceremonies,
although it was most apparent in funeral or
memorial potlatches when the deceased were
called by name to share the food and tobacco.
One of the most important ceremonies among
the Bella Coola, as among the Kwakiutl, was the
return of the bride price to the son-in-law,
"repurchasing the wife," essential for all re-
spectable marriages. This handsome payment
was made to the husband at the beginning of a
potlatch he was giving and was added to the
wealth he distributed. The potlatch raised the
status of his children and "strengthened the
seat." Moreover, it also smoothed the way of
the donor after death, when his spirit had to
retrace the path of his predecessors back to the
mountain where the ancestor first came to earth,
there to don the discarded bird or animal garment of the ancestor and ascend to heaven. The
most dramatic moment in the potlatch was the
visit of a deceased relative, played by a secret
society member disguised in an elaborate costume made by the "carpenters" (supernaturally
endowed artists) to represent the ancestral animal or bird and accompanied by the whistles
of the secret society. After imitating the animal

through clever acting and manipulation of strings
controlling the costume, the figure left the house,
and the host threw down a copper behind it or
into the fire, thereby destroying its value but
"making bone for the dead." At a Kwakiutl
memorial potlatch, the masked figure of the
dead chief might appear, escorted by living
colleagues.

The original winter ceremonial may have been
like the Coast Salish winter dances, simply a
way to appease the spirits that were troubling
their human partners. This malaise could be
relieved only by a "power sing" sponsored by
someone with ceremonial powers. While he
fasted, each spirit-inspired person danced in
turn to his or her own song, accompanied by
singers and drummers and followed by dancing
helpers. This continued every night until all the
powers were satisfied, the sponsor rendering
the last song, and ended with a distribution of
gifts to the audience. Unlike the Salish, whose
ceremonial powers had no definite shape and
who danced in stylized fashion, the originators
of the secret society performances were probably inspired by animals and imitated them in
their dances and costumes. One might also see
animal mimicry at a Tlingit potlatch, when a
young man danced behind a curtain with only
his crest hat visible and moving like the Raven
or Halibut it represented. Those possessed by
an animal spirit became "crazy" and acted like
animals, gradually losing their human appearance. This transformation is shown in masks of
the Land Otter Man (worn by shamans) or of
the Wild Man or Wild Woman (worn by secret
society dancers). The loss of humanity is most
evident in the loss of appetite for human food
and the craving for the raw flesh devoured by
animals.

The most widely known and probably one of
the oldest societies was that of persons inspired
by supernatural wolves, who in consequence bit
live dogs and ate them—a horrible act, since
dog flesh was believed poisonous. Dog-Eaters
were known to all the tribes but the Nootka.
Among the latter, the supernatural wolves, impersonated by the secret society members, simply kidnapped initiates to teach them their inherited rights. The Bella Bella surpassed the
Dog-Eaters by creating the worst monsters of
all—eaters of human flesh, inspired by the
"Cannibal at the North End of the World." Their
act was the most terrifying, since a corpse was
the object of horrified aversion and was believed
to be the source of power for the witch or killing
shaman.

The Cannibal Dancer as initiate was essential
to the Kwakiutl winter ceremonial, a role filled
by the son of the chief who had inherited the

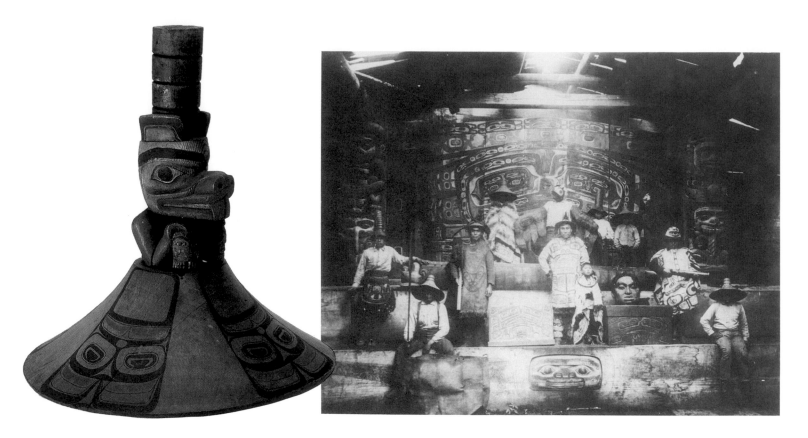

right. His daughter became the Cannibal's female attendant. Associated with them were many other characters who were being initiated into the society: Grizzly Bears, Warriors, Fools, the Fire-Thrower, the Smasher of Property, and those who had to be restrained by ropes passed through slits in their flesh. In addition, there were the already initiated, some of whom were active in handling the novices, and the older members who controlled the society. Although the latter acted in their sacred capacity with their sacred names, they were the same persons as the secular chiefs. Among the Tsimshian, there was the society of the Dancers and the society of the Dog-Eaters, but only certain chiefs held the right to be Cannibals or Smashers. The Bella Coola combined the Cannibal and Dog-Eater as one character in their most important society.

The Cannibal initiate actually bit people in the arm—those who had inherited the right to be bitten and who were paid for their pain by the initiate's sponsor—just as other performers would run amok through the houses, smashing things, if taboos were broken—again on purpose and with restitution. But it is not entirely clear whether the Cannibal actually ate a corpse, although it is known that the flesh he bit (usually cut by sleight of hand) from a living person was not swallowed—it would be too poisonous. Still, there is some evidence that the female attendant of the Cannibal novice carried a mummified body in her arms as she danced to pacify the Cannibal and that he actually ate some of it. It is said too that slaves were once sacrificed for

his food. Yet all this could easily have been faked.

The penalty for revealing the secrets of the society was death—death to the performer who stumbled and exposed the hoax, for it would be too expensive to initiate the whole audience; death to the Tsimshian artificers if their wonderful mechanical contraptions broke just when the chief tried to display his sacred powers; and death to the Bella Coola member who betrayed his society's secrets and who was thrown to the ground and strangled by two men who sat on a pole across his neck.

But the most extraordinary feature about all these winter ceremonial acts is that they were knowingly performed as frauds and tricks.

385. Crest Headdress
Haida: NMNH 89036

Wooden crest hats were carved in imitation of woven basketry hats. On this hat the crest is a beaver holding two humans with his claws and wearing as his hat a column of four cylinders that rises between his formline ears. The four formline figures painted on the brim probably represent coppers. The brilliant red pigment is vermillion, made in China and acquired by trade.

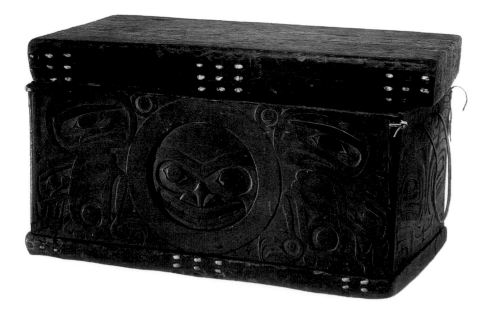

Art and Culture Change at the Tlingit-Eskimo Border

Bill Holm

386. Whale House

SI neg. 74-3623, Winter and Pond photo

The right to own and display crest objects commemorating the real or mythological origins, history, or events of the clan was vested in the chief and could be transferred only by inheritance or sale. At important occasions, the clan's valuable crest objects were put on display for all to marvel at. This photograph shows the interior of the Whale House at Klukwan, with members of the Ganaxtedi clan wearing crest objects in front of the Raven screen, flanked by the Woodworm post at the left, and the Raven post at the right.

387. Chief's Chest

Tlingit: NMNH 60176

Crest objects and clan regalia were stored in bentwood chests, themselves decorated with crests and clan designs. A circular face surrounded by a corona and flanked by birds decorates the front of this chief's chest, rather than the usual stylized formline figure. It was probably a specific crest, the moon. Much of the original paint has worn away, but enough remains to show that it was painted in the traditional manner. The two profile birds are elegantly rendered in formlines. Inlay of snail opercula in the broad front edge of the lid is common on carved chests, but less so in the edge of the bottom board.

The cultural continuum extending along the arch of the North Pacific Rim, and, with some logic, reaching southward on the American side as far as northern California, links peoples of myriad languages and physical shapes. Those cultural links are amazingly strong over certain long stretches of the Pacific shore. The linguistically diverse groups occupying the 1,200-mile coastline between the Columbia River and Yakutat Bay share among them so many features of environment and culture that they are universally described as making up the Northwest Coast culture area. Within this larger continuity there are numerous culturally diverse sectors, shading more or less imperceptibly with one another at their junctures. The similarities of their resource bases, the relative uniformity of climate (given the 15° increase in latitude between the south and north ends of the region), and especially the almost continuous network of waterways allowing easy contact between these sectors were factors in the development and maintenance of a high degree of cultural homogeneity along the whole Northwest Coast.

The northernmost of these Northwest Coast people, the Yakutat Tlingit, were expanding westward along the mainland shore of the Gulf of Alaska into Eyak territory in the years just preceding the first European sea voyages to the region. The coast from Cape Spencer, at the mouth of Cross Sound, to the northwest all the way to Prince William Sound is a nearly unbroken shore open to the prevailing southeasterly winter storm winds. Nearly midway in that 300-mile shore is Yakutat Bay, one of only half a dozen refuges available and the only one relatively safe to enter in storm conditions.

The western shores of the Gulf of Alaska were home to Pacific Yupik-speaking people, the Chugach of Prince William Sound, and the Koniag of Kodiak Island. Their use of framed, skin-covered boats, gutskin parkas, throwing boards, stone oil lamps, semisubterranean sod-roofed houses, and many other Eskimo features established them clearly to be part of that arcticwide cultural continuum. The country they lived in supported that culture well, with an abundance of sea mammals, fish, shellfish, and birds. But it also differed markedly from most other Eskimo lands in its vegetation and its mountainous inlet- and island-broken character—the westernmost extension of the glaciated, forest-covered Northwest Coast.

In spite of the intervening and forbidding open waters, the Chugach and Koniag had contact with the Tlingit of the eastern shores of the gulf, but it was more often than not an unfriendly and even violent contact, to judge by the traditions of both peoples and the record of their actions during the early historic period (de Laguna 1972:158–75). They were, in fact, mutual enemies. Some of this contact and exchange took place secondhand, through the intermediary Eyak, with whom the Yakutat Tlingit had frequent and friendly relations. So in spite of the difficulties posed by differing cultures, ancient enmities, and intervening open sea, there was considerable interchange of ideas, and the Northwest Coast overlay on Pacific Eskimo culture is obvious and universally recognized.

Influences in the other direction, although less overt, were nonetheless present. These exchanges certainly increased after the arrival of fleets of Aleut and Pacific Eskimo *baidarka*s in the service of the Russian fur hunters, but evidence for intercultural borrowing in pre-European times is convincing.

The most obvious Pacific Eskimo import among the Tlingit (specifically the Yakutat and Huna) was the sea otter harpoon-arrow and probably the surround technique with which it was used (de Laguna 1971:381, plates 108–12; Emmons and de Laguna in press: ms. pp. 310–12). All the details of the sea otter arrow—the tapered, red-painted shaft, the gracefully proportioned bone foreshaft and its method of hafting, the cut of the eagle-feather fletching, and the decorated, braided-sinew line—are completely Eskimo in character (fig. 76). Use of a cylindrical, bell-mouthed wooden quiver was shared by north-

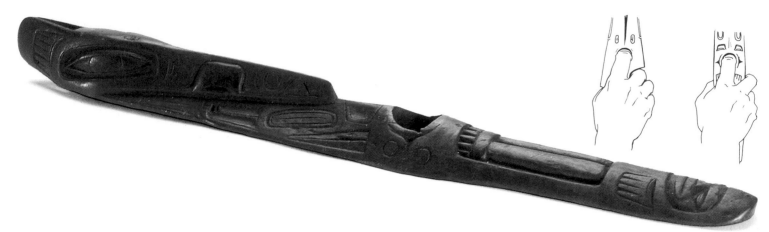

western Tlingit and Pacific Eskimo sea hunters, but on which end of the gulf it originated is not clear. Several known quivers from Prince William Sound are decorated with Tlingit-like designs modified in typically Chugach ways.

Although the Pacific Eskimo harpoon-arrow was adopted intact by Tlingit hunters, the throwing board was not. Retention of this ancient implement by the Eskimo is understandable for people hunting sea mammals from kayaks and *baidarkas*. For a hunter balancing a narrow, decked boat there were clear advantages to the throwing board that could be grasped, fitted with its dart, brought into throwing position, and cast with one hand while holding a steadying paddle with the other. Pacific Eskimo and Aleut hunters also used the bow, but apparently only from the two-man boat, with the paddler in the stern cockpit and the archer in the bow. Tlingit sea hunters, in open dugout canoes with two-man crews, had no need for the special attributes of the throwing board—the bow was just as convenient and perhaps more accurate.

If Tlingit hunters failed to adopt the throwing board, how can the existence in present-day collections of a dozen or so throwing boards, heavily decorated with true northern Northwest Coast figures, be explained (fig. 388)? It has been suggested that they were made by Tlingit carvers in imitation of examples brought to their country by Aleut sea otter hunters in the early fur trade days, and that their rarity, and the lack of knowledge of their use by latter-day Tlingits, must be the result of their failure to catch on among the local hunters. That they were derived from a Pacific Eskimo or Aleut prototype seems likely, but that they were ever intended for hunting use does not. Although many of them show signs of venerable age and wear and have a grooved upper face and a lug to engage the socket of the harpoon, they do not seem suitable for hunting. Every Aleut and Eskimo throwing board, from Greenland to the end of the Aleutian chain, has a shaped grip that fits the hand, placing the fingers and thumb in the natural

position to grasp the shaft of the dart. The typical Tlingit throwing board is extremely short between the forefinger hole and the socket lug (averaging just over half the length on a typical Pacific Eskimo board, fig. 193) and has a straight, tapered handle with the index finger hole centered, resulting in a cramped, insecure and ungainly grip. Even though it would be inefficient and awkward to throw a harpoon with the Tlingit board, those extant are nearly all well worn. Their decorations, which closely resemble the carvings on shamans' amulets, wands, and rattles, suggest that they were used as weapons in the struggles against malevolent supernatural beings rather than as practical hunting implements (Holm and Vaughan 1982:76–79). George Emmons, in a note accompanying a Tlingit throwing board in the American Museum of Natural History (cat. no. 19-1164), described it as "elaborately carved to represent an old Yakutat spirit of a celebrated Shaman 'Sick-kearkow' with a spirit head dress on at one end, in the centre a legendary spirit from Yakutat country, 'Shem' and at the other end a hair seal" (Emmons n.d.b:90). Stylistically they are old, and this, along with their patination, apparent shamanic use, and later Tlingit unfamiliarity, suggests that the throwing-board concept was around for a long time, perhaps preceding the historic arrival of the *baidarka* flotillas of Aleut, Koniag, and Pacific Eskimo sea otter hunters (see page 76).

A number of object types that resemble typical Tlingit artifacts but were made and used by the Koniag and Chugach have been collected as early as Cook's third expedition, in 1778. They illustrate varying degrees of influence primarily from east to west, although some of the similarities may actually represent Eskimo concepts that have been incorporated in Tlingit and other northern Northwest Coast design traditions. Carved wooden grease bowls from both areas, in the form of animals (most often seals) and birds, share a number of features. The bowl of such a vessel (fig. 389) is typically broad and

388. Spear Thrower
Tlingit: NMNH 20771

The very few Tlingit spear throwers, or throwing boards, that survive are all carved with figures that resemble those on shaman's rattles and amulets. Although completely functional, they are poorly shaped for efficient use (*right*) compared to Pacific Eskimo throwing boards (*left*). It is possible that they were all shamans' instruments, weapons to be used in war with the spirits. Whichever is the case, they are often beautifully carved. A long-beaked, crested bird (a kingfisher or merganser) bites an asymmetrically rendered sea creature on the shaft of this board. The legs, hands, and face of a man, with closed eyes, emerge from recesses in the grip. Although collected in the late 19th century, its early style, heavy wear and patination indicate a much earlier origin.

389. Grease Bowl
Chugach Eskimo: NMNH 168623
(above right)

Pacific Eskimo carved grease bowls resemble Tlingit bowls in their principal form, but are generally shallower and with more naturalistic treatment of the animal or bird heads. They often include Tlingit-like treatment of the details, such as the ovoid wing joints of this merganser. Another decorative feature favored by the Chugach artists was an inlay of rows of small, white, glass beads rather than the opercula typical of Tlingit bowls. This is a fine example of a Pacific Eskimo bowl, with sweeping form, upraised head, bead inlay and deep color, the result of long years of oil saturation.

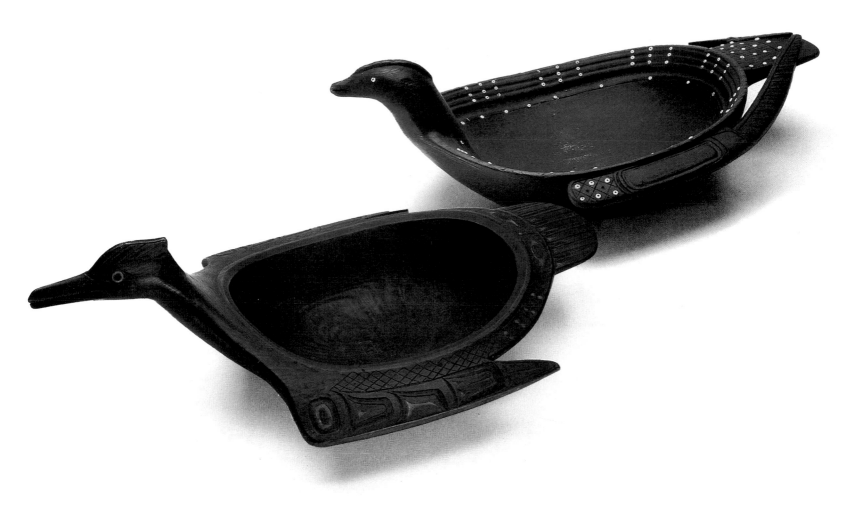

390. Grease Bowl

Chugach Eskimo: MAE 536-4 (above left)

Even more Tlingit in style than fig. 389, but still identifiable as Pacific Eskimo in origin, is this unused grease bowl in the form of a merganser. The formline details of the wings and tail joint are close approximations of northern Northwest Coast designs, but certain anomalies in their structure suggest that they are from outside the tradition. As in the case of painted hats, the degree of adherence to the introduced design tradition varies from piece to piece. The flat form of the vessel, the naturalistic head, and the rows of dots analogous to bead inlay are all features of Chugach and Koniag bowls. The bird's feet are delicately and naturalistically carved in relief on the body under the tail. Its pristine state suggests that it was made for sale. On the Northwest Coast, the tourist trade was well advanced at the beginning of the 19th century.

round with the ends, in the form of the creature's head and tail, raised and the inner surface fluted with one or more shallow grooves paralleling the rim. The heads of Prince William Sound and Kodiak Island bowls tend to be represented in a simplified, naturalistic style consistent with other Alaskan Eskimo sculpture, while comparable Tlingit bowls have the heads, as well as other anatomical parts, carved and detailed according to the well-known stylistic conventions of the region. A number of Pacific Eskimo bowls, including some collected in the first years of the 19th century, show detailing of tail and wings or flippers that is clearly derived from Tlingit designs. Some of these (fig. 390) follow the Northwest Coast conventions so closely that if the bowls themselves were not so obviously Pacific Eskimo in style they could be taken for Tlingit work. In almost every case, however, there are clues in the details of the designs that indicate their non-Tlingit origin.

Other objects with Tlingit-like decoration come from the Pacific Eskimo. Some of the wooden quivers, mentioned above, combine geometrically detailed bands around the tubular body, with modified form-line ovoids and U-shaped feather or fin designs on the expanded end. Two of them (Taylor Museum 4999 and Berlin Museum IV A 6608, Birket-Smith 1953:fig. 13) are

so nearly identical they may be the work of the same maker. Another from Kodiak Island (Lowie Museum 2-6570, Clark 1984:fig. 4) shows more geometrization of the decorated area, a tendency seen in some other adaptations of Northwest Coast design in the region.

Several small boxes, Eskimo-like in construction but with surface decoration in modified form-line style, were collected in the early 19th century. Some of these may have been made for sale to collectors. An elaborate example (National Museum of Finland, 62) fitted with drawers and perhaps designed as a writing box, was collected by (and may have been made for) Arvid Adolf Etholen, chief manager of the Russian American Company from 1840 to 1845. Etholen's service in Alaska had begun in 1818, so it is possible that the writing box and several other similar boxes from his collection (all now in the National Museum of Finland) were collected earlier than 1840. The decoration on these small boxes varies from generalized and Tlingit-like patterns to designs that follow many of the conventions of northern Northwest Coast two-dimensional art, exemplified by a small chest in the Museum of Anthropology and Ethnography in Leningrad (fig. 391) attributed to the Lisianskii collection of 1805–06. Although the design on the long face of this chest appears at first glance to be of Tlingit origin, the resemblance is superficial, as explained in the analysis of hat painting below. The designs on the sides of the chest are nearly identical to those on the wooden quivers described earlier and can be considered a typical Pacific Eskimo adaptation of Tlingit art. Geometric detail, crosshatching, and zigzag and dentate lines also resemble the details of decoration on Chugach horn spoons.

Mountain goats, the most important large land animal in the Chugach economy (Birket-Smith 1953:37), furnished black horns from which the Pacific Eskimo made spoons very much like those so well known from the Northwest Coast tribes. The ready availability of the material and its special suitability for spoons probably would have led to their manufacture even without the influence of Tlingit usage, and their superficial resemblance to Tlingit spoons probably resulted as much from the natural (and continentwide) technology of horn spoon-making as it did from any attempt to imitate a Northwest Coast model. The carving of the handles, however, seems to have been heavily influenced by Tlingit spoons, with heads of humanoid beings, birds, and even whole figures sculpted on the tapering, curved horn (fig. 393). In style, however, they differ markedly from Northwest Coast carving (figs. 61 and 393 right). The carving on the Pacific Eskimo examples is angular, with flat, angled planes often detailed with parallel incised lines. The invariable large head at the juncture of bowl and handle is sometimes shown with the upper lip overhanging the spoon bowl, giving it the appearance of an enormously broad, extended tongue. The usual upright ears over this head are often flared out, an effect achieved by carving them free of the spoon handle and bending the steam-softened ears outward.

Unlike the typical Northwest Coast one-piece goat-horn spoon, the bowl forms a distinct, oval unit, sharply demarked from the handle, which extends in a raised, rectangular ridge halfway down the underside of the bowl. The ridge is decorated with incising, sometimes in modified formline design. The inner surface of the bowl (or tongue) is always incised with a narrow median oval flanked by groups of parallel, sometimes dentate lines and dashes joining it to the bowl edge. On the more elaborate examples the median oval is inlaid with white beads or dentalium shells, inlay material rarely found on Northwest Coast pieces but common on Eskimo carvings. Another feature differentiating Pacific Eskimo spoons from their Tlingit counterparts is the lack of recurve to the handle, an almost universal characteristic of Northwest Coast goat-horn spoons. The three illustrated by Kaj Birket-Smith (1953:fig. 32) are almost certainly Tlingit

spoons that have made their way through trade to Prince William Sound.

Living as they were between the grass-twining Aleut and the spruce-root-twining Tlingit, it would be surprising if the Chugach and Koniag women weren't also expert makers of twined baskets. Spruce root was the available material, and the twined basketry of the Pacific Eskimo is almost indistinguishable from that of their eastern neighbors. Given the enormous production of spruce-root basketry all over southeastern Alaska, the complexity and elaboration of the techniques used there, and the importance of

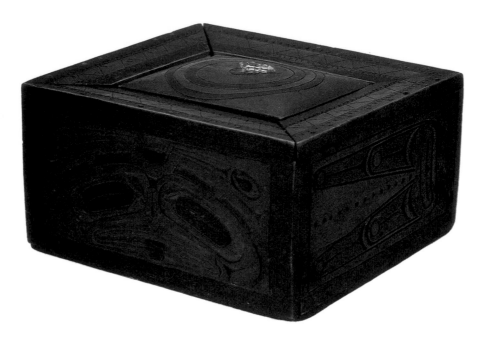

391. Painted Chest
Koniag or Chugach: MAE 2915-1a,b
This little chest, Eskimo in construction but Tlingit-like in decoration, appears to have been broken and repaired. Originally it had been made with shallow drawers at the bottom of the ends. Long ago the drawers were disassembled and the fronts pegged in place with yew wood pins. The chest was probably made for sale, perhaps as a writing box. Pacific Eskimo variants of Tlingit designs decorate all four sides.

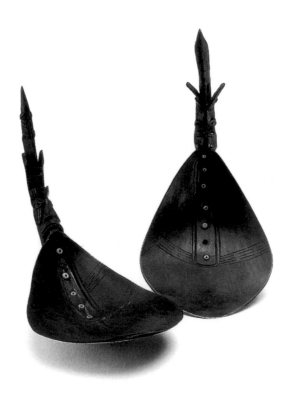

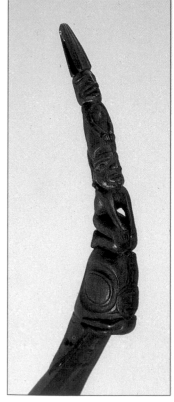

392. Basket

Chugach Eskimo: MAE 4291-7

Tlingit spruce-root basketry has three broad bands of false embroidery below the rim, the upper and lower having the same design. Pacific Eskimo baskets, like this one, have many narrow bands of alternating designs.

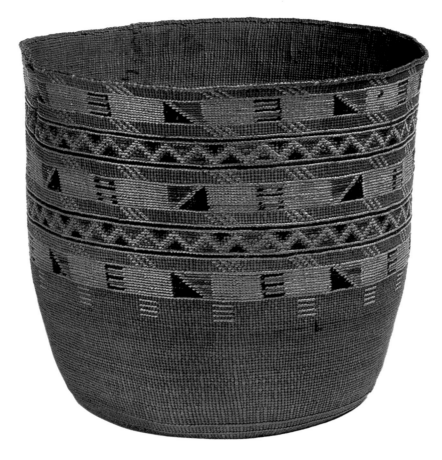

393. Horn Spoons

Chugach Eskimo: MAE 518-1a,b
Haida: NMNH 89167 (detail, right)

Like their Tlingit neighbors, the Chugach Eskimo made spoons of mountain goat horn. Unlike the Tlingit, the Chugach never recurved the handles. Angled planes, geometric incising, flaring ears, and parallel chevrons engraved on the bowl are common features of Chugach spoons. White beads and sections of dentalium shells are often inlaid into the bowls. The handle (detail) of the Haida spoon features a dragonfly holding a man in its mouth. Though collected from the Haida in the Queen Charlotte Islands, the treatment is reminiscent of Tlingit work, in which representations of the dragonfly also occur.

basketry to Tlingit culture, it seems certain that the Pacific Eskimo twined spruce-root basketry tradition has its roots in contact with the Tlingit.

Pacific Eskimo spruce-root baskets (fig. 392) have often been mistaken for Tlingit work. The techniques and materials used were nearly identical, and the general effect of the geometrically detailed bands of false embroidery in dyed grass is much alike in the two basketry traditions. Add to that the confusion resulting from baskets of Pacific Eskimo type having been collected at Sitka and the misidentifications are understandable. Molly Lee (1981:66–73) has defined their characteristics. Repeated bands of false embroidery using a limited vocabulary of design units (contrasted to the Tlingit style of three complex bands with the upper and lower alike), a secondary design field on the lower half consisting of Aleut-like rows of false embroidered designs on the twined root background,

and concentric reinforcing rings of three-strand twining on the base are the most significant recognition features. The decoration of a unique bell-mouthed quiver of traditional form but made of twined spruce-root basketry rather than carved wood in the Lowie Museum (cat. no. 2-6594a, b) combines three-strand twining and false embroidery in grass and red and dark blue woolen yarn, a material use also reminiscent of Aleut basketry decoration. Although this is the only Pacific Eskimo basketry quiver known to me, Lisianskii (1814:181) mentioned their use by the Koniag in 1805.

It is in the making and decorating of painted spruce-root hats that the Koniag-Chugach-Tlingit connection is most graphically displayed. In "A Man of Prince William's Sound," drawn in 1778 by John Webber, the official artist on Cook's third expedition, the subject wears a very Eskimo gutskin parka, nose pin, and peglike labrets, but on his head is a Northwest Coast–type twined spruce-root hat decorated with beads and a painted design in black and red. This was the first of many 18th- and early-19th-century depictions of Chugach and Koniag men wearing conical hats of Northwest Coast type. Martin Sauer, in his journal of the Billings Expedition of 1787–92, illustrated a Koniag man wearing a spruce-root hat (Sauer 1802: plate 6), and those hats often appear in early drawings of Pacific Eskimo men in their *baidarka*s, and are worn as well by the crewmen in model skin boats in early collections. Interestingly, although the evidence for exclusive male use of spruce-root hats among the Pacific Eskimo is overwhelming, Lisianskii wrote of the Koniag in 1805, "Both sexes wear . . . hats, of the fine roots of trees, platted" (Lisianskii 1814:194). Probably the most detailed and convincing of the early-19th-century depictions are in three watercolor paintings by Mikhail Tikhanov, an artist who accompanied the Golovnin Expedition around the world in the *Kamchatka* in 1817–19. One of these depicts two views of a Koniag man wearing a broad, low, painted hat (Golovnin 1979:34); a second shows two hat-wearing hunters (labeled "Aleuts"[1]), one with a throwing board and harpoon-dart and the other with a bow (Golovnin 1979:32); and the third is a portrait, also labeled "Aleut," with a detailed representation of a typical Pacific Eskimo painted hat (USSR Academy of Art, Tikhanov portfolio, no. 15). All four of these hats seem surprisingly large and shallow, but a number of early hats still in existence resemble them (figs. 206 and 396). A fine Tlingit hat of nearly these proportions was collected by Alejandro Malaspina at Yakutat in 1791 (Weber 1976:fig. 11), and others illustrated by the expedition artists José Cardero and Tomas de Suría are of

285

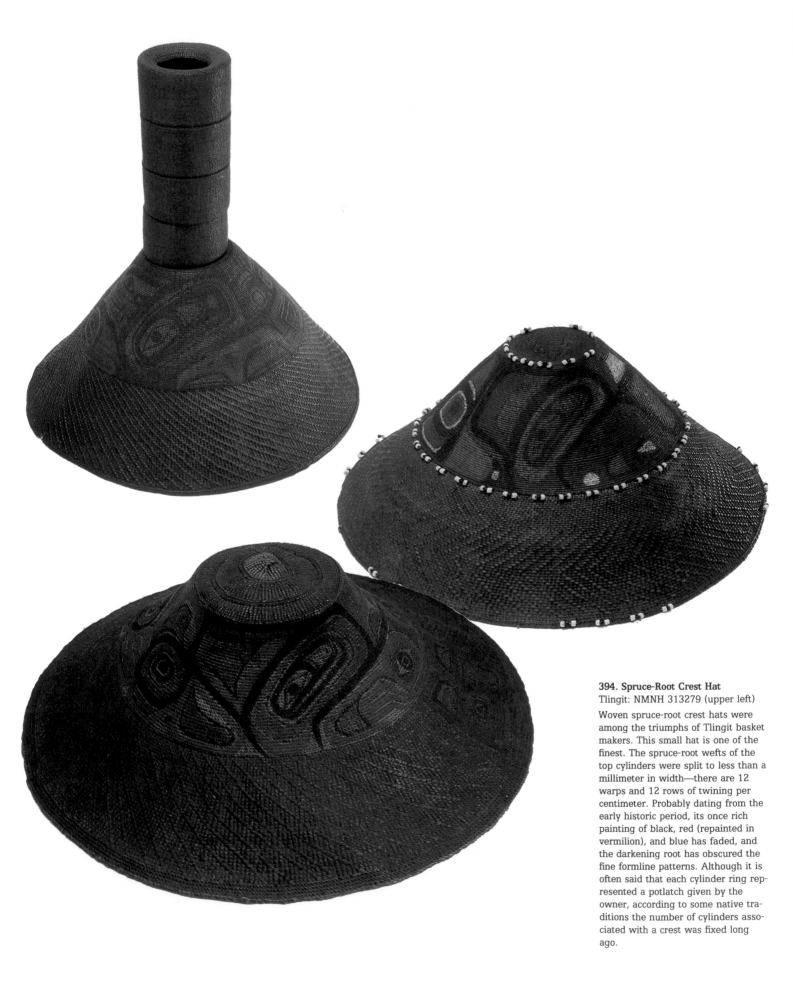

394. Spruce-Root Crest Hat

Tlingit: NMNH 313279 (upper left)

Woven spruce-root crest hats were among the triumphs of Tlingit basket makers. This small hat is one of the finest. The spruce-root wefts of the top cylinders were split to less than a millimeter in width—there are 12 warps and 12 rows of twining per centimeter. Probably dating from the early historic period, its once rich painting of black, red (repainted in vermilion), and blue has faded, and the darkening root has obscured the fine formline patterns. Although it is often said that each cylinder ring represented a potlatch given by the owner, according to some native traditions the number of cylinders associated with a crest was fixed long ago.

395. Beaded Spruce-Root Hat

Tlingit: MAE 2520-21 (center left)

Although the painting on this early hat is classic Tlingit in composition and detail, it appears to have been partially repainted in a way that suggests use by non-Tlingits, perhaps Pacific Eskimo. Orange-and-white paint have been applied over some tertiary areas that would have been properly painted blue, and white also appears over two black inner ovoids and in some background areas. Bead decorations are also atypical for Tlingit hats. Since no information accompanies the hat which could tell us more, the assumption must be that here is a Tlingit piece acquired and modified by a Chugach or Koniag, before its purchase by a Russian collector. It is good evidence for intertribal contact and exchange.

396. Painted Spruce-Root Hat

Tlingit: MAE 2520-14 (lower left)

Very similar in its proportions, weaving techniques, and arrangement of painted design to early hats of the Chugach and Koniag, this hat can be identified as of Tlingit origin on the basis of the close adherence of its painting to the formline design system followed by Tlingit artists. Both black primary and vermilion secondary formlines show the continuity and structure of a typical early Northwest Coast hat design. The principal figure cannot be positively identified, but in his wide mouth he holds an animal, apparently a frog, delineated in red formlines. A rectangular panel of painting extending to the front edge of the hat shows a faint, facelike design apparently once overpainted with blue.

similar form. Two other beautifully woven and painted hats much like the Malaspina example in basketry technique, form, and painting style were also collected early in the historic period. (They are now in the Anthropological Museum of the Lomonosov State University, in Moscow, and the Institute für Völderkunde der Universität, in Göttingen.) The painting on all three of these hats is in classic Tlingit style, although the hats themselves have basketry details similar to those of documented Pacific Eskimo baskets. The close relationship of Koniag and Chugach painted basketry hats to those of the Tlingit is obvious even at a casual glance.

Contact-period twined spruce-root hats of the northern Northwest Coast and the Pacific Eskimo region share many structural and formal features. They usually have a truncated conical form with little or no concavity to the slope of the sides, unlike later 19th-century hats. The flat top and the sides as far down as the inner headband were typically woven in three-strand twining, producing a regular texture similar to a tight coil of finely plied cord, well suited as a painting surface. On a few hats from both areas the flat circular top was elaborated with concentric rings of alternating single or multiple rows of two- and three-strand twining. Below the smooth three-strand section the weavers changed techniques, twining two weft strands over single warps, resulting in a radiating texture. This was elaborated by enclosing two warps at regular intervals, producing raised lines on the surface in diagonal, zigzag, or concentric diamond designs. On some of the finest hats these patterns were divided by spaced, concentric lines of three-strand twining.

There is no way to know whether the custom of painting only the top of the hat determined the placement of the smoothly twined, three-strand surface at the top, or vice versa. In any case, most early hats follow that arrangement. On Pacific Eskimo hats the painted designs were clearly derived from Tlingit prototypes. Kaj Birket-Smith wrote of them, "[That] the elaborate *designs* in carving and painting are derived from Northwest Coast art is so obvious that it needs no further documentation" (1953:221) (emphasis added). What is not so obvious is just how the two design traditions differ and in what ways Pacific Eskimo painters modified the parent style to suit their own aesthetic.

If a twined spruce-root hat in the form of a truncated cone and painted with formline-like designs on the upper, three-strand half is decorated with bundles of sea lion whiskers, it is certainly a Chugach or Koniag hat, and if it has glass beads sewn on the outer surface, the chances are also very good that it is one. Of the 46 hats examined for this study attributed to the Pacific Eskimo,[2] 23 were decorated with beads and 12 of those also with dentalium shells. Of the 24 old Tlingit-attributed hats examined (comparable in shape and style of decoration to the Chugach and Koniag hats) only 3 had bead decoration (fig. 395). One of those has unusual painting that may have been redone. A number of early accounts mention the use of beads on the basketry hats. David Samwell, with Cook at Prince William Sound in May of 1778, wrote,

They wear two sorts of Caps, one of which is exactly like those of George's Sound & variously painted, the other sort have a kind of Pyramid built on top of them & are worn only by the Men of the first Consequence among them; they paint all their Caps with various figures and some who can afford it have them ornamented with beads of different colors (Cook 1967:1112).

The Cook expedition had come directly from Nootka (King George's) Sound to Prince William Sound and had not met any Tlingits, otherwise Samwell would probably have recognized the "kind of Pyramid" as the stack of basketry cylinders topping the hats of high-ranking men. Among the Tlingit and other northern Northwest Coast people the number of these cylinders on a crest hat had specific significance (fig. 394), whereas it appears that those on the hats of the "Men of the first Consequence" at Prince William Sound and Kodiak (fig. 405) had only a general reference to high status since there was no developed sense of crests or inherited rank there. A Chugach-style hat in the British Museum, apparently collected by Cook (King 1981a:50 no. 10, 1981b:fig. 11), is surmounted by four large "potlatch rings," and another (King 1981a:no. 9) has bead decorations of the kind mentioned by Samwell.

Although the forms of the hats and the material and techniques used in making them are nearly identical to those of Tlingit hats, the painted designs on Pacific Eskimo hats show interesting differences from their Tlingit prototypes. Those differences are most apparent if the design system followed by Tlingit painters is well understood, and for that reason it would be useful to briefly review its structure (Holm 1965). This system is a remarkably organized and logical one, followed closely by artists of the northern Northwest Coast from some ancient time long before the historical period and extending through the 19th century. After a period of decline, it was revived in the mid-20th century and is again widely and closely adhered to by native artists. The principles of form and structure were clearly defined. Designs were representations, often depicting creatures with crest significance, the display of which was the main motivation for art production. The system of design was flexible enough to allow the artists to fit those figures in any given space, to depict them with varying degrees of naturalism, and to develop individual styles (Holm 1981).

The basic element of the design system was the formline (figs. 397 and 398), a broad linelike figure, most often black in painting, which delineated the main features of the depicted creature. It varied in width according to set principles and formed design units (most characteristically the ovoid and the U shape) that had the attributes of semiangularity and continuity; that is, they were joined in a continuous network across the design field. There were a number of ways that formlines could be merged to avoid abrupt or awkward junctures. Some of these junctures were relieved by tapering the joining formline, and others were broadened at their points of attachment and relieved by a narrow crescent or T-shaped opening that defined the edge of the joined formline. The proper or improper use of these reliefs and their precise shapes and positions are clues to the artist's understanding of the design system. The one exception to the continuity of formlines is in the free-floating character of inner ovoids, the eye irises or centers of joints, which almost never touch their surrounding formline ovoids.

Joining these black, primary formlines and filling in many of the remaining spaces were secondary formlines painted in red. Most of the spaces still unpainted were developed into tertiary designs (not formlines) that were outlined with narrow black, or sometimes red, true lines. If these outlined spaces were painted, it was in blue.

Since the designs were representations of creatures, heads (as well as other body parts that were often conventionalized as heads) were almost always shown, and there were a few standard structures developed for their depiction. Most easily recognized is a rather naturalistic face, either full-face or profile, with a mouth with teeth, nostrils, small round eyes with eyelids, and eyebrows. This form of face seldom represents the head of the depicted animal but typically was used for joints or sometimes the trunk of the animal. It frequently appears on both Tlingit and Pacific Eskimo hat paintings and never as the principal head. The usual way of representing the head of the depicted creature was with a large formline design that with few exceptions takes one of two structural arrangements. The simpler of the two, and the most common on hat paintings, can be called the one-step structure (Holm 1965:fig. 36) (figs. 395–397). The one-step structure can be used for a profile face, but on hats the main creature's head is always bilaterally symmetrical. A peculiarity of paintings on early

hats (and on some other objects) is that the lower edge of the three-strand twining (designed) section acts as the lower formline of the face, which is omitted from the painting itself. The primary formline representing the outer rim of the head begins at this edge. It runs upward and then turns, in a semiangular bend, toward the upper front of the hat, forming the upper edge of the head or forehead in a gentle arch. At the inner edge of the eye socket it turns downward, again with a semiangular bend, until it reaches the upper lip. It then turns outward, with a somewhat more angular bend, and continues nearly parallel with the forehead formline until it reaches the end of the mouth, where it turns downward and joins the lower edge of the design. This is usually a tapered juncture and

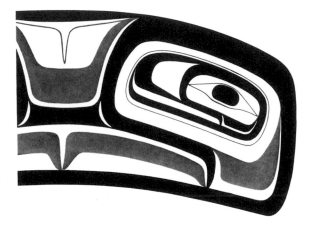

forms the corner of the mouth. The term "one-step" chosen for this structure refers to this single "step" from the corner of the mouth to the eye socket. The second side of the face is a mirror image of the first. A space is left between the two eyes at the front of the hat, and they are joined by a formline that is a continuation of the upper line of the mouth. It may make either straight, tapered junctures with the eye ovoids, or swelling junctures with appropriate reliefs. In any case, the eye ovoid formline is the proper joined formline, while the bridging formline is the joining one.

Joining the formlines of the upper lip and outer edges of the face are red secondary designs that form the cheeks, completing the ovoids of the eye sockets. Within those sockets float the eyes, often elaborated inner ovoids, surrounded by tertiary lines. The space between the tertiary eyelid line and the surrounding formlines is a tertiary area and, if painted, is blue. Within the mouth are more formline designs, usually in secondary red, although sometimes a primary black snout or incisors appear in the center (fig. 396). The space between the eyes is also elaborated with secondary designs and may be bridged by a primary formline at the top.

A somewhat less common and more elaborate arrangement of the facial parts is sometimes seen (figs. 398, 399), which can be called a two-step structure (Holm 1965:fig. 38). In this variant, the formline of the forehead dips sharply between the eyes and continues across the top of the head. A separate formline defines the upper lip, and another formline complex depicts two long nostrils and the bridge of the nose. The nostrils form the second "step" between the corners of the mouth and the eye sockets. These sockets are longer and narrower than those in the one-step form, and they are usually much more angular. Generally the eyes in a two-step face are surrounded by a tertiary line with extended, eyelidlike points. Long cheek designs extend over the top of the upper lip to join the corners of the nostrils, and the inside of the mouth is often elaborated with teeth and a red, secondary tongue.

These large head designs spread at least halfway around the hat. The remaining space is devoted to the rest of the creature in highly abstracted form (fig. 400). A typical arrangement includes a pair of large ears, represented by horizontal formline U's, attached to the outer edges of the head. The upper leg of each U is joined to the forehead formlines along the top

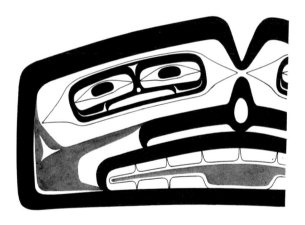

398. Diagram of Two-Step Structure

rim of the hat, and the lower legs join the head at or near its outer corners. At the back of the hat are usually placed a pair of formline ovoids with their enclosed inner ovoids, representing joints, probably of the pelvis of the represented creature. Extending forward from these joints and filling the spaces between the U-form ears and the lower edge of the painting are U complexes representing feathers or fins, or feet with extended claws. The majority of hat paintings follow some variation on this composition. The differences come in the way the rear ovoids are joined and in the elaborations of the secondary spaces. Some of these differences have to do with the meaning of the design; others are the result of the individual artist's choices.

Painted spruce-root hats of the Chugach and Koniag were seen, described, pictured, and collected by many of the earliest European explorers of the North Pacific. In 1805 Lisianskii noted that "on the upper part of these hats some whimsical figures are generally painted" (Lisianskii 1814:194). Although it is typical of early commentators to write condescendingly of the unfamiliar cultures with which they came in contact, and to misjudge the meaning of objects, Lisianskii's characterization of Koniag hat painting as whimsical may not have been too far off the mark. Certainly the designs on Pacific Eskimo hats were derived from Tlingit models without any of the burden of crest significance. There is no direct evidence that any Koniag or Chugach man could not have such a painted hat. Samwell's comments of 1778 suggest only that hat rings denoted a man of "first Consequence" and that bead decorations were limited to those who could afford them.

Little sense can be made of the documentation for these existing painted hats in determining any pattern of styles in relation to age or source. Many hats that are clearly Pacific Eskimo in style have been labeled Tlingit, often by a later cataloger. Hardly any have original collection information to indicate whether they came from Kodiak or Prince William Sound.[3] Because of the many ambiguities in the record, for the purposes of this study I have identified hat paintings as Tlingit or Pacific Eskimo according to their adherence or lack of adherence to the formline system[4] and have not differentiated between Chugach and Koniag examples. Neither am I going to try to relate dates to changes in style over the century from Cook in 1778 to William Fisher in 1884, during which these hats were collected. The three hats in this study believed to have been collected on the Cook expedition in 1778 exhibit a range of styles as great as can be seen in the whole collection.

Some of the Pacific Eskimo hat designs are so much changed from their Tlingit prototype that only a vestige of face structure remains to tell of their origins. On the other hand, a number of hat paintings are so like Northwest Coast designs that it takes careful examination to be sure that they are not. A beautiful hat with elaborately false-embroidered, hair-fringed top cylinders in the Etholen collection (fig. 401; National Museum of Finland 45c; Collins et al. 1973:no. 253) is a good example. The formlines have the same continuity and semiangularity of Tlingit work, the facelike elaboration of the eye is nearly correct, and the red secondary designs are convincing at first glance. A second look reveals many discrepancies. Many of the secondary designs are outlined in black, and all of them,

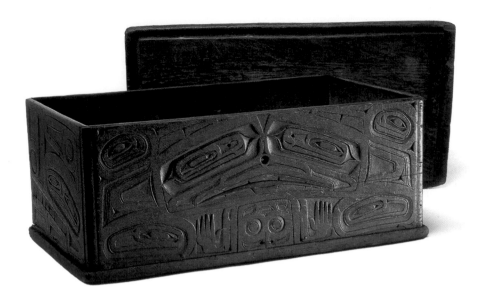

399. Carved Chest
Tlingit: FM 78703
This long, low chest covered with formlines beautifully executed in low relief was once painted, but long use and wear have darkened it until none of the original colors are visible. The old style of the heavy, angular formlines corroborates its age. Standard, symmetrical chest compositions fill the front and back sides, while asymmetrical figures were used on the ends. Later chests were seldom carved on the ends, but were painted only. Although the maker of this chest strictly followed the rules of the formline tradition, the arrangement of the formlines, especially on the end designs, is unique.

including the cheek, float; that is, they do not join the primary formlines at their corners. Many formline junctures are unrelieved by tapering or relief slits. The structure of the eye ovoid is not according to formline principles, and the outline of the secondary U between the eyes merges with the formline bridge at the top. All of these details are unlike classic Tlingit formline design, and their occurrence on a hat with Pacific Eskimo techniques of basketry elaboration clinches the identification. Another equally beautiful hat, in the Turku (Finland) Historical Museum (cat. no. 82 [255]), collected in the 1850s, is almost identical in style and detail. Almost certainly by the same painter, it is decorated with dentalium shells and glass beads in Pacific Eskimo style.

Many Pacific Eskimo hats follow the basic composition of the one-step structure but vary the forms and details so much that they are easily distinguishable from their Tlingit counterparts. An example is a hat in the Museum of Anthropology and Ethnography (fig. 402). The primary formline outlines the upper part of the eye socket but joins the lip rather than continuing under the eye (a common Pacific Eskimo variant). The upper lip formline parallels the lower edge of the design rather than the upper formline. It then angles sharply down instead of following the semiangular form of the prototype. There is a red, secondary cheek design that repeats the angle of the lip, giving the eye socket an unusual, angular bottom. Three circles connected by a horizontal line in the eye is a very Eskimo, geometric suggestion of the formline detail of the Northwest Coast elaborated inner ovoid. A humanoid face fills the rear joint area, like many Tlingit hats in concept but unlike them in style. Geometrization of the claws, limbs, and U forms are further indicators of Pacific Eskimo origin.

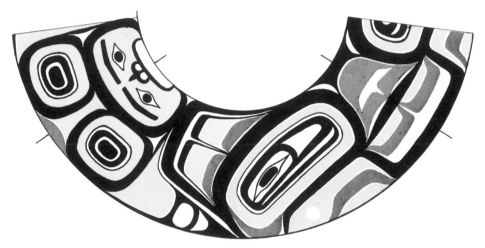

400. Diagram of Tlingit Hat
Fm 53024-1

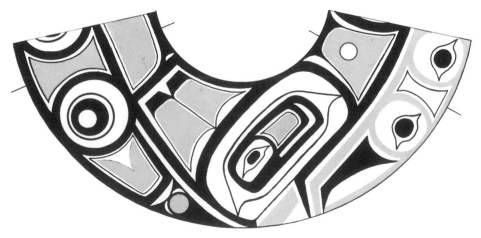

401. Diagram of Pacific Eskimo Hat
National Museum of Finland 45c

402. Painted Spruce-Root Hat
Chugach?: MAE 2520-16

Broad conical hats, expertly woven of split spruce-root, were among the Northwest Coast culture features adopted by the Pacific Eskimos sometime before the arrival of Europeans on the coast. Many, like this one, show their Northwest Coast heritage clearly in the painted designs on the crown. But even though the artist kept close to traditional Tlingit arrangement and color use (black-and-red formlines with blue tertiary areas), the formline shapes and junctures are recognizably different from those in Tlingit painting. They have become adapted to the Pacific Eskimo aesthetic and are beautiful in their own right.

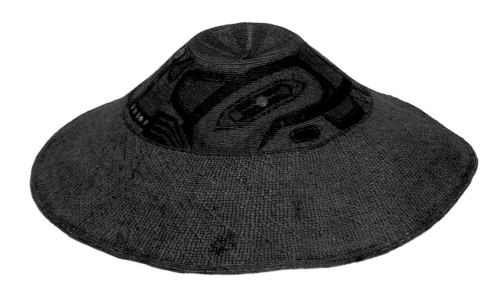

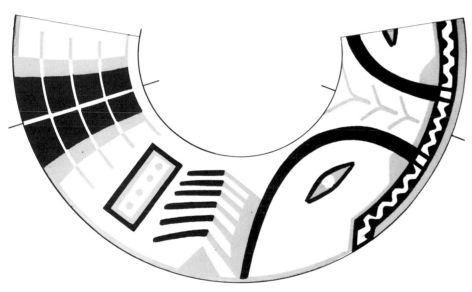

403. Diagram of Pacific Eskimo Hat
MAE 536-12

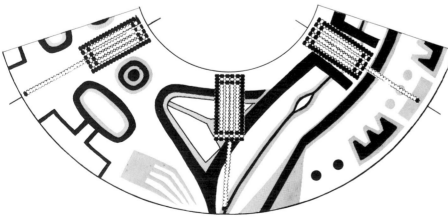

404. Diagram of Eskimo Hat
Koniag? MAE 5795-23

Another fine Pacific Eskimo hat illustrates another version of the one-step composition (fig. 206). The formlines are very angular, with a right-angle juncture at the lip relieved by a small, square gap. The ear formlines are rounded with sudden tapers at their points of joining the head. The lower juncture strikes the corner of the eye ovoid, rather than turning and fairing into its side according to formline conventions. Many Pacific Eskimo hat paintings use an eye and eyelid like this one, with a small, narrow iris and long, constricted eyelid points reaching to the edge of the socket. The tertiary split U in the ear is open and angular. Although the clawed foot is similar to the Tlingit form, the lack of an attached limb and the red paint between the claws is another indication of its nonconformity. And finally, the ovoid complex at the rear of the hat has become completely geometric—a pair of black-bordered rectangles separated by a crosshatched space and flanked by small rectangular projections.

The hat worn by Webber's ''Man of Prince William's Sound'' in 1778 has a peculiar design on the front. It is much like the back of this hat. I'm convinced that Webber has drawn the back rather than the front. Perhaps his sketch was finished in his cabin onboard the *Discovery*, with the hat, newly purchased for a few blue beads, on the table before him—backwards.[5] Webber's drawing is even more like the back of another hat in Leningrad (fig. 403). The design has become even more geometric. The formline has been reduced to an arc looping over the eye, joining a long, toothed mouth. The secondary cheek designs have disappeared. The claws are reversed and have become multiple, narrow chevrons. The ovoid joints in the back are now floating, narrow rectangles lined with a row of

291

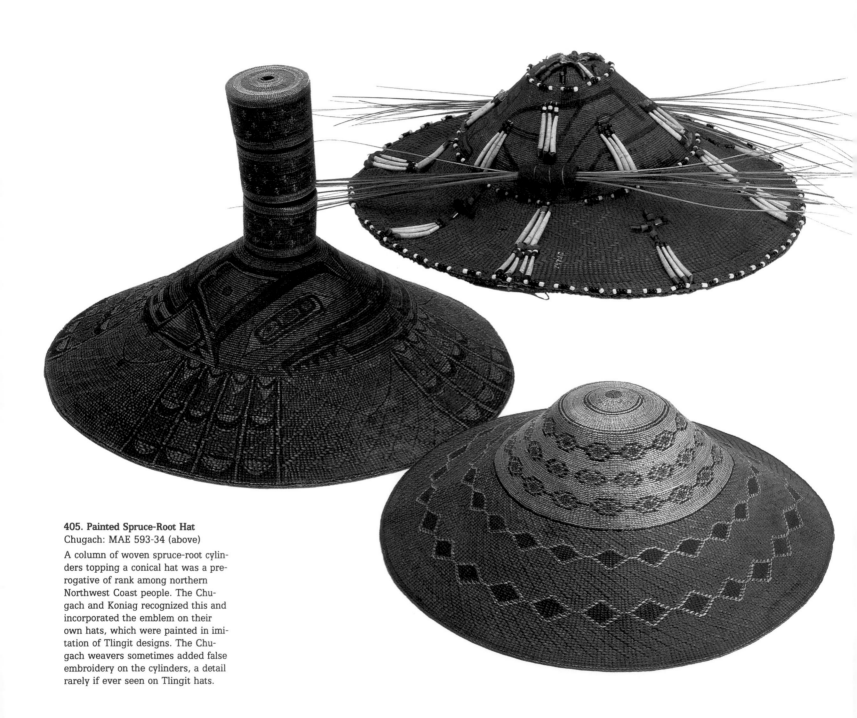

405. Painted Spruce-Root Hat
Chugach: MAE 593-34 (above)

A column of woven spruce-root cylinders topping a conical hat was a prerogative of rank among northern Northwest Coast people. The Chugach and Koniag recognized this and incorporated the emblem on their own hats, which were painted in imitation of Tlingit designs. The Chugach weavers sometimes added false embroidery on the cylinders, a detail rarely if ever seen on Tlingit hats.

406. Decorated Spruce-Root Hat
Koniag: NMNH 74720 (left)

Koniag spruce-root hats of the 19th century often carried a spectacular array of beads, dentalia, and sea lion whiskers, arranged in symmetrical patterns right over, and seemingly without regard to, the painted designs on the crown. The spruce root and whiskers were local products, the beads and probably the shells were acquired in trade. Dentalia grew here and there off the coast, but the best-known fisheries were on the west coast of Vancouver Island. Nootka and west coast Kwakiutl harvested the shells and sold them to traders, who spread them over western North America. No doubt many were traded intertribally before the Euro-American fur trade, and they were highly prized everywhere.

407. Diagram of Pacific Eskimo Spruce-Root Hat
Pacific Eskimo: MAE 344-73

408. Woven Spruce-Root Hat
Chugach: MAE 633-18 (left)

Most Pacific Eskimo spruce-root hats are painted with Tlingit-like designs. A few incorporate *grass false embroidery* (fig. 405). This elegant and unique hat uses false embroidery decoration, in patterns like those seen on Pacific Eskimo baskets. Painting in dark red and blue sets off the grass embroidery, now nearly a uniform gold but probably once dyed in bands of color.

dots. And the stripe up the back has lost all semblance of a Northwest Coast formline design.

A group of hats all heavily decorated with beads, dentalia, and bundles of sea lion whiskers share design characteristics that are even further removed from their formline roots but that still can be traced back to them (fig. 404). Although a hat in the U.S. National Museum of Natural History (fig. 406) was collected in 1884 on Kodiak Island, it is nearly identical with others collected much earlier. Most of these hats are, or were, painted entirely blue, with the design over-painted in red and black. The formlines have become very narrow and open and have lost nearly all continuity. Long eyelids—black, red-bordered lines opening to tiny, diamond eyes in their centers, a frequent convention in Eskimo art—reach from the lower border to the abrupt inner ends of the eye sockets. In the mouth two short bars, each with three upright projections, suggest teeth. Ears form long, split loops, and the claws have become tiny, geometric vestiges. The rear joints are now pairs of rectangles over flat bars with upright, round-headed knobs. The spidery, meandering paintings of this group of hats are overwhelmed by their spectacular clusters of dentalium shells and beads and the thrust of the flanking sprays of sea lion whiskers.

A group of 13 hats using the two-step configuration is very uniform in detail. Many of them are decorated with beads and a few with dentalium shells and whiskers. Three of them have top cylinders, and two of those are elaborated with false embroidery. Five of them have four painted panels extending to the outer rim of the hat. Classic formline two-step designs tend to

be somewhat angular, and these all share that characteristic. They all have the separate mouth and nostril formlines (with resulting long, angular cheek designs) typical of two-step structures. Large, angular U-shaped ears extend back from the head. At the rear of the hat, complexes of formline ovoids and U forms fill the space, extending out under the ears in the form of feathers or claws. Human faces fill the space between the ends of the ears on six of these hats (figs. 405, 407). The eyes on eight of the hats resemble elaborated formline inner ovoids, the rest are decorated with two or three ovals in a row. An interesting hat in the U.S. National Museum originally was painted with a standard Pacific Eskimo version of the two-step structure and was later overpainted with a design typical of hats decorated with dentalia, beads, and sea lion whiskers (figs. 404 and 406). Unfortunately this hat has no documentation, so all we know is that on this particular hat the one style preceded the other.

At the end of the 18th century, when the first of these hats were noted and collected, the Pacific Eskimo were already in the grip of a powerful acculturative force. Russian fur hunters dominated them and their Aleut neighbors, and the continuing development of their distinctive way of life was diverted. The assimilation of a foreign style of hat and its decoration was in progress just at the time when native lifestyle and art production were about to disappear. Fortunately a good number of examples of this interesting product of diffusion were collected and preserved in the museums of the world.

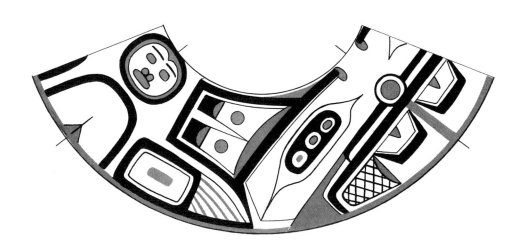

Comparative Art of the North Pacific Rim

William W. Fitzhugh

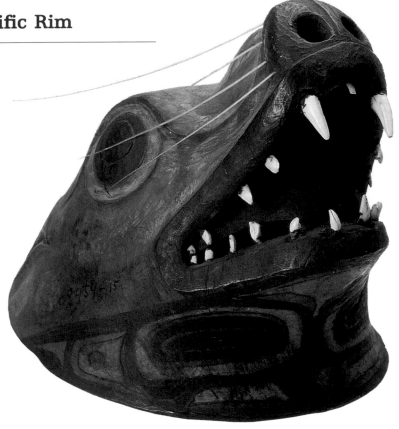

"There is in New York a magic place where all the dreams of childhood hold a rendezvous, where century old tree trunks sing or speak, where indefinable objects lie in wait for the visitor with an anxious stare; where animals of superhuman gentleness press their uplifted little paws, clasped in prayer for the privilege of constructing for the chosen one the palace of the beaver, of guiding him into the realm of the seals, or of teaching him, with a mystic kiss, the language of the frog and kingfisher" (Lévi-Strauss 1943:175).

For more than 50 years the native arts of the Northwest Coast and Alaska have been recognized as being among the finest in the Americas. Originally seen at the Philadelphia Centennial Exposition of 1876 as "repellant curiosities" (Cole 1985:30), its obscure, fantastic forms and primal energy remained unappreciated by most Western viewers until the 1940s when it was discovered by the Surrealists (Cowling 1978). Today, following a generation of "primitive" art exhibitions, native arts are increasingly seen in the context of the cultures that produced them. While the arts of the Northwest Coast and North Pacific–Bering Sea region typically have been studied from a regional or local (ethnographic) perspective, few studies address the problem of broader comparative analysis. This study is a preliminary attempt to reveal patterns, relationships, and historical processes in the arts of North Pacific peoples.

Early anthropologists believed that high-quality art resulted from settled agricultural life, market economy, craft specialization, and centralized political control. Somehow, Caucasians could imagine exceptions in the European Paleolithic but not among peoples of the Far North. Yet the discoverers of North Pacific peoples found the inhabitants of the foggy, windswept, often icebound North Pacific and Bering Sea

coasts in possession of elaborate works of art. Apparently, productive maritime economies offered alternative routes to aesthetic excellence, even under harsh environmental conditions.

Geographically, the artistic panorama of the North Pacific consists of two distinct groups, one American and the other Siberian. Only in the cases of Asian and Inupiat Eskimo, who share opposite sides of Bering Strait, and the Eskimo-influenced Maritime Chukchi is there evidence of significant overlap. Quintessentially American, the great carved memorial (totem) posts of the Haida, the elaborate winter ceremonial masks of the Kwakiutl, the elegant formline art of the Tlingit, and the less well known but equally artistic clothing, carved ivory, and ceremonial arts of the Aleut, Athapaskan, and Eskimo peoples have added immeasurably to the world's great art traditions. Less well known to North Americans are the works of Northeastern Siberian peoples: the formal elegance of Amur fishskin clothing, the embroidered and beaded costumes of Even shamans, the stunning design of Koryak funeral coats, and the sculptural work of Koryak and Chukchi ivory carvers. Though less elaborate than Native American arts, Northeastern Siberian art represents a large and cohesive body of material. Yet, despite two centuries of collecting, exhibition, and publica-

409. Ceremonial Raven Pipe
Tlingit: NMNH 337354

This pipe, carved as mythical Raven in partly human form, is monumental in concept but only eight centimeters high. Animal ears top his head, but human ears and tiny feet show him in a state of transformation. He grasps a human head with raven's claws. His formline wing and tail carvings cover him like a painted robe. Few objects epitomize the ceremonial, social, and aesthetic concepts of Tlingit art as well as this.

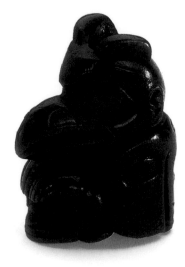

410. Sea Lion War Helmet
Tlingit: MAE 2454-15

Animal-based art, characteristic of hunting cultures, was a dominant theme on the Northwest Coast and in Alaska. Tlingit artists carved many animals on war helmets, but perhaps the most common was the bull sea lion. Among the largest, strongest and most aggressive mammals encountered by the Tlingit, the Steller sea lion was a fitting subject for warrior's regalia. The bull's habitual pose, head thrust upward, roaring, lent itself to helmet art. Real sea lion teeth and whiskers, sweeping back from the nostrils, gave added realism.

411. Ritual Hunting Helmet
Alaska Peninsula?: MAE 2868-40

The blending of artistic traditions that often occurs at the boundaries between cultures is clearly seen in this hunting helmet. In basic form the hat is Aleut: shape, construction, ivory side volutes, rear plaque, Thunderbird crest carving, beaded sea lion whiskers, and multicolor horizontal banding (cf. fig. 204). However, a Koniag or Bering Sea Eskimo origin is likely for its detailed pictographic panels of Thunderbird mythology and linear narratives of hunting expeditions.

412. Killer Whale Fish Club
Tlingit: NMNH 224419

Clubs of hardwood, sometimes elaborately carved as animals or spirit allies, were used to kill halibut and salmon. Seals and sea otters were killed the same way. Very often these carvings took the form of predators like sea lions or killer whales—animals that feed on salmon and seals.

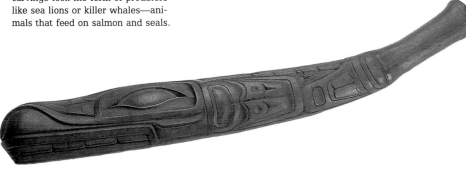

tion, the arts of the greater Beringian region have never been viewed within a single comparative perspective.

On one level, the reasons for this neglect are understandable. The arts of the North Pacific are heterogeneous, and the effects of different histories, environments, and beliefs on the traditions of Asian and American cultures are evident. Unquestionably, there are more similarities within Asian and American groups than between them. There are also more similarities between Asia and America in prehistoric times than in the 19th century. But at a deeper level, both regions share structures, themes, and artistic patterns that betray common heritage.

Within Siberian and American regional traditions, the function of art varied according to economic and social conditions. Four basic types are found in the North Pacific. Hunting art is most widely known from the European Paleolithic but among ethnographic peoples is exemplified best by 19th-century Native Alaskan art. In hunting art, images of game and weapons,

helping spirits, and animal controllers were used to influence, and sometimes to help overcome, animal spirits; in itself, a man's own powers were considered weak and ineffectual. South of the Bering Sea, where communal exploitation of the large, relatively stable fish resources replaced the hunting of marine mammals, different religious views and artistic representations were found. Here, art was used primarily to communicate social values through heraldic crests and insignia. Although art functioned also as hunting magic on the Northwest Coast, its primary role was in expressing social rank, social (totemic) organization, and rights of possession. In Siberia these types of religious and ceremonial art were less important than in America. Siberian art was primarily directed at the design and decoration of clothing. In this regard, it intersected a fourth function common to both regions, as an indication of ethnicity or group membership in ethnic styles of clothing, headgear, and artifact decoration.

The role of history is everywhere apparent in North Pacific art. In medieval Europe, hunting art lingered on the periphery of Western civilization in Celtic and early Norse art, but otherwise one must revert to paleolithic times in Europe to find common ground with artistic traditions of 18th- and 19th-century North Pacific societies. This is what stunned the Surrealists.

But even in the remote North Pacific, historical processes modified ancient artistic patterns. This did not begin with Vitus Bering or James Cook—although it was accelerated by European contacts—nor was it geographically symmetrical. In northwestern North America, hunting art was still dominant everywhere at the time of discovery, as the collections in this exhibition attest. Archeological data indicate its former presence in Siberia, but by the time of the first historical accounts in the 16th century, few traces remained. This process had begun at least 2,000 years ago when reindeer pastoralism and technological developments (especially metalworking) and their economic and social consequences began to transform Siberian hunting cultures into more specialized, production-oriented (as opposed to subsistence-oriented) societies. The economic and religious basis for hunting art was incompatible with the ascendant philosophy of human manipulation of the natural world. These changes were manifested in Siberian art by reduction of animal-based themes and increased use of strictly anthropomorphic forms (see Serov, p. 245 in this volume). In North America, where Siberian production economies never gained a foothold, ancient masking traditions and animal-based hunting art prevailed.

Apart from these larger historical patterns, native cultures of the North Pacific developed and changed partly according to their own dynamics and partly in relation to cultures, peoples, and events around them. They created distinctive cultural and regional styles, shared artistic themes, and interpreted their religions and social beliefs in a multitude of artistic forms.

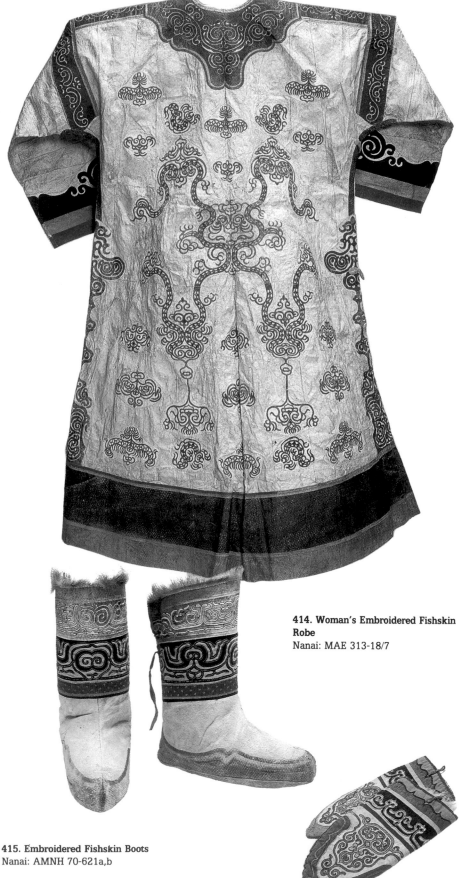

414. Woman's Embroidered Fishskin Robe
Nanai: MAE 313-18/7

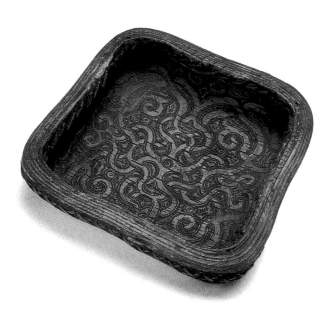

413. Embossed Birchbark Tray
Nivkhi (Gilyak): AMNH 70-876
This tray epitomizes Nivkhi band design, cryptic zoomorphism, and interplay between positive and negative fields.

415. Embroidered Fishskin Boots
Nanai: AMNH 70-621a,b

416. Woman's Embroidered Mittens
Nanai: AMNH 70-620a,b

417. Tasseled Shaman's Coat
Yukaghir: AMNH 70-5620a
Bird features of this shaman's coat
include a winglike shoulder band and
"light world" crosses (birds); also
seen are "dark world" spirits and an
adapted Orthodox cross as a vertebral element.

Siberian Cultures

The Lower Amur

Peoples of the Lower Amur, like those of the
Northwest Coast, created one of the most distinctive art styles of the region (Laufer 1975;
Okladnikov 1981; Shrenk 1883–1903; Schurtz
1896). Fishskin garments, wood utensils and
bowls, birchbark vessels, harpoon heads, fishing
equipment, and metalwork were decorated with
designs based on interlocking bands and spirals,
sometimes hiding beastly animal faces similar
to those known as *t'ao-t'ieh* images on ancient
Chinese sculptures. Bilteral symmetry and use
of "split" design was common. Symmetry, and
the use of negative fields (also shared by the
Ainu), and motifs like roosters, fish, and dragons
also occurred in Chinese art (figs. 21, 413, and
414; Laufer 1975). Amur-style decoration im-
parted a distinctive stamp to nearly all items of
material culture. Embellishment of even the
smallest items, like needlecases (fig. 273), was
de rigueur.

Even

Differences in culture, history and language
between Amur groups and their northern neighbors were expressed also in artistic traditions.
Even ethnic style was seen primarily in clothing;
other material culture was relatively unelabor-
ate. Even clothing decoration was rectilinear and
decorative rather than, as among the Amur
groups, curvilinear, cryptic, and animal-based.
Open coats, aprons, and boots displayed such
patterns as linear and zigzag patterns of brightly
contrasting glass beads; welted seams of light
and dark skin; linear bands of alternating light
and dark panels created by weaving light-colored
skin through slits in a dark skin base; rectangular
panels of decorated skin; and framing of clothing
borders by bead, welted seam, fringe, and fur
trim (figs. 270 and 418). Shamans' clothing,
often acquired from Evenk or Yukaghir shamans,
who were considered more powerful, was decorated with emblematic human forms, amulets,
fur tassels, and various power insignia, including
syncretic adaptations of the Orthodox cross (fig.
417). Dyed moose hair or reindeer hair embroidery (occurring also in North America; Turner
1976), in rectilinear patterns, was applied to
coats, hats, mitts, and gloves, sometimes in
skeletal patterns (fig. 295). Even clothing and
jewelry styles closely resembled those of the
Evenk because of close historical ties.

418. Decorated Cradle Back
Yukaghir: AMNH 70-5200

419. Embroidered and Beaded Pouch
Even: MAE 1799-1

297

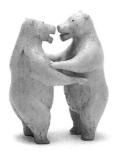

Koryak

Koryak ethnic arts (Jochelson 1975:646–732) were somewhat similar to those of the Even and Evenk, probably because of influence from these groups, but Koryak styles also displayed features derived from Itelmen, Amur, Russian, and local sources. Koryak knives and weapons carried the curvilinear designs of Amur metalsmiths. Similarly, equipment used in reindeer transportation, a technology borrowed from the Even, was decorated with beaded designs familiar to those interior Siberian groups (fig. 232). Despite this evidence of regional craft specialization, Koryak iron jewelry, which was produced from metal traded from Amur sources through the Evenk, featured whaletail imagery.

As with other Siberian groups, it was in their clothing that the most distinctive features of Koryak ethnicity was noted. Emphasizing bold, contrasting forms enhanced by light-dark contrasts, Koryak seamstresses produced striking garments for everyday, festival, and funeral use (figs. 29 and 278); their designs contrasted dark and light geometric patterning in fur appliqué that was offset, occasionally, by equally striking asymmetry (fig. 293) and included fringes and

beaded tassels (fig. 421). Parka hem friezes of quilted reindeer fur and of multicolor embroidered silk were especially distinctive. Skin garments were decorated with stamped geometric designs made with woodcut blocks that, like floral patterns (fig. 293), seem to have been stimulated by designs on Russian calico.

Animal and human subjects were represented in both sacred and secular art. Whale imagery was used in jewelry and in ritual vessels used in the Whale Festival. Anthropomorphic stick-figure charms (''masters'')—dressed and masked in grass—took the same form as masters among other Northeastern Siberian groups. Particularly striking was the elaboration of these designs in ceremonial art, as on Evenk shaman costumes, and in old ritual designs, sometimes disguised, like those on Koryak quivers and on ''masters'' of nets (figs. 182 and 227). Koryak art also included freestanding ivory and wood sculpture depicting animals and people engaged in everyday activities, used both for toys and for sale to outsiders (fig. 420). Coiled baskets with designs similar to late-19th-century Alaskan types were also produced.

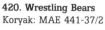

420. Wrestling Bears
Koryak: MAE 441-37/2

Jochelson (1908:646-68) commented on the high quality of Maritime Koryak ivory and bone carving, which he likened to Magdelenian art and to Alaskan Eskimo and Chukchi art. He contrasted it with the lack of carved art among the Yakut, Evenk, and Even, noting that even the Reindeer Koryak produced little in the way of realistic carvings. Jochelson attributed this to the lack of permanent winter settlement and the requirements of nomadic life. Similar differences in art exist between sedentary coastal and nomadic interior hunting peoples of northwestern North America.

These wrestling bears, a subject commonly portrayed in Koryak and Chukchi carving, reflect market developments. In producing illustrative, freestanding art severed from its previous religious and technological functions, Koryak carvers drew on traditional themes and skills to produce works that pleased whalers, traders, and scientists. Similar changes occurred, for similar reasons, in Alaskan Eskimo art after the whaling era began in 1848.

421. Siberian Design Sampler
(top to bottom) Koryak: MAE 956-54; Chukchi: MAE 1791-174; Kamchadal: AMNH 70-2203; Koryak: MAE 1059-85

This set of Siberian designs begins with a slit-embroidered man's funeral belt (*top*) of white dog skin against dark hide, creating rhythmic color contrasts. Chukchi created a similar effect in a belt using dyed appliqué against bleached sealskin. Plant ornamentation, seen in the embroidered Kamchadal belt, was not native to Siberia, but was stimulated by designs on Russian calico. Floral designs also spread around the world in the other direction, reaching Siberia from the east (fig. 323). Both geometric and floral designs were used in the elaborate appliqué and colored silk embroidery on Koryak dance and funeral coats.

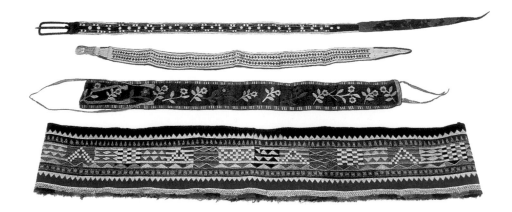

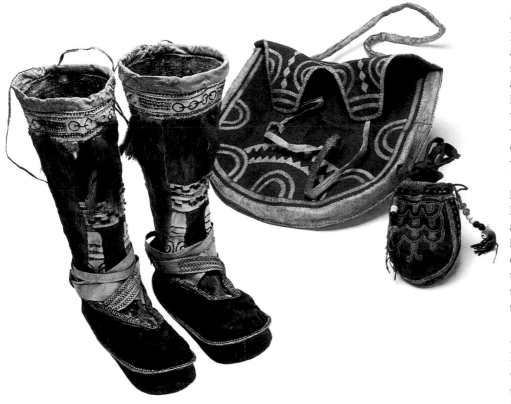

422. Winter Boots

Asian Eskimo: AMNH 60-3552a,b

These Asian Eskimo winter boots have tasseled uppers like Alaskan boots, but the foot construction is a strictly Siberian style. Soles are crimped out rather than in, as in Eskimo fashion; toes are square; and the boot has a high, loose vamp of curried leather that provided room for grass insoles. This pair is embroidered with spurred line and barred circle motifs, executed in colored wool.

423. Pouch Design

Asiatic Eskimo: AMNH 60-3678 (left); Koryak: 70-1951 (right)

These St. Lawrence Island Eskimo and Koryak bags display similar patterns even though based on different traditional design systems. The larger bag uses bleached sealskin appliqué of doubled pendant "U" and bar motifs and an arcing toothed mouth design to create the face of a stylized beast. Rows of similar pendant "U" forms embroidered in white reindeer hair create a fishscale pattern in the tasseled Koryak bag.

Chukchi

Proceeding toward Bering Strait, a trend of declining artistic production was evident in the 19th century. The inhabitants of this region were not noted for their art but for trade, war, and independence. Among Reindeer Chukchi, the requirements of reindeer nomadism were not conducive to artistic production, especially for the men; consequently, their utensils, tools, and ivory carvings were simple and unelaborated. (Later, in the 20th century a skilled engraving art developed among the Maritime Chukchi; fig. 327.) The finest artworks were those of Chukchi women, who excelled at needlework, producing bold and elegant appliqué designs on skin bags and finely embroidered boots, mitts, quivers, and emblematic plaques on hide shields. These designs included interlocked circles, doubled and spurred lines reminiscent of ancient Old Bering Sea and Punuk art (pp. 121–29), and appended U forms with interlocked semicircular and arch (sometimes toothed) motifs (figs. 38, 40, 227, and 297).

Men's art was largely figurative. Complex painted illustrations representing cosmological concepts appeared on ritual paddles (fig. 344), but most common were simple illustrations, sometimes using perspective, depicting spirits, myths, animals, hunting scenes, and encounters with other people, including Westerners (fig. 443). The most elaborate creation of this type is a sealskin hide painting illustrating Chukchi life, environment, and history (fig. 444).

Siberian Overview

Except when used as pictographic art on wood and ivory, as effigy figures on the clothing of shamans, as simple leather and wooden masks, and as zoomorphic forms of ritual containers, humans and animals appeared infrequently in the art of Northeastern Siberians and rarely were presented in abstracted rendition. The exception to this pattern was in the Amur region, where zoomorphic representation, often in "cryptic" form, was common. Here, masked beasts, semihuman faces, and even simple forms like roosters, fish, and dragons appear and disappear from the tracery of lines alternating between positive and negative fields. Artisans of the Amur abhorred blank surfaces and filled them with complex curvilinear designs and cryptic imagery reminiscent of ancient art styles of the northern steppes, China, and the Bering Sea.

Elsewhere in Northeastern Siberia, an entirely different type of art predominated. Among the Even, Evenk, Koryak, and Chukchi, the most elaborate form of artistic expression was a rigidly geometric decorative style of fine beadwork, embroidery, and piecework patterning in clothing. The dominance of this Northeast Siberia geometric style, flanked to the south by a highly ornamental animal-style tradition, raises questions of its origins and history. The geometric style had more affinities with northern Eurasian art than with southern Siberian and Asiatic forms. One wonders what became of Scytho-Siberian art, once distributed from southern Siberia to Bering Strait (see below). The replacement (except in figurative shamanistic art) of the early Eurasian animal-type cryptic art by a largely decorative geometric art north of the Amur marks a major cultural change in eastern Siberia.

These general remarks also note the weak development of masking in Northeast Siberian traditions (cf. Ivanov and Stukalov 1975). The Chukchi did not use masks. The Asian Eskimo used simple masks to depict *Kasak*, Master of the Sea Animals, in annual ceremonies. Elsewhere, the Koryak (including Aliutor and Kerek), Even, Evenk, and Yukaghir used simple hoodlike leather masks in masquerades to scare children and to cover the face of the deceased in funeral rites; Yukaghir men used masks when dissecting the corpses of shamans. Grass masks were worn by the Koryak in the Whale Festival (fig. 346). Few of these Asian masks were named beings (Great Raven being one). In this part of Asia, wood masks were used only by the Koryak and were of simple construction, depicting gaunt-faced men with straw, fur, or patches of black paint to indicate facial hair (fig. 424). Animal masks or masks of semihuman beings, so widely used in North America, were not known. Waldemar Jochelson noted the reduced importance of masking in Northeastern Siberia as compared with northwestern America and saw Koryak masks as most similar to masks from Barrow, Alaska (fig. 425).

In Siberia, mask distribution was spotty, social support for masking was weak or even banned, and the art of masking was of poor quality. The impression created by this general pattern is of a dying tradition, once more widespread, only remnants of which survived into the 19th century. This contrasts strongly with the highly visible and dynamic masking traditions of America and of eastern and southeastern Asia.

Finally, the weak masking complex and lack of animal and human forms in general contrasts with the widespread use of stylized human representations in religious contexts. Stylized anthropomorphic designs were used on shamans' clothing (fig. 417) and as schematic stick-figure masters throughout Northeastern Siberia. Taking human rather than animal or semihuman form as in America, these masters reflect changes in Siberian beliefs from a worldview in which men were dominated by animal spirits and semihuman controlling deities to one in which men exerted significant influence over their destiny. Sacrifice of dogs (fig. 342), bears, and reindeer was one manifestation of this change; depicting gods in human form was another.

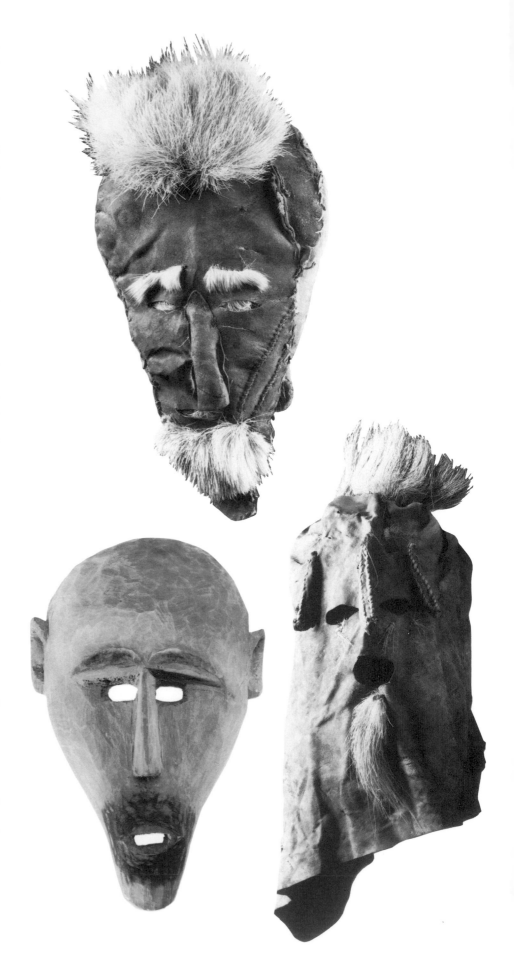

424. Siberian Wood and Leather Masks
Koryak: AMNH 70-3938 (left), 70-3130(right); Chukchi: AMNH 70-6325 (upper)

Grass masks and wood masks were used among the Maritime Koryak, the former in the Whale Festival (fig. 346), and the latter in a Masquerade Festival intended to purge *kalas* (evil spirits) from their winter houses. The mask figured here is typical of Koryak wood masks, whose only elaboration is the marking of facial hair. Reindeer Koryak donned leather hood masks (*right*) representing cannibal *kalas* to scare children. Chukchi used a similar type of mask called "hairy face" (*above*) to represent an evil spirit who carried off naughty children. Except as beastly faces on Chukchi and Asian Eskimo eye shades (Bogoras 1904-09:260), animals were not represented in the rudimentary Siberian masking complex.

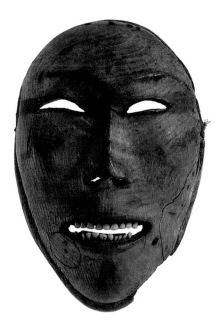

425. Eskimo Mask

North Alaskan Eskimo: NMNH 64230

The American masks most similar to Koryak masks are those from Barrow, Alaska. This mask has a grooved outer rim for securing a hood, a ruff, human teeth, a mustache, and black marks on its chin and across its eyes, which Murdoch (1892:368) called the "whale man's mark." It was worn with a gorget featuring the whale-holding giant *Kikamigo* (fig. 444; cf. fig. 350).

426. Skeletized Animals

Bering Sea Eskimo?: NMNH 168626 (otter). Bering Sea Eskimo: NMNH 1076 (bowl),38637 (spoon)

X-ray views of skeletons and lifelines are seen on this sea otter carving used as a kayak charm; in a hunting magic scene in a bowl showing three "x-rayed" caribou pierced by an arrow and encircled by a thunderbird; and in a similarly portrayed seal encircled by pierced (*tunghak?*) palms.

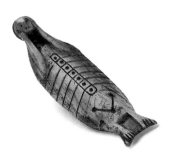

Alaskan Eskimo

The ethnic arts of northwestern North America, as known during the 18th and 19th centuries, surpassed those of Northeastern Siberia in complexity, range, and originality. Not only was stylistic diversity greater between these adjacent regions of Asia and North America overall, but also diversity within Eskimo culture alone (see Himmelheber 1953; Ray 1967b, 1977, 1981) possibly surpassed that of all Northeast Asian groups combined.

The Inupiat Eskimo were renowned for their skill in ivory carving. Tools and personal ornaments were decorated with carvings of arctic species like polar bears, seals, and whales; with various types of line engraving; and with frequent use of the Y motif, usually thought to symbolize a whale's tail but identical also to the image of Siberian anthropomorphic charms (figs. 210, 260). Many Inupiat (and some Yupik) designs were derived from the engraved art of the Punuk archeological culture (A.D. 800–1500) of Bering Strait. Ivory drillbow narrative art portrayed pictographic scenes of hunting activities, village and ceremonial life, hunting tallies, and even encounters with Chukchi and Europeans (fig. 17). Pictographic art was also used in hunting magic (fig. 445). Masking was poorly developed by comparison with Alaskan Yupik peoples (pp. 306–7), but garment transformation styles included walrus symbolism (fig. 71), seen also in doll effigies (fig. 350). Overall, the art of Inupiat Eskimos emphasized decorative and figurative (pictographic) art and lacked abstract qualities.

Alaskan Yupik art was more diverse, abstract, and symbolic than that of Inupiat peoples. Talismans and charms; decoration to beautify hunting gear (figs. 47, 181, and 191); delicately carved ornaments; tools, utensils, and grasswork; exceptional engraved and painted art in ivory and wood; masks of originality and imagination; and finely tailored fur clothing all attest to the exceptional artistic skills of Yupik Eskimos. Although West Alaskan Yupik culture was still largely unacculturated in the mid to late 1800s, glass beads were favored over earlier ivory and jet beads; metal, also a trade item, was still rare.

Whales, polar bears, and walrus dominated the iconography of Eskimo art north of Norton Sound, while seals, fish, and birds dominated along the Bering Sea coast, where these northern fauna were not found. Similarly, Inupiat engraved decoration was derived from earlier Punuk geometric art, whereas engraved styles south of Norton Sound tended toward animal themes, often imbued with spiritual concepts of power and transformation indicated by masked images, joint marks, skeletal designs, and other motifs with specific religious meanings.

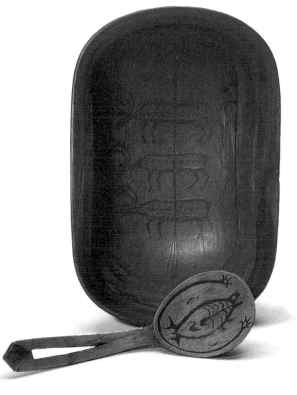

Throughout much of western Alaska, Eskimo art utilized a combination of figurative animal-style and geometric art in both narrative (as in boxlid and drillbow art) and emblematic form. In these areas, the Yupik animal-style art owes more to Old Bering Sea ancestry, with its many cryptic and masked designs, than to Punuk art, whose geometric styles influenced Inupiat art more strongly. Outstanding examples of Yupik art include human and animal effigy bowls and containers (figs. 44 and 94), boxlid art (figs. 444 and 445), illustrated bowls and spoons (figs. 267 and 426), and an imaginative mask-making tradition (see below).

This description applies generally to the Yupik-speaking Pacific Eskimo of the Alaska Peninsula, Kodiak, and Prince William Sound, where clothing, mask types, weapon decoration, and other categories blend elements of Bering Sea Eskimo, Aleut, and Tlingit artistic traditions.

Aleut

Aleut art (Black 1982; Ray 1981) is more difficult to characterize because few traditional artifact types have survived from this region. Aleut material culture is renowned for its attention to detail and its elegance, style, and general fineness. These qualities are noted across all artifact classes. Its kayaks were the fastest and most technologically advanced of any in the arctic world (Dyson 1986), its gutskin clothing the most elegant, its grasswork the finest, and its ritual hunting headgear the marvel of all who viewed them. These paper-thin bentwood hats, festooned with beaded sea lion whiskers, ivory carvings, and flowing scrolls or pictographic painted designs (figs. 181, 203, 204), represented the artistic pinnacle of the type and were so highly abstracted that their probable development from animal-effigy hats (Ivanov 1930; Black 1982, and in press) is almost unrecognizable. This history, not yet proven archeologi-

cally, is suggested by preservation of putative stages in its evolution seen in ethnographic specimens. The sequence begins with Chukchi animal-effigy leather visors and Eskimo decoy hats of identifiable animal head form (fig. 200), followed by intermediate Eskimo forms with abstracted eyes, mouths, and limbs (figs. 201 and 202) and highly abstracted Aleut helmets illustrated with multicolor scrolls, rosettes, spirals, and pictographs. The abstracted band designs are so striking and so unlike other art forms in the North Pacific that one suspects Russian folk art influence. Yet, nearly all of these motifs can be found elsewhere in the Bering Sea—Aleut region in less refined form, even in Old Bering Sea and Aleutian archeological cultures. High social status was a condition of ownership and display of the finest Aleut hats and garments.

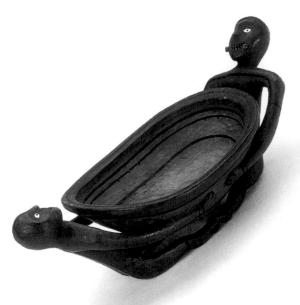

427. Effigy Dish
Bering Sea Eskimo: MAE 593-45

Effigy figures were popular on bowls and dishes made by Eskimos of the Bering Sea coast and Yukon-Kuskokwim Delta. These men wear labrets (beads) and are posed holding the dish in their arms, with their feet braced beneath. Painted bands encircle their wrists and knees as well as the interior of the dish, whose rim is carved with an encircling groove. Encircling marks, characteristic of bowl art and found on most items of material culture, are basic to Bering Sea Eskimo religious beliefs (cf. Fienup-Riordan p. 266). The occurrence of effigy containers among Bering Sea, Koniag, and Chugach Eskimos, and among Northwest Coast Indians, suggests a common North Pacific origin.

428. Painted Hunting Visor
Aleut: MAE 4270-96

Double scrolls, rosettes, and composite forms bordered with dots decorate this thin bentwood visor. The restriction of sea lion whiskers to the left side of the hat kept the hunter's right casting arm free of obstruction. The meaning and origin of the designs are not known. Similar motifs are seen in the 2000-year-old art of the old Bering Sea culture, and they also occur in early historic Aleut art. However, similarities with Eurasian folk art designs and lack of Aleut archeological antecedents render the history of the style ambiguous (cf. fig. 203).

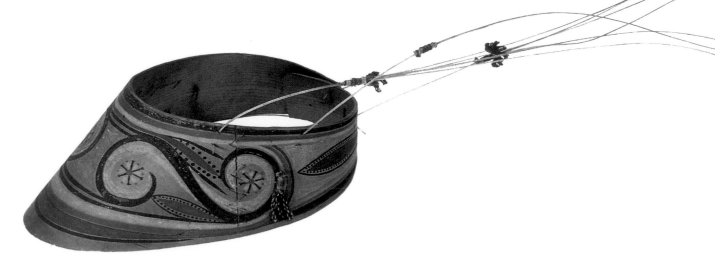

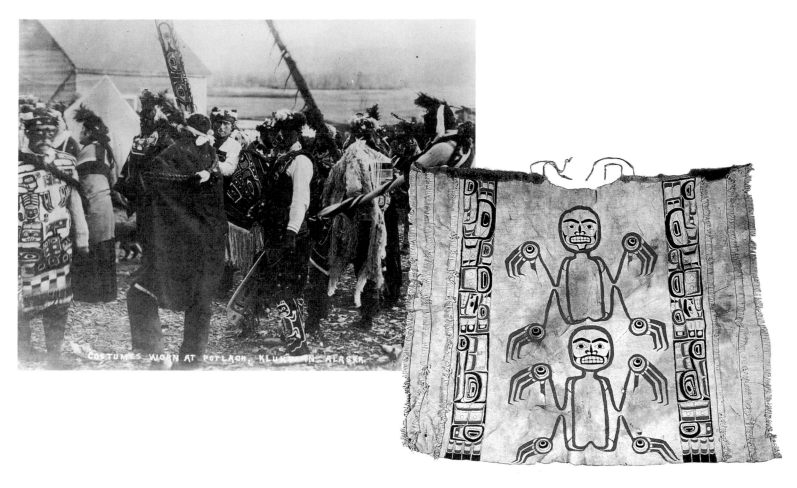

Tlingit and Other Northwest Coast Groups

429. Klukwan Potlatch Costumes
SI neg. 209288, Eric A. Hegg, 1898

Art played an important role in Northwest Coast ceremonial costume and regalia. This photograph shows Tlingit men in potlatch costumes, including Chilkat blankets and leggings ornamented with skeletized birds, bears, and other creatures. Ceremonial headdresses and staffs were also on display.

430. Painted Skin Robe
Haida: NMNH 20807

The squatting semihuman beings painted on this fringed skin robe have toothed mouths, clawed hands, and pierced (or eyed) palms—features also seen in Eskimo and Tlingit art. The border design, probably a sea lion, is a bilaterally symmetrical split image of a single beast. Axial symmetry, also seen in the central figures, is an important principle in Northwest Coast and Old Bering Sea art. Skin robes of this type may have been the predecessors of the appliquéd button blanket, their ornamented borders equivalent to the latter's red flannel, button-decorated borders.

Northwest Coast art is even more difficult to characterize than Eskimo art (Carlson 1983; Holm 1965, 1987; Jonaitis 1986). Regional styles abound, but the practice of owning rights to the use and display of crests, the acquisition of such objects outside their areas of origin, and the commissioning of works from acclaimed artists whose fame had spread outside their own group, produced homogenizing and diversifying elements that complicate regional stylistic patterning. For instance, Chilkat blankets, made among the Tlingit, became highly prized as ceremonial garments throughout the northern and central coast, and canoes made in one place were painted in another and sold to men living in a third.

A differentiating feature of Northwest Coast art, compared with the art of most other North Pacific peoples (except Pacific Eskimo and Aleuts), is its association with social life. Art was used as crests to illustrate and signify social rights and prerogatives, and the social function of Northwest Coast art is emphasized more strongly than is its use in hunting magic or shamanism, which were primary concerns of northern cultures.

Tlingit art was among the most elegant and, in some ways, the most restricted of Northwest Coast art, being expressed primarily on baskets, crest figures, boxes and bowls, blankets, hats, and shaman masks. As in the case of the Amur peoples, Tlingit artisans utilized a single, dominant Northern style that was applied to clothing, painting, and sculpture in a wide variety of media, though not in basketry. Using the visual principle of the formline (Holm 1965 and essay in this volume), Tlingit artists developed codes to present real and mythical beings in highly complicated and abstracted forms. In the fashion of Amur artists, their figures are composed by ingenious modification of a few basic graphic elements within a complex field design; figures and background design wrap around curves and corners on hats and boxes, on spoons and halibut hooks, on helmets, rattles, and other items. The use of cryptic art (hiding animal forms within overall design patterns, creating multiple or alternative images, making figures within figures) and frequent portrayal of semihuman beings were also common. One type of motif, an ovoid face composed of human and bearlike features, is so standardized and so dominates Tlingit art that it must represent an important supernatural concept of character (figs. 281 and 449). This being, used as a repetitive border figure, as a joint mark, as a whale blowhole, and for other

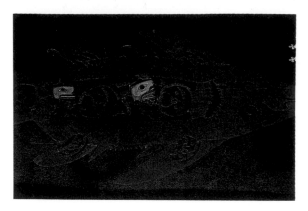

purposes, has an iconlike function in Tlingit art that is similar to the use of face charm motifs in Bering Sea Eskimo art (fig. 198).

Northwest Coast artists utilized a wide range of standardized motifs or codes to communicate information about their subject matter. Since a major function of this art was to represent mythological beings and crest animals, character identification was important. Species were rendered with diagnostic features—dorsal fin for Killer Whale; thick, curved beak for Raven; bulging eyes for Frog. The original key was worked out by Franz Boas (1897), but even Tlingit artists argue about the identity of problem pieces. Other widely used motifs in Tlingit art include joint marks, pierced palms, thumbless hands, the skeletized or "x-ray" views, crouched figures, and use of such techniques as split and splayed figures, cryptic art, and negative fields. Portrayal of humans per se, except in shamans' masks, is rare, nor is gender indicated, except in prehistoric art (Duff 1983).

Tlingit art also included certain styles outside the formline system. A highly developed twined basketry tradition employed geometric and non-curvilinear styles that had little, if any, zoomorphic content. In some respects Tlingit art was more restricted in scope than that of central and southern Northwest Coast groups or of western Alaskan Eskimos. Although formline art seems to have spread south from the northern coast, this style only slightly influenced the art of the neighboring Chugach and Kodiak Island peoples and was, in turn, little influenced by them, except as noted by Bill Holm elsewhere in this volume. Perhaps relevant to its artistic traditions, origin myths tell of Tlingit people arriving on the coast from the interior, and linguists link Tlingit language with Athapaskan rather than with the languages of other Northwest Coast groups.

Athapaskan

Athapaskan art, like that of interior Siberian peoples, is primarily expressed in clothing design and decoration. Created by seminomadic hunters and fishermen without permanent winter villages, who lacked any means of transportation other than by foot or dogsled, Athapaskan material culture was restricted in size and weight and consisted of a relatively few artifact types. Most outstanding was their skinwork, which employed dyed porcupine quill and moosehair embroidery in its early stages and, later, glass beads, dentalium shell, and other trade goods.

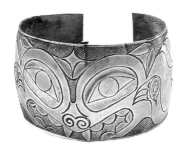

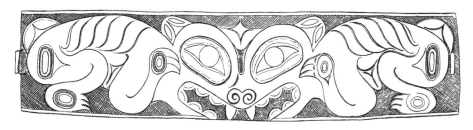

Early contact designs employed bands of checkered pattern quillwork and quill-wrapped fringes as margin and chest decorations on fine, bleach-tanned buckskin tunics (figs. 67 and 298). By the mid-1800s floral patterns introduced into eastern North American Algonquian Indian culture by Europeans reached the Yukon Territory and Alaska overland. These patterns replaced the earlier styles and evolved into elaborate designs on both traditional tunics and European-style "chief's" coats (fig. 433) and on beaded bags. One particular bag made by the Great Lakes Ojibway found its way across North America to the Chukchi, where it was collected by Waldemar Bogoras (fig. 323). The appearance of the floral design among the Chukchi via North America and among the Itelmen via Russian sources (fig. 421) completed its spread around the globe, much like that of tobacco.

431. Button Blanket
Haida: NMNH 89198b

Squatting skeletized humanoids (cf. fig. 430), with wood dorsal fins emerging from their chests, cover the back of this appliquéd dogfish button blanket. The dogfish, a clan crest, is recognized by its arched head and downturned, toothed mouth. Humanoid faces mark the joints of the fins, tail, and dorsal fins. A double row of buttons edges the red flannel border that frames three sides of the robe. The design is particularly bold, and the three dimensional wooded fins add a dynamic note to the flat, appliquéd dogfish.

432. Silver Bracelet
Haida: NMNH 20251b

Khoots, the grizzly bear, a crest of the Raven moiety, is seen on this fine silver bracelet. He has a skeletized back and perforated (or joint-marked) paws and tail rendered in the split form that allows both sides of an animal to be shown on a two-dimensional surface. Nuggets of copper had been used by Northwest Coast peoples for jewelery in prehistoric times. When silver coins came into common use in the mid-19th century, they were hammered into bracelet form, and artists translated formline principles and native designs to the popular new medium.

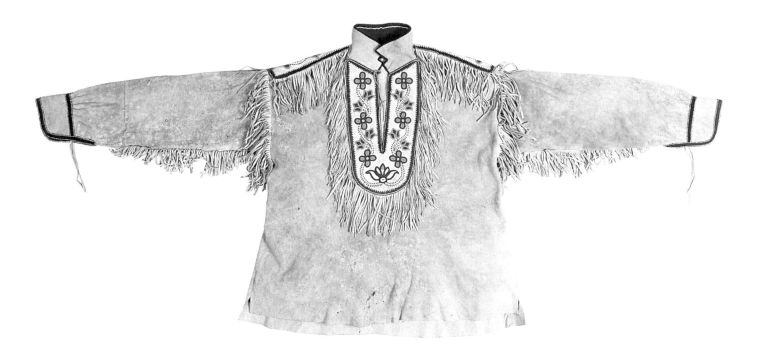

North American Overview

433. Beaded Shirt
Ingalik: NMNH 129824

By the mid-19th century quill-embroidered geometric designs (fig. 298) on Athapaskan buckskin clothing were being replaced by beaded designs, and European cuts were becoming popular. Both fringes, a native tradition also prevalent among Siberian groups, and the use of decorated panels were carried over into the newer styles. The floral design of tendrils, leaves and flowers, derived ultimately from European folk patterns via eastern North America, reached Alaska through a chain of Indian-White and native trade contacts spanning the North American subarctic.

434. Raven's Footprint
Norton South Eskimo: NMNH 393156

For the Eskimos of western Alaska, Raven, Creator of the World and its beings and spirits, was also an untrustworthy trickster. Perhaps for this reason his image was studiously avoided in Eskimo art, in contrast with the frequent representations of Thunderbird, and masks portraying puffins, owls, and other birds and animals. Raven appears in western Eskimo art only as a telltale footprint on the bottom of serving bowls, and occasionally in ivory engravings.

Sometimes confused with Raven's footprint is the "Y" motif, used frequently in prehistoric and ethnographic art of Bering Strait and Northwest Alaska, where it represents a whaletail. Siberian groups use the same motif, in inverted form, to represent two-legged anthropomorphic guardian spirits (fig. 331).

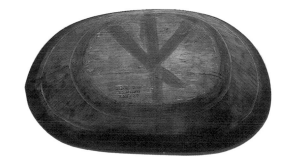

As a group, the arts of the Northwest Coast and Alaska share a number of general and specific features that cut across the distinctive stylistic signatures of individual cultures. As was noted for the Siberian cultures, there are more similarities shared by the American cultures than between these cultures and Siberia. The exception is the Inupiat, whose close cultural connections with Siberian Eskimo represent a special case.

What is most distinctive about American art is the manner in which it expressed spiritual beliefs. Eskimo, Aleut, and Tlingit hunting and fishing implements displayed high-quality craftsmanship, used helping-spirit carvings, and were supported by technologically advanced watercraft and hunting costumes designed to honor the spirits of the animals. Stylistic features varied from group to group, but the underlying theme of showing respect for animal spirits was dominant throughout. Although shamans were also important, individuals retained primary responsibility for relationships with animals they

hunted by virtue of making and maintaining their own equipment and performing necessary rituals.

The social manifestation of these beliefs was expressed in elaborate festivals and ceremonials. Among Alaskan Yupiks, ferocious *tunghak* masks (figs. 180, 436) portrayed semihuman spirit controllers whose superhuman predatory capabilities were moderated by thumbless hands and whose pierced palms signified a role as gatekeeper of the animals' spirit passage between the sky world and the earth. *Tunghak* masks frequently took on phantasmagoric dimensions: twisted "Old Man in the Moon" faces (fig. 353); hoops and feathers signifying the stars and galaxies; and devilishly grinning beastly faces festooned with severed body parts, blood-stained mouths, skeletized views, and panoplies of animal prey. Transformation masks, common in the central Northwest Coast, were relatively rare in Southwest Alaska, but some occur, having grinning heads that turn with strings and bellies that swing open to reveal *inuas,* spirit beings, *tunghak,* animals, and people in grisly encounters (fig. 435). Even masks portraying gentle animals were imbued with vibrant power (fig. 347). Animal spirit and controller masks of similar form and iconography were used by Kodiak Eskimo and Ingalik Indians (figs. 437 and 439). It appears that some Aleut used masks with frames, hoops, and appendages similar to those of Bering Sea Eskimo, but their heavy-featured masks (figs. 164 and 440) are more similar to some Kodiak and Chugach types and to ancient Old Bering Sea forms (fig. 146).

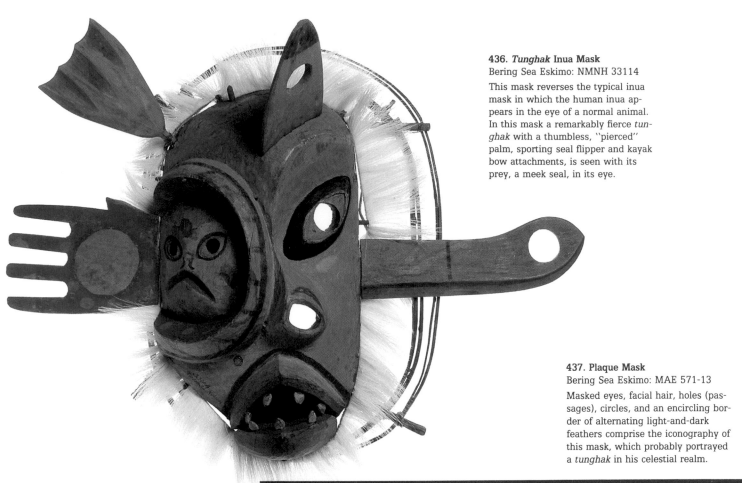

436. *Tunghak* **Inua Mask**
Bering Sea Eskimo: NMNH 33114
This mask reverses the typical inua mask in which the human inua appears in the eye of a normal animal. In this mask a remarkably fierce *tunghak* with a thumbless, "pierced" palm, sporting seal flipper and kayak bow attachments, is seen with its prey, a meek seal, in its eye.

437. Plaque Mask
Bering Sea Eskimo: MAE 571-13
Masked eyes, facial hair, holes (passages), circles, and an encircling border of alternating light-and-dark feathers comprise the iconography of this mask, which probably portrayed a *tunghak* in his celestial realm.

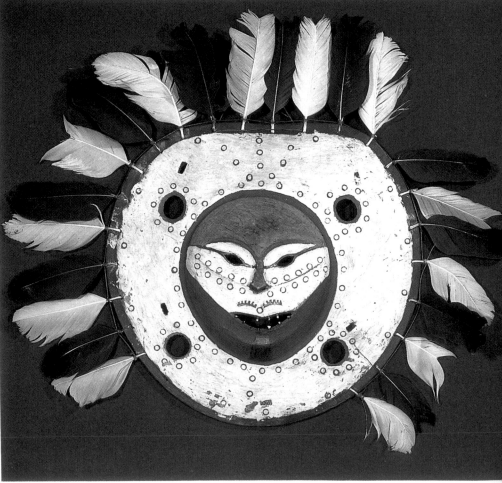

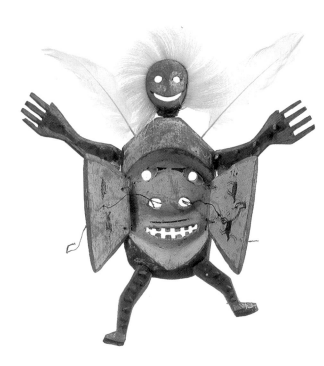

435. Transformation Mask
Bering Sea Eskimo: NMNH 64260
Theatrical surprise enhanced the transformational aspect of this mask figure, whose hinged belly opens to reveal a thumbless, semihuman *tunghak*, framed by fleeing, defecating caribou.

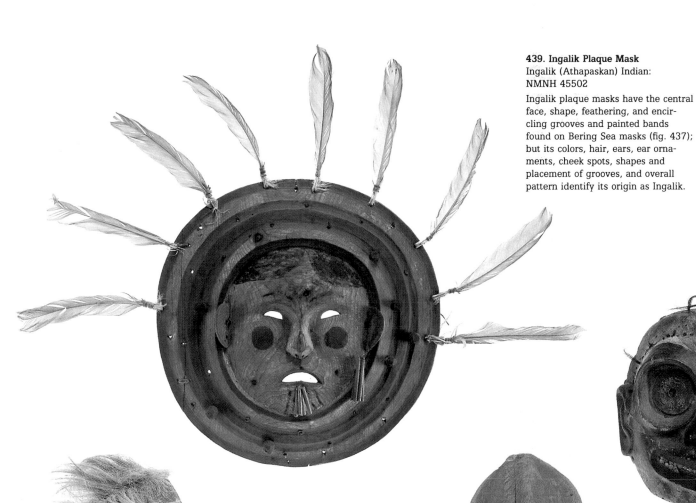

439. Ingalik Plaque Mask
Ingalik (Athapaskan) Indian:
NMNH 45502

Ingalik plaque masks have the central face, shape, feathering, and encircling grooves and painted bands found on Bering Sea masks (fig. 437); but its colors, hair, ears, ear ornaments, cheek spots, shapes and placement of grooves, and overall pattern identify its origin as Ingalik.

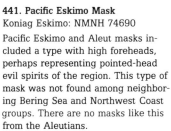

442. Shaman's Mask
Tlingit: NMNH 76855

The staring eyes in this old shaman's mask are made of large bronze Chinese "temple coins" embossed with dragon and foliate forms. The coins could have come from a junk cast ashore on the coast. Disabled junks drifted to North America by ocean currents during the historic period and probably did so periodically over thousands of years (Quimby 1985). But other sources of the coins are possible, including native intertribal trade or the 19th-century maritime fur trade between Canton and the Northwest Coast. In any case, they do well as mystic eyes in the round, hollow sockets of a beaked humanoid spirit face, grinning with power.

440. Death Mask
Aleut: MAE 538-2

Documentation indicates this mask was found in a shaman's grave on Atka Island. Like the similar Ekven burial mask (fig. 146), lack of eyeholes probably protected the corpse from spirit possession.

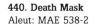

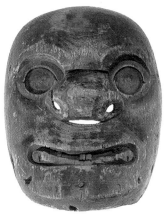

438. Spirit Mask
Ingalik (Athapaskan) Indian: NMNH 339831

While utilizing elements of Eskimo iconography like "spectacles" and spots, this mask from Anvik, upstream from Eskimo territory on the Yukon River, has the long face, hair, and ear ornaments that distinguish Ingalik Indian masks.

441. Pacific Eskimo Mask
Koniag Eskimo: NMNH 74690

Pacific Eskimo and Aleut masks included a type with high foreheads, perhaps representing pointed-head evil spirits of the region. This type of mask was not found among neighboring Bering Sea and Northwest Coast groups. There are no masks like this from the Aleutians.

307

Many features of the Bering Sea masking tradition are found also among various Northwest Coast groups. Transformation masks and circular masks resembling the *tunghak* type were made by various central and southern Northwest Coast groups. More specific are the co-occurrence in western and southern Alaska and the Northwest Coast of motifs such as pierced palms (passage imagery), muzzled jaws, thumbless hands, skeletal views, split images, lifelines, joint marks, "shaman's teeth," eye symbolism (closed, blinded, inset), and semi-human controller images. These similarities are paralleled also by depictions of mythological themes: Thunderbird, Raven (seen only by his footprint in Yupik art; fig. 434), and the drag-onlike illustrations painted on Northwest Coast dugout canoes and Kuskokwim kayaks (*palrai-yuk*). Northwest Coast *sisiutl* serpents or drag-onlike creatures and various wormlike forms, which sometimes assume gigantic proportions, are found in both areas as well. Other similarities between Eskimo and Northwest Coast material culture include effigy bowls, box drums, "house-wives" (sewing kits), and pictographic art.

Asia and America

In their published reports of the Jesup Expedition, Boas, Bogoras, Jochelson, and Laufer had little to say about Siberian-American contacts in art and material culture; instead, they based their "Americanoid" theory—the purported expansion of American cultures west into Siberia—primarily on mythology and linguistic ties. The absence of more extensive parallels (other than harpoons, skin boats, armor, the sinew-backed bow, and a few other elements) was explained by an intrusion of Eskimo into western Alaska from Canada that severed preexisting links between the peoples of Asia and North America. Since the Jesup Expedition, a number of comparisons have been made, but comparisons between Siberian and American art have been rare or nonexistent.

As noted previously, the differences between 19th-century Siberian and American art are more apparent than their similarities and are greater than differences within the Asian or Alaskan groups. The similarities fall into several distinct categories: Eskimo-Chukchi parallels, pictography, and animal art.

Eskimo-Chukchi Parallels

Similarities between Alaskan and Asian Eskimo art exist in clothing, ivory sculpture and engraving, pictographic art, and use of simple human and animal image masks. Resulting from common ancestry and extensive interaction across Bering Strait, these 19th-century parallels are to be expected but would become more interesting should future archeological work demonstrate a deeper and more widespread Eskimo penetration in Asia. Chukchi-Eskimo parallels also exist because of their recent expansion into the Bering Strait coastal region and contacts with Eskimo.

Pictographic Art

Pictographic art (Hoffman 1897; Ivanov 1954) is not confined to the Bering Strait but was noted among Reindeer and Maritime Chukchi, Inupiat and Yupik Eskimo of Alaska, Aleut, Athapaskan, and southern Northwest Coast groups, especially the Nootkan and Salishan groups. Mythological Thunderbird scenes and hunting narratives are a frequent subject both in Siberia and Alaska (figs. 51, 411, and 446). The inherent nature of pictographic art makes it difficult to determine if this art belongs to one or several traditions. Nevertheless, its distribution and its possible relation to North Pacific petroglyphs, which occur widely in northern Eurasia and America, suggest that careful study of this art form is needed.

Even superficial study, however, reveals significant differences between Siberian and Alas-

The arts of northwestern American cultures therefore share common features of various strengths and degrees. These similarities exist both at the level of exchange between neighboring cultures and also at larger scales. At the deepest level are parallels that stem from their common roots in hunting magic and the hunter-prey relationship; the specific artistic forms these parallels take are less similar across cultural boundaries than those, such as Thunderbird, that have a specific (though perhaps ancient) mythological base. Consideration of both general and specific traits reveals a closer relationship between Bering Sea Eskimo and central and southern Northwest Coast art than between Bering Sea or Pacific Eskimo and Tlingit art.

While emphasizing similarities, one must also note the many differences in art styles among American cultures. The shared features noted above signify only modest interchange between cultures whose arts are quite distinct and obviously developed largely independently over the course of thousands of years. Ultimately, only archeological investigation can provide answers to these problems.

443. "History of a Year of the Chukchi"
Chukchi?: Pitt Rivers Museum 1966-19-1

A note attached to this remarkable painted sealskin reads: "A Chukchi drawing on sealskin brought by the Captain of an Arctic Whaler from the Behring Straits, given by him to the late Edward Goodlake, by Mr. Goodlake to Thomas Lord Walsingham, and by Lord Walsingham to me Alfred Denison, 1882." Its published history is equally complex (Hildebrand 1883; Hoffman 1897:938; Ivanov 1954:449). Although alleged to be of Chukchi origin, it may be Asian Eskimo, whose style and cultural activities it more closely resembles.

According to Hoffman, the painting depicts the events of one year on the Chukchi Peninsula coast, whose shoreline outlined in black around the margin, can be identified as Plover Bay, Chaplino, Michigme, and St. Lawrence Bay. Its depictions include whale and walrus hunts, fishing, caribou hunts, sled travel, encounters with European whalers and traders, armored warriors, village and camp life, dancing, sexual encounters, spirits, religious symbols, and a *Kasak* ceremony (equivalent to the Chukchi *Keretkun* ceremony). The two discs in the middle of the drawing probably represent the "Moon-Man" and the "Moon-Man's wife" (cf. Bogoras 1904-0909:313).

444. Pictographic Board and Gorget
Chukchi: AMNH 70-7891; North Alaskan Eskimo: NMNH 64230

Most Chukchi paintings are simple, but this illustration on a plank illustrates a sexual scene in a Chukchi house *polog*, Chukchi women (*left*) and men (*right*) in a line, and Europeans, with a dog, receding behind in convincing perspective. Cranes (*right*) and raptors or ravens (*left*) are shown as profiled in the sky above a viewer.

The notched-edged gorget from Point Barrow is part of a ceremonial mask and gorget set (fig. 209) depicting whaling scenes and birds (crosses) surrounding a giant man holding whales in his hands, probably the North Alaskan equivalent to the Chukchi Master of the Sea, *Keretkun*.

445. Box Sculpture and Pictographic Art
Bering Sea Eskimo: NMNH 36246, 24350

This lid from a box representing a seal monster features hunting art and defecating caribou pursued by mythic Thunderbirds, which hold caribou, whales, and men in kayaks in their talons. A hatted European and a pregnant woman are shown in red.

446. Box Lid Art

Bering Sea Eskimo: NMNH 36242
Bering Sea Eskimo men decorated
the inside lids of their workboxes
with illustrations and pictographic
designs relating to hunting magic,
travel, sex, and encounters with Europeans (cf. Fitzhugh and Kaplan
1982:172-77). Occasionally these designs took on a more formal aspect,
as in this stylized illustration of a
whiskered and masked predator spirit
with a pierced ("passage") belly and
flipperlike extremities.

kan pictographic traditions. Generally, these parallel the patterns previously noted in animal-
and human-style art. Asian and Inupiat Eskimo
pictographs frequently illustrate narrative scenes
and images of animal masters or controllers that
take (often gigantic) human form (fig. 444).
Anthropomorphic controllers are absent in Yupik
art and other Alaskan pictographic art; when
shown, usually only in ceremonial masks, these
deities have a beastly or only semihuman form
(fig. 346). A rare exception is the lunar and
human transformation image seen on a Bering
Sea Eskimo float board (fig. 360).

Animal Art

Animal and semihuman cryptic or "masked" art
occurs most prominently in Northern style (Tlingit) formline art and among Amur groups. Both
employ negative fields, complex backgrounds,
bilateral symmetry, composite motif systems,
cryptic masks or *t'ao-t'ieh* faces of semihuman
beasts, and other forms. Despite differences, the
underlying structures of some Pacific art styles
are similar enough to have had related ancestry.
More specific arguments have been made regarding the similarities between Northwest Coast

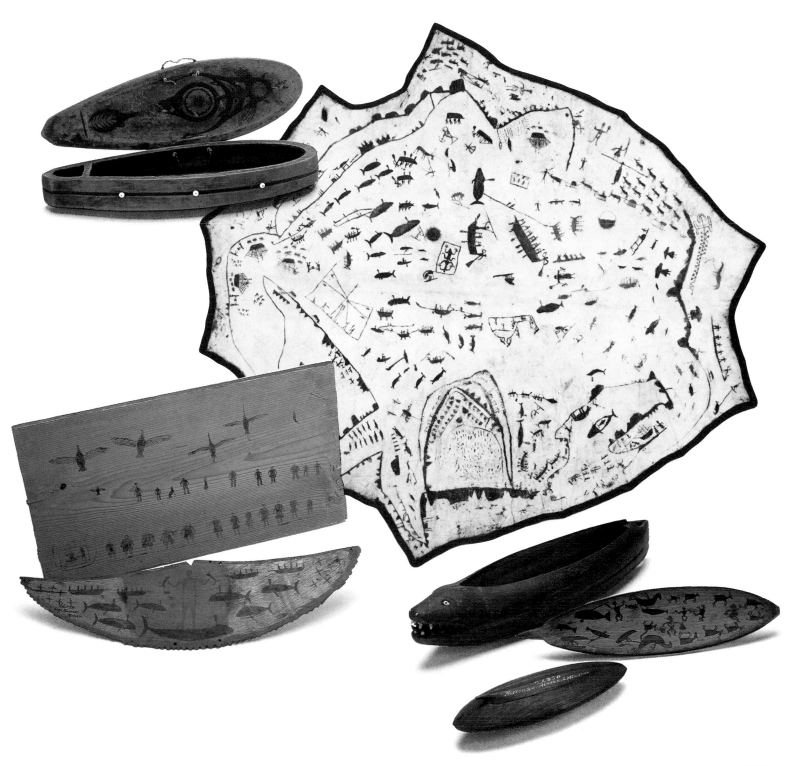

309

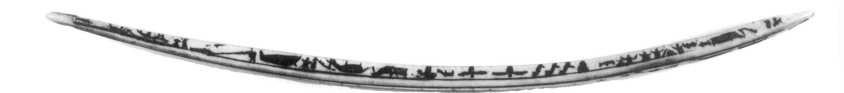

Chilkat blanket designs and *t'ao-t'ieh* faces in the art of Shang China (Covarrubias 1954). The work of Schuster, who extended the study of joint marks, skeletal art, animal styles, and other motifs around the Pacific Ocean, long ago raised the question of the survival of Eurasian animal-style art in Eskimo culture (Schuster 1951a,b).

Asian clothing does not mimic animals as explicitly as does that of Alaskan Eskimo, nor are there Asian equivalents (except among Asian Eskimo) for the animal-style visors or helping-spirit engravings on hunting weapons. Among hunting equipment, the only areawide decorative tradition noted is the decoration of quivers, which in Siberia was present only on the oldest ethnographic specimens. More important is the

widespread use of serpent and dragonlike beings on Eskimo and Northwest Coast boats, and *sisiutl*-type images on masks, clothes, transformation masks, and soul catchers (fig. 45). Serpents are known in Amur iconography, along with the rooster and the fish, which Berthold Laufer thought were derived from Chinese influence. Beastly faces are widespread in Amur, Bering Sea Eskimo, and Northwest Coast art (figs. 287, 435, and 449).

Hunting art is conspicuously absent among Northeastern Siberian cultures. Except for harpoon technology among the Koryak and Amur groups and hunting spear decoration (figs. 195, 307), Asian hunting equipment is unelaborated, as are utensils relating to reindeer herding.

447. Pictographic Drillbow
North Alaskan Eskimo?: MAE 4291-50

Bering Sea Eskimos did not use engraved ivory bows for drilling holes or starting fires as did the Eskimos of Norton Sound, Bering Strait, and Kotzebue Sound, the most likely origin for this specimen. Pictographic art first appears in Punuk culture about A.D. 800 and becomes more elaborate through time, culminating in the richly illustrative art of the historic period. Whether or not this style began in the Bering Strait region is not known. Petroglyphic art, which is distributed widely in the Eurasian and North American subarctic (de Laguna 1975; Dikov 1972; Lundy 1983), is probably linked with the pictographic tradition in North Pacific cultures. This drillbow depicts various scenes from Eskimo daily life, including seal hunting (*left*) and a dance scene outside a tent (*right*). The center panel shows caribou feeding and dancers wearing dance gauntlets.

forehead lozenge   crest   eyebrows or C-horn of ram   tail   quill

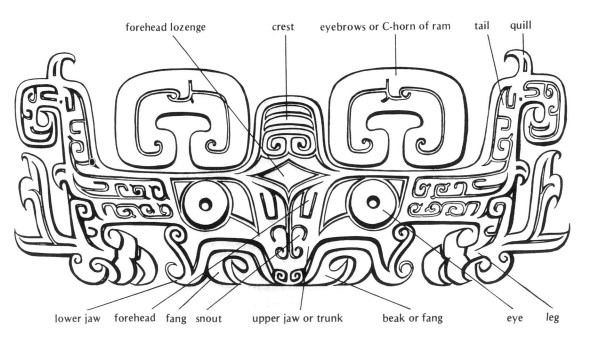

lower jaw   forehead   fang   snout   upper jaw or trunk   beak or fang   eye   leg

Throughout Asian technology one finds little to complement the detailed attention paid by the hunters of northwestern North America to the aesthetic features of their equipment, either in beautification of technology or in application of spirit helpers. Among Asian groups this function remained in the realm of special anthropomorphic hunting charms representing masters of animals or places, carried on one's belt or clothing rather than, as among New World groups, carved into the hunting implements themselves.

Differences between Asian and Alaskan figurative art also extend to the illustration of man's relationship to animals in pictographic and fig-

urative art. Chukchi and Siberian Eskimo artists frequently depicted scenes of men hunting animals with firearms in ways that emphasize the power of the weaponry and the role of man as a manipulator of technology (fig. 236). In North America, where firearms were rare or absent in early contact periods, painted and pictographic art displayed hunting encounters with less attention to technology and more attention to social and spiritual aspects of the hunt, emphasizing the personal relationship between hunter and prey (fig. 181). Here, hunting art, the ornamentation of weapons, and use of ritual hunting clothing were the hunter's way of asking for

448. *T'ao-T'ieh* Mask
Shang Dynasty, 16th-11th Century B.C.

Beastly faces of predators or mythological beings appear frequently on ritual bronze vessels and in bone, jade, and ivory carvings in Shang Dynasty China. The similarity of these "masks" suggest that they represent a single mythological creature or being. These conventionalized mask-like faces are composed of discrete anatomical elements—fangs, eyes, horns/eyebrows, claws, tails—as shown in this diagram (Davis and Davis 1974:21). These elements alternate between a positive and negative field of ornamental fill consisting of delicate spirals, curls, and U-forms. The overall design is always symmetrical, showing both sides of the creature in "split" form.

449. Chilkat Blanket
Tlingit: NMNH 357445

Early in the 19th century Tlingit weavers began to make dancing robes completely covered with formline patterns derived from their painted art. The figures represented were crest animals, but they were often so conventionalized that their identity is not clear. A creature like this one on a nearly identical blanket was described to George Emmons as a "sea bear," while to Franz Boas it was identified as a "standing eagle."

Although Chilkat blankets in this style are of recent age, they, and other types of Tlingit art, exhibit intriguing parallels with *t'ao-t'ieh*-type designs of ancient China: prominence of masklike images of fanged beasts or semihuman forms, split images, and reduction of figures to elemental forms with stylized rearrangement of their parts. With little archeological evidence available, the significance of these parallels cannot be ascertained.

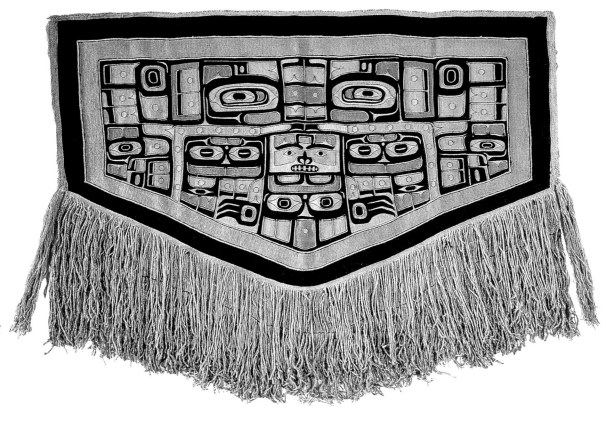

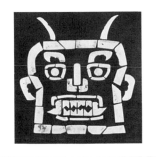

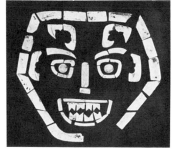

450. Composite Shell Mask
Shang Dynasty, 16th-11th century B.C.: Royal Ontario Museum 2300

These fragments of a single mask have been reconstructed in two possible configurations based on intact finds (Hsio-Yen Shih 1963). The fragments from a Shang tomb at K'aifeng, near An-yang (White 1945), represent a demonic creature with both human and animal traits. Similar masks were used as horse and chariot ornaments in burials. The latter were known as *fang-hsiang*, an ancient Chinese name for exorcists who performed at times of death or disaster. Similarities between Chinese burial masks and composite masks from Ipiutak (fig. 149) have been noted (Collins 1971).

the gift of an animal rather than overpowering it physically or spiritually. These differences also extend to the depiction of spirits: Siberian spirits were often shown as stylized humans, either as Y-shaped stick figures, as in the common spirit effigies, or with human likenesses (fig. 417); among most American groups spirits took explicitly nonhuman or semihuman form, their status indicated by goggles, spiked appendages, and beastly forms (figs. 435–438).

Prehistoric Ties

For many years, arguments supporting Asian-American contact (e.g., Covarrubias 1954; Gladwin 1947; Heine-Geldern 1966; Rivet 1943) relied on the intriguing but frustrating evidence compiled from different regions and chronological periods. Among a larger group of parallels, traits such as squatting ("hocker") figures, double-headed serpents, figures with protruding tongues, bilateral symmetry, split and splayed figures, and semihuman beastly faces seemed to link ethnographic arts of the Pacific Islands and Northwest Coast Indians to the ancient art of Mesoamerica, China, and southern Siberia. For the most part, lack of rigorous standards and presence of large geographic and chronological gaps in data caused scholars to question the validity of these observations.

However, there is reason to give consideration to Northwest Coast and Alaskan parallels with Asian cultures. Although similarities in ethnographic art styles are not extensive, significant parallels in underlying structures exist, especially in Northwest Coast and Amur art. More important, archeological evidence suggests that greater similarities existed in the past than during the historical period. Although archeological data from the region are sparse, there are suggestions that North Pacific and Bering Sea art may once have been more unified than it was during the past millennium and that related forms of animal-style hunting art may have existed throughout the region. Divergence between Siberian and American art may have occurred relatively recently as a result of changes in Siberian cultures stimulated by economic, social, and technological innovation—reindeer breeding and metallurgy; by attendant demographic shifts toward the northeast; and by influence from Scytho-Siberian and other cultures. Perhaps it is too early to discount the presence of a modified Old Pacific style (Heine-Geldern 1966) in North Pacific coastal regions.

The existence of northward- and eastward-flowing ocean currents, which not only carried Asian flotsam but also are known to have delivered many disabled Japanese vessels and their crews to the western coast of North America, provides an obvious mechanism for direct contact, with or without geographically intermediate links (Quimby 1985; Brooks 1876).

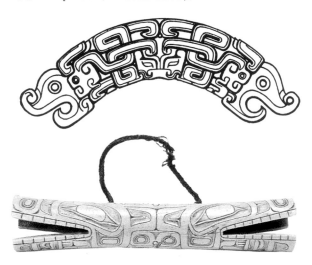

The possibility that cultures of the North Pacific may have been in contact should not come as a surprise to readers at this stage. Two-thousand-year-old Old Bering Sea, Okvik, and Ipiutak art has long been suspected of having been influenced by Shang, Chou, and Scytho-Siberian cultures (Collins 1937, 1971; Larsen and Rainey 1948). The cryptic animal-based art of these early arctic cultures with its interplay of image and field pattern, its transformational quality, and its motif systems—all occurring within a North Pacific hunting art tradition—calls for combined ethnographic and archeological solutions to the question of Asian-American relationships. Boas's original goals for the Jesup Expedition are still valid and still need attention. As we have seen, interrelated patterns of culture and culture history do emerge when archeological and ethnographic data are viewed in larger, trans-Beringian perspective.

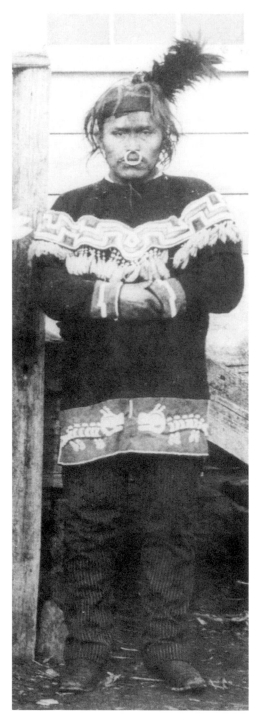

451. Serpent, Soul Catcher, and *Sisiutl*
Tsimshian: NMNH 10983. Chou Dynasty illustration: Freer Gallery of Art. SI neg. 736821, Winter and Pond, 1894-95

Like most soul catchers, this one (*bottom*) has large, toothed, wolflike heads at each end and a humanoid face in the middle, only partly visible here. It resembles the Kwakiutl supernatural being, *Sisiutl*, whose usual form is a serpent with a head at each end of his body and a humanoid face in the center (Holm 1983:55-57). Serpent figures were also used as motifs on ceremonial clothing, as seen here on a Chilkat (Tlingit) Indian's shirt.

Compositions identical to the *Sisiutl* occur in Chou Dynasty art (*top*). Although stylistic features differ, there are similarities in concept and organization. In these respects, and others, intriguing parallels exist between Shang, Chou, Old Bering Sea Ipiutak, and ethnographic Amur River and Northwest Coast culture art.

Opposite:
"Tamaima, an Inhabitant of Kodiak Island" (Mikhail Tikhanov, 1817, RIPSA 2117)

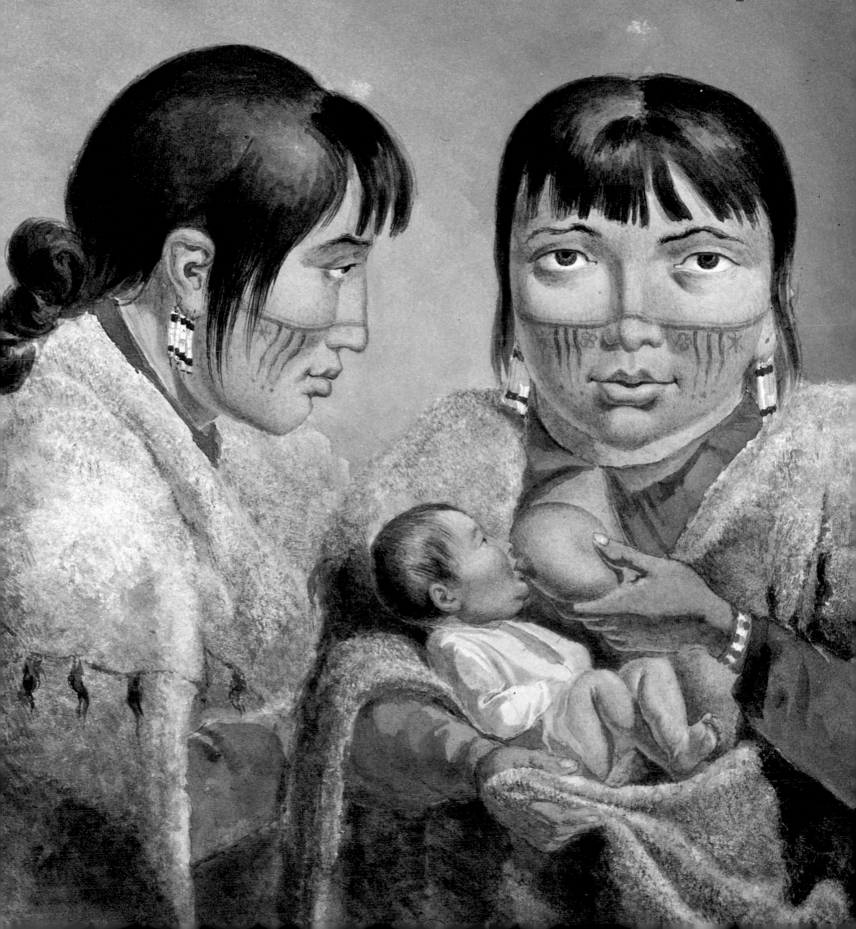

Siberian Peoples: A Soviet View

V. V. Lebedev

The cultures of the native peoples of Kamchatka and Chukotka, along with other peoples of northern Siberia, underwent dramatic changes in the 20th century. In 70 years of Soviet administration, these groups advanced from patriarchal social and economic organization to contemporary socialism.

As early as the 1920s, the Soviet government's attention was drawn to the difficult situation of the native peoples of the northern provinces of Russia, who often underwent famine when hunting and fishing activities were unsuccessful. Periodic epidemics also resulted in dramatic losses of population.

In 1925, at the initiative of the two Siberian ethnographers, Waldemar Bogoras and L. Ia. Sternberg, the Soviet government organized the Committee of the North to study the economy, social relations, culture, and way of life of northern peoples and to determine what should be done to improve their situation. The following year, the committee instituted a population census, which was part of a larger program of development. The census collected data not only on demography but also on northern economy, on the structure of population in the economic (hunting) territories, on relations between individual households and between households and markets, and on many other subjects. This census was an important source of scientific data, which were the basis for decisive steps toward socialist reconstruction in 1930.

In the 1920s a network of trading posts was organized to provide the northern natives with food and consumer goods. One of these posts served the Chukchi, Chuvantsy, Yukaghir, and Even, whose reindeer pastures and hunting territories were located in the middle Anadyr River region.

In 1930 the boundaries of the Chukchi and Koryak national districts were set by the Soviet government, which gave the Chukchi, Eskimo, Koryak, Itelmen, Chuvantsy, Even, Kerek, Yukaghir, and Aleut, like all the other Soviet north-

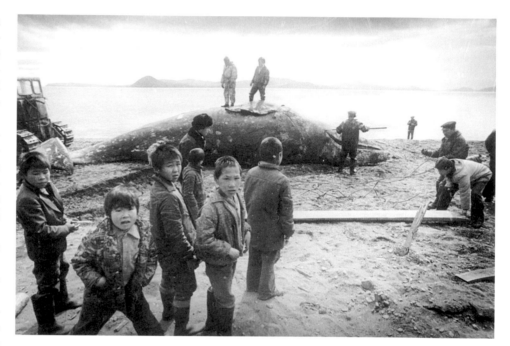

ern groups, a national autonomy with their own local governmental representatives. At this time local cultural centers and "Red Iaranga" were created. The centers taught reading and writing and provided medical care, veterinary and herding advice, and economic and scientific expertise. The Red Iaranga, a political information office housed in a nomadic dwelling, played an important role in the struggle against illiteracy. In the early 1930s six schools opened in Chukotka, where P. Ia. Skorik, I. S. Vdovin, A. G. Menovshchikov, and others worked as teachers before they became renowned ethnographers and linguists. Many of the children they taught went on to higher education in Moscow, Leningrad, or Khabarovsk. As adults, they became leaders of the local soviets (councils) and Communist Party organizations, specialists in reindeer herding, physicians, teachers, poets, and writers, such as L. G. Tynel', N. P. Otke, A. Kymytval', and Iu. Rytkheu.

452. Butchering a Whale at Uelen/ Yanrakynnot, Chukotka

In the early 1930s in Chukotka and Kamchatka the construction of *kolkhoz,* or collective farms, began. At first, these Chukchi and Koryak *kolkhoz* were oriented toward only a single economic activity; workers were organized in brigades of communal fishermen, sea mammal hunters, or reindeer herders. Later, the *kolkhoz* became more complex, each encompassing two or three economic activities.

The 1930s marked the beginning of systematic geological study of Chukotka. It was already obvious that future economic development of the region depended on mining. Consequently, a special Chukchi trust was created by the Soviet government in 1935, under the General Direction of the Northern Sea Route, which had been founded in 1932 after the passage of the icebreaker *Sibiriakov* along the Soviet Arctic Ocean coast. All the economic and cultural units of Chukotka above the 62nd parallel were transferred to the administration of the Chukchi trust. This administration had an influence on the natives as well, improving the supply of goods, conditions of life, and medical care. Airlines were also organized for the transportation of goods and passengers between Anadyr and Petropavlovsk-Kamchatskii, between Anadyr and the northern Chukchi coast, between Chaun and Ostrovnoe, and between Markovo and Belaiia. The rescue mission to relieve the steamer *Cheliuskin* in 1934 demonstrated the need for aircraft bases in the North.

In 1932 the First Pan-Russian Conference on the Development of Languages and Script of the Peoples of the North voted to create the Committee of the New Alphabet, which worked in all regions of the North, recruiting professional linguists and northern school teachers. An alphabet was created for the languages of Chukotka and Kamchatka in 1937. It should be noted that just prior to this, Tynevil', a Reindeer Chukchi, had created his own pictographic writing system, which he had taught to his relatives. National art also received much attention at that time, with an exhibition of 11 cases of engraved ivory tusks from Uelen at the Tretiakov Gallery in Moscow.

During World War II, a significant contribution was made by the peoples of Chukotka and Kamchatka by producing meat, fish, and fur needed for foreign currency for the war effort. The economic organization within *kolkhoz* grew during and after the war, so that by the end of the 1950s northern villages became centers of large *kolkhoz* territories.

In 1957 the ministers of the USSR and the Central Committee of the Communist Party decreed further improvement in all spheres of economic and social life of the northern natives.

This decree provided concrete measures for herding, hunting, and fishing, with an emphasis on the living conditions in the northern settlements. Among other measures, it gave native families a 50 percent subsidy for new housing and provided for improved medical care, education, and cultural enlightenment.

In the 1960s, a new step was taken to reinforce collective farms by reorganizing some of them into *sovkhoz* (state farms), a more developed form of socialist economy. The present *sovkhoz* organization of Kamchatka and Chukotka was formed by the mid-1970s and today consists of large state reindeer herding, fishing, sea mammal hunting, and fur hunting enterprises. Some *sovkhoz* also include farms for fur breeding and milk production, and even greenhouse vegetable production in some areas. The *sovkhoz* budgets provided for purchase of machinery, tractors, whaleboats, motorboats, and for airplane charter.

With the formation of committees of agronomists, many areas of Chukotka and Kamchatka started to produce not only raw but also processed products from traditional industries. Processing increased the value of food materials and improved social conditions substantially.

The central villages of the *sovkhoz* are now in the process of modernization, shifting from one- or two-story wooden houses, which are not very suitable to arctic and subarctic climates, to four- to five-story modern concrete apartment buildings equipped with appropriate sanitary and heating systems. These settlements, although considered villages, look urban. They include Palana, the center of the Koryak District; Tilichiki, Ossora, Beringovskii, Egvekinot, Provideniia, Lavrentiia, and other regional centers of the Koryak and Chukchi districts; and the *sovkhoz* villages of Amguema, Lorino, Srednie Pakhachi, and Konergino.

The *sovkhoz* villages were designed to meet the social and cultural needs of the workers and their families. Lorino, the center of the Lenin *sovkhoz* in northern Chukotka, is one example. The activities of this *sovkhoz* include reindeer breeding, sea mammal hunting, fishing, fur animal breeding, milk animal breeding, skin and fur processing, and clothing manufacture. The higher governmental representatives at the *sovkhoz* level are the people's deputies of the village soviet, or council. The deputies are elected by secret vote by all the village inhabitants above age 18. Lorino village includes a medical center, a kindergarten, an elementary school with a dormitory for the children of nomadic families, public baths, a barber shop, and stores for groceries, pharmaceutical products, and hardware. The village cultural center is in charge of cultural enlightenment and has a mobile brigade serving nomadic workers. The construction of tall concrete apartment buildings has transformed Lorino into a small town. Today, radio has entered the life of even the most remote villages, and some also have television reception.

The economic reorganization and development of central villages has led to a completely different social organization among the peoples of the North. One third of the native population of Chukotka and Kamchatka is now employed in traditional reindeer breeding, hunting, fishing, and sea mammal hunting activities. Another third works in medicine, education, culture, administration, and economic planning—disciplines that require elementary and higher education or special training. The third group includes service workers, nurses, unskilled *sovkhoz* workers, guards, and others. All men older than age 55 and women older than 50 receive retirement pension. All workers are paid, without exception, according to a regional income standard, to which is added the northern bonus. The result is that workers in Chukotka and Kamchatka receive a salary two to three times higher than workers in the same positions in European parts of the Russian Republic.

One tenth of the native population of Kamchatka and Chukotka is considered urban. These are the inhabitants and workers of the large regional centers such as Petropavlovsk-Kamchatskii, Magadan, Anadyr, and Pevek, who are employed in medical, educational, and scientific sectors but also, especially the young, as miners and mechanics. The growth of urban centers was determined by local economic conditions—in Kamchatka by the fish industry and in Chukotka by mining. Before World War II Petropavlovsk-Kamchatskii and Magadan were only small towns with wooden houses. Today they are major industrial centers comparable to European Russian cities. The same can be said of the other regional centers, which shelter regional political and economic administrations. These regional centers are important seaports and have airports. Hospitals, schools (one or two in each city), a regional cultural center and mobile brigade, and a branch of the State Bank are present in each regional center. A soviet of people's deputies with representatives from the soviets of every village constitutes the higher political organization at this level.

A characteristic of Chukotkan and Kamchatkan industrialization is that state enterprises such as fish industry and mining, although located on native territories, occupy relatively small geographic areas and therefore do not damage reindeer pasture or the *sovkhoz* fishing and hunting territory, except in the case of gold mining, which requires dredging the riverbeds

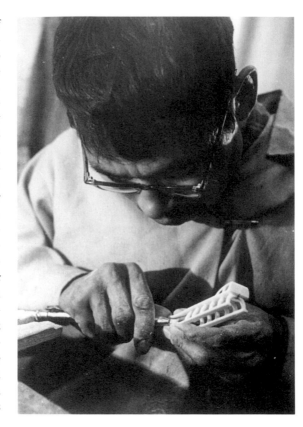

453. Ivan Segutegin, a Chukchi Ivory Carver Working at the Uelen Workshop

of the lower Kolyma drainage. In most cases, the ecological balance has been preserved, while industrial development has facilitated urbanization and village reconstruction.

The settlement of Iul'tin in Chukotka, for example, was built for the workers of a mining complex, and roads were constructed to join Iul'tin to Egvekinot, the regional center and seaport, which necessitated the construction of a factory to make concrete housing buildings. This factory, in its turn, permitted the construction of urban architecture in the reindeer herding villages of Amguema and Konergino.

Two other centers, Anadyr and Palana, shelter many administrative and political organizations, including the agronomic committees of the Chukchi and Koryak districts; regional medical and education services; radio and television, which broadcast programs in native language; district newspapers in Russian and in native language; and schools of music, art, and teaching. In Provideniia, a technical and professional training school was built to train workers in the traditional sectors of the economy (i.e., mechanics and radio monitors as well as herders and hunters). Therefore, training of native specialists at the elementary level remains a local activity. After graduation, young people who want higher education leave to study in Khabarovsk, Leningrad, Moscow, Iakutsk, and Irkutsk.

The highest political organization at the district level is the District Soviet of the People's Deputies, which is composed of deputies from the different regions of each district. Special deputies represent the districts at the Soviet of the People's Deputies of the Russian Republic (Siberia being part of it) and at the Soviet of the People's Deputies of the USSR. Representatives of the Chukchi and Koryak districts are also part of the special division of the Soviet of Ministers in Charge of Social and Economic Development of the Peoples of the North; for example, V. M. Tototto, a Chukchi born in the village Inchoun by the Arctic Ocean, is in charge of the Chukchi District. Consequently, the native population of Chukotka and Kamchatka is represented at every level of political and administrative organization of the country.

The art of Kamchatka and Chukotka natives received an important stimulus after World War II. The Uelen ivory engraving workshop (fig. 327) produced many remarkable artists, such as Vukvutagin, Tukkai, Khukhutan, and Emkul', who engraved scenes from the lives of their people on walrus and mammoth tusks and on reindeer antlers. Many of these artists are members of the Artists' Union of the Russian Republic, and some have been honored as Master Artists of the Russian Republic.

Ethnic music and dance also experienced a revival such that today practically every village has its own amateur singing and dancing ensemble with participants from both younger and older generations, the latter imparting to the former their knowledge of traditional music and dance. These performing groups tour nomadic settlements and perform at regional, district, and provincial amateur festivals. The Koryak professional ensemble Mengo and the Chukchi professional ensemble Ergyron, which began as amateur ensembles, are now world famous. Although performing in many cities of the Soviet Union and abroad, they perform primarily for nomadic herders, even in the most remote regions.

One of the most important contemporary issues is that of native languages. An Institute of Native Schools has been created under the Ministry of Education of the Russian Republic to publish school books for native-language teaching up to the eighth grade in the ten-grade Soviet school system. More and more books in native languages are being published, mainly works of contemporary native writers and poets such as, to name the most famous, the writer Iurii Rytkheu and the poet Antonina Kymytval'.

The 1978 Constitution of the USSR gave the national districts of the peoples of the North the status of autonomous districts, providing them with greater national autonomy—i.e., higher political representation. The Constitution guaranteed that the social and economic levels of the formerly backward peoples of the North were now equal to that of the rest of the Union.

New ethnic processes emerged as a result of these social, economic, and cultural changes in Chukotka and Kamchatka in the 20th century. At the beginning of the 20th century, the Chuk-

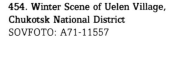

454. Winter Scene of Uelen Village, Chukotsk National District
SOVFOTO: A71-11557

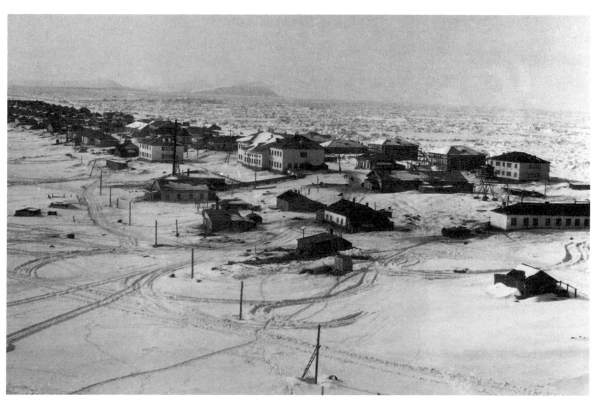

chi, Koryak, Eskimo, Kerek, Itelmen, Even, Yukaghir, and Chuvantsy occupied territories that were ethnically distinct. A person's ethnic identity was based on the person's territorial group. The folklore of these groups is filled with stories of conflicts and raids, both between and within ethnic groups. For example, there are stories from the Meinypyl'ginskii Chukchi about the warrior Kunleliu and his brothers, who fought against the Reindeer Koryak over reindeer pastures, and stories from the Karaginskii Koryak about raids against their neighbors to capture women.

In the Soviet period, during economic reconstruction and the creation of the *kolkhoz* and *sovkhoz*, the various ethnic groups began working together in brigades, and a process of unification commenced. Installation of the Soviet political system also brought these groups together to participate in important regional social and economic decisions. Growth of larger settlements, modern social structures, and the development of education allowed previously separated groups to interrelate freely.

Interethnic marriages are a useful indicator of the closer relations between peoples of Kamchatka and Chukotka. Such marriages were practically absent at the beginning of the 20th century. A few were recorded in the 1940s; they became significant in the 1960s and have increased steadily to this day.

In villages such as Kanchalan, Amguema, Karaga, Enurmino, and Neshkan, where the native population is represented by one group only, many mixed marriages with the European emigrant population have been recorded also. The ethnic composition of mixed villages such as Vaegi and Tavaivaam in Chukotka or Srednie Pakhachi and Achaivaiam in Kamchatka is particularly interesting. In Vaegi, for example, on the bank of the Main River, near the Vaezhskii Mountains, children of mixed marriages consisted of 21.4 percent of the young (age 0 to 20) population in 1960. Today the population of Vaegi includes 313 Chukchi, 21 Koryak, 81 Even, 31 Chuvantsy, 1 Yukaghir, and 1 Eskimo, which represents 123 families in which one or both parents are native. These families include 69 Chukchi couples, 12 Even couples, 6 Chuvantsy couples, and 4 Koryak couples; mixed couples number 3 Chukchi-Koryak, 2 Chukchi-Even, 4 Koryak-Chukchi, 2 Chuvantsy-Chukchi, 3 Even-Chukchi, 1 Even-Chuvantsy, 1 Yukaghir-Even, 1 Eskimo-Chukchi, 1 Koryak-Russian, 2 Even-Russian, 2 Russian-Chukchi, 2 Russian-Even, 2 Ukrainian-Even, and 2 Buriat-Chukchi. In most of these marriages, the spouses have similar professions, as in the example of a 30-year-old couple consisting of a Chukchi reindeer herder husband and his Russian zoo-technician wife. Children from mixed marriages represent 46.5 percent of the young generation. It is interesting to note that mixed families have almost twice as many children as monoethnic families. Finally, we should note that during the 20th century the native population of Chukotka and Kamchatka increased more than 30 percent.

455. Asiatic Eskimo Dance Group "Uelen" Performing "Dance of Joy"

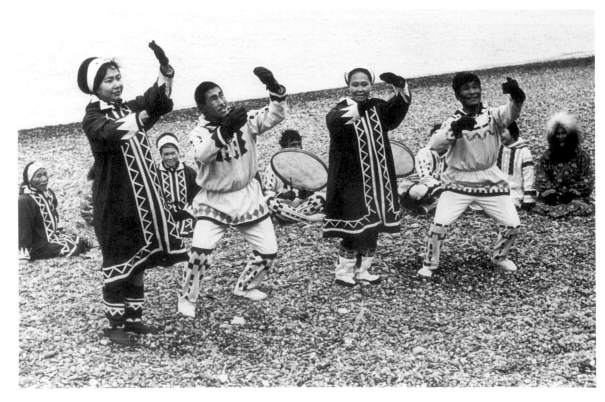

Alaska Natives Today

Rosita Worl

As contact with Western influences intensified throughout the 20th century, sociocultural change among Alaska's indigenous population was rapid and extensive. The five distinct cultural groups, the Inupiat (Northern Eskimo) and Yupik (Southern Eskimo), the Aleuts, the Athapaskans, and the Tlingit and Haida are collectively referred to as Alaska Natives. By the mid-1900s, the last hunters and fishermen had abandoned their nomadic way of life. Alaska Natives entered the cash economy initially through fur trading ventures and later through participation in seasonal wage jobs. However, villagers continued to depend on hunting and fishing resources throughout the contemporary period. Western religions suppressed many of the traditional ceremonial activities, but by the 1970s a cultural revitalization movement was apparent. The five cultural groups united under a single statewide organization to seek protection of their aboriginal claims of ownership to their land. As the impacts of Western diseases to which the Natives had proven to have little immunity subsided during the first half of the 1900s, they were replaced by a host of acute social problems. The aboriginal population, which had been estimated to be 80,000, had declined to 25,000 in 1909. By the 1980s alcoholism and suicide had reached epidemic proportions. During the most recent period, two separate and seemingly conflicting movements emerged among the Native American population. One is led by the more assimilated Natives who are working to administer land and financial resources under the corporate structure mandated by the Alaska Native Claims Settlement Act (ANCSA) of 1971. The second movement began with the more traditional Natives who are seeking to protect their land base and their hunting and fishing lifestyle as well as to obtain greater control and autonomy over their communities.

Village Alaska

By the 1950s the last remaining nomadic groups had settled into permanent communities. This ended the process that had begun initially with the establishment of fur trading posts, schools, and missions, first by the Russians in the 1780s and followed by the Americans 100 years later. The Inupiat hunters of northeastern Alaska who established the communities of Kaktovik and Anaktuvuk Pass in the Brooks Range were the last of the indigenous population in Alaska to abandon a nomadic lifestyle. The new communities were generally established in sites that were formerly occupied as semipermanent habitation areas.

By 1960 approximately 70 percent of the total Alaska Native population, which numbered 53,000, was living in 178 villages that were predominantly inhabited by Alaska Natives. These villages, which were scattered across the half-million square miles of the state, ranged in size from 25 to 2,500. An additional 50 sites were occupied by less than 25 inhabitants, usually comprising one or more Native families. Only 6 communities that were predominantly Native had populations larger than 1,000. The median size of the villages was 155 persons (Federal Field Committee 1968). These larger communities served as regional centers to the smaller villages.

The remainder of the Native population lived in communities that were predominantly non-Native. The non-Native communities were often established in areas that had traditionally been inhabited by Natives. Beginning in the 1950s, a migration of Natives from village Alaska to urban centers began and is continuing into the present period. An estimated 16,000 Natives live in Alaska's urban centers. Anchorage is the largest Native "village," with an estimated Native population of 10,000. However, a high degree of circular migration is found among the urban Natives. Many return seasonally to their village each year to participate in subsistence activities.

Most all Native villages remain fairly isolated from the urban communities. Fewer than a dozen of the villages are accessible on the state's limited road system. Access to the majority of the villages is only by air and seasonally by boat or snowmobile. In the last decade, the state's ferry system was expanded to several villages in southeastern Alaska. Communication with most villages was by mail or radio transmitters and receivers until the 1970s, when telephones were finally installed. Television was only recently introduced into most villages, but its continued presence is uncertain because of the lack of state funds available to support the TV satellite system.

Traditional housing has been replaced by modern-style houses in all villages. Both the federal and state governments implemented housing construction projects in village Alaska, but Native housing is still considered to be substandard. In most villages in western Alaska, modern water and sanitation systems are lacking. Villagers continue to carry water from nearby rivers or lakes. In the winter months, water is obtained by melting ice blocks cut from the frozen lakes. By the mid-1970s, water systems or water delivery trucks had been introduced into the larger regional communities. The "honey bucket" system to dispose of human waste is still prevalent in most villages.

Education

The education of Alaska Natives was slow in coming, and it was often initiated as a result of Native action. In 1877, a Puget Sound newspaper carried the report of three Tlingit Stikine chiefs who requested that schools be established in their communities.

Education began with missionary educators. During the late 1800s, several Protestant denominations divided Alaska among themselves, and they agreed not to proselytize in one another's territory. The church schools were initially supported by the federal government. Federal subsidization enabled the establishment of schools in Native villages and hastened the arrival of mission groups.

The official educational policy of the United States government was to "civilize" and assimilate the Natives, and leadership was to be developed through vocational training (Ray 1958). English was to replace Native languages, and students were often punished for speaking their own language.

In communities where both Natives and non-Natives lived, segregated schools were established. The federal government assumed responsibility for the education of Alaska Natives while local governments and later the territorial government assumed responsibility for educating white children. The Nelson Act of 1905 authorized the two separate systems of education in Alaska but also allowed "children of mixed blood who lead a civilized life" to attend the white schools.

The requisites for leading a civilized life were tested in court in 1908, when six children of

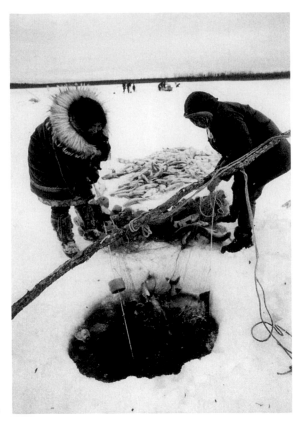

456. Eskimo Women Fishing for Whitefish on the Kobuk River, Alaska
National Park Service neg. 100023

mixed blood attempted to enroll in the Sitka territorial school. When they were refused, the Southeast Tlingits brought the issue to court in *Davis* v. *Sitka School Board* (Alaska 481. 1908). The judge concluded that the children were mixed blood but ruled that they were not civilized. Although the judge accepted the facts that the parents spoke, read, and wrote English, wore the white man's style of clothing, resided in houses separate from other Natives, paid business taxes and rented post office boxes and were members of the Presbyterian Church, he concluded that these were not the requisites to lead a civilized life. Native children were barred from attending public schools until they were integrated in 1949, which was four years after the Southeast Natives had successfully lobbied for the passage of the Anti-Discrimination Act in the Territorial Legislature (Drucker 1958).

The village elementary school became the focal point for the federal government's program for the social improvement of Alaska Natives. In addition to education, the teachers' responsibilities included those of a social worker, physician, business manager, and general advisor. After 1920, the federal government established vocational schools in various regions of the territory. The brightest students were sent to these vocational boarding schools after they completed their elementary training.

Until the late 1970s, most Alaska Native high school students were required to leave their homes to attend state and federally operated boarding schools and high schools in urban and regional centers. The famous Molly Hootch case settled the civil class action suit brought against the State of Alaska on behalf of Alaska Native children of secondary school age who lived in communities without a high school. The consent decree that was signed in 1976 called for the establishment of high schools in 126 small rural communities (Barnhardt et al. 1979). During the next decade, high school facilities were constructed in these rural villages.

Post-secondary educational opportunities and success are even more limited for Alaska Natives. Although the number of Natives receiving higher academic degrees is increasing, the actual number receiving degrees remains low. In a five-year period from 1967 to 1972, an average of 22 Natives per year received bachelor degrees (Kohout and Kleinfeld 1974). The 1970 census reveals that only 235 Natives had college degrees and 73 had graduate training (Kleinfeld et al. 1973). A differential rate of change between Native men and Native women has also been found in the trend toward a greater number of females receiving bachelor degrees. In the spring of 1981, a 4 to 1 ratio of female to male graduates was apparent, and indications are that the difference in the ratio is increasing.

Although educational opportunities for Alaska Natives expanded throughout the 1900s, the overall record reveals that success has been limited. The implications of poor educational attainment among Alaska Natives are far-reaching. The new institutions that have been introduced in rural communities require educational and professional skills that cannot always be found among Alaska Natives. A 1973 study projected the manpower needs of Native corporations established under ANCSA and found that the professional, technical, and clerical needs would intensify existing manpower shortages among Alaska Natives (Kleinfeld et al. 1973). The implication is that non-Natives would continue to dominate these positions.

Mixed Economies

Although the aboriginal hunting and gathering economies of Alaska Natives were independent and autonomous, contemporary village economies are dependent on both cash and hunting and gathering resources. In Alaska, the term "subsistence" has been adopted to refer to traditional hunting and gathering of natural resources. Throughout the 1900s, Alaska Natives adapted strategies to combine and maximize both subsistence and cash pursuits. Numerous social scientific studies conducted during the last decade indicate that subsistence-based economies also continue to play a significant role in the cultural and social realm of Alaska Native societies.

Modern subsistence hunters and fishermen require cash to purchase tools, equipment, and supplies. Items such as snowmobiles, outboard motors, fuel, rifles, and ammunition improved the efficiency of subsistence production and altered traditional subsistence harvest methods. The adoption and need for the new hunting equipment as well as other goods and services necessitated the cash income.

The infusion of cash into the subsistence-based economy is derived from wage employment, the sale of subsistence goods, and in some instances governmental transfer payments. Members of the traditional social group or extended families will often alternate among themselves in either working in wage jobs or subsistence activities. Wives also seek employment to obtain cash to support subsistence activities. The elderly and other welfare recipients also bring cash into the subsistence economy through their transfer payments. These individuals often contribute cash or purchase supplies and equipment for the hunters in exchange for a share in the harvest. Arts and crafts production or the sale of surplus subsistence resources is also another means to obtain cash to support subsistence pursuits. Cash also circulates through the subsistence economy by other means, for example, as compensation for specialized services such as sewing skins and covering the frame of a boat. Individuals may also receive cash as a ceremonial gift in rituals, as in the Tlingit potlatches.

Kinship continues to dictate the membership of a subsistence production unit. Generally the household or extended family members comprise the basic producing unit, but these smaller units will join with others to form larger groups to engage in communal hunts, such as those associated with bowhead and beluga hunting. Kin members who live in urban centers often return to participate in seasonal subsistence activities.

Distribution systems continue to be governed by traditional customs. However, the movement of Alaska Natives into urban centers has added new dimensions to the distribution and exchange of subsistence goods. Some villages have adopted formal codes to ensure that relatives living in urban centers receive shares of subsistence resources. For example, the Inupiat community of Kaktovik has formally designated portions of the bowhead whale to be exported to relatives living in urban centers.

Alaska Natives moved to regulate their own hunting and fishing activities. In the late 1970s, the Inupiat and Yupik hunters formed the Alaska Eskimos Whaling Commission and the Eskimo Whaling Commission. They developed regulation based on biological principles as well as their own customary laws to regulate their hunting activities.

Although the ANCSA of 1971 extinguished aboriginal hunting and fishing rights of Alaska Natives, other federal legislation (the Marine Mammal Protection Act of 1972, the Endangered Species Act of 1973, the American Indian Religious Freedom Act of 1978, and the Alaska National Interest Lands Conservation Act of 1980) as well as numerous judicial decisions continue to recognize the subsistence rights and needs of Alaska Natives. In 1978, the state enacted a law that established a subsistence priority over sports and commercial hunting and fishing but made no distinction between Natives and non-Natives. However, an increasing non-Native population in Alaska and competing use by commercial fishermen and sports hunters and fishermen have made subsistence a point of bitter and continuing conflict between Natives and non-Natives.

The cash economy in village Alaska is largely dependent on the public rather than the private sector. In most rural communities, local, state, and federal government expenditures account for 62 percent of earned income, and the private sector accounts for 38 percent. The reverse characterizes urban Alaska, where governmental expenditures account for 33 percent and the private sector accounts for 67 percent of earned income.

Village residents have a per capita income that is considerably less than for all Alaskans. The average per capita income for all of Alaska is $18,018, whereas the average per capita income for rural residents is $8,389. When the regional centers are removed, the average per capita income for villagers is $5,364 (Alaska Department of Labor 1986). Villagers also receive welfare payments that are about four times as much per capita as urban Alaskans'.

Village economies are dependent on a subsistence-based economy and governmental expenditures and are fundamentally different from urban economies. They are extremely sensitive to governmental action. Restrictive governmental hunting and fishing regulations and decreases in governmental revenues severely impact rural economies.

During 1986 and 1987, governmental expenditures in rural Alaska decreased dramatically as a consequence of declining oil prices and revenues available to the state government. The great construction boom in which schools and other public facilities had been built in rural

communities ended. By late 1987, a rural economic crisis was apparent. Rural experts had predicted that a rural migration to the urban centers would occur. In September 1987, the Anchorage School District reported that more than 250 new Native students had enrolled in the Anchorage schools. The State of Alaska developed a rural recovery program in response to the crisis, but the remedies offer no hope for long-range solutions for economic development in village Alaska.

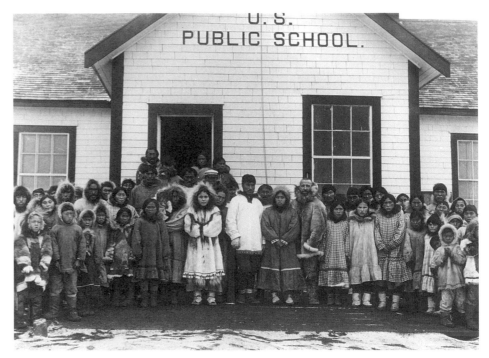

457. Eskimos at Government School, Wainwright, Alaska
Photo: Denver Museum of Natural History BA21-091, A.M. Bailey

The Land Claims Movement

The reduction of the furbearing sea mammals in Alaska, a diminished profit return, and the demands of the Crimean War were among the reasons the Russian government agreed to sell Alaska to the United States. The general American public believed Alaska to be a land mass of ice and snow and labeled the purchase Seward's Folly, after the Secretary of State who supported the purchase. However, the economic potential of Alaska had been evident to the Committee on Foreign Affairs, which had access to reports describing the rich fisheries and other natural resource potential.

The transfer of Alaska from Russian rule to the United States occurred at Sitka in Southeast Alaska on October 18, 1867. Jeff Davis, who was a career soldier who had made his reputation fighting Indians, accepted Alaska on behalf of the United States (Miller 1967). The 1867 Treaty of Cession guaranteed that the ''uncivilized tribes,'' which included those groups that had remained independent from Russian domination, would have the same protection of the laws and regulations that applied to the tribes of the United States. The most important of these protections to Native people was recognition of their possessory land rights.

The Tlingit and Haida Indians were not allowed to watch the ceremony in which their land was transferred from one nation to another, but they immediately voiced their objections. They argued that Alaska was sold without their consent and that the $7 million purchase price should have been paid to them (Bancroft 1886). Their objections were to go unheeded until they brought their claims to court.

While the 1867 Treaty of Cession and the 1884 Organic Act recognized the land rights of Alaska Natives, Congress did little to restrict non-Native occupation of Native lands. The gold rush, followed by salmon fisheries, commercial whalers, trappers, and the military, brought a large population of whites to the territory, and everywhere they began to encroach on Native land.

The Jurisdictional Act was passed by Congress in 1935, allowing the Tlingit and Haida Indians of Southeast Alaska to sue the United States for the loss of their lands. The creation of the Tongass National Forest, Glacier Bay National Monument, and the Metlakatla Reservation for the Tsimshian Indians who had moved into Alaska from Canada had eroded much of the land base of the Southeast Indians.

The Hydaburg Reservation, which had been created for the Haida Indians, was invalidated by a 1952 court decision. The judge ruled that the reservation had not been validly created. In contrast to earlier judicial decisions in which Natives had been determined to be uncivilized, the judge in this case ruled that the Haida Indians were assimilated. He further reasoned that the 101,000-acre reservation would be created at the expense of the whites who had nothing to do with the exploitation of the Indians (Gruening 1968).

It was not until 1968 that the Indian Court of Claims awarded the Tlingit and Haida Indians a $7.5 million judgment, far short of the $80 million value claimed by the Indians. The award did not provide for a land base, and the remainder of the Tlingit's land in the northern region of their territory was to be included in the statewide Native claims.

The Statehood Act of 1958 granted the State of Alaska the right to select 103 million acres, and at the same time it recognized the rights of Natives to lands they used and occupied. The state's proposed selection of land initiated a series of protests by Alaska Natives. Native people were most concerned that their hunting,

fishing, and trapping grounds would be taken by the state. Village after village began to file protests with the federal government. In early 1963, nearly 1,000 Natives from 24 villages petitioned the Secretary of the Interior to impose a land freeze, to halt all transfer of land ownership until the Native land rights had been resolved. The Secretary did not respond to this petition (Arnold et al. 1976).

The Southeast Natives were the first group to organize on a regional basis. The Alaska Native Brotherhood (ANB) was organized in 1912, and it claims to be the oldest organization among American Indians. The ANB had attempted to organize local "camps" in communities outside of the Southeast but had met with only limited success. It was not until the 1960s that other regional associations were formed to advocate for land and political rights of Alaska Natives. In 1963, several of the regional organizations discussed the possibility of organizing a state-wide organization, but deeply rooted mistrust that persisted among the different cultural groups deterred its formation.

A growing awareness of the need to take concerted action to protect Native land ownership finally prompted the formation of the state-wide organization, the Alaska Federation of Natives (AFN). AFN adopted three recommendations relating to land protection: a land freeze until Native claims were resolved, Congressional legislation to settle the claims, and Congressional consultation with Natives before the enactment of land claims legislation. Before the year ended, Secretary of the Interior Udall had imposed a land freeze until the land claims issue could be resolved.

With the formation of AFN, the legislative land claims battle began. The Natives' claims to their ancestral lands were adamantly opposed by the state. The Prudhoe Bay oil lease sales in the North Slope brought the State of Alaska $900 million, and it brought support to the Natives for the settlement of the land claims. It was clear that no permit for a pipeline that would carry oil from the North Slope to a southern terminus could be granted until the claims of Natives to land were settled. The assistance of the oil companies and other business interests assured the passage of a land claims bill.

ANCSA was signed into law on December 18, 1971. The statewide Native newspaper, *Tundra Times*, hailed its passage as "the beginning of a great era for Native people of Alaska."

The basic provisions of the act were land, money, and corporations. Under the terms of the act, Congress agreed that Alaska Natives would be compensated $962.5 million for the extinguishment of aboriginal title to 330 million acres of land and that they would retain ownership to 44 million acres of land under fee-simple title. Congress also authorized that corporations rather than traditional Native groups or clans would hold title to the land and assets. The land was to be divided among 12 regional and 200 village corporations. (The act was later amended to allow for the formation of a 13th regional corporation for those Alaska Natives living in the lower 48 states). The regional corporations would hold subsurface title to village corporation land. The act allowed individuals who were alive on December 18, 1981, and who were one fourth Alaska Native to enroll as shareholders.

ANCSA was heralded as a monumental piece of legislation. Alaska Natives were to receive more land than land held in trust for all other American Indians, and the compensation for lands surrendered was nearly four times the amount all Indian tribes had won from the Indian Claims Commission over its 25-year lifetime. The settlement was also a clear departure from previous Indian settlements. Under ANCSA, lands would be held by corporations under fee simple title rather than as reservations held in trust by the federal government. Congress clearly intended that ANCSA would provide the means for economic development and assimilation of Alaska Natives.

Alaska Natives were initially elated over ANCSA, but it took only a few years before they would completely understand the complexities and problems associated with the settlement act. Corporations would have to wait up to ten years before they received title to their land, and the cost of implementing the settlement used most of their financial award. They also came to realize that perpetual ownership of their lands could not be assured under the corporate structure, and they found that the shareholder system did not allow for the enrollment of Alaska Natives born after 1971.

The corporations have met with varying success. Several regional corporations and village corporations have been extremely successful, but for the most part, a greater number of corporations have been less than successful, and several are on the verge of bankruptcy. Alaska Natives have proposed a series of amendments to ANCSA that they are hopeful will resolve many of the corporate problems.

The Tribal Movement

The tribal movement in Alaska began with Natives who feared that they could lose their ancestral lands, which are held by ANCSA corporations. The concern of the tribal Natives is that without their land they will lose their culture.

They contend that their cultural survival is based on hunting and gathering of wildlife resources. They also fear that with a growing non-Native population in Alaska, they will lose control over their communities. They are concerned that the proliferation of modern institutions in the villages, including the tribal council, city council, corporation, school, and other organizations, has been a source of conflict. They also express opposition to jurisdiction exercised by a state government and judicial system in which they are not represented. They maintain that the state systems enact laws and regulations and render decisions that often conflict with their needs and do not always represent their best interest.

Thomas R. Berger, a former Canadian Supreme Court jurist who is an internationally recognized advocate of Native rights, was invited by the Inuit Circumpolar Conference (ICC) to head the Alaska Native Review Commission. The ICC is an international organization composed of Alaskan, Canadian, and Greenlandic Inuit dedicated to maintaining Inuit culture. The ICC established the commission to assess the impacts of ANCSA. Judge Berger traveled to 62 villages to receive testimony from Alaska Natives on ANCSA and reported his findings in a 1985 publication *Village Journey*.

More often Judge Berger found that villagers believed that ANCSA represented a cultural encounter between two different societies. They reported that the concept of buying or selling land was alien to Alaska Natives and that land was communally held by a group rather than individual stockholders. They expressed concern that the 10,000 to 12,000 Alaska Native children who were born after the passage of ANCSA were not given automatic membership in the corporation as they were in their traditional social groups or clan by virtue of their birth. They talked about their subsistence activities and how the sharing of resources under their traditional customs established social obligations and reinforced bonds among them.

Congress amended the Indian Reorganization Act (IRA) in 1936 to allow Alaska Native villages to form tribal governments. Seventy villages organized themselves under the IRA council, and many other villages are governed by traditional councils. A common assumption in Alaska is that ANCSA extinguished tribal sovereignty. However, an increasing number of villages, particularly in western Alaska and the interior regions, are beginning to reassert their sovereign rights under their tribal government and judicial councils. Akiachak, which has been on the forefront of the tribal movement, was the first community to dissolve its local government established under state laws in favor of the tribal government and to organize its own judicial council.

In 1985, a number of the tribal governments organized themselves under the Alaska Native Coalition (ANC). ANC was not successful in obtaining an amendment to ANCSA that would allow corporations to transfer their lands to the tribal governments. A number of tribal governments in southwestern Alaska have united under the Yupiit Nation to strengthen tribal governments and rights further.

The tribal movement was also in response to the growing concerns over the social problems that plague Native villages. Alcoholism and self-destructive behavior have been a destructive force in many villages. The suicide rate has been reported to be the highest in the country, particularly among young Native males. Alienation, loss of family, low income, and alcohol abuse are cited as factors related to suicide. In an effort to control alcohol abuse, many tribal governments have prohibited the importation of alcohol into their communities.

Associated with the movement towards self-determination has been a cultural resurgence. Many communities in which traditional dancing and ceremonies were prohibited by the local churches have reinstituted Native dance and many of the traditional ceremonies. Native leaders and elders organized cultural camps in which young children would be immersed in Native culture. Children spend a period of time in these camps learning about traditional ways and beliefs. The elders have reasserted their traditional authority in many villages. They participate in formal elders' conferences to record traditional knowledge. The continuing political efforts to protect their land bases and subsistence hunting and fishing have become the rallying point to protect the survival of Native cultures.

While the Native languages have been incorporated into the educational systems, the policy has been to instill English language usage as quickly as possible. Dr. Michael E. Krauss (1983), the foremost Alaska Native linguist, believes that by the year 2055 only 5 of the 20 Native languages will be spoken. He suggests that Western Aleut, Kutchin, Central Yupik, and Siberian Yupik might conceivably survive indefinitely under ideal conditions. Dr. Krauss predicts that the first half of the 21st century will see the death of most Alaska Native languages. Tlingit is expected to become extinct with the death of the oldest Tlingit-speaking population in the year 2030. The Athapaskan language will survive only in the communities of Venetie and Arctic Village.

Conclusion

Whether the Inupiat, Yupik, Aleuts, Athapaskans, and the Tlingit and Haida will survive as distinct cultural groups remains to be determined. It is well accepted that the Native cultures have changed dramatically since the time of their contact with Western societies. However, it is well recognized that they retain elements and values of their traditional cultures that distinguish them from one another and set them apart from non-Natives.

Alaska Natives are on a collision course with non-Natives who oppose the tribal sovereignty movement and their subsistence rights. The mere increasing numbers of non-Natives, with their expansion into rural communities, set up competing uses for the wildlife resources. Alaska Natives have become accustomed to and dependent on goods and services that can be obtained only from the capital economy, but the prospects for economic development in the rural regions of Alaska are uncertain. The lack of economic opportunities in rural communities will undoubtedly accelerate the migration to urban centers.

Native corporations continue to hold all Native land except in two villages that turned over their lands to the tribal government. It is unlikely that the corporations will reconvey their lands to the tribal governments, but Alaska Natives are currently pursuing a number of amendments to ANCSA that they believe will ensure the continued ownership of Native land. The record is clear that the Native people have made a firm commitment to ensure the survival of their cultures.

Alaska Native Arts in the Twentieth Century

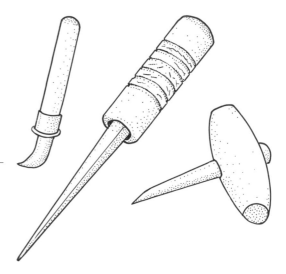

Margaret B. Blackman and Edwin S. Hall, Jr.

In the late 20th century, Alaska Native arts are flourishing, for reasons perhaps best expressed by Tlingit artist Jim Schoppert:

The exquisite work of our ancestors teaches us to create work suited for the day in which we live. By taking the old, breathing new life into it, and developing a new creation, the spirit of our people lives (Institute of Alaska Native Arts 1984).

We [native artists] carry with us fragments of our culture and are now bringing those elements into the much broader scope of world civilization. We cannot return to the old ways, but we must retain the old ways and reflect them in our attitudes and in our art. This will be our contribution (Alaska State Council on the Arts 1981).

By the turn of the twentieth century, relatively few of Alaska's native peoples were making objects that might be classed as art for their own use, either for utilitarian or ceremonial purposes. This is not to say that native ceremonies and accompanying artistic symbols were entirely moribund; for example, a Tlingit totem pole was set up on Pennock Island opposite Ketchikan in 1902 (Keithahn 1963:61), numerous works of art were made for the famous 1904 Tlingit potlatch at Sitka, and the participants in the 1915 Tanana Chiefs Conference wore beaded jackets as a sign of power and prestige (Duncan 1984:22–23). Nor were native peoples no longer manufacturing objects of practical use, as demonstrated by the production of utilitarian goods of Western design by the natives of Kodiak Island. However, it was primarily in northern Alaska that a significant number of art and craft pieces were derived from traditional native designs and made from traditional materials using ancient techniques; these objects were created by the Inupiat almost entirely for sale (Ray 1981:58).

The course of artistic production by Alaska native artisans from 1900 until the present day has proceeded in different ways and at different paces, depending upon the geographical area and the cultural group involved, tempered by a myriad of outside influences, including the arts and crafts market and the efforts of governmental agencies and interested non-native individuals. Table 4 indicates some of these factors that have influenced the development of native arts in Alaska over the past 87 years. The effects of these and other influences on native art are best known for the Eskimo and Aleut areas because of the extensive research conducted by Dorothy Jean Ray (1977, 1981, n.d.), but briefer studies and scattered references in the literature allow a general understanding of similar events among the Athapaskan, Tsimshian, Haida, and Tlingit peoples.

In the north, the Inupiat had long sold objects of everyday use, and items created specifically for sale, to the occasional explorer, whaler, and other outsiders who arrived by ship. It was the Nome gold rush, however, that prompted a permanent market for "Eskimo art" as the thousands of goldrushers and their tourist successors sought a souvenir of their sojourn in the Arctic (Ray 1977:42–43). Art produced for the market during the late years of the 19th century focused on the engraving of naturalistic scenes and geometric forms on a variety of ivory objects including bow drills, bag handles, cribbage boards, pipes, and whole walrus tusks and whale teeth. Ray has distinguished four engraving styles spanning the years from the mid-1800s to the present. In general, the progression was from minimal, rather schematic figures carved on bow drills and pipes at the beginning of the period to intricately detailed pictorial-style engravings on whole tusks and teeth or on cribbage boards proffered by some Inupiat artists (most notably Happy Jack) during and after the late 1890s; subsequently, the market popularity of engraved objects declined in favor of smaller sculptural items, and correspondingly, the quality of the engraving also declined (Ray n.d.:26). The market also prompted the carving of nontraditional objects ranging from napkin rings to the still popular billiken, which was first produced by Happy Jack in 1909 (Ray 1974). Small animal

458. Aleut Ivory Carver's Tools

This drawing was made from memory by Agagangel Stepetin of Unalaska to represent the ivory carving tools of his father, German Stepetin, of St. Paul Island and Unalaska. These tools include a carving knife that can be fitted with blades of different curvature and shape for different tasks. The tool with the T-handle is a drill. A long, thin file, this one with an ivory handle, completed the kit.

Table 4
20th-Century Alaska Native Arts: Significant Events and Influences

1900   Alaska Historical Library and Museum is founded (Juneau)

1914–18   First baleen basket is made at Barrow

1920s   Development of ivory bracelets, "Nunivak tusk" carvings, small ivory bird and animal figurines

1937   Alaska Native Arts and Crafts Clearing House is established through auspices of Indian Arts and Crafts Board

1930s   Teacher participation in native arts and crafts programs in schools becomes mandatory

1938–42   Civilian Conservation Corps totem pole restoration project

1940s   Twelve Alaska Natives take part in workshop at silver studio in Taxco, Mexico

late 1940s   First miniature ivory masks are carved

1951   Caribou skin masks first made at Anaktuvuk Pass

1952   Alaska Native Service and Indian Arts and Crafts Board begin Shungnak Jade Project

1956   Clearing House reorganizes as Alaska Native Arts and Crafts (ANAC) with board of directors composed largely of natives

1961   ANAC opens first retail shop in Juneau

1962   Eighteen Alaska Natives enroll in the Institute for American Indian Arts in Santa Fe

1962   Indian Arts and Crafts Board establishes experimental demonstration workshop in Sitka to develop native arts and crafts

1964   Toksook Bay Arts and Crafts Co-op, Inc., is formed

1964–65   Manpower and Development Training Act Designer-Craftsman workshops in Nome and Port Chilkoot

1965   Extension Center for Arts and Crafts at University of Alaska, Fairbanks, is established (later to become the Native Arts Center)

1966   Alaska Eskimo Arts and Crafts Association is organized in Nome

1966   Juried Alaska Festival of Native Arts begins (Anchorage)

1968   Anchorage Historical and Fine Arts Museum opens

1969   Beginnings of Musk Ox Producers' Cooperative

1970   Division of Statewide Services of UAF begins Village Art Upgrade program

1971   Community Enterprise Development Program begins program to stimulate production of fine art at Shishmaref

1971   Alaska Native Claims Settlement Act (ANCSA)

1971   Development of "Silver Hand" emblem by Alaska Division of Economic Enterprise to denote nativemade products

1972   Visual Arts Center (Anchorage) is established

1973   First Festival of Alaska Native Arts is held (Fairbanks)

1974   ANAC store opens in Anchorage

1975   Artist-in-Residence Program in Alaska schools is begun by State Council on the Arts

1975   State Percent for Art Program is initiated

1976   Institute of Alaska Native Arts is founded (Fairbanks)

1976   Artist-controlled collective Raven's Bones Foundation is formed

1976   Totem Heritage Center opens in Ketchikan

1978   First "Alaskameut" exhibit of native art

1978   First exhibition of contemporary Alaskan art at the National Collection of Fine Art of the Smithsonian Institution

1979   Exhibition of contemporary native art at the Anchorage Historical and Fine Arts Museum

1980–87   Traditional Native Arts program of the Alaska State Council on the Arts

1981   "Seeing with the Native Eye" statewide conference on native arts and cultural heritage programs is sponsored by the Alaska State Council on the Arts

1983   First Athapaskan Fiddling Festival is held (Fairbanks)

1984   Exhibition of Alaska Native Arts and artist demonstrations at the Smithsonian Folklife Festival

1985   Calista Corporation conducts a survey of arts and crafts opportunities in the Yukon-Kuskokwim area

1986   First Southeast Alaska Native Juried Art Exhibit (Sitka)

1986   First Annual Howard Rock Poetry Competition, for Alaska Natives

carvings and ivory jewelry also were produced for sale early and have maintained their popularity, comprising the bulk of carved ivory pieces sold today.

The Inupiat also worked in other media. Baskets woven from the baleen of the bowhead whale were first created sometime around 1914 at the behest of Charles Brower, the Barrow trader; later the manufacture of these baskets spread to other North Slope villages (Lee 1983). The supply of good baleen baskets has never equaled the demand, and thus relatively poorly made specimens sell for high prices today in Alaskan curio shops; meanwhile the corpus of skilled weavers declines steadily. Other North Alaska Inupiat arts made for sale have included dolls, skin clothing, caribou jaw sleds, skin, bone and wood masks, objects made from jade and caribou hoof, and paintings, drawings, and prints.

In South Alaska, that area of the coast and adjacent hinterland stretching from the Yukon-Kuskokwim delta area to Prince William Sound, the development of Eskimo and Aleut art differed from region to region. The Yupik-speaking peoples in the delta region are today best known for their coiled basketry. Though there is some evidence for greater antiquity, the production of coiled baskets appears to have been stimulated by the influx of outsiders into Alaska as a result of the Nome gold rush (Ray 1981:51). A rise in market popularity began in the 1930s and continues today; in general the salability of well-made baskets, juried competitions, and the efforts of interested individuals have led to increasing excellence in production and innovation in design. Yupik artisans have worked at ivory carving, graphic arts, mask carving, and skin sewing for many years; in recent years mask carving in particular has attracted attention of both artists and the market.

In the Aleut area, the activity of basket weaving almost entirely disappeared after World War II, but there has been a revival of late as a number of younger Aleut and Pacific Eskimo women have participated in formal basketry classes and workshops (Ray 1981:61). Mask making died out in both the Aleutians and Pacific Eskimo territory, but at least two modern Aleut artists include masks in their repertoire. Today Aleut artists have also achieved prominence in painting, sculpture, and jewelry.

Since the mid-19th century, beadwork has been the most prominent art form among most Alaskan Athapaskan groups, and the woman's role as beadworker for her family continues to be important today (Duncan 1984, 1988). Since gold rush days, outside markets have also been significant, so that now items such as moccasins and mitts are commonly made for both family and for sale, while others such as the baby-carrying straps once used by the Kutchin are now beaded primarily for sale. The women of several Kutchin and Tanana communities have also worked together to bead elaborate altar cloths for their churches. Contemporary beadwork designs show continuity with older ones, but motifs tend to be bolder and less detailed. Today's beads are slightly larger than old ones, more restricted in color range, and bolder in color. Among the Athapaskans, manufactured containers have now replaced birchbark storage baskets, although women continue to make small versions of the latter for sale and as knickknacks for their own use. Coiled willow baskets have become increasingly decorative as they have been manufactured for sale.

Artistic production, primarily for local use, continued on the Northwest Coast after the turn of the century, despite depopulation and exposure to Christianity and other outside influences. This was particularly true for the Tlingit; totem poles were adzed and raised, Chilkat blankets woven, beaded garments sewn, and masks carved. Silver bracelets, miniature wooden totem poles, spruce-root basketry, and beaded items such as moccasins and small bags were produced for a tourist market, and older pieces continued to command high prices. Beginning in the 1930s, a number of totem pole restoration and duplication projects both employed and informed a new generation of artists; for example, approximately 250 natives worked on the Civilian Conservation Corps project (Keithahn 1963:116). Despite this impetus and that of various workshops, it was not until recently that artists began to produce quality work in wood and silver and other media. Chilkat weaving is experiencing a small revival, and beadwork continues to appear on the market. Bracelets and other jewelry, beadwork, button blankets, and some masks continue to be made for native use. At Totem Heritage Center in Ketchikan and the National Historical Park at Sitka, training and instruction in traditional Northwest Coast arts are regularly offered.

By the 1960s Alaska Native art had for several generations been predominantly made for sale. As a largely tourist art it provided a source of income for many natives—the only cash income for some. At the same time, the classification of native art as tourist art seriously hampered creativity, for most important to the purchaser was the ethnic identity of the artist and what the piece represented, not the artistic merit of the work. At the same time, the tourist market for Alaska Native arts has helped keep the art alive by making art production financially rewarding for native artisans. In the early 1960s attempts were made to redirect the course of Native Alaska art away from the souvenir art market. Alaska Native Arts and Crafts (ANAC) experimented with the workshop as a setting for introducing new design concepts, new materials, and up-to-date production methods in Eskimo arts; it was hoped that the scope of the art could be broadened while native arts yet remained within the bounds of ethnic subject matter. The first pilot workshop was held in Nome in 1963. It was followed in 1964–65 by the Designer-Craftsman Training Project organized under the federally funded Manpower Development and Training Act. The act's intent was to provide vocational training, which in Alaska included training in the arts and crafts. Workshop classes were held at various locations throughout the state where training was provided in the local arts. The Nome workshop was attended by Bering Strait men (and one woman) and supervised by Ronald Senungetuk, an Eskimo from Wales whose formal art training included a year on a Fulbright scholarship in Norway and degrees from the American School of Craftsmen at Rochester Institute of Technology. Participants in the Nome project took classes in basic drawing and drafting, sculpture, metalwork, printmaking, and lapidary (Ray 1967b). Assessing the project, Dorothy Jean Ray commented: "The results were mixed. The older participants returned home to continue the same kind of work they had done before entering the program, but several of the younger ones moved from the Nome area to participate in newly-established artists-in-residence programs in villages or to take further training in other programs that were underway" (Larsen and Dickey 1982:39).

One of the programs under way in the mid-1960s evolved out of the Designer-Craftsman project. Extension classes at the University of Alaska in Fairbanks in native arts were begun under the direction of Ron Senungetuk. For two decades now, native students, regardless of educational background, have been able to get formal training in art at what has since become the university's Native Arts Center. Beginning in the 1960s aspiring Alaska Native artists also traveled outside the state for formal training. In the first year of its operation (1962) the Institute of American Indian Arts in Santa Fe enrolled 18 Native Alaskans.

In addition to the educational opportunities that opened up in the 1960s for Alaska Native artists, other organizations within the state have nurtured and directed the course of recent native arts. The Alaska State Council on the Arts provides fellowships and travel grants for native artists, offers project grants and master artist and apprentice grants in traditional native arts, supports the Visual Arts Center in Anchorage at which native artists have studied, and operates an artist-in-residence program that places established artists in school classrooms throughout Alaska. Until fiscal 1987 the council had a Director of Traditional Native Arts, but budget cuts have eliminated this position as well as other programs within the council. Arts Council funds also support a variety of other arts organizations in the state that affect native arts. The most important of these is the Institute of Alaska Native Arts (IANA), founded in 1976 and devoted to promoting and providing services for native visual, literary, and performing arts. In addition to organizing and funding exhibits and festivals, the institute has regularly sponsored workshops for native artists on topics as diverse as Chilkat weaving, basketry, beadwork, carving, bentwood technology, a sculpture study tour of San Francisco, and survival as an artist. Also important are the regional arts organizations within the state that have been instrumental in advertising and promoting local native arts (see Table 4 for examples).

Since 1971 several of the native regional corporations formed as a result of the Alaska Native Claims Settlement Act have been actively involved in native arts. Sealaska, the southeastern regional corporation, for example, has a nonprofit cultural heritage foundation that biennially hosts a gathering of Tlingit, Haida, and Tsimshian peoples; the several-day event includes performances by dance groups, oratory and presentations by elders, storytelling, traditional feasts, and theater productions (*Alaska State Council on the Arts Bulletin*, November 1986). Cook Inlet Regional Corporation, representing the native groups in the area surrounding Anchorage, allocated a large sum of money to the Anchorage Historical and Fine Arts Museum to commission major Alaska Native artists to produce works of art in both contemporary and traditional styles; those collected works are now on permanent display at the museum. Calista Corporation, serving natives in the Yukon-Kuskokwim area, in an attempt to expand the market for the indigenous arts of its people recently funded a study of those arts and their potential markets (Calista Professional Services 1985).

The collection and exhibition of 20th-century native art has been significant in recent years both in educating the larger resident and tourist public and in bringing art to village Alaska. The exhibit "Eskimo Dolls," organized by the Traditional Native Arts Program of the State Council on the Arts in 1982, exemplifies the attention given to traditional arts still being practiced (Jones 1982). Like many exhibits it was not only shown in major population centers but also traveled to village Alaska. Workshops sponsored by various institutions have often resulted in exhibits or juried competitions of native art. The "*Alaskameut*" ("from Alaska") exhibits of native art in 1978, 1980, and 1986 all grew out of workshops, as did "Interwoven Expressions," a 1985 exhibit of contemporary native basketry, and "New Traditions," a 1984 native sculpture exhibit. In 1980 the Alaska State Museum and the State Council on the Arts joined to organize a juried native art woodworking competition. This was followed in 1981 by a juried competition in wood, ivory, and bone. Regional native art competitions such as the annual Beaver Roundup, Barrow's Suliavut, and the Kivetoruk Moses Art Show are popular and draw significant numbers of participants. The juried competitions, like recent exhibits, have included both traditional and contemporary native arts, reflective of the two major directions Alaska native art has taken since the 1960s. Other special exhibits of 20th-century native art include the University of Alaska Museum's exhibits of modern Alaska Eskimo ivory carving (Larsen and Dickey 1982), Athapaskan beadwork (Duncan 1984), and the lifework of four traditional Alaska Native artists (Jones 1986). In addition to the two larger museums in Anchorage and Fairbanks, regional museums such as the Yugtarvik Museum in Bethel have also played an important role in exhibiting and nurturing native arts.

Publications have done much to promote and educate the public about Alaska Native art; Dorothy Jean Ray's (1961, 1967b, 1977, 1981) work on Eskimo art, in particular, is internationally known. The widely publicized and traveled "Inua" exhibit of Smithsonian material from the Bering Sea area brought 19th-century Yupik Eskimo art to the attention of the general public. The "Inua" catalog (Fitzhugh and Kaplan 1982) included a chapter on modern Eskimo art. In addition, there are a number of less widely distributed catalogs and other works published within the state that have documented little-known art forms (Jones 1982; Lee 1983), provided new perspectives on well-known traditional arts (Larsen and Dickey 1982), brought together contemporary and traditional art forms in a visual display and given voice to their creators (Steinbright 1986), provided an in-depth look at the artists behind the work (Jones 1986), and showcased the works of individual artists (O'Brien 1986). For a number of years the Institute of Alaska Native Arts has published a bimonthly journal distributed to over 4,000 people featuring Alaska Native arts through staff interviews with artists, native poetry, and news of artists, exhibits, conferences, and workshops.

Much could be written of the changes in Alaska Native arts in the 20th century. One can readily visualize some of them by comparing the photographs of native art accompanying this essay with the photographs of traditional native art shown in several of the bibliographic sources. Several recent trends are noteworthy. As elsewhere in native North America today, increasing numbers of women are working in art forms that were once a strictly male domain, many native artists have broadened their artistic horizons to include contemporary design and media, and, although over 90 percent of Alaska Native art is made for sale, an increasing amount is being made for native use. Art made for native consumption is not art for art's sake; rather, the masks, ceremonial blankets, beadwork, drums, dance fans, and other paraphernalia are made for native ceremonies. These works of art speak to the growth of native performing arts, which, like the visual art forms, are expressive of a newfound pride in native heritage and identity and, like the visual arts, have been supported by the institutions discussed above. Native dancing is performed regularly in the summer in the larger native communities such as Barrow and Kotzebue for tourists; dances are part of the Christmas celebrations in many villages and are performed on other occasions particular to individual ethnic groups. Native dance groups from throughout the state gather to dance and compete at the annual summer World Eskimo-Indian Olympics and at the spring Native Arts Festival, both held in Fairbanks. Native theater is also flourishing in several localities. Native arts have received added visibility through numerous public commissions during the last decade under the state's Percent for Art Program. Sullivan Arena and the Egan Convention Center in Anchorage as well as the Anchorage Airport prominently display examples of such commissioned works. A massive example of native-inspired public art can be seen in the interior decoration of the Anchorage Sheraton Hotel; the columns in the lobby are painted to represent Kodiak Eskimo arrow quivers, the floor tiles mimic Tlingit rattle basket tops, and the wallpaper motif is taken from Yupik coiled basketry.

Although the focus in this essay has been on the visual arts, native literary arts have burgeoned in recent years, receiving public attention through publication and the institutions supporting them. Oral traditions have been carefully committed to the written word (e.g., Dauenhauer and Dauenhauer 1987), native writers have participated in several writers' workshops offered in native communities, and an annual native poetry competition, inaugurated in 1986, has drawn talented native writers.

Several people provided invaluable help in putting together this essay, offering critical comments on our first draft, providing data and photographs, and interviewing some of the artists. We extend our thanks to Janet Brower, Pete Corey, Kate Duncan, Ann Fienup-Riordan, Rose Atuk Fosdick, Suzi Jones, Dave Libbey, Jim Schoppert, and Lynn Wallen. Special thanks to all the artists, who are identified with their works in the plates accompanying this article.

Twenty Contemporary Alaskan Artists

Lawrence Ullaaq Aviaq Ahvakana   (Inupiat, b. 1946) received his training at the Institute of American Indian Arts (Santa Fe), the Rhode Island School of Design, the Cooper Union School of Art, and the Pilchuck Glass Center. His work with various media, including sculpture in alabaster, metal, wood and blown, cast, and fused glass has led to positions as artist in residence at Barrow and at the Visual Arts Center in Anchorage and as art instructor in 1977 at the Institute of American Indian Arts. Ahvakana's pieces have been exhibited in many galleries and shows, including the Heard Museum Invitational in Phoenix (1967–69), Brooklyn Fine Arts Museum (1971), Smithsonian Portrait Gallery (1972), All-Alaska Juried Arts Show (1974–75), Alaska State Museum (solo exhibit 1977), Smithsonian Institution (''Alaskan Art'' 1978), Sacred Circle Gallery in Seattle (1981), the Field Museum in Chicago (''Exhibition of Contemporary Pacific Rim Art'' 1982), and the Contemporary Art Center in New Orleans (''Other Gods: Containers of Belief'' 1986). Numerous permanent collections (the Atlantic Richfield Corporation, the North Slope Borough, and the Alaska State Council on the Arts, for example) include his work. Major commissions can be seen at the North Slope Borough High School (bronze sculpture), the Alaska State Court building in Anchorage (welded wall relief), the Institute of American Indian Arts (welded sculpture), and the Rainier Bank in Anchorage (stone sculpture).

''My culture is a living culture. It is not a static or dead way of life but an ever-changing metamorphosis of adaptation. My grandfather Ahvakan was among the generation to first experience the beginning of adaptation. He showed me that change was not the death of a culture. Ahvakan, like many elders, was a composer of songs. He used singing as a tool to pass on many of these insights and personal interpretations of life as it changed around him. Being an Inupiat is not bound by landscape. I live away from my ancestral home but retain the essence of my ancestors. It is this basic nature of our way of life which I capture in my artwork. The tools may be modern, the material perhaps foreign to my grandfather, but the final statement would be the same.

''The spirit of my peoples' identity and its evolution [up] to today are expressed within the songs and dances. The drummer is the caretaker of this spirit.''

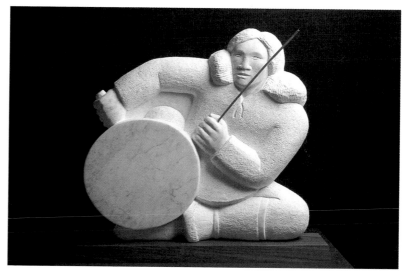

459. *Drummer*
Marble relief
2' × 2' × 4"

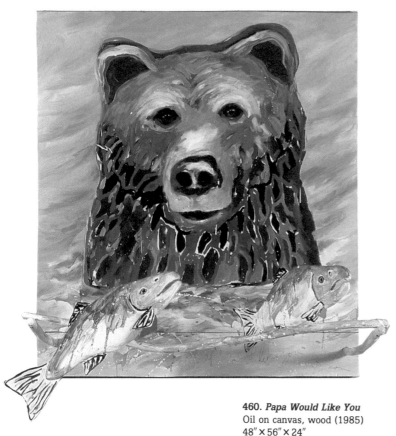

Alvin Eli Amason   (Aleut, b. 1948) has worked for the past 17 years in mixed-media paintings and sculpture, lithographs, and silk-screen prints. His training includes an M.A. from Central Washington University and an M.F.A. from Arizona State University. Amason's artistic creations, however, come from his past: ''I like to make things out of memories and sometimes out of things I'd like to see. Being raised in a colorful land with colorful people gave me attitudes that help me make these things. . . . Like Bill de Kooning, I believe the ultimate high occurs when you feel you're walking in your own landscape.'' Paintings resulting from Amason's memories have been seen at the National Collection of Fine Art (Smithsonian Institution), Nordjyllands Kunstmuseum (Aalborg, Denmark), American Indian Arts and Crafts Board (Washington, D.C), Alaska State Museum, Anchorage Historical and Fine Arts Museum, and many galleries. Important commissions have included the U.S. Federal Art in Architecture Program (U.S. Federal Building, Anchorage) and the Alaska Percent for Art Program (Anchorage International Airport).

''I like this one because of the youth and the hope it expresses.''

460. *Papa Would Like You*
Oil on canvas, wood (1985)
48″ × 56″ × 24″

Sylvester Ayek   (Inupiat, b. 1940s) has been working for more than 25 years in ivory, hardwoods, metal, and stone. He was born on King Island, the center of ivory carving in Alaska, and sought training at the Extension Center for Alaska Native Arts (Fairbanks), Alaska Pacific University, the University of Alaska, and the Visual Arts Center of Alaska. Ayek's pieces have been displayed at the Anchorage Historical and Fine Arts Museum, the Visual Arts Center of Alaska, and numerous Anchorage and Fairbanks galleries. Purchasers include the above institutions as well as many private collectors. For Ayek, the message of his art is ''Possibilities for growth are unlimited if you are unafraid to experiment with new forms and materials.''

461. *Day and Night Journey to the Spawning Grounds*
Wood, ivory, and braided nylon
5′3″ × 4′ × 6″

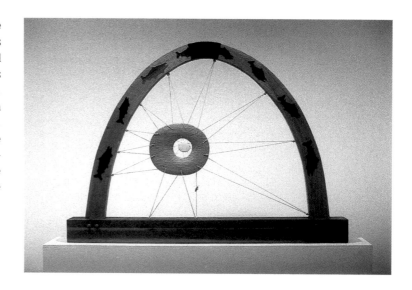

Larry J. Beck (Yupik, b. 1938) has long made large-scale abstract fabricated steel and cast-metal sculptures, but in 1981 he turned to making masks of what he calls "found" materials. Beck's walruses, polar bears, and other creatures are fashioned from hubcaps, auto mirrors, kitchen utensils, and similar materials. His work has met with great acceptance, having been shown in almost 100 exhibitions since 1964 and having received many awards and honors. Pieces by Beck grace many major public and private collections: the U.S. Department of the Interior, Calista Corporation (Anchorage), the University of Alaska Museum (Fairbanks), and the Heard Museum (Phoenix) being examples. Larry Beck's artistic training includes a B.A. in painting from the University of Washington in 1964 and a M.F.A. in sculpture from the same institution the next year; in turn, he has taught and lectured at universities throughout the west and in England. But just as Beck's artistic creations reflect his training, they also speak of his Yupik heritage.

"I am an Eskimo, but I'm also a 20th-century American. I live in a modern city where my found materials come from junk yards, trash cans, and industrial waste facilities, since the ancient beaches where my ancestors found driftwood and washed-up debris from shipwrecks are no longer available to me. But my visions are mine, and even though I use Baby Moon hubcaps, pop rivets, snow tires, Teflon spatulas, dental pick mirrors, and stuff to make my spirits, this is a process to which the old artists could relate. Because, below these relics of your world, reside the old forces familiar to the Inua."

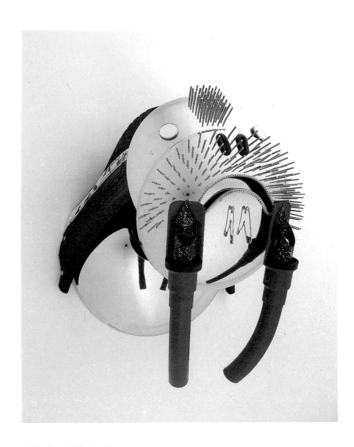

462. *Punk Walrus Inua*
Mixed media (1986)

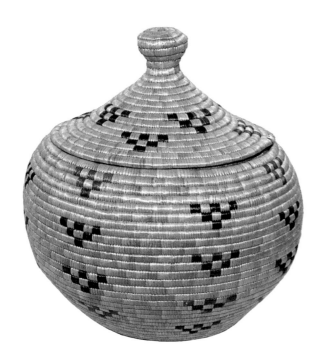

Rita Pitka Blumenstein (Yupik, b. 1933) is best known as a basketmaker, though she lists skin sewing, beading, dancing, and storytelling on mud (drawing of figures with a special knife in the illustration of girls' stories). She has been working in these media since her teens. Her woven baskets are on display in the Alaska State Museum, the University of Alaska (Fairbanks), and the Smithsonian. Blumenstein has demonstrated her craft at the Anchorage Historical and Fine Arts Museum, the Sheldon Jackson Museum in Sitka, and the Smithsonian Folklife Festival (1984), among other places. For ten years she has taught basketry and other Alaska Native arts at Matanuska-Susitna Community College at the University of Alaska. Of her weaving, she says, "Since it's a fast-disappearing art, I would like to keep it from disappearing."

463. Grass Basket

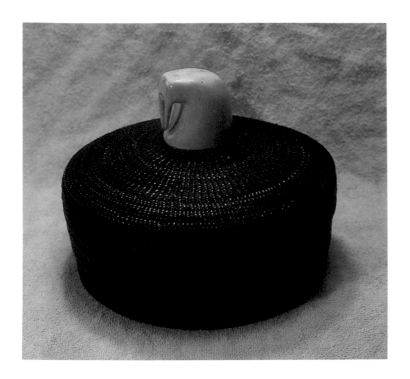

Archie K. Brower (Inupiat, b. 1929) learned how to make baleen baskets at the Bureau of Indian Affairs school in Barrow sometime in the 1940s but did not work actively at the craft until about ten years ago. When asked what philosophy guided his basketmaking, Brower concluded, ''I just try to do the best I can.'' Most of Archie's baskets have been sold through gift shops in Fairbanks.

This basket won $1000 for best of show in Suliavut, Barrow's annual arts and crafts show. Brower entered it in Suliavut because ''I just wanted to try it out and see how I would do.''

464. Baleen Basket
Baleen and ivory
$7\frac{1}{2}'' \times 6''$

Nicholas Charles, Sr. (Yupik Eskimo, b. 1910), was born on Nelson Island but has lived, with his wife, in Bethel since 1943. As a young boy he learned the carving skills in the village men's house from his father and other men that would later make him known to a larger world as an extraordinary mask maker. Today his masks not only sell in Anchorage shops but, more important, are also made for local native use. What is important to Charles is not the finished product but the process of making the mask and the performance of it in the dance. Today Charles and his wife, Elena, are active teaching dancing and carving throughout the Yukon-Kuskokwim delta region. His exquisite pieces can be found at Yugtarvik Museum in Bethel, the University of Alaska Museum in Fairbanks, and the Smithsonian, as well as in numerous private collections. In 1982 Charles was one of several participants in a mask-making workshop in Bethel sponsored by the State Council on the Arts; in 1984 he traveled to Washington to participate in the Smithsonian Folklife Festival; and in 1985 he participated in the Native Art Festival at the Anchorage Historical and Fine Arts Museum. In 1986 he was one of four native artists featured in the exhibit ''The Artists behind the Work,'' organized by the University of Alaska Museum, Fairbanks. The double-headed hawk mask shown here won him a merit award at the 1980 Statewide Native Woodworking competition.

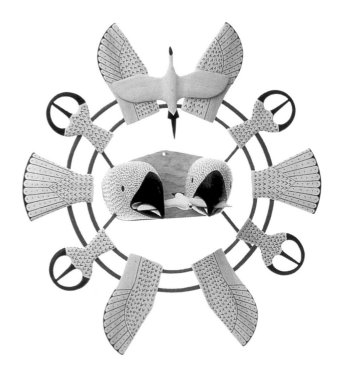

465. Double-headed Hawk Mask

Delores Churchill (Haida, b. 1929) has been weaving baskets since 1972, having learned Haida basketry from her mother, Selina Peratrovich, a well-known Haida weaver. Churchill has also trained in Tlingit, Tsimshian, and Aleut basketry and in Athapaskan birchbark basketmaking. More recently she has studied Chilkat and raven's tail (geometric) weaving under Cheryl Samuel. From Jennie Thlunaut, the last traditional Chilkat weaver from Klukwan, Churchill learned more than weaving. "Her humility, grace, and wonderful sense of humor . . . I strive to emulate." Delores's works have been exhibited in Honolulu in "Pacific Basketmakers: A Living Tradition" (1983), at the Smithsonian Folklife Festival in Washington, D.C. (1984), at the Anchorage Historical and Fine Arts Museum (1977–86), and at the Stonington Gallery in Seattle (1986), among other places. She has taught numerous workshops in basketry and received several awards for her work, including the Alaska State Legislative Award, in recognition of her commitment to native art.

"This basket cup and cover are symbolic of the interwoven tradition of basketry spanning several thousand years. My mother, Selina Peratrovich, saw her uncles drink salt water from a similar container to purify themselves when fasting before going hunting, fishing, or trapping. The uncles would not drink the salt water until they had blown it in all the directions from which the prevailing winds blew; this insured them good fortune in their endeavors. These glimpses into the past weave me culturally to my ancestry and help me to maintain stability in the present but are also the driving force which convinces me that this wonderful tradition must survive in the future."

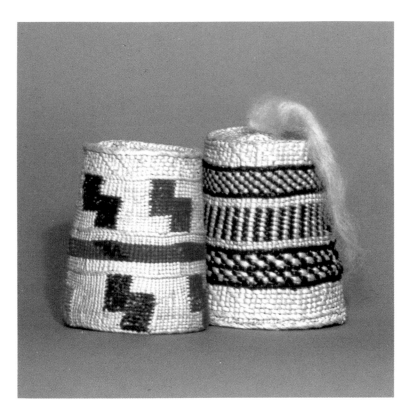

466. Basket Cup and Cover

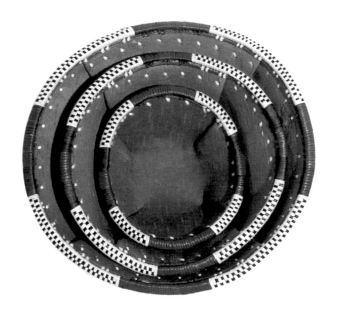

Belle Deacon (Athapaskan, b. 1905) is originally from Anvik but now lives in Grayling, Alaska. She learned birchbark basketmaking from her grandmother when she was young. "I watched her, used her scraps, and that's how I learned." Deacon isn't certain where all her finished pieces have gone, noting, "I think I've got lots of baskets all over, some in Anchorage, Fairbanks, and Ketchikan." In 1984 Deacon participated in the Smithsonian Folklife Festival, and on a number of occasions she demonstrated her art at the Anchorage Historical and Fine Arts Museum. She has also taught birchbark basketry in a workshop in Ketchikan. Speaking of her basketry, Deacon says, "I invent lots of things. I use mostly old-style stitches that my grandmother was using. I taught my daughter Daisy to do basketmaking. Now my little granddaughter age seven wants to make baskets. She doesn't make fancy stitches like I do, but she made a pretty good basket and sold it for seven dollars."

467. Basket

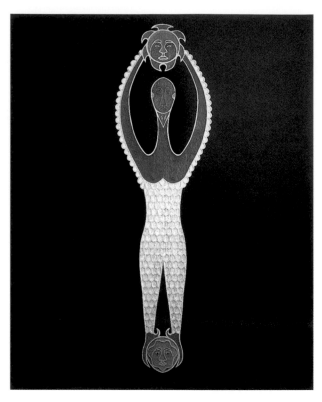

468. *Raven the Creator*
Paint and wood
6′ high

John J. Hoover (Aleut, b. 1919) specializes in wood, bronze, and stone sculpture, though in the early part of his more than 40 years as an artist he mostly worked in oils. His formal training included work at the Fine Art School of Painting and Design in Seattle and stints as artist in residence at the Institute of American Indian Arts (Santa Fe) and in Asia (Japan, Formosa, Philippines) with the Air Force school system. However, his artist inspiration also draws on his life-long experiences as a fisherman and his extensive reading about his native heritage. The roster of galleries and museums that have displayed and purchased Hoover's pieces is extensive and includes: the Horniman Museum (London), Heard Museum (Phoenix; "Sculpture I" 1973; first-place awards in 1975 and 1978), Museum of the Plains Indian (Browning, Montana; one-man show in 1975), Philbrook Art Center (Tulsa; awards in 1974 and 1975), Anchorage Historical and Fine Arts Museum (1979 and 1985), Smithsonian Institution (1982), and Portland Art Museum (1987). Large commissions have been forthcoming as various Percent for Art projects and from corporate clients like ARCO.

"You know, shamans, who influenced the workings of good and evil spirits, made symbols of primitive man's fears. And when they could see their fears take form, they often were no longer afraid. The idea of the spirit world, trances, the close relationship of man, animals, and nature, seemed so real and meaningful I tried to fathom these mysteries."

Edna Davis Jackson (Tlingit, b. 1950) received a B.F.A. from Oregon State University in 1980 and a M.F.A. from the University of Washington three years later. Additionally, she completed an apprenticeship with Cheryl Samuel in Chilkat weaving and worked with Chilkat weaver Jennie Thlunaut and basketmaker Delores Churchill. Selected exhibitions of Jackson's mixed-media works in handmade cast cedar paper include Anchorage Historical and Fine Arts Museum ("Earth, Fire, and Fibre XI" 1980), Sacred Circle Gallery (Seattle: "Indian Artists of the 1980s" 1983), Native American Arts Gallery (Los Angeles: "Native American Artists—California and the West Coast" 1984), Gallery of the American Indian Community House (New York: "Women of Sweetgrass, Cedar and Sage" 1985), and Institute of Alaska Native Arts ("Alaskameut" 1986). Important commissions have come from the Alaska State Museum, the Anchorage Historical and Fine Arts Museum, and the American Indian Arts and Crafts Board. For Jackson, "My artwork marks events in my life. I have a respect for native traditions, but I refuse to be bound by them in my artwork or my life. My life has been spent crossing boundaries: one of the first half-breed kids in the village, obtaining advanced degrees in art, one of the few contemporary Alaska Native artists who have returned to village living rather than urban. I like crossing boundaries in my artwork: making mask forms out of cast cedar paper, taking traditional geometric basket designs to make large pieces of artwork using hand-manipulated paper techniques, weaving traditional patterns in cedar and wool to use in my mixed-media pieces.

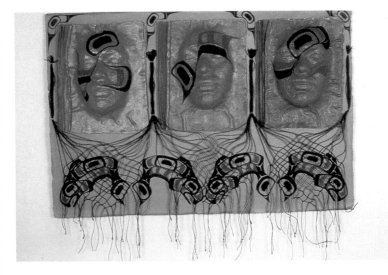

469. *Ka-oosh and Coho Salmon*
Cast cedar paper
32″ × 40″ × 5″

"*Ka-oosh and Coho Salmon* is a portrait of my husband. It marks twelve years of marriage, as symbolized by the twelve pages of cedar behind the faces. My husband belongs to the Coho Salmon Clan, which is marked by the four leaping salmon on the bottom of the piece."

Nathan P. Jackson (Tlingit, b. 1938) draws much of his artistic inspiration from his heritage as a member of the Sockeye Clan on the Raven side of the Chilkoot-Tlingit people. He began creating woodcarvings and jewelry in traditional Tlingit style in 1962, but it was not until 1967, after completing courses at the Institute of American Indian Arts in Santa Fe and working with Alaska Indian Arts, Inc., that he became a full-time artist. Nathan has taught many classes in wood carving and design at the Alaska State Museum, the Ketchikan Arts Council, the Juneau-Douglas Community College, the Sheldon Jackson College, the Totem Heritage Center, and in public schools, as well as classes in dancing at Klawock, Ketchikan, and in British Columbia. Additionally, he has worked as a consultant for the Alaska State Museum's totem restoration project and the University of Alaska Native Arts Upgrade program and has worked with several apprentices. Nathan's work has been shown in many places, including the New York World's Fair (1964), the Alaska State Museum (1971), the University of Alaska Museum, and various galleries. In particular, he has excelled in the creation of larger pieces such as restored and original totem poles and carved panels and screens. His poles are found in locations throughout Alaska, in Kobe (Japan), Salt Lake City, London, and New York, and his panels adorn the Ketchikan International Airport, Peabody Museum of Harvard, Daybreak Star Arts Center in Seattle, Sealaska Corporation building in Juneau, Hendrickson Building at the University of Alaska,

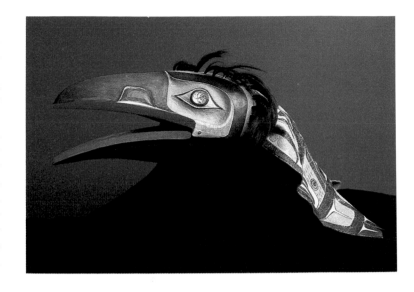

470. *Raven Mask*
Wood, abalone, and hair (1979)

Ketchikan Totem Heritage Center, and Anchorage Historical and Fine Arts Museum, among other places.

"My goal is to produce high-quality traditional Tlingit work, staying within the boundaries of the old-style artform."

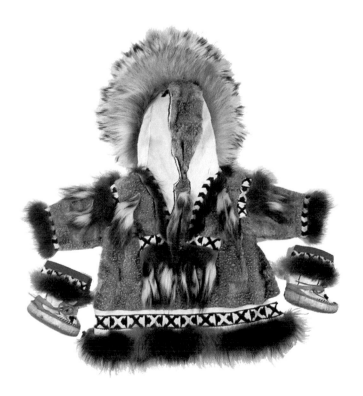

Bertha Leavitt (Inupiat, b. 1912) of Barrow has been skin sewing since she was a little girl and making fancy parkas and boots for the last 15 or 16 years. She regularly teaches a skin sewing class in Barrow and is often called upon to give demonstrations of her craft. All of her work has been made for native use. In regard to the skin clothing and boots she makes, Leavitt notes, "I make them the old-fashioned style from long, long ago." The squirrel parka and mukluks shown here won first place in Suliavut, Barrow's annual arts and crafts show; they were originally made to be worn in the town's annual baby contest.

The child's parka is made from the skins of arctic ground squirrels. The cuffs, bottom trim, and hanging pieces on the parka are wolverine. The black and white design is calfskin. The hood ruff is composite; the inner part (not shown) is wolverine and the outer sunburst is wolf. The mukluks have crimped soles of bleached ugruk hide with a seal leather border and seal leather gasket as the seam. The mukluk uppers are calfskin with a ring of wolverine and a band of red felt around the top. Vertical lines of red felt trim separate the pieces comprising the upper boot. A narrow band of black and white rickrack borders the upper boot where it joins the top of the ugruk soles. The ties are leather.

471. Squirrel Parka, Calfskin Mukluks

James Schoppert (Tlingit, b. 1947) describes the work he has been producing as an artist since 1973 as "modern minimalist and abstracted Northwest Coast art, pictographic image paintings, and masks inspired by Northwest Coast and Eskimo art traditions." He began carving on his own but soon began to take college courses to increase his knowledge of art and improve his technique; in 1981 he was awarded a M.F.A. degree in sculpture from the University of Washington. Schoppert's work has appeared in many exhibitions and galleries, including the Philbrook Art Center (Tulsa: "What Is American Art?" 1986), Heard Museum (Phoenix: Second Biennial Invitation, 1985), American Contemporary Indian Arts Gallery (San Francisco, 1985), Alaska State Museum (1985), Yellowstone Arts Center (Billings: "New Ideas from Old Traditions" 1985), G. N. Gorman Museum (Davis, California: 1984), and Sacred Circle Gallery (Seattle: 1982). His artistic creations grace many permanent collections: Alaska Mutual Bank (Bellevue, Washington), Alaska State Council on the Arts, Anchorage Community College, Anchorage Historical and Fine Arts Museum, Calista Corporation (Anchorage), Sheraton Hotel (Anchorage), the Newark Museum, the University of Alaska (Fairbanks), and the Washington State Arts Commission Arts Bank. Also, he has been awarded numerous Percent for Art commissions for pieces to be displayed in public facilities as varied as the Alaska State Troopers building, the Sullivan Sports Arena (Anchorage), and the Ketchikan Pioneer Home.

"My inspiration is drawn from both the Eskimo and Tlingit art traditions. In using the idiom of Northwest Coast art conventions, I've divested it of cultural intent, social meaning,

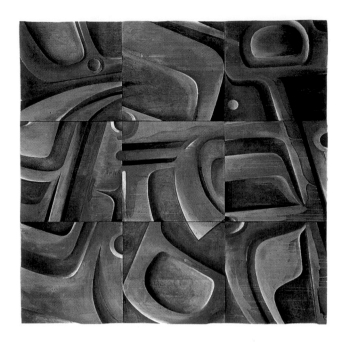

472. *Blueberries*
Wood, paint (1986)
72" × 72"

and accustomed appearances and substituted freedom of color, fragmentation, abstraction, and minimalization. It's from this point I've arrived at these creations, which are both modern and speak directly to the continuance and maintenance of the Tlingit cultural identity."

Joseph E. Senungetuk (Inupiat, b. 1940) began producing artistic creations in 1964 and has worked in both sculpture (wood, stone, and metal) and woodcut printmaking. His training was primarily at the San Francisco Art Institute. Numerous galleries have exhibited Senungetuk's work, including the Anchorage Historical and Fine Arts Museum, the Chicago Field Museum ("Exhibition of Contemporary Pacific Rim Art" 1982), the Visual Arts Center of Alaska, and the Stonington Gallery (Anchorage). Commissions have come from the New York Metropolitan Museum of Modern Art, the Bellingham Whatcom Museum, the University of Alaska (Fairbanks), the Seattle-Tacoma International Airport, the Alaska State Museum, the Bethel Corrections Center, the American Indian Arts and Crafts Board, and the San Francisco American Indian Historical Society.

"Innovation and resourcefulness, care and skill, craftsmanship and originality, are my big concerns in everything I do."

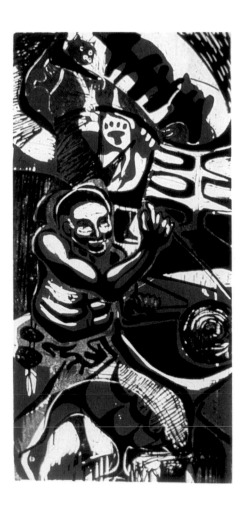

473. *The Shaman Beckons*
Woodcut (1971)
11" × 16"

Delores Sloan (Athapaskan, b. 1938) identifies herself as Irish-Athapaskan and lives in Fairbanks. She has been doing beadwork since childhood, having learned from her mother, who was always busy sewing for the family. Her work has been exhibited at the University of Alaska Museum, in the Athapaskan beadwork exhibit "Some Warmer Tone" (1984) and in "A Child Is Born" (1987–88), an exhibit of art in recognition of children. Sloan has also shown her beadwork at the Alaska State Fair, where in 1981 and 1982 she was a grand champion winner. Her work received national recognition when she was elected to the Homemakers Hall of Fame in Ralston, Virginia. Sloan is especially proud of her beaded stole that was presented to Pope John Paul II when he visited Alaska in 1984. That piece now resides in the Vatican Museum. Sloan's experimentation with beadwork has led to beaded portraits of famous individuals—John F. Kennedy, Richard Nixon, and Alaska governor William Egan. Sloan has taught beadworking at the Anchorage Historical and Fine Arts Museum, and for the last six years she has taught beadworking to children in the Fairbanks School District's Alaska Indian Education Program.

"I would love to have younger people carry on the tradition and get ideas from the elders before they all leave us. That's the most important thing. The elders have so much to teach us."

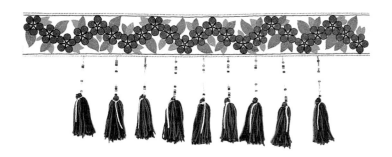

474. Baby Belt

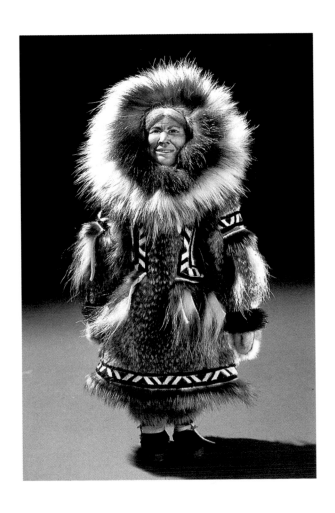

Dolly Spencer (Inupiat, b. 1930) is well known as a maker of exquisite, detailed traditional-style Eskimo dolls. Originally from Kotzebue and now a resident of Homer, she learned skin working and sewing from her mother when she was eight years old and made her first doll at government school in 1941 or 1942. Spencer uses all traditional materials in her dolls—carved birchwood heads, skin bodies stuffed with caribou hair, fur and skin garments sewn with sinew. The right materials are important. She says, "I want my people to go back to using sinew when they sew. I would like someone to teach the younger generation to learn to strand sinew and twist the sinew for sewing skin and also how to prepare the skin different ways. There are five different ways to tan a hide to use. This I tell to my people in the villages, not to use dental floss [for thread]. It cheapens their work." Spencer's works have been exhibited in Homer, Juneau, Fairbanks, Anchorage, and Cincinnati, and her dolls are in several museums as well as private collections. Spencer has demonstrated doll-making at the Smithsonian and taught doll-making to her own people in the village schools.

"This doll represents an Eskimo woman from above the arctic circle dressed in a fancy parka made of ground squirrel with badger, coyote, and wolverine ruff and pieced calfskin fancy work. This lady doll was said by my husband to be 'the best doll you ever made.' She's traveling in a doll show somewhere."

475. "Above the Arctic Circle Lady Doll" (1982)

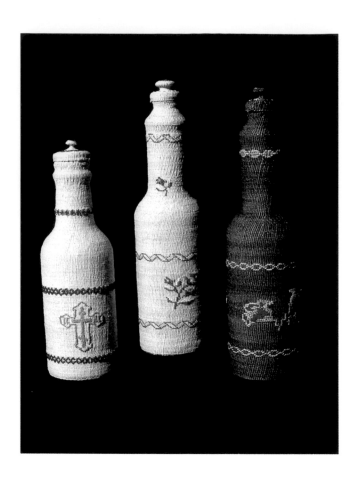

Agnes Thompson (Aleut, b. 1947) learned basketmaking from her mother in Atka and has been weaving for some 15 years. She has participated in basketry workshops in Fairbanks and Kodiak and regularly demonstrates her weaving at the annual Native Arts Festival at the Anchorage Historical and Fine Arts Museum. In 1985 she was one of the curators of the Institute of Alaska Native Arts basketry exhibit "Interwoven Expressions." Thompson's work is in the Anchorage Museum's collection and has been exhibited outside the state at Snow Goose Associates Gallery in Seattle. Most of her baskets are sold either to private collectors or through Alaska Native Arts and Crafts in Anchorage.

"Aleut basketry is considered along with [that of the] Pomo to be one of the most finely woven of the world. It takes a very long time to weave one. I like to weave, and I'm trying to keep the Aleut art of basketweaving alive. There are only a handful left who are weaving on a regular basis."

476. Baskets

Appendix I

BEADS AND BEAD TRADE IN THE NORTH PACIFIC REGION

Peter Francis, Jr.

Beads are the universal personal adornment, the oldest and most widespread art form. In use since the beginning of the modern human race, beads and bead materials have long been trade items. When explorers ventured into unfamiliar areas or encountered strange peoples, they invariably took beads. Despite their relative isolation, the Alaskans and Siberians received glass trade beads from around the world: Venice (Italy), Bohemia (now part of Czechoslovakia), China, and possibly Central Asia. Trade beads were quickly adpated to decorate the human body and were sewn or fastened onto articles of everyday and ceremonial use.

Yet it was not always so. Before Europeans entered the region, beads were made of natural materials: soft stones, bone, ivory and other teeth, shells, and amber, some of which are preserved on objects in this volume. They were relatively rare. Trade beads accelerated the use of beads until nearly every class of object from quiver to labret was decorated with them.

The Russians first brought their beads for this trade from Europe across Siberia and from China through the Mongolian border town of Kiakhta, where they charged no import duties upon them (Coxe 1780:241). By 1811 they were buying beads from Yankee (mostly Bostonian) skippers and the American Fur Company, and by 1839 from the Hudson's Bay Company. After the sale of Alaska to the United States, the beads in Siberia still came across land and from China, while those of Alaska were furnished exclusively by Americans.

Beads served many functions. Vitus Bering and other early explorers gave them away as gifts, to break down initial shyness, and as symbols of respect. Almost as early, they were used to barter for essential food and, above all, for pelts. Soon they became a quasicurrency and played an important economic role in the fur trade. In time, they were so common that they were devalued, although the older beads were always considered special by the Alaskans and Siberians.

There is a great variety of glass beads, and many ways to make them. Some particular methods can help us identify certain beadmakers, but others are virtually universal and not diagnostic of one locale.

Venice has been the world's leading beadmaker for 500 years, and her beads were taken on virtually all European voyages of discovery. Most early Venetian beads were made by forming a glass tube, cutting it into short segments, and agitating them over heat to smooth their sharp edges. These drawn beads have their fabric and inclusions running parallel to their perforations. The most common of these are small "seed" beads, up to 5 millimeters in diameter, used for most of the beadwork on the objects illustrated here.

The Bohemians began to outsell the Venetians in the mid 19th century. They made beads by several methods, most notably by molding glass in two-part molds and either leaving the resulting seam on or grinding it off.

The oldest and most universal way to make beads is to wind glass around a wire or metal rod. This can be done by dipping a rod into hot glass in a crucible or by melting glass and allowing it to drip around a wire. Wound beads have their fabric and inclusions encircling the perforations. Most wound beads illustrated in this volume appear to be Chinese, with typical bubbly glass, large perforations, and uneven outlines.

Most beads in this collection divide into four groups based upon museum accession dates and regions: those from the 1840s, those from 1874 to 1886, those from Alaska between 1897 and 1902, and those from Siberia also from 1897 to 1902. The accession date of an object only hints at its age. It cannot be more recent than that date, but how much older it may be is quite another matter.

Each of these groups has distinctive beads. Those from the 1840s are similar to the ones excavated at early (pre-1810) Russian contact sites in Alaska. They are dominated by irregular seed beads of semitranslucent medium blue and white ones coated with clear glass. The larger beads are all wound and most likely of Chinese manufacture (figs. 193, 204, 395).

In the next period (1874–86) the seed beads persist, with the addition of opaque red over translucent green or other colors (*cornaline* d'Allepos) from Venice. The larger beads are also mostly European: drawn hexagonal beads with the corners ground off in solid blue, blue on white, and amber (commonly but inappropriately called Russian beads) from Bohemia, and wound beads of translucent blue or red that have been crudely pressed into facets (figs. 48, 202, 203, 406). A few simple wound Chinese beads are also found at this time.

In the 1897–1902 period there is a divergence between the Alaskan and Siberian beads. Both areas have drawn translucent red over whites (also called *cornaline* d'Allepos; figs. 213, 299 top right) and cornerless hexagonals, especially in blue (fig. 62). They also have seed beads, but they have changed; the older types are now outnumbered by deep opaque blues, pure whites, and a variety of other colors, all quite uniform in size (figs. 315, 341 boots, 418,419). However, the Siberians had many Chinese wound beads (fig. 232) and beads wound in a series of four and later cut apart, often left as doubles (fig. 325 center). Beads are made this way in Herat, Afghanistan, by a family who migrated from Bukhara, Uzbekistan, in the early 20th century; the Siberian beads may have come from Central Asia.

There is a time lag between the appearances of most bead types elsewhere in America or Africa and in the North Pacific. Cornerless hexagonals were first made in the 1820s but are not found here until 1874–86. Translucent red-over-white beads were made from about 1830 but did not reach the North Pacific until 1897–1902. Bohemian molded biconical beads with conical holes and many ground facets were being made by the 1820s but are listed here only in 1897–1902. Uniform seed beads resulted from the inventions of automatic cutting and sorting machines in Venice in 1867 but are dated here only in the 1897–1902 period. Why? Alaska and Siberia were still relatively isolated in the 19th century, and beaded objects were in use for some time before they were acquired by museums.

The reuse of old beads is an interesting phenomenon, especially evident on beadwork. Many newer pieces have a mixture of older blue and clear-over-white seed beads alongside new blues and whites. The older ones often decorated a distinctive place, such as an outer border. In some cases, entire beaded panels were cut from their original garments and added whole onto a new one, as with the top panel of the apron in figure 270.

The most historically significant bead of the region is a medium-sized opaque blue one, crudely wound into a sphere. These were in the area very early and may well have been first brought by Vitus Bering in the 1740s. Three members of his crew wrote that the beads they had were Chinese (Golder 1922:99, 147, 272). They reached Prince William Sound, Alaska, before the Russians did. Capt. James Cook purchased a few in 1778 to satisfy himself they were glass, and Capt. James King described them: "They set a very great Value [upon them] . . . They are about the size of a large current berry, & intended to be (but are not) round" (Cook 1967:365, 1418). The same bead was in demand all along the Northwest Coast, as far south as the Columbia River, and enjoyed long-lasting popularity. It is found on a number of objects, usually accorded a place of honor (figs. 204, 232, 296).

Another bead with possible historical references was roughly wound and pressed into facets (figs. 324 earrings, 361). It is found on a few American sites from 1700 to 1890 (Brain 1979:111, type WIIA7) and answers best to those called garnets by Carl Merck of the Billings Expedition of 1788–92.

Among the most notable specimens of bead use in this exhibit is the beaded cap from Kodiak Island (fig. 48), with its wealth of beads that reflect nearly the whole later trade of the region. The triple belt of 363 caribou front teeth alternating with two rows of the prized old wound blue beads (fig. 296) was purchased in 1939 but was even then recognized as an outstanding older piece (a Seattle dealer sold it for $125).

Appendix II

LIST OF ILLUSTRATIONS

Fig | Page | Caption title / (culture/artist)

Crossroads of Continents: Beringian Oecumene
1 10 Cultures of the North Pacific
2 13 Alaskan Native Costumes (Postels?)
3 13 Anthropological Collecting, 1840)1901
4 14 Bentwood Hunting Hat (Bering Sea Esk.)
5 14 Quivers and Arrows (Chukchi/ Athapaskan)
6 15 Koryak Egg Gatherers
7 15 Koryak Shaman
8 16 Chilkat Tunic (Tlingit)
9 16 Eskimo Trade Fair
10 16 Engraved Winged Object (Old Bering Sea)
11 16 Lime Mortar (Haida)

Ethnic Connections Across Bering Strait
12 17 Birdskin Parka (St. Lawr. Is. Eskimo)
13 17 Ivory Bolas (Norton Sound Eskimo)
14 18 "Summer/Winter Habitations. . ." (Webber)
15 18 Snow Goggles (Koryak/Bering Sea Esk.)
16 19 "Natives of Oonalaschaka. . ." (Webber)
17 20 Trade and War: Drillbow (C. Nome Esk.)
18 20 Tobacco Pipe and Pouch (Even)
19 21 Tobacco Pipe (Chukchi)
20 21 Siberian Curios (Siberian Native)

Peoples of the Amur and Maritime Regions
21 24 Nanai Woman's Coat
22 25 Nanai Family Group
23 26 Wood Box (Nivkhi)
24 27 Nivkhi Woodworking
25 27 Knife and Sheath (Nivkhi)
26 29 Bear Festival Bowl (Nivkhi)
27 29 Festival Spoon and Amulet (Nivkhi)

Koryak and Itelmen: Dwellers of the Smoking Coast
28 31 Imported Technology (Koryak)
29 33 Koryak Dancer
30 33 Koryak Winter Village
31 34 Spinner (Koryak)
32 34 Koryak Jewelry

Even: Reindeer Herders of Eastern Siberia
33 35 Pendants (Even)
34 36 Even Woman
35 37 Apron (Even)

Chukchi: Warriors and Traders of Chukotka
36 38 Chukchi Woman and Child
37 40 Chukchi Travelers
38 40 Pouch (Chukchi)
39 41 "Tchouktchis. . ." (Choris)
40 41 Embroidered Summer Boots (Chukchi)

Eskimos: Hunters of the Frozen Coasts
41 42 Eskimo Dancer
42 44 Baleen Basket (N. Alaskan Eskimo)
43 45 Asian Eskimo Village (Plover Bay)
44 46 Retrieval Hook (Bering Sea Eskimo)
45 47 Personal Ornamentation (Ber. Sea Esk.)
46 47 "Beautiful Things" (Bering Sea Eskimo)
47 48 Ritual Hunting Headgear (Ber. Sea Esk.)
48 49 Beaded Dance Headdress (Koniag Eskimo)
49 49 "Woman of Ykamoka Island. . ." (Tikhanov)
50 50 "Happy Fellow" (Koniag Eskimo)
51 51 Gunnelboard and Paddle (Koniag Eskimo)

Aleut: Islanders of the North Pacific
52 53 Aleut Hunter
53 54 "Oonalashka Native Codfishing" (Elliott)
54 55 Kayak Suction Pump (Aleut)
55 55 Aleut Man and Assemblage (Levashev)
56 56 Gutskin Raincoat (Aleut)
57 56 Grass Basket (Aleut)
58 57 Gutskin Hat (Aleut)

Tlingit: People of the Wolf and Raven
59 58 Tlingit Chief
60 59 Trap Sticks (Tlingit)
61 59 Goathorn Spoons (Tlingit/Haida)
62 60 Personal Ornaments (Tlingit)
63 61 "Cape and Rattle of Kolosh.." (Mikhailov)
64 61 Tobacco Pipes (Tlingit)
65 62 Raven Rattle (Tlingit)
66 63 Sea Lion Headdress (Tlingit)

Northern Athapaskans: People of the Deer
67 65 Athapaskan Hunter
68 66 Fort Yukon Indian

The Story of Russian America
69 70 "Barabaras. . .Koloshi. . ." (Voznesenskii)
70 70 Russian Double-headed Eagle Crest
71 71 North Alaskan Eskimos, Cape Smith
72 72 Map of. . .First Bering Exp. (1725-30)
73 72 Ivory Sea Otter with Pup (Aleut)
74 73 Early Voyages of Exploration to Alaska
75 73 War Shield (Aleut)
76 73 Harpoon Arrow for Sea Otters (Koniag)
77 74 Grigorii Shelikov (1747-1795)
78 74 Aleks. Baranov (Tikhanov)
79 74 "View of Pavlovskii Harbor. . ." (Shields)
80 76 "Portrait of. . .Katlian. . ." (Tikhanov)
81 77 War Helmet (Tlingit)
82 77 Painted Hide Armor (Tlingit)
83 76 Baranov's Chain Mail Shirt (Russian)
84 79 Novo-Arkhangel'sk Harbour (Mikhailov)
85 79 "Inhabitants of the Aleut. . ." (Choris)
86 79 Gutskin Cape. . .(Aleut or Koniag)
87 80 Orthodox Traveling Icon (Even)
88 80 Woven Grass Purse (Aleut)
89 80 Triptych Icon (Russ. fr. Aleutian Is.)
90 82 Notched Calendar (Even)

Treasures by the Neva: The Russian Collections
91 83 Museum of Anthr. and Ethnog., Leningr.
92 84 Iu. Lisianskii; ivory fig.(Koniag/BSE)
93 85 Tlingit Sketch (I. Vozn.); pouch (Aleut)
94 86 L. A. Zagoskin; tobacco box (BSE)
95 87 Rattle Panel (Tlingit)
96 88 "Sand Piper/Woodcock" Mask (Koniag Esk.)
97 88 Woman's Dance Coat (Koryak)

Baird's Naturalists: Smithsonian Collectors in Alaska
98 89 Spencer F. Baird
99 90 Robert Kennicott
100 90 Sealing Stool (Anderson River Eskimo)
101 91 William H. Dall
102 92 James G. Swan
103 92 Crest Hat (Haida)
104 93 Sketch of a Tlingit House (Swan)
105 93 Shaman's Whale Tooth Amulet (Tlingit)
106 94 Edward W. Nelson
107 94 Man's Ground Squirrel Parka (BSE)

The American Museum's Jesup North Pacific Expedition
108 96 Morris K. Jesup
109 96 Franz Boas
110 98 Haida Village (Swanton)
111 98 Shaman's Apron (Yukaghir)
112 99 Bogoraz on the Kolyma River
113 100 Bogoraz, the Revolutionary; telegram
114 101 Sled Travel in Siberia
115 101 Jochelson Camp in Stanovoi Mountains
116 102 Dina Brodsky in Native Hut
117 103 Expedition Freight at Mariinsky Post
118 103 Rafting Down the Korkodon

Young Laufer on The Amur
119 104 Berthold Laufer

Beringia: An Ice Age View
120 107 Vegetation History in Alaska (pollen)
121 108 The Bering Land Bridge. . .(map)
122 108 Composite Lance Head (Upper Paleolithic)
123 110 Yukon-Kuskokwim Delta

Ancient Peoples of The North Pacific Rim
124 111 Arctic Dentition (McKenzie Eskimo)
125 114 Old World—New World Dental Relationship
126 115 Western North Amer. Dental Relationships
127 115 North Pacific Dental Relationships

Prehistory of Siberia and The Bering Sea
128 117 Cultures and Sites of the N. Pacific. . .
129 118 Early Man in Siberia (Upper Paleolithic)
130 118 Takoe II: Proto-Paleoindian?
131 119 Early Man in Alaska (Clovis/Folsom)
132 119 Paleoarctic Tradition (Denali Complex)
133 120 "Nefertiti" of the Amur (Siber. Neol.)
134 120 Sakhalin Harpoons (Neolithic)

135 121 Boat Model (Old Bering Sea Culture)
136 121 Hat Ornaments (Old Bering Sea Culture)
137 122 Old Bering Sea Harpoon
138 122 Winged Objects (Old Bering Sea Culture)
139 123 Ancient Hunting Magic (Old Bering Sea)
140 123 Style Shift in Eskimo Art
141 124 Containers and Float Gear (OBS Culture)
142 124 Women's Work (Old Bering Sea Culture)
143 125 Pottery (Old Bering Sea Culture)
144 125 Shaman's Pottery Paddles (OBS Culture)
145 126 Shaman's Burial (Old Bering Sea Culture)
146 126 Burial Mask (Old Bering Sea Culture)
147 126 Antler Soul Catcher (Ipiutak Culture)
148 127 Masked Spirits (Old Bering Sea Culture)
149 127 Ipiutak Burial Mask
150 128 Ivory Ornaments (Old Bering Sea Culture)
151 128 Wrist Guards (Punuk Culture)
152 129 Tattooed Maskette (Old Bering Sea/ Punuk)
153 129 Pegtymel' Rock Art (Prehistoric Chukotka)

Prehistory of Alaska's Pacific Coast
154 130 Seated Figure Bowl (Prehist. Br. Columb.)
155 131 Bone Ornament (Prehistoric, Alaska)
156 132 Ornamented Stone Lamp (Kachemak Culture)
157 133 Kachemak Carvings (Kodiak Island)
158 134 Prehistoric Koniag Villages. . .Kodiak Is.
159 134 A Koniag Settlement on the Karluk River
160 134 Koniag Masks and Figurines
161 135 Koniag Labrets
162 135 Pebble People (Koniag)
163 136 Miniature Masks (Koniag)
164 136 Dance Mask and Attachments (early Aleut)
165 136 Birthing Amulet (Koniag)
166 137 Harpoon Head (Prehistoric Aleut)
167 138 Eye Amulet (British Columbia)
168 138 Raven Amulet (British Columbia)
169 138 Prehistoric Carvings from Pr. Rupert Hbr.
170 139 Late Prehistoric NWC Stone Carving
171 140 Petroglyph (Cast) (Tsimshian)
172 140 Whale Bone Club (Prince Rupert)

Raven's Creatures
173 141 Biological Productivity in the N. Pacific
174 142 Walrus Herd on the Chukotka Coast

Many Tongues—Ancient Tales
175 145 Languages of the Greater N. Pacific
176 145 Na-Dene Language Group
177 146 Eskimo-Aleut Language Family
178 147 Chukotko-Kamchatkan Language Group
179 148 Tungusic Language Family

Maritime Economies of the North Pacific Rim
180 150 Tunghak, Keeper of the Game (B.S. Esk.)
181 152 Hunting Magic; hunt. hat (Aglemiut/ Aleut)
182 152 Guardian of the Nets (Koryak)
183 153 Sculpin Headdress (Tlingit)
184 154 Ocean Fishing (Tlingit; Elliott)
185 155 Ice-Fishing (Koryak/Chukchi)
186 155 Lures (Western Alaska Eskimo)
187 156 Canoe Model (Tlingit)
188 156 Northwest Coast Canoe and Aleut Kayaks
189 156 War Canoe (Tlingit)
190 157 Steering Paddle (Haida)
191 157 Sea Mammal Magic (Koniag?)
192 159 Kayak Models (Koryak/Nort. Sd. Esk./ Ale.)
192a 158 Kayak Construction Diagram
192b 159 Distribution Map
193 160 Throwing Boards (BSE/Aleut/Koniag)
194 160 Throwing Darts (Aleut/Bering Sea Eskimo)
195 161 Harpoon Technology (W. Alaskan Eskimo)

196	161	Lances (W. Alaskan Eskimo)
197	162	Hunting on the Ice (W. Alaskan Eskimo)
198	162	"Wife" and "Husband" Charms (BS Eskimo)
199	162	Walrus and Sealing Harpoons (W. Ak. Esk.)
200	164	Seal and Pike Spirit Hats (Koniag/BSE)
201	164	Bering Sea Hunting Hats (BS Eskimo)
202	164	Katmai Hunting Hat (Koniag Eskimo?)
203	165	Painted Visor (Aleut)
204	165	Painted Hunting Hat (Aleut)
205	165	Bentwood Hunting Hat (Ber. Sea Eskimo)
206	165	Spruce-Root Hunting Hat (Chugach or Kon.)
207	167	Spring-Summer Ranges of Whale Species
208	167	The Umialik: N. Ak. Esk. Whaling Captain
209	168	Ceremony and Magic: the Esk. Whale Cult
210	168	Koryak and Eskimo Whaling
211	168	Line Weight and Blade. . .(N. Ak. Esk.)
212	169	Ceremonial Baleen Bucket (N. Ak. Esk.)
213	169	Umialik's Headband (N. Ak. Esk.)
214	169	Whaling Charms (N. Ak. Esk.)
215	170	Whaling Canoe Model (Makah)
216	170	Whaling Float (Makah)
217	171	Nootka Whaler's Shrine
218	172	"Aleutians Striking Humpback Whales. . ."
219	172	Whale Dart (Aleut)

Hunters, Herders, Trappers, and Fishermen

220	173	Caribou Spirit (Bering Sea Eskimo)
221	174	Button Blanket (Tsimshian)
222	174	"Interior or 'Stick' Indians. . ." (Elliot)
223	175	A Tsimshian Shaman's Outfit
224	175	Grease Bowl (Tlingit)
225	176	Arrows and Shaft Straightener (Chuk/Esk)
226	176	Bows (Koniag/Chugach Esk.)
227	177	Siberian Quivers
228	178	Reindeer Herders of Siberia
229	179	Alaskan Reindeer Herders
230	180	Dog Sledding
231	181	Skis (Itelmen)
232	182	Reindeer Riders (Evenk or Yukaghir)

Economic Patterns in Northeastern Siberia

233	183	Economic Systems of Siberia and Alaska
234	184	Koryak Bringing Home a Beluga Whale
235	185	Chukchi Duck Hunters at Cape Wankarem
236	186	Russian Firearms (Koryak/Chukchi)
237	187	Fox Trap (Chukchi)
238	188	Koryak Women Cleaning Fish
239	189	Home of a Rich Reindeer Koryak
240	190	Markovo Post (Russian settlement)

Economic Patterns in Alaska

| 241 | 192 | "Eskimo Whaling and Walrus Camp. . ." |
| 242 | 193 | Ivory Drill Bow (Alaskan Eskimo) |

Dwellings, Settlements, and Domestic Life

243	194	The Koryak Home and. . .Sacred Fireboard
244	195	Northern Simplicity: Whale Bone Bucket
245	195	Northwest Coast Elaborations (Tli./Hai.)
246	196	Eskimo Graves at Razboinski, Lower Yukon
247	197	North Alaskan Eskimo Winter House
248	198	Ulu (Woman's Knife) (Bering Sea Eskimo)
249	198	Bering Sea Eskimo Winter House
250	198	Toys for Learning
251	199	Aleut Winter House
252	200	Aleut Grass Wallets
253	200	Koryak Winter House Interior
254	201	Maritime Koryak Winter House
255	202	Summer Camp at Cape Lisburne
256	202	North Alaskan Eskimo Skin Tent
257	202	The Even Tent
258	203	The Iaranga . . .Sleeping Chamber (Chuk.)
259	203	Toys (Chukchi/Tlingit)
260	204	Master of the Herd (Reindeer Koryak)
261	205	Nivkhi Summer House on the Amur River
262	205	Athapaskan Indian House
263	205	Gambling Sticks (Tlingit)
264	206	Tlingit Winter House
265	206	Grease Bowl (Haida)
266	207	House Screen (Haida)
267	207	Spoons (Tlingit)

Needles and Animals: Women's Magic

268	209	Koniag Birdskin Coat (Koniag Eskimo)
269	210	Snow Beater (Chukchi)
270	210	Beaded and Embroidered Apron (Even)
271	211	Reindeer Koryak Mother and Children. . .
272	211	Infant's Combination Suit (Chukchi)
273	212	Needlecases
274	213	Tools of the Seamstress
275	213	Beaded Boots and Leggings (Koryak)
276	214	Eskimo Woman's Parka (North Alaskan Esk.)
277	214	Eskimo Dress Boots (North Alaskan Esk.)
278	214	Koryak Funeral Coat
279	215	Clothing Patterns
280	216	Eskimo Sewing Bag (Bering Sea Eskimo)
281	216	Chilkat Blanket
282	216	"Indian of Mulgrave" (Tomas de Suria)
283	216	Eskimo Labrets
284	217	Geometric Woven Blanket (Tlingit)
285	218	Bark Shredder (Tlingit)
286	218	Tlingit Blanket Weaving. . .at Klukwan
287	219	Paper Appliqué Pattern (Nivkhi)
288	219	Amur River Fishskin Coat (Nanai)
289	219	Tunic (Tlingit)
290	219	Dance Apron and Leggings (Tlingit)
291	220	A Close Look at Decorative Techniques
292	221	From Guts to Garment (St. Lawr. Is. Esk.)
293	222	Koryak Coat Styles
294	223	Beaded Bands
295	223	Joints and Skeletal Motifs
296	224	Caribou Teeth Belt (Bering Sea Eskimo)
297	224	Tattoos of Womanhood
298	225	Athapaskan Tunic
299	225	Koryak and Eskimo Ornaments
300	226	Dress Gloves (Even)
301	226	Girls Dancing (Chukchi)

War and Trade

302	227	Asiatic Eskimo Warrior
303	228	Provisional Political Map. . .(1800-1825)
304	229	Athapaskan Indian Weaponry
305	230	"Battlefield Near Point Barrow"
306	230	Plate and Rod Armor (N. Ak. Eskimo/Aleut)
307	231	The Art of the Armorer (Koryak/Nivkhi)
308	231	Tlingit Armor
309	232	"A Kolosh Warrior. . ." (Tikhanov)
310	232	Tlingit Helmets and Visor
311	232	Tlingit Daggers
312	232	Spear (Tlingit)
313	234	War Club (Tsimshian ?)
314	235	"Tuski and Mahlemuts Trading for Oil"
315	235	Tobacco Pipes (Chukchi/Bering Sea Eskimo)
316	236	North Pacific Trade Systems (1775-1900)
317	237	Pipe Inlaid with Abalone (Tlingit)
318	238	Aniui Trade Fair
319	238	Tea Brick (Chinese)
320	238	Tobacco and Snuff Boxes (N. Ak./BSE Esk.)
321	239	Koryak Tobacco Paraphernalia
322	239	American Whalers (Scammon)
323	240	A 2,000 Mile Journey (Northern Ojibwa)
324	240	Alaskan Bead and Dentalium Shell Jewelry
325	240	Chukchi Beads

Guardians and Spirit-Masters of Siberia

326	241	Igor Shamanov, Shaman (Yukaghir)
327	242	Kelet Myth—tusk (Chukchi)
328	242	Ancestor Guardian and Sacr. Bowl (Chuk.)
329	242	The Koryak Raven Game
330	243	Koryak Child's Cremation
331	244	Chukchi Guardians
332	245	Man's Funeral Cap (Koryak)
333	246	Tasseled Shaman's Hat (Yukaghir)
334	247	Hat of a "Transformed" Shaman (Yukaghir)
335	247	Antlered Shaman's Hat (Evenk)
336	248	Toy Drum (Chukchi)
337	248	Magic Surgery (Chukchi)
338	249	Sun-Worm and Divining Guardian (Kor/Chuk)
339	249	Shaman's Leggings (Even)
340	249	Divining Pouch (Chukchi)
341	251	Man's Cremation Costume (Koryak)
342	252	Koryak Dog Sacrifice
343	253	Eider Duck Ceremony
344	253	Keretkun Net and Prayer Paddle (Chukchi)
345	254	Whale Festival Altar Objects (Koryak)
346	255	Masked Koryak Women

Eye of the Dance: Spiritual Life of the Bering Sea Eskimo

347	256	Black Bear Inua Mask (Bering Sea Eskimo)
348	257	Grizzly Bear Spirit Realm (BS Esk.)
349	258	Fish Club (Bering Sea Eskimo)
350	258	Walrus-Man (North Alaskan Eskimo)
351	259	Transformation Mask (Bering Sea Eskimo)
352	259	Seal Inua Ornaments (Bering Sea Eskimo)
353	260	Lunar Tunghak (Bering Sea Eskimo)
354	261	Conventionalized Animal Face (BS Esk.)
355	261	Ornamented Sewing Gear (BS Eskimo)
356	262	Child's Doll (Bering Sea Eskimo)
357	262	Storyknife (Bering Sea Eskimo)
358	263	Reality, Masked—Spirit Ornaments (BSE)
359	263	Ivory Kayak Ornaments (Bering Sea Eskimo)
360	264	Eskimo Floatboard and Paddles (BS Eskimo)
361	265	Beaded Ermine Dance Headdress (Koniag)
362	265	Dance Fans (Bering Sea Eskimo)
363	266	Spotted Mask (Bering Sea Eskimo)
364	266	Nucleated. . .Dance Fans (Bering Sea Esk.)
365	268	Festival Dress (Bering Sea Eskimo)
366	268	The Bladder Festival (Norton Sound Esk.)
367	268	Festival Masks (Norton Sound Eskimo)
368	270	Bird Mask (Koniag Eskimo)
369	270	Dance Rattle (Koniag Eskimo)

Potlatch Ceremonialism on the Northwest Coast

370	271	Shaman's Rattle (Tlingit)
371	271	Tlingit Curing Ceremony/Rattle
372	272	Shaman's Masks (Tlingit)
373	272	Club and Necklace Amulets (Tlingit)
374	273	Pendant Amulets (Tlingit)
375	274	Bear and Duck Rattles (Haida/Tlingit)
376	275	Shaman's Bow (Tlingit)
377	275	"Kolosh Indians..Sitka" (Voznesenskii)
378	275	Shaman's Rattle (Haida)
379	277	Potlatch Gathering (Tlingit)
380	277	Copper (Tlingit)
381	277	Appliquaa Tunic (Haida)
382	278	Crest Headdress (Tlingit)
383	278	Nagunaks Crest Hat—killer whale (Tsim.)
384	279	"The Funeral of the One-Armed Kolosh. . ."
385	280	Crest Headdress (Haida)
386	281	Whale House (Tlingit)
387	281	Chief's Chest (Tlingit)

Art and Culture Change at the Tlingit-Eskimo Border

388	282	Spear Thrower (Tlingit)
389	282	Grease Bowl (Chugach Eskimo)
390	283	Chugach Grease Bowl
391	284	Painted Chest (Koniag or Chugach)
392	285	Basket (Chugach Eskimo)
393	285	Horn Spoons (Chugach Eskimo/Haida)
394	286	Spruce-Root Crest Hat (Tlingit)
395	287	Beaded Spruce-Root Hat (Tlingit)
396	287	Painted Spruce-Root Hat (Tlingit)
397	288	Diagram of One-Step Structure
398	289	Diagram of Two-Step Structure
399	290	Carved Chest (Tlingit)
400	290	Diagram of Tlingit Hat
401	290	Diagram of Pacific Eskimo Hat
402	291	Painted Spruce-Root Hat (Chugach?)
403	291	Diagram of Pacific Eskimo Hat
404	291	Diagram of a Eskimo Hat (Koniag?)
405	292	Painted Spruce-Root Hat (Chugach Eskimo)
406	293	Decorated Spruce-Root Hat (Koniag Eskimo)
407	293	Diagram of Pacific Eskimo Spruce Root Hat
408	293	Woven Spruce-Root Hat (Chugach Eskimo)

Comparative Art of the North Pacific Rim

409	294	Ceremonial Raven Pipe (Tlingit)
410	295	Sea Lion War Helmet (Tlingit)
411	295	Ritual Hunting Helmet (Alaska Peninsula?)
412	295	Killerwhale Fish Club (Tlingit)
413	296	Embossed Birchbark Tray (Nivkhi)
414	296	Woman's Embroidered Fishskin Robe (Nanai)
415	296	Embroidered Fishskin Boots (Nanai)

416	296	Woman's Embroidered Mittens (Nanai)
417	297	Tasseled Shaman's Coat (Yukaghir)
418	297	Decorated Cradle Back (Yukaghir)
419	297	Embroidered and Beaded Pouch (Even)
420	298	Wrestling Bears (Koryak)
421	298	Siberian Design Sampler
422	299	Winter Boots (Asian Eskimo)
423	299	Pouch Design (Asiatic Eskimo/Koryak)
424	300	Siberian Wood and Leather Masks
425	301	Eskimo Mask (North Alaskan Eskimo)
426	301	Skeletized Animals (Bering Sea Eskimo)
427	302	Effigy Dish (Bering Sea Eskimo)
428	302	Painted Hunting Visor (Aleut)
429	303	Klukwan Potlatch Costumes
430	303	Painted Skin Robe (Haida)
431	304	Button Blanket (Haida)
432	304	Silver Bracelet (Haida)
433	305	Beaded Shirt (Ingalik Athapaskan)
434	305	Raven's Footprint (Norton Sound Eskimo)
435	306	Transformation Mask (Bering Sea Eskimo)
436	306	*Tunghak* Inua Mask (Bering Sea Eskimo)
437	306	Plaque Mask (Bering Sea Eskimo)
438	307	Spirit Mask (Ingalik Athapaskan)
439	307	Ingalik Plaque Mask (Athapaskan)
440	307	Death Mask (Aleut)
441	307	Pacific Eskimo Mask (Koniag Eskimo)
442	307	Shaman's Mask (Tlingit)
443	308	"History of a Year of the Chukchi"
444	308	Pictographic Board and Gorget
445	308	Box Sculpture and Pictographic Art
446	309	Boxlid Art (Bering Sea Eskimo)
447	310	Pictographic Drillbow (Bering Sea Esk.?)
448	310	*T'ao-T'ieh* Mask (Shang Dynasty, China)
449	311	Chilkat Blanket (Tlingit)
450	311	Composite Shell Mask (Shang, China)
451	312	Serpent, Soul Catcher, *Sisiutl* (Tsim.)

Siberian Peoples: A Soviet View

452	314	Butchering a Whale at Uelen, Chukotka
453	316	Ivan Segutegin, a Chukchi Ivory Carver
454	317	Winter Scene of Uelen Village
455	318	Asiatic Eskimo Dance Group "Uelen"

Alaska Natives Today

456	320	Eskimo Women Fishing for Whitefish
457	322	Eskimos at Government School

Alaska Native Arts in the Twentieth Century

458	328	Aleut Ivory Carver's Tools

(459 to 476: Native Alaskan Artists)

Appendix III

Exhibition Checklist

AMNH: American Museum of Natural History (New York)

0-239
Fig. 228, Reindeer harness, Chukchi
acc. 1894, Bering Sea coast, Siberia
18 cms (l; bit), bone, leather

16-9930
Fig. 217, Human figure, Nootka
Hunt, acc. 1904, Vancouver Island, B.C.
99 cms (h), wood (red cedar)

16-9968
Fig. 217, Whale carving, Nootka
Hunt, acc. 1904, Vancouver Island, B.C.
149 cms (l), wood (red cedar)

60-3552a,b
Fig. 422, Boots, Asiatic Eskimo
Bogoras, col. 1900-01, Indian Point, Siberia
40 cms (h), dehaired sealskin, caribou leg fur, leather, yarn

60-3678
Fig. 423, Bag, Asiatic Eskimo
Bogoras, col. 1900-01, St. Lawrence Island, Alaska
34 cms (w), sealskin, cloth

60.1-453
Fig. 147, Shaman's sucking tube, Ipiutak
Larsen and Rainey, col. 1939-41, Pt. Hope, Alaska
38 cms (l), antler

60.1-7713a-k
Fig. 149, Burial mask, Ipiutak
Larsen and Rainey, col. 1939-41, Pt. Hope, Alaska
31 cms (h), ivory

70-387
Fig. 333, Shaman's hat, Yukaghir
Cottle, acc. 1907, Siberia
61 cms (h), reindeer skin, dyed seal pup fur, beads, textile, dog(?) fur trim, brass, hair embroidery

70-620a,b
Fig. 416, Mittens, Nanai
Laufer, col. 1898-99, Amur River region, Siberia
26 cms (l), cloth, fur, thread, brass buttons

70-621a,b
Fig. 415, Fishskin boots, Nanai
Laufer, col. 1898-99, Amur River region, Siberia
33 cms (h), reindeer skin, dyed fishskin, cotton cloth, cotton thread

70-628
Fig. 288, Fishskin coat, Nanai
Laufer, col. 1898-99, Amur River region, Siberia
104 cms (l), dyed and undyed fishskin, thread

70-870a,b
Fig. 23, Wood box, Nivkhi
Laufer, col. 1898-99, Amur River region, Siberia
17 cms (h), wood, leather

70-871
Fig. 24, Tray, Nivkhi
Laufer, col. 1898-99, Amur River region, Siberia
51 cms (l), wood

70-876
Fig. 413, Birchbark tray, Nivkhi
Laufer, col. 1898)99, Amur River region, Siberia
25 cms (w), embossed birchbark

70-881
Fig. 24, Drill, Nivkhi
Laufer, col. 1898-99, Amur River region, Siberia
56 cms (l), wood, iron

70-891
Fig. 27, Bear festival spoon, Nivkhi
Laufer, col. 1898-99, Amur River region, Siberia
28 cms (l), wood

70-1205
Fig. 27, Amulet, Nivkhi
Laufer, col. 1898-99, Amur River region, Siberia
9 cms (l), wood

70-1936b
Fig. 287, Paper pattern, Nivkhi
Laufer (?), Amur River region, Siberia
36 cms (l), painted paper

70-1951
Fig. 423, Bag, Koryak
Bogoras, col. 1900-01, Northern Kamchatka, Siberia
12 cms (l), Tanned hide, beads, fur, cloth, hair, thread

70-2203
Fig. 421, Embroidered belt, Itelmen
Bogoras, col. 1900-01, Sedanka, Siberia
82 cms (l), leather, leather appliqué

70-2723
Fig. 15, Snow goggles, Koryak
Jochelson, 1900-01, Gizhiga, Siberia
15 cms (w), wood, leather

70-2737
Fig. 210, Whaling harpoon head, Koryak
Jochelson, col. 1900-01, Siberia
38 cms (l), chert blade, antler head, larch gum, walrus thong, wood

70-2752
Fig. 182, "Guardian of Nets" figure, Koryak
Jochelson, col. 1900-01, Siberia
22 cms (l), wood, grass

70-2856
Fig. 345, Whale Festival dish, Koryak
Jochelson, col. 1900-01, Kuel, Siberia
17 cms (l), wood

70-2859
Fig. 243, Sacred fireboard, Koryak
W. Jochelson, col. 1900-01, Siberia
43 cms (l), wood

70-2860a,b,c
Fig. 243, Spindle, bow, mouthpiece of fireboard, Koryak
Jochelson, col. 1900-01, Siberia
46 cms (l:spindle), wood, leather, bone

70-2887a,b
Fig. 341, Cremation boots, Koryak
Jochelson, col. 1900-01, Mikino, Siberia
24 cms (l), reindeer fawn legskins, dyed hide, trade cloth, sinew, beads

70-2888
Fig. 341, Cremation coat, Koryak
Jochelson, col. 1900-01, Mikino, Siberia
132 cms (l), reindeer skin, dyed seal pup fur, sealskin, yarn, hair embroidery, silk thread, bead, dog fur

70-2992
Fig. 345, Whale carving, Koryak
Jochelson, col. 1900-01, Kamenskoe, Siberia
23 cms (l), wood

70-3040
Fig. 115, Doll, Koryak
Jochelson, col. 1900-01, Kamenskoe, Siberia
22 cms (h), wood, skin

70-3150
Fig. 293, Carved pattern stamp, Koryak
Jochelson, col. 1900-01, Kamenskoe, Siberia
8 cms (l), wood

70-3151
Fig. 293, Carved pattern stamp, Koryak
Jochelson, col. 1900-01, Kamenskoe, Siberia
6 cms (l), wood

70-3152
Fig. 293, Carved pattern stamp, Koryak
Jochelson, 1900-01, Kamenskoe, Siberia
7 cms (l), wood

70-3153
Fig. 293, Carved pattern stamp, Koryak
Jochelson, col. 1900-01, Kamenskoe, Siberia
7 cms (l), wood

70-3187
Fig. 293, Reindeer skin coat, Koryak
Jochelson, 1900-01, Kamenskoe, Siberia
115 cms (l), reindeer skin, designs stamped in dye

70-3216a,b
Fig. 299, Beaded earrings, Koryak
Jochelson, col. 1900-01, Talovka, Siberia
28 cms (l), iron, beads, sinew

70-3234a,b
Fig. 341, Leggings of cremation suit, Koryak
Jochelson, col. 1900-01, Talovka, Siberia
63 cms (l), reindeer leg skins, sealskin, yarn, dyed seal pup fur, beads, cloth, sinew

70-3240
Fig. 210, Boat charm, Koryak
Jochelson, col. 1900-01, Kamenskoe, Siberia
21 cms (h), wood

70-3246
Fig. 345, Figure, Koryak
Jochelson, col. 1900-01, Kamenskoe, Siberia
10 cms (h), wood, grass

70-3278
Fig. 192, Kayak model, Koryak
Jochelson, col. 1900-01, Greater Itkana, Siberia
45 cms (l), gutskin, wood, sinew

70-3314
Fig. 185, Ice-fishing rod, Koryak
Jochelson, col. 1900-01, Greater Itkana, Siberia
86 cms (l), wood, sinew, ivory, bone, lead

70-3441
Fig. 28, Knife, Koryak
Jochelson, col. 1900-01, Kushka, Siberia
28 cms (l), iron, wood

70-3543
Fig. 236, Cutting board, Koryak
Jochelson, col. 1900-01, Kushka, Siberia
42 cms (l), wood

70-3590
Fig. 299, Beaded headband, Koryak
Jochelson, col. 1900-01, Kushka, Siberia
18 cms (l), leather, beads, brass, sinew

70-3594
Fig. 338, "Sun Worm" charm, Koryak
Jochelson, col. 1900-01, Kushka, Siberia
11 cms (h), hide, fur, beads, cloth

70-3655a,b
Fig. 28, Large knife and sheath, Koryak
Jochelson, col. 1900-01, Kushka, Siberia
53 cms (l:knife), iron, brass, whalebone, sealskin sheath

70-3684
Fig. 32, Iron pendant, Koryak
Jochelson, col. 1900-01, Kushka, Siberia
6 cms (dia), iron

70-3753a,b
Fig. 299, Ear ornaments with whale tails, Koryak
Jochelson, col. 1900-01, Kushka, Siberia
18 cms (l), iron, leather

70-3822
Fig. 307, Helmet, Koryak
Jochelson, col. 1900-01, Kushka, Siberia
13 cms (h), iron

70-3846
Fig. 319, Tea brick, Chinese
Jochelson, col. 1900-01, Kushka, Siberia
23 cms (l), compressed tea powder

70-3892
Fig. 293, Ceremonial coat, Koryak
Jochelson, col. 1900-01, Kushka, Siberia
96 cms (l), dyed seal pup fur, dyed reindeer skin, hair embroidery, cotton thread, cloth, dog fur trim, leather

70-3938
Fig. 424, Mask, Koryak

Jochelson, col. 1900-01, Kushka, Siberia
36 cms (h), wood, sinew, pigment (charcoal?)

70-5123
Fig. 321, Pipe, Koryak
Jochelson, Col. 1900-01, Naiachan, Siberia
21 cms (L), inlaid brass

70-5185a,b
Fig. 275, Fur leggings, Koryak
Jochelson, col. 1900-01, Naiachan, Siberia
71 cms (l), Reindeer leg skins, beads

70-5200
Fig. 232, Cradle, Evenk or Yukaghir
Jochelson, col. 1900-01, Naiachan, Siberia
60 cms (l), hide, beads, wood, cloth

70-5222
Fig. 232, Saddle bag, Evenk or Yukaghir
Jochelson, col. 1900-01, Naiachan, Siberia
127 cms (w), reindeer skin, beads, hair embroidery

70-5260a,b
Fig. 275, Boots, Koryak
Jochelson, col. 1900-01, Kushka, Siberia
38 cms (h), reindeer skin, beads, cloth

70-5264
Fig. 232, Reindeer saddle, Evenk or Yukaghir
Jochelson, col. 1900-01, Naiachan, Siberia
44 cms (L), leather, wood, beads, cordage

70-5601a
Fig. 34, Jacket, Even
Bogoras, col. 1900-01, Markovo, Siberia
99 cms (l), reindeer skin, beads, hair embroidery, dyed seal
and dog fur trim

70-5601c,d
Fig. 34, Boots, Even
Bogoras, col. 1900-01, Markovo, Siberia
86 cms (h), tanned leather, red yarn, sinew, beads

70-5601e
Fig. 34, Cap, Even
Bogoras, 1900-01, Markovo, Siberia
27 cms (h), reindeer skin, hair embroidery, fur trim

70-5601f
Fig. 270, Apron, Even
Bogoras, col. 1900-01, Markovo, Siberia
81 cms (l), reindeer skin, beads, hair embroidery, fur trim

70-5601g,h
Fig. 300, Gloves, Even
Bogoras, col. 1900-01, Markovo, Siberia
24 cms (l), reindeer skin, beads, red flannel

70-5620a
Fig. 417, Shaman's coat, Yukaghir
Bogoras, col. 1900-01, Markovo, Siberia
96 cms (l), reindeer skin and fur, leather appliqué, hair
embroidery, sinew, fur trim, red flannel

70-5620b
Fig. 111, Shaman's apron, Yukaghir
Bogoras, col. 1900-01, Markovo, Siberia
94 cms (l), reindeer skin and fur, hair embroidery, red flannel,
sinew

70-5620c
Fig. 334, Shaman's hat, Yukaghir
Bogoras, col. 1900-01, Markovo, Siberia
91 cms (l), reindeer skin, hair embroidery, dyed seal pup fur
tassels, sinew

70-5623a,b
Fig. 18, Tobacco pipe and pouch, Even
Bogoras, col. 1900-01, Markovo, Siberia
22 cms (l), brass bowl and chain, leather, wood, iron, beads

70-5623c
Fig. 34, Beaded pouch, Even
Bogoras, col. 1900-01, Markovo, Siberia
11 cms (l), leather, beads, brass, stone (charm inside)

70-5695
Fig. 236, Flintlock with stand and powder kit, Chukchi
Bogoras, col. 1900-01, Markovo, Siberia
99 cms (l), wood, metal, skin

70-5698
Fig. 236, Gun kit, Chukchi
Bogoras, col. 1900-01, Markovo, Siberia
33 cms (l), leather, metal, bone, ivory, wood

70-5773a,b
Fig. 339, Shaman's boots, Even or Evenk
Bogoras, col. 1900-01, Markovo, Siberia
70 cms (h), reindeer suede, hair emboidery, dog fur, dyed seal
pup fur tassels, beads, leather, sinew, red flannel

70-5796a,b
Fig. 87, Orthodox traveling icon with pouch, Even
Bogoras, col. 1900-01, Markovo, Siberia
13 cms (w; icon), wood, paper, lacquer, leather

70-5873b
Fig. 323, Beaded pouch, Ojibwa
Jesup Exp., col. 1900-01, Siberia
28 cms (h), cloth, beads

70-6303
Fig. 31, Spinning game/sinew twister, Koryak
Bogoras, col. 1900-01, Baron Korff's Bay, Siberia
17 cms (l), walrus ivory, sinew, iron

70-6453
Fig. 237, Fox trap, Chukchi
Bogoras, col. 1900-01, Marinskii Post, Siberia
74 cms (l), wood, leather, bone, sinew, iron nails

70-6548
Fig. 336, Toy drum with beater, Chukchi
Bogoras, col. 1900-01, Marinskii Post, Siberia
25 cms (l), Wood, walrus stomach, baleen beater

70-6566
Fig. 344, Keretkun ceremonial net, Chukchi
Bogoras, col. 1900-01, Marinskii Post, Siberia
157 cms (l), fiber, baleen, painted wood pendants

70-6620
Fig. 325, Necklace, Chukchi
Bogoras, col. 1900-01, Marinskii Post, Siberia
41 cms (l), beads, fiber

70-6690
Fig. 328, Sacrificial bowl, Chukchi
Bogoras, col. 1900-01, Marinskii Post, Siberia
54 cms (l), wood

70-6691
Fig. 340, Divining pouch, Chukchi
Bogoras, col. 1900-01, Marinskii Post, Siberia
23 cms (h), reindeer skin, graphite pendant

70-6792
Fig. 337, Shaman's knife, Chukchi
Bogoras, 1900-01, Marinskii Post, Siberia
26 cms (l), iron, wood, leather cut-out figures, bead, sinew

70-6793
Fig. 337, Shaman's knife, Chukchi
Bogoras, col. 1900-01, Marinskii Post, Siberia
17 cms (l), ivory, leather cut-out figures

70-6932
Fig. 344, Keretkun prayer paddle, Chukchi
Bogoras, col. 1900-01, Marinskii Post, Siberia
74 cms (l), painted wood

70-6979A
Fig. 228, Reindeer training club, Chukchi
Bogoras, col. 1900-01, Marinskii Post, Siberia
80 cms (l), wood, leather

70-6980a
Fig. 227, Quiver, Chukchi
Bogoras, col. 1900-01, Marinskii Post, Siberia
85 cms (l), wood, leather, hair emboidery, seal fur trim

70-6980b
Fig. 225, Arrow, Chukchi
Bogoras, col. 1900-01, Marinskii Post, Siberia
83 cms (l), wood, feather, bone tip

70-6980d
Fig. 225, Arrow, Chukchi
Bogoras, col. 1900-01, Marinskii Post, Siberia
wood, iron tip

70-6980e
Fig. 225, Arrow, Chukchi
Bogoras, col. 1900-01, Marinskii Post, Siberia
wood, feathers, iron tip, leather

70-7267a,b
Fig. 36, Earrings, Chukchi
Bogoras, col. 1900-01, Cape Anannon, Siberia
19 cms (l), leather, beads, dyed seal pup fur, dog fur, brass
cartridge ends

70-7435
Fig. 325, Necklace, Chukchi
Bogoras, col. 1900-01, Marinskii Post, Siberia
40 cms (l), glass beads, brass navy buttons

70-7455
Fig. 325, Bracelet, Chukchi
Bogoras, col. 1900-01, Marinskii Post, Siberia
9 cms (w), glass beads, hide, fiber, button

70-7684
Fig. 228, Reindeer whip, Chukchi
Bogoras, col. 1900-01, Middle Anadyr River, Siberia
148 cms (l), wood, ivory or bone

70-7689a,b
Fig. 231, Fur-covered skis, Itelmen
Bogoras, col. 1900-01, Anadyr River, Siberia
150 cms (l), wood, sealskin, leather thongs

70-7781a,b
Fig. 325, Braid ornaments, Chukchi
Bogoras, col. 1900-01, Marinskii Post, Siberia
39 cms (l), glass beads, leather, brass bottons, sinew

70-7810
Fig. 331, Charm string, Chukchi
Bogoras, col. 1900-01, Marinskii Post, Siberia
91 cms (l), wood, sinew, leather, fiber

70-7861a
Fig. 302, Spear, Chukchi
Bogoras, col. 1900-01, Markovo, Siberia
153 cms (l), wood, iron

70-7888
Fig. 230, Dog sled model, Chukchi
Bogoras, col. 1900-01, Marinskii Post, Siberia
39 cms (l), wood, sinew, hide, fur

70-7891
Fig. 444, Pictograph drawing on board, Chukchi
Bogoras, col. 1900-01, Marinskii Post, Siberia
48 cms (l), wood

Uncataloged
Fig. 113, Telegram
20 cms (l), paper

Uncataloged
Fig. 116, Tea pot
25 cms (h), brass

Uncataloged
Fig. 116, Compass
5 cms (dia), brass, glass

CMC: Canadian Museum of Civilization (Ottawa)

GbTo-23: 850
Fig. 169, Comb, prehistoric
MacDonald, col. 1960s, Garden I. site, Prince Rupert Hbr. B.C.
6 cms (l), bone

GbTo-31: 211
Fig. 169, Miniature wa club, prehistoric
MacDonald, col. 1960s, Boardwalk site, Prince Rupert Hbr.,
B.C.
18 cms (l), bone

GbTo-31: 522
Fig. 172, Club, prehistoric
MacDonald, col. 1960s, Boardwalk site, Prince Rupert Hbr.,
B.C. 43 cms (l), whalebone

GbTo-31:2178
Fig. 168, Raven amulet, prehistoric
MacDonald, col. 1960s, Boardwalk site, Prince Rupert Hbr.,
B.C.
5 cms (l), schist

GbTo-31:X717
Fig. 169, Segmented stone, prehistoric
MacDonald, col. 1960s, Boardwalk site, Prince Rupert Hbr.,
B.C.
8 cms (l), stone

GbTo-34:1805
Fig. 169, Comb, prehistoric
MacDonald, col. 1960s, Kitandach site, Prince Rupert Hbr.,
B.C.
9 cms (l), bone

Uncataloged
Fig. 171, Petroglyph (cast), Tsimshian
Skeena River, B.C., Canada

VII-A-360
Fig. 289, Tunic, Tlingit
Powell, col. 1879, Lynn Canal, Alaska
80 cms (l), mountain goat wool, red wool cloth, cotton print
cloth

VII-B-1000
Fig. 9, Lime mortar, Haida
Mackenzie, col. 1884, Masset, British Columbia, Canada
9 cms (l), sperm whale tooth

VII-B-1527
Fig. 266, House screen, Haida
Bossom, col. c. 1900, Howkan, Long Island, Alaska
380 cms (w), painted wood (cedar)

VII-B-908
Fig. 170, Maul/ tobacco pestle, Haida
Aaronson, acc. 1899, Queen Charlotte Is., B.C.
21 cms (h), stone

VII-C-1766a-j
Fig. 383, Crest hat, Tsimshian
Bossom, col. ca. 1900, Port Simpson, B.C., Canada
59 cms (l), painted wood

VII-C-271
Fig. 167, Eye amulet, Tsimshian
Newcombe, col. 1905, Kitladamiks, British Columbia, Canada
4 cms (h), stone

VII-C-339,340
Fig. 375, Rattles, Tsimshian
Powell, col. ca. 1879, Bella Coola (?), B.C., Canada
28 cms (h), painted wood (maple?), human hair, pebbles

XII-B-1798
Fig. 154, Seated figure bowl, prehistoric
Alouette River, B.C., Canada
21 cms (h), steatite

XII-B-317
Fig. 170, Tobacco mortar (frog), Haida
Powell, col. 1879, British Columbia, Canada
28 cms (l), stone

XII-B-560
Fig. 170, War club (fish), prehistoric
Powell, col. 1879, Metlakatla, British Columbia, Canada
20 cms (l), stone

FM: Field Museum of Natural History (Chicago)

13747
Fig. 285, Bark shredder, Tlingit
Emmons (?), acc. 1921, Upper Nass River, British Columbia
46 cms (w), wood (yew)

14937
Fig. 67, Quiver, Athapaskan
acc. 1894, Yukon River, Alaska
59 cms (l), buckskin, beads, sinew

19022
Fig. 380, Copper, Tlingit
acc. 1913, Queen Charlotte Is., B.C. (?)
76 cms (h), painted copper

53420
Fig. 211, Container for endblades, North Alaskan Eskimo
Bruce, col. 1897, King Island, Alaska
27 cms (l), ivory, bone, leather, bead

53423
Fig. 209, Whale charm for umiak bow, North Alaskan Eskimo
Bruce, col. 1897, Pt. Hope, Alaska
35 cms (w), wood, quartz crystal, beads

53453
Fig. 197, Meat sled, North Alaskan Eskimo
Bruce, col. 1897, Pt. Hope, Alaska
28 cms (l), wood, ivory, leather, iron

78703
Fig. 399, Chest, Tlingit
Emmons, acc. 1902, Admiralty Island, Alaska
63 cms (w), Wood (yellow and red cedar)

177368
Fig. 212, Ceremonial baleen bucket, North Alaskan Eskimo
Borden, col. 1927, Cape Prince of Wales, Alaska
12 cms (h), baleen, ivory, iron

Koniag, Inc. (Kodiak, Alaska)

UA84.193. 889
Fig. 161, Labret, Koniag
Jordan, col. 1984, Karluk 1 site, Kodiak Island, Alaska
7 cms (w), wood

UA84.193. 893
Fig. 161, Labret, Koniag
Jordan, col. 1984, Karluk 1 site, Kodiak Island, Alaska
7 cms (w), wood

UA84.193.1044
Fig. 160, Owl mask, Koniag
Jordan, col. 1984, Karluk 1 site, Kodiak Island, Alaska
23 cms (h), wood

UA84.193.2475
Fig. 161, Labret, Koniag
Jordan, col. 1984, Karluk 1 site, Kodiak Island, Alaska
4 cms (w), bone

UA85.193.3406
Fig. 161, Labret, Koniag
Jordan, col. 1985, Karluk 1 site, Kodiak Island, Alaska
4 cms (l), wood

UA85.193.3455
Fig. 160, Mask, Koniag
Jordan, col. 1985, Karluk 1 site, Kodiak Island, Alaska
16 cms (h), wood

UA85.193.3695
Fig. 160, Figurine, Koniag
Jordan, col. 1985, Karluk 1 site, Kodiak Island, Alaska
16 cms (h), wood

UA85.193.3733
Fig. 160, Figurine with labrets, Koniag
Jordan, col. 1985, Karluk 1 site, Kodiak Island, Alaska
17 cms (h), wood

UA85.193.4026
Fig. 163, Maskette, Koniag
Jordan, col. 1985, Karluk 1 site, Kodiak Island, Alaska
4 cms (h), wood

UA85.193.4063
Fig. 160, Figurine with labrets, Koniag
Jordan, col. 1985, Karluk 1 site, Kodiak Island, Alaska
16 cms (h), wood

UA85.193.4188
Fig. 161, Labret, Koniag
Jordan, col. 1985, Karluk 1 site, Kodiak Island, Alaska
4 cms (l), bone

UA85.193.4372
Fig. 161, Labret, Koniag
Jordan, col. 1985, Karluk 1 site, Kodiak Island, Alaska
2 cms (w), walrus ivory

UA85.193.6311
Fig. 163, Maskette, Koniag
Jordan, col. 1985, Karluk 1 site, Kodiak Island, Alaska
4 cms (h), wood

UA85.193.6459
Fig. 161, Labret, Koniag
Jordan, col. 1985, Karluk 1 site, Kodiak Island, Alaska
6 cms (w), wood

Uncataloged
Fig. 161, Labret, Koniag
Jordan, col. 1987, Karluk 1 site, Kodiak Island, Alaska
3 cms (l), ground slate

Uncataloged
Fig. 999, Maskette, Koniag
Jordan, col. 1987, Karluk 1 site, Kodiak Island, Alaska
13 cms (h), wood

Uncataloged
Fig. 165, Birthing amulet, Koniag
Jordan, col. 1987, Karluk 1 site, Kodiak Island, Alaska
16 cms high, wood, human(?) hair

Uncataloged
Fig. 161, Labret, Koniag
Jordan, col. 1987, Karluk 1 site, Kodiak Island, Alaska
2 cms (w), limestone

MAE: Museum of Anthropology and Ethnography (Leningrad)

11-167
Fig. 360, Float board, Eskimo
Alaska
74 cms (l), wood, baleen

36-162a
Fig. 25, Knife, Nivkhi
Schrenk, acc. 1857, Sakhalin Island, Siberia
44 cms (l), iron, lead, copper, brass

36-162b
Fig. 25, Sheath for knife, Nivkhi
Schrenk, acc. 1857, Sakhalin Island, Siberia
33 cms (l), sturgeon skin

138-42
Fig. 273, Needlecase, Oroch
Poliak, acc. 1883, Sakhalin Island
12 cms (l), ivory, wood, leather strip

147-4
Fig. 90, Calendar, Even
Bunge, acc. 1884, Siberia
14 cms (l), incised ivory, pigment

202-102
Fig. 307, Spear point, Nivkhi
Suprunenko, acc. 1890, Sakhalin Island, Siberia
43 cms (l), iron, brass

211-2
Fig. 371, Oyster catcher rattle, Tlingit
Chudnovskii, col. 1891, Admiralty Island, Alaska
31 cms (l), painted wood, sinew, hide

256-17
Fig. 36, Boots, Chukchi
Shklovskii, acc. 1894, Nizhne-Kolymsk, Siberia
44 cms (h), reindeer skin, red yarn

313-18/7
Fig. 414, Fishskin coat, Nanai
acc. 1896, Amur River region, Siberia
109 cms (l), dyed fishskin, brass buttons

337-18
Fig. 245, Beaver bowl, Tlingit
Doroshin, acc. 1897, Alaska
19 cms (l), painted wood (alder?, red cedar), operculum shell, spruce root

395-8b
Fig. 36, Woman's combination suit, Chukchi
Gondatti, acc. 1898, Anadyr district, Siberia
100 cms (l), reindeer fur, dog fur trim, fiber cords

395-11
Fig. 272, Infant's combination suit, Chukchi
Gondatti, acc. 1898, Anadyr district, Siberia
58 cms (l), reindeer fawn fur, dyed leather thong, sinew

408-71
Fig. 227, Chukchi quiver, Chukchi
Gondatti, acc. 1898, Anadyr district, Siberia
58 cms (l), reindeer skin, hair and sinew embroidery, wood

422-59
Fig. 338, Divination charm, Chukchi
Gondatti, acc. 1898, Anadyr district, Siberia
9 cms (h; figure), wood, skin, sinew

422-77
Fig. 328, Ancestor guardian amulet, Chukchi
Gondatti, acc. 1898, Anadyr district, Siberia
15 cms (h), wood, skin

434-17/2
Fig. 195, Harpoon head, Chukchi
Gondatti, acc. 1898, Anadyr district, Siberia
37 cms (l), bone, walrus ivory, iron, rawhide

434-21d
Fig. 185, Jig fishing outfit, Chukchi
Gondatti, acc. 1898, Anadyr district, Siberia
49 cms (l), wood, baleen, ivory, leather thong, iron

434-38/1
Fig. 315, Pipe, Chukchi
Gondatti, acc. 1898, Anadyr district, Siberia
48 cms (l), wood, lead

434-7
Fig. 269, Snow beater, Chukchi
Gondatti, acc. 1898, Anadyr district, Siberia
51 cms (l), antler

434-80d
Fig. 259, Doll, Chukchi
Gondatti, acc. 1898, Anadyr district, Siberia
38 cms (h), reindeer skin, cotton cloth, beads, sinew

434-83
Fig. 259, Leather kick ball, Chukchi
Gondatti, acc. 1898, Anadyr district, Siberia
17 cms (dia), sealskin, seal hair

441-37/2
Fig. 420, Carving of bears, Koryak
Gondatti, col. 1890s, Anadyr River region, Siberia
6 cms (h), walrus ivory

442-6-5
Fig. 32, Earrings, Koryak
Gondatti, col. 1890s, Siberia
5 cms (l), brass

442-7-5
Fig. 32, Bracelet, Koryak
Gondatti, col. 1890s, Siberia
9 cms (w), iron, tin

442-7-7
Fig. 32, Bracelet, Koryak
Gondatti, acc. 1898, Paren' or Kuel, Anadyr district, Siberia
8 cms (dia), iron, tin

442-25/2
Fig. 19, Ivory pipe, Chukchi
Gondatti, acc. 1898, Anadyr district, Siberia
11 cms (l), walrus ivory, lead

445-1-13a.b
Fig. 295, Gloves, Even
Gondatti, acc. 1898, Anadyr district, Siberia
23 cms (l), leather, hair embroidery

445-6/1
Fig. 33, Pendant, Even

Gondatti, acc. 1898, Anadyr district, Siberia
15 cms (w), brass, leather

445-6/3
Fig. 33, Pendant, Even
Gondatti, acc. 1898, Anadyr district, Siberia
17 cms (w), brass, leather

454-3
Fig. 35, Woman's apron, Even
Bogdanovich, acc. 1899, Kamchatka, Siberia
90 cms (l), dyed and tanned leather, hair embroidery, beads, sinew

518-1a
Fig. 393, Spoon, Chugach Eskimo
Kashevarov, acc. 1840s, Southeastern Alaska
16 cms (l), mountain goat horn, beads

518-1b
Fig. 393, Spoon, Chugach Eskimo
Kashevarov, acc. 1840s, Southeastern Alaska
18 cms (l), mountain goat horn, beads

536-4
Fig. 390, Grease bowl, Chugach Eskimo
Lisianskii, acc. 1807, Alaska
19 cms (l), painted wood (spruce?)

537-4a
Fig. 46, Three-cylinder box, Bering Sea Eskimo
Zagoskin, col. 1842-44, Lower Yukon River, Alaska
11 cms (w), painted wood, ivory, beads

537-4b
Fig. 94, Carved tobacco box, Bering Sea Eskimo
Zagoskin, col. 1842-44, Lower Yukon River, Alaska
12 cms (l), painted wood, beads, ivory

538-2
Fig. 440, Death mask, Aleut
Archimandritov, acc. 1857, Atka Island, Aleutians, Alaska
31 cms (h), painted wood

539-1
Fig. 206, Spruce root hat, Chugach or Koniag Eskimo
Golovnin, col. 1818, Kodiak Island (?), Alaska
24 cms (dia), painted twined spruce root

568-1
Fig. 193, Throwing board, Aleut
Romanovskii, Aleutian Islands, Alaska
52 cms (l), painted wood, ivory hook

571-6
Fig. 50, Mask, Koniag
Voznesenskii, col. 1842, Kodiak Island, Alaska
painted wood, feathers

571-12
Fig. 368, Mask, Koniag
Voznesenskii, col. 1840s, Kodiak Island, Alaska
43 cms (h), painted wood, rawhide, sinew

571-17
Fig. 310, Helmet, Tlingit
Voznesenskii, col. 1840s, Southeastern Alaska
22 cms (h), painted wood, human hair, abalone shell, hide ties

571-19
Fig. 382, Headdress, Tlingit
Voznesenskii, col. 1840s, Southeastern Alaska
41 cms (w), painted wood, sea lion whiskers, copper eyebrows, painted hide, iron nails, baleen

571-52
Fig. 242, Drill bow, North Alaskan Eskimo
Voznesenskii, col. 1840s, Kotzebue Sound, Alaska
43 cms (l), walrus ivory, leather

571-60
Fig. 93, Pouch, Aleut
Voznesenskii, col. 1840s, St. George Island, Pribilof Is., Alaska
20 cms (w), painted skin, sinew thread, cormorant feathers, hair

571-63
Fig. 46, Tobacco box (wolf head), Bering Sea Eskimo
Voznesenskii, col. 1840s, Probably lower Yukon River, Alaska
11 cms (w), painted wood, ivory, beads, hair, bone "teeth"

571-79
Fig. 58, Gutskin hat, Aleut
Voznesenskii, col. 1840s, St. George Island, Pribilof Is., Alaska
30 cms (dia), colored esophagus, yarn, hair, hair embroidery

593-16
Fig. 47, Hunting hat, Koniag Eskimo
Voznesenskii, col. 1840s, Katmai, Alaska Peninsula, Alaska
28 cms (h), painted wood, ivory, hair

593-18
Fig. 52, Ceremonial kameleika, Aleut
Voznesenskii, col. 1844, Unalaska Island, Aleutian Is., Alaska
125 cms (h), gutskin, cormorant feathers, colored skin strips, sinew thread embroidery, hair, woven grass

593-34
Fig. 405, Spruce root crest hat, Chugach Eskimo
Voznesenskii, col. 1840s, Southeastern Alaska
20 cms (dia), painted spruce root, grass, wool, metal wire

593-45
Fig. 427, Effigy dish, Bering Sea Eskimo
Voznesenskii, col. 1840s, Yukon River, Alaska
22 cms (l), painted wood, beads

593-51
Fig. 201, Hunting hat, Bering Sea Eskimo
Voznesenskii, col. 1840s, Prob. Norton Sound, Alaska
50 cms (l), painted wood, walrus ivory, leather, oldsquaw feathers, grass, bone

593-53
Fig. 187, Canoe model, Tlingit
Voznesenskii, col. 1840s, Southeastern Alaska
102 cms (l), painted wood
593-64
Fig. 226, Bow, Koniag Eskimo
Voznesenskii, col. 1840s, Katmai, Alaska Peninsula, Alaska
131 cms (l), painted wood (red and black mineral paint),
  sinew, red yarn, ivory
593-67
Fig. 193, Throwing board, Bering Sea Eskimo
Voznesenskii, col. 1840s, Nunivak Island, Alaska
43 cms (l), wood, glass beads, walrus ivory
593-93a
Fig. 51, Kayak paddle, Koniag Eskimo
Voznesenskii, col. 1840s, Probably Kodiak Island, Alaska
147 cms (l), painted wood
611-79/1a,b
Fig. 40, Summer boots, Chukchi
Miagkov, col. 1900, Provideniia, Siberia
40 cms (h), dehaired sealskin, tanned and dyed leather, sinew,
  reindeer hair embroidery
620-40a
Fig. 298, Tunic, Holikachuk
Voznesenskii, col. 1840s, Upper Innoko River, Alaska
140 cms (l), tanned skin, dyed porcupine quills, seeds
633-12
Fig. 252, Pouch, Aleut
Admiralty Dept, acc. 1826, Aleutian Islands, Alaska
19 cms (w), grass, thread
633-14
Fig. 252, Pouch, Aleut
Admiralty Dept, acc. 1826, Aleutian Islands, Alaska
15 cms (w), painted linen, painted leather, gutskin thread,
  hair, yarn
633-18
Fig. 408, Spruce root hat, Chugach Eskimo
Admiralty Dept, acc. 1826, Southeastern Alaska
38 cms (dia), painted spruce root
633-8
Fig. 81, War helmet, Tlingit
Lisianskii, col. 1802, Southeastern Alaska
23 cms (h), wood (maple?), hide ties, human hair, red turban
  snail opercula
656-42
Fig. 195, Harpoon head, Oroch
Sternberg, col. 1902, Sakhalin Island, Siberia
28 cms (l), ivory, iron, rawhide
666-15b
Fig. 273, Needlecase, Chukchi
Litke, col. 1828, Chukchi Peninsula, Siberia
27 cms (l), ivory, leather
668-2
Fig. 197, Ice scratcher for sealing, Chukchi
Litke (?), Chukchi Peninsula, Siberia
32 cms (l), wood, ivory, seal claws, leather, sinew
668-6
Fig. 273, Needlecase, Chukchi
Chukchi Peninsula, Siberia
10 cms (l), ivory, leather
668-17
Fig. 244, Bucket, Asiatic Eskimo
Chukchi Peninsula, Siberia
25 cms (dia), whalebone, wood
699-1
Fig. 92, Figurine, Koniag Eskimo
Lisianskii, col. 1804-05, Kodiak Island, Alaska
10 cms (h), ivory, sinew, beads
864-1
Fig. 230, Dog sled model, Itelmen
acc. 1784, Prob. Kamchatka Peninsula, Siberia
44 cms (l), wood, sealskin, cloth, reindeer skin, antler toggles,
  metal chains
956-54
Fig. 421, Belt for funeral costume, Koryak
Jochelson, col. 1900-01, Anadyr district, Okhotsk coast,
  Siberia
139 cms (l), sealskin, iron buckle, hair embroidery, yarn
956-65a,b
Fig. 321, Tobacco box with beaded pouch, Koryak
Jochelson, col. 1900-01, Anadyr River, Siberia
11 cms (w; box), leather, birch bark, wood, metal hinges, skin,
  beads
956-82
Fig. 332, Funeral hat, Koryak
Jochelson, col. 1900-01, Kushka, Siberia
27 cms (h), reindeer fawn skin, sealskin, dyed seal pup fur,
  hair embroidery, sinew
956-87
Fig. 227, Funeral quiver, Koryak
Jochelson, col. 1900-01, Kushka, Siberia
75 cms (l), reindeer skin, cloth, wood, silk thread, hair and
  sinew embroidery, red-dyed fur
956-92
Fig. 307, Spear point, Koryak
Jochelson, col. 1900-01, Kushka, Siberia
46 cms (l), iron, brass
1059-85
Fig. 421, Embroidered hem, Koryak

Jochelson, col. 1900-01, Anadyr district, Siberia
216 cms (l), leather, wool, silk, reindeer hair, sinew
1791-174
Fig. 421, Belt, Chukchi
Tolmachev, col. 1909, Mouth of Kolyma River, Siberia
102 cms (l), Dyed and bleached sealskin, bone buckle, cotton
  thread
1791-186
Fig. 38, Pouch, Chukchi
Tolmachev, col. 1909, Mouth of Kolyma River, Siberia
26 cms (w), sealskin, leather appliquaa
1799-1
Fig. 419, Pouch, Even
Tolmachev, col. 1909, Siberia
24 cms (l), fur, appliquaad leather, hair, beads, red wool,
  leather thong, bone
2442-3
Fig. 192, Three-hole kayak model, Aleut
acc. 1915, Aleutian Islands, Alaska
62 cms (l), gutskin, wood, sinew, beads, yarn, pigment, ivory,
  cord
2448-24
Fig. 65, Raven rattle, Tlingit
Voznesenskii, col. 1840s, Southeastern Alaska
30 cms (l), painted wood (maple?), pebbles, hide thong
2448-26
Fig. 245, Paint brush, Tlingit
Voznesenskii, col. 1840s, Southeast Alaska
30 cms (l), wood (yellow cedar), porcupine guard hair, spruce
  root
2448-28
Fig. 245, Paint brush, Tlingit
Voznesenskii, col. 1840's, Southeast Alaska
19 cms (l), wood (yew?), porcupine guard hair, spruce root
2448-30
Fig. 95, Rattle panel, Tlingit
Voznesenskii(?), Southeast Alaska
78 cms (l), painted wood, pebbles
2448-9
Fig. 372, Mask, Tlingit
Voznesenskii(?), Southeast Alaska
22 cms (h), painted wood
2454-10
Fig. 82, Leather armor shirt, Tlingit
Sitka, Alaska
101 cms (l), tanned, painted hide
2454-15
Fig. 410, Helmet, Tlingit
Southeast Alaska
25 cms (h), painted wood, sea lion teeth and whiskers, hide
  ties
2454-17
Fig. 310, Helmet, Tlingit
Southeast Alaska
26 cms (h), painted wood, human hair, red turban snail
  opercula, heavy hide
2454-8
Fig. 308, Slat armour cuirass, Tlingit
Southeast Alaska
103 cms (l), painted wood (crabapple?), sinew, heavy hide
2520-2
Fig. 189, Canoe model, Tlingit
Southeast Alaska
78 cms (l), painted wood, human hair
2520-14
Fig. 396, Spruce root hat, Tlingit
Voznesenskii(?), Southeast Alaska
42 cms (dia.), painted spruce root, leather straps
2520-16
Fig. 402, Woven spruce root hat, Chugach (?) Eskimo
Voznesenskii(?), Southeast Alaska
45 cms (dia), painted spruce root
2520-21
Fig. 395, Spruce root hat, Tlingit
Voznesenskii(?), Southeast Alaska
34 cms (dia), painted spruce root, glass beads, sinew
2520-6
Fig. 284, Geometric woven blanket, Tlingit
Cook (?), Southeast Alaska
166 cms (w), mountain goat wool, fur trim
2539-3
Fig. 184, Halibut hook, octopus design, Tlingit
Voznesenskii(?), Southeast Alaska
31 cms (l), wood, spruce root, iron
2539-17
Fig. 224, Grease dish, Tlingit
Southeast Alaska
25 cms (l), wood (alder?), red turban snail opercula
2539-30
Fig. 374, Shaman's hair fastener, Tlingit
Voznesenskii, col. 1840s, Southeast Alaska
11 cms (w), wood (yew?)
2667-14
Fig. 304, Club, Ahtna
Voznesenskii, col. 1840s, Copper River, southeast Alaska
56 cms (l; with fringe), antler, leather, beads, hair embroidery,
  sinew, ocher
2868-40
Fig. 411, Hunting hat, Aleut or Eskimo

Voznesenskii, col. 1840s, Alaska Peninsula?, Alaska
98 cms (l; incl. whiskers), painted wood, ivory, beads, sea lion
  whiskers, sinew, hair, grass
2868-76
Fig. 86, Gutskin cape in Russian style, Aleut (?)
Aleutian Is. or Kodiak I., Alaska
140 cms (l), dyed gutskin, hair embroidery, cormorant
  feathers, sinew
2868-82
Fig. 204, Hunting hat, Aleut
Voznesenskii, col. 1840s, Aleutian Islands, Alaska
103 cms (l; incl. whiskers), painted wood, walrus ivory, beads,
  sealion whiskers, dyed grass, yarn, sinew, hair, leather
2868-83
Fig. 181, Hunting hat, Aleut
Voznesenskii, col. 1840s, Aleutian Is. (?), Alaska
80 cms (l; incl. whiskers), painted wood, walrus ivory, sea lion
  whiskers
2888-30
Fig. 193, Throwing board, Koniag Eskimo
Voznesenskii, col. 1840s, Kodiak Island, Alaska
51 cms (l), wood, ivory, beads
2888-84
Fig. 268, Cormorant coat, Koniag
Voznesenskii, col. 1840s, Kodiak Island, Alaska
121 cms (l), cormorant neck skins, dyed skin and gutskin, hair
  embroidery, ermine fur trim, cloth, puffin beaks
2888-89
Fig. 200, Seal hunting helmet, Koniag Eskimo
Voznesenskii, col. 1840s, Kodiak Island, Alaska
29 cms (l), painted wood, leather
2888-93
Fig. 88, Woven pouch, Aleut
Voznesenskii, 1840s, Aleutian Islands (?), Alaska
15 cms (w), grass, silk, wool, cotton thread
2913-20
Fig. 226, Bow, Chugach Eskimo
Southeast Alaska
138 cms (l), painted wood, sinew
2915-1a,b
Fig. 391, Chest, Koniag or Chugach
Southeast Alaska
22 cms (l), painted wood, woolen string, glass beads
2938-2
Fig. 92, Doll, Bering Sea Eskimo
Voznesenskii, col. 1840s, Norton Sound, Alaska
19 cms (h), walrus ivory
2938-6
Fig. 73, Sea otter carving, Aleut
Voznesenskii, col. 1840s, Aleutian Islands, Alaska
17 cms (l), ivory
3235-14
Fig. 205, Hunting hat, Bering Sea Eskimo
Nunivak Island (?), Alaska
38 cms (l), painted wood, walrus ivory, leather thong
3896-1
Fig. 97, Dancecoat, Koryak
Stebnitskii, col. 1928, Gizhiga, Siberia
168 cms (w), alder-dyed reindeer skin, fur patchwork, dog fur
  trim, leather fringes, beads, sinew
4087-10
Fig. 193, Throwing board, Koniag Eskimo
acc. 1930, Kodiak Island (?), Alaska
49 cms (l), wood, sea otter teeth
4104-26
Fig. 252, Pouch, Aleut
Aleutian Islands, Alaska
18 cms (w), grass
4104-38
Fig. 192, Kayak model, Aleut
acc. 1930, Aleutian Islands, Alaska
55 cms (l), wood, sealskin, gutskin, sinew, ivory, baleen, yarn,
  cord, pigment
4104-5
Fig. 203, Hunting visor, Aleut
acc. 1931, Aleutian Islands, Alaska
31 cms (l; incl. whiskers), painted wood, sea lion whiskers,
  glass beads, walrus ivory, sinew
4105-1
Fig. 372, Mask, Tlingit
acc. 1930, Southeast Alaska
25 cms (h), painted wood (alder?)
4105-2
Fig. 372, Mask, Tlingit
acc. 1930, Southeast Alaska
22 cms (h), painted wood, hide ties
4270-44
Fig. 219, Whale dart, Aleut
acc. 1931, Aleutian Islands, Alaska
141 cms (l), painted wood, ivory, sinew, chert blade
4270-96
Fig. 428, Hunting visor, Aleut
Aleutian Islands, Alaska
80 cms (l), painted wood, sea lion whiskers, yarn
4291-7
Fig. 392, Spruceroot basket, Chugach Eskimo
Southeast Alaska
36 cms (h), spruce root, dyed grass

4291-50
Fig. 447, Drill bow, North Alaskan Eskimo
Alaska
28 cms (l), walrus ivory

5031-1
Fig. 195, Harpoon head, Koryak
Bilibin, acc. 1933, Paren', Siberia
31 cms (l), wood, ivory, chert, rawhide

5536-165
Fig. 26, Bear festival bowl, Nivkhi
Kozin, col. 1934,
100 cms (l), wood

5795-12
Fig. 66, Sea lion headdress, Tlingit
acc. 1938, Southeast Alaska
34 cms (h), painted wood (alder?), hide, teeth

5795-26
Fig. 372, Mask, Tlingit
acc. 1938, Southeast Alaska
23 cms (h), painted wood, iron, human hair, red turban snail
    opercula

5795-31
Fig. 372, Mask, Tlingit
Southeast Alaska
23 cms (h), painted wood (red cedar), hair

5795-9
Fig. 310, Visor, Tlingit
acc. 1938, Southeast Alaska
25 cms (dia), wood, hide

5801-2
Fig. 5, Quiver, Athapaskan
64 cms (l), tanned leather, glass beads, porcupine quill, seeds

6010-38
Fig. 327, Engraved tusk showing kelets, Chukchi
acc. 1951, Uelen, Siberia
65 cms (l), walrus tusk, pigments

6479-17-582
Fig. 139, Harpoon socket piece, Old Bering Sea
Arutiunov, col. 1960s, Ekven site, Chukotka, Siberia
31 cms (l), walrus ivory

6479-269
Fig. 139, Harpoon head, Old Bering Sea
Arutiunov, col. 1960s, Ekven site, Chukotka, Siberia
19 cms (l), walrus ivory

6479-552
Fig. 152, Maskette, Old Bering Sea
Arutiunov, col. 1960s, Ekven site, Chukotka, Siberia
3 cms (h), walrus ivory

6479-612
Fig. 138, Winged object, Old Bering Sea
Arutiunov, col. 1960s, Ekven site, Chukotka, Siberia
18 cms (w), walrus ivory

6479-9-205
Fig. 139, Socket piece, Old Bering Sea
Arutiunov, col. 1960s, Ekven site, Chukotka, Siberia
35 cms (l), walrus ivory

6479-9-208
Fig. 138, Winged object, Old Bering Sea
Arutiunov, col. 1960s, Ekven site, Chukotka, Siberia
23 cms (w), walrus ivory

6479/11-407
Fig. 135, Carving of boat, Old Bering Sea
Arutiunov, col. 1960s, Ekven site, Chukotka, Siberia
14 cms (l), walrus ivory

6508-547
Fig. 144, Pottery paddle, Old Bering Sea
Arutiunov, col. 1960s, Ekven site, Chukotka, Siberia
33 cms (l), walrus ivory

6508-562
Fig. 142, Needle case, Old Bering Sea
Arutiunov, col. 1960s, Ekven site, Chukotka, Siberia
8 cms (l), walrus ivory

6561-1000
Fig. 148, Gorget/maskette, Old Bering Sea
Arutiunov, col. 1960s, Ekven site, Chukotka, Siberia
13 cms (h), walrus ivory

6561-1014a,b
Fig. 143, Pottery fragments, Old Bering Sea
Arutiunov, col. 1960s, Ekven site, Chukotka, Siberia
8 and 11 cms (w), clay

6561-126
Fig. 139, Socket piece, Old Bering Sea
Arutiunov, col. 1960s, Ekven site, Chukotka, Siberia
23 cms (l), walrus ivory

6561-256
Fig. 140, Winged object, Old Bering Sea
Arutiunov, col. 1960s, Ekven site, Chukotka, Siberia
14 cms (w), walrus ivory

6561-329
Fig. 140, Winged object, Okvik
Arutiunov, col. 1960s, Ekven site, Chukotka, Siberia
13 cms (w), walrus ivory

6561-419
Fig. 142, Boot creaser, Old Bering Sea
Arutiunov, col. 1960s, Ekven site, Chukotka, Siberia
9 cms (l), walrus ivory

6561-516
Fig. 142, Ulu, Old Bering Sea
Arutiunov, col. 1960s, Ekven site, Chukotka, Siberia
11 cms (w), walrus ivory, ground slate

6561-722
Fig. 148, Plaque, Old Bering Sea
Arutiunov, col. 1960s, Ekven site, Chukotka, Siberia
9 cms (w), walrus ivory

6587-298
Fig. 136, Hunting hat ornament, Old Bering Sea
Arutiunov, col. 1960s, Ekven site, Chukotka, Siberia
12 cms (l), walrus ivory

6587-300
Fig. 136, Hunting hat ornament, Old Bering Sea
Arutiunov, col. 1960s, Ekven site, Chukotka, Siberia
10 cms (l), walrus ivory, jet

6587-564
Fig. 144, Pottery paddle, Old Bering Sea
Arutiunov, col. 1960s, Ekven site, Chukotka, Siberia
28 cms (l), walrus ivory

6588-118
Fig. 148, Dance goggles, Old Bering Sea
Arutiunov, col. 1960s, Ekven site, Chukotka, Siberia
11 cms (w), wood

6588-119
Fig. 146, Burial mask, Old Bering Sea
Arutiunov, col. 1960s, Ekven site, Chukotka, Siberia
23 cms (h), wood, bone

6588-12
Fig. 141, Vessel, Old Bering Sea
Arutiunov, col. 1960s, Ekven site, Chukotka, Siberia
54 cms (l), wood

6588-139
Fig. 139, Harpoon head, Old Bering Sea
Arutiunov, col. 1960s, Ekven site, Chukotka, Siberia
11 cms (l), walrus ivory

6588-233
Fig. 141, Float nozzle, Old Bering Sea
Arutiunov, col. 1960s, Ekven site, Chukotka, Siberia
4 cms (l), walrus ivory

6588-241
Fig. 142, Sinew twister weight, Old Bering Sea
Arutiunov, col. 1960s, Ekven site, Chukotka, Siberia
9 cms (l), walrus ivory

6588-33
Fig. 142, Ulu handle, Old Bering Sea
Arutiunov, col. 1960s, Ekven site, Chukotka, Siberia
5 cms (w), walrus ivory

6588-36
Fig. 142, Knife handle, Old Bering Sea
Arutiunov, col. 1960s, Ekven site, Chukotka, Siberia
7 cms (w), walrus ivory

6588-38
Fig. 150, Openwork carving, Old Bering Sea
Arutiunov, col. 1960s, Ekven site, Chukotka, Siberia
11 cms (w), walrus ivory

6588-39
Fig. 142, Carving of foot, Old Bering Sea
Arutiunov, col. 1960s, Ekven site, Chukotka, Siberia
8 cms (h), walrus ivory

6588-40
Fig. 150, Ivory chain, Old Bering Sea
Arutiunov, col. 1960s, Ekven site, Chukotka, Siberia
41 cms (l), walrus ivory

6588-41
Fig. 142, Ulu handle, Old Bering Sea
Arutiunov, col. 1960s, Ekven site, Chukotka, Siberia
11 cms (w), walrus ivory

6588-61
Fig. 141, Float plug, Old Bering Sea
Arutiunov, col. 1960s, Ekven site, Chukotka, Siberia
4 cms (dia.), wood

6588-63
Fig. 141, Wound plug, Old Bering Sea
Arutiunov, col. 1960s, Ekven site, Chukotka, Siberia
13 cms (l), wood

6588-69
Fig. 141, Baleen pail, Old Bering Sea
Arutiunov, col. 1960s, Ekven site, Chukotka, Siberia
13 cms (l), baleen, wood bottom

6588-72
Fig. 139, Harpoon head, Old Bering Sea
Arutiunov, col. 1960s, Ekven site, Chukotka, Siberia
13 cms (l), walrus ivory

6588-74
Fig. 143, Pottery paddle, Old Bering Sea
Arutiunov, col. 1960s, Ekven site, Chukotka, Siberia
25 cms (l), walrus ivory

6588-80
Fig. 141, Float plug stopper, Old Bering Sea
Arutiunov, col. 1960s, Ekven site, Chukotka, Siberia
13 cms (l), wood

6750-16
Fig. 260, Sacred fireboard, Koryak
Antropova and Taksami, col. 1960s, Penzhina River area,
    Siberia
58 cms (l), wood, fiber, leather, beads, fur

MIHPP: Museum of History and Culture of the Peoples of
    Siberia and the Far East (Novosibirsk)
Kn-53-48090
Fig. 133, Statuette (reproduction), Neolithic
Okladnikov, col. 1965, Kondon site, Khabarovsk, Siberia
11 cms (h), fired clay

NMAH: National Museum of American History (Washington,
    D.C.)
25819.130
Fig. 89, Icon (triptych), Russian
Swan, acc. 1876, Aleutian Islands, Alaska
10 cms (l), brass

56334a
Fig. 322, Whale gun, American
Lewis, acc. 1882, New Bedford, Massachusetts
84 cms (l), iron stock, steel barrel

237848
Fig. 83, Chain mail cuirass, Russian
Kostrometinoff, acc. 1906, Sitka, Alaska
iron rings

420307
Fig. 70, Double eagle plaque, Russian
Krieger, col. 1934, Lower Mamaloose Island, Oregon
23 cms (h), brass

NMNH: National Museum of Natural History (Washington,
    D.C.)
1076
Fig. 426, Bentwood bowl, Bering Sea Eskimo
Alaska
29 cms (l), painted wood

1857
Fig. 67, Tunic, Kutchin
Ross, col. 1860, Yukon River, Alaska
114 cms (l), caribou skin, beads, dentalium shells, ocher,
    sinew

1857
Fig. 67, Leggings, Kutchin
Ross, col. 1860, Yukon River, Alaska
100 cms (l), caribou skin, beads, ocher, sinew

2024
Fig. 304, Knife, Athapaskan
Ross, acc. 1866, Arctic coast, Alaska or Canada
67 cms (l), iron, split bark wrapping on handle

2128
Fig. 56, Gutskin cape, Aleut
Wilkes, acc. 1866, Aleutian Islands, Alaska
153 cms (l), gutskin, painted skin, hair, and sinew thread
    embroidery, cormorant feathers, yarn, hair

3978
Fig. 100, Sealing stool, Canadian Eskimo
McFarlane, acc. 1867, Anderson River, Canada
14 cms (l), wood

6014
Fig. 317, Pipe, Haida
Bulkley, acc. 1868, British Columbia, Canada
21 cms (l), wood, abalone shell, sheet copper

9257
Fig. 370, Shaman's rattle, Tlingit
Hoff, acc. 1870, Sitka, Alaska
25 cms (h), painted wood, human hair, sinew, leather, pebbles

9273
Fig. 61, Spoon, Tlingit
Hoff, acc. 1870, Sitka, Alaska
27 cms (l), mountain goat horn

9288
Fig. 311, Dagger, Tlingit
acc. 1870, Southeast Alaska
72 cms (l), iron, copper, tanned hide

9813
Fig. 374, Amulet, Nishga
Ring, acc. 1870, Ft. Simpson, British Columbia, Canada
19 cms (l), bone, abalone shell

10313
Fig. 62, Hair ornament, Tsimshian
Ring, acc. 1871, British Columbia, Canada
17 cms (l), iron, abalone shell

10983
Fig. 451, Soul catcher, Tsimshian
Ring, acc. 1872, Ft. Simpson, British Columbia, Canada
23 cms (l), bone, braided wool cord

13002
Fig. 164, Mask, Aleut
Dall, acc. 1873, Unga Island, Aleutian Is., Alaska
23 cms (h), painted wood

13002n
Fig. 164, Mask fragment, Aleut
Dall, acc. 1873, Unga Island, Aleutian Is., Alaska
24 cms (l), painted wood

13082r
Fig. 164, Model of harpoon head, Aleut
Dall, acc. 1873, Unga Island, Aleutian Is., Alaska
20 cms (l), painted wood

13082r
Fig. 164, Mask fragment, Aleut
Dall, acc. 1873, Unga Island, Aleutian Is., Alaska
23 cms (l), painted wood

16089
Fig. 155, Whale-man ornament

Dall, col. 1870s, Hot Springs site, Port Moller, Alaska
4 cms (l), bone
16140
Fig. 355, Bag fastener, Bering Sea Eskimo
Dall, acc. 1874, Nunivak Island, Alaska
18 cms (l), walrus ivory
16204
Fig. 283, Labret, Bering Sea Eskimo
Dall, acc. 1874, North Alaska
3 cms (w), ivory, bead, wood
16407
Fig. 76, Harpoon arrow, Koniag Eskimo
Dall, acc. 1874, Kodiak Island, Alaska
90 cms (l), painted wood, bone, sinew cord, feathers
17249
Fig. 306, Rod armour, Aleut
Dall, acc. 1875, Kagamil Island, Aleutian Is., Alaska
60 cms (h), painted wood, leather, sinew cord
18912
Fig. 64, Pipe, Tlingit
Swan, acc. 1875, Sitka, Alaska
11 cms (l), wood (walnut), copper bowl
20251b
Fig. 432, Silver bracelet, Haida
Swan, acc. 1876, Queen Charlotte Is., British Columbia
7 cms (dia), silver
20573
Fig. 183, Sculpin back mask, Tlingit
Swan, acc. 1876, Southeastern Alaska
114 cms (l), painted wood, copper, iron, muslin, grass, leather,
  sinew
20610
Fig. 313, War club, Tsimshian
Swan, acc. 1876, Fort Simpson, British Columbia
64 cms (l), wood (yew?)
20633
Fig. 59, Nose ring, Tsimshian
Swan, acc. 1876, Fort Simpson, British Columbia
4 cms (w), abalone shell
20771
Fig. 388, Throwing stick, Tlingit
Swan, acc. 1876, Sitka, Alaska
39 cms (l), wood (yew?), iron lug
20807
Fig. 430, Painted robe, Haida
Swan, acc. 1876, Prince of Wales Island, Alaska
painted skin, fur
20828
Fig. 375, Rattle, Tlingit
Swan, acc. 1876, Klawock, Prince of Wales I., Alaska
54 cms (l), painted wood (red cedar?), tufted puffin beaks,
  buckskin, sinew
20844
Fig. 64, Pipe, Tlingit
Swan, acc. 1876, Hootsnuwoo, Alaska
9 cms (l), wood (walnut), copper pipe bowl and tail
23387
Fig. 216, Painted whaling float, Makah
Swan, acc. 1876, Neah Bay, Washington
122 cms (l), painted seal skin, whale sinew, wood, and cedar
  bark rope
23409
Fig. 265, Grease bowl, Haida
Swan, acc. 1876, Massett, Queen Charlotte Is., Alaska
27 cms (l), wood (alder?)
24350
Fig. 445, Box, Bering Sea Eskimo
Turner, acc. 1876, Norton Sound, Alaska
21 cms (l), wood
24436
Fig. 274, Copper needlecase, Bering Sea Eskimo
Turner(?), acc. 1876(?), St. Michael(?), Alaska
40 cms (l), leather, copper, ivory
30764
Fig. 274, Woman's tool box, Bering Sea Eskimo
Turner, acc. 1877, Norton Sound, Alaska
23 cms (l), wood, ivory, leather
33013
Fig. 320, Snuff box and tube, Bering Sea Eskimo
Nelson, col. 1878, St. Michael, Norton Sound, Alaska
10 cms (l; box), leather, baleen, bird bone, leather thong
33060
Fig. 354, Bentwood bowl, Bering Sea Eskimo
Nelson, col. 1878, St. Michael, Norton Sound, Alaska
49 cms (l), painted wood
33106
Fig. 367, Mask, Bering Sea Eskimo
Nelson, col. 1878, Kigiktauik, Norton Sound, Alaska
52 cms (h), painted wood, sinew, feathers, leather strap
33114
Fig. 436, Mask, Bering Sea Eskimo
Nelson, col. 1878, Yukon River near Magemut, Alaska
66 cms (h), painted wood, caribou fur, split root binding
33136
Fig. 200, Hunting visor, Bering Sea Eskimo
Nelson, col. 1878, St. Michael, Norton Sound, Alaska
36 cms (l), wood, beads, teeth
33700
Fig. 273, Needlecase, North Alaskan Eskimo

Nelson, col. 1878, Norton Sound, Alaska
11 cms (l), walrus ivory
33956
Fig. 194, Seal dart, Bering Sea Eskimo
Nelson, col. 1878, Yukon River mouth, south of Magemut
131 cms (l), wood, bone, feathers, rawhide
36057
Fig. 360, Kayak paddles (pair), Bering Sea Eskimo
Nelson, col. 1878-79, Kushunuk, Alaska
150 cms (l), painted wood
36058
Fig. 196, Repeating lance, Bering Sea Eskimo
Nelson, col. 1878-79, Anogogmut, Alaska
175 cms (l), wood, walrus ivory, fiber cordage
36242
Fig. 446, Box with illustrated lid, Bering Sea Eskimo
Nelson, col. 1878-79, Sfugunugumut, Alaska
34 cms (l), wood, ivory, rawhide
36246
Fig. 445, Box with illustrated lid, Bering Sea Eskimo
Nelson, col. 1878-79, Pastolik, Yukon River mouth, Alaska
40 cms (l), painted wood, ivory
36316
Fig. 248, Ulu, Bering Sea Eskimo
Nelson, col. 1878-79, Kongigunogumut, Alaska
8 cms (l), ivory, iron blade
36859
Fig. 45, Earrings, Bering Sea Eskimo
Nelson, col. 1878-79, Kushunuk, Alaska
2 cms (l), walrus ivory
37063
Fig. 359, Line fastener, Bering Sea Eskimo
Nelson, col. 1878-79, Askinuk, Alaska
2 cms (w), walrus ivory
37120
Fig. 46, Painted spoon, Bering Sea Eskimo
Nelson, col. 1878-79, Chalitmut, Alaska
25 cms (l), painted wood
37127
Fig. 364, Dance fan, Bering Sea Eskimo
Nelson, col. 1878-79, Lower Kuskokwim River, Alaska
14 cms (l), painted wood
37413
Fig. 186, Tom cod hook, Bering Sea Eskimo
Nelson, col. 1878-79, Askinuk, Alaska
15 cms (l), bone
37571
Fig. 195, Harpoon head, Bering Sea Eskimo
Nelson, col. 1878-79, Anogogmut, Alaska
27 cms (l), leather, sinew, bone, ivory, copper blade
37648
Fig. 186, Fish hook, North Alaskan Eskimo
Nelson, col. 1878-79, Port Clarence, Alaska
6 cms (l; hook), stone, sinew, auklet beaks, bone, iron
37663
Fig. 283, Labret, North Alaskan Eskimo
Nelson, col. 1878-79, Norton Sound, Alaska
2 cms (h), limestone, split glass bead
37745
Fig. 358, Hair ornament, Bering Sea Eskimo
Nelson, col. 1878-79, Kongigunogumut, Alaska
7 cms (w), walrus ivory
37763
Fig. 352, Belt buckle, Bering Sea Eskimo
Nelson, col. 1878-79, Kuskokwim Bay, Alaska
5 cms (w), ivory
38444
Fig. 13, Bolas, Bering Sea Eskimo
Nelson, col. 1878-79, Shaktolik, Norton Sound, Alaska
89 cms (l), walrus ivory, rawhide, feather
38451
Fig. 364, Dance fans (pair), Bering Sea Eskimo
Nelson, col. 1878-79, Big Lake, Alaska
14 cms (l; without feathers), painted wood, feathers
38635
Fig. 46, Wooden spoon, Bering Sea Eskimo
Nelson, col. 1878-79, Sfugunugumut, Alaska
29 cms (l), painted wood
38637
Fig. 426, Painted spoon, Bering Sea Eskimo
Nelson, col. 1878-79, Sfugunugumut, Alaska
22 cms (l), painted wood
38645
Fig. 353, Tunghak mask, Bering Sea Eskimo
Nelson, col. 1878-79, Pinuit, Alaska
23 cms (h), painted wood, leather thong
38649
Fig. 364, Dance fan, Bering Sea Eskimo
Nelson, col. 1878-79, Lower Koskokwim River, Alaska
14 cms (l), painted wood
38717
Fig. 4, Hunting hat, Bering Sea Eskimo
Nelson, col. 1878)79, Kaiuhgumut, Alaska
31 cms (l), painted wood, root lashing, cotton cloth, bone or
  ivory
38734
Fig. 348, Bear mask, Bering Sea Eskimo
Nelson, col. 1878-79, Rasboinsky, Yukon River, Alaska
57 cms (h), oldsquaw and swan feathers, quill, painted wood,
  leather thong, sinew, split root binding

38754
Fig. 197, Drag handle, Bering Sea Eskimo
Nelson, col. 1878-79, Shaktolik, Alaska
21 cms (l), walrus ivory, leather, sinew, beads
38800
Fig. 283, Labret, Bering Sea Eskimo
Nelson, col. 1878-79, Pinuit, Alaska
2 cms (l), ivory, bead
38855a,b
Fig. 362, Dance fans, Bering Sea Eskimo
Nelson, col. 1878-79, Rasboinsky, Alaska
15 cms (l), painted wood, feathers
38871
Fig. 41, Woman's boots, Bering Sea Eskimo
Nelson, col. 1878-79, Nushugak, Alaska
45 cms (h), caribou skin, sealskin, red yarn, sinew
43352
Fig. 5, Arrows, Athapaskan
Nelson, col. 1878-80, Fort Reliance, Upper Yukon River,
  Alaska
69 - 80 cms (l), wood, feathers, iron points, cordage
43509
Fig. 359, Float plug, Bering Sea Eskimo
Nelson, col. 1878-80, Cape Vancouver, Alaska
5 cms (h), walrus ivory, wood
43535
Fig. 355, Awl, Bering Sea Eskimo
Nelson, col. 1878-80, Cape Vancouver, Alaska
14 cms (l), walrus ivory, wood and hair plugs
43538
Fig. 359, Spearguards (pair), Bering Sea Eskimo
Nelson, col. 1878-80, Cape Vancouver, Alaska
4 cms (w), walrus ivory, hair
43661
Fig. 355, Boot creaser, Bering Sea Eskimo
Nelson, col. 1878-80, Cape Vancouver, Alaska
7 cms (l), walrus ivory
43670
Fig. 358, Earring, Bering Sea Eskimo
Nelson, col. 1878-80, Cape Vancouver, Alaska
2 cms (l), walrus ivory
43720
Fig. 45, Pendant, Bering Sea Eskimo
Nelson, col. 1878-80, Nunivak Island, Alaska
5 cms (l), walrus ivory
43727
Fig. 352, Earrings, Bering Sea Eskimo
Nelson, col. 1878-80, Nunivak Island, Alaska
2 cms (l), ivory
43746
Fig. 194, Bird dart, Bering Sea Eskimo
Nelson, col. 1878-80, Nunivak Island, Alaska
147 cms (l), wood, walrus ivory, sinew
44399
Fig. 17, Drill bow, North Alaskan Eskimo
Nelson, col. 1878-80, Cape Nome, Alaska
44 cms (l), walrus ivory, leather thong
44457
Fig. 20, Cap box, Siberian
Nelson, col. 1878-80, Cape Nome, Alaska
13 cms (l), wood, leather thong
44709
Fig. 359, Line fastener, Bering Sea Eskimo
Nelson, col. 1878-80, Sledge Island, Alaska
2 cms (h), walrus ivory
44906
Fig. 283, Labret, North Alaskan Eskimo
Nelson, col. 1878-80, Sledge Island, Alaska
3 cms (l), glass
45475
Fig. 199, Walrus harpoon, North Alaskan Eskimo
Nelson, col. 1878-80, Cape Nome, Alaska
174 cms (l), wood, ivory, bone, antler, iron, rawhide, beads,
  baleen
45502
Fig. 439, Mask, Athapaskan
Nelson, col. 1878-80, Anvik, Alaska
54 cms (h), painted wood, leather, feathers
45524
Fig. 250, Toy bird arrow, North Alaskan Eskimo
Nelson, col. 1878-80, Cape Nome, Alaska
29 cms (l), wood, feather, thread, bone
46349
Fig. 184, Halibut hook (salmon design), Tlingit
Bean, acc. 1880, Sitka, Alaska
26 cms (l), wood, split root binding, cedar bark line
48384
Fig. 211, Whale-shaped line sinker, North Alaskan Eskimo
Nelson, col. 1878-80, Sledge Island, Alaska
30 cms (l), graphite
48986
Fig. 347, Inua mask, Bering Sea Eskimo
Nelson, col. 1878-81, Sabonitsky, Alaska
24 cms (h), painted wood, hair
48996
Fig. 15, Snow goggles, Bering Sea Eskimo
Nelson, col. 1878-81, Sabotnisky, Alaska
16 cms (w), painted wood, leather strap

49060
Fig. 365, Feather dance wand, Bering Sea Eskimo
Nelson, col. 1878-81, Rasboinsky, Alaska
67 cms (l), golden eagle feather, wood stick, leather
49061
Fig. 365, Feather dance wand, Bering Sea Eskimo
Nelson, col. 1878-81, Rasboinsky, Alaska
63 cms (l), golden eagle feather, wood stick, leather
56026
Fig. 220, Caribou spirit carving, Bering Sea Eskimo
McKay, acc. 1882, Bristol Bay, Alaska
26 cms (l), painted wood, sinew cord, (human?) hair
56045
Fig. 250, Top and launcher, Bering Sea Eskimo
McKay, acc. 1882, Bristol Bay, Alaska
Top, 12 cms (h), painted wood, leather thong
56070
Fig. 324, Earrings, Bering Sea Eskimo
McKay, acc. 1882, Bristol Bay, Alaska
10 cms (l), glass beads, dentalium shells, brass wire, sinew,
  leather
56512
Fig. 320, Tobacco box (caribou), North Alaskan Eskimo
Ray, col. 1881-82, Point Barrow, Alaska
15 cms (l), caribou antler, wood, beads
56703
Fig. 214, Whale amulet, North Alaskan Eskimo
Ray, col. 1881-82, Pt. Barrow, Alaska
9 cms (l), glass
60144
Fig. 267, Painted spoon, Tlingit
McLean, acc. 1882, Hoonah, Alaska
34 cms (l), painted wood (alder?)
60147
Fig. 267, Soapberry spoon, Tlingit
McLean, acc. 1882, Hootznahoo, Alaska
37 cms (l), wood (yew?)
60176
Fig. 387, Chest, Tlingit
McLean, acc. 1882, Hoonah, Baranoff Island, Alaska
64 cms (w), painted wood (yellow and red cedar), red turban
  snail opercula
60241
Fig. 308, Leather tunic, Tlingit
Mclean, acc. 1882, Hoonah, Baranoff Island, Alaska
76 cms (l), painted heavy hide, Chinese coins, carved bone
  ''shark teeth''
63514
Fig. 197, Ice creepers, Asiatic Eskimo
Nelson, col. 1878-81, St. Lawrence Island, Alaska
10 cms (l), walrus ivory, iron nails, leather straps
63876
Fig. 197, Net weight, North Alaskan Eskimo
Nelson, col. 1878-81, Diomede Islands, Alaska
23 cms (l), walrus ivory
64218
Fig. 349, Fish club, North Alaskan Eskimo
Nelson, col. 1878-81, Diomede Islands, Alaska
21 cms (l), wood, walrus ivory
64230
Fig. 444, Gorget, North Alaskan Eskimo
Nelson, col. 1878-81, Point Barrow, Alaska
48 cms (w), painted wood
64230
Fig. 425, Mask, North Alaskan Eskimo
Nelson, col. 1878-81, Point Barrow, Alaska
22 cms (h), painted wood, teeth, sinew
64241
Fig. 180, Tunghak mask, Bering Sea Eskimo
Nelson, col. 1878-81, Kuskokwim River, Alaska
72 cms (w), painted wood, teeth, feathers
64260
Fig. 435, Transformation mask, Bering Sea Eskimo
Nelson, col. 1878-81, Kuskokwim River, Alaska
44 cms (h), painted wood, sinew, feathers
72842
Fig. 295, Gloves, Athapaskan
Petroff, acc. 1883, Copper River, Alaska
33 cms (l), tanned leather, dyed porcupine quills, yarn, ocher,
  sinew
72936
Fig. 215, Whaling canoe model, Makah
Swan, acc. 1883, Neah Bay, Washington
97 cms (l), painted wood (alder), spruce root, cedar bark,
  mussel shell, sinew
72993
Fig. 62, Ear ornaments, Tlingit
Swan, col. 1876, Admirality Island, Alaska
6 cms (l), shark teeth, red yarn
73544
Fig. 190, Paddle, Haida
Gould, acc. 1884, Haida Mission, Jackson, Alaska
173 cms (l), painted wood (yellow cedar)
73831
Fig. 373, Shaman's club, Tlingit
Bolles, acc. 1884, Hoonah, Alaska
67 cms (l), painted wood (alder?), human hair
74041
Fig. 276, Parka, North Alaskan Eskimo

Ray, col. 1881-83, Point Barrow, Alaska
110 cms (l), caribou, reindeer, and mountain sheep skin, wolf
  and marten fur trim, dyed leather, red yarn, sinew
74690
Fig. 441, Mask, Koniag
Fisher, col. 1884, Douglas, Alaska
61 cms (h), painted wood
74720
Fig. 406, Spruce root hat, Koniag Eskimo
Fisher, col. 1884, Karluk, Kodiak Island, Alaska
38 cms (dia), painted spruce root, beads, dentalium shells, sea
  lion whiskers, sinew, woolen cloth
74926
Fig. 64, Pipe, Tlingit
McLean, acc. 1884, Sitka, Alaska
12 cms (l), wood, iron musket barrel section
74990
Fig. 105, Amulet, Tlingit
McLean, acc. 1884, Sitka, Alaska
13 cms (l), sperm whale tooth
75419
Fig. 312, Spear, Tlingit
McLean, acc. 1884, Sitka, Alaska
155 cms (l), wood (yellow cedar), steel bayonet blade, brass
  ferrule
75423
Fig. 263, Gambling sticks in leather pouch, Tlingit
Mclean, acc. 1885, Sitka, Alaska
21 cms (w; pouch), hardwood, abalone shell, hide
76855
Fig. 442, Shaman's mask, Tlingit
Bolles, col. 1883, Chilkat River, Alaska
24 cms (h), painted wood, human hair, opercula, bronze
  Chinese coins
88900
Fig. 62, Ear pendants, Haida
Swan, col. 1884, Massett, Queen Charlotte Is., B.C.
15 cms (w), abalone shell
88924
Fig. 61, Spoon, Haida
Swan, acc. 1884, Massett, Queen Charlotte Is., B.C.
22 cms (l), mountain goat horn, mountain sheep horn
88961b
Fig. 103, Spruce root hat, Haida
Swan, col. 1884, Massett, Queen Charlotte Is., B.C.
61 cms (dia), painted spruce root, wood, buckskin ties, metal
  buttons
89022
Fig. 245, Paint dish, Haida
Swan, col. 1884, Fort Simpson, British Columbia
24 cms (l), stone
89036
Fig. 385, Crest hat, Haida
Swan, col. 1884, Skedans, British Columbia
50 cms (h), painted wood (red cedar, alder)
89052
Fig. 378, Shaman's rattle, Haida
Swan, col. 1884, Queen Charlotte Is., British Columbia
30 cms (h), painted wood
89079
Fig. 102, Raven rattle, Haida
Swan, col. 1884, Skidegate, Queen Charlottes Is., B.C.
33 cms (l), painted wood (maple?), leather cord
89167
Fig. 61, Spoon, Haida
Swan, col. 1884, Skidegate, Queen Charlotte Island, B.C.
43 cms (l), mountain goat horn, cow horn
89194
Fig. 381, Appliquaa tunic, Haida
Swan, col. 1884, Skidegate, Queen Charlotte Is., B.C.
96 cms (l), blue wool blanket, red wool flannel, glass beads
89198b
Fig. 431, Button blanket, Haida
Swan, col. 1884, Skidegate, Queen Charlotte Is., B.C.
173 cms (w), blue woolen blanket, red flannel, pearl buttons,
  painted wood
89418
Fig. 210, Harpoon rest, North Alaskan Eskimo
Ray, col. 1881-83, Point Barrow, Alaska
21 cms (h), ivory, leather
89552
Fig. 186, Fish hook, North Alaskan Eskimo
Ray, col. 1881-83, Point Barrow, Alaska
14 cms (l), bone, iron, sinew
89577
Fig. 214, Whale amulet, North Alaskan Eskimo
Ray, col. 1881-83, Point Barrow, Alaska
5 cms (l), red chert
89761
Fig. 195, Harpoon head, North Alaskan Eskimo
Ray, col. 1881-83, Point Barrow, Alaska
33 cms (l; with thong), walrus ivory, wood, skin cord, brass
  blade
89800
Fig. 250, Bullroarer, North Alaskan Eskimo
Ray, col. 1881-83, Point Barrow, Alaska
35 cms (l; handle), painted wood, sinew
89817
Fig. 209, Mask and gorget, North Alaskan Eskimo

Ray, col. 1881-83, Point Barrow, Alaska
47 cms (w; gorget), painted wood, sinew, baleen
89827
Fig. 350, Walrus man doll, North Alaskan Eskimo
Ray, col. 1881-83, Point Barrow, Alaska
45 cms (h), wood, gutskin, fur, sinew cord, ivory, bone, hair
90420
Fig. 51, Kayak gunnelboard, Koniag Eskimo
Fisher, col. 1884, Orlova, Kodiak Island, Alaska
101 cms (l), painted wood
90438
Fig. 369, Puffin beak rattle, Koniag
Fisher, col. 1884, Uganik Island (Kodiak), Alaska
25 cms (dia), wood, sinew, tufted puffin beaks
90444
Fig. 202, Hunting hat, Koniag (?) Eskimo
Fisher, col. 1884, Katmai, Alaska
20 cms (h), painted wood, woven grass and yarn tassels,
  beads, ivory, sea lion whiskers
90451
Fig. 361, Dance hat, Koniag
Fisher, col. 1884, Ugashik, Alaska
38 cms (h), pelagic cormorant skins, ermine skins, beads,
  wool, hair, leather
90453
Fig. 48, Beaded headdress, Koniag
Fisher, col. 1884, Ugashik, Bristol Bay, Alaska
51 cms (h), beads, leather strips, sinew
127353
Fig. 280, Sewing bag (''housewife''), Bering Sea Eskimo
Applegate, acc. 1886, Nassianmute, Alaska
28 cms (l), caribou or reindeer skin, fur, leather strap, cotton
  cloth, bone handle, red yarn, sinew embroidery
127403
Fig. 357, Storyknife, Bering Sea Eskimo
Applegate, acc. 1886, Togiak River, Alaska
18 cms (l), walrus ivory
127473
Fig. 299, Earrings, Bering Sea Eskimo
Applegate, acc. 1886, Tuniakput, Togiak River, Alaska
6 cms (l), ivory, beads, sinew
127766
Fig. 181, Harpoon socket piece, Aglegmiute Eskimo
Fisher, col. 1885-86, Koggiung, Alaska
19 cms (l), walrus jaw bone, wood, leather
127777
Fig. 181, Barbed point, Aglegmiute Eskimo
Fisher, col. 1885-86, Koggiung, Alaska
12 cms (l), bone
129219
Fig. 20, Needle case, Bering Sea Eskimo
Turner, acc. 1887, St. Michael, Norton Sound, Alaska
34 cms (l), ivory, leather, beads, sinew
129236
Fig. 356, Doll, Bering Sea Eskimo
Turner, acc. 1887, St. Michael, Alaska
15 cms (h), walrus ivory, reindeer skin, fur
129824
Fig. 433, Beaded shirt, Ingalik
Hazen, acc. 1888, Yukon River, Alaska
81 cms (l), tanned (moose?) skin, trade cloth, beads
153428
Fig. 67, Knife, Athapaskan
Russell, acc. 1892, Upper Yukon River, Alaska
28 cms (l), iron, leather
153623
Fig. 367, Mask, Bering Sea Eskimo
Turner, acc. 1892, Norton Sound (?), Alaska
42 cms (h), painted wood, feathers, leather thong
153627
Fig. 363, Mask, Bering Sea Eskimo
Turner, acc. 1892, Norton Sound (?), Alaska
49 cms (h), painted wood, feathers, quills, teeth, baleen
153659
Fig. 250, Toy bow, Bering Sea Eskimo
Turner, acc. 1892, Norton Sound (?), Alaska
32 cms (l), painted wood, sinew, leather
153727
Fig. 199, Sealing harpoon, Bering Sea Eskimo
Turner, acc. 1892, Norton Sound (?), Alaska
170 cms (l), wood, bone, iron, sinew, rawhide
153731
Fig. 196, Lance, North Alaskan Eskimo
Turner, acc. 1892, Norton Sound (?), Alaska
182 cms (l), wood, chert, sinew
153734
Fig. 208, Fur parka, North Alaskan Eskimo
Turner, acc. 1892, Norton Sound (?), Alaska
123 cms (l), reindeer and caribou skin, wolf and wolverine fur,
  fox trim, dyed leather, sinew
153892
Fig. 277, Boots, North Alaskan Eskimo
Ray, col. 1881-83, Point Barrow, Alaska
53 cms (h), reindeer skin, sealskin, fur trim, yarn, leather
  strings
160564
Fig. 302, Leather armor shield, North Alaskan Eskimo
acc. 1910, Alaska
78 cms (l), sealskin, wood, bone toggles, dyed seal pup fur
  tassel, hair embroidery

168157
Fig. 310, Helmet, Tlingit
Ogden, acc. 1893, Taku, Alaska
25 cms (h), painted wood

168372
Fig. 373, Shaman's necklace, Tlingit
Emmons, acc. 1894, Gonaho, Alaska
43 cms (l), bone, ivory, leather, pigment

168569
Fig. 54, Kayak bailer, Aleut
acc. 1894, Unalaska Island, Aleutian Is., Alaska
58 cms (l), painted wood, fiber

168623
Fig. 389, Grease bowl, Chugach Eskimo
Fisher, acc. 1894, Prince William Sound, Alaska
38 cms (l), wood, glass beads

168625
Fig. 195, Harpoon head, Bering Sea Eskimo
Fisher, acc. 1894, Bristol Bay, Alaska
42 cms (l), ground slate, antler, wood, leather, bark, sinew

168626
Fig. 426, Sea otter charm, Bering Sea Eskimo
Fisher, acc. 1894, Bristol Bay, Alaska
10 cms (l), walrus ivory

175668
Fig. 44, Boat hook, Bering Sea Eskimo
Nelson, col. 1878-81, Nunivak Island, Alaska
185 cms (l), wood, ivory, rawhide

175825
Fig. 194, Sea otter dart, Aleut
acc. 1896, Unalaska Island, Aleutian Is., Alaska
129 cms (l), painted wood, sea mammal bone, ivory head, sinew cord, seal throat skin, red yarn

176104
Fig. 107, Fur parka, Bering Sea Eskimo
Nelson, col. 1878-81, Alaska
118 cms (h), ground squirrel skins, caribou skin, dyed leather, wolf and wolverine fur

176105
Fig. 41, Fur parka, Bering Sea Eskimo
Nelson, col. 1878-81, Alaska
131 cms (h), arctic ground squirrel skins, reindeer and marmotskin, red-dyed leather, wolf and wolverine fur trim

176142
Fig. 355, Thread reel, Bering Sea Eskimo
Nelson, col. 1878-81, Cape Vancouver, Alaska
10 cms (l), walrus ivory, wood plugs

176145
Fig. 359, Float plug, Bering Sea Eskimo
Nelson, col. 1878-81, Cape Vancouver, Alaska
5 cms (h), walrus ivory, beads

176207
Fig. 47, Hunting visor, Bering Sea Eskimo
Nelson, col. 1878-81, Pastolik, Alaska
49 cms (l), painted wood, ivory, oldsquaw feathers, leather, grass

176229
Fig. 273, Needlecase, Bering Sea Eskimo
Nelson, col. 1878-81, Cape Vancouver, Alaska
15 cms (l), bone, wood, hair

176232
Fig. 45, Hair clasps (pair), Bering Sea Eskimo
Nelson, col. 1878-81, Cape Vancouver, Alaska
5 cms (w), walrus ivory

176304
Fig. 315, Pipe, Bering Sea Eskimo
Nelson, col. 1878-81, Nunivak Island, Alaska
40 cms (l), wood, metal, beads, leather, sinew

203720
Fig. 208, Boots, North Alaskan Eskimo
Gilbert, acc. 1899, Port Clarence, Alaska
44 cms (h), ring seal skin, sinew, dehaired sealskin

209550
Fig. 62, Bead necklace, Tlingit
Emmons, acc. 1901, Southeastern Alaska
43 cms (l), glass beads

209567
Fig. 259, Doll, Tlingit
Emmons, acc. 1901, Southeastern Alaska
25 cms (h), marble, hair, cloth, buckskin

209841
Fig. 213, Dall sheep tooth headband, North Alaskan Eskimo
Marsh, acc. 1901, Point Barrow, Alaska
18 cms (dia), leather, beads, Dall sheep teeth, sinew

209941
Fig. 67, Bow, Athapaskan
Emmons, acc. 1901, Southeastern Alaska
148 cms (l), wood, leather string and wrappings

219504
Fig. 281, Chilkat blanket, Tlingit
Landsberg, acc. 1903, Southeastern Alaska
191 cms (w), mountain goat wool, cedar bark, skin, sinew

220185
Fig. 170, Tobacco mortar, Tsimshian
Emmons, acc. 1903, Skeena River, British Columbia
19 cms (h), stone

221184
Fig. 311, Dagger, Tlingit
Emmons, acc. 1903, Killisnoo, S.E. Alaska
67 cms (l), iron, copper, tanned hide, abalone shell

224419
Fig. 412, Club, Tlingit
Emmons, acc. 1904, Fort Wrangell, Alaska
47 cms (l), wood (yew?)

229546b
Fig. 374, Killer whale amulet, Tlingit
acc. 1904, Fort Tongass, Alaska
14 cms (l), walrus ivory

229789
Fig. 8, Chilkat tunic, Tlingit
Emmons, acc. 1904, Southeastern Alaska
100 cms (l), mountain goat wool, cedar bark, hide headline, sinew

260384
Fig. 192, Kayak model, North Alaskan Eskimo
acc. 1910, Norton Sound, Alaska
75 cms (l), wood, sealskin, sinew, ivory

260441
Fig. 250, Toy harpoon, North Alaskan Eskimo
acc. 1910, Kotzebue Sound, Alaska
46 cms (l), wood, bone, ivory, rawhide, fiber cordage

260531
Fig. 230, Dog sled model, Bering Sea Eskimo
acc. 1910, Norton Sound
32 cms (l), wood, leather, ivory runners

274433
Fig. 59, Ceremonial staff, Tlingit
Harriman, acc. 1912, Southeastern Alaska
208 cms (l), painted wood, hair

274676
Fig. 221, Button blanket, Tsimshian
Brady, acc. 1912, Souteastern Alaska
168 cms (w), wool trade blanket, flannel, pearl buttons, glass beads

280111
Fig. 208, Pants, Asiatic Eskimo
Moore, col. 1912, St. Lawrence Island, Alaska
77 cms (h), sealskin, caribou fur, sinew

280117
Fig. 258, Leather briefs, Asiatic Eskimo
Moore, col. 1912, St. Lawrence Island, Alaska
38 cms (l), tanned leather, cotton thread, sealskin, caribou hair

280200
Fig. 302, Leather hoop armour, Asiatic Eskimo
Moore, col. 1912, St. Lawrence Island, Alaska
70 cms (h), sealskin, bone toggles

313279
Fig. 394, Spruce root crest hat, Tlingit
acc. 1920, Southeastern Alaska
27 cms (h), painted spruce root basketry

316777
Fig. 355, Bone needle blank, Aleut
acc. 1921, Unalaska Island, Aleutian Is., Alaska
10 cms (l), bird bone

316851
Fig. 186, Set of small fish hooks, North Alaskan Eskimo
acc. 1921, King Island, Alaska
45 cms (l), fossil ivory, gull tendons, iron hooks, ground stone, beads, bird beak fragments

324930
Fig. 376, Shaman's bow, Tlingit
Stephens, acc. 1923, Chilkat, Alaska
271 cms (l), painted wood (yellow cedar), human hair, gut bowstring

337354
Fig. 409, Pipe, Tlingit
Forsyth, acc. 1927, Southeastern Alaska
8 cms (h), wood (walnut)

339831
Fig. 438, Mask, Athapaskan
acc. 1928, Anvik, Yukon River, Alaska
59 cms (h), painted wood, fur, string

339833
Fig. 151, Wrist guard, Punuk
Collins, acc. 1928, St. Lawrence Island, Alaska
10 cms (l), walrus ivory

340331
Fig. 324, Necklace, Bering Sea Eskimo
Collins, acc. 1927, Nunivak Island, Alaska
64 cms (l), beads, ivory, leather

340332
Fig. 299, Necklace, Bering Sea Eskimo
Collins, acc. 1927, Nunivak Island, Alaska
32 cms (l), beads, ivory, metal

340373a
Fig. 198, Charm plaques (pair), Bering Sea Eskimo
Collins, acc. 1927, Nunivak Island, Alaska
17 cms (h), painted wood

341202
Fig. 290, Dance apron, Tlingit
Popenoe, acc. 1928, Southeastern Alaska
111 cms (w), mountain goat wool, cedar bark, trade blanket cloth, cotton cloth, buckskin, tufted puffin beaks, sinew

341202a,b
Fig. 290, Leggings, Tlingit
Popenoe, acc. 1928, Southeastern Alaska
39 cms (h), mountain goat wool, cedar bark, trade blanket cloth, cotton cloth, bucksin, tufted puffin beaks, sinew

344677
Fig. 140, Winged object, Punuk

Collins, acc. 1929, Punuk Islands, Alaska
7 cms (h), walrus ivory

356126
Fig. 140, Winged object, Punuk
Collins, col. 1930, St. Lawrence Island, Alaska
13 cms (w), walrus ivory

356128
Fig. 140, Winged object, Punuk
Collins, col. 1930, St. Lawrence Island, Alaska
9 cms (h), walrus ivory

357445
Fig. 449, Chilkat blanket, Tlingit
Evans, acc. 1938, Lynn Canal, Alaska
172 cms (w), moutain goat wool, yellow cedar bark, sinew

358255
Fig. 296, Caribou teeth belt, Bering Sea Eskimo
Evans, acc. 1938, Alaska
103 cms (l), leather, caribou teeth, glass beads, sinew, cordage

363740
Fig. 157, Maskette, Kachemak
Hrdlicka, acc. 1931, Uyak site, Kodiak Island, Alaska
9 cms (h), bone

365592
Fig. 157, Plaque, Kachemak
Hrdlicka, acc. 1932, Uyak Site, Kodiak Island, Alaska
19 cms (w), walrus ivory

372080
Fig. 142, Needle case, Punuk
Chambers, acc. 1933, Gambell, St. Lawrence Island, Alaska
7 cms (l), walrus ivory

372667
Fig. 42, Baleen basket, North Alaskan Eskimo
Walcott, acc. 1935, Point Barrow, Alaska
10 cms (h), baleen, ivory, fossil ivory

375349
Fig. 156, Lamp, Kachemak
Hrdlicka, acc. 1935, Uyak site, Kodiak Island, Alaska
30 cms (l), stone

378054
Fig. 139, Harpoon socket piece, Old Bering Sea
Jones, acc. 1937, St. Lawrence Island, Alaska
22 cms (l), walrus ivory

381859
Fig. 214, Amulet (human figure), North Alaskan Eskimo
Henderson, acc. 1940, Alaska
5 cms (l), black chert

382259
Fig. 196, Lance tip, North Alaskan Eskimo
acc. 1942, King Island, Alaska
43 cms (l), wood, chert, fiber

383300
Fig. 225, Arrow shaft straightener, North Alaskan Eskimo
Stanley-Brown, acc. 1943, Point Hope, Alaska
14 cms (l), antler

389861
Fig. 75, Shield, Aleut
Hrdlicka, col. 1936, Kagamil Island, Aleutian Is., Alaska
70 cms (h), painted wood, leather

391806
Fig. 131, Projectile point, Clovis)Folsom
Thompson, acc. 1948, Utukok River site, Alaska
6 cms (l), black chert

393152
Fig. 351, Mask, Bering Sea Eskimo
Eastman, acc. 1955, Stebbins, Norton Sound, Alaska
33 cms (h), wood, fur, nails

393156
Fig. 434, Bowl, Bering Sea Eskimo
Eastman, acc. 1955, Stebbins, Norton Sound, Alaska
25 cms (l), painted wood

395958
Fig. 166, Harpoon head, Prehistoric Aleut
Hrdlicka, acc. 1938, Umnak Island, Aleutian Is., Alaska
26 cms (l), sea mammal bone

395999
Fig. 166, Endblade, Prehistoric Aleut
Hrdlicka, acc. 1938, Umnak Island, Aleutian Is., Alaska
4 cms (l), chert

398238
Fig. 210, Whaling harpoon head, North Alaskan Eskimo
Fellows, acc. 1960, Icy Cape, Alaska
29 cms (l), bone, obsidian, sinew

398246
Fig. 274, Skin scraper, North Alaskan Eskimo
Fellows, acc. 1960, Icy Cape, Alaska
15 cms (l), wood, chert blade, iron wire

398408
Fig. 60, Trap stick, Tlingit
Toner, acc. 1961, Southeastern Alaska
23 cms (l), whalebone

398409
Fig. 60, Trap stick, Tlingit
Toner, acc. 1961, Southeastern Alaska
26 cms (l), whalebone

398410
Fig. 60, Trap stick, Tlingit
Toner, acc. 1961, Southeastern Alaska
28 cms (l), whalebone

417767
Fig. 57, Grass basket, Aleut
Hutchinson, , Attu Island, Aleutian Is., Alaska
10 cms (h), split woven grass

418612
Fig. 12, Auklet parka, Asiatic Eskimo
Moore, col. 1912, St. Lawrence Island, Alaska
111 cms (l), auklet breasts, fur trim, sinew

T-717
Fig. 184, Black cod hook, Tlingit
Southeastern Alaska
15 cms (l), wood, spruce root

T-1611
Fig. 41, Woman's fur pants, Bering Sea Eskimo
Alaska
73 cms (l), caribou skin, dyed leather, fox(?) fur, sinew

T-1676
Fig. 292, Gutskin parka, Asiatic Eskimo
Moore, col. 1912, St. Lawrence Island, Alaska
99 cms (h), walrus gut, auklet beaks and feathers, sinew

T-1886
Fig. 306, Armor vest, North Alaskan Eskimo
Alaska
39 cms (w), heavy hide, bone plates, leather thong, sinew

T-16626
Fig. 302, Boots, Asiatic Eskimo
Moore, col. 1912, St. Lawrence Island, Alaska
33 cms (h), caribou skin, sealskin, yarn, hair embroidery, fur
    trim, sinew

T-16634
Fig. 302, Fur pants, Asiatic Eskimo
Moore, col. 1912, St. Lawrence Island, Alaska
85 cms (l), sealskin, hair embroidery, dyed seal fur trim

T-23244
Fig. 151, Wrist guard, Punuk
acc. 1988, St. Lawrence Island, Alaska
7 cms (h), walrus ivory

Uncataloged
Fig. 122, Composite lance head, Paleolithic
Dennis Stanford facsimile
23 cms (l), bison bone, chert microblades, pine pitch

PMS: Peabody Museum (Salem, Massachusetts)

E7344
Fig. 999, Gutskin cape, Aleut
Barker, acc. 1835, Aleutian Islands, Alaska
seal intestine, colored skin and sinew thread embroidery

SA: Smithsonian Archives (Washington, D.C.)

Uncataloged
Fig. 101, Field notebook, 1866-7,
19 cms (h), leather cover, paper, ink

SKRM: Sakhalin Regional Museum (Iuzhno)Sakhalinsk,
    U.S.S.R.)

3670-44
Fig. 130, Microblade, Paleolithic
Shubin, col. 1973, Takoie II site, Sakhalin Island, Siberia
4 cms (l), obsidian

3670-45
Fig. 130, Sidescraper, Paleolithic
Shubin, col. 1973, Takoie II site, Sakhalin Island, Siberia
6 cms (l), obsidian

3670-52
Fig. 130, Microblade, Paleolithic
Shubin, col. 1973, Takoie II site, Sakhalin Island, Siberia
3 cms (l), obsidian

3670-54
Fig. 130, Triangular endblade, Paleolithic
Shubin, col. 1973, Takoie II site, Sakhalin Island, Siberia
3 cms (l), obsidian

3670-83
Fig. 130, Endblade, Paleolithic
Shubin, col. 1973, Takoie II site, Sakhalin Island, Siberia
5 cms (l), obsidian

3670-99
Fig. 130, Microblade fragment, Paleolithic
Shubin, col. 1973, Takoie II site, Sakhalin Island, Siberia
3 cms (l), obsidian

3670-107
Fig. 130, Triangular endblade, Paleolithic
Shubin, col. 1973, Takoie II site, Sakhalin Island, Siberia
3 cms (l), obsidian

3670-109
Fig. 130, Pointed microblade, Paleolithic
Shubin, col. 1973, Takoie II site, Sakhalin Island, Siberia
2 cms (l), obsidian

3670-113
Fig. 130, End scraper, Paleolithic
Shubin, col. 1973, Takoie II site, Sakhalin Island, Siberia
6 cms (l), chert

3670-194
Fig. 130, Microblade core, Paleolithic
Shubin, col. 1973, Takoie II site, Sakhalin Island, Siberia
4 cms (l), chert

4072-1
Fig. 129, Microblade core, Paleolithic
Shubin, col. 1981, Sokol site, Sakhalin Island, Siberia
8 cms (l), obsidian

4072-2
Fig. 129, Sidescraper, Paleolithic
Shubin, col. 1981, Sokol site, Sakhalin Island, Siberia
6 cms (l), obsidian

4072-3
Fig. 129, Triangular endblade, Paleolithic
Shubin, col. 1981, Sokol site, Sakhalin Island, Siberia
4 cms (l), obsidian

4072-4
Fig. 129, Retouched blade, Paleolithic
Shubin, col. 1981, Sokol site, Sakhalin Island, Siberia
4 cms (l), obsidian

4072-7
Fig. 129, Flake knife, Paleolithic
Shubin, col. 1981, Sokol site, Sakhalin Island, Siberia
6 cms (l), obsidian

4072-9
Fig. 129, Burin, Paleolithic
Shubin, col. 1981, Sokol site, Sakhalin Island, Siberia
4 cms (l), chert

4072-14
Fig. 129, Microblade, Paleolithic
Shubin, col. 1981, Sokol site, Sakhalin Island, Siberia
4 cms (l), obsidian

4072-15
Fig. 129, Microblade, Paleolithic
Shubin, col. 1981, Sokol site, Sakhalin Island, Siberia
3 cms (l), obsidian

4072-16
Fig. 129, Microblade, Paleolithic
Shubin, col. 1981, Sokol site, Sakhalin Island, Siberia
3 cms (l), obsidian

4072-18
Fig. 129, Microblade, Paleolithic
Shubin, col. 1981, Sokol site, Sakhalin Island, Siberia
3 cms (l), obsidian

70-213
Fig. 134, Toggling harpoon head, Neolithic
Kozyrev, col. 1957, Nevelsk II site, Sakhalin I., Siberia
8 cms (l), bone

70-214
Fig. 134, Toggling harpoon head, Neolithic
Kozyrev, col. 1957, Nevelsk II site, Sakhalin I., Siberia
11 cms (l), bone

70-216
Fig. 134, Barbed harpoon head, Neolithic
Kozyrev, col. 1957, Nevelsk II site, Sakhalin I., Siberia
9 cms (l), bone

70-219
Fig. 134, Toggling harpoon head, Neolithic
Kozyrev, col. 1957, Nevelsk II site, Sakhalin I., Siberia
9 cms (l), bone

795-3764-1
Fig. 130, Core, Paleolithic
Shubin, col. 1973, Takoie II site, Sakhalin Island, Siberia
4 cms (l), flint

795-3764-2
Fig. 130, Conical core, Paleolithic
Shubin, col. 1973, Takoie II site, Sakhalin Island, Siberia
4 cms (l), obsidian

UAFM: University of Alaska Museum (Fairbanks)

DCr73-13
Fig. 132, Microblade, Paleoarctic
Powers, col. 1973-77, Dry Creek site, Alaska
3 cms (l), chert

DCr73-24
Fig. 132, Microblade core, Paleoarctic
Powers, col. 1973-77, Dry Creek site, Alaska
4 cms (l), rhyolite

DCr73-46
Fig. 132, Microblade, Paleoarctic
Powers, col. 1973-77, Dry Creek site, Alaska
3 cms (l), rhyolite

DCr73-47
Fig. 132, Microblade, Paleoarctic
Powers, col. 1973-77, Dry Creek site, Alaska
3 cms (l), rhyolite

DCr73-48
Fig. 132, Microblade, Paleoarctic
Powers, col. 1973-77, Dry Creek site, Alaska
3 cms (l), rhyolite

UA76-155-3269
Fig. 132, Burin, Paleoarctic
Powers, col. 1973-77, Dry Creek site, Alaska
3 cms (l), chert

UA76-155-4097
Fig. 132, Blade core/scraper, Paleoarctic
Powers, col. 1973-77, Dry Creek site, Alaska
3 cms (l), chert

UA77-44-1591
Fig. 132, Elliptical knife, Paleoarctic
Powers, col. 1973-77, Dry Creek site, Alaska
9 cms (l), rhyolite

UA77-44-2659
Fig. 132, Spall scraper, Paleoarctic
Powers, col. 1973-77, Dry Creek site, Alaska
9 cms (l), rhyolite

UA77-44-3884
Fig. 132, Elliptical biface, Paleoarctic
Powers, col. 1973-77, Dry Creek site, Alaska
12 cms (l), rhyolite

UBCMA: University of British Columbia, Museum of
    Anthropology (Vancouver, B.C.)

A-150
Fig. 223, Soul catchers, Tsimshian
Burnett, col. 1920-27, Post Essington, British Columbia
each 7 cms (w), ivory, red ocher, cord

A-151
Fig. 223, Soul catcher, Tsimshian
Burnett, col. 1920-27, Port Essington, British Columbia
15 cms (l), ivory, grass, leather, cord, ocher

A-152
Fig. 223, Fish effigy, Tsimshian
Burnett, col. 1920-27, Port Essington, British Columbia
37 cms (l), wood, ocher

A-153
Fig. 223, Fish effigy, Tsimshian
Burnett, col. 1920-27, Port Essington, British Columbia
36 cms (l), wood, ocher

A-157
Fig. 223, Wooden canoe model with figure, Tsimshian
Burnett, col. 1920-27, Port Essington, British Columbia
31 cms (l), wood, ocher

Bill Holm

Uncataloged
Fig. 326, Shaman's drum, Yukaghir
Facsimile by Bill Holm
85 cms (l), hide, wood, iron, sinew

Uncataloged
Fig. 67, Nosepin, Athapaskan
Facsimile by Bill Holm

Uncataloged
Fig. 67, Dentalium shell hairband, Athapaskan
Facsimile by Bill Holm

Uncataloged
Fig. 67, Dentalium shell earrings, Athapaskan
Facsimile by Bill Holm

Notes

The American Museum's Jesup North Pacific Expedition

1. For related information see two additional articles by Stanley A. Freed, Ruth S. Freed, and Laila Williamson: "Scholars Amid Squalor," *Natural History*, March 1988, pp. 60–68; and "Capitalist Philanthropy and Russian Revolutionaries: The Jesup North Pacific Expedition (1897–1902)," *American Anthropologist*, vol. 90(1), pp. 7–25 (1988). The authors thank Douglas Cole, May Ebihara, Richard Gould, Aldona Jonaitis, Laurel Kendall, Vittorio Maestro, Jill Neitzel, and David Hurst Thomas for commenting on various drafts of the foregoing papers, Karen Pedersen and Geraldine Santoro for research assistance, and Renate Khambatta for her translations from German to English.

The sources of the letters cited in this essay are identified as follows: DA for the archives of the Department of Anthropology of the American Museum of Natural History; AMNH for the archives of the American Museum of Natural History; and BPP for the Boas Professional Papers at the American Philosophical Society. The authors used a microfilm version of the BBP at the American Museum. We thank archivist Belinda Kaye, Department of Anthropology archives, for her assistance.

Ancient Peoples of the North Pacific Rim

1. Siberian, Alaskan, Canadian, and Japanese data for figs. 2 and 3 were collected and analyzed with aid from the National Geographic Society, National Science Foundation, IREX (International Research and Exchanges Board), USSR Academy of Sciences, and Arizona State University Research Committee. Linda Nuss Watson handled much of the computer analysis; Jacqueline and Korri Dee Turner helped with some data gathering. Collections were examined, and assistance provided by many individuals: Smithsonian Institution, National Museum of Natural History, Washington, D.C. (J.L. Angel, D. Ubelaker, T.D. Stewart, B.J. Meggers); American Museum of Natural History, New York (I. Tattersall, H.L. Shapiro, D.H. Thomas); Peabody Museum, Harvard University, Cambridge (W.W. Howells, E. Trinkhaus); National Museum of Man, Ottawa (J. Cybulski); Field Museum, Chicago (G. Cole); Lowie Museum, Berkeley (F. Norick); Provincial Museum, Victoria (G. Boehm); Simon Fraser University, Burnaby (R. Shutler, R. Carlson); Institute of Ethnography, Moscow (A.A. Zubov, S.A. Arutiunov, A. Pestriakov, V.P. Alekseev), Institute of Ethnography, Leningrad (I.I. Gokhman, A. Kozintsev); Moscow State University (V.P. Chtetzov, S. Efimova); University of Oregon, Eugene (D. Dumond); University of Alaska, Anchorage (W. and K. Workman); Panam Institute, Copenhagen (B. Jorgensen, P.O. Pedersen, P. Bennike); Musée de l'Homme, Paris (R. Gessain, J. Robert-Lamblin); University of Tokyo (K. Hanihara).

Art and Culture Change at the Tlingit-Eskimo Border

1. Russian writers frequently included the Koniag and the Chugach in their term "Aleut," so that early captions and labels may use it in that generic sense. These two hunters were more likely Chugach or Koniag, since there seems to be no evidence for true Aleut use of spruce-root hats.

2. Documentation on early collections is often poor or nonexistent. In many cases tribal attributions were added years after collection, often by people who had little idea of what the material was. Where documentation was questionable or nonexistent, I have attributed hats to Tlingit or Pacific Eskimo origin based on my understanding of early historic period Tlingit design conventions and the degree to which the designs on the hats conform to them. In a few cases the choice was very difficult, but usually the hats seemed to be clearly one or the other.

3. A hat in the Museum of Anthropology and Ethnography in Leningrad, documented as Koniag and collected by Illia Voznesenskii (593-34), is identical in style and nearly in detail to one in the National Museum of Finland (45b), collected about the same time by Arvid Adolph Etholen and cataloged as Tlingit. There is, of course, always the possibility that some hats collected from the Tlingit could have been acquired by them from the Chugach or Koniag, but I believe that it is usually possible to identify their origin on the basis of style.

4. A hat in the Billings collection in Leningrad (562-5) is identified as Tlingit (Razumovskaia 1967:plate VI, 3), but details of the design clearly violate the principles of the formline system. Since the Billings Expedition in 1790 reached only as far east as the mouth of the Copper River, it is more likely that this hat is Pacific Eskimo in origin, as the character of its painting implies. Razumovskaia's paper (1967) on Northwest Coast basketry includes diagrams and descriptions of thirteen spruce-root hats from the Tlingit and Pacific Eskimo. Each hat is shown in a plan view and a front or rear elevation. Although the drawings are impressive, they omit or distort many details, making it impossible to determine from them the degree of adherence to formline principles.

5. Interestingly, the Tlingit man in Alexander Postels' watercolor of an Aleut, a Koniag, and a Tlingit (Fig. 2; Collins et al. 1973:280; Henry 1984:plate 4) is also wearing his hat backwards, perhaps for the same reason. The hat and the rest of his regalia are now in the Anthropological Museum of the Lomonosov State University, Moscow.

Pacific Eskimo painted hats examined:

One-step structure
British Museum VAN 191
British Museum Van 190
British Museum 2239
British Museum NWC 8
Cambridge University Museum 49.205
Leiden Museum 1-1410
Leiden Museum 1-1411
Museum of America, Madrid 191
Museum of America, Madrid 194

Museum of Anthropology and Ethnography, Leningrad 536-12
Museum of Anthropology and Ethnography, Leningrad 539-1
Museum of Anthropology and Ethnography, Leningrad 562-5
Museum of Anthropology and Ethnography, Leningrad 633-16
Museum of Anthropology and Ethnography, Leningrad 2520-16
Museum of Anthropology and Ethnography, Leningrad 2520-18
Museum of Anthropology and Ethnography, Leningrad 2520-20
Museum of Anthropology and Ethnography, Leningrad 5795-19
Museum of Anthropology and Ethnography, Leningrad 5795-21
National Museum of Finland 45c
Turku Historical Museum 82(255)

One-step with beads and whiskers
Denver Art Museum YT1-149
Museum of Anthropology and Ethnography, Leningrad 5795-23
Museum of the American Indian, Heye Foundation
Museum of the American Indian, Heye Foundation
National Museum of Finland 90
National Museum of Finland 5307
National Museum of Natural History 11378
National Museum of Natural History 74720
National Museum of Natural History 360,667
Washington State Historical Society

Two-step structure
British Museum NWC 4
Museum of Anthropology and Ethnography, Leningrad 344-73
Museum of Anthropology and Ethnography, Leningrad 593-34
Museum of Anthropology and Ethnography, Leningrad 2520-19
Museum of Anthropology and Ethnography, Leningrad 2520-27
Museum of Anthropology and Ethnography, Leningrad 5795-22
Museum of Ethnography, Berlin IV A 6174
Museum of Ethnography, Berlin IV A 9380
Museum of Ethnography, Munich 134
National Museum of Finland 45
National Museum of Finland 45b
National Museum of Finland 4911:6
Oakland Museum White Loan 16

Other
Museum of Anthropology and Ethnography, Leningrad 633-17
Museum of Ethnography, Vienna 279

References

Ackerman, Robert E.
1982   The Neolithic-Bronze Age Cultures of Asia and the Norton Phase of Alaska Prehistory. *Arctic Anthropology* 19(2):11–38.
1984   Prehistory of the Asian Eskimo Zone. *Handbook of North American Indians* 5 (Arctic). Washington, D.C.: Smithsonian Institution. pp. 106–118.

Ackerman, R. E.; Hamilton, T. D.; and Stuckenrath, R.
1979   Early Culture Complexes on the Northern Northwest Coast. *Canadian Journal of Archaeology* 3:195–209.

Acosta, José de
1598   *Historia Natural y Moral de las Indias.* Enchuysen: Jacob Lenaertsz Meyn [reprinted Madrid 1792, 2 volumes].

Aigner, Jean S.
1978   Activity Zonation in a 4,000-year-old Aleut House, Chaluka Village, Umnak Island, Alaska. *Anthropological Papers of the University of Alaska* 19(1):11–25.

Aigner, Jean S., and Veltre, Douglas
1976   The Distribution and Pattern of Umqan Burial on Southwest Umnak Island. *Arctic Anthropology* 13(2):113–127.

Alaska Department of Labor
1986   *Alaska Economic Trends.* November. Juneau, Alaska: State of Alaska.

Alaska State Council on the Arts
1981   *1981 Native Art Competition: Wood, Ivory, and Bone.* Anchorage, Alaska.

Alexseev, Valeri P.
1979   Anthropometry of Siberian Peoples. *The First Americans: Origins, Affinities, and Adaptations.* Edited by William Laughlin and Albert B. Harper. New York: Gustav Fisher. pp. 57–90.

American Anthropologist
1930   Anthropological Notes and News. *American Anthropologist* 32:375–377.
1938   Notes and News: Recent Deaths. *American Anthropologist* 40:345.

Ames, Kenneth M.
1981   The Evolution of Social Ranking on the Northwest Coast of North America. *American Antiquity* 46(4):789–805.

Anderson, D. D.
1974–75 Trade Network among the Selawik Eskimos, Northwest Alaska, during the Late Nineteenth and Early Twentieth Centuries. *Folk* 16/17:63–72.

Antropova, V. V., and Kuznetsova, V. G.
1964   The Chukchi. *The Peoples of Siberia,* edited by M. G. Levin and L. P. Potapov. Chicago: University of Chicago Press. pp. 799–835. (Translated from Russian edition, 1956.)

Arnold, R., et al.
1976   *Alaska Native Land Claims.* Anchorage, Alaska: Alaska Native Foundation.

Arsen'ev, V. K.
1926   *Lesnye liudi—Udekheitsy* [The forest people: The Udegey]. Vladivostok.

Arutiunov, S. A., and Sergeev, D. A.
1975   *Problemy etnicheskoi istorii Beringomor'ia (Ekvenskii mogil'nik)* [Problems of ethno-history of the Bering Sea region (Ekven burial site)]. Moscow: Nauka.

Arutiunov, S. A.; Krupnik, I. I.; and Chlenov, M. A.
1982   *"Kitovaia Alleia"; Drevnosti ostrovov proliva Seniavina.* [The "Whale Alley"; antiquities of the Seniavin Strait islands]. Moscow; Institut Etnografii Nauka.

Bancroft, H. H.
1886   *History of Alaska.* New York: McGraw-Hill Book Co.

Barnhardt, Ray, et al.
1979   Small High School Programs for Rural Alaska. *A Preliminary Report of the Small High school Project* 1. Fairbanks, Alaska: Center for Cross-Cultural Studies, School of Education, University of Alaska.

Barratt, Glynn
1981   *Russia in Pacific Waters, 1715–1825. A Survey of the Origins of Russia's Naval Presence in the North and South Pacific.* Vancouver/London: University of British Columbia Press.

Beechey, F. W.
1831   *Narrative of a Voyage to the Pacific and Bering's Strait, to Co-operate with the Polar Expeditions; Performed in His Majesty's Ship "Blossom" . . . in the Years 1825, 26, 27.* London: Colburn & Bently.

Belov, M. I.
1955   *Semen Dezhnev* [Simon Dezhnev]. Moscow: Morskoi Transport.
1956   Arkticheskoe moreplavanie s drevneishikh vremen do serediny XIX veka. *Istoriia otkrytiia i osvoeniia Severnogo Morskogo Puti* T.1 [Arctic navigation from the ancient times to the mid-nineteenth century. Vol. 1 of the history of the discovery and navigation of the Northern Sea route]. Moscow: Morskoi Transport.
1973   *Podvig Semena Dezhneva.* [Simon Dezhnev's exploit]. Moscow.

Berger, Thomas
1985   *Village Journey.* New York: Hill and Wang.

Birket-Smith, Kaj
1953   The Chugach Eskimo. *Nationalmuseets Skrifter, Etnografish Raekke* 6. Copenhagen.

Black, Lydia
1973   The Nivkh (Gilyak) of Sakhalin and the Lower Amur. *Arctic Anthropology* 10(1):1–110.
1982   *Aleut Art.* Anchorage, Alaska: Aleutian/Pribilof Islands Association.
In press. *The Bentwood Hats of Alaska: Symbols of Power and Identity.* Juneau: Alaska State Museum.

Boas, Franz
1897   The Decorative Art of the Indians of the North Pacific Coast. *Bulletin of the American Museum of Natural History* 9:123–176.
1903   The Jesup North Pacific Expedition. *American Museum Journal* 3(5):72–119.
1905   The Jesup North Pacific Expedition. *Proceedings of the International Congress of Americanists, 13th Session, New York 1902.* pp. 91–100.
1910   Ethnological Problems in Canada. *Journal of the Royal Anthropological Institute of Great Britain and Ireland,* 40:529–539.
1916   Tsimshian Mythology. *31st Annual Report of the Bureau of American Ethnology 1909–1910.* Washington, D.C.: U.S. Government Printing Office. pp. 29–1037.
1925   America and the Old World. *Proceedings of the 21st Congress of Americanists* II:21–38. Göteborg.
1927   *Primitive Art.* Oslo: Institutet for Sammenlig-
[1955] nende Kulturforskning. (Reprinted 1955, New York: Dover Publications.)
1933   Relationships Between North-west America and North-east Asia. In: *The American Aborigines: Their Origin and Antiquity,* edited by Diamond Jenness, pp. 357–370. University of Toronto Press.
1937   Waldemar Bogoras. *American Anthropologist* 39:314–315.

Bockstoce, J. R.
1986   *Whales, Ice, and Men: The History of Whaling in the Western Arctic.* Seattle: University of Washington Press.

Bogoras, Waldemar (see also Bogoraz)
1901   The Chukchi of Northeastern Asia. *American Anthropologist* 3:80–108.
1902   Folklore of Northeastern Asia as Compared with that of Northwestern America. *American Anthropologist* 4:577–683.
1904–09 The Chukchee. *The Jesup North Pacific Expe-
[1975] dition* 7, *Memoirs of the American Museum of Natural History.* Leiden/New York. (Reprinted 1975, New York: AMS Press.)
1910   Chukchee Mythology. *The Jesup North Pacific
[1975] Expedition* 8(1), *Memoirs of the American Museum of Natural History.* Leiden/New York. (Reprinted 1975, New York: AMS Press.)
1913   The Eskimo of Siberia. *The Jesup North Pacific
[1975] Expedition* 8(3), *Memoirs of the American Museum of Natural History.* Leiden/New York. (Reprinted 1975, New York: AMS Press.)

Bogoraz, Vladimir Germanovich (see also Bogoras)
1901b   Ocherk material'nago byta olennykh chukchei sostavlennyi na osnovanii kolletsii N. L. Gondatti, nakhodiashchikhcia v Etnograficheskom Muzee Imperatorskoi Akadimii Nauk [Sketch of the Reindeer Chukchi material culture based on the Gondatti collection at the Museum of Ethnography of the Imperial Academy of Sciences]. *Sbornik Muzeia Antropologii i Etnografii* 2. St. Petersburg.
1934   *Chukchi* [The Chukchi]. Part 1. Leningrad.
1935   Drevneishie elementy v iazyke aziatskikh Eskimosov [Ancient elements in the language of the Asiatic Eskimo]. *Sbornik AN SSSR* 16.
1939   *Chukchi* [The Chukchi]. Part 2. Leningrad.

Bolles, Lt. T. Dix
1883   Chinese Relics in Alaska. *Proceedings of the U.S. National Museum* 15(899):221–222.
1889   Preliminary Catalogue of the Eskimo Collections in the U.S. National Museum. *U.S. National Museum Annual Report for 1887.* pp. 335–365.

Borden, Charles E.
1983   Prehistoric Art of the Lower Frazer Region. *Indian Traditions of the Northwest Coast,* edited by Roy L. Carlson. Burnaby, British Columbia: Simon Frazer University. pp. 130–165.

Briggs, Jean L.
1970   *Never in Anger: Portrait of an Eskimo Family.* Cambridge, Mass.: Harvard University Press.

Brooks, Charles Wolcott
1876   Report of Japanese Vessels Wrecked in the North Pacific Ocean, from the Earliest Records to the Present Time. *Proceedings of the California Academy of Sciences,* 6.

Burch, E. S., Jr.
1974   Eskimo Warfare in Northwest Alaska. *Anthropological Papers of the University of Alaska* 16:1–14.
1978   Traditional Eskimo Societies in Northwest Alaska.
[1980] in *Alaska Native Culture and History,* edited by Y. Kotani and W. B. Workman. *National Museum of Ethnology, Senri Ethnological Series* 4. Osaka, Japan. pp. 253–304. (Reprinted 1980.)
1979   Indians and Eskimos in North Alaska, 1816–1977: A Study in Changing Ethnic Relations. *Arctic Anthropology* 16:123–151.
1981   *The Traditional Eskimo Hunters of Point Hope, Alaska: 1800–1875.* Barrow, Alaska: North Slope Borough.
1984   Kotzebue Sound Eskimo. *Handbook of North American Indians* 5 (Arctic). Washington, D.C.: Smithsonian Institution. pp. 303–319.

Burch, E. S., Jr., and Corell, T. C.
1972   Alliance and Conflict: Inter-regional Relations in North Alaska. *Alliance in Eskimo Society,* edited by D. L. Guemple. Seattle: University of Washington Press. pp. 17–39.

Calista Professional Services, Inc.
1985   *Yukon-Kuskokwim Region Arts and Crafts Opportunities Study.*

Cannizzo, Jeanne
1983   George Hunt and the Invention of Kwakiutl Culture. *Canadian Review of Sociology and Anthropology* 20:44–58.

Carlson, Roy L.
1979   The Early Period on the Central Coast of British Columbia. *Canadian Journal of Archaeology* 3:211–228.
1983   Prehistory of the Northwest Coast. *Indian Art Traditions of the Northwest Coast,* edited by Roy L. Carlson. Burnaby, British Columbia: Simon Frazer University. pp. 13–32.

Carpenter, Edmund
1973   Some Notes on the Separate Realities of Eskimo and Indian Art. *The Far North, 2,000 Years of American Eskimo and Indian Art,* edited by Henry Collins, Frederica de Laguna, Edmund Carpenter, and Peter Stone. Washington, D.C.: National Gallery of Art. pp. 281–289.

Chlenov, Mikhail A., and Krupnik, Igor I.
1984   Whale Alley: A Site on the Chukchi Peninsula, Siberia. *Expedition* 26(2):6–15.

Chowning, Ann
1962   Raven Myths in Northwestern North America and Northeastern Asia. *American Anthropologist* 1(1):1–6.

Clark, Donald W.
1970   The Late Kachemak Tradition at Three Saints and Crag Point, Kodiak Island, Alaska. *Arctic Anthropology* 6(2):73–111.

1974   Koniag Prehistory: Archaeological Investigations at Late Prehistoric Sites on Kodiak Island, Alaska. *Tubinger Monographien sur Urgeschite* 1. Stuttgart.

1979   Ocean Bay: An Early North Pacific Maritime Culture. *National Museum of Man. Mercury Series. Archaeological Survey of Canada*, Paper no. 86. Ottawa.

1984   Pacific Eskimo: Historical Ethnography. *Handbook of North American Indians* 5 (Arctic). Washington, D.C.: Smithsonian Press.

Clark, Gerald H.
1977   Archaeology on the Alaska Peninsula: The Coast of Shelikof Strait. *University of Oregon Anthropological Papers* 13.

Cole, Douglas
1985   *Captured Heritage: The Scramble for Northwest Coast Artifacts*. Seattle/London: University of Washington Press.

Collins, Henry B.
1937   The Archeology of St. Lawrence Island. *Smithsonian Miscellaneous Collections* 96(1). Washington, D.C.: Smithsonian Institution.

1946   Wilderness Exploration and Alaska's Purchase. *The Living Wilderness*. December. The Wilderness Society.

1971   Composite Masks: Chinese and Eskimo. *Anthropologica* n.s. 13(1–2):271–278.

Collins, Henry B.; de Laguna, Frederica; Carpenter, Edmund; and Stone, Peter
1973   *The Far North, 2,000 Years of American Eskimo and Indian Art*. Washington, D.C.: National Gallery of Art.

Cook, James
1967   The Voyage of the "Resolution" and "Discovery". 1776–1780. *The Journals of Captain James Cook on His Voyages of Discovery*, edited by J. C. Beaglehole (in 4 vols., 1955–1974), vol. 3, pt. 2. Cambridge: Cambridge University Press. (Selections from original by Cook: *A Voyage to the Pacific Ocean . . . in the Years 1776, 1777. . . .* London: W. and A. Strahan, 1784.)

Count, Earl W.
1949   The Earth-Diver and the Rival Twins: a Clue to Time Correlation in North-Eurasiatic and North American Mythology. *Selected Papers of the 29th International Congress of Americanists* III:55–62, edited by Sol Tax. University of Chicago Press.

Covarrubias, Miguel
1954   *The Eagle, the Jaguar, and the Serpent: Indian Art of the Americas; North America: Alaska, Canada, and the United States*. New York: Alfred A. Knopf, Inc.

Cowling, Elizabeth
1978   The Eskimos, the American Indians, and the Surrealists. *Art History* 1(4):484–500.

Coxe, William
1780   *Account of the Russian Discoveries between Asia and America*. London: Cadell and Davies.
[1966]   (Reprinted 1966, *March of America Facsimile Series* 40. Ann Arbor, Michigan: University Microfilms.)

Cracroft, Sophia
1981   *Lady Franklin Visits Sitka, Alaska 1870: The Journal of Sophia Cracroft, Sir John Franklin's Niece*. Edited by R. N. DeArmond. Anchorage, Alaska: Alaska Historical Society.

Curtis, Edward S.
1930   *The North American Indian* 20. Norwood, Mass.:
[1976]   Plimpton Press. (Reprinted 1976, New York/San Francisco/London: Johnson Reprint Corporation.)

Dall, William Healy
1870   *Alaska and Its Resources*. Boston: Lee and She-
[1970]   pard. (Reprinted 1970, New York: Arno Press, Inc.)

1873   Notes on the Pre-historic Remains in the Aleutian Islands. *Proceedings of the California Academy of Sciences* 4:283–287. San Francisco.

1876   On the Remains of Later Pre-Historic Man Obtained from Caves in the Catherina Archipelago, Alaska Territory, and Especially from the Caves of the Aleutian Islands. pp. 1–40. Published in 1880 in *Smithsonian Contributions to Knowledge* 22(318). Washington, D.C.

1877   On Succession in the Shell-Heaps of the Aleutian Islands. *in* Tribes of the Extreme Northwest, edited by W. H. Dall and G. Gibbs. *Contributions to North American Ethnology* 1, *U.S. Geographical and Geological Survey*. Washington, D.C.

1881   On the So-called Chukchi and Namollo People of Eastern Siberia. *American Naturalist* 15(10):857–868.

1884   On Masks, Labrets, and Certain Aboriginal Customs. *Third Annual Report of the Bureau of American Ethnology for the Years 1881–1882*. Washington, D.C. pp. 67–203.

Dauenhauer, Nora Marks, and Dauenhauer, Richard (Editors)
1987   *Haa Shuká, Our Ancestors: Tlingit Oral Narratives*. Juneau, Alaska: Sealaska Heritage Foundation.

Davis, Barbara Starr, and ·Davis, Richard
1974   *Tongues and Totems: Comparative Arts of the Pacific Basin*. Anchorage: Alaska International Art Institute.

Davydov, Gavriil Ivanovich
1977   *Two Voyages to Russian America, 1802–1807*, edited by Richard Pierce. Kingston, Ontario: Limestone Press. (Translated by Colin Bearne from *Dvukratnoe puteshestvie v Ameriku morskikh ofitserov Khvostova i Davydova, pisannoe sim poslednim* in two parts. St. Petersburg, 1810–1812.)

Debets, G. F.
1948   Paleoantropologiia SSSR [Paleoanthropology of the U.S.S.R.] *Trudy Instituta Etnografiia* n.s.4. Moscow/Leningrad: ANSSSR.

de Laguna, Frederica
1934   *The Archaeology of Cook Inlet, Alaska*. Univer-
[1975]   sity of Pennsylvania Museum. (Reprinted with introduction, 1975, Anchorage: Alaska Historical Society.)

1972   Under Mount Saint Elias: The History and Culture of the Yakutat Tlingit. *Smithsonian Contributions to Anthropology* 7 (in 3 parts). Washington, D.C.: Smithsonian Institution Press.

Dikov, N. N.
1965   The Stone Age of Kamchatka and the Chukchi Peninsula in the Light of New Archaeological Data. *Arctic Anthropology* 3(1):10–25. (Translated from *Trudy Severo-Vostochnogo Kompleksnogo Nauchno-Issledovatel'skogo Instituta* 8:5–27. Magadan, 1964.)

1968   The Discovery of the Palaeolithic in Kamchatka and the Problem of the Initial Occupation of America. *Arctic Anthropology* 5(1):191–203. (Translated from Istoriia i kul'tura narodov severa Dal'nego Vostoka, *Trudy Severo-vostochnogo Kompleksnogo Nauchno-Issledovatel'skogo Instituta* 17:16–31. Moscow, 1967.)

1972   Les Petroglyphes de Pegtymel' et leur Appartenance Ethnique. *Inter-Nord* 12:245–261.

1977   *Arkheologicheskie pamiatniki Kamchatki, Chukotki i Verkhnei Kolymy* [Archeological sites of Kamchatka, Chukotka, and the Upper Kolyma]. Moskow: Nauka.

Dmytryshin, B.; Crownhart-Vaughan, E.A.P.; and Vaughan, T. (Editors)
1985   Russia's Conquest of Siberia, 1558–1700: A Documentary Record. *To Siberia and Russian America: Three Centuries of Russian Eastward Expansion*. Vol. 1. Portland, Oregon: Western Imprints.

Doig, Ivan
1980   *Winter Brothers: A Season at the Edge of America*. New York: Harcourt Brace Jovanovich.

Drucker, Phillip
1951   The Northern and Central Nootkan Tribes. *Bureau of American Ethnology, Bulletin* 144. Washington, D.C.: Smithsonian Institution.

1958   The Native Brotherhoods. Modern Inter-Tribal Organization of the Northwest Coast. *Bureau of American Ethnology, Bulletin* 168. Washington, D.C.: Smithsonian Institution.

Duff, Wilson
1964   The Indian History of British Columbia. *Anthropology in British Columbia*, Memoir 5, Vol. 1, The Impact of the White Man.

1975   *Images: Stone: B.C.: Thirty Centuries of Northwest Coast Indian Sculpture*. Saanichton, British Columbia: Hancock House Publishers.

1981   The World Is as Sharp as a Knife: Meaning in
[1983]   Northwest Coast Art. *The World Is as Sharp as a Knife: An Anthology in Honour of Wilson Duff*, edited by Donald W. Abbott. Victoria, British Columbia: British Columbia Provincial Museum. pp. 209–224. (Reprinted in *Indian Art Traditions of the Northwest Coast*, edited by Roy L. Carlson, 1983, Burnaby, British Columbia: Simon Frazer University. pp. 47–66.)

1981a   Thoughts on the Nootka Canoe. *The World Is as Sharp as a Knife: An Anthology in Honour of Wilson Duff*, edited by Donald W. Abbott. Victoria, British Columbia: British Columbia Provincial Museum. pp. 201–6.

Dumond, Don E.
1981   Archaeology on the Alaska Peninsula: The Naknek Region. *University of Oregon Anthropological Papers* 21.

1984   Prehistory: Summary. *Handbook of North American Indians* 5 (Arctic). Washington, D.C.: Smithsonian Institution. pp. 72–79.

1987   A Reexamination of Eskimo-Aleut Prehistory. *American Anthropologist* 89:32–56.

Duncan, Kate
1984   *Some Warmer Tone: Alaska Athabascan Bead Embroidery*. Fairbanks, Alaska: University of Alaska Museum.

1988   *Northern Athapaskan Art: A Beadwork Tradition*. Seattle: University of Washington Press.

Dyson, George
1986   *Baidarka*. Edmonds, Washington: Alaska Northwest Publishing Company.

Elliott, Henry W.
1881   *The Seal Islands of Alaska*. U.S. Department of
[1976]   the Interior. Washington, D.C.: U.S. Government Printing Office. (Reprinted 1976, Kingston, Ontario: Limestone Press.)

Emmons, George T.
n.d.a.   *Notes on Tlingit*. British Columbia Provincial Archives.

n.d.b   *Collection Notes*. Unpublished. American Museum of Natural History.

1907   The Chilkat Blanket. *Memoirs of the American Museum of Natural History* 3(4):229–277.

1916   The Whale House of the Chilkat. *Anthropological Papers of the American Museum of Natural History* 19, pt. 1. pp. 1–33.

Emmons, G. T., and de Laguna, F.
In press   *The Tlingit Indians*. Seattle: University of Washington Press.

Fagan, Brian M.
1987   *The Great Journey: The Peopling of Ancient America*. New York/London: Thames and Hudson.

Federal Field Committee for Development Planning in Alaska.
1968   *Alaska Natives and the Land*. Anchorage, Alaska.

Fienup-Riordan, Ann
1983   *The Nelson Island Eskimo*. Anchorage: Alaska Pacific University Press.

1986   Nick Charles, Sr.: Worker in Wood. *The Artist Behind the Work*, edited by Suzi Jones. Fairbanks: University of Alaska Museum. pp. 25–57.

1987   The Mask: The Eye of the Dance. *Arctic Anthropology* 24(12):40–55.

Fisher, Raymond H.
In press   Early Russian Aspirations for an American Empire. Paper presented at the 2d International Conference on Russian America, Sitka, Alaska, August 19, 1987. *Conference Proceedings*. Kingston, Ontario: Limestone Press,

Fisher, William J.
1883   Catalogue of a Collection of Ethnological Specimens Obtained from the Ugashagmut Tribe, Ugashak River, Bristol Bay, Alaska. *Proceedings of the U.S. National Museum* 7(11):161–165.

Fitzhugh, William W.
1975   Introduction. In: *Prehistoric Maritime Adaptations of the Circumpolar Zone*, edited by William W. Fitzhugh, pp. 1–18. The Hague: Mouton.

1984   Images from the Past: Thoughts on Bering Sea Eskimo Art and Culture. *Expedition* 26(2):24–39.

Fitzhugh, William W., and Kaplan, Susan A.
1982   *Inua: Spirit world of the Bering Sea Eskimo*. Washington, D.C.: Smithsonian Institution Press.

Fitzhugh, William W., and Selig, Ruth O.
1981   The Smithsonian's Alaska Connection: Nineteenth Century Explorers and Anthropologists. *Alaska Journal: A 1981 Collection*. Alaska Northwest Publishing Company. pp. 193–208.

Fladmark, Knut R.
1975   A Paleoecological Model for Northwest Coast Prehistory. *National Museum of Man. Mercury Series. Archeological Survey of Canada* Paper no. 43. Ottawa.

Frachtenberg, Leo J.
1921   The Ceremonial Societies of the Quileute Indians. *American Anthropologist* 23:320–52.
Friday, Joe
1984   Interview, August 7, Chevak, Alaska. 14(h)(1) Site Survey. Anchorage, Alaska: Bureau of Indian Affairs Realty Office.
1985   Interview, Feburary 19, translated by Louise Leonard. San Francisco: Lansburg Productions.
Frost, O. W. (Editor)
1970   *Cross-Cultural Arts in Alaska.* Anchorage, Alaska: Alaska Methodist University Press.
Gerasimov, M. M.
1964   The Paleolithic Site Mal'ta: Excavations of 1956–1957. *The Archaeology and Geomorphology of Northern Asia,* edited and translated by H. Michael. Toronto: Arctic Institute of North America. pp. 3–32.
Gjessing, Gutorm
1944   The Circumpolar Stone Age. *Acta Archaeologica* 2.
Gladwin, Harold S.
1947   *Men Out of Asia.* New York: McGraw-Hill Book Co.
Golder, Frank
1914   *Russian Expansion on the Pacific 1641–1850.* Cleveland: Arthur H. Clark Co.
Golovnin, Vasilii Mikhailovich
1979   *Around the World on the "Kamchatka," 1817–1819.* Honolulu: University Press of Hawaii. (Translated from *Puteshestvie vokrug sveta,* 1822.)
Greenberg, Joseph H.
1987   *Language in the Americas.* Stanford: Stanford University Press.
Greenberg, Joseph H.; Turner, Christy G., II; and Zegura, Stephen L.
1986   The Settlement of the Americas: A Comparison of the Linguistic, Dental, and Genetic Evidence. *Current Anthropology* 27(5):477–497.
Gruening, Ernest
1968   *The State of Alaska.* New York: Random House.
Gurvich, I. S.
1987   Novye dannye po traditsionnoi obriadnosti koriakov. *Traditsionnye verovaniia i byt narodov Sibiri* [New data on the traditional rituals of the Koriak, *in* Traditional beliefs and life of the peoples of Siberia]. Novosibirsk.
Gurvich, I. S. (Editor)
1980   *Semeinaia obriadnost' narodov Sibiri* [Family rituals of the peoples of Siberia]. Moscow: Nauka.
Hallowell, A. I.
1926   Bear Ceremonialism in the Northern Hemisphere. *American Anthropologist* 28:1–173.
Hamilton, Thomas D.; Reed, Katherine M.; and Thorson, Robert M.
1986   *Glaciation in Alaska: The Geologic Record.* Alaska Geological Society.
Hatt, Gudmund
1934   North American and Eurasian Culture Connections. *Proceedings of the Fifth Pacific Science Congress,* pp. 2755–2763. University of Toronto Press.
1949   Asiatic Influences in American Folklore. *Det. Kgl. Danske Videnskabernes Selskab, Historisk-Filologiske Meddelelser* 31(6):1–122. Copenhagen.
1969   Arctic Skin Clothing in Eurasia and America: An Ethnographic Study. *Arctic Anthropology* 5(2):1–132. (Translated from J. H. Schultz, *Forlagsboghandel Graebes Bogtrykkeri,* 1914.)
Haven, Samuel F.
1856   Archaeology of the United States. *Smithsonian Contributions to Knowledge.* Washington, D.C. pp. 1–168.
Healy, Michael A.
1887   Report of the Cruise of the Steamer "Corwin." *Report of the Cruise of the Revenue Marine Steamer "Corwin" in the Arctic Ocean, 1885.* Washington, D.C.: U.S. Government Printing Office. pp. 5–20.
1889   *Report of the Cruise of the Revenue Marine Steamer "Corwin" in the Arctic Ocean in the Year 1884.* Washington, D.C.: U.S. Government Printing Office.
Heine-Geldern, Robert
1966   A Note on Relations between the Art Styles of the Maori and of Ancient China. *Weiner Beitrage zur Kulturgeschichte und Linguistik,* Band XV:47–68. Wein.
Heizer, Robert F.
1943   Aconite Poison Whaling in Asia and America: An Aleutian Transfer to the New World. *An-*

thropological Papers 24, *Bureau of American Ethnology Bulletin* 133:415–468. Washington, D.C.
1956   Archaeology of the Uyak Site, Kodiak Island, Alaska. *University of California Anthropological Records* 17(1). Berkeley.
Henry, John F.
1984   *Early Maritime Artists of the Pacific Northwest Coast, 1741–1841.* Seattle: University of Washington Press.
Hildebrand, Hans
1883   De lägre naturfolkens knost, *Studier och forskningar. . . ., by Nordenskiöld. pp. 303–402. (Translated as Kunst der niedern Naturvölker, in* Nordenskiöld, 1885).
Himmelheber, Hans
1938   *Eskimokünstler: Teilergebnis einer Ethnographischen Expedition in Alaska von Juni 1936 bis April 1937.* Stuttgart: Strecker and Schröder.
1953   *Eskimolünstler; Ergebnisse einer Reise in Alaska.* 2d ed. Eisenach, Germany: Erich Roth-Verlag.
Hoffman, Walter J.
1897   The Graphic Art of the Eskimos, Based upon
[1974]   the collections in the National Museum. *Annual Report of the United States National Museum for 1895.* Washington, D.C. pp. 739–968. (Reprinted 1974, Seattle, Washington: Shorey Book Store.)
Holm, Bill
1965   *Northwest Coast Indian Art: An Analysis of Form.* Seattle: University of Washington Press.
1981   Will the Real Charles Edensaw Please Stand Up? The Problem of Attribution in Northwest Coast Indian Art. *The World Is as Sharp as a Knife.* Victoria, British Columbia: British Columbia Provincial Museum. pp. 175–200.
1983   *The Box of Daylight: Northwest Coast Indian Art.* Seattle/London: University of Washington Press.
1983a   *Smoky-Top: The Art and Times of Willy Seaweed.* Seattle: University of Washington Press.
1987   *Spirit and Ancestor: A Century of Northwest Coast Indian Art at the Burke Museum.* Seattle: University of Washington Press.
Holm, Bill, and Reid, William
1975   *Form and Freedom: A Dialogue on Northwest Coast Indian Art.* Houston: Institute for the Arts, Rice University.
Holmberg, Henrik Johan
1855–63 Ethnographische Skizzen Ueber die Volker des
[1985]   Russischen Amerika, *Acta Scientiarum Fennicae.* (Republished as *Holmberg's Ethnographic Sketches,* translated by Fritz Jaensch, 1985, University of Alaska Press.)
Hooper, Calvin L.
1881   *Report of the Cruise of the U.S. Revenue Steamer "Corwin" in the Arctic Ocean, November 1, 1880.* Washington, D.C.: U.S. Government Printing Office.
1884   *Report of the Cruise of the U.S. Revenue Steamer "Thomas Corwin," in the Arctic Ocean, 1881.* Washington, D.C.: U.S. Government Printing Office.
1897   A Report on the Sea-Otter Banks of Alaska, U.S. Treasury Department Document No. 1977. Washington, D.C.: Office of the Secretary, Division of Revenue Cutter Service.
Hrdlicka, Ales
1944   *The Anthropology of Kodiak Island.* Philadelphia: Wistar Institute of Anatomy and Biology.
1945   *The Aleutians and Commander Island and Their Inhabitants.* Philadelphia: Wistar Institute of Anatomy and Biology.
Hsio-Yen Shih
1963   A Chinese Shell-Inlay Motif, *1962 Annual,* Toronto: Art and Archaeology Division, Royal Ontario Museum, University of Toronto.
Huggins, Eli Lundy
1981   *Kodiak and Afognak Life, 1868–1870.* Kingston, Ontario: Limestone Press.
Hughes, Charles C.
1984   Asiatic Eskimo: Introduction. *Handbook of North American Indians* 5 (Arctic). Washington, D.C.: Smithsonian Institution. pp. 243–246.
Institute of Alaska Native Arts
1984   *New Traditions: An Exhibition of Alaska Native Sculpture.* Fairbanks, Alaska.
Iokhel'son, Vladimir Il'ich (see also Jochelson)
1907   Etnolingvisticheskie problemy na severnykh beregakh Tikhogo okeana. *Izvestiia Russkogo Geograficheskogo Obshchestva* 13 [Ethno-linguistic problems of the Northern Coasts of the Pacific Ocean, *in* Bulletin of the Russian Geographical Society 13].

Ivanov, S. V.
1930   Aleut Hunting Headgear and Its Ornamentation. *International Congress of Americanists 23d Session.* pp. 477–509.
1937   Medved' v religioznom i dekorativnom iskusstve narodnostei Amura. *Pamiati V. G. Bogoraza (1865–1936)* [The bear in the religious and decorative art of the peoples of the Amur, *in* In memory of W. G. Bogoras (1865–1936)]. Moscow/Leningrad: Institut Etnografii. pp. 1–45.
1954   Materialy po izobrazitel'nomu iskusstvu narodov Sibiri XIX-nachala XX v [Material on the depictive art of the peoples of Siberia, nineteenth and early twentieth centuries]. *Trudy Instituta Etnografii* n.s.22. Moscow/Leningrad: ANSSSR.
1963   Ornament narodov Sibiri kak istoricheskii istochnik [Ornamentation of the peoples of Siberia as a historical source]. *Trudy Instituta Etnografii,* n.s.81. Moscow/Leningrad: ANSSSR.
Ivanov, S. and V. Stukalov
1975   *Ancient Masks of Siberian Peoples.* Leningrad: Aurora Publishers.
Ivashintsov, N. A.
1980   *Russian Round-the-World Voyages, 1803–1849.* Edited by Richard Pierce. Kingston, Ontario: Limestone Press. (Translated by Glynn R. Barratt from *Russkie krugosvetnyia puteshestviia, s 1803 po 1849 g.,* first published as *Zapiski gidrograficheskago departamenta 7–8,* St. Petersburg, 1848 and 1849.)
Jacobson, Steven A.
1984   *Yup'ik Eskimo Dictionary.* Fairbanks, Alaska: Alaska Native Language Center, University of Alaska.
James, James Alton
1942   The First Scientific Exploration of Russian America and the Purchase of Alaska. *Northwestern University Studies in the Social Science* 4. Evanston/Chicago.
Jefferson, Thomas
1787   *Notes on Virginia.* Richmond: Bibliotheca Americana.
Jenness, D.
1929   Little Diomede Island, Bering Strait. *Geographic Review* 19:78–86.
Jensen, Doreen, and Sargent, Polly
1986   Robes of Power, Totem Poles on Cloth. *Museum Note* 17. Vancouver: University of Columbia Press/UBC Museum of Anthropology.
Jochelson, Waldemar (see also Iokhel'son)
1907   Past and Present Subterranean Dwellings of the Tribes of Northeastern Asia and Northwestern America. *Congrès International des Américanistes, 15ème Session, Québec.* pp. 115–128.
1908   The Koryak. *The Jesup North Pacific Expedition*
[1975]   6, *Memoirs of the American Museum of Natural History.* Leiden/New York. (Reprinted 1975, New York: AMS Press.)
1926   The Yukaghir and the Yukaghirized Tungus.
[1975]   *The Jesup North Pacific Expedition 9, Memoirs of the American Museum of Natural History.* Leiden/New York. (Reprinted 1975, New York: AMS Press.)
1926a   The Ethnological Problems of Bering Sea. *American Museum Journal* 26(1):90–95.
1928   *Peoples of Asiatic Russia.* New York: American Museum of Natural History.
1933   *History, Ethnology, and Anthropology of the Aleut.* Washington, D.C.: Carnegie Institution of Washington.
Jonaitis, Aldona
1986   *The Art of the Northern Tlingit.* Seattle: University of Washington Press.
Jones, Susan (Editor)
1982   *Eskimo Dolls.* Anchorage, Alaska: Alaska State Council on the Arts.
1986   *The Artists Behind the Work.* Fairbanks, Alaska: University of Alaska Museum.
Jordan, Richard H., and Knecht, Richard A.
1986   Archaeological Research on Western Kodiak Island, Alaska: The Development of Koniag Culture. *in* Late Prehistoric Development of Alaska's Native People, edited by Robert D. Shaw; Roger K. Harritt; and Don E. Dumond. *Alaska Historical Commission Studies in History* 190. Anchorage. pp. 356–453.
Kaplan, Susan A.; Jordan, Richard H.; and Sheehan, Glenn W.
1984   An Eskimo Whaling Outfit from Sledge Island, Alaska. *Expedition* 26(2):16–23.
Keithahn, Edward L.
1963   *Monuments in Cedar.* New York: Bonanza Books.
Kendall, Laurel
1986   Berthold Laufer and the Amur River Collection at the American Museum of Natural History.

Unpublished Ms. American Museum of Natural History.

Khlebnikov, Kirill T.
1979   *Russkaia America v neopublikovannykh zapis-kakhakh Khlebnikova* [Russian America in Khlebnikov's unpublished manuscripts], edited and annotated by R. G. Liapunova and S. G. Fedorova. Leningrad: Nauka.
1985   *Novo-Arkhangel'sk* [Novo-Arkhangelsk], edited and annotated by S. G. Fedorova. Moscow: Nauka.

King, Jonathan C. H.
1981a   *Artificial Curiosities from the Northwest Coast of America.* London: British Museum Publications, Ltd.
1981b   Eighteenth Century Pacific Collections in the British Museum. *American Indian Art Magazine* 6(2):32–39.

Kleinfeld, Judith, et al.
1973   *Land Claims and Native Manpower Staffing Regional and Village Corporations under Alaska Native Settlement Act of 1971.* Anchorage, Alaska: Alaska Native Foundation and Institute of Social, Economic, and Government Research, University of Alaska.

Kohout, Karen, and Kleinfeld, Judith
1974   *Alaska Natives in Higher Education.* Fairbanks, Alaska: Institute of Social, Economic, and Governmental Research, University of Alaska.

Kos'ven, M. O.
1962   Iz istorii etnografii koriakov v XVIII v. [History of the ethnography of the Koryak in the eighteenth century]. *Sibirskii Etnograficheskii Sbornik 4. Trudy Instituta Etnografii* n.s. 74. Moscow: ANSSSR. pp. 276–291.

Kotzebue, O. V.
1821   *A Voyage of Discovery into the South Sea and Beerings Straits, for the Purpose of Exploring a North-East Passage, Undertaken in the Years 1815–1818....* London: Longman, Hurst, Reese, Orme, and Brown.

Krader, Lawrence
1968   Bogoraz, Vladimir G.; Sternberg, Lev Y.; and Jochelson, Vladimir. *International Encyclopedia of the Social Sciences* 2:116–119. New York: Free Press.

Krasheninnikov, Stepan P.
1755   *Opisanie Zemli Kamchatki.* St. Petersburg.
1972   *Exploration of Kamchatka.* Portland: Oregon Historical Society. (Translated with introduction and notes by E. A. P. Crownhart-Vaughan from *Opisanie Zemli Kamchatki,* 1755.)

Krauss, Michael E.
1983   Survival or Extinction for Alaska Native Languages. *Alaska Native News,* February. Anchorage, Alaska.

Krushanov, A. I. (Editor)
1987   *Istoria i kul'tura chukchei* [Chukchi history and culture]. Leningrad: Nauka.

Lantis, Margaret
1938   The Alaska Whale Cult and Its Affinities. *American Anthropologist* n.s.40:438–464.
1947   Alaskan Eskimo Ceremonialism. *Monographs of the American Ethnological Society,* (New York) 11. New York: J. J. Augustin.
1954   Edward William Nelson. *Anthropological Papers of the University of Alaska* 3(1):4–16. Fairbanks.
1970   The Aleut Social System, 1750 to 1810, from Early Historical Sources. *Ethnohistory in Southwestern Alaska and the Southern Yukon,* edited by M. Lantis. The University Press of Kentucky. pp. 139–302.
1984a   Nunivak Eskimo. *Handbook of North American Indians* 5 (Arctic). Washington, D.C.: Smithsonian Institution. pp. 209–223.
1984b   Aleut. *Handbook of North American Indians* 5 (Arctic). Washington, D.C.: Smithsonian Institution. pp. 161–184.

Larsen, Dinah, and Dickey, Terry
1982   *Setting It Free: An Exhibition of Modern Alaska Eskimo Ivory Carving.* Fairbanks, Alaska: University of Alaska Museum.

Larsen, Helge E., and Rainey, Froelich G.
1948   *Ipiutak and the Arctic Whale Hunting Culture. Anthropological Papers of the American Museum of Natural History,* 42. New York.

Laufer, Berthold
1902   The Decorative Art of the Amur Tribes. *The*
[1975] *Jesup North Pacific Expedition* 4, *Memoirs of the American Museum of Natural History.* Leiden/New York. (Reprinted 1975, New York: AMS Press).

Laughlin, William S.
1951   The Alaska Gateway Viewed from the Aleutian Islands. *The Physical Anthropology of the American Indian.* New York: Viking Fund. pp. 98–126.
1967   Human Migration and Permanent Occupation in the Bering Sea Area. *The Bering Land Bridge,* edited by David M. Hopkins. Stanford: Stanford University Press. pp. 409–450.
1980   *Aleuts: Survivors of the Bering Land Bridge.* New York: Holt, Rinehart, and Wilson.

Laughlin, W. S., and Reeder, G. (Editors)
1966   Studies in Aleutian-Kodiak Prehistory, Ecology, and Anthropology. *Arctic Anthropology* 3(2).

Lee, Molly
1981   Pacific Eskimo Spruce Root Baskets. *American Indian Art Magazine* 6(2):66–73.
1983   *Baleen Basketry of the North Alaska Eskimo.* Barrow, Alaska: North Slope Borough Planning Department.

Lee, Molly, and Graburn, Nelson H. H.
1986   *Commerce and Curios.* Berkeley: Lowie Museum of Anthropology.

Leont'ev, V. V.
1983   *Etnografiia i folklor kerekov* [Kerek ethnography and folklore]. Moscow.

Leroi-Gourhan, André
1946   Archéologie du Pacifique-Nord. Matériaux pour l'étude des Relations entre les Peuples Riverains d'Asie et d'Amérique. *Travaux et Mémoires de l'Institut d'Éthnologie* 42. Paris: Institut d'Éthnologie.

Levin, M. G.
1958   *Etnicheskaia antropologiia i problemy etnogeneza narodov Dal'nego Vostoka* [Ethnic anthropology and problems of ethnogenesis of the peoples of the Far East]. Moscow.
        Anthropological Types of the Northeastern Paleoasiatics and Problems of Ethnogenesis. *Proceedings of the 32nd Congress of Americanists,* pp. 607–616.

Levin, M. G., and Potapov, L. P.
1961   *Istoriko-etnograficheskii atlas Sibiri* [Historico-ethnographic atlas of Siberia]. Moscow-Leningrad: ANSSSR.
1964   *The Peoples of Siberia.* Stephen Dunn, translation editor. Chicago and London: University of Chicago Press (Orig. Publ. *Narody Sibiri,* 1956, Moscow: ANSSSR.)

Lévi-Strauss, Claude
1943   The Art of the Northwest Coast at the American Museum of Natural History. *Gazette des Beaux-Arts* pp. 175–182.

Liapunova, Roza Gavrilovna
1975   *Ocherki po etnografii Aleutov: konets XVIII-pervaia polovina XIX v.* [Essay on the ethnography of the Aleut. Late eighteenth to mid-nineteenth centuries]. Leningrad: Institut Etnografii, ANSSSR.

Lipshits, B. A.
1955   O kollektsiiakh Muzeia antropologii i etnografii ... na Alaske i v Kalifornii [On the collections in the Museum of Anthropology and Ethnography ... from Alaska and California]. *Sbornik Muzeia Antropologii i Etnografii* 16:358–69. Leningrad: ANSSSR.

Lisiansky, Urey (Lisianskii, Iurii)
1814   *A Voyage Round the World in the Years 1802,*
[1968] *4, 5, and 6 ... in the Ship "Neva".* London. (Reprinted in Bibliotheca Australiana No. 42, 1968, Amsterdam/New York.)

Lomonosov, M.
1763   *Kratkoe opisanie raznyky puteshestvii po severnym moriam i pokazanie vozmozhnogo pro-*
[1952] *khodu sibirskim okeanom* [Short Description of several travels on the northern seas and demonstration of the possibility of a passage to the Siberian Ocean]. (Reprinted in Vol. 6 of Complete Works, 1952, Moscow: Nauka.)

Lopatin, Ivan A.
1922   Gol'dy amurskie, ussuriiskie i sungariiskie. *Zapiski Obshchestva izucheniia Amurskogo kraia Vladivostokskogo otdeleniia Priamurskogo Otdela Russkogo geograficheskogo obshchestva* T.17 [The Gold of the Amur, Ussuri, and Sungari in Documents of the Society for the study of the Amur region, Vladivostok bureau of the Amur branch of the Russian Geographic Society, Vol. 17]. Vladivostok.
1925   Orochi—sorodichi Man'chzhur [Oroch: Kinsmen of the Manchu]. *Vestnik Manzhurii* 8–10. Kharbin.

Low, Jean
1977   George Thornton Emmons. *Alaska Journal* 7(1): 2–11.

Lundy, Doris
1983   Styles of Coastal Rock Art. *Indian Art Traditions of the Northwest Coast,* edited by Roy Carlson. Burnaby, British Columbia: Simon Frazer University. pp. 89–97.

Lütke, Frederic (Litke, Fedor Petrovich)
1835–36 *Voyage autour du Monde 1826–1829.* Paris:
[1971] Didot Frères. (Reprinted 1971, Bibliotheca Australiana no. 62. Amsterdam: N. Israel; New York: Da Capo Press.)

MacDonald, George
1983   Prehistoric Art of the Northern Northwest Coast. *Indian Art Traditions of the Northwest Coast,* edited by Roy L. Carlson. Burnaby, British Columbia: Simon Frazer University. pp. 99–121.

Majors, H. M.
1983   Early Russian Knowledge of Alaska, 1701–1730. *Northwest Discovery* 4:84–152.

Mather, Elsie
1985   *Cauyarnariuq.* Bethel, Alaska: Lower Kuskokwim School District Bilingual-Bicultural Department.

Meletinskii, E. M.
1963   *Proiskhozhdenie geroicheskogo eposa* [Origins of the heroic epic]. Moscow.
1979   *Paleoasiatskii mifologicheskii epos* (Paleoasiatic mythological epic]. Moscow.

Menovshchikov, G. A.
1964   The Eskimos. *The Peoples of Siberia,* edited by M. G. Levin and L. P. Potapov. (Orig. publ. 1956). Chicago: University of Chicago Press. pp. 836–850.
1987   *Materialy i issledovaniia po iazyku i fol'kloru naukanskikh eskimosov* [Data and research on the language and folklore of the Naukansky Eskimo]. Leningrad: Nauka/ANSSSR.

Merck, C. H.
1978   (see Titova)
1980   *Siberia and Northwestern America 1788–1792: The Journal of Carl Heinrich Merck...* Kingston, Ontario: Limestone Press.

Michael, Henry, and James W. VanStone, editors
1983   *Cultures of the Bering Sea Region: Papers from an International Symposium.* International Research and Exchanges Board. New York.

Miller, Polly
1967   *Lost Heritage of Alaska.* Cleveland/New York: World Publishing Company.

Moberg, Carl-Axel
1960   On Some Circumpolar and Arctic Problems. *Acta Arctica* 12:67–74.

Mochanov, Iurii A.
1969   The Ymyiakhtakh Late Neolithic Culture, translated by R. Powers. *Arctic Anthropology* 6(1):115–118.

Moore, Riley D.
1923   Social Life of the Eskimo of St. Lawrence Island. *American Anthropologist* 25(3):339–375.

Morrow, Phyllis
1984   It Is Time for Drumming: A Summary of Recent Research on Yup'ik Ceremonialism. *Etudes/Inuit/Studies* 8 (Special Issue):113–140.

Murdoch, John
1892   Ethnological Results of the Point Barrow Expe-
[1988] dition. *9th Annual Report of the Bureau of American Ethnology for the Years 1887–1888.* Washington, D.C. (Reprinted with introduction by William W. Fitzhugh, Classics of Smithsonian Anthropology Series, 1988, Washington, D.C.: Smithsonian Institution Press).

Nagishkin, Dmitrii
1980   *Folktales of the Amur: Stories from the Russian Far East.* New York: Harry N. Abrams, Inc./Leningrad: Aurora Art Publisher.

Nelson, Edward William
1882   A Sledge Journey in the Delta of the Yukon, Northern Alaska. *Proceedings of the Royal Geographical Society and Monthly Record of Geography,* n.s. 4:660–670.
1887   *Report upon Natural History Made in Alaska between the Years 1887–1881.* Washington, D.C.: Arctic Series of Publications. U.S. Army Signal Service, III.
1899   The Eskimo about Bering Strait. *Bureau of Amer-*
[1983] *ican Ethnology Annual Report* 18:1–518. Washington, D.C.: Smithsonian Institution. (Reprinted with introduction by William W. Fitzhugh, Classics of Smithsonian Anthropology Series, 1983, Washington, D.C.: Smithsonian Institution Press.)

Niblack, Ensign Albert P.
1890   The Coast Indians of Southern Alaska and Northern British Columbia. pp. 225–386. *U.S. National Museum Annual Report for 1888.*

Nordenskiöld, Adolf E. F. von
1882   *The Voyage of the Vega Round Asia and Europe, with a Historical Review of Previous Journeys along the North Coast of the Old World.* New York: Macmillan and Co. (Translated by Alexander Leslie.)
1883   *Studier och forskningar föranledda af mina resor i höga Norden. Ett populärt vetenskapligt bihang till "Vega färd kuing Asien och Europa".* Stockholm: F. & G. Beijer.
1885   *Studien und Forschungen veranlasst durch meine Reisen im hohen Norden. Ein populär-wissenschaftliches Supplement zu die Umsegelung Asiens und Europas auf der Vega.* Leipzig: F. A. Brockhuas.

Nuligak
1966   *Nuligak.* Toronto: P. Martin Associates.

Nute, Grace Lee
1943   Kennicott in the North. *The Beaver* Outfit 274 (September):28–32.

O'Brien, Irma
1986   *Sam Fox: The Life and Art of a Yup'ik Eskimo.* Dillingham, Alaska: Samuel K. Fox Museum.

Okladnikov, A.
1981   *Ancient Art of the Amur Region.* (Also entitled: *Art of the Amur, Ancient Art of the Russian Far East.*) Leningrad: Aurora.

Okladnikova, E. A.
1987   Science Education in Russian America. In: *Russia's American Colony,* edited by S. Frederick Starr, pp. 218–248. Raleigh: Duke University Press.

Olson, R. L.
1936   The Quinault Indians. *University of Washington Publications in Anthropology* 6(1).

Oquilluk, W. A.
1973   *People of Kauwerak: Legends of the Northern Eskimo.* Anchorage, Alaska: Alaska Methodist University.

Orlova, N. S. (Compiler)
1951   *Otkrytiia russkikh zemleprokhodtsev i poliarnykh morekhodov XVII veka na severo-vostoke Azii. Sbornik dokumentov* [Discoveries of the Russian explorations and polar navigations in northeastern Asia in the seventeenth century. Collection of documents]. Moscow.

Pierce, Richard A.
1975   Voznesenskii: Scientist in Alaska. *Alaska Journal* 5(1):11–15.

Pinart, Alphonse L.
1875   *La caverne d'Aknañh, Ile d'Ounga (Archipel Shumagin, Aliaska).* Paris: E. Leroux.

Popova, U. G.
1981   *Eveny Magadanskoi oblasti; ocherki istorii i kul'tury evenov Okhotskogo poberezh'ia 1917–1977 gg* [The Magadan District Even; sketch of the history and culture of the Okhotsk Sea coast Even, 1917–1977]. Moscow: Nauka.

Price, T. Douglas, and Brown, James A. (Editors)
1985   *Prehistoric Hunter-Gatherers: The Emergence of Cultural Complexity.* Orlando, Florida: Academic Press.

Prokof'eva, E. D.
1971   Shamanskie kostiumy narodov Sibiri. [Shamanistic costumes of the peoples of Siberia] *Sbornik Muzeia Antropologii i Etnografii* 27:5–100. Leningrad: ANSSSR.

Prytkova, N. F.
1976   Odezhda chukchei, koriakov i itel'menov. *Material'naia kul'tura narodov Sibiri i severa.* [Chukchi, Koryak, and Itelmen clothing, *in* The material culture of the peoples of Siberia and the North]. Leningrad: Nauka. pp. 5–88.

Quimby, George I.
1985   Japanese Wrecks, Iron Tools, and Prehistoric Indians of the Northwest Coast. *Arctic Anthropology* 22(2):7–15.

Rasmussen, K. J. V.
1927   *Across Arctic America: Narrative of the Fifth Thule Expedition.* New York: G. P. Putnam's Sons.
1931   The Netsilik Eskimos: Social Life and Spiritual Culture. *Report of the Fifth Thule Expedition 1921–24* 8(1–2). Copenhagen.

Ray, Charles K.
1958   *A Program of Education for Alaska Natives.* Fairbanks, Alaska: University of Alaska.

Ray, Dorothy Jean
n.d.   Graphic Arts of the Alaska Eskimo. *Native American Arts* 2. Indian Crafts Board, U.S. Department of the Interior.
1961   *Artists of the Tundra and the Sea.* Seattle: University of Washington Press.
1964   Nineteenth Century Settlement and Subsistence Patterns in the Bering Strait. *Arctic Anthropology* 2:61–94.
1967a   Land Tenure and Polity of the Bering Strait Eskimos. *Journal of the West* 6:371–394.
1967b   Alaskan Eskimo Arts and Crafts. *The Beaver* (Autumn):80–91.
1974   The Billiken. *The Alaska Journal* 4(1):25–31.
1975   *The Eskimo of the Bering Strait, 1650–1898.* Seattle/London: University of Washington Press.
1977   *Eskimo Art: Tradition and Innovation in North Alaska.* Seattle/London: University of Washington Press.
1981   *Aleut and Eskimo Art. Tradition and Innovation in South Alaska.* London: C. Hurst & Company.
1984   Bering Strait Eskimo. *Handbook of North American Indians* 5 (Arctic). Washington, D.C.: Smithsonian Institution. pp. 285–302.

Ray, Dorothy Jean, and Blaker, Alfred A.
1967   *Eskimo Masks: Art and Ceremony.* Seattle/London: University of Washington Press.

Ray, Patrick Henry
1885   Ethnographic Sketch of the Natives of Point Barrow. *U.S. Signal Service Report of the International Polar Expedition to Point Barrow, Alaska.* Washington, D.C.: U.S. Government Printing Office.

Razumovskaia, R. S.
1967   Pletenye izdeliia severo-zapadnykh indeitsev. [Woven objects of the Northwest Coast Indians]. *Sbornik Muzeia Antropologii i Etnografii* 24:93–123. Leningrad: ANSSSR.

Rivet, Paul
1943   *Les Origines de l'Homme Américain.* Montréal, Québec: Les Éditions de l'Arbre.

Robert-Lamblin, Joëlle
1980   Le Kayak Aléoute—Vu Par Son Constructeur et Utilisateur—et la Chasse à la Loutre de Mer. *Objets et Mondes* 20(1):5–20.

Rohner, Ronald P. (Editor)
1969   *The Ethnography of Franz Boas.* Chicago: University of Chicago Press.

Sapir, Edward
1915   The Na-Dene Languages: A Preliminary Report. *American Anthropologist* 17:534–558.
1916   Time Perspective in Aboriginal American Culture: A Study in Method. *Canada Department of Mines. Geological Survey Memoir 90, Anthropological Series* 13. Ottawa.

Sarychev, G. A.
1806–07 *Account of a Voyage of Discovery to the Northeast of Siberia, the Frozen Ocean and the Northeast Sea.* London: Richard Phillips.

Sauer, M.
1802   *An Account of a Geographical and Astronomical Expedition to the Northern Parts of Russia . . . in the Years 1785, etc. to 1794.* London: T. Cadell.

Scammon, Charles M.
1874   *The Marine Mammals of the North–Western Coast of North America.* San Francisco: John H. Carmony and Co.

Schurtz, H.
1896   Zur Ornamentik der Aino. *Internationales Archiv für Ethnography* 9:233–251.

Schuster, Carl
1951a   A Survival of the Eurasiatic Animal Style in Modern Alaskan Eskimo Art. *Selected Papers of the 29th Congress of Americanists,* edited by Sol Tax. Chicago: University of Chicago Press. pp. 35–45.
1951b   Joint Marks: A Possible Index of Cultural Contact between America, Oceania, and the Far East. *Royal Tropical Institute* 39:4–51. Amsterdam.

Shapsnikoff, Anfesia T., and Hudson, Raymond
1974   Aleut Basketry. *Anthropological Papers of the University of Alaska* 16(2):41–61.

Sherwood, Morgan
1965   *Exploration of Alaska, 1865–1900.* New Haven: Yale University Press.

Shirokogoroff, S. M.
1929   *Social Organization of the Northern Tungus.* Shanghai, China: Commercial Press, Ltd.
1935   *Psychomental Complex of the Tungus.* London: Kegan et al.

Shotridge, Louis, and Shotridge, Florence
1913   Indians of the Northwest. *The Museum Journal* 4(3). Philadelphia: University Museum.

Shrenk, L. I. (Schrenk)
1883–   *Ob Inorodtsakh Amurskogo Kraia* [The natives
1903   of the Amur region] Vol. 1 1883, Vol. 2 1899, Vol. 3 1903. St. Petersburg. (Translated from *Reisen und Forschungen im Amur-Lande,* 3 vols. 1881–1892.)

Shternberg, Lev Ia. (Sternberg)
1930   *Giliaki, Orochi, Gol'dy, Negidal'tsy, Ainy* [The Gilyak, Oroch, Gold, Negidal, and Ainu]. Khabarovsk.
1931   Ornament iz olen'ego volosa i igl dikobraza [Reindeer hair and porcupine quill ornamentation]. *Sovetskaia Etnografiia* (3–4):103–121.

Shur, L. A., and Pierce, R. A.
1976   Artists in Russian America: Mikhail Tikhanov (1818). *The Alaska Journal* 6(1):40–49.
1978   Pavel Mikhailov, Artist in Russian America. *The Alaska Journal* 8(4):360–363.

Siebert, Erna V.
1980   Northern Athapaskan Collections of the First Half of the Nineteenth Century. *Arctic Anthropology* 17(1):49–76.

Smithsonian Institution
        Annual Reports of the Smithsonian Institution. Washington, D.C.

Smoliak, A. V.
1966   *Ul'chi: khoziaistvo i byt v proshlom i nastoiashchem* [The Ul'chi: Economy and way of life in the past and present]. Moscow: Nauka.

Spencer, Robert F.
1959   *The North Alaskan Eskimo: A Study in Ecology and Society.* Washington, D.C.: Smithsonian Institution.

Stanyukovich, T. V.
1970   *The Museum of Anthropology and Ethnography Named After Peter the Great.* Leningrad: Nauka/ANSSSR.

Starr, S. Frederick (Editor)
1987   *Russia's American Colony.* Durham, North Carolina: Duke University Press.

Steinbright, Jan (Editor)
1985   *Interwoven Expressions: Works by Contemporary Alaska Native Basketmakers.* Fairbanks, Alaska: Institute for Alaska Native Arts.
1986   *Alaskameut '86: An Exhibit of Contemporary Alaska Native Masks.* Fairbanks, Alaska: Institute for Alaska Native Arts.

Stejneger, Leonhard H.
n.d.   Ms. report on 1882–83 expedition. Smithsonian Institution Archives.
1936   *Georg Wilhelm Steller: The Pioneer of Alaskan Natural History.* Cambridge: Harvard University Press.

Sternberg (see Shternberg)

Stewart, T. D.
1973   *The People of America.* New York: Charles Scribner's Sons.

Stoney, George M.
1890   *Naval Explorations in Alaska: An Account of Two Naval Expeditions to Northern Alaska, with Official Maps of the Country Explored.* Annapolis: U.S. Naval Institute.

Swadesh, Morris
1962   Linguistic Relations across Bering Strait. *American Anthropologist* 64:1262–1291.

Swan, James G.
1869   The Indians of Cape Flattery at the Entrance to the Strait of Fuca, Washington Territory. *Smithsonian Contributions to Knowledge* 16. Washington, D.C.: Smithsonian Institution.

Swanton, John R.
1908   Social Condition, Beliefs, and Linguistic Relationship of the Tlingit Indians. *Annual Report, Bureau of American Ethnology, 1904–1905* 26:391–485.

Szathmary, Emöke J. E.
1984   Human Biology of the Arctic. *Handbook of North American Indians* 5 (Arctic). Washington, D.C.: Smithsonian Institution.

Szathmary, E. J. E., and Ossenberg, N. S.
1978   Are the Biological Differences between North American Indians Truly Profound? *Current Anthropology* 19:673–701.

Tennant, Edward A., and Bitar, Joseph N. (Editors)
1981   *Yupik Lore: Oral Traditions of an Eskimo People.* Bethel, Alaska: Lower Kuskokwim School District.

Thalbitzer, William
1908   The Heathen Priests of East Greenland. *Verhand Lungen des XVI Amerekanisten-Kongresses, Wien 1908.* pp. 447–464.

Titova, Z. D. (Compiler)
1978   *Etnograficheskie materialy severo-vostochnoi*

geograficheskoi ekspeditsii 1785–1795 [Ethnographic material of the north-eastern geographic expedition of 1785–1798]. Magadan.

Townsend, Joan B.
1980 Ranked Societies of the Alaskan Pacific Rim. *in* Alaska Native Culture and History. *Senri Ethnological Studies* 4:123–156. Osaka: National Museum of Ethnology.

Turner, Christy G., II
1985 The Dental Search for Native American Origins. *Out of Asia: Peopling the Americas and the Pacific,* edited by Robert Kirk and Emöke Szathmary. Canberra: Australian National University. pp. 31–78.

Turner, Christy G. II; Aigner, Jean S.; and Richard, Linda R.
1974 Chaluka Stratigraphy, Umnak Island, Alaska. *Arctic Anthropology* 11(Supplement):125–142.

Turner, Geoffrey
1976 Hair Embroidery in Siberia and North America. *Pitt Rivers Museum, University of Oxford, Occasional Papers on Technology* 7.

Turner, Lucien
1894 Ethnology of the Ungava District, Hudson Bay Territory. Edited by John Murdoch. *11th Annual Report of the Bureau of American Ethnology.* Washington, D.C. pp. 159–350.

U.S. Congress
1868 Russian America. *House of Representatives, Executive Document* 177. Washington, D.C.: Government Printing Office.

U.S. Department of the Interior, Indian Arts and Crafts Board,
1966 Alaska. *Smoke Signals,* 50/51 (Fall–Winter).

Usugan, Frances
1984 Interview, July 20, Toksook Bay, Nelson Island, Alaska. 14(h)(1) Site Survey. Anchorage, Alaska: Bureau of Indian Affairs Realty Office.

VanStone, J. W.
1983 Protective Hide Body Armor of the Historic Chukchi and Siberian Eskimos. *Etudes/Inuit/Studies* 7:3–24.

Vasil'evskii, R. S.
1969 The Origin of the Ancient Koryak Culture on the Northern Okhotsk Coast. *Arctic Anthropology* 6(1):150–164.
1971 *Proiskhozhdenie i drevniaia kul'tura koriakov* [Origin and ancient culture of the Koryak]. Novosibirsk: ANSSSR/Nauka.

Vaughan, Thomas, and Holm, Bill
1982 *Soft Gold, the Fur Trade and Cultural Exchange on the Northwest Coast of America.* Portland: Oregon Historical Society.

Vaughan, Thomas; Crownhart-Vaughan, E. A. P.; and Palau de Iglesias, Mercedes
1977 *Voyages of Enlightenment: Malaspina on the Northwest Coast, 1791/1792.* Portland, Oregon: Oregon Historical Society.

Vdovin, I. S.
1961 Eskimosskie elementy v kul'ture chukchei i koriakov [Eskimo elements in the Chukchi and Koryak cultures]. *Sibirskii Etnograficheskii Sbornik* 3. *Trudy Instituta Etnografii* 64. Moscow: ANSSSR. pp. 27–63.
1973 *Ocherki etnicheskoi istorii koriakov* [Ethno-history of the Koryak]. Leningrad.

Veniaminov, Ivan
1984 *Notes on the Islands of the Unalashka District.* Edited by R. Pierce. Kingston, Ontario: Limestone Press. (Translated by Lydia T. Black and R. H. Geoghegan from *Zapiski ob ostrovakh Unalashkinskago otdela,* St. Petersburg, 1840.)

Wardwell, Allen
1978 *Objects of Bright Pride: Northwest Coast Indian Art from the American Museum of Natural History.* New York: Center for Inter-American Relations and American Federation of Arts.

Wauchope, Robert
1962 *Lost Tribes and Sunken Continents.* Chicago: University of Chicago Press.

Weber, Michael
1976 Artifacts from the Northwest Coast. *El Palacio: Quarterly Journal of the Museum of New Mexico* 82(4):4–18.

West, Frederick Hadleigh
1981 *The Archaeology of Beringia.* New York: Columbia University Press.

Weyer, Edward Moffat, Jr.
1929 An Aleut Burial. *Anthropological Papers of the American Museum of Natural History* 31:219–238.
1932 *The Eskimos, Their Environment and Folkways.* New Haven, Conn.: Yale University Press. (Reprinted 1962, Hamden, Conn.: Archon Books.)
[1962]

White, William C.
1945 Bone Culture of Ancient China. *Museum Studies* 4. Toronto: University of Toronto Press.

Woodbury, Anthony C.
1984 Eskimo and Aleut Languages. *Handbook of North American Indians* 5 (Arctic). Washington, D.C.: Smithsonian Institution.

Wrangell, F. P.
1980 *Russian America: Statistical and Ethnographic Information.* Kingston, Ontario: Limestone Press.

Zagoskin, Lavrentii Alekseevich
1967 *Lieutenant Zagoskin's Travels in Russian America 1842–1844,* edited by Henry N. Michael. University of Toronto Press, for the Arctic Institute of North America. (Orig. *Puteshestvie i otkrytiia leitenanta L. Zagoskina v Russkoi Amerike,* Publ. 1847–48, reprinted under editorship of M. B. Chernenko, 1956 Moscow.)

Zimmerly, David W.
1986 *Qajaq: Kayaks of Siberia and Alaska.* Juneau, Alaska: Division of State Museums.

CREDITS

Original Maps and Drawings: Jo Ann Moore (except as noted below).

Russian manuscript translation and Russian literature research: Valérie Chaussonnet

Photo credits:

Unless otherwise credited, all photographs of objects in this book were taken by Smithsonian staff photographers under the direction of Richard Hoffmeister: Eric Long, Laurie Minor, Dane A. Penland, Richard Strauss, Jeff Tinsley, and Rick Vargas; additional contribution by staff photographers Chip Clark and Victor Krantz.

Most ethnographic photographs in this book are from the photo archives at the American Museum of Natural History (primarily from the Jesup Expedition), and at the National Museum of Natural History, Smithsonian Institution.

Other credits to individuals and organizations are listed below, with figure or page numbers.

American Museum of Natural History, Photographic Department: fig. 149.
Academy of Sciences, Leningrad: figs. 63, 69, 84, 96, 188, 191, 193, 377, 384, 437.
Aurora Press, Leningrad: figs. 49, 80.
James H. Barker: p. 2–3.
Bancroft Library, University of California-Berkeley: fig. 247.
Joel Breger: fig. 366.
British Columbia Provincial Museum, Victoria, George T. Emmons: fig. 379.
Edmund Carpenter: fig. 2.
Denver Museum of Natural History, A. M. Bailey: p. 22–23, fig. 457.
William W. Fitzhugh: fig. 91.
Glenbow Museum, Calgary, Lomen Brothers: fig. 229; p. 143.
Grove National Historic Landmark, Glenview Park District, Illinois: fig. 99.
Institute of Alaska Native Art: figs. 467, 474.
S. N. Ivanov: figs. 452, 453, 455.
Limestone Press: figs. 77, 78, 79, 92, 93, 309.
Robert E. Mates: fig. 2.
Michigan State University Archives and Historical Collections, Charles C. Hughes: fig. 297.
Museo de America, Madrid: fig. 282.
NASA—Goddard Spaceflight Center: fig. 173.
National Museum of Denmark, Department of Ethnography, Leo Hansen: fig. 305.

National Park Service, Robert Belous: fig. 456.
Novosti from Sovfoto, R. Zviagel'skii: p. 313; fig. 454.
Peabody Museum, Harvard University: fig. 16.
Pitt Rivers Museum, Oxford, England: fig. 443.
Ken Pratt: fig. 123.
Nicholas Rokitiansky (Collection), photo courtesy of John Blair: p. 69.
Royal Library, Stockholm: fig. 72.
Andres Slapinsh: figs. 174, 331.
Christie G. Turner II: fig. 124.
University Museum, University of Pennsylvania, William B Van Valin: fig. 212.
University of Alaska Museum: fig. 465.
University of Washington Libraries, Special Collections Division: fig. 55.
Dan Wheeler: fig. 462.

Special thanks are due to the following:
Alaska Geological Society (Hamilton et al. 1986): fig. 121.
Alaska International Art Institute (Davis and Davis, 1974: fig. 16); fig. 448.
American Museum of Natural History, Anthropological Papers (Larsen and Rainey 1948): fig. 147.
Lydia Black: fig. 458.
Paula Brizee, research: fig. 316.
Ernest S. Burch, Jr., illustration: fig. 303.
Donald Cavallieri, Gene Fieldman, and Per Gloersen (NASA—Goddard Spaceflight Center): fig. 173.
Christopher Donta, illustration: fig. 162.
Bill Holm, facsimiles: earrings, hairband, and nosepin fig. 67, drum fig. 326; illustrations: figs. 388, 397, 400, 401, 403, 404, 407.
Inter-Nord (Dikov, 1972): fig. 153.
Alfred A. Knopf (Covarrubias 1954: fig. 18, 40): figs. 140, 451.
Michael Krauss, research: fig. 175.
Nauka press (Arutiunov and Sergeev, 1975): fig. 145.
Julie Perlmutter, illustration: figs. 139, 153, 458.
Royal Ontario Museum: fig. 450.
V. O. Shubin and N. N. Dikov (USSR Academy of Sciences, Siberian Branch): fig. 134.
Jessica Sloane, research: figs. 247, 249, 251, 254, 256, 257, 258, 262.
Dennis Stanford, Smithsonian Institution, facsimile: fig. 122.
University of Washington Press (Dauenhauer and Dauenhauer 1987): p. 69.

Acknowledgments

Crossroads of Continents has been an enormous undertaking. Since its inception in 1977, scores of institutions and hundreds of individuals have been swept into its vortex, which deepens and widens with every passing day. Nevertheless, the time has thankfully come to call a halt and repay debts, which are really too substantial to be squared fairly in these few lines. Note, however, that many credits will be found in the captions, credit lists, and appendices.

Our first acknowledgment is to the peoples of the North Pacific and Bering Sea region whose genius created the remarkable materials illustrated in this book and exhibition; to those who collected these materials; and to the museum curators in whose care they have been entrusted for so many years. The fact that the most important Siberian collections reside in New York and the most important Alaskan collections reside in Moscow and Leningrad emphasizes the reciprocal interests in conservation of these and other collections.

Crossroads was conceived in 1977 in discussions between Iu. V. Bromlei, Director of the Institute of Ethnography of the Soviet Academy of Sciences, and William W. Fitzhugh and William C. Sturtevant of the Smithsonian Institution. While the operational aspects of the project have been managed respectively on each side by the Institute and the Smithsonian, general sponsorship involving scholarly exchanges has been by the American Council of Learned Societies (ACLS) and its operational arm, the International Research and Exchanges Board (IREX). Stanley Katz (ACLS), and Allen Kassof, Wesley Fisher, Arlen Hastings, and Karen Kiesel of IREX have been invaluable in this intermediary role. Also deserving special thanks are staffs of the American and Soviet embassies in Washington and Moscow, and the USIA and the Department of State staff, especially Tom Simons.

On the Soviet side, the project was managed by the Institute of Ethnography under the direction of Iu.V. Bromlei, assisted by L.P. Kuzmina and V.A. Tishkov. Scientific direction of the Soviet curatorial team was provided by S.A Arutiunov, assisted by S.Ia. Serov. Support for exhibition aspects within the Academy came from the Council on Exhibitions, headed by A.P. Kapitsa, assisted by M. Martianova. We are especially indebted, however, to the Museum of Anthropology and Ethnography, a branch of the Institute of Ethnography in Leningrad, directed by R.F. Its, assisted by E.G. Fedorova and I.D. Vasil'eva. This revered institution contributed virtually all of the Soviet-owned objects in the exhibition with the exception of a small group of Siberian Paleolithic artifacts loaned by the Sakhalin Regional Museum, directed by V.O. Shubin. Other Soviet institutions contributing illustrative materials included the Academy of Arts in Leningrad (courtesy of L.S. Poliakova and D. Safor-Alieva), Museum of History and Culture of the Peoples of Siberia and the Far East in Novosibirsk, the I.W. Repin Institute of Leningrad, and the State Russian Museum in Leningrad (courtesy of E.M. Petrova and L.P. Rybakova). Thanks are also due to Vladmir Gusev of Aurora Press.

Crossroads has, from its inception, been based on the principle of Soviet-American reciprocity. This principle has governed curatorial exchanges, selection of objects, and even exhibition venues. Thus, when *Crossroads* completes its tour of North America in 1992, it will begin a Soviet tour under joint auspices of the Soviet Academy of Sciences and the Ministry of Culture. It is with great pleasure that we note the Ministry's collaboration. On the American side, the exhibition has been supported by a wide group of museums, institutions, and individuals. Among the many cooperating institutions (noted in individual credits for loans and illustrations), one organization stands out: the American Museum of Natural History. Without its collections of early Siberian ethnography and the generous assistance of its staff, Barbara Conklin, Stanley Freed, Laurel Kendall, David Hurst Thomas, Anibal Rodriguez, Belinda Kaye, Judith Levinson, and Bill Weinstein, *Crossroads* would have been still-born.

The third major body of material in this exhibition and book comes from the Smithsonian's Department of Anthropology and its subunits, the National Anthropological Archives, Processing and Conservation Laboratories, Human Studies Film Archive, and Handbook of North American Indians. As part of the Smithsonian's Museum of Natural History/Museum of Man, we have received strong support for over ten years from directors Richard Fiske, Stanwyn Shelter, James Tyler and Robert Hoffmann, all of whom have contributed important administrative, financial, and moral support, as have two anthropology Department Chairs, Douglas Ubelaker and Adrienne Kaeppler. Within the National Musuem of Natural History, special thanks are due to the Office of Special Exhibits, directed by Sheila Mutchler, assisted by Marjory Stoller, Constance Lee, Pat Douglas, Cissy Anklam. This exhibition and publication would not have been possible without their tireless efforts at coordinating research, design, and production. Advertising and publicity were expertly handled by Vicky Moeser and the Office of Public Affairs. The task of artifact conservation fell to Michelle Austin, Gabrielle Browne, Edith Dietze, Vera Espinola, Sonja Fogle, Natalie Firnhaber, Greta Hansen, Ingrid Neuman, and Catherine Valentour. Artifact photography was done under the direction of Richard Hofmeister by Harold E. Dougherty, Eric Long, Laurie Minor, Dane Penland, Richard Strauss, Jeff Tinsley, and Rick Vargas, and by Chip Clark and Victor Krantz. Our fine manikins were designed by Barbara Charles based upon research by Aron Crowell and Valérie Chaussonnet, sculpted by Frances H. Moore, and fabricated and dressed by Virginia Heaven. Casting volunteers included JoAllyn Archambault, Mitchell L. Bush, Jr., Monica Carver, Aron Crowell, Frank Ducheneaux, Natalie Firnhaber, Francis Harjoe, Robert Holden, and Kebin Nephew, Exhibition planning and design has been by Barbara Charles, Jeff Jones, and Bob Staples of Staples and Charles, Ltd. Sanders Design did the bracket and installation work.

Most of our fine illustrations are the work of Jo Ann Moore, with some contributions by Julie Perlmutter. Veteran *Inua* book designers Alex and Caroline Castro performed miracles in fitting *Crossroads* attractively into too few pages, edited by Jeanne Sexton and Lorraine Atherton. Alex Castro was also the artistic director for catalog photography. Publication has been managed by Kathleen Brown, with project direction by Daniel Goodwin and Felix Lowe of Smithsonian Press. Among those contributing research information were Robert Ackerman, Phil Angle, Marjorie Balzer, Lydia Black, Edmund Carpenter, Richard and Nora Dauenhauer, James E. Dixon, Bernadette Driscoll, Don E. Dumond, Kate Duncan, Vera Espinola, Charles Handley, Richard H. Jordan, Richard A. Knecht, Oleg Kobtzeff, Roxie Laybourne, Molly Lee, Michael Ostrogorsky, Richard Pierce, Roger Powers, Susan Rowley, Dwight Schmidt, Dennis Stanford and staff of the Canadian Museum of Civilization and its Archeological Survey of Canada, coordinated by Sandra Gibb. The Smithsonian National Museum of Natural History's Education Office staff, Laura Lou McKie, Debby Rothberg, and Caroline Sadler, provided assistance in many ways, as did interns Paula Brizee, Christina Burke, Tess Freidenburg, John Nissenbaum, Jessica Sloan, Curtis Thrapp, Kimberly Wageman, Sonja Webb, Alexia Bloch, and Audrey Porsche.

Crossroads has been assembled by a joint curatorial team of Soviet, American, and Canadian anthropologists. Project direction has been by William W. Fitzhugh, assisted by Aron Crowell (Smithsonian). Additional curatorial team members for American cultures included Bill Holm (Burke Museum, Seattle), who wrote the Northwest Coast captions and fabricated the shaman's drum (fig. 326) and various other props; George MacDonald (Director, Canadian Museum of Civilization, Ottawa); Jean-Loup Rousselot (Museum für Völkerkunde, Munich); William C. Sturtevant (Smithsonian), James VanStone (Field Museum of Natural History, Chicago). The Soviet curatorial team worked under the direction of Sergei A. Arutiunov, assisted by Sergei Ia. Serov, with contributions by I.S. Gurvich, Igor Krupnik, and Vladimir Vasil'ev of the Institute of Ethnography in Moscow, and G.I. Dzeniskevich, Rosa G. Liapunova, Larisa Pavlinskaia, and Sergei Poliakov of the Institute's Museum of Anthropology and Ethnography in Leningrad. In addition, we heartily thank our other volume contributors and Alaska Native artists, listed in the table of contents and in the final chapter. Except for Northwest Coast portions, captions were written by Aron Crowell and William W. Fitzhugh. Ted Timreck produced the exhibition films, with special assistance from Rosita Worl and Soviet filmmaker Andres Slapinsh, and other filmmakers, especially Sarah Elder and Leonard Kammerling.

Crossroads of Continents received enthusiastic support from Smithsonian officials ex-Secretary S. Dillon Ripley and ex-Assistant Secretary for Museum Programs, Paul Perrot. Later, their torches were passed to different leaders, including Secretary Robert McC. Adams, and Assistant Secretaries Thomas Freudenheim, Ralph Rinzler, and Robert Hoffmann. *Crossroads* was funded by a major grant from the Smithsonian's Special Exhibition Fund; but this in itself was not sufficient without supplemental contributions from museums cooperating in the North American tour following the Washington opening, notably the American Museum of Natural History, Indiana State Museum, Anchorage Museum of History and Art, Canadian Museum of Civilization, and two others, as yet undecided. We thank Martha Cappelletti and the Smithsonian Traveling Exhibition Service staff in advance for management of the touring program. Pan American Airlines has agreed to provide exhibition shipment to and from the Soviet Union. We also thank Gretchen Ellsworth, Lauren Grant, and Kennedy Schmertz for their assistance in the "great protocol effort," and Wilton Dillon, Carla Borden, and Cheryl LaBerge for symposia coordination.

Finally we give special thanks to our collaborator and friend for the past two difficult years, Valérie Chaussonnet, for her methodical work as Russian ethnographic literature researcher, Russian language translator (assisted by Sergei Arutiunov, James Bernhardt, and Muriel Joffre), bibliographer, illustrations researcher, proof-reader, and volume contributor.

We would like to dedicate this volume to our 'widowed' wives, Dee Crowell and Lynne Fitzhugh, for their support and forbearance. Quoth the Raven, "Nevermore."